Revision Total Hip Arthroplasty

Springer Science+Business Media, LLC

James V. Bono
Joseph C. McCarthy
Thomas S. Thornhill
Benjamin E. Bierbaum
Roderick H. Turner

Editors

Revision Total Hip Arthroplasty

Foreword by Eduardo A. Salvati, M.D.

With 572 Illustrations, 49 in Full Color

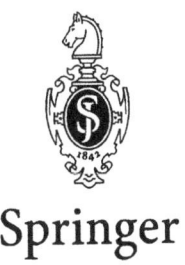

Springer

James V. Bono, M.D., New England Baptist Hospital, Boston, MA 02120, USA

Joseph C. McCarthy, M.D., New England Baptist Hospital, Boston, MA 02120, USA

Thomas S. Thornhill, M.D., Brigham and Women's Hospital, Boston, MA 02115, USA

Benjamin E. Bierbaum, M.D., New England Baptist Hospital, Boston, MA 02120, USA

Roderick H. Turner, M.D., New England Baptist Hospital, Boston, MA 02120, USA

On the Cover: The cover illustration is a representative cutaway view of a left total hip revision depicting acetabular reconstruction with structural and particulate allograft and jumbo socket and long-stem femoral component with femoral strut onlay allografts. The illustration was airbrushed and painted in acrylic by William Thomas Stillwell, M.D., and is used by permission.

Library of Congress Cataloging-in-Publication Data
Revision total hip arthroplasty / James V. Bono . . . [et al.] .
   p. cm.
  Includes bibliographical references and index.
  ISBN 978-1-4612-7131-4   ISBN 978-1-4612-1406-9 (eBook)
  DOI 10.1007/978-1-4612-1406-9
   1. Total hip replacement—Reoperation.   2. Total hip replacement—
Complications.   I. Bono, James V.
   [DNLM: 1. Hip Joint—surgery.   2. Hip Prosthesis.   3. Reoperation.
4. Arthroplasty, Replacement, Hip.   WE 860 R4535 1998]
RD549.R443   1998
f617.5'810592—dc21   97-42562

Printed on acid-free paper.

© 1999 Springer Science+Business Media New York
Softcover reprint of the hardcover 1st edition 1999
Originally published by Springer-Verlag New York, Inc. in 1999
All rights reserved. This work may not be translated or copied in whole or in part without the written permission of the publisher Springer Science+Business Media, LLC.
except for brief excerpts in connection with reviews
or scholarly analysis. Use in connection with any form of information storage and retrieval, electronic adaptation, computer software, or by similar or dissimilar methodology now known or hereafter developed is forbidden.
The use of general descriptive names, trade names, trademarks, etc., in this publication, even if the former are not especially identified, is not to be taken as a sign that such names, as understood by the Trade Marks and Merchandise Marks Act, may accordingly be used freely by anyone.
While the advice and information in this book are believed to be true and accurate at the date of going to press, neither the authors nor the editors nor the publisher can accept any legal responsibility for any errors or omissions that may be made. The publisher makes no warranty, express or implied, with respect to the material contained herein.

Production coordinated by WordCrafters Editorial Services, Inc., and managed by Lesley Poliner; manufacturing supervised by Jacqui Ashri.
Typeset by Matrix Publishing Services, Inc., York, PA.

9 8 7 6 5 4 3 2 1

ISBN 978-1-4612-7131-4

Dedication

This book is dedicated to Otto E. Aufranc, the New England Baptist Hospital, and the New England Baptist Bone and Joint Institute. This brilliant surgeon and these unusual institutions have made possible an academic climate and a staff of orthopedic surgeons working in concert with their institutional colleagues and with colleagues across North America. Otto E. Aufranc was a man who always wanted to be remembered by the things he created and the surgeons he trained rather than by the honors or plaudits that were bestowed upon him during his lifetime. He was a generous, humble, unselfish, caring physician who lived by standards that we all strive for but never achieve. In a thoughtful eulogy, Ben Bierbaum states:

> Otto was critical of the surgery he performed and carefully analyzed every operation. He stressed that an orthopedic surgeon should be creative and offer preventive and restorative surgery.... Otto has been described as an unusually quiet, dignified man with a remarkable capacity for work and exceptional devotion to the care of his patients.... The life of many patients and surgeons were touched by his gentleness, attention to detail, his understanding and loyalty. Otto was an innovator, a master surgeon, and a master friend.

Otto Aufranc looked upon the training of surgeons as the single most important responsibility in his life. He felt that such training was his opportunity to upgrade the practice of his surgery on a very broad basis and to touch the lives of many more patients than he could reach with his own hands and his own practice. He was clearly the most admired and most productive teacher of reconstructive hip surgeons of his era. His contributions to orthopedic surgery were extensive in their scope and their impact on his chosen field of reconstructive hip surgery. The Aufranc Joint Fellowship at the New England Baptist Hospital is a fitting legacy to his teaching, patient care, and emphasis on meticulous surgical technique.

It is a measure of the man that he closed his own reflections on his life with the following statement: "I have found that over the years I have made all the mistakes that are necessary to be made about hip surgery and I hope that I have passed all of these lessons along. It is never too late to change one's mind or to perhaps abandon a prejudice in the continual changes made in our surgery, as long as it is based on sound principles and not just for change."

The New England Baptist Hospital was a truly great and compassionate institution even before it joined forces with Otto E. Aufranc in 1969. However, the efforts of this man and this institution were both greatly strengthened in combination. The New England Baptist Hospital shared Otto's deep-felt beliefs about preserving patient care and patient dignity. Dr. Aufranc worked closely with the innovative nurse/administrator of NEBH, the late Elinor Kirby, RN, in the initial establishment of an Orthopedic Department at NEBH. It was my great pleasure and honor to work closely with Doctors Aufranc, Bierbaum, Smith-Petersen, Potter, Nalebuff, and others to build a teaching service both at the fellowship and residency levels.

The mentioned services were put together in the early 1970s with consistent academic support from Professors Henry Banks of Tufts University School of Medicine and Arthur Pappas of University of Massachusetts Medical School. These institutions and their leaders were eager to affiliate with NEBH largely because of their respect for Otto E. Aufranc.

The reputations of Dr. Aufranc and the great institutions mentioned above were likewise important in the evolution and birth of the Bone and Joint Institute. This Institute came about due largely to the shared vision and cooperation between NEBH medical staff and the NEBH administration and trustees, especially the Institute's first two leaders, Dr. Thomas Thornhill and Dr. Benjamin Bierbaum.

The Board of Directors of the Bone and Joint Institute consists of the following outstanding physicians and administrators:

Benjamin E. Bierbaum, M.D.

Arthur Bond, Jr.

Robert R. Foster, M.D.

Michael J. Goldberg, M.D.

Steven R. Goldring, M.D.

Mark E. Haffenreffer, M.D.

Paul P. Harasimowicz, III, M.D.

Stepehn J. Lipson, M.D.

David A. Mattingly, M.D.

Joseph C. McCarthy, M.D.
John M. Mulroy, M.D.
Edward A. Nalebuff, M.D.
Alan H. Robbins, M.D.
Patricia M. Roberts
Arnold D. Scheller, Jr., M.D.
Richard D. Scott, M.D.
Steven M. Wetzner, M.D.
Louis J. Woolf
Alexander M. Wright, M.D.

Excepting members working in closely related orthopedic disciplines, all of these board members regard Otto E. Aufranc as the major role model of their orthopedic career. The Bone and Joint Institute is currently headed by Dr. Bierbaum and is fortunate to have Patty Roberts as its director. The Institute carries on the tradition and philosophy of Dr. Aufranc in that it has an equal commitment to patient care, teaching, and musculoskeletal research.

The history of reconstructive hip surgery in America in the second half of the twentieth century starts solidly with the teaching and exemplary leadership of Otto E. Aufranc. Tragically, his surgical career was significantly shortened by myasthenia gravis. He fought that disease with courage and dignity for two decades.

Dr. Aufranc's principal legacy lives as he wished: in the patient care, the teaching, and the research of the hundreds of men and women whom he trained and/or influenced by his excellence, his integrity, and his compassion for patients.

RODERICK H. TURNER, M.D.
New England Baptist Hospital
Boston, Massachusetts
September 1998

Foreword

It gives me great pleasure to write a foreword for this book, which represents the culmination of a remarkable, fertile, and dedicated career in hip surgery by Dr. Roderick H. Turner. Dr. Turner continued, expanded, and advanced the art and science of total hip replacement, following the work of his distinguished and legendary teacher, Dr. Otto Aufranc. During the three decades of Dr. Turner's tenure, the New England Baptist Hospital established itself as a preeminent center for postgraduate education, particularly in the area of hip joint replacement surgery and complex revision surgery. Legions of fellows competed for a position to work at his side. Those promising young doctors who were fortunate enough to be selected had the privilege to learn the intricacies of hip surgery, the devotion to patient care, and the discipline of basic and clinical research directly from a natural-born educator and innovator.

This new volume expands and updates Dr. Turner's acclaimed 1983 publication *Revision Total Hip Arthroplasty* and is a valuable reference for the orthopedic surgeon particularly interested in revision joint replacement hip surgery. With outstanding contributions by world leaders with vast experience, Dr. Bono, et al., *Revision Total Hip Arthroplasty* places particular emphasis on the importance of preoperative clinical, radiological, and laboratory evaluation. The various areas that need to be covered to assure a complete preoperative plan are described in detail. In fact, most operations become simple if the surgeon has given adequate thought, time and preparation, and has all the necessary information and armamentarium available, prior their execution.

Several chapters address, in depth, different avenues of access to the artificial hip joint, the intraoperative management of severe anatomical abnormalities and bone loss, and the complex subject of bone grafting and its intricacies. They are all described extensively by master surgeons. Unfortunately, the complex nature of revision surgery increases the perioperative morbidity and chances of complications. Some of these patients, depressed by the occasional unsatisfactory outcome, may seek legal compensation. A thoughtful chapter on medical malpractice adds a welcome dimension to this book.

The editors, Doctors Bono, McCarthy, Thornhill, Bierbaum and Turner, should be complimented for their efforts in this successful endeavor. Having had the pleasure of reading all the chapters prior to publication, I am assured that this new volume will be received enthusiastically by our orthopedic community, and particularly by those seriously interested in revision surgery.

EDUARDO A. SALVATI, M.D.
Professor of Orthopedic Surgery
Cornell University Medical College
Director, Hip and Knee Surgery
The Hospital for Special Surgery
New York, New York

A History of Hip Replacement Surgery

William Thomas Stillwell

Revision total hip arthroplasty has emerged as a necessary response to the failures of primary total hip replacement. Surgical techniques and implants for revision procedures have been developed to compensate for the loss of the optimal conditions of index surgery. The purpose of revision surgery is to recapture the goal of the failed primary total hip arthroplasty: to reconstruct the arthritic hip so as to reproduce, as closely as possible, the form and function of the natural joint. To this end, surgery in intended to relieve pain, restore function, and correct deformity.

The fundamental principles of joint replacement have been identified over time, largely through intuitive mimicry of nature and analysis of our failures. To fully appreciate the foundations of current thought in revision hip surgery, it is helpful to reexamine the underlying biological and physical principles of reconstruction as they were discovered, by tracing the evolution of replacement arthroplasty of the hip.

Osteotomy Arthroplasty

In an effort to provide some motion and correct significant deformity associated with ankylosis of the hip, osteotomy or resection of the proximal femur was one of the earliest attempts at arthroplasty.[1] Based on the concept of the planned pseudoarthrosis, these procedures were effective but unstable. The latest incarnation of this concept is the Girdlestone resection arthroplasty,[2] used today as a salvage procedure for intractable infection, or as a temporizing procedure in two-stage revisions.

Interpositional Arthroplasty

Stability was regained and motion preserved with the advent of the interpositional arthroplasty. The principle was to insert a mechanical spacer between the raw bone surfaces of a transected ankylosis to prevent refusion. The first known interpositional arthroplasty was performed in 1840 in New York by Carnochan, who inserted a wooden block between the resected ends of an ankylosed temperomandibular joint. Various materials, biological and foreign, were used for the interpositional membrane, including skin, fascia, muscle, chromicized pig bladder, and gold foil.[3] All met with unpredictable and often stiff and painful results. Interpositional arthroplasty was elevated to a serious surgical option, however, by the introduction of the mould arthroplasty of Marius Smith-Petersen in 1923.[4]

Inspired by the reactive synovial-like membrane investing a piece of glass embedded in a workman's back, the original cups were fashioned of glass and were bell shaped. Designed to stimulate a regeneration of articular cartilage in the hip, the cup was meant to mold the fibrin layer of clotted blood on the congruously reshaped articular surfaces on either side of the new joint. Under the conditions of gentle motion and prolonged limited weight-bearing, the initial fibrin clot would undergo metaplasia to fibrocartilage.[4] The mold or cup was originally intended for retrieval after the cartilage surfaces had been restored. The impressive clinical results after surgery, however, discouraged their removal, and thereafter the cups were left in the joint by design.

Glass proved too fragile a material for the joint forces in the hip, often fracturing during use. Molds were fashioned from a variety of other materials, including Viscaloid (a celluloid derivative, 1925), Pyrex (1933), Bakelite (1939), and–later that year—the chrome-cobalt alloy Vitallium, which was used thereafter. Vitallium was durable, unlike glass, Pyrex, and Bakelite, and it was inert, unlike Viscaloid.

The original bell-shaped cup was intended to provide a measure of stability within the bony acetabulum. The brim of the bell, however, often became fixed by fibrous tissue, leading to entrapment, impingement, and erosion of the underlying regenerated cartilage in painful "corns," which led to failure. The removal of the brim and congruous inner and outer contours were features of the hemispherical True-Arc cup design, developed by Otto E. Aufranc (Fig. 1), Smith-Petersen's protégé.[5] Employing meticulous surgical techniques, a reverence for soft tissue, and an appreciation of the importance of progressive rehabilitation, Dr. Aufranc elevated the art of the cup arthroplasty to its apex, reporting 82% successful results in 1000 arthroplasties[6] and demonstrating the reformation of hyaline cartilage by histologic sections, a feat never duplicated by other investigators.[7]

For all its good results, however, cup arthroplasty was a demanding procedure, requiring exacting surgical technique, an appreciation of the underlying biological principles, and complete patient compliance. Because it was reliant upon biological response, its success was unpredictable. For these reasons, the average success rate was about 50% and it was used only by experienced hip surgeons. Still, cup arthroplasty represented a milestone in hip surgery, and its principles foreshadowed later developments.

The occasional entrapment of the Smith-Petersen bell-shaped cup within the acetabulum, thereby permitting motion on the femoral interface alone, was the antecedent for deliberate pelvic fixation of a cup: the hip socket arthroplasty. Gaenslen (1952), McBride (1955), and Urist (1957) all developed variations on the theme of a mobile, reshaped femoral head articulating with a highly polished metal hip socket.[8] These procedures failed to become popular, despite reports of good results.

The intra-articular situation was reversed in the Aufranc mold variant, with motion mainly between the cup and acetabular surface, suggestive of the femoral head prosthesis, although this line of development had an independent pedigree.

Femoral Head Replacement Arthroplasty

Efforts at prosthetic femoral replacement date from the experimental carved ivory joint substitutes of Gluck in 1890. A reinforced rubber femoral head was used to treat transcervical hip fractures by Delbet in 1919. Hey Groves used an ivory "nail" in 1926 to replace the articular surface of the femoral head, a design that was a model for the short-stemmed femoral prostheses that followed.[3]

A short-stemmed Vitallium femoral head replacement was developed and used by Harold Bohlman in patients with nonunited femoral neck fractures (1939). Thereafter, Bohlman collaborated with Austin T. Moore in the fabrication and implantation of a custom, 12-inch-long Vitallium proximal femoral replacement in a patient with recurrent giant cell tumor (1939).[9] This prosthesis functioned well for 2½ years, until the patient's death from unrelated causes, and it was retrieved at autopsy.[9,10] This procedure was an historic milestone in hip surgery and the mode for later long-stemmed femoral prostheses. Thus, based on the early prototypes of Hey Groves and Bohlman, two basic patterns of femoral prostheses emerged: the short-stem femoral head prosthesis and the long-stem head/neck implant.

The Short-Stem Prosthesis

The Judet acrylic femoral head arthroplasty was developed by the Judet brothers in 1946 for the treatment of osteoarthritis, intracapsular fracture nonunions, nontuberculous ankylosis, and the dislocated hip. Designed after the Hey Groves "nail," the Judet prosthesis was fashioned of polymethylmethacrylate, with a head that was two-thirds of a sphere attached to a short stem, meant to transfix the axis of the femoral neck, after resection of the femoral head.[11] Although the initial clinical results were dramatic, they rapidly yielded to loosening, wear, and inflammatory reactions to acrylic debris. Later versions of the Judet and other similar designs were made of Vitallium, because the earlier failures had been attributed to acrylic. These, too, failed, as

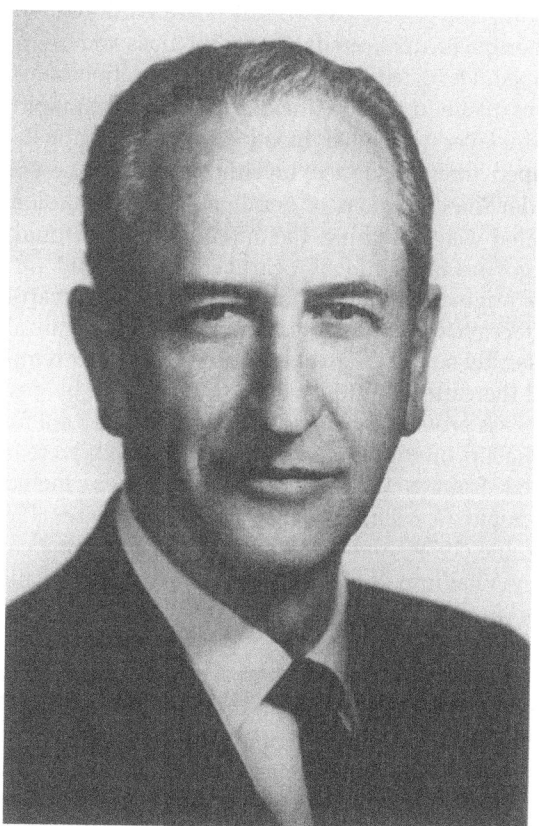

Figure 1. Otto E. Aufranc, master of the cup arthroplasty.

they all succumbed to the shared intrinsic flaw in the short-stem transcervical designs, the excessive shear stresses at the prosthetic–bone interface.

The Long-Stem Prosthesis

The second basic pattern of femoral prosthesis utilized a round head mounted on a long stem, for insertion down the axis of the femoral canal. Although a number of surgeons designed such prostheses, two emerged as clear leaders in the field: F.R. Thompson and Austin T. Moore. The prototypes of both prostheses were introduced at about the same time in 1950, and both designs attracted adherents. The Thompson prosthesis was a head/neck design with an oblique neck flange that required partial resection of the femoral neck.[12] This feature made it useful in cases of low neck fracture, nonunion, avascular necrosis, and with resorption of the femoral neck, as often occurred with failed Judet prostheses. The Austin Moore prosthesis head sat on a more horizontal collar, designed to preserve more of the femoral neck. Its broader proximal stem made it somewhat less likely to subside, its dorsal vane less likely to rotate, and its stem fenestrations for "self-locking" were a foreshadowing of later efforts in the 1980s for biological fixation.[13] Later modifications of both designs lent their use to cement fixation and extended their benefits to patients with osteoporosis and severe arthritis. The intrinsic merit in these designs is evident in that both are still used today.

Long-stem femoral prostheses were successful because they used a relatively long intramedullary stem to transmit the stresses of weight-bearing along the physiological axis of the femoral shaft. This minimized the shear stresses that were the source of failure in the short-stem implants of Judet and others and induced instead prosthetic–bone compression stresses that were far better tolerated.

Despite the clinical success of the femoral replacement arthroplasty in cases of femoral neck fracture, nonunion, and avascular necrosis, its extension to the arthritides was less uniformly successful. It soon became evident that the femoral prosthesis was far more effective in cases in which disease was more pronounced on the femoral side of the joint. The attempt to use the uncemented femoral prosthesis as a mold within a reamed acetabulum was unpredictable at best, and by the late 1960s the cup arthroplasty was preferred to the femoral endoprosthesis for the treatment of arthritis.

Total Hip Arthroplasty

The relative failure of the femoral prosthesis to address the acetabular side of the joint, combined with the emerging problems of the cup arthroplasty and the failure of hip socket arthroplasty to attract a following, led to the empirical combination of a femoral prosthesis with an acetabular cup. Phillip Wiles is generally credited with the first "total hip" arthroplasty in 1938: a metal-on-metal stainless steel ball-in-cup design. The polished steel head was fastened through the axis of the femoral neck with a bolt, like the Judet prosthesis. The socket was a flanged cup, mechanically ground for an accurate fit with the head, fixed to the acetabulum by screws through the peripheral flange.[14] Wiles improved on his initial implants in the early 1950s, in response to the failures of the Judet, but the intrinsic design was flawed and the implants failed by loosening. Similar efforts mated Gaenslen acetabular sockets with Austin Moore femoral prostheses, with similar results.

McKee-Farrar Total Hip

In 1951, an F.R. Thompson prosthesis was used in conjunction with a polished metal socket by McKee and his associate, Watson-Farrar of Norwich, England. Initially fabricated in stainless steel, the implants loosened within a year. The next model used cast chrome cobalt implants and lasted for three years, until the stem fractured. Subsequent modifications to the system included fixation by means of dental acrylic cement, a true spherical head with a suppressed undercut neck, to allow an increased arc of motion before impingement on the socket rim, and a redesigned acetabular cup, featuring multiple posterior metal studs, to increase surface area and therefore fixation, and ensure an even mantle of acrylic cement.[15]

Acrylic Cement Fixation

Acrylic cement, previously used by dentists, was introduced to orthopedics by Sven Kiaer in 1950, when he used it to bond a plastic prosthesis to bone. Haboush used it to implant total hip prostheses later that year at the Hospital for Joint Diseases in New York.[16] It was subsequently incorporated into the McKee-Farrar procedure to improve durability and fixation of the implants.

Charnley Low-Friction Arthroplasty

The major conceptual breakthrough that defined the modern era of total hip replacement was the advent of the Charnley low-friction arthroplasty. Sir John Charnley (Fig. 2), of Wrightington, England, pioneered the concept of the metal-on-plastic total hip replacement as a result of his analysis of lubrication of animal joints.[17] His experiments suggested that a cartilage substitute was necessary to allow artificial joints to function close to the extremely low-friction state found in nature. His first effort was the Teflon on PTFE (polytetrafluoroethylene) arthroplasty, in which thin Teflon shells resurfaced the femoral and acetabular sides of the hip joint.

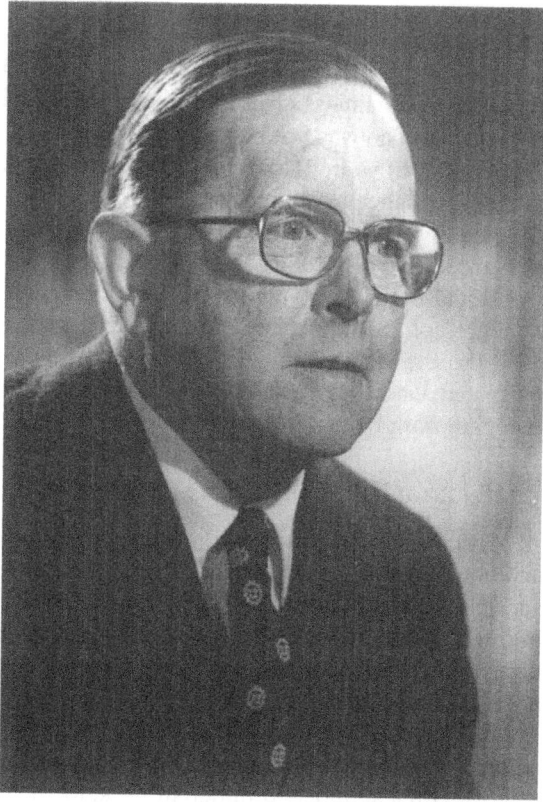

Figure 2. Professor Sir John Charnley, father of total hip arthroplasty.

The failure of this initial effort led to the adoption of a new design: a small-diameter femoral head mounted at an offset on an intramedullary stem, fixed within the femoral canal with acrylic cement to resist torsional forces, and articulating with a thick-walled Teflon socket. This new design, the low-friction arthroplasty, was based upon the engineering principle of low frictional torque, which resulted from the differential radii of the small femoral head and the larger-diameter socket. The small head generated relatively low torque at the outer margin of the socket, thereby reducing shear stresses and favoring fixation.[18]

Although the material Teflon was an excellent intuitive choice for its extremely low coefficient of friction, in practice it had poor wear properties, which provoked massive inflammatory reactions and early failures of the first series of low-friction arthroplasties. It is a measure of Charnley's greatness that he was not deterred by this disheartening turn of events. Where a lesser man might have been discouraged, he analyzed his failures and concluded that they might be prevented by the use of a bearing material of greater wear properties. Teflon was abandoned and the next generation of hip replacements utilized a socket of ultrahigh molecular weight polyethylene, a polymer with wear properties 500 to 1000 times greater than those of Teflon.

The original Charnley procedure called for the implantation of the cemented femoral stem and socket through a transtrochanteric approach. This was deemed by Charnley to be an integral part of the operation. The initial implants were all one size and had but one neck length. Accordingly, stability and restoration of the abductor moment arm were dependent on trochanteric advancement, which remained an important principle of this procedure.[19]

Muller Total Hip

The dramatic clinical success of the low-friction arthroplasty inspired other surgeons to attempt their own variations on the concept. Maurice Muller of Berne, Switzerland, developed a system incorporating several innovations that differed from Charnley's original precepts. His femoral component featured a 32-mm-diameter head instead of the 22-mm head of the Charnley LFA, to allow greater range of motion of the hip, increase stability, and resist wear of the polyethylene socket. The Muller stem was gracefully curved (often called the *banana stem*) to allow easy insertion into the femoral canal without trochanteric osteotomy, with a variety of neck sizes to allow adjustment of leg lengths and abductor tension without trochanteric advancement.[20] All subsequent implant designs were based on one or the other of these two prototypes. In Exeter, Robin Ling, working with A.J.C. Lee, introduced a pointed, wedge-shaped design for the stem.[21] In the United States, Otto E. Aufranc (of cup arthroplasty fame) and his associate Roderick H. Turner introduced one of the most influential total hip systems, the Aufranc-Turner.

Aufranc-Turner Total Hip

Taking note of stem fractures reported with the initial Charnley and Muller stems, the Aufranc-Turner stem design addressed the perceived flaws of the other earlier designs with several innovative modifications. It presented a broader proximal profile, a more valgus orientation, and a more horizontal collar—all intended to decrease bending moments and shear forces on the stem, and increase compression forces under the collar. Its neck had an elliptical cross section, intended to increase the excursion of the neck before impingement with the socket, and thereby increase range of motion. The head diameter was also 32 mm, to provide stability and increased motion and to appeal to the surgeons who found the Muller design attractive. The socket was machined from ultrahigh molecular weight polyethylene like the others, but it had an eccentric introitus, with additional material in the superior portion of the cup, in anticipation of wear.[22]

Its defects were apparent only in hindsight: its diamond-shaped cross section, like that of a knife, provided a less-than-optimal distribution of metal and its sharp edges and corners, like those of the Muller, served as stress risers to the cement mantle. Since it was quite successful in its day, the Aufranc-Turner design, in turn, served as inspiration for other implants, such as the New England Baptist Hip, which was a slightly longer version of the Aufranc-Turner, but which shared the suppressed AP diameter of the elliptical neck and the Trapezoidal, or TR-28, design.

TR-28 Total Hip

The TR-28 design introduced the 28-mm head size. Its stem had a rectangular cross section and a trapezoidal neck, narrower in the AP dimension, which accomplished much the same thing as the elliptical neck with regard to increased arc of motion and decreased impingement. Like other stems of this second generation, the TR-28 also had sharp edges and was initially made of cast metal—first steel, then chrome–cobalt alloy.[23]

Initial Failures Influence Design

Total hip replacement became more common after the introduction and FDA approval of methylmethacrylate bone cement in the United States in 1971. Cement techniques of that time were based on the original finger-packing method described by Charnley. Introduction of cement by mechanical means, such as syringes and caulking guns, was introduced in the late 1970s. Due to the primitive fixation techniques and the stem designs of that time, aseptic loosening was the most common cause of failure. Although the cemented metal-on-plastic articulation had proven itself superior to other forms of arthroplasty, the relatively unsophisticated metallurgy of the times, combined with stems that were designed intuitively rather than scientifically, led to an unacceptably high rate of stem deformation and fracture. Specific modes of failure leading to loosening and stem fracture were identified, based on the concept that loosening was primarily a mechanical phenomenon.[24]

CAD Design

In 1974, the field of total hip arthroplasty changed forever with the introduction of the CAD, or computer-assisted design stem. Though made of cast Vitallium, it was the first time that engineering principles had been deliberately applied to the design of an implant stem. This provided for the optimal distribution of metal for maximum strength, featuring a "teardrop" depression on either side of the stem that resulted in an I-beam cross section, to address the problem of stem fracture.[25] Like the Aufranc-Turner, it had a valgus orientation and more horizontal collar, but it also had a broad medial border, rounded contours, and no sharp edges, which served to minimize stresses in the cement mantle to prevent cement fracture. It was also the first stem offered in several sizes. Its excessive bulk, however, limited its usefulness in the smaller femur.

Superalloys

An alternative approach to the problem of stem fracture was the introduction of high-strength metals with superior tensile strength and fatigue properties—the so-called "superalloys." These were produced by special treatments of temperature and pressure to decrease the grain size of the alloy. The first of these was Protosol, a chrome-cobalt-nickel alloy from Protek (MP35N). Originally applied to existing stem designs prone to stem fracture, such as the Muller, the superalloy concept was expanded with the introduction of forged Vitallium from Howmedica, and HIP (hot isostatically pressed) Zimaloy from Zimmer, both chrome-cobalt variations. Subsequently, forging was extended to titanium (Ti-6Al-4V) alloy stems to provide superior strength and fatigue resistance in a stem with a significantly lower modulus of elasticity. It was soon realized that the combination of superalloys and scientific design of stems in accord with engineering principles would allow greater approximation of the normal geometry of the hip, with greater offsets, thinner stems, and more physiological head–neck angles.[26]

HD-2 Total Hip

Most of these features were incorporated into subsequent efforts. Designed by William H. Harris, the HD-2 shared many similarities with the CAD, but its forged Vitallium construction allowed a curve in the stem to provide a greater, more anatomical offset, and it was not nearly as bulky as its predecessor.

Socket Designs

Similar engineering principles were applied to socket design. The initial eccentric introitus in the polyethylene socket, to concentrate a thicker layer of plastic in the superior weight-bearing portion, was an intuitive concept shared by the Aufranc-Turner, Harris, New England Baptist Hospital and other systems that did not stand up to scientific scrutiny. Bench testing revealed that the eccentricity set up torsional moments in the cement mantle, and that these moments were likely to contribute to socket loosening. The eccentric concept was subsequently abandoned.

Based on the work of Crowninshield and others, Harris was the first to apply a metal backing shell to the polyethylene socket.[27] Highly controversial at first and rejected by Charnley, Ling, and others, the concept gradually was accepted as a means of diminishing peak stresses in the cement mantle and providing for a more even distribution of forces about the periphery.[28] Harris also pioneered the replaceable socket liner, in anticipation of polyethylene wear problems. Initially conceived as a means to enhance cement fixation, the metal socket shell with its replaceable liner was to become the first of the modular implants, and would become the standard pattern for the generation of cementless sockets that followed in the mid to late 1980s.

Another socket modification, an anterior 40° cutaway to allow clearance for the psoas tendon, was adopted from the St. Georg (Buccholz) total hip by the Buck-32 and ATS (Aufranc-Turner-Scheller) systems in the United States. It never became popular, however, and the modification was abandoned.

Iowa Total Hip

The Iowa Total Hip was designed by Crowninshield and his associates specifically to reduce the stresses in the proximal cement mantle.[29] To this end, the stem was composed of HIP Zimaloy with a proximal tapered wedge cross section, broader at the lateral surface, enhanced by anterior and posterior flanges, like the hood of a cobra. The chrome–cobalt superalloy permitted a more pronounced proximal stem curvature and physiological head offset than the HD-2. The proximal flanges and tapered wedge shape were intended to apply compression stresses to the cement mantle and enhance proximal load transfer. The stems were designed in longer lengths to decrease peak tensile and compressive strains within the cement. The system included a titanium-backed socket with a fine porous coated surface enhancement for acrylic fixation (TiBac). A later improved version included acrylic spacer pods on the posterior surface to ensure an even cement mantle (TiBac II). This system was well designed and well received and inspired other designs to mimic its taper wedge cross section and/or lateral cement flanges, including the Spectron, ATS, Precision, and Charnley cobra stems. Other designs used different methods to accomplish the same end: the Omnifit stem (Osteonics) used "normalization curves," a series of inverted perpendicular steps cut into the anterior and posterior surfaces of the proximal stem, to convert hoop stresses into compression stresses within the cement mantle.

Surface Replacement Arthroplasty

In the late 1970s and early 1980s there was a flurry of interest in Surface Replacement Arthroplasty (SRA), sometimes called the "double cup." Based on the work of Wagner, this procedure attempted to preserve the femoral head beneath a polished shell of chrome–cobalt alloy, articulating with a thin polyethylene socket.[30] Various American modifications on the theme were attempted, including the Aufranc, the THARIES[31] and the TARA.[32] All shared the same intrinsic defect: the necessarily thin socket shell of polyethylene wore rapidly, producing large volumes of particulate debris and subsequent early loosening, often with massive acetabular osteolysis. The procedure failed to achieve its purpose as a conservative arthroplasty; it was, in fact, the very opposite, and was rapidly abandoned.

Cementless Total Hip Arthroplasty

The early failures of cemented total hip arthroplasty, chiefly on the femoral side, led many to believe that cement was the "weak link" in the fixation composite. This supposition led some to seek alternatives to acrylic fixation in an effort to eliminate that element. Others felt that the answer lay in improving the quality and the use of cement. These two opposing schools of thought diverged and evolved along separate paths simultaneously.

Interest in various forms of cementless fixation of total hip components had flourished in Europe for many years. All involve intrinsically stable geometry and/or some means of surface treatment for biologic implant stabilization. The depressions along the stem of Mittelmeier's Autophor hip and the multiple irregularities of the Judet stem and the Madreporic of Lord all increase surface area and provide recesses for ingrowth of endosteal bone. Press-fit stems and press-fit all-polyethylene sockets were featured in the systems promoted by MAR Freeman in England and Bombelli in Italy.

The major area of investigation in the United States has been porous-coated metallic implants, which promote fixation by bony ingrowth into a three-dimensional network of surface-communicating interstices, applied to a solid substrate of the same metal. More recently, interest has developed in Europe and North America in implants fixed by hydroxylapatite (HA) coatings, which induce active bone ongrowth to metal without an intervening fibrous membrane.[33]

AML Total Hip

The first of the porous-coated implants for biologic fixation to achieve widespread use was the AML (Anatomic Medullary Locking) system, developed and popularized by Charles Engh and Dennis Bobyn. A modified Austin Moore stem, with a collar and a round distal cross section, was extensively porous-coated by sintering small beads of chrome cobalt onto the solid metal substrate.[34] This device initially was a one-piece component, with a 32-mm head. It was mated with the Lunceford socket, a hemispherical metal shell, porous-coated on its backside, with three short prongs extended rearward for impaction into the bony acetabulum. The socket was one piece also, lined with polyethylene.

The AML was designed for a diaphyseal interference fit. Later models were modular, with replaceable femoral heads, and for a time were available porous-coated only on the upper third of the stem to permit easier extraction, should removal become necessary. The basic design, however, has not changed to date.

PCA Total Hip

The PCA (Porous Coated Anatomic) was developed by David Hungerford and his associates and became available in 1983.[35] The anatomically curved chrome–cobalt femoral stem was proximally porous-coated with sintered beads and was designed for a line-to-line fit within the endosteal envelope of the femur. This stem depended on metaphyseal fixation, obtained by optimal "fit and fill" of the canal. Its average pore size was larger than that of the AML, but both pore sizes were demonstrated to support bony ingrowth. It was the first of the American implants to incorporate modularity, for intraoperative adjustment of leg lengths and abductor tension, and the first to use the femoral rasp as a trial component, to which trial head–neck assemblies could be applied. These features were rapidly co-opted by other systems. This stem pattern was the inspiration for other "anatomic" designs, including the Zimmer Anatomic and the Intermedics APR.

The PCA socket was initially offered in one piece, but later it was available with modular polyethylene liners. The hemispherical chrome–cobalt shell was fully porous-coated, with two tangential studs at the superior margin of the cup, to stabilize the socket and prevent rotation.

HGP (Harris-Galante) Total Hip

The Harris-Galante Porous (HGP) total hip system made by Zimmer was designed through the collaboration of Jorge Galante and William H. Harris.[36] Unlike the other popular systems of the time, the HGP was manufactured in forged titanium alloy substrate with porous coating of commercially pure titanium wire pads applied by a process called *diffusion bonding*. The resultant porous surface had an average porosity of around 50%, compared with about 35% for the beaded surfaces of the PCA and AML coatings. However, initially it could be applied only to flat surfaces in porous pads, compared with the circumferential coating of sintered beaded surfaces. This defect was responsible for a number of failures, manifesting as subsidence or loosening, due to disassociation of the pads from their receptor sites, osteolysis due to fretting, and inadequate surface area for stabilization by bony ingrowth. Similar problems beset the long-stem BIAS stem design of Raymond Gustilo,[37] initially used for cementless revision, which shared these design flaws.

If the stems had inherent problems, however, the HGP sockets proved superior. The hemispherical titanium alloy shell was fully porous-coated with titanium wire, with multiple fenstrations for supplemental screw fixation. The shell supported a modular hemispherical polyethylene liner. Both animal and human studies demonstrated evidence of excellent stabilization by bony ingrowth.

Evolution of Cement Technique

While cementless implant design was evolving, cement technology was improving. Harris and his coworkers described and codified the elements of cementing technique common to successful results. Charnley's original finger-packing method was deemed first generation technique. The second generation was distinguished by the use of a distal femoral plug to obturate the femoral canal and create a closed proximal cylinder; femoral preparation with brush and pulsatile irrigation to skeletonize the endosteal cancellous bone for improved cement penetration; retrograde injection of low-viscosity cement with a long-barreled cement gun to decrease voids; and pressurization of the cement before implantation, a technique pioneered by Robin Ling and perfected by Jo Miller.[38] The addition of porosity reduction by either centrifugation or vacuum mixing to enhance the fatigue life of cement, and surface enhancement of implants by PMMA precoating, macrotexturing, or both, are the hallmarks of the third and current generation of cement technique.

Modes of Failure Influence Later Designs

Debonding between the implant and the cement was identified as the first step in the process of loosening. Efforts were directed at increasing the durability of this interface. Newer implant designs incorporated macrotexturing and finer surface enhancement, such as bead blasting, to increase surface area and thereby strengthen the cement–implant bond. Bench studies demonstrated that thinner areas or voids in the cement mantle were sites of cement fracture propagation about the stem. Efforts were therefore directed at preventing this problem by ensuring an even, concentric mantle of adequate thickness everywhere about the stem. Optimal positioning of the stem and proportionality were required to accomplish this.

Precision Total Hip

Anthropomorphic studies by Noble and his coworkers led to the creation of the Precision hip, a system that provided proportional increases in stem length and girth based on anatomical variations. These stems were shot-blasted and proximally macrotextured for improved cement bonding. Implanted with a precise reaming technique, this design ensured an even cement mantle about the entire stem. Alignment with the neutral axis of the femur was provided by proximal and distal modular acrylic centralizers, which would chemically bond with cement at surgery.

Precoat Total Hip

The latest refinement of the stem design of Harris, the Precoat femoral stem, featured a unique, industrially applied film of methylmethacrylate about the proximal third of the stem. This film allowed the formation of a chemical bond with cement applied at surgery to enhance durability of the implant–cement interface.

In response to this development, the Precision hip was soon modified to the Strata stem, which used the same basic stem design but added a proximal industrially applied wedge of solid acrylic instead of a thin film, to both bond with and pressurize the cement injected at surgery. The Precoat was, in turn, modified to the Centralign, which included small teardrops of acrylic both proximally and distally on the stem to provide neutral alignment and an even cement mantle, as well as its own version of proximal macrotexturing and precoating both proximally and distally. The competition between manufacturers led to cross-pollination of concepts and similar features began to appear on stems of various companies.

The most recent implant designs have incorporated the knowledge that a minimum thickness of cement must be maintained at all points to prevent fragmentation and subsequent loosening. Thinner, tapered distal stems, with napkin-ring centralizers of acrylic and more physiological head–neck offsets, are common features of the Definition stem from Howmedica and the Versys system from Zimmer.

Hybrid Total Hip

Long-term studies documented superior results with second generation cement technique. It became apparent that to compete with cemented clinical results, the new generation of cementless implants had to equal or better the results achieved with the newer implant designs and modern cement fixation methods. While it was true that both cemented and cementless implants could yield successful results, it was observed that cemented sockets tended to loosen in a linear fashion, with time. Cementless sockets offered a potential advantage for durability of fixation, and were proved clearly superior to cemented sockets for revisions.[39] On the other hand, although a number of successful results were observed with cementless stems, they were associated with a higher incidence of stress shielding, periprosthetic osteolysis, and thigh pain than their cemented counterparts. This observation led to the combination of both forms of fixation in one joint, the hybrid total hip replacement: a cementless socket with a cemented stem.[40]

The Consequences of Wear Debris

The bioactive membrane at the bone–cement interface has been found to elaborate enzymes and local factors, leading to macrophage-mediated dissolution of bone, or osteolysis, in response to polyethylene wear debris.[41] Whereas fixation was once the primary problem in joint replacement, the clinical response to polyethylene wear debris has now emerged as the major factor in failure, responsible for both prosthetic loosening and loss of bone stock. This realization has had major implications for implant design and fixation techniques. It is now believed that an intact cement mantle and circumferential porous or HA coating may prevent or delay the insinuation of wear particles into the interfaces. Current investigations are now focused on means to minimize wear within the joint and the attendant ills that wear promotes. Ceramic on plastic, ceramic on ceramic, and metal on metal arthroplasties are being evaluated. The recent development of IMS (Irradiated in the Molten State) polyethylene, with a wear rate eight to ten times that of standard gamma-irradiated polyethylene, as reported by Jasty and his associates,[42] opens entire new vistas for arthroplasty of the hip. If its promise is fulfilled, such a bearing surface will allow the benefits of hip replacement to be extended to the very young and may offer the prospect of an implant that will last the lifetime of the patient. Most of all, if the products of wear can be reduced to tolerable levels and the problems of osteolysis and loosening can be eliminated, save for trauma or infection, then revision total hip arthroplasty may well become but a footnote in the history of hip replacement surgery.

References

1. Shands AR, Jr. Historical milestones in the development of modern surgery of the hip joint. In: Tronzo RG ed. *Surgery of the Hip Joint*. Philadelphia: Lea and Febiger, 1973:1–26.
2. Girdlestone GR. Acute pyogenic arthritis of the hip. An operation giving free access and effective drainage. *Lancet*. 1943:1:419–421.
3. Fielding JW, Stillwell WT. Evolution of total hip arthroplasty. In: Stillwell WT. *The Art of Total Hip Arthroplasty*. Orlando: Grune and Stratton, 1987:1–23.
4. Smith-Petersen MN. Evolution of mould arthroplasty of the hip joint. *J Bone Joint Surg Br*. 1948;30:59–75.
5. Aufranc OE. Constructive hip surgery with mold arthroplasty. In: *Instructional Course Lectures*. Am Academy Orthopaedic Surgeons. Ann Arbor: J.W. Edwards, 1954:11:163–176.
6. Aufranc OE. Constructive hip surgery with the vitallium mold. A report on 1000 cases of arthroplasty of the hip over a fifteen-year period. *J Bone Joint Surg Am*. 1957;39:237–248.
7. Aufranc OE *Constructive Surgery of the Hip*. St. Louis, C.V. Mosby, 1962:96–126.

8. Urist MR. The principles of hip-socket arthroplasty. *J Bone Joint Surg Am.* 1957;39:786–810.
9. Moore AT, Bohlman HR. Metal hip joint. A case report. *J Bone Joint Surg.* 1943;25:688–692.
10. Moore AT. The self-locking metal hip prosthesis. *J Bone Joint Surg Am.* 1957;39:811–827.
11. Judet J, Judet R. The use of an artificial femoral head for arthroplasty of the hip joint. *J Bone Joint Surg Br.* 1950;32:166–173.
12. Thompson FR. Vitallium intramedullary hip prosthesis: preliminary report. *NY State J Med* 1952;52:3011–3020.
13. Moore AT. Metal hip joint: A new self-locking vitallium prosthesis. *Southern Med J.* 1952;45;1015–1019.
14. Wiles P. The surgery of the osteoarthritic hip. *Brit J Surg* 1958;45:488–497.
15. McKee GK, Watson-Farrar J. Replacement of arthritic hips by the McKee-Farrar prosthesis. *J Bone Joint Surg Br.* 1966;48:245–259.
16. Haboush EJ. A new operation for arthroplasty of the hip based on biomechanics, photoelasticity, fast-setting dental acrylic and other considerations. *Bul Hosp Joint Dis.* 1953;14:242.
17. Charnley J. The lubrication of animal joints. *New Scientist.* 1959;6:60.
18. Charnley J. Arthroplasty of the hip. A new operation. *Lancet.* 1961;1:1129.
19. Charnley J. Low friction arthroplasty of the hip joint. *J Bone Joint Surg Br.* 1971,53:149.
20. Muller ME. Total hip prostheses. *Clin Orthop.* 1970;72:46–68.
21. Ling RSM. Total hip replacement using a collarless femoral prosthesis. In: *The Hip*. St. Louis: C.V. Mosby, 1980:82–111.
22. Aufranc OE, Turner RH. Total replacement of the arthritic hip. *Hospital Practice.* 1971;6(10):66.
23. Amstutz, HC. Trapezoidal-28 total hip replacement. *Clin. Orthop.* 1973;95:158.
24. Gruen TA, McNeice GM, Amstutz HC. "Modes of failure" of cement stem-type femoral components: A radiographic analysis of loosening *Clin. Orthop.* 1979;141:17–27.
25. Walker PS. *Human Joints and Their Artificial Replacements*. Springfield: Charles C. Thomas, 1977.
26. Stillwell WT. Implant selection for total hip arthroplasty. In: Stillwell WT, ed. *The Art of Total Hip Arthroplasty*. Orlando: Grune and Stratton, 1987:69–96.
27. Carter DR, Harris WH, Vasu R. Stress distributions in the acetabular region. II. Effects of cement thickness and metal backing in total hip acetabular component. *J Biomech.* 1982;15:165–170.
28. Pedersen DR, Crowninshield RD, Brand RA, Johnston RC. An axisymmetric model of acetabular components in total hip arthroplasty. *J Biomech.* 1982;15:305–315.
29. Crowninshield RD, Brand RA, Johnston RC, Milroy JC. The effect of femoral stem cross-sectional geometry on cement stresses in total hip reconstruction. *Clin Orthop.* 1980;146:71–77.
30. Wagner H. Surface replacement arthroplasty of the hip. *Clin Orthop.* 1978;134:102–130.
31. Amstutz HC, Graff-Radford A, Gruen TA, Clarke IC. THARIES surface replacements: A review of the first 100 cases. *Clin Orthop.* 1978;134:87–101.
32. Townley CO. Hemi and total articular replacement arthroplasty of the hip with the fixed femoral cup. *Orthop Clin North Am.* 1982;13:869–894.
33. Geesink RGT. Hydroxylapatite coated toatl hip replacement. Five year clinical and radiological results. In: Geesink RGT, Manley MT. ed. *Hydroxylapatite Coatings in Orthopaedic Surgery*. New York: Raven, 1993:171–208.
34. Engh CA, Bobyn JD, Matthews JG II. Biologic fixation of a modified Moore prosthesis. I. Evaluation of early clinical results. In: *The Hip*. St. Louis: C.V. Mosby, 1984.
35. Hungerford DS, Borden LS, Hedley AK, Habermann ET, Kenna RV. Principles and techniques of cementless total hip arthroplasty. In: Stillwell WT, ed. *The Art of Total Hip Arthroplasty*. Orlando, Grune and Stratton, 1987:293–316.
36. Harris WH, Krushell RJ, Galante JO. Results of cemented total hip arthroplasties using the Harris-Galante prosthesis. *Clin Orthop.* 1988;235:120–126.
37. Gustilo RB, Pasternak HS. Revision total hip arthroplasty with titanium ingrowth prosthesis and bone grafting for failed cemented femoral component loosening. *Clin Orthop.* 1988;235:111–119.
38. Miller J, Johnson JA. Advances in cementing techniques in total hip arthroplasty. In: Stillwell WT, ed. *The Art of Total Hip Arthroplasty*. Orlando: Grune and Stratton, 1987;277–291.
39. Harris WH, Davies JP. Modern use of modern cement for total hip replacement. *Orthop Clin North Am.* 1988;19(3): 581–589.
40. Harris WH, Maloney WJ. Hybrid total hip arthroplasty. *Clin Orthop.* 1989;249:21–29.
41. Goldring SR, Schiller AL, Roelke M, Rourke CM, O'Neil DA, Harris WH. The synovial-like membrane at the bone-cement interface in loose total hip replacements and its proposed role in bone lysis. *J Bone Joint Surg Am.* 1983;65:575–584.
42. Jasty M, Bragdon C, O'Connor D. Wear performance of a new form of ultra high molecular weight polyethylene. Presented at the 26th Annual Harvard Hip Course: Total hip replacement. Polyethylene: where are we now? Cambridge, MA. Oct. 3, 1996.

Contents

Dedication	v
Roderick H. Turner	
Foreword	vii
Eduardo A. Salvati	
A History of Hip Replacement Surgery	ix
William Thomas Stillwell	
Contributors	xxv

Part 1. Mechanisms of Failure of Total Hip Arthroplasty 1
Thomas S. Thornhill

1. Prosthetic Loosening in Total Hip Replacements 3
   Murali Jasty

2. Polyethylene Wear 11
   James V. Bono and George Faithfull

3. Osteolysis in Total Joint Arthroplasty: Basic Science 21
   W.A. Jiranek and S.R. Goldring

4. Dislocation Following Total Hip Arthroplasty 32
   Douglas A. Dennis

5. Fracture 40
   Mitchell Geiger, Merrill A. Ritter, and John B. Meding

Part 2. Evaluation of the Painful Total Hip Arthroplasty 45
Thomas S. Thornhill

6. Evaluation of the Painful Total Hip Arthroplasty 47
   Robert J. Carangelo and Arnold D. Scheller

7. Radiographic Evaluation of the Painful Total Hip Arthroplasty 59
   Arthur H. Newberg, Steven M. Wetzner, and John M. Ellis

8. Pain Syndromes in Revision Total Hip Arthroplasty 78
   Ross J. Muscomeci

Part 3. Preoperative Planning 89
James V. Bono and Joseph C. McCarthy

9. Bone Stock Loss and Allografting: Acetabulum 93
   Wayne G. Paprosky, Michael S. Bradford, and Todd D. Sekundiak

10. Bone Stock Loss and Allografting: Femur 100
    Donald B. Longjohn and Lawrence D. Dorr

11. Bone Stock Loss and Allografting: Trochanter 112
    Geoffrey H. Westrich

12. Blood Management in Revision Total Hip Arthroplasty 118
    THOMAS P. SCULCO AND DAVID E. TATE

13. Anesthesia Considerations: Hypotension and Hemodilution 124
    NIGEL E. SHARROCK

14. Preoperative Templating in Revision Total Hip Arthroplasty 129
    KENNETH B. MATHIS, PHILIP C. NOBLE, AND HUGH S. TULLOS

15. Biomechanics of Revision Hip Replacement 135
    PHILIP C. NOBLE

16. Equipment Overview 142
    JAMES C. SLATER

17. Use of the Cup-Out® Device for Difficult Acetabular Revisions 149
    PAUL F. LACHIEWICZ

18. Hand Tools 150
    JAMES V. BONO

19. Ultrasonic Cement Removal 152
    RICHARD L. WIXSON

20. Drill and Excavation 154
    FRANK B. GRAY

21. Bone Bank/Bone Graft 155
    JAMES C. SLATER

22. Implant Inventory 160
    GEOFFRY VAN FLANDERN

Part 4. Surgical Techniques in Revision Total Hip Arthroplasty 165

        Section 1. Femur 165
                JOSEPH C. MCCARTHY AND JAMES V. BONO

23. Reconstruction of Cavitary Defects: Bone Grafting 167
    JAMES P. JAMISON

24. Reconstruction of Cavitary Defects: Endosteal Grafting 176
    JAMES J. ELTING

25. Reconstruction of Segmental Defects: Onlay Allografting 185
    ROGER H. EMERSON, JR. AND WILLIAM C. HEAD

26. Use of Femoral Allografts in Reconstruction of Major Segmental Defects .. 189
    HUGH P. CHANDLER AND ROBERT J. CARANGELO

27. Revision of the Femoral Component Using Cement Fixation 204
    JOHN J. CALLAGHAN

28. Cement within Cement Femoral Revision 214
    FRANK V. ALUISIO AND DAVID A. MATTINGLY

29. Distal Fixation 217
    CHARLES A. ENGH AND CHARLES A. ENGH, JR.

30. Modularity in Total Hip Arthroplasty: The S-ROM Prosthesis 224
    ROBERT J. CARANGELO AND JAMES V. BONO

31. Femoral Component Using the Impact Modular Total Hip Implant 234
    LEO A. WHITESIDE

32. Cemented Long-Stem Femoral Components in Revision Total Hip Arthroplasty 239
    DAVID A. MATTINGLY

    Section 1. Conclusions **243**

    Section 2. Surgical Approaches **245**

33. Posterolateral Approach 247
    DAVID A. MATTINGLY

34. The Direct Lateral and Vastus Slide Approach 251
    HUGH P. CHANDLER AND ROBERT J. CARANGELO

35. Modified Dall Approach 263
    DESMOND M. DALL

36. Conventional Trochanteric Osteotomy 266
    BENJAMIN E. BIERBAUM AND RUSSELL G. TIGGES

37. The Anterolateral Surgical Approach 270
    THOMAS H. MALLORY

38. Trochanter Slide Surgical Approach 274
    JOSEPH C. MCCARTHY

39. Extended Trochanteric Osteotomy 277
    ROGER H. EMERSON, JR. AND WILLIAM C. HEAD

40. Extended Lateral Femoral Osteotomy 280
    WAYNE G. PAPROSKY, TODD D. SEKUNDIAK, AND TERRY I. YOUNGER

41. The Cameron Anterior Osteotomy 285
    HUGH U. CAMERON

42. Retroperitoneal Approach 287
    STEVEN J. CAMER AND JOSEPH C. MCCARTHY

    Section 3. Acetabulum **291**
                JOSEPH C. MCCARTHY

43. Management of Cavitary Deficiencies 293
    RICHARD D. SCOTT AND CHRISTOPHER W. OLCOTT

44. Management of Acetabular Deficiency with a Bipolar Prosthesis at Revision THA 298
    STEVEN ROBERT WARDELL

45. Management of Segmental Deficiencies 302
    WAYNE G. PAPROSKY, MICHAEL S. BRADFORD, AND TODD D. SEKUNDIAK

46. Use of Structural Allografts in Hip Reconstruction 309
    HUGH P. CHANDLER AND ROBERT J. CARANGELO

47. Determination of the Hip Center 320
    EDWARD C. BROWN III AND SCOTT S. KELLEY

48. Use of Oblong or Modular Cups 326
    PHILIP A. G. KARPOS

49. Management of Medial Deficiencies 330
    CHRISTOPHER W. OLCOTT

50. Management of Posterior Acetabular Deficiencies 339
    VIKTOR E. KREBBS, JOSEPH C. MCCARTHY, AND LESTER S. BORDEN

51. Use of Cages 349
    WILLIAM N. CAPELLO, EDWARD J. HELLMAN, AND JUDY R. FEINBERG

Part 4. Conclusions 357

Part 5. Evaluation and Prevention of Postoperative Complications 359
RODERICK H. TURNER

52. Neurological Injury 361
    PETER P. ANAS AND BRENT FELIX

53. Postoperative Infection 371
    GEOFFREY H. WESTRICH, EDUARDO A. SALVATI, AND BARRY BRAUSE

54. Dislocation Following Total Hip Arthroplasty 391
    JOHN P. MCCABE, PAUL M. PELLICCI, AND EDUARDO A. SALVATI

55. Prevention of Deep Venous Thromboembolism Following Primary and
    Revision Hip and Knee Arthroplasty 401
    JAY R. LIEBERMAN

56. Anesthetic Complications 418
    MICHAEL SMALKY AND DONALD FOSTER

57. Cardiac Complications 425
    GERARD A. SWEENEY AND CHARLES J. DOW

58. Broken Femoral Stems 431
    JAMES P. JAMISON AND ST. GEORGE TUCKER AUFRANC

59. Surgical Complications in Revision Arthroplasty 438
    STEVEN J. CAMER

60. Genitoruinary Complications 448
    GARY P. KEARNEY AND CHRISTOPHER J. DOYLE

61. Postoperative Wound Problems 459
    LEONARD B. MILLER

62. Heterotopic Ossification 464
    DOUGLAS E. PADGETT

Part 6. Special Considerations 475
BENJAMIN E. BIERBAUM

63. Total Hip Replacement Following Prior Surgeries 477
    MICHAEL H. HUO, PETER R. JAY, AND ROBERT L. BULY

64. Leg Length Inequality Following Total Hip Replacement 492
    JOSÉ A. RODRIGUEZ AND CHITRANJAN S. RANAWAT

65. Metastatic Disease of the Hip 498
    STEPHEN M. HOROWITZ AND ARNOLD T. BERMAN

66. Conversion of Girdlestone Arthroplasty to Total Hip Replacement 505
    ERIC MASTERSON, BASSAM A. MASRI, AND CLIVE P. DUNCAN

67. Conversion of the Fused Hip to Total Hip Arthroplasty 517
    BENJAMIN E. BIERBAUM AND RUSSELL G. TIGGES

68. Motor Deficits 522
    RUSSELL G. COHEN AND AARON G. ROSENBERG

69. Fractures after Total Hip Replacement 530
    MITCHELL H. GEIGER, MERRILL A. RITTER, JOHN B. MEDING, AND PHILIP M. FARIS

70. Protrusio Acetabuli 538
    MICHAEL J. CHMELL AND RICHARD D. SCOTT

Part 7. Making Revision Hip Surgery Work **543**
    JOSEPH C. MCCARTHY AND JAMES V. BONO

71. Maximizing Efficiency in Revision Total Hip Surgery 545
    JOSEPH C. MCCARTHY AND NANCY L. HILTZ

72. Physical Rehabilitation 549
    DONNA DINARDO

73. Outcome Studies 553
    RICHARD IORIO AND WILLIAM L. HEALY

74. Looking Forward: Implant Research 562
    HAROLD ABERMAN, MICHAEL BUSHELOW, LARRY GUSTAVSON, CAS STARK, D.C. SUN,
    AIGUO WANG, AND KATHY WANG

75. Robotically Assisted Cement Removal 576
    BILL WILLIAMSON, WILLIAM BARGAR, AND ALAN KALVIN

Part 8. Medical Malpractice in Revision Hip Surgery **581**
    DOUGLAS DANNER AND RODERICK H. TURNER

76. Medical Malpractice in Revision Hip Surgery 583
    DOUGLAS DANNER AND RODERICK H. TURNER

Index 599

Contributors

Harold Aberman, DVM
Howmedica Corporation
359 Veterans Blvd.
Rutherford, NJ 07070

Frank V. Aluisio, MD
Greensboro Orthopedic Center
P.O.Box 38008
Greensboro, NC 27438-8008

Peter P. Anas, MD
New England Baptist Hospital
125 Parker Hill Ave.
Boston, MA 02120

St. George Tucker Aufranc, MD
New England Baptist Hospital
125 Parker Hill Ave.
Boston, MA 02120

William Bargar, MD
UC Davis, School of Medicine,
Sutter General Hospital
1020 29th Street, #450
Sacramento, CA 95816

Arnold T. Berman, MD
Allegheny University Hospital, Center City
Broad and Vine Street
Philadelphia, PA 19102

Benjamin E. Bierbaum, MD
New England Baptist Hospital
125 Parker Hill Avenue
Boston, MA 02120

James V. Bono, MD
New England Baptist Hospital
125 Parker Hill Avenue
Boston, MA 02120

Lester S. Borden, MD
Cleveland Clinic Foundation
9500 Euclid Avenue
Cleveland, OH 44195

Michael S. Bradford, MD
Sunrise Medical Center
Las Vegas, NV 89106

Barry Brause, MD
The Hospital for Special Surgery
535 E. 70th Street
New York, NY 10021

Edward C. Brown III, MD
University of North Carolina Hospitals,
Chapel Hill
242 Burnett Womack Bldg., CB 7055
Chapel Hill, NC 27599

Robert L. Buly, MD, MS
The Hospital for Special Surgery
535 E. 70th Street
New York, NY 10021

Michael Bushelow
Howmedica Corporation
359 Veterans Blvd.
Rutherford, NJ 07070

John J. Callaghan, MD
University of Iowa College of Medicine
Iowa City, IA 52242

Steven J. Camer, MD
New England Baptist Hospital
125 Parker Hill Avenue
Boston, MA 02120

Hugh U. Cameron, MD, ChB, FRCSC
University of Toronto
43 Wellesley St. E., Suite 318
Toronto, Ontario
Canada M4Y 1H1

William N. Capello, MD
Indiana University School of Medicine
541 Clinical Drive - CL600
Indianapolis, IN 46202-5111

Robert J. Carangelo, MD
New Britain Hospital
New Britain, CT 06052

Hugh P. Chandler, MD
Harvard Medical School
15 Parkman Street
Boston, MA 02114

Michael J. Chmell, MD
University of Illinois College of Medicine
5668 East State Street
Rockford, IL 61108

Russell G. Cohen, MD
Rush-Presbyterian-St. Lukes Medical Center
1725 W. Harrison Street, Suite 1063
Chicago, IL 60612

Desmond M. Dall, MCh. Orth. FRCS
University of Southern California
1975 Zonal Avenue
Los Angeles, CA 90033

Douglas Danner, Esq.
of the Boston Bar
Duxbury, MA 02332

Douglas Dennis, MD
Medical Director, Rose Musculoskeletal Laboratory
Denver Orthopedic Specialists, PC
1601 E. 19th Ave., Suite 5000
Denver, CO 80218

Donna Dinardo, BS, RPT
New England Baptist Hospital
125 Parker Hill Avenue
Boston, MA 02120

Lawrence D. Dorr, MD
Center for Arthritis & Joint Implant Surgery
University of Southern California
School of Medicine
1450 San Pablo Street
Los Angeles, CA 90033

Charles J. Dow, MD
One Brookline Place
Brookline, MA 02146

Christopher J. Doyle, MD
319 Longwood Avenue
Boston, MA 02115

Clive P. Duncan, MD, FRCS
Vancouver Hospital & Health Science Center
90 West 10th Avenue
Vancouver, British Columbia
Canada V5Z 4E3

John M. Ellis, MD
New England Baptist Hospital
125 Parker Hill Avenue
Boston, MA 02120

James J. Elting, MD
Department of Orthopedics
Bassett Healthcare
Oneonta, NY 13820

Roger H. Emerson, Jr., MD
University of Texas Southwestern Medical School
6300 West Parker Road
Plano, TX 75053

Charles A. Engh, MD
Anderson Orthopaedic Research Institute
2501 Parker's Lane
Alexandria, VA 22306

Charles A. Engh, Jr., MD
Anderson Orthopaedic Research Institute
2501 Parker's Lane
Alexandria, VA 22306

George Faithfull
Howmedica Corporation
359 Veterans Blvd.
Rutherford, NJ 07070

Philip M. Faris, MD
1199 Hadley Road
Mooresville, IN 46158

Judy R. Feinberg, PhD
Indiana University School of Medicine
541 Clinical Drive - CL600
Indianapolis, IN 46202-5111

Brent Felix, MD
Salt Lake Orthopedic Clinic
1160 E. 3900 South
Salt Lake City, UT 84124

Contributors

Donald Foster, MD
New England Baptist Hospital
125 Parker Hill Ave.
Boston, MA 02120

Mitchell H. Geiger, MD
770 Magnolia, Suite 1D
Corona, CA 91719

S.R. Goldring, MD
New England Baptist Bone and Joint Institute
Boston, MA

Frank B. Gray, MD
Knoxville Orthopedic Clinic
1128 Weisgarber
Knoxville, TN 37909

Larry Gustavson
Howmedica Corporation
359 Veterans Blvd.
Rutherford, NJ 07070

William C. Head, MD
6300 W. Parker Road, Suite 220
Plano, TX 75093

William L. Healy, MD
Lahey Hitchcock Medical Center
41 Mall Road
Burlington, MA 01805

Edward J. Hellman, MD
Indiana University School of Medicine
541 Clinical Drive - CL600
Indianapolis, IN 46202-5111

Nancy L. Hiltz, MS, RN, ONC
New England Baptist Hospital
125 Parker Hill Ave.
Boston, MA 02120

Stephen M. Horowitz, MD
Allegheny University Hospital, Center City
Broad and Vine Street
Philadelphia, PA 19102

Michael H. Huo, MD, MS
Arthritis Center
6550 Fannin, Suite 2625
Houston, TX 77030

Richard Iorio, MD
Lahey Hitchcock Medical Center
41 Mall Road
Burlington, MA 01805

James P. Jamison, MD
Youngstown Orthopedic Assn.
6470 Tippecanoe
Canfield, OH 44406

Murali Jasty, MD
Massachusetts General Hospital
Boston, MA 02114

Peter R. Jay, MD
Johns Hopkins Univ. School of Medicine
Johns Hopkins Bayview Medical Center
4940 Eastern Avenue
Baltimore, MD 21224

W.A. Jiranek, MD
Medical College of Virginia
Virginia Commonwealth University
Richmond, VA

Alan Kalvin, PhD
Thomas J. Watson Research Center
Yorktown Heights, NY 10674

Philip A.G. Karpos, MD
Tennessee Orthopaedic Alliance
St. Thomas Hospital
Nashville, TN 37203

Gary P. Kearney, MD
319 Longwood Avenue
Boston, MA 02115

Scott S. Kelley, MD
University of North Carolina Hospitals, Chapel Hill
242 Burnett-Womack Bldg, CG 7055
Chapel Hill, NC 27599

Viktor E. Krebbs, MD
Cleveland Clinic Foundation
9500 Euclid Avenue
Cleveland, OH 44195

Paul F. Lachiewicz, MD
Univ. of North Carolina School of Medicine, Chapel Hill
242 Burnett-Womack Bldg., CB 7055
Chapel Hill, NC 27599

Jay R. Lieberman, MD
UCLA Medical Center
10833 LeConte Avenue
Los Angeles, CA 90095

Donald B. Longjohn, MD
Center for Arthritis and Joint Implant Surgery
University of Southern California School of Medicine
1450 San Pablo Street
Los Angeles, CA 90033

Thomas H. Mallory, MD, FACS
Joint Implant Surgeons, Inc.
720 Broad Street
Columbus, OH 43215

Bassam A. Masri, MD, FRCS
Vancouver Hospital & Health Science Center
90 West 10th Avenue
Vancouver, British Columbia
Canada V5Z 4E3

Eric Masterson, Bsc, Mch, FRCS
Vancouver Hospital & Health Science Center
90 West 10th Avenue
Vancouver, British Columbia
Canada V5Z 4E3

Kenneth B. Mathis, MD
11914 Astoria
Houston, TX 77089

David A. Mattingly, MD
New England Baptist Hospital
125 Parker Hill Avenue
Boston, MA 02120

John P. McCabe, MMSC, Mch, FRCSI
The Hospital for Special Surgery
535 E. 70th Street
New York, NY 10021

Joseph C. McCarthy, MD
New England Baptist Hospital
125 Parker Hill Avenue
Boston, MA 02120

John B. Meding, MD
1199 Hadley Road
Mooresville, IN 46158

Leonard B. Miller, MD
One Brookline Place
Brookline, MA 02146

Ross J. Muscomeci, MD
New England Baptist Hospital
125 Parker Hill Road
Boston, MA 02120

Arthur H. Newberg, MD
New England Baptist Hospital
125 Parker Hill Avenue
Boston, MA 02120

Philip C. Noble, PhD
Methodist Hospital
6565 Fannin, MS, F102
Houston, TX 77030

Christopher W. Olcott, MD
University of Rochester Medical Center
601 Elmwood Ave.
Rochester, NY 14648

Douglas E. Padgett, MD
Hospital for Special Surgery
535 East 70th Street
New York, NY 10021

Wayne G. Paprosky, MD
Rush-Presbyterian-St. Luke's Medical Center
Chicago, IL 60612

Paul M. Pellicci, MD
The Hospital for Special Surgery
535 E. 70th Street
New York, NY 10021

Chitranjan S. Ranawat, MD
Center for Total Joint Replacement
Lenox Hill Hospital
130 East 77th Street
New York, NY 10021

Merrill A. Ritter, MD
1199 Hadley Road
Mooresville, IN 46158

José A. Rodriguez, MD
Center for Total Joint Replacement
Lenox Hill Hospital
130 East 77th Street
New York, NY 10021

Aaron G. Rosenberg, MD
Rush-Presbyterian-St. Lukes Medical Center
1725 W. Harrison Street, Suite 1063
Chicago, IL 60612

Eduardo A. Salvati, MD
The Hospital for Special Surgery
535 E. 70th Street
New York, NY 10021

Arnold D. Scheller, MD
New England Baptist Hospital
125 Parker Hill Avenue
Boston, MA 02120

Richard D. Scott, MD
New England Baptist Hospital
125 Parker Hill Avenue
Boston, MA 02120

Contributors

Thomas P. Sculco, MD
The Hospital for Special Surgery
535 E. 70th Street
New York, NY 10021

Todd D. Sekundiak, MD
University of Manitoba
St. Boniface Hospital
Winnipeg, Canada R2H 3C3

Nigel E. Sharrock, MD, BhB
The Hospital for Special Surgery
535 E. 70th Street
New York, NY 10021

James C. Slater, MD
Arthritis Surgical Center of Oklahoma
1919 South Wheeling, Suite 500
Tulsa, OK 74104

Michael Smalky, MD
New England Baptist Hospital
125 Parker Hill Avenue
Boston, MA 02120

Cas Stark
Howmedica Corporation
359 Veterans Blvd.
Rutherford, NJ 07070

William Stillwell, MD, FACS
St. John's Episcopal Hospital
Smithtown, NY 11787

D.C. Sun, PhD
Howmedica Corporation
359 Veterans Blvd.
Rutherford, NJ 07070

Gerard A. Sweeney, MD
One Brookline Place
Brookline, MA 02146

David E. Tate, MD
Christine M. Kleinert Institute
225 Abraham Flexner Way
Louisville, KY 40202

Thomas S. Thornhill, MD
Brigham and Women's Hospital
75 Francis Street
Boston, MA 02115 USA

Russell G. Tigges, MD
100A Fulton Avenue
Poughkeepsie, NY 12603

Hugh S. Tullos, MD
6550 Fannin Street
Houston, TX 77030

Roderick H. Turner, MD
New England Baptist Hospital
125 Parker Hill Ave.
Boston, MA 02120

Geoffry Van Flandern, MD
New England Baptist Hospital
125 Parker Hill Ave.
Boston, MA 02120

Aiguo Wang, PhD
Howmedica Corporation
359 Veterans Blvd.
Rutherford, NJ 07070

Kathy Wang, PhD
Howmedica Corporation
359 Veterans Blvd.
Rutherford, NJ 07070

Steven Robert Wardell, MD
Parkview Orthopaedic Group, S.C.
Palos Heights, IL 60463

Geoffrey H. Westrich, MD
The Hospital for Special Surgery
535 E. 70th Street
New York, NY 10021

Steven M. Wetzner, MD
New England Baptist Hospital
125 Parker Hill Avenue
Boston, MA 02120

Leo A. Whiteside, MD
Biomechanical Research Laboratory
Missouri Bone & Joint Center
Barnes-Jewish West County Blvd.
12634 Olive Blvd.
St. Louis, MO 63141

Bill Williamson
1850 Research Park Drive
Davis, CA 95616

Richard L. Wixson, MD
Northwestern University Medical School
676 North St. Clari St., Suite 450
Chicago, IL 60611

Terry I. Younger, MD
University of Illinois
Chicago, IL 60612

Part 1
Mechanisms of Failure of Total Hip Arthroplasty

Thomas S. Thornhill

The path to a successful revision total hip arthroplasty begins with a thorough understanding of the mechanism(s) of failure of the index arthroplasty. The treatment paradigm and the timing of revision surgery are based on the biomechanic and biologic aspects of the failure mechanism. This section deals with three important mechanisms of failure: (1) wear with subsequent loosening and osteolysis, (2) dislocation, and (3) fracture. Other failure mechanisms such as infection, heterotopic ossification, component breakage, and thigh pain will be covered in other sections.

Although any textbook dedicated to revision hip arthroplasty must focus on failure, it is clear that total hip arthroplasty has been one of the major advances in medicine in the 20th century. The American Rheumatological Association lists total joint arthroplasty as the major improvement in the care of the arthritic patient, and literally hundreds of thousands of people have been spared the pain and functional limitation that characterizes patients with hip arthritis. As we push the envelope of this procedure to include younger, more active patients, we unfortunately also increase the risks of failure. Using our current metallurgy and fixation methods, we are not able to offer hip replacement for the young, active patient. The metals currently in use—cobalt chrome and titanium alloys—do not have an elastic modulus that reproduces bone. This creates a modulus mismatch and, hence, relative motion between the implant and the adjacent bone. Methylmethacrylate has the serendipitous property of an elastic modulus between cortical and cancellous bone and, therefore, can offer an implant composite modulus that more closely mimics the bony substrate.

Investigators have attempted to use hollow implant designs with conventional metals, or even composite designs that have a modulus similar to bone. The isoelastic hip is one such design that gained fleeting popularity. Unfortunately, most attempts at radical change from the cemented Charnley design have proven to be inferior and have been abandoned. This learning curve in design has left a legacy of failed hips requiring revision arthroplasty. Threaded cups, surface arthroplasty, carbon-impregnated polyethylene, Teflon™, Delrin™, and, more recently, Hyalmer™ have all proven to be inferior compared to standard design with ultra-high molecular weight high-density polyethylene (UHMWHDP). Moreover, these failures have left a generation of skeptical surgeons wary of radical design changes. This has both a healthy effect as well as a potential negative effect that may delay incorporation of a beneficial evolutionary change. The renewed interest in metal-on-metal articulations is mollified by a concern over systemic metal toxicity. Recent reports have extolled the benefits of hydroxyapatite in primary uncemented fixation. Its osteoconducive properties leading to a potentially stronger implant bond have been borne out in early clinical studies. Concerns over its inflammatory potential as a particulate material, the critical parameters for application, and its bond to the substrate material have prevented the widespread acceptance of this material.

Wear debris particle formation and osteolysis remain the singular most common cause of failure in total hip arthroplasty. This has led to the rekindling of interest in alternate bearing surfaces such as metal-to-metal articulations and ceramic bearing surfaces on ceramic or polyethylene, as well as attempts to strengthen polyethylene. The zirconia ceramics are purported to reduce polyethylene wear, resist scratching, and be of sufficient strength to withstand the loads of hip arthroplasty. Unfortunately, the unacceptable fracture rate with aluminum ceramics coupled with short follow-up of ceramic designs has prevented widespread acceptance of this material.

There are, however, some clearcut issues of design and surgical technique that can minimize wear debris formation. Titanium should not be used as a bearing surface. Acetabular polyethylene inserts should be a minimum of 6 mm thick. An uncemented acetabular component must have a sound locking mechanism with full backsided contact to prevent wear. An uncemented femoral component should be circumferentially porous-coated to prevent propagation of wear debris to the distal portions of the femoral component. Cemented femoral components should be designed to facilitate transfer of load from the prosthesis to the cement to the adjacent bone.

In the past few years there has been a great deal of controversy as to the optimal design for a cemented femoral component. It is generally accepted that the implant material should be cobalt chrome rather than titanium. Proponents of a collared implant stress the importance of load transfer to the adjacent calcar, while those who advocate collarless implants feel that subsidence of the prosthesis in the cement mantle occurs and is beneficial. The most recent controversy in cemented femoral components involves the surface finish on the implant. Opinions of experts vary, from those who advocate a polished surface to allow subsidence of the implant, to those who recommend a rougher surface to facilitate bonding of the prosthesis to the cement. Moreover, preferences of this latter group vary from a satin finish, a matte finish, or a grit-blasted surface, to a precoat prosthesis. Unfortunately current data are not sufficient to clearly determine which surface finish is ideal. Part of this difficulty is due to confounding variables such as cement mantle thickness, position of the implant within the mantle, cement preparation and pressurization, and quality of the host bone. Wear in hip arthroplasty can also be decreased by attention to technical detail such as proper cleaning of the bearing surface, avoidance of scratching either the femoral head or the polyethylene insert, and placement of the acetabular component in a proper position. A vertically oriented acetabular component tends to wear more rapidly secondary to the increased forces in the weight-bearing area.

Ultra-high molecular weight high density polyethylene has been used as a bearing material for many years. Attempts to modify this material by carbon reinforcement and physical manipulation have increased strength, but have also increased wear. In recent years the adverse effects of gamma sterilization of polyethylene in air have led investigators to modify the manufacturing process. Many controversial aspects of polyethylene preparation and sterilization will be covered in this section. Should the material be calcium stearate free? Should it be ram extruded or compression molded? Is gamma sterilization in a vacuum or inert gas preferable to ethylene oxide sterilization? Will highly cross-linked polyethylene be more resistant to wear? Can we develop a new polyethylene or modify existing stock to limit or even prevent accumulation of polyethylene wear debris?

While manufacturers, engineers, and materials scientists concentrate on the implant design aspects to increase longevity, biologists are now beginning to understand the host response to wear debris material. Can we understand the mechanisms by which wear debris stimulates macrophages, fibroblasts, synoviocytes, and other cells to produce cytokines, eicosinoids, and pro-inflammatory mediators to cause bone resorption, inflammation, and recruitment of cells to amplify the local response? Is the osteoclastic stimulation the common pathway leading to osteolysis and, if so, can it be blocked by the bisphosphonates? Is osteolysis that simple, or is a complex combination of adverse mechanical event and elaboration of mediators that leads to bone resorption? Can we identify at-risk patients based upon their nonspecific immune reactivity? Can we, by understanding the mechanism of host response to wear debris, modify the response and increase implant longevity?

The next generation of orthopedic surgeons will consider our current technologies as arcane, just as we consider arcane bloodletting, amputation for fractures, and treatment of infected wounds in the preantibiotic era. Our successors will repair cartilage, induce new bone formation, and develop inert materials that will osteointegrate with bone and mimic its mechanical properties. Tissue engineering will allow us to repair damaged joints, and newer medical interventions will prevent joint destruction. For now, however, we must deal with the present. We have an obligation to the hundreds of thousands of patients with functioning implants to carefully study these mechanisms of failure, to recognize that we have created a new disease called *implant failure disease,* and to master the techniques of revision hip arthroplasty. In so doing, we will allow our patients to continue to enjoy the relief from pain and return to function afforded by total hip arthroplasty.

1
Prosthetic Loosening in Total Hip Replacements

Murali Jasty

Total replacement of arthritic joints with artificial metal and plastic materials has provided dramatic relief of pain and improvement in function for millions of patients with end-stage arthritis.[1] It has also revolutionized the surgical treatment of arthritis for the past 30 years. Despite the enormous success of these procedures, however, aseptic loosening of the components—often associated with periprosthetic osteolysis and frequently necessitating revision surgery—remains the major problem. The THAs done in the 1970s had loosening rates of 30% to 40% by 10 years after surgery.[2,3] Improvements in surgical techniques, prosthetic designs, and biomaterials[1,4-6] have subsequently improved the longevity of the prosthesis, with only 3% of the femoral components and 10 percent of the acetabular components of THAs now requiring revision surgery at 10 to 15 years.[7] Even though these results appear satisfactory for the vast majority of the elderly patients, continuously increasing life expectancy of the population in developed countries and demands for making these procedures available for younger, heavier, and more active patients necessitate continued investigation to extend the longevity of these procedures even further.

Revision surgery for aseptic loosening is, unfortunately, not an acceptable alternative, as it is technically much more challenging than the primary arthroplasty and is associated with both markedly higher costs and markedly lower success rates. Loosening of the prosthetic components is frequently associated with marked bone loss, necessitating the use of special components and surgical techniques.[8-11] In some cases, bone loss occurs to such an extent as to preclude revision surgery altogether.

Much of the research in this area of orthopedics for the past 2 decades has therefore focused on the elucidation of the mechanisms involved in prosthetic loosening and periprosthetic bone loss, so that improvements in the prosthetic designs and surgical techniques can be made to improve the longevity of these devices. Most of the past data on the mechanisms of failures has come from long-term clinical and radiographic studies or experimental simulations using animals or mechanical models.[5,8,12] More recently, biomechanical and morphologic studies of whole specimens retrieved at autopsy from patients with successful and unsuccessful total joint arthroplasties have considerably expanded knowledge of the usual mechanisms involved in late prosthetic loosening.[13-15] These advances are discussed in this chapter.

Symptom Complex of Aseptic Loosening

Aseptic loosening of prosthetic components is usually, but not always, manifested as pain. New onset of hip pain in a previously painfree joint indicates either loosening or infection. Pain persisting since surgery should raise suspicion of infection. The pain from loosening is usually aggravated by weight bearing. Certain movements, such as internal and external rotation or axial push on the bent knee, may aggravate the pain and point to aseptic loosening. An antalgic gait and positive Trendelenburg's sign are clinical signs that the prostheses may be loose.

Acetabular component loosening usually gives rise to pain in the groin, whereas femoral component loosening usually gives rise to pain in the thigh. However loosening of either component can be manifested by pain either in the groin or thigh, or both. Pain in the buttock, when associated with either pain in the groin or pain in the thigh, indicates that the pain may be from prosthetic loosening, whereas pain in the buttock alone is a nonspecific indicator of prosthetic loosening.

It is important to recognize other causes for pain, such as disc disease, hernia, intra-abdominal disorders, bone tumors, trochanteric bursitis, and iliopsoas bursitis. In general, pain in the groin and anterior thigh aggravated by weight bearing is the most reliable sign of loosening or infection.

Infection must be suspected in every case of loosening. Fever, chills, and relentless pain even at rest are symptoms that suggest infection. Infection should also be suspected when early prosthetic loosening occurs without an obvious cause. Periosteal reaction and unexplained osteolysis on radiographs also suggest infection. It is best to rule out infection, however, by appropriate laboratory studies, culture of the joint fluid, and intraoperative frozen section pathology.

Not all loose components will lead to pain. Loose femoral components cause pain more often than do loose acetabular components. Loose acetabular components may be entirely asymptomatic. In one 15-year follow-up study, 52% of cemented acetabular components were loose, while only 10% were symptomatic enough to warrant revision surgery.[7] While femoral component loosening often leads to pain, a debonded loose femoral component with intact cement–bone interface may be asymptomatic for several years.

Radiographic Signs of Loosening

Postoperative follow-up radiographs should include an anteroposterior view of the pelvis with the radiographic source centered on the pubic symphysis, an anteroposterior view of the hip to include the entire femoral component, a true lateral view of the hip, and a frog lateral view of the hip. Oblique views of the pelvis may be helpful if loosening of the acetabular component is suspected but not obvious on the anteroposterior views.

An obvious change in the position of the components between serial radiographs is pathognomonic of loosening. This applies to cemented as well as cementless components. However, subtle loosening cannot be detected by this method. Furthermore, it may not be possible to obtain comparable radiographs with the patient in the same position. There are several other radiographic clues that are helpful in evaluating prosthetic loosening. These may depend on whether the implant is cemented or uncemented and whether it involves the acetabular component or the femoral component.

Radiolucencies at the cement–bone interface of cemented implants and at the porous coating–bone interface of uncemented components are helpful in evaluating the status of fixation of the implant. A continuous radiolucency that surrounds the entire interface and that measures greater than 2 mm in thickness is used as a criterion for loosening of the acetabular component,[16] and the same criteria can be applied to the femoral component. It is important to note, however, that radiolucencies, particularly around cemented femoral components, can be caused by osteoporosis of the cortical bone in the absence of loosening. A radiological line of demarcation at the cement–bone interface and at the porous coating–bone interface is a more reliable indicator for loosening (Fig. 1.1), particularly if it is greater than 2 mm thick, is progressive, and surrounds the entire interface. The demarcation line is characterized by a radiolucency surrounded by a radiodense line of sclerosis. The presence of the demarcation line that is 2 mm or greater in thickness and that occupies the entire interface is a strong indicator that the implant is loose, whether it is cemented or uncemented and whether it affects the acetabular component or the femoral component.

In the case of cemented femoral components, development of a new radiolucency at the cement–metal interface indicates that the prosthesis is subsided and loose.[7] This lucency is best seen on the proximal anterolateral aspect of the prosthesis on the frog lateral view. Cement fractures are also pathognomonic of loosening in both cemented femoral and acetabular components, but may be too small to be seen on radiographs. When either of these criteria is met, the prosthesis is definitely loose.

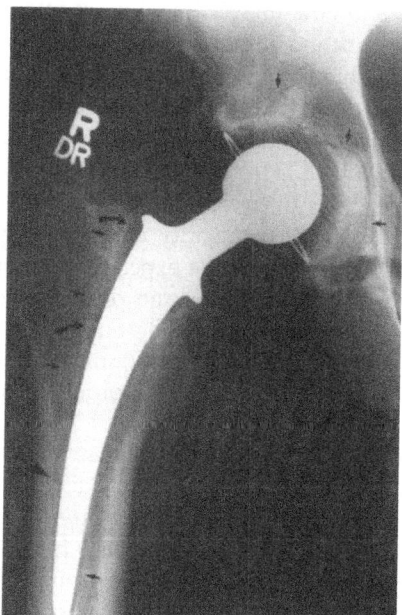

Figure 1.1. Anteroposterior radiograph of cemented acetabular and femoral components, both of which are loose. The demarcation lines (radiolucent line at the cement–bone interface adjacent to the radiodense line) located circumferentially around the acetabular component (small arrows) indicates that it is loose. The femoral component has separated from the femoral cement (large arrows), indicating that the femoral component is loose. Note also the demarcation lines (small arrows) at the femoral cement–bone interface.

Loosening of uncemented components may be more difficult to detect on radiographs. Separation of the porous coating from the metal substrate or broken screws used to fix the acetabular component may indicate loosening. In rare cases, the components may be loose without any radiographic evidence of loosening. If loosening is suspected with negative radiographs, additional studies may be necessary.

Arthrography may be helpful if loosening is strongly suspected but the radiographs are negative.[17,18] However, it is difficult to perform accurately, and interpretation of the test requires considerable experience. The procedure should be done under meticulous sterile conditions. Preliminary scout radiographs are taken with a 22-gauge spinal needle in the hip joint. Hip fluid is then aspirated and sent for culture. Radio-opaque dye is then injected and the films are repeated with no change in position. The needle is withdrawn and the patient is walked for 10 to 15 minutes. Delayed films are then taken with the hip in the same position. Presence of dye in the bone–implant interface at least 2 to 3 cm away from the joint strongly indicates loosening.

Mechanisms of Prosthetic Loosening

Clinical and radiographic studies of the past two decades have indicated that different patterns of loosening may occur depending on material, design, site, and host-specific factors. The mechanisms of prosthetic loosening may be different on the acetabular and femoral sides of a total hip replacement. Both the loosening rates and the time course of the loosening have been shown to be different at these two sites.[7]

A small subset of femoral components become loose early, but the remainder function well over the long term. In contrast, the loosening rates of the acetabular components steadily increase with time. The radiographic patterns of loosening also appear to be different at these two sites, with the femoral components usually showing cement fractures and separation at the cement–metal interface,[19] but the acetabular components usually demonstrating separation at the cement–bone interface without cement fractures. Some designs of femoral components have a markedly higher rate of loosening than others, suggesting the importance of design specificity. The rate of acetabular component loosening is also higher in components with thinner polyethylene and large inner diameter. The high failure rates with devices using polytetrafluoroethylene[20] and polyester[10] materials, and the high failure rates in femoral components with titanium femoral heads[21,22] indicate the importance of material specificity. The development of aggressive periprosthetic osteolysis, appearing as large cystic lesions in bone in some patients but not others, and the high rate of loosening in young, active, heavy patients suggest host specificity. Since all total joint arthroplasties involve creating a composite interface between artificial materials and the skeleton, it is not surprising that many complex mechanical and biologic interactions occur between the devices and the host bone over time, and that loosening may depend on the interaction of many design, material, site, and host-specific factors.

Morphologic studies of hips harvested at autopsy from patients who were functioning well for varying time periods after undergoing cemented total hip arthroplasty have improved understanding of the usual mechanisms initiating late aseptic loosening of cemented total hip arthroplasties.

Cemented Femoral Components

Post-mortem studies of femoral arthroplasties have shown that the cement–bone interface is virtually intact over the long term, with rare or no fibrous tissue formation.[15] Serial sections of the femurs showed that the bone-remodeling process creates a dense shell of new bone around the cement mantle, resembling a new inner cortex attached to the outer cortex by new trabecular struts. This shell of new bone is intimately associated with the cement mantle and supports the prosthetic components over the long term. These remodeling changes, and not fibrous tissue formation, produce the appearance of radiolucent lines at the cement–bone interface in most specimens.[23]

In spite of the excellent cement–bone interface, partial separation of the cement–prosthesis interface and fractures in the cement mantle were frequent findings in one study and indicated that last aseptic loosening of the femoral components is initiated by mechanical causes prior to clinical or radiographic evidence of failure.[13] The initial mechanisms of mechanical failure of cemented femoral components were predicted by experimental and analytical mechanical engineering studies, but did not receive appropriate recognition. By far the most common early features of failure were debonding of the cement from the metal prosthesis and cement mantle fractures (Fig. 1.2). The debonding started at the most proximal and the most distal ends of the prosthesis and progressed to involve the entire component over time. Circumferential fractures in the cement near the cement–metal interface and radial fractures extending from the cement–metal interface into the cement and to the cement–bone interface were common and were associated with progressive loosening. The most extensive cement fractures arose from the corners of those prostheses with sharp corners and in the areas where the cement mantles were thin or incomplete. Cement fractures also arose from the voids in the cement. Rarely did they occur at the cement–bone interface.

Some specimens were particularly valuable in elucidating the sequence of events involved in the loosening

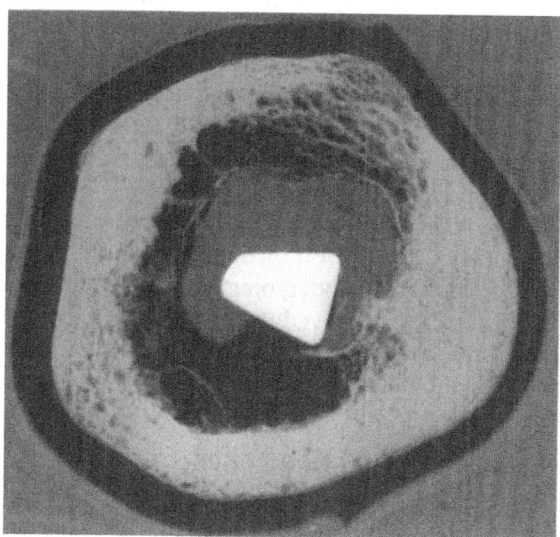

Figure 1.2. Microradiograph of a transverse section of a femur retrieved postmortem from a patient who had a total hip arthroplasty 17 years earlier. The prosthesis had debonded from the cement mantle and shifted into retroversion. The cement had cracked at the sharp corner of the prosthesis and fragmented. The cement–bone interface is disrupted in some areas, but intact in other areas.

process. The specimen that was radiographically loose with radiolucency at the cement–metal interface (retrieved at 156 months) showed that the prosthesis was completely debonded from the cement mantle and was surrounded by a layer of fibrous tissue at the cement–metal interface, in spite of an excellent cement–bone interface. There were numerous radial fractures within the cement mantle, and the prosthesis had subsided into retroversion by opening these cement fractures. Even though the prosthesis met the radiographic criteria for loosening and was confirmed to be grossly loose on manual palpation, the patient was not experiencing pain at the time of death, and the cement–bone interface was intact.

Another specimen with focal osteolysis at the tip of a rigidly fixed femoral component showed the relationship between acrylic fragmentation and development of osteolysis. Localized debonding of the tip of the prosthesis from the cement mantle had occurred. This debonding, combined with a thin cement mantle in this region, led to numerous fractures through the voids in the cement at this area of high stress. The focal osteolysis was restricted to only this area of acrylic fragmentation, while the rest of the cement–bone interface was intact. All of these findings suggest that mechanical events preceded the biologic events in the loosening process on the femoral side and that the destruction of the cement–bone interface was a late event in the loosening process.

Thus, late aseptic loosening of the femoral components of total hip arthroplasty is initiated by predictable mechanical causes, namely acrylic fragmentation, and mechanical failures at the cement–metal interface and within the cement precede the biological failures at the cement–bone interface.

Cemented Acetabular Components

In contrast to the usual pattern of femoral component loosening, the findings on the acetabular side showed that late aseptic loosening of cemented acetabular components is governed by the progressive, three-dimensional resorption of the bone immediately adjacent to the cement mantle due to particulate material prior to acrylic fragmentation.[24] The mechanical causes leading to the production of the particulate material and the sites where the loosening is initiated are different for the acetabular components than for the femoral components. However, even the failure of the acetabular components is usually initiated by mechanical causes, namely polyethylene wear, while the process is governed by the biologic responses to the polyethylene wear particles. This process of loosening begins circumferentially at the intra-articular margin and progresses toward the dome to the implant. Microscopic evidence of bone resorption at the cement–bone interface is present even in the most well-fixed implants, before the appearance of lucent lines on standard radiographic views. The mechanical stability of the implant depends on the three-dimensional extent of bone resorption and fibrous membrane formation at the cement–bone interface.

Of special importance is the transition between the regions of the membrane interposition and regions of intimate cement–bone contact. Histologic examination of this region has shown that the progressive bone resorption is due to the ingress of small particles of polyethylene wear debris migrating along the cement–bone interface (Fig. 1.3). The areas of bone resorption are characterized by the macrophage inflammatory responses to the particulate polyethylene and the formation of a fibrous tissue. There is a correlation between the amount of polyethylene wear visible at the articulation and the degree of acetabular component loosening.

Thus, late aseptic loosening of the acetabular components is related to the wear of the polyethylene articulating surfaces. The adverse biological responses to the polyethylene wear debris leads to the late aseptic loosening of the acetabular components from the skeleton.

Osteolysis Around Cemented Components

As early as 1976, it was reported that aggressive osteolysis occurs at the bone–implant interface in some cases

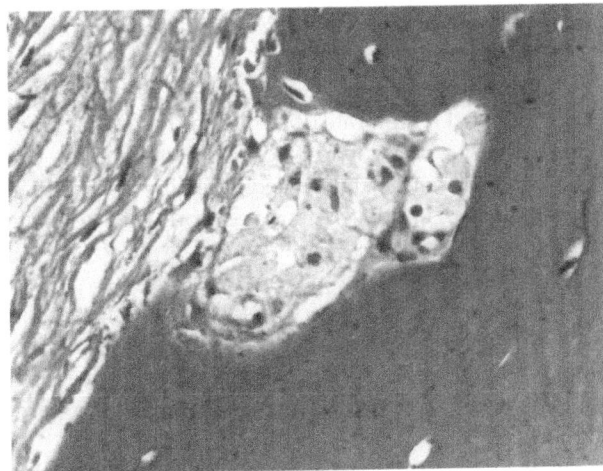

Figure 1.3. Tissue from the cement–bone interface of an acetabular component retrieved postmortem from a patient who had a total hip arthroplasty 14 years earlier. Fibrous tissue was found at the interface. Foamy macrophages containing particulate polyethylene debris were found in the resorption cavities of adjacent bone.

of total joint arthroplasty.[9] While osteolysis is more common in instances in which the components are loose, in many instances, particularly the acetabular component, it contributes to loosening in some cases due to the loss of supporting bone. These lesions were originally thought to be related to sepsis, but detailed clinical, bacteriologic, and histologic studies have ruled out sepsis. The focal aggressive periprosthetic osteolysis occurs in some cases around prostheses that were not loose based on clinical, radiographic, or mechanical criteria. In both instances, these lesions appear as generalized or focal areas of osteolysis at the cement–bone interface surrounded occasionally by a thin rim of reactive new bone formation.

Histologic analysis of this tissue from the areas of bone lysis at the cement–bone interface of both loosened and well-fixed prostheses retrieved at revision surgery has provided much valuable information on the causes and the nature of the lesions.[25–28] Numerous macrophages and giant cells are interspersed in a fibrous stroma. The tissue is usually thick (1–4 m) and markedly cellular. The surface of the tissue adjacent to the cement often has a synovial-like appearance with villous projections and polarization of the nuclei at the surface layer of cells. The intermediate layer is primarily cellular and contains numerous macrophages/giant cells with plump granular cytoplasm. Deeper to this layer, adjacent to the bone, the tissue contains fibrous marrow infiltrated with sheets of macrophages. Areas of active bone resorption and adjacent new bone formation were seen in these regions. In some areas, large numbers of osteoclasts were present in the resorption cavities in bone, whereas in other areas only mononuclear macrophages were present in the resorption cavities. Adjacent to these areas, occasionally areas of active bone formation were present, presumably formed in an attempt to wall off the invading tissue.

The tissue in the osteolytic lesions contains large amounts of particulate cement and polyethylene debris, varying widely in size from less than 1 μm to several hundred micrometers. These particles are usually phagocytosed by the macrophages and giant cells in the tissue.[14] Smaller particles of polyethylene are difficult to see under normal light, but their presence can be determined by their birefringence when viewed under polarized light.[24] Cement particles are also difficult to see because the vast majority of them are dissolved away during slide processing, although their presence can be inferred by the visualization of the barium granules in the empty spaces (Fig. 1.4). Upon examination by electron microscopy, numerous implant particles that are light to medium in electron density and lined by double-layer membranes are identified in the cells. The particles occupy up to 70% of the cytoplasm in some cells. Signs of cell degeneration and necrosis are found frequently, and many of the macrophages contain myeloid bodies.

Thus the foreign body granulomatous tissue reaction consisting of macrophages and giant cells within a fibrous stroma occurring either focally or extensively at the bone–cement interface of cemented implants is associated with osteolysis, and the liberation of the particulate implant materials into the interface is responsible for its production.

Biochemical studies of tissue from the areas of bone lysis at the cement–bone interface of loosened prosthe-

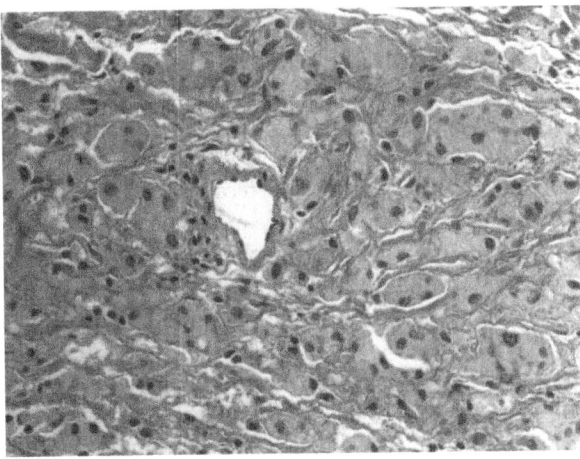

Figure 1.4. Tissue from the cement–bone interface of a loose cemented femoral component with osteolysis. Note sheets of foamy macrophages and giant cells. In the middle is an empty space that had been occupied by acrylic debris but that had been dissolved during the tissue processing.

ses have provided important insights on the etiology of bone destruction and loosening.[27,28] A variety of biochemical mediators of bone resorption, such as prostaglandin-E_2, metalloproteases, and collagenase, have been identified in this tissue. Additional evidence for the mediation of bone resorption by this tissue was provided by experiments in which conditioned medium from explants of the granulation tissue caused resorption of radiolabelled mouse calvarium in vitro.[29]

Recent advances in molecular biology techniques have furthered the elucidation of the biochemical processes that are involved in loosening and periprosthetic osteolysis.[30] A variety of cytokines are now known to be present in this tissue, and they mediate tissue destruction, repair, and remodeling in a host of disease states. Several interlukens, tumor necrosis factors, platelet-derived growth factors, and transforming growth factors have been identified in this tissue, and they are capable of causing osteoclast activation, bone resorption, chemotaxis of other inflammatory cells, and fibrinogenesis.[31]

Osteolysis and Loosening with Uncemented Components

Progressive bone loss due to nonseptic osteolysis observed around cemented components of total hip arthroplasty led to the widespread use of uncemented porous-coated components, especially in young and active patients. It was initially hoped that loosening and periprosthetic osteolysis would be eliminated by using prostheses that do not require bone cement for fixation. At that time, it was thought that cement invariably would undergo fracture and that particulate cement debris would invariably cause extensive foreign-body reaction and progressive lysis of adjacent bone.

Initial designs of uncemented porous-coated components had a slightly higher rate of loosening within the first 2 to 3 years as compared with cemented components.[32–34] In vitro mechanical testing has indicated that initial stability of early-design cementless components was not as good as for cemented components.[12] The failures were related to the early experience with the design of the components and techniques used to implant them. The stability of the uncemented femoral components depends on their fit and fill in the femoral canal. Poor tolerances between the implants and broaches have led to femoral fractures or undersizing of the components in some cases. This, in turn, has led to large micromotions at the porous coating–bone interfaces and inhibition of bone ingrowth. The availability of better designs of prostheses, selection of the proper type of prosthesis for the particular type of femoral canal (tapered stem for tapered canal, cylindric diaphyseal filling stem for cylindrical diaphysis, and cemented stem for the older osteoporotic femur), and incorporation of more extensive porous coatings have largely eliminated this problem.[35,36]

Some early designs of the acetabular components have also had a high rate of failure in the first few years after surgery.[32,37] Nonporous-coated hemispherical components and nonporous-coated threaded rings are examples of such failures. Extensively porous-coated hemispherical components, either press fit or fixed with adjunctive fixation devices such as screws, pegs, or spikes, have performed very well over the short and intermediate term. In one study of porous-coated hemispheric acetabular components fixed with supplemental screws, none were revised at a mean follow-up period of 7 years.[38]

In the early series of cementless components there was a high incidence of thigh pain. While it usually resolved in 1 or 2 years, in some cases it persisted, necessitating revision surgery. In one study, pain in the thigh was found in 27% of hips at 5 years following cementless arthroplasty. The pain was new (occurring between 2 and 5 years) in 14%, unchanged in 8%, increased in 4%, and decreased in 1%.[39] It is now appreciated that the thigh pain is related to either unstable fixation or to differences in the stiffness between the implant and bone, particularly at the distal end of prostheses.[36,40] Prosthetic designs are currently modified to reduce the stiffness at the distal end through such techniques as tapering the distal end or splitting the distal end.

It was noted in the late 1980s that osteolysis can also occur around radiographically well-fixed and loose cementless porous-surfaced femoral components. Subsequent reports have shown that not only is osteolysis not prevented by eliminating the cement from total joint re-

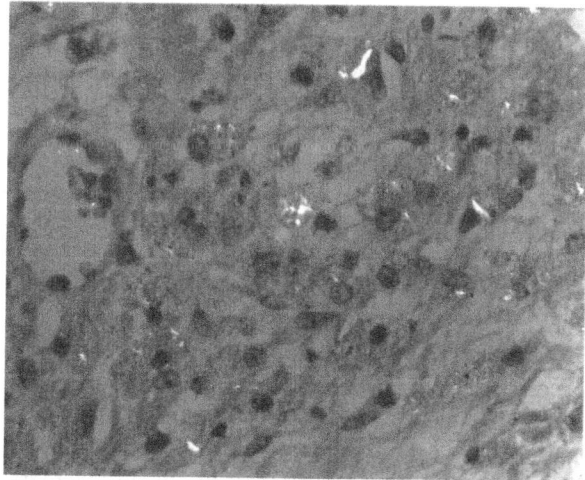

Figure 1.5. Particulate polyethylene and metal debris in the macrophages from the tissue in the osteolytic lesion around a cementless component. The debris is very small, measuring a few micrometers or less.

placements, but also that it might be a more significant problem with cementless arthroplasty than with cemented arthroplasty, as evidenced by the early onset, high incidence, and severity of the lesions.[41] Studies in the past few years have provided many insights into the etiology of osteolysis around uncemented components. Tissues from the regions of osteolysis around uncemented components are virtually identical to the tissues from the regions of osteolysis around cemented components, and they contain sheets of macrophages and giant cells (Fig. 1.5). An abundant amount of submicron-size polyethylene debris has been found to be ingested by these cells, along with some metallic debris. The polyethylene liners in these cases also show higher wear rates than do conventional cemented components. Fretting corrosion at the head–neck junction and burnishing of the stem against the bone is found in some cases. Arthrography in selected cases shows a communication between the joint space and the implant–bone interface, a means whereby the metal debris generated at the implant–bone interface can gain access to the articulation and the polymeric debris generated at the articulation can gain access to the implant–bone interface.[42]

Thus it appears that a large amount of fine particulate debris of polyethylene is liberated into the tissues around these cementless prostheses from the articulating surface by abrasive or adhesive wear mechanisms, probably accelerated by third body wear from metal particles. The abundant fine polymeric debris found universally in all cases plays an important role in the production of osteolysis around these uncemented components by giving rise to an aggressive foreign body granulomatous reaction (Fig. 1.6). The loss of supporting bone can lead to fatigue failure of remaining bone and prosthetic loosening.

References

1. Harris WH, Sledge CB. Medical progress: total hip and total knee replacement. *N Engl J Med*. 1990;323:725–731.
2. Stauffer RN. Ten year follow-up study of total hip replacement. *J Bone Joint Surg Am*. 1982;64:983–990.
3. Sutherland CJ, Wilde AH, Borden LS, Marks KE. A ten year follow-up of one hundred consecutive Muller curved-stem total hip replacement arthroplasties. *J Bone Joint Surg Am*. 1982;64:970–982.
4. Ahmed AM, Raab A, Miller JE. Metal/cement interface strength in cemented stem fixation. *J Orthop Res*. 1984;2:105–118.
5. Crowninshield RD, Brand RA, Johnston RC, Milroy JC. The effect of femoral stem cross-sectional geometry on cement stresses in total hip reconstruction. *Orthopedics*. 1980;146:71–77.
6. Engh CA, Hooten JP Jr, Zettl-Schaffer KF, Ghaffarpour M, McGovern TF, Macaling GE, et al. Porous-coated total hip replacement. *Clin Orthop*. 1994;298:89–96.
7. Mulroy RD, Harris WH. The effect of improved cementing techniques on component loosening in total hip replacement. *J Bone Joint Surg Br*. 1990;72:757–760.
8. Amstutz HC, Markolf KL, McNeice GM, Gruen TA. Loosening of total hip components: cause and prevention. In: *The Hip: Proceedings of the Fourth Open Scientific Meeting of the Hip Society*. St Louis, Mo: CV Mosby, Inc; 1965.
9. Harris WH, Schiller AL, Scholler JM, Freiberg RA, Scott R. Extensive localized bone resorption in the femur following total hip replacement. *J Bone Joint Surg Am*. 1976;58:612–618.
10. Weber BG. Total hip replacement revision surgery: surgical technique and experience. *Hip*. 1981;XX:3–14.
11. Willert HG, Bertram H, Buchhorn GH. Osteolysis in alloarthroplasty of the hip: the role of bone cement fragmentation. *Clin Orthop*. 1990;258:108–121.
12. Burke DW, O'Connor DO, Zalenski EB, Jasty M, Harris WH. Micromotion of cemented and uncemented femoral components. *J Bone Joint Surg Br*. 1991;73:33–37.
13. Jasty M, Maloney WJ, Bragdon CR, O'Connor DO, Haire T, Harris WH. The initiation of failure in cemented femoral components of hip arthroplasties. *J Bone Joint Surg Br*. 1991;73:551–558.
14. Jasty M, Jiranek WJ, Harris WH. Acrylic fragmentation in total hip replacements and its biologic consequences. *Clin Orthop*. 1992;285:116–128.
15. Jasty M, Maloney WJ, Bragdon CR, Haire T, Harris WH. Histomorphological studies of the long-term skeletal responses to well fixed cemented femoral components. *J Bone Joint Surg Am*. 1990;72:1220–1225.
16. Hodgkinson JP, Shelley P, Wroblewski BM. The correlation between the roentgenographic appearance and oper-

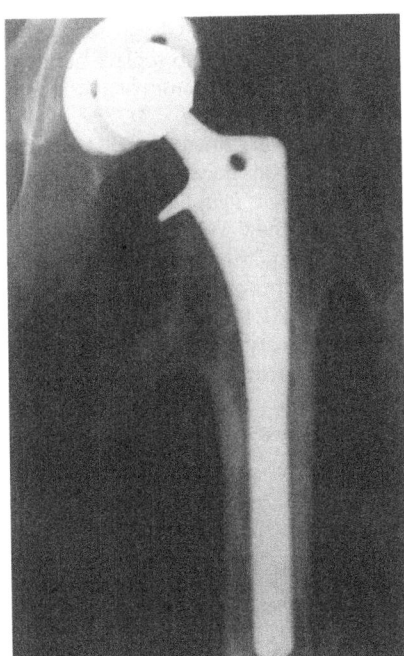

Figure 1.6. Extensive osteolysis leading to femoral component loosening in a patient who underwent cementless total hip arthroplasty 7 years earlier.

ative findings at the bone–cement junction of the socket in Charnley low friction arthroplasties. *Clin Orthop.* 1988;228:105–109.
17. Barrack RI, Tanzer M, Kaltapuram SV, Harris WH. The value of contrast arthrography in assessing loosening of symptomatic uncemented total hip components. *Skeletal Radiol.* 1994;23:37–41.
18. Hardy DC, Reinus WR, Totty WG, Deyser CK. Arthrography after total hip arthroplasty: utility of postambulation radiographs. *Skeletal Radiol.* 1988;17:20–23.
19. Fornasier VL, Cameron HU. The femoral stem/cement interface in total hip replacement. *Clin Orthop.* 1976;116:248–253.
20. Charnley J. Low friction arthroplasty of the hip. New York: Springer-Verlag; 1979:6–7.
21. Agins HJ, Alcok NW, Bansal M, et al. Metallic wear in failed titanium-alloy total hip replacements. *J Bone Joint Surg Am.* 1988;70:347–356.
22. Lombardi AV, Mallory TH, Vaughn BK, Drouillard P. Aseptic loosening in total hip arthroplasty secondary to osteolysis induced by wear debris from titanium-alloy modular femoral heads. *J Bone Joint Surg Am.* 1989;71:1337–1342.
23. Kwong L, Jasty M, Mulroy R, Maloney W, Bragdon C, Harris WH. "Radiolucencies" in cemented femoral total hip replacements: a correlation of radiographic and histologic findings after in vivo service. *J Bone Joint Surg Br.* 1992;74:67–73.
24. Schmalzried TP, Kwong LM, Jasty M, et al. The mechanism of loosening of cemented acetabular components. *Clin Orthop.* 1992;274:60–78.
25. Athanasou NA, Quinn J, Bulstrode CJK. Resorption of bone by inflammatory cells derived from the joint capsule of hip arthroplasties. *J Bone Joint Surg Br.* 1992;74:57–62.
26. Anthony PP, Gie GA, Howie CR, Ling RS. Localised endosteal bone lysis in relation to the femoral components of cemented total hip arthroplasties. *J Bone Joint Surg Br.* 1990;72:971–979.
27. Goldring SA, Schiller AL, Roelke M, Rourke CM, O'Neill DA, Harris WH. The synovial-like membrane at the bone–cement interface in loose total hip replacements and its proposed role in bone lysis. *J Bone Joint Surg Am.* 1983;65:575–584.
28. Goldring SR, Jasty M, Roelke M, Rourke CM, Harris WH. Factors responsible for formation of synovial-like membrane after total hip replacement (THR): its role in prosthesis loosening. *Arthritis Rheum.* 1985;28:S36.
29. Goldring SR, Jasty M, Roelke MS, Rourke CM, Bringhurst FR. Formation of a synovial-like membrane at the bone–cement interface: its role in bone resorption and implant loosening after total hip replacement. *Arthritis Rheum.* 1986;29:836–842.
30. Jiranek WA, Michado M, Jasty M, et al. Production of cytokines around loosened cemented acetabular components. *J Bone Joint Surg Am.* 1993;75:863–879.
31. Santivirta S, Hoikka V, Esokola A, Konttinen YT, Paavilainen T. Aggressive granulomatous lesions in cementless total hip arthroplasty. *J Bone Joint Surg Br.* 1990;72:980–984.
32. Astion DJ, Saluan P, Stulberg BN, Rimnac CM, Li S. The porous-coated anatomic total hip prosthesis: failure of the metal-backed acetabular component. *J Bone Joint Surg Am.* 1976;78:755–766.
33. Hedley AK, Gruen TAW, Baden LS, Hungerford DS, Haberman E, Kenna RV. Two year follow-up of the PCA noncemented total hip replacement. In: *The Hip: Proceedings of the Fourteenth Open Scientific Meeting of The Hip Society.* St Louis: CV Mosby, Inc; 1987:225–250.
34. Martell JM, Pierson RH, Jacobs JJ, Rosenberg AG, Maley M, Galante JO. Primary total hip reconstruction with a cementless titanium fiber coated prosthesis inserted without cement. *J Bone Joint Surg Am.* 1993;75:554–571.
35. Cameron HU. The 3–6 year results of a modular noncemented low-bending stiffness hip implant: a preliminary study. *J Arthroplasty.* 1993;8:239–243.
36. Engh CA, Glassman AH, Suthers KE. The case for porous-coated hip implants: the femoral side. *Clin Orthop.* 1990;261:63–81.
37. Bruijn JD, Seelen JL, Feenstra RM, Hansen BE, Bernoski FP. Failure of the mecring screw-ring acetabular components in total hip arthroplasty. *J Bone Joint Surg Am.* 1995;77:760–766.
38. Latimer HA, Lachiewicz PF. Porous-coated acetabular components with screw fixation. *J Bone Joint Surg Am.* 1976;78:975–981.
39. Bourne RB, Rorabeck CH, Ghazal ME, Lee MH. Pain in the thigh following total hip replacement with a porous-coated anatomic prosthesis for osteoarthrosis. *J Bone Joint Surg Am.* 1994;77:1464–1470.
40. Barrack RL, Jasty M, Bragdon C, Haire T, Harris WH. Thigh pain despite bone ingrowth into uncemented femoral stems. *J Bone Joint Surg Br.* 1992;74:507–510.
41. Tanzer M, Maloney WJ, Jasty M, Harris WH. The Progression of femoral cortical osteolysis in association with total hip arthroplasty without cement. *J Bone Joint Surg Am.* In press. 1992;74:404–410.
42. Schmalzried TP, Jasty M, Harris WH. Periprosthetic bone loss in total hip arthroplasty: polyethylene wear debris and the concept of the effective joint space. *J Bone Joint Surg Am.* 1992;74:849–863.

2
Polyethylene Wear

James V. Bono and George Faithfull

Ultrahigh molecular weight polyethylene (UHMWPE) possesses a unique blend of toughness, wear resistance, and biocompatibility.[1,2] It has been the articular-bearing surface of choice against metal or ceramic since 1962.[3] To date, it is still the best polymer available for joint implant use.[4] However, with respect to long-term function and durability, just like the cartilage it replaces, its resistance to wear can be limited by the effects of aging and degradation. Failed total hip arthroplasties can occur as the result of infection, instability, component fracture, implant loosening, and prostheses malalignment. Polyethylene wear has become the limiting factor to long device lifetime in total hip arthroplasty, and it is becoming an increasing concern. The average long-term wear rate of Charnley acetabular cups, measured radiographically, has been reported to be 0.07 to 0.15 mm/year.[5–12] Charnley and Halley[13] described the average wear rate for a 22-mm stainless steel head against an all-polyethylene acetabular component.[13]

The advent of cemented metal-backed acetabular components, developed by Harris in 1970 to address the problem of polyethylene wear, allowed replacement of the worn polyethylene insert without removal of the existing methacrylate.[14] The replacement of Charnley's all-polyethylene acetabular component with a metal-backed design (composed of a metal shell and a polyethylene-bearing insert), although providing stress benefits, reduced the available polyethylene thickness for a given outside cup diameter, often to an alarming extent in the 1980s.[15] In the 1990s this has been addressed by utilization of smaller head sizes, thicker polyethylene choices, and designs that allow greater conformity to the metal backing.

Polyethylene Wear
Particulate Debris

Because of continued improvements and clinical success, joint replacements are remaining in service longer, and surface wear—even in well-functioning implants—increases with time.[16] Wear of polyethylene results in the generation of particulate debris, which in certain circumstances can cause adverse tissue reactions and may ultimately accelerate prosthetic loosening.[17] This has become a dominant factor compromising the long-term results of total joint replacement.[18] Further, it is now recognized that the smallest polyethylene particles are the most insidious, and only recently have techniques been developed to identify the presence, size, and number of these particles in cells.[19]

Metal-on-Metal Design

Metal-on-metal design has been put forward as creating wear volume magnitudes of order less than PE–metal bearings. However, characterization analysis has indicated that retrieved metal particles can be so much smaller than typical retrieved PE particles that the calculated number of metal particles results in a figure a magnitude of order higher than the number of PE particles.[20] It should not be forgotten that, in comparison with metal-on-metal implants, UHMWPE implants have performed very successfully in long-term clinical survival studies.[21]

Not a New Issue

Polyethylene wear is not a new issue. More than 20 years ago, Willert discussed the consequences of polyethylene debris,[22] and more than 10 years ago, Bartel and Wright defined the effect of conformity and PE thickness on material stresses.[23] In fact, 35 years ago, Sir John Charnley turned to UHMWPE as an alternative to a form of Teflon™ he originally used when severe granulomatous reactions to the Teflon™ wear debris began to appear in the 300 patients he had used it in. A salesperson selling plastic gears introduced him to UHMWPE by chance, and Charnley's primitive wear tests demonstrated it to be a good candidate. However, Charnley was so concerned about not repeating his mistake that he inserted some of this new material into his thigh and observed it over a 6-month period. Only when no adverse reaction occurred was he prepared to use UHMWPE in patients.[24]

Multiple Factors

Polyethylene wear is a complex mechanism involving several factors. These include design aspects, such as bearing surface finish, surface-contact area, and PE thickness; clinical aspects, which include attention to technique, careful ligament balancing, stability of the implant, and patient activity; and finally, characteristics of the PE material itself.[3,25] The first two aspects possibly account for the greatest effect on wear, outweighing the material factors alone. However a greater understanding of the polyethylene material is emerging and should be carefully considered in the quest to reduce the potential of wear debris generation.

Structure of UHMWPE

Scanning electron micrographs of UHMWPE powder particles at the 1-μm level shows a dense network of spherulites and fibrils. Breakdown of these structures can create the submicron debris particles typically seen within cells. Several orders of magnitude closer, down to the angstrom level, the UHMWPE microstructure shows that the long linear polyethylene chains are folded into highly organized crystalline regions. Sometimes chains continue from one crystallite to another through the amorphous region between, and these bridges are called tie molecules. They act as cross-links and provide load bearing, stress transfer, and physical and chemical strength.[26] The major morphological difference between UHMWPE and high density polyethylene (HDP), a less wear-resistant polyethylene, is in the number of tie molecules, and this characteristic is why UHMWPE exhibits high resistance to creep, notch impact, chemical attack, stress cracking, and wear.[26] A process such as chain-extension—which results in higher modulus or stiffness, a greater degree of crystallinity and fewer tie molecules—may also result in embrittlement, a lower impact strength, and lower tensile toughness.[27,28]

Manufacture and Processing of UHMWPE

Resin

Ultrahigh molecular weight polyethylene is formed from resin powder by the low-pressure modified Ziegler process, which was developed at the Max Planck Institute in the early 1950s.[27] Worldwide, there are several suppliers of PE resin for medical applications. Hoechst, who supplies various versions of GUR412 and GUR415, and Himont, who makes the 1900 resins, are the largest suppliers in the United States and Europe. The grades differ in average molecular weight (eg, 412 being an average of roughly 2 million; 415, roughly 5 million), and in the inclusion or exclusion of calcium stearate, a chemical added at the powder stage to prevent degradation of the processing equipment. There have been conflicting studies as to the effect of calcium stearate on wear and oxidation. The synthesis of the powder occurs by feeding ethylene molecules onto catalyst particles of titanium and aluminum, and a chain polymerization then occurs. When the chain reaches a certain length, structural changes occur in the molecule that impart not only high impact strength, but also very high abrasion resistance and a low coefficient of friction. The resulting powder particles range from 60 to 250 μm in diameter.

Consolidation

Ram extrusion and compression molding are the two major processes used to form UHMWPE resin into rods or sheets that can then be machined into the final component. Both processes involve heating the UHMWPE powder to a temperature above the melting temperature and applying pressure until the entrapped air is forced out of the mass. In ram extrusion, pressure is applied horizontally as the sintered powder is forced through a die, whereas in compression molding pressure is applied vertically as the UHMWPE powder is sintered in a mold. A less frequently used process called direct compression molding, in which the component is molded directly into an implant shape from the PE powder, is still sometimes used, although on a more limited basis.

Compression-Molded Versus Ram-Extruded

One source of controversy is whether compression-molded material is inherently better than ram-extruded material. At the 1995 American Academy of Orthopedic Surgeons meeting Hungerford presented a clinical series of 96 implants of the same design monitored for 7 to 10 years showing a revision rate of 19% with compression-molded PE versus only 1.5% using ram-extruded material.[29] Other studies have suggested the opposite. It is apparent that one cannot draw general conclusions as to which process is inherently superior. In a definitive study by Lykins and Evans,[30] mechanical properties were measured to evaluate the degree of consolidation achieved by ram extruding or compression molding the same UHMWPE resin. The results showed identical values, and the investigators concluded that either process with carefully controlled conditions can produce well-consolidated UHMWPE free of fusion defects.

Fusion Defects

Fusion defects, or nonconsolidated powder particles, are considered to be indicators of poor quality control and are still described in reports on polyethylene raw material. But over the last few years, because of processing control improvements, consolidators of the raw material now offer consistent, high-quality, virtually defect-free UHMWPE. One orthopedic supply company even took the step of consolidating in house to improve upon previous quality and claims to have achieved the same improvements. Reports of high variability in PE properties throughout the industry have certainly not been reflected in recent material received and inspected, possibly because of a combination of careful internal quality control procedures and the general process improvements.

General Issues Influencing Polyethylene Wear

Over the last two decades, different issues have emerged to be addressed with regard to polyethylene wear. Design factors, such as thickness, conformity, and surface finish, were first to emerge, and they have been largely addressed by most prosthetic manufacturers. Next came quality issues pinpointing process variability and fusion defects, and it appears that these quality issues have also been addressed by both prosthesis manufacturers and polyethylene consolidators. The latest issues revolve around material property factors, most recently concentrating on oxidation.

Oxidation—The "White Band"

Oxidation of UHMWPE causes property changes in the material, which makes it more susceptible to damage. Although it has been reported in the literature, the exact mechanisms of oxidation and how it affects the properties of polyethylene have not been well understood. The microscopic changes brought about by oxidation occur over time and can be seen in the form of a subsurface white band, presented by Sun.[31,32] This white band is actually a visual effect seen on sectioning a highly oxidized area that is more brittle than the surrounding material. This highly oxidized area appears over time and, although it does not occur universally, the band seems to be enhanced by gamma irradiation.

Clinical Relevance of Oxidation

There is conflicting research on the frequency and clinical correlation of the white bands seen in implants. Collier's group reported that 71% of air-irradiated implants that had been on the shelf a minimum of 3 years showed the white band.[32] Dr. Steven Li,[33] in a similar retrieval study, reported that only 6% of air-irradiated implants that had been on the shelf a minimum of 3 years showed the white band. These are significantly different findings. The analysis of the results also differs in that Collier saw a correlation with clinical wear modes, whereas Li showed no clinical correlation at all, in fact noting that cups with the white band survived longer than those without. Further research presented by Li at the 1997 Society for Biomaterials suggests that, although oxidation occurs on the shelf, it appears to occur far more slowly in vivo.[34]

Oxidation Mechanism

Oxidation occurs when gamma radiation reacts with the polymer chains, catalyzing the formation of free radicals. These free radicals are capable of combining with each other in a mechanism called cross-linking or, as occurs more frequently, with oxygen if it is present. The two processes of cross-linking and oxidation compete with each other. When oxygen combines with these free radicals, as time continues, the polymer chain can split in two at that location in a process called *chain scission*, resulting in a lower average molecular weight. This can affect PE wear performance by reducing the ultimate tensile strength and the ductility of the material. These alterations in chemical and mechanical properties tend to occur slowly but progressively.

Cross-Linking

Although gamma irradiation triggers the formation of free radicals with a future possibility of oxidation, it also has a major beneficial effect due to the cross-linking of those free radicals. Streicher has previously described cross-linking as "the ideal condition for a wear-resistant material."[35] McKellop[36] described oxidation as detrimental, in part because it competes with the wear resistance improvement brought about by cross-linking. At the 1997 meeting of the Society for Biomaterials there was a clear acceptance of cross-linking as a highly desirable factor for improving polyethylene by increasing its resistance to wear and creep.[37–40] The recently published long-term clinical follow-up from Oonishi, describing the use of highly cross-linked polyethylene, seems to endorse this point.[41]

Wear—The Clinically Relevant Test

Mechanism of Wear

The most clinically relevant test for polyethylene is wear. However, in the laboratory, there are several types of wear testing devices, and they differ in complexity, ranging from simple pin-on-disk to more complex screening machines. Devices that use only a uniaxial motion are often used to make wear comparisons. These so-called wear testers do not generate debris by means of the same multiaxial stresses seen in vivo. The recent recognition of the concept of cross-shear[42] and the importance of the molecular orientation of the implant material as it is loaded[43] have allowed a better understanding of UHMWPE wear mechanisms. This work, published by Wang and others, demonstrates that the load pattern of wear in a uniaxial linear motion forces the PE chains to orient themselves, so that any stress breakage can only occur down the main molecular chains. But the actual physiological motion of wear in a joint implant is multiaxial, which creates stresses *between* the chains. Cross-linkages provide strength between the chains and can reduce the subsequent bond breakage and thus wear. Hence, joint simulators that test actual prostheses in a physiological multiaxial (cross-shear) load situation correlate far better with clinical reality. A cross-shear hip-type wear simulator such as that developed by Wang[44] can consistently result in clinically equivalent wear rates, wear particles, and even wear modes. Similarly, a cross-shear wear machine simulating the geometry and motion of the knee joint has also been developed.

Clinical Experience

A variety of factors affect the rate of polyethylene wear in total joint arthroplasty.[47–59] Examination of retrieved implants can provide valuable information regarding mechanical performance of the prosthesis. Clinically it appears that several factors, including age, gender, level of activity, implant design, size, and position, can influence the rate of acetabular polyethylene wear.[60] In many series, there is a subset of patients with early failure.[61–69] Accelerated polyethylene wear is more prevalent in young active patients[61–65] with thin polyethylene liners. Other risk factors noted include obesity and cup abduction angle.[65] Deficiencies in polyethylene thickness, congruency, and locking mechanism have all been implicated in accelerated polyethylene wear and failure.

The surgeon is responsible for certain variables in the wear equation. In selecting cup and head size, the surgeon should keep in mind the patient's age, activity level, and weight. Component alignment should avoid excessive abduction when anatomy permits. The one variable that is directly controlled by the surgeon is head size. A 32-mm head has been favored historically in many parts of the world. The advantages of a 32-mm head over a 22-mm head are that stability is enhanced (by virtue of a greater head:neck ratio) and contact stresses are lowered. However, given a fixed outer diameter, the thickness of the polyethylene decreases as the head size increases. Stresses tend to increase as the polyethylene becomes thinner. Despite lower contact stresses with a 32-mm head, overall stress may increase if the polyethylene is of insufficient thickness.[46] Finite element analysis by Bartel in a knee model demonstrated that as polyethylene thickness decreases to less than 6 mm, stress begins to dramatically increase.[46] Therefore, it is reasonable to suggest that a minimum plastic thickness of 6 mm should be maintained for metal-backed components.

The results of first and second generation modular acetabular designs have not been uniformly successful. Premature failure has been noted with numerous designs in varied patient populations. There exists a com-

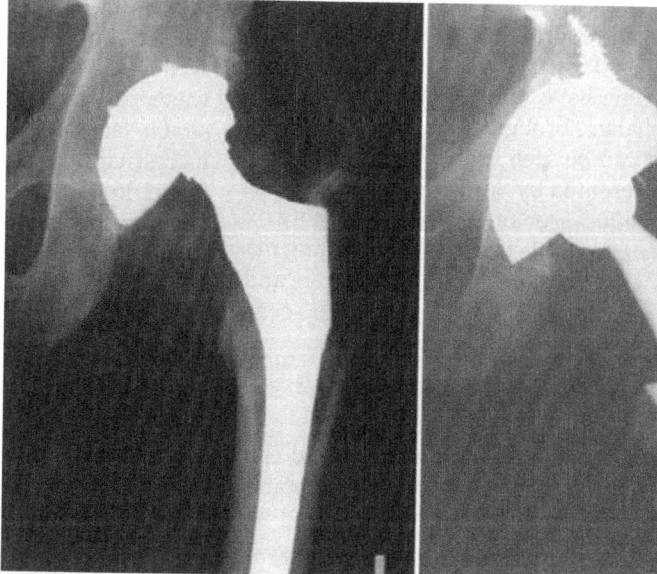

Figure 2.1. Radiograph showing failed DePuy anatomic medullary locking cup with acetabular cup system liner. Extensive acetabular and femoral osteolysis was noted preoperatively.

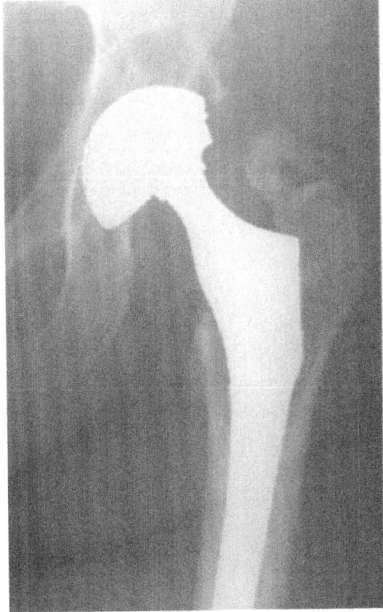
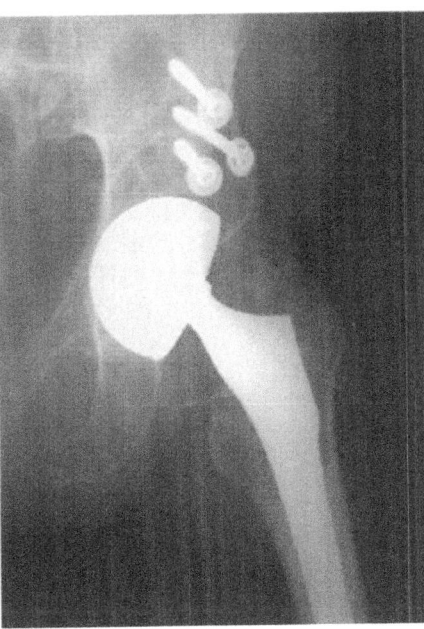

Figure 2.2. Radiograph showing eccentric polyethylene wear requiring major structural allografting.

mon pathway leading to failure amongst all modular designs: accelerated polyethylene wear leading to osteolysis[62–69] and eventual component loosening.[67] Accelerated polyethylene wear has been reported with various implant designs (Fig. 2.1 to 2.5).[64–66]

Implant design has been shown to have an adverse effect on acetabular wear. With certain designs, a gap may be found between the polyethylene liner and the metal acetabular component. Implants are manufactured with exact dimension in mind. In the manufacturing process, reproduction of the exact dimensions of the implant, both plastic and metal, is not always achieved. At best, the implant is manufactured within a narrow range (ie, tolerance). In fact, the actual implant may be slightly smaller or larger than the design specifications. Thus if the tolerance stack-up at the interface between the polyethylene liner and the acetabular cup were to exceed a certain level, a gap would occur between the liner and the metal cup. In effect, the liner would be unsupported over the weight-bearing dome of the prosthesis and would transfer stresses to the rim. This creates a trampoline effect. Vertical positioning of the acetabular component, which places increased stress at the rim (Fig. 2.6), compounds this problem.

Unfortunately, with certain designs[65] the polyethylene is thinnest at the rim, thereby transferring the greatest implant stresses to the thinnest polyethylene. Over time, the yield strength (Fig. 2.7) of the polyethylene at the rim is exceeded, leading to fracture of the polyethylene liner at the rim with eventual fracture and penetration of the femoral head against the metal acetabular shell.

Fortunately, many liners in this scenario manufactured with a gap do not fail. With time many liners "bottom out" because of creep or cold flow, thus rendering the liner fully supported by the metal shell, reducing stresses, and eliminating fatigue failure at the rim. In effect there is a race between the liner bottoming out and the rim fracturing.

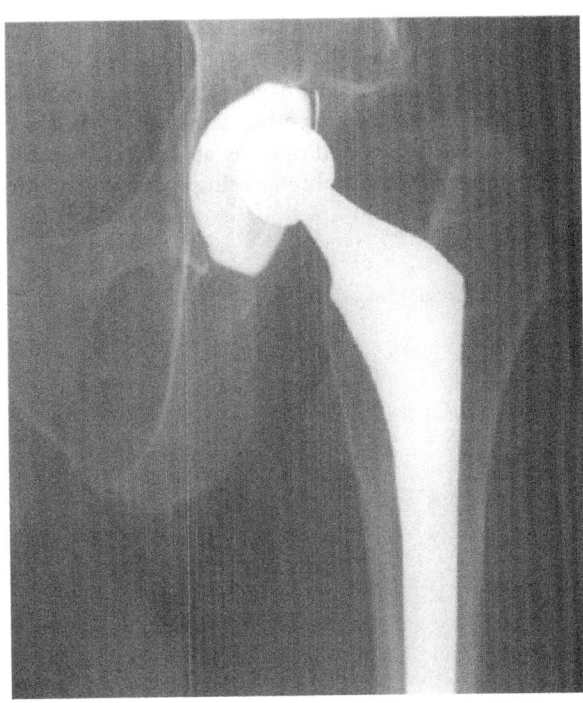

Figure 2.3. Radiograph showing accelerated polyethylene wear noted with Osteonics dual-geometry cup.

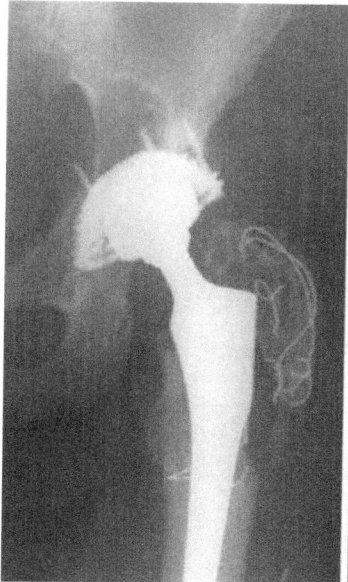
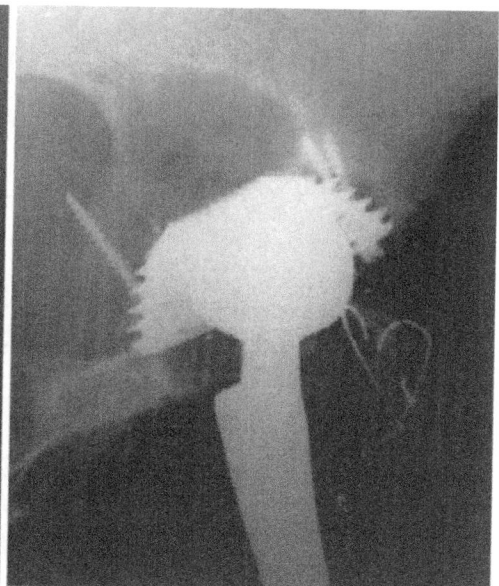

Figure 2.4. Radiograph showing extensive zone II acetabular lysis with asymmetric polyethylene wear in an Anderson cup.

In addition to the possibility of fracture or cracking of a polyethylene liner from severe wear, there is concern of osteolysis and granulomatous destruction due to the release of large quantities of polyethylene debris.[11,12,22,70–75] The amount of osteolysis and resorption correlate positively with the extent of linear wear. The potential for loss of particulates through holes in modular cups allows direct access to the pelvis. Because osteolysis from polyethylene debris is an insidious three-dimensional process, the actual effect of massive polyethylene wear may not manifest for years.

Patients with accelerated wear of a polyethylene liner should be assessed for the need of revision surgery. In the symptomatic patient, the decision to revise is straightforward. Surgical options at this point include revising the cup or simply replacing the liner. In either case, a complete synovectomy should be performed to eradicate as much polyethylene and metal debris as possible. If only the liner is replaced, a smaller inner diameter (ID) liner may be used, providing that the femoral component is modular. This would allow for increased polyethylene thickness, but would not change implant geometry, nor allow for osteolytic areas beneath the cup to be completely debrided. If the decision is made to revise the cup, which may be firmly ingrown, an implant of another design may be reimplanted. In

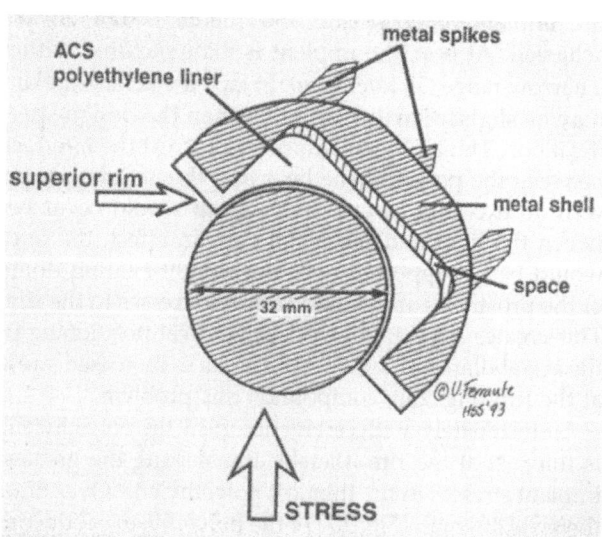

Figure 2.5. Radiograph showing premature polyethylene failure of Harris–Galante component.

Figure 2.6. The cylindric geometry of the acetabular cup system (ACS) liner predisposes the polyethylene to increased stress at the superior rim if a gap exists between the liner and the shell.

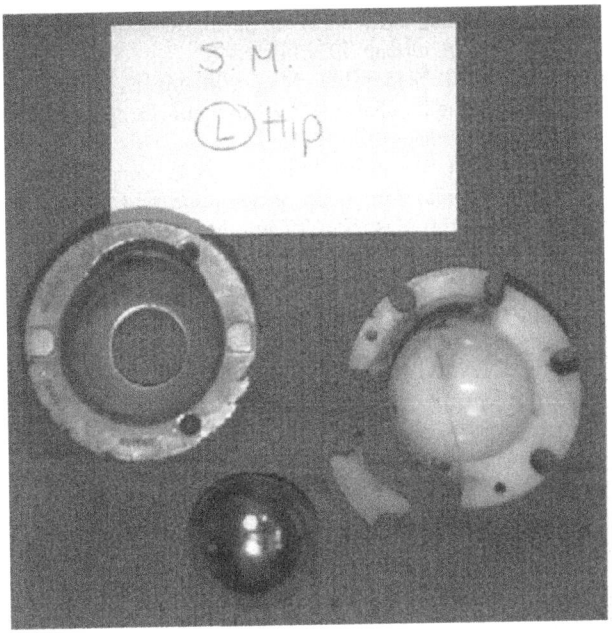

Figure 2.7. Polyethylene insert failure with fracture at the rim.

our experience, the amount of osteolysis at revision is far more extensive than noted radiographically. Intraoperative inspection of exposed acetabular bone seen through the implant's large central hole is inadequate to determine the extent of osteolysis. Therefore for most patients we recommend acetabular implant removal and thorough curettage of osteolytic defects at revision. Many implants, however, are rigidly fixed despite massive amounts of osteolysis. In these cases, one has to consider the potential harm of removing a well-fixed component and the possibility of poor fixation of the revision acetabular component. Retention of a well-fixed acetabular component with limited debridement and grafting of the osteolytic defects and liner exchange may be considered in this case. This approach allows the bone to recover and represents a less invasive reconstruction with a speedier recovery period.

The decision to revise in the asymptomatic patient is difficult. If the femoral head is allowed to penetrate through the polyethylene and against the metal shell, there will be gross metallosis and polyethylene contamination. This, no doubt, will affect future reconstructive procedures and preclude the option of isolated liner replacement. It is also difficult to convince the asymptomatic patient with accelerated polyethylene wear that revision is indicated, especially in light of current expectations of total hip arthroplasty.

Orthopedic surgeons should be aware of the importance of adequate polyethylene thickness and component position. The potential exists for accelerated polyethylene wear in asymptomatic patients following modular acetabular total hip arthroplasty. All patients with modular total hip arthroplasties, regardless of implant size, should be carefully observed for evidence of polyethylene wear. Continued surveillance of accelerated polyethylene wear in the asymptomatic patient is warranted.

Alternative Sterilization Methods

Avoiding Gamma Irradiation: Ethylene Oxide (ETO) and Gas Plasma

In comparison with components that have been gamma-sterilized in air, gas plasma and ethylene oxide-sterilized components demonstrate much lower oxidation over time, sharing similar properties to those of unirradiated PE. Long-term they tend to appear pristine, despite long periods of shelf aging. However, there are some concerns that need to be carefully investigated prior to considering these alternatives. Most importantly, because gas plasma and ethylene-oxide sterilized components are unirradiated material, free radicals are not produced, and so cross-linking cannot occur. Several centers have demonstrated increased wear with unirradiated material, which further increases when exposed to third-body type environments. Clearly, if one could reduce or eliminate the oxidation of PE while maintaining the benefits of cross-linking from gamma irradiation, it could achieve the best of both worlds.

Inert Packaging

Inert packaging of the polyethylene components prior to gamma irradiation retards contact of free radicals with oxygen and still allows some of the benefit of cross-linking to be maintained. This method has been chosen by the larger orthopedic supply companies and usually involves packaging implants in an oxygen-free environment such as nitrogen, argon, or a vacuum. Although this is a positive step and it precludes oxidation in the absence of oxygen short term, free radicals are long-lived, and oxidation can still occur over the long term, during seepage into the packaging while on the shelf or on exposure after opening. Vacuum foil packaging can allow the hydrogen gas, given off from the formation of free radicals, to reenter the polyethylene and "replug" the free radicals. This could reduce the free radicals, but it permits less chance for increased cross-linking as a result.

Stabilization of UHMWPE

Stabilization of UHMWPE is a patented sterilization process that essentially eliminates oxidation while improving and then stabilizing the mechanical properties of the polyethylene. The stabilization process consists of three steps: initial packaging of the implant in nitrogen, gamma irradiation, and then a final stabilization step. This process essentially eliminates the free radicals capable of reacting with oxygen by cross-linking them, which then removes the ability for oxidation to occur, both in the short term and over time. Meticulous testing of the resulting stabilized polyethylene, by using clinically relevant state-of-the-art laboratory test methods, has been performed, and the scientific results have been replicated and validated independently at several centers.[38,76] Further testing shows no detrimental effects on the chemical, mechanical, physical, biological, or morphological properties of the polyethylene. These results have been published and they demonstrate that virtually no oxidation occurs over time, even in the presence of oxygen, and that a substantial improvement in wear resistance is achieved. Other properties such as ultimate tensile strength, impact strength, and modulus of elasticity, are maintained.[77]

Conclusion

It is essential that the previously little known science of PE be demystified, especially as the issues surrounding it continue to become more complex and more distorted. Past attempts by industry to improve UHMWPE have been hampered by an imperfect understanding of polyethylene and its properties. Small pieces of the research puzzle acted on in isolation may sometimes lead to solutions being put forward in answer to the wrong issues. Failure to apply clinically relevant state-of-the-art laboratory testing to such proposed solutions may compound this further. Despite a greater understanding of UHMWPE, the application of modern sophisticated multiaxial joint simulators, and the ability to speed up the future by means of accelerated aging methods, we can never replace a 10-year prospective clinical follow-up, and so we must be cautiously optimistic in the meantime. But no matter how great or small the improvements prove to be clinically, optimism must be built on a thorough research program based on a carefully reviewed foundation of science.

References

1. Kurth M, Eyerer P, Ascherl R, Dittel K, Holz U. An evaluation of retrieved UHMWPE hip joint cups. *J Biomat Applic.* 1988;3:33–51.
2. Roe RJ, Grood ES, Shastri R, Gosselin CA, Noyes FR. Effect of radiation sterilization and aging on UHMWPE. *J Biomed Mater Res.* 1981;15:209–230.
3. Livermore JT. Polyethylene wear in total hip arthroplasty. *Semin Arthroplasty.* 1993;4:136–142.
4. Clarke IC. Role of ceramic implants. *Clin Orthop.* 1992;282:19–30.
5. Bartel DL, Wright TM, Edwards D. The effect of metal backing on stresses in polyethylene acetabular components. In: *The Hip: Proceedings of the 18th Open Scientific Meeting of the Hip Society.* St Louis, MO: CV Mosby, Inc; 1989.
6. Cupic Z. Long term follow-up of Charnley arthroplasty of the hip. *Clin Orthop.* 1979;141:28–43.
7. Griffith MJ, Seidenstein MK, Williams D, Charnley J. Socket wear in Charnley low friction arthroplasty of the hip. *Clin Orthop.* 1978;137:37–47.
8. McCoy TM, Salvati EA, Ranawat CS, Wilson PD Jr. A fifteen year follow-up study of one hundred Charnley low friction arthroplasties. *Orthop Clin North Am.* 1988;19:467–476.
9. Rimnac CM, Wilson PD, Fuchs MD, Wright TM. Acetabular cup wear in total hip arthroplasty. *Orthop Clin North Am.* 1988;19:631–636.
10. Salvati EA, Wilson PD Jr, Jolley MN, Vakili F, Aglietti P, Brown GC. A ten year follow-up study of our first one hundred consecutive Charnley total hip replacements. *J Bone Joint Surg Am.* 1981;63:753–767.
11. Wroblewski BM. Direction and rate of socket wear in Charnley low-friction arthroplasty. *J Bone Joint Surg Br.* 1985;67:757–761.
12. Wroblewski BM. Fifteen to twenty-one-year results of the Charnley low-friction arthroplasty. *Clin Orthop.* 1986;211:30–35.
13. Charnley J, Halley DK. Rate of wear on total hip replacements. *Clin Orthop.* 1975;112:170–179.
14. Harris WH. A new total hip implant. *Clin Orthop.* 1971;81:105–113.
15. Collier JP, Mayer MB, Jensen RE, Surprenant VA, Suprenant HP, McNamar JL, et al. Mechanisms of failure of modular prostheses. *Clin Orthop.* 1992;285:129–139.
16. Wright TM, Bartel DL, Rimnac CM. Surface damage in polyethylene total joint components. American Academy of Ortho-paedic Surgeons Kappa Delta award paper, presented at Hospital for Special Surgery; 1989.
17. Landy MM, Walker PS. Wear of UHMWPE components of 90 retrieved knee prostheses. *J Arthroplasty.* 1988;(suppl):S73–S85.
18. Jasty M et al. Wear of PE cups in THR: analysis of 159 cups retrieved at revision surgery or autopsy. *Trans Orthop Res Soc.* 1993;18:291.
19. Campbell, et al. Histological analysis of tissues suggests that "metallosis" may really be "plasticosis." *Trans Orthop Res Soc.* 1992;17:393.
20. Doorn, et al. Characterization of metal wear particles from metal on metal total hip replacements. *Trans Soc Biomater.* 1997;10:192.
21. Malchau, Herberts. Prognosis of total hip replacement. Presented at scientific exhibit, 64th meeting of the American Academy of Orthopaedic Surgeons; February 1996.
22. Willert HG. Reactions of the articular capsule to wear products of artificial joint prostheses. *J Biomed Mater Res.* 1977;11:157–164.
23. Bartel DL, Burstein AH, Toda MD, Edwards DL. The effect of conformity and plastic thickness on contact stresses in metal-backed plastic implants. *J Biomech Eng.* 1985;107:193–199.
24. Waugh W. In: *John Charnley: The Man and the Hip.* New York, NY: Springer-Verlag; 1990:120–121.
25. Maloney WJ, Jasty MJ. Wear debris in THA. *Semin Arthroplasty.* 1993;4:125–135.
26. Lustiger A. *Tie Molecules in Polyethylene.* Gas Research Institute; 1985. Report GRI-85/0129.

27. Lupton JM, Regester JW. Physical properties of extended-chain high-density polyethylene. *J Appl Poly Sci.* 1974;18:2407.
28. Eyerer P, et al. UHMWPE for replacement joints. Translated from *Kunstoffe German Plastics*. 1987;77:617–622.
29. Alexander N, Hungerford DS, Jones LC, Mont MA. Correlation of acetabular failure to polyethylene manufacturing techniques in total hip arthroplasty. Presented at 62nd meeting of the American Academy of Orthopaedics; February 1995; Paper 121.
30. Lykins CL. A comparison of extruded and molded UHMWPE. *Trans Soc Biomater*. 1995;18:385.
31. Sun DC, Stark C, Dumbleton J. The origin of the white band observed in direct compression molded UHMWPE inserts. *Trans Soc Biomater*. 1994;17:121.
32. Sutula LC, Collier JP, Saum KA, Currier BH, Currier JH, Sanford WM, et al. Impact of gamma sterilization on clinical performance of polyethylene in the hip. *Clin Orthop*. 1995;319:28–40.
33. Li S. Radiation damage in polyethylene. Presented at Second Annual Midwest Conference on UHMWPE; October 1995; Warsaw, Ind.
34. Gillis A, Furman B, Perone J, Lefebvre F, Reish T, Li S. Oxidation of in vivo vs. shelf life aged gamma sterilized total knee replacements. *Trans Soc Biomater*. 1997;20:73.
35. Streicher. The behavior of UHMW-PE when subjected to sterilization by ionizing radiation. In: Willert HG, Buchhorn G, Eyerer P, eds. *UHMWPE as Biomaterial in Orthopedic Surgery*. Toronto, Canada: Hogrefe & Huber; 1991:66–73.
36. McKellop HA, Shen FW, Yu YJ, Lu B, Salovey R, Campbell P. Effect of sterilization method and other modifications on the wear resistance of UHMWPE cups. Presented at Polyethylene Wear in Orthopaedics Implants Workshop, 23rd annual meeting of the Society for Biomaterials; 1997.
37. McKellop H, Shen F, Ota T, Lu B, Wiser H, Yu E. The effect of sterilization method, calcium stearate, and molecular weight on wear of UHMWPE acetabular cups. *Trans Soc Biomater*. 1997;20:43.
38. McKellop H, Shen F, Ota T, Lu B, Wiser H, Yu E. Wear of UHMWPE acetabular cups after gamma sterilization in nitrogen, thermal stabilization, and artificial aging. *Trans Soc Biomater*. 1997;20:45.
39. Clarke IC, Good V, Williams P, Oparaugo P, Oonishi H, Fujisawa A. Simulator wear study of high-dose gamma-irradiated UHMWPE cups. *Trans Soc for Biomater*. 1997;20:71.
40. Muratoglu OK, Bragdon CR, O'Connor DO, Merrill EW, Jasty M, Harris WH. Electron beam cross-linking of UHMWPE at room temperature: a candidate bearing material for total joint arthroplasty. *Trans Soc Biomater*. 1997;20:74.
41. Oonishi H. The low wear of cross-linked polyethylene socket in total hip prostheses. *Encyclopaedia of Biomaterials and Bioengineering*. Part A, vol 2. New York, NY: Marcel Dekker, Inc; 1995:1853.
42. Ramamurti BS, Bragdon CR, Harris WH. Loci of selected points on the femoral head during normal gait. *Trans Soc Biomater*. 1995;18:347.
43. Wang A, Sun DC, Stark C, Dumbleton J. Factors affecting wear screening. Presented at the American Society for Testing and Materials Workshop on Characterization and Performance of Articular Surfaces; May 1995; Denver, Colo.
44. Wang A, Essner A, Polineni VK, Sun DC, Stark C, Dumbleton J. Wear mechanisms and wear testing of ultra-high molecular weight polyethylene in total joint replacements. Presented at Polyethylene Wear in Orthopaedics Implants Workshop, 23rd annual meeting of the Society for Biomaterials; 1997.
45. Amis AA, Seedhorn BB. Design factors for polyethylene prosthesis components with particular reference to Sheehan knee implant. *J Bone Joint Surg Br*. 1983;65:367.
46. Bartel DL, Bicknell VL, Wright TM. The effect of conformity, thickness and material on stresses in ultra-high molecular weight components for total joint replacement. *J Bone Joint Surg Am*. 1986;68:1041–1051.
47. Cameron HU, Hunter GA. Failure in total knee arthroplasty: mechanisms, revisions, and results. *Clin Orthop*. 1982;170:141–146.
48. Elbert KE, Kurth M, Bartel DL, Eyerer P, Rimnic CM, Wright TM. In vivo changes in material properties of polyethylene and their effects on stresses associated with surface damage of polyethylene components. Presented at the Orthopaedic Research Society 34th annual meeting; February 1–4, 1988; Atlanta, Ga.
49. Engh GA. Failure of the polyethylene bearing surface of a total knee replacement within four years. *J Bone Joint Surg Am*. 1988;70:1093–1096.
50. Ewald FC, Jacobs MA, Miegel RE, Walker PS, Poss R, Sledge CB. Kinematic total knee replacement. *J Bone Joint Surg Am*. 1984;66:1032–1040.
51. Eyerer P, Ke YC. Property changes of UHMW polyethylene hip cup endoprostheses during implantation. *J Biomed Mater Res*. 1984;18:1137–1151.
52. Mirra JM, Marder RA, Amstutz HC. The pathology of failed total joint arthroplasty. *Clin Orthop*. 1982;170:175–183.
53. Rose RM, Crugnola A, Ries M, Cimino WR, Paul I, Radin EL. On origins of high in vivo wear rates in polyethylene components of total joint prostheses. *Clin Orthop*. 1979;145:277–286.
54. Rose RM, Nusbaum HJ, Schneider H, Ries M, Paul I, Crugnola A, et al. On the true wear rate of ultra high-molecular-weight polyethylene in the total hip prosthesis. *J Bone Joint Surg Am*. 1980;62:537–549.
55. Walker PS, Hsieh HJ. Conformity in condylar replacement knee prostheses. *J Bone Joint Surg Br*. 1979;59:222–228.
56. Wright TM, Astrin DJ, Bansal MK, Rimnac CM, Green T, Insall JN, et al. Failure of carbon-fiber reinforced polyethylene total knee replacement components. *J Bone Joint Surg Am*. 1988;70:926–932.
57. Wright TM, Bartel DL. The problem of surface damage in polyethylene total knee components. *Clin Orthop*. 1986;205:67–74.
58. Wright TM, Hood RW, Burstein AJ. Analysis of material failures. *Orthop. Clin North Am*. 1982;13:33–44.
59. Wright TM, Rimnac CM, Faris PM, Bansal M. Analysis of surface damage in retrieved carbon fiber–reinforced and plain polyethylene tibial components from posterior stabilized total knee replacements. *J Bone Joint Surg Am*. 1988;70:1312–1319.

60. Wright TM, Rimnac CM, Stulberg SD, Mintz L, Tsao AK, Klein RW, et al. Wear of polyethylene in total joint replacements. *Clin Orthop.* 1992;276:126–134.
61. Nashed RS, Becker DA, Gustilo RB. Are cementless acetabular components the cause of excess wear and osteolysis in total hip arthroplasty? *Clin Orthop.* 1995;317:19–28.
62. Jasty M, Bragdon C, Jiranek W, Chandler H, Maloney W, Harris WH. Etiology of osteolysis around porous-coated cementless total hip arthroplasties. *Clin Orthop.* 1994;308:111–126.
63. Wan Z, Dorr LD. Natural history of femoral focal osteolysis with proximal ingrowth smooth stem implant. *J Arthroplasty.* 1996;11:718–725.
64. Perez R, Deshmukh R, Ranawat CS. Polyethylene wear and periprosthetic osteolysis in acetabular components with cylindrical inserts. *Orthop Trans.* 1995;19:319.
65. Bono J, Sanford L, Toussaint J. Polyethylene wear in total hip arthroplasty: observations from retrieved AML plus hip implants with ACS polyethylene liner. *J Arthroplasty.* 1994;9:119–125.
66. Bierbaum B, Mattingly D, Leone A, Karpos P, Van-Flandern G, Gomes S. Fixation, polyethylene wear, and osteolysis with the press-fit dual geometry acetabulum at minimum seven years follow-up. *Orthop Trans.* 1995–96;19:753.
67. Dorr LD, Lewonowski K, Lucero M, Harris M, Wan Z. Failure mechanisms of anatomic porous replacement/cementless total hip replacement. *Clin Orthop.* 1997;343:157–678.
68. Kim YH, Kim VE. Cementless porous-coated anatomic medullary locking total hip prostheses. *J Arthroplasty.* 1994;9:243–252.
69. Owen T, Moran C, Smith S, Pinder I. Results of uncemented porous-coated anatomic total hip replacement. *J Bone Joint Surg Br.* 1994;76:258–262.
70. Dall DM, Grobbelaar CJ, Learmonth ID, Dau G. Charnley low-friction arthroplasty. *Clin Orthop.* 1986;211:85–90.
71. Johanson NA, Bullough PG, Wilson PK Jr, Salvati EA, Ranawat CS. The microscopic anatomy of the bone–cement interface in the failed total hip arthroplasty. *Clin Orthop.* 1987;216:123–135.
72. Johanson NA, Callaghan JJ, Salvati EA, Merkow RL. Fourteen year follow-up study of a patient with massive calcar resorption: a case report. *Clin Orthop.* 1986;213:189–196.
73. Remagen W, Morschler E. Histologic results with cement-free implant hip sockets of polyethylene. *Arch Orthop Trauma Surg* 1984;103:145–151.
74. Wilson PD Jr, Rimnac CM, Wright TM. Wear as a cause of failure in total hip arthroplasty. In: Noble J, Galasko CBS, eds. *Recent Developments in Orthopaedic Surgery.* Manchester, England: Manchester University Press; 1987.
75. Wroblewski BM. Wear of high density polyethylene on bone and cartilage. *J Bone Joint Surg Br.* 1979;61:498–500.
76. Blunn GW, Bell CJ. The effect of oxidation on the wear of untreated and stabilized UHMWPE. *Trans Orthop Res Soc.* 1996;21:482.
77. Sun DC, Wang A, Stark C, Dumbleton J. Development of stabilized UHMWPE implants with improved oxidation resistance via crosslinking. Presented at Scientific Exhibit, 63rd annual meeting of the American Academy of Orthopaedic Surgeons; February 1996.

3
Osteolysis in Total Joint Arthroplasty: Basic Science

W.A. Jiranek and S.R. Goldring

Osteolysis is a radiographic term used to describe loss of preexisting bone. As early as 1975 this term was used to characterize the loss of bone adjacent to prosthetic orthopedic implants.[1,2] Three radiographic patterns of periprosthetic bone resorption have been described[3,4] (Table 3.1): linear osteolysis, expansile osteolysis, and so-called stress-shielding. The existence of these distinct radiographic patterns implies that different underlying mechanisms may be involved in their pathogenesis. In considering these mechanisms it is essential to first define the radiologic patterns.

Linear osteolysis is characterized by a slow, uniform pattern of bone resorption, which is commonly 5 mm or less. One example of linear osteolysis is the common form seen around cemented acetabular components with linear radiolucencies beginning at the periphery and progressively moving to the dome.

Aggressive or *expansile osteolysis* is characterized by a focal cystic or balloon-like pattern of bone resorption. This pattern of osteolysis tends to develop more rapidly than linear osteolysis and is often associated with irregular borders and larger areas of bone destruction. It is apparent, however, that the bone resorption process adjacent to prosthetic joints is a continuum, and as such, both forms may be found within the same patient.

Whereas these two forms of bone resorption are characterized by an alteration in the normal bony architecture, *stress-shielding* refers to a more generalized loss of bone that involves attrition, but not destruction, of normal bone architecture. This phenomenon is believed to be a manifestation of Wolff's law, in which a stiff prosthetic construct shields bone from its normal stress, leading to a net bone resorption through the process of bone remodeling. Whereas the term osteolysis implies complete bone loss in a specific region, stress-shielding implies partial trabecular bone loss, which is radiographically described as osteopenia. Stress shielding occurs most commonly around extensively coated cementless femoral components, but it also may be seen around cemented femoral components and metal-backed acetabular components.

Stress-shielding has also been documented around well-functioning cemented femoral components retrieved at autopsy.[5] In this situation, apparent linear radiolucencies develop adjacent to the prosthesis. This process differs radiographically from linear osteolysis in that there are still trabecular elements in the radiolucency that are merely thinned. Although the differences in the two processes are clearly visible in cross-section, they also can be distinguished by careful inspection of plain radiographs.

An additional form of stress-related remodeling around cementless prostheses involves the development of linear fibrous radiolucencies adjacent to the prosthesis surrounded by a thin layer of condensed bone (neocortex). This phenomenon can be distinguished from linear osteolysis by its early formation (1 year) and the presence of a neocortex.

Analysis of the histologic and radiographic findings associated with stress-shielding and linear and aggressive peri-implant osteolysis provides strong evidence that these conditions are produced by different pathophysiologic processes (Table 3.1). Examination of the skeletal tissues associated with stress-shielding suggests that this condition more likely reflects an adaptation of the normal bone-remodeling unit to the unique biomechanical environment adjacent to the implant. In contrast, the skeletal tissues adjacent to implants in individuals with linear or expansile osteolysis have been replaced by a membranous connective tissue that contains cellular features of a chronic inflammatory reaction. The cellular and connective tissue organization of the membrane associated with these forms of osteolysis demonstrates distinct features that reflect the influences of additional environmental factors, including the presence of implant wear products. The pathogenesis and functional significance of this distinct tissue reaction are addressed in the subsequent discussion.

Table 3.1. Correlation of radiographic features and mechanism of bone loss in different patterns of osteolysis after total joint replacement.

Pattern of bone loss	Mechanism	Radiographic features
Stress-shielding	Biomechanical effect on bone remodeling; bone architecture maintained	Generalized regional bone loss; not associated with loss of fixation; decreased radiodensity (osteopenia)
Linear osteolysis	Both mechanical effect (increased micromotion related to loss of fixation) and biologic effect (low-grade chronic inflammation)	Progressive regional bone loss with zones of complete radiolucency; smooth borders with primarily loss of trabecular bone
Aggressive osteolysis	Fragmented particulate implant wear debris with localized foreign body granulomatous inflammation	Focal radiolucency with irregular borders; both trabecular and cortical bone losses

Incidence of Osteolysis

Determination of the true incidence of osteolysis has been difficult, in part related to differences in the definition of osteolysis used by individual investigators. Much of the recent literature on this subject has concentrated on the aggressive, expansile balloon-like form of osteolysis. In effect, this form represents one end of a continuum, with a slower, more linear form of osteolysis representing the other end.[6] In addition, osteolysis has been described around apparently well-fixed, as well as loose total hip prostheses, and the pathogenetic processes in these two conditions may be quite different.[3,7–9]

Linear osteolysis has been implicated as a sign of prosthetic loosening.[10] For example, Hodgkinson et al.[11] have shown an association between the extent of linear acetabular osteolysis and the presence of component loosening. A potential role for implant wear debris in the pathogenesis of this process has been suggested by many investigators, including Schmalzreid et al.,[12] who correlated the degree of linear osteolysis around cemented acetabular components with the presence of particulate debris, especially polyethylene. Linear osteolysis also has been described around cementless acetabular components.[13] Other factors that have made it difficult to define the true incidence of linear osteolysis include the problem of distinguishing linear osteolysis from remodeling associated with stress shielding.[10] There also is a lack of consensus among researchers on what constitutes minor versus major osteolysis.

The reported incidence of osteolysis around cemented acetabular components has ranged from 8% to 44% at mean follow-ups of 5 to 15 years.[14,15] Alsema et al.[16] reported a 33% incidence of lysis around cemented acetabular components at 15 year follow-up in their series of Stanmore total hip replacements. This osteolysis progresses with time and is associated with loosening[11] and, in general, linear osteolysis is the most common form seen around cemented acetabular components.

Osteolysis around cementless acetabular components appears to occur earlier than in cemented components. Reports of pelvic osteolysis, independent of the need for revision, have ranged from 14% to 49% for cementless components.[17–20] Rorabeck et al.[14] reported an incidence of 14% at 4.8 years in their randomized prospective trial, and Capello et al.[17] reported an incidence of 14% at 5 year follow-up with a different type of cementless acetabular component. Bettin et al.[21] reported a 24% incidence of acetabular osteolysis in their series of 83 Judet prostheses at 10.8 year follow-up. In all of these series, the incidence of osteolysis appears to increase with time, and with cementless acetabular components aggressive osteolysis is the most common radiographic pattern.

To some extent, the pattern and incidence of osteolysis are influenced by the design of the components and the surgical techniques. For example, the incidence of lysis around cementless acetabular components may be lower in the hybrid constructs in which the femoral component is cemented. Goldberg et al.[22] reported a 4% incidence of pelvic osteolysis in their series of hybrid total hip replacements at 5 year follow-up. Woolson and Haber[23] reported minimal acetabular osteolysis in their series of 121 hybrid hip replacements at 6 year follow-up.

At longer follow-up, however, the incidence of osteolysis may equalize. Zicat et al.[3] compared the rates of osteolysis in 74 cemented and 63 cementless acetabular components inserted by the same surgeon using the same uncemented femoral component. At a mean follow-up of 8.8 years (range, 4.5–11.8 years), the incidence of osteolysis was 18% around uncemented acetabular components and 37% around cemented acetabular components. They reported that cemented cups were associated primarily with linear osteolysis, whereas cementless cups were primarily associated with aggressive osteolysis.

The incidence of lysis around cemented femoral prostheses has been reported as 0% to 12%. In general, these data have been based on assessments obtained at a longer time of follow-up.[24,25] Mulroy and Harris[25] found a 6% incidence of small, focal osteolysis around stable cemented femoral components at 11 year follow-up. The incidence of osteolysis increases with unstable femoral components, and also in areas of incomplete or deficient cement mantles.[26]

The reported incidence of lysis around cementless femoral components has ranged from 7% to 56%[27-30] at a mean follow-up of 5.5 years. In one matched pair analysis comparing cemented versus cementless femoral prostheses, there was a significantly greater incidence of femoral lysis in the cementless group.[24]

In summary, osteolysis has been observed in association with both cemented and cementless hip components. Integration of the findings from all the studies provides strong evidence that osteolytic lesions are seen at earlier follow-up periods in individuals with cementless hip arthroplasties, compared with patients with cemented arthroplasties. Cemented prostheses are more commonly associated with linear osteolysis, whereas aggressive osteolysis is more often seen in patients with cementless components, although either pattern of osteolysis can be observed in patients with cemented or cementless designs. Of particular clinical relevance is the observation that once osteolysis has been identified, it will almost surely progress over time. For example, one study has documented a progression in the size of osteolytic lesions in 84% of patients.[31] These findings suggest that, over time, an increasing number of patients with osteolysis will eventually require revision surgery.[32]

Wear Debris and Osteolysis

Numerous early investigations established a relationship between the incidence of implant wear and high rates of osteolysis. For example, in Charnley's series of patients in which the acetabular-bearing surface was composed of Teflon™, there was evidence of rapid deterioration of the Teflon™ surface with generation of large quantities of wear debris. The presence of these wear particles was associated with extensive bone destruction, leading to premature clinical failure.[33-35] The Monk soft top prosthesis, which consisted of an all-polyethylene prosthetic head articulating with articular cartilage, was associated with very high rates of polyethylene wear leading to catastrophic peri-implant osteolysis.[36,37] Surface replacement types of prostheses, which have a higher polyethylene wear rate than conventional prosthetic devices, also are associated with higher rates of osteolysis.[38] Total hip replacement constructs with titanium femoral head bearing surfaces have also been associated with high wear rates and elevated levels of osteolysis in both cemented and cementless constructs.[39,40]

Many investigators have observed a relationship between osteolysis and regions of particle generation and collection. For example, Schmalzreid et al.[41] have noted the onset of progressive osteolysis in areas that are contacted by synovial fluid containing particulate debris. They have shown that joint fluid can penetrate regions that are distant from the actual joint cavity, thus promoting the concept of the effective joint space. Other investigators have noted the onset of focal osteolysis in areas distant from the articulation, in areas of localized particulate debris generation, such as fragmentation of cement mantles.[42-44]

To gain insights into the mechanisms by which particulate wear debris induces the different patterns of osteolysis, investigators have analyzed retrieved peri-implant tissues from patients undergoing revision surgery for aseptic loosening[45-51] (Fig. 3.1). These studies document the presence of a connective tissue membrane corresponding to the radiographic zones of osteolysis in subjects with linear and aggressive patterns of osteolysis. The tissue exhibits features of a so-called foreign body granuloma associated with the particulate implant wear debris. The granulomatous response is similar to that seen with other particulate materials, such as silica, asbestos, or a variety of other environmental particulates. In individuals with cemented implants, particles of polymethylmethacrylate and polyethylene, many of which have been internalized by the resident cell populations, can be readily identified. In noncemented implants, metal wear debris and presumed corrosion products can be detected. The presence of particles provides definitive evidence that fragmentation of the prosthetic implant materials has occurred, presumably as a consequence of mechanical factors associated with cyclic loading.

Macrophages are the predominant cell type within the granuloma (Fig. 3.2). They make up 40% to 70% of the cells. Most of the macrophages express the MAC3 cell marker, indicating that they are activated.[52] *Macrophage activation* has been experimentally defined as the process by which macrophages become more mobile and phagocytic, show many more lysosomes, and produce cytokines such as tumor necrosis factor and other interleukins. Some regions of the granuloma contain macrophages that exhibit morphologic features of apoptosis. These cells can be identified by their loss of pseudopods, and rounding out of the cell membrane, with a more eosinophilic cytoplasm and pycnotic nuclei. In vitro studies have confirmed the potential cytotoxic effects of polymeric and metal implant debris. The finding of cells with apoptotic features indicates that the particles may also induce a specific program of cell death.[53,54]

Fibroblasts are seen throughout the membrane, but are more numerous in the linear form of osteolysis.[32] They make up 20% to 50% of the cells in some specimens. Many of these cells contain internalized particulate wear debris and, although traditionally viewed as facultative phagocytes, they may respond directly to wear particulates by upregulating many of their biologic activities, including the production of collagen and biologically active molecules such as prostaglandins.[55-58]

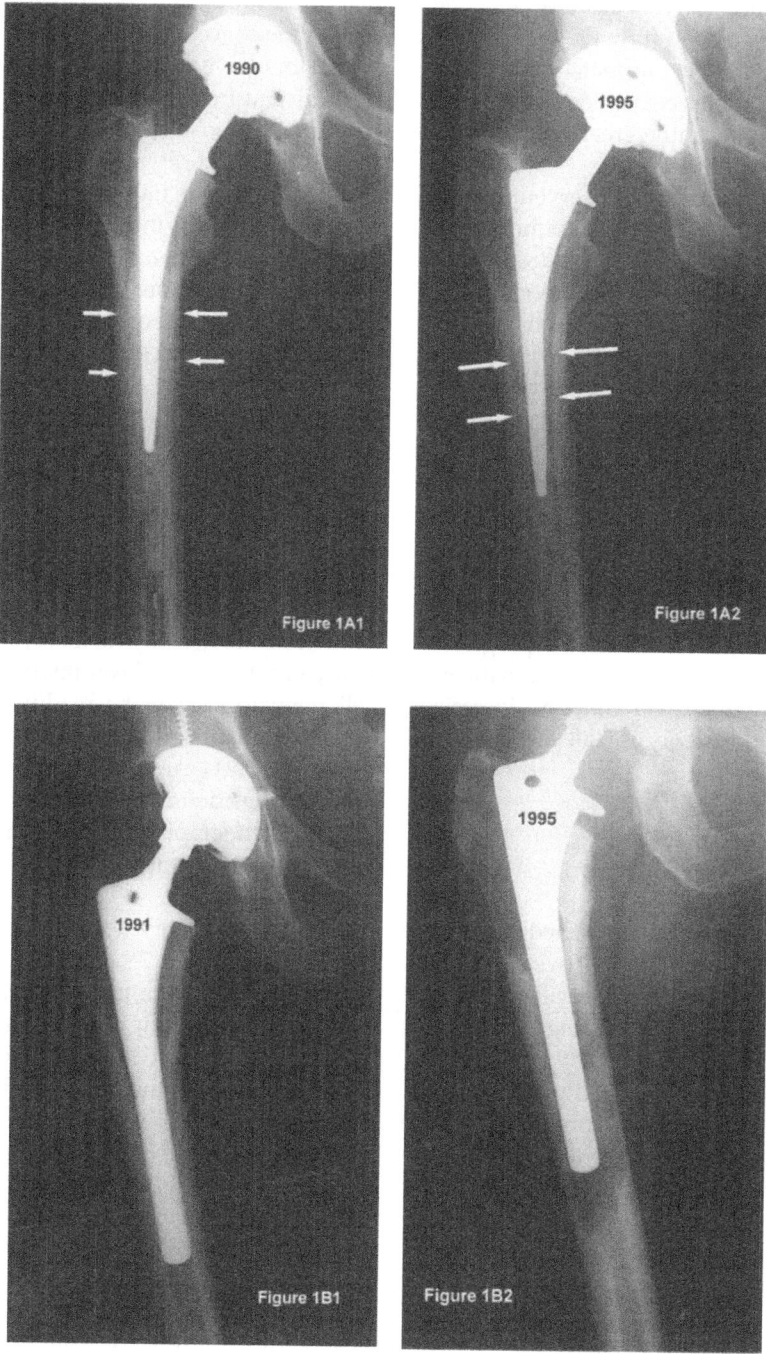

Figure 3.1. 1A1. Cemented femoral component in early postop period. 1A2. The same femoral component at 5-year follow-up showing the development of linear 2–3 mm radiolucent line. 1B1. Cementless femoral component in early postop period. 1B2. The same femoral component at 5-year follow-up showing the development of erosive large lytic lesions (*arrows*). 1C1. Extensively coated cementless femoral component in the early postop period. 1C2. The same femoral component at 6-year follow-up showing considerable attrition of the cortical density and thickness (*arrows*). (*Photos 1C1 and 1C2 courtesy of Dr. Charles A. Engh, Anderson Orthopaedic Clinic, Alexandria, VA*)

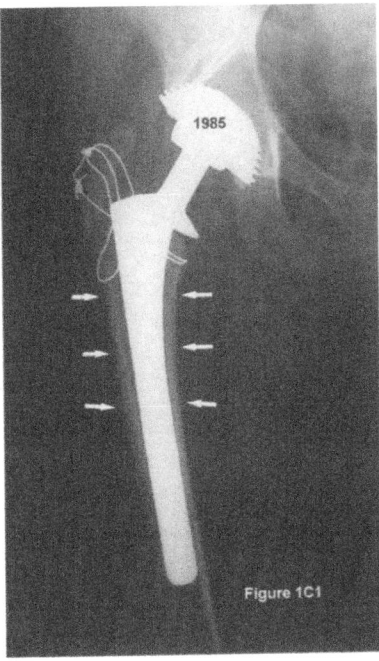 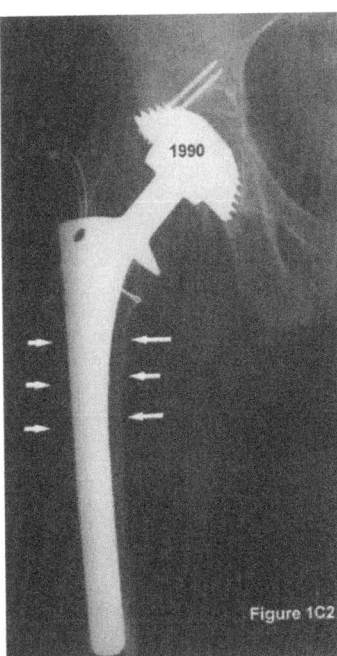

Figure 3.1. Continued

Foreign body giant cells are commonly seen within the granuloma, but they make up less than 5% of the total cells. They are often associated with larger particles (>10 μm), although many of these cells also contain internalized wear debris. Analysis of these multinucleated giant cells indicates that they express functional markers that are distinct from osteoclasts.[59]

Lymphocytes are often seen within the membrane, but they generally make up less than 5% of the cell population,[52,60] although one study has shown a greater concentration.[61] These cells express functional characteristics of T lymphocytes. Their role in the pathogenesis of peri-implant osteolysis is controversial. Two studies of immunodeficient animal models have shown that lymphocytes are not required for the generation of a foreign body response to particulate debris, and that this response is similar to the response mounted by immunocompetent animals.[62,63] Another study, however, has suggested lymphocyte activation in patients with loose total hip replacements.[64] The aggregate information, however, suggests that the response to particulate debris is one of a nonimmune granuloma in which the tissues fail to show histologic evidence of a hypersensivity reaction. In support of this conclusion is the absence of clear-cut systemic signs or symptoms of hypersensitivity to the implant materials in the vast majority of patients with failed prosthetic devices.

In our own experience, the presence or absence of histologic evidence of hypersensitivity may relate more to the patient's underlying clinical rheumatic disorder and immunologic state. We have identified a subgroup of patients, namely patients with rheumatoid arthritis, in whom the peri-implant tissues demonstrate histologic features of an immune granuloma. In these patients, the peri-implant tissues are heavily infiltrated with lymphocytes, suggesting that in individuals with an underlying disturbance in immune regulation the inflammatory reaction to particulate wear debris may exhibit features of an immune granuloma.[65] It is of interest that Caplan[66] described a similar *immune* granulomatous reaction in the lungs of individuals with rheumatoid arthritis who were exposed to particulate coal dust. It is likely, however, that even in individuals without an obvious underlying immune disorder there is a spectrum of reactivity to particulate implant materials and that, in some individuals, the more aggressive clinical course may be attributed to an enhanced cellular and tissue reaction to the wear debris, even in the absence of an identifiable hypersensitivity phenomenon. Identification of this subset of patients and development of strategies to attenuate the tissue reaction are of tremendous clinical importance.

The layer of tissue adjacent to the peri-implant bone surface exhibits evidence of active bone remodeling, including resorption lacunae and isolated zones of new bone formation. Many of the cytokines released by macrophages in the interface membrane inhibit osteoblast synthetic activity,[67–69] and this may in part account for the absence of a more active bone formation response in individuals with aseptic loosening. The os-

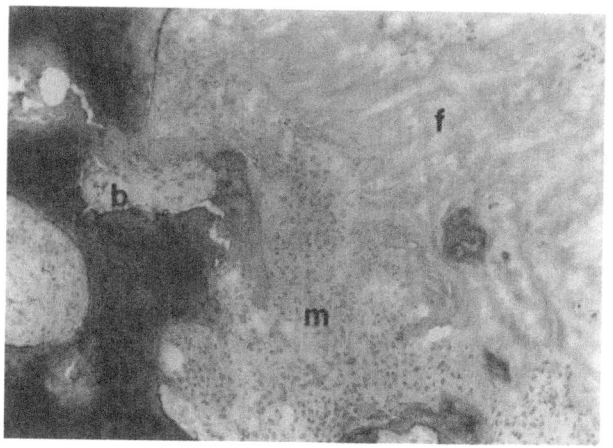

Figure 2A

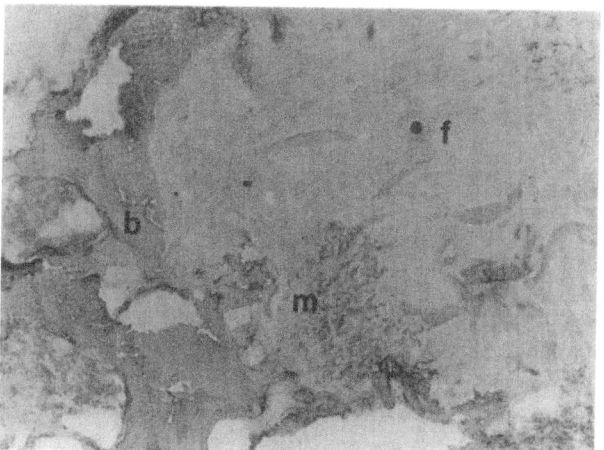

Figure 2B

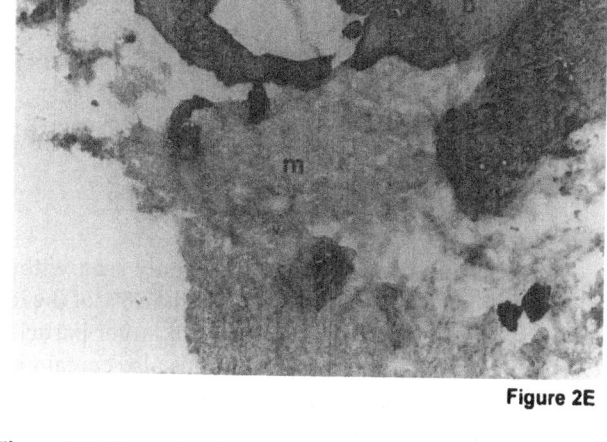

Figure 2D

Figure 2E

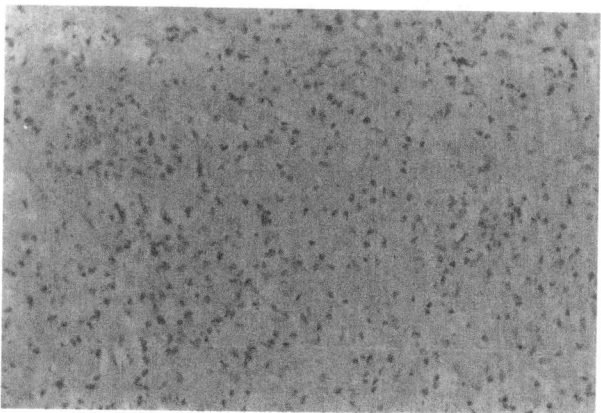

Figure 2C

Figure 3.2. (See color insert.) 2A. Linear osteolysis demonstrating the three layers: trabecular bone to the left (*b*), a macrophage infiltrate in the center (*m*), and the reparative fibrous layer to the right (*f*). X200, H&E. 2B. Linear osteolysis: a serial section to A treated with MAC 3 antibody (*red staining*) showing pockets of macrophages adjacent to bone but no staining in the fibrous tissue. X100, Hematoxylin. 2C. Transitional osteolysis, from a case of moderate erosive osteolysis around a cementless titanium component. The cells are primarily macrophages, there is less fibrous tissue (*pink*) and it is disorganized, and there is a large amount of titanium debris. 2D. Transitional osteolysis: a serial section from C taken under polarized light showing a large number of birefringent polyethylene particles. 2E. Aggressive osteolysis. This section is treated with MAC 3 antibody (specific for activated macrophages) showing virtually all cells are macrophages, with little reparative fibrous tissue response. There is a large amount of cell necrosis. X100, Hematoxylin.

teoblasts, or related osteoblast-like cells on the bone surfaces, may also function as intermediates in modulating the activity of osteoclasts by transducing the effects of cytokines produced by activated macrophages.[70]

The resorption lacunae are frequently lined by multinucleated giant cells that morphologically resemble osteoclasts. Critical to the understanding of the mechanisms underlying the pathogenesis of peri-implant focal osteolysis is the definition of the relationship between the so-called foreign body giant cells that are associated with the particulate wear debris and the multinucleated cells that are presumably mediating the bone resorptive process. Current evidence would favor that the resorbing cells are indeed osteoclasts, and that they are recruited to the bone surface and induced to resorb the bone by factors (cytokines and other soluble mediators) released from the adjacent inflammatory tissues. It is of interest that cells with phenotypic features of osteoclasts are seen in greater numbers on the bone surfaces in individuals with aggressive osteolysis.[59]

Athanosou and Quinn[59] have investigated the relationship between macrophage polykaryons and osteoclasts in peri-implant tissues. These two multinucleated cell types, which are derived from a common lineage, exhibit a variety of distinct functional properties that distinguish them from each other.[71] Both cell types, however, have the capacity to directly resorb bone, although the osteoclast is considerably more effective. Several investigators have suggested that at least a component of the bone resorption associated with osteolysis may be mediated by cells other than osteoclasts, including particle-stimulated macrophages and foreign body giant cells.[72,73]

Other cell types identified within the membrane include mast cells and endothelial cells. Although mast cells are commonly seen, they are not present in large numbers.[74] These cells are seen in a variety of inflammatory conditions and could play a role in modulating the response to particulate debris, particularly in relationship to the processes of bone resorption.

In many cases, analysis of the tissue adjacent to loosened implants reveals an organized lining layer with features of a synovial-like lining. This layer contains large polygonal cells with nuclei polarized away from the cement or metal surfaces. Convoluted folds in this tissue resembling villous projections are often present. The synovial-like lining is most likely formed in response to the local forces (shear) at the membrane surface abutting the prosthetic components.

Wear Debris and Osteolysis: In Vitro Experiments

A number of investigators have used in vitro organ culture systems to gain insights into the mechanisms responsible for the enhanced bone resorption associated with osteolytic lesions.[20,75–77] These studies confirm that the membranes release abundant cytokines and other biologically active molecules that have the capacity to stimulate osteoclast-mediated bone resorption.

More recently, the techniques of in situ hybridization and immunohistochemistry have been used to examine directly the relationship between particulate wear debris and cell and tissue responses.[78] These analyses have shown that macrophages containing particulate debris express increased messenger RNA levels for a number of growth factors and cytokines that have potent effects on bone resorption and connective tissue remodeling. The techniques of immunohistochemistry have been used in parallel to confirm that the actual translated protein products of these genes are being synthesized and released by the particle-stimulated cells. These analyses have shown a correlation between zones of macrophage and debris accumulation and the production of interleukin-1, tumor necrosis factor, and interleukin 6 (Fig. 3.3). These cytokines have been implicated in osteoclast recruitment and activation in a variety of pathologic states of bone resorption.[79,80]

In situ hybridization techniques have provided preliminary insights into potential differential mechanisms

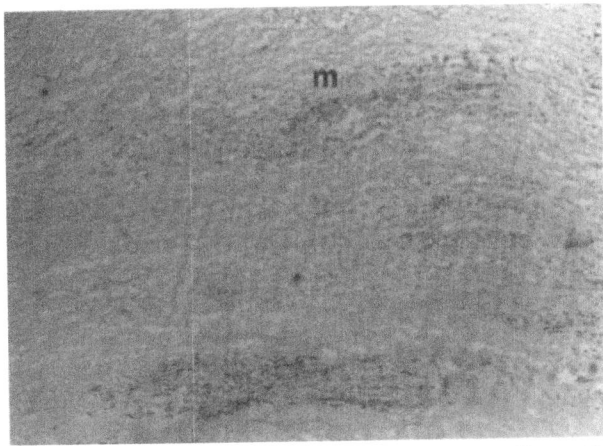

Figure 3A

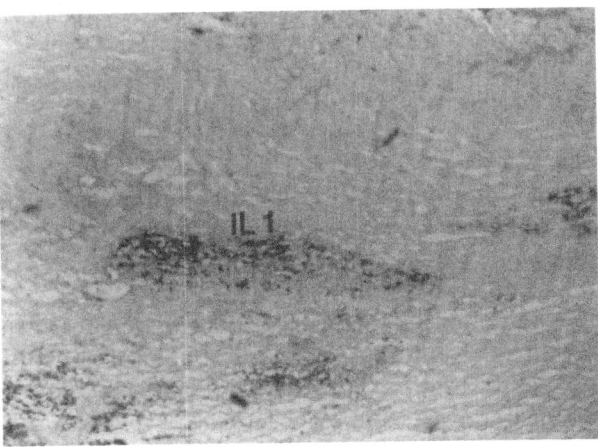

Figure 3B

Figure 3.3. (See color insert.) A. From a case of linear osteolysis, treated with MAC3 antibody showing collections of macrophages (*red staining*) contained within well organized fibrous tissue. X40, H&E. B. A serial section, treated with a probe specific for interleukin 1B messenger RNA (*purple color*), showing that IL1 is being produced by the macrophage populations.

involved in the pathogenesis of the pattern of slow linear osteolysis and more aggressive focal or expansile osteolysis (Fig. 3.4). Analysis of retrieved tissues reveals that interleukin-6 is preferentially expressed in regions of aggressive osteolysis, indicating a possible pivotal role for IL-6 in this condition.[81] Clearly, more studies are needed to dissect the factors that are responsible for these patterns of osteolysis. It is likely that the specific radiographic pattern and clinical course will reflect a complex interplay among biomechanical, biologic, and individual host factors.

The results of organ culture studies and tissue analyses described earlier provide strong evidence that particle-mediated cell stimulation plays a critical role in the biologic events associated with osteolysis. To test this hypothesis more rigorously, investigators have developed in vitro cell culture models that have permitted direct assessment of the effects of particulate implant wear debris on various target cell systems.[51] These studies have established that polymeric or metal particulate wear debris can stimulate macrophages or fibroblasts to release a variety of proinflammatory products with the capacity to induce osteolysis.[53–56,82]

Comparison of the effects of wear debris in these in vitro cell culture models reveals that the particles exhibit considerable differences in their capacity to modulate the activity of target cells.[51,83] These observations are consistent with the results of investigations involving other particulate materials that have demonstrated that particle size and shape, relative hydrophobicity or hydrophilicity, surface charge, and composition all influence the pattern and magnitude of the cellular and tissue response. Particle size is among the factors that appears to be of particular importance, with 10 μm being the apparent threshold for phagocytosis.[84] Particles larger than 10 μm are usually sequestered by fibroblasts and giant cells and appear to produce less of a mediator response. Goodman et al.[85–87] have shown a clear difference in the degree of response to bulk versus particulate forms of certain biomaterials. Other studies have looked at the effect of morphology and surface area of particles on the inflammatory response.[88,89]

An additional factor that affects the cell and tissue response to wear debris relates to the influence of particle load and the chronicity of the stimulus. In the case of failed implants, there is a sustained delivery of particulate wear debris to the peri-implant zones. Although the granulomatous response may initially sequester the wear debris in a fibrous capsule, the continued release of additional materials perpetuates the local inflammatory reaction and contributes to the expansion of the focal bone resorptive process. Interruption of this cycle by removal of the source of the wear debris would be expected to interrupt these events and attenuate the progressive osteolysis.

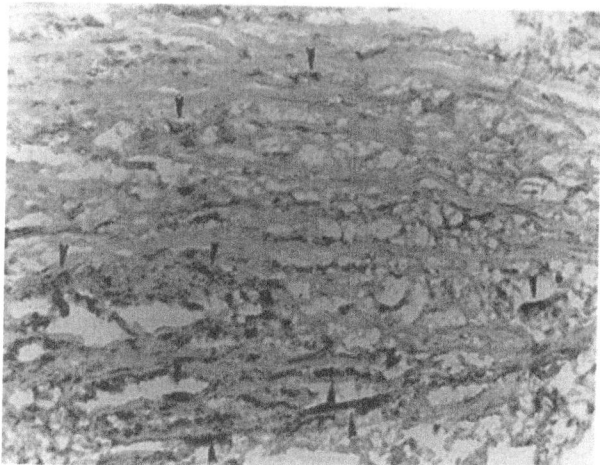

Figure 4A

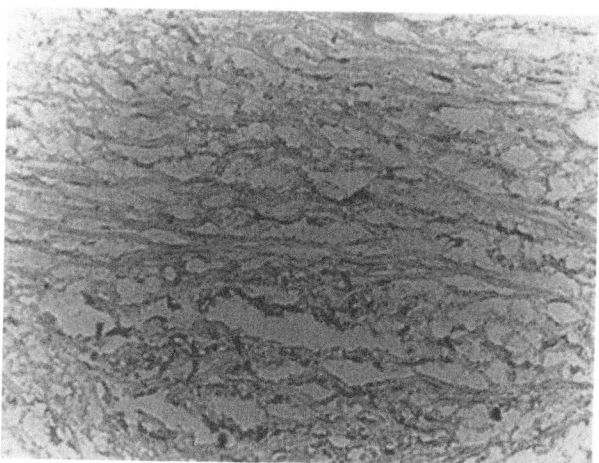

Figure 4B

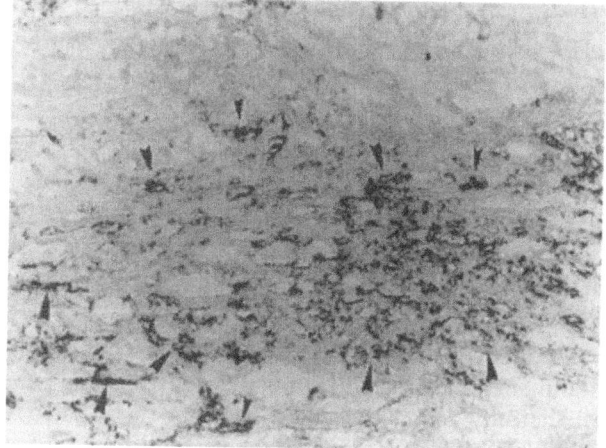

Figure 4C

Figure 3.4. (See color insert.) A. Specimen from linear osteolysis treated with antifibroblast antibody, demonstrating a preponderance of positive cells. (AEC chromagen, X100). B. Serial section from Figure 4A, hybridized with Interleukin 1B probe, showing limited localization to fibroblasts. (X100). C. Serial section from Figure 4A, hybridized with Interleukin 6 probe, showing large amount of localization to fibroblasts. (X100).

Table 3.2. Explanations for different patterns of peri-implant osteolysis.

Differences in physical-chemical wear debris properties (biomaterial factors)
Distinct patterns of particle distribution (biomechanical factors) related to
—implant design
—biomechanical loading pattern
Differences in host responses to implant wear debris (biologic factors)

Conclusion

Analysis of retrieved tissues from zones of osteolysis and correlation of the results with the distinct radiographic patterns of osteolysis have provided important insights into the pathogenesis of aseptic loosening. These events clearly represent an intimate interplay among biomechanical, biologic, and individual host factors. Fragmentation of the original implant components and generation of particulate wear debris appear to be critical initiating events in the formation of osteolysis associated with linear and aggressive expansile bone resorption, whereas stress-shielding represents an adaptation of peri-implant bone through cellular remodeling to the local mechanical environment. Particulate wear debris has the capacity to induce a granulomatous inflammatory reaction, and particle-mediated stimulation of macrophages and fibroblastic cells within the granuloma provides a rich source of proinflammatory products with the capacity to induce osteoclastic bone resorption. In addition, these activated inflammatory cells may themselves have the capacity to resorb the adjacent skeletal tissues. As summarized in Table 3.2, a better understanding of the specific cellular events associated with the host reaction to particulate wear debris, and insights into the interplay between biomechanical and biologic factors, should lead to more effective strategies for preventing osteolysis.

References

1. Willert BJ, Ludwig J, Semlitsch M. Reaction of bone to methylmethacrylate after hip arthroplasty. *J Bone Joint Surg Am.* 1974;56:1368–1382.
2. Charnley J. Fractures of femoral prostheses in total hip replacement: a clinical study. *Clin Orthop.* 1975;222:105–110.
3. Zicat B, Engh CA, Gokcen E. Patterns of osteolysis around total hip components inserted with and without cement. *J Bone Joint Surg Am.* 1995;77:432–439.
4. DeLee JG, Charnley J. Radiological demarcation of cemented sockets in total hip replacement. *Clin Orthop.* 1976;121:20–32.
5. Kwong LM, Jasty M, Mulroy RD, Maloney WJ, Bragdon C, Harris WH. The histology of the radiolucent line. *J Bone Joint Surg Br.* 1992;74:67–73.
6. Harris WH. The problem is osteolysis. *Clin Orthop.* 1995;311:46–53.
7. Maloney WJ, Jasty M, Rosenberg A, Harris WH. Bone lysis in well-fixed cemented femoral components. *J Bone Joint Surg Br.* 1990;72:966–970.
8. Maloney WJ, Jasty M, Harris WH, Galante JO, Callaghan JJ. Endosteal erosion in association with stable uncemented femoral components. *J Bone Joint Surg Am.* 1990;72:1025–1034.
9. Jasty MJ, Floyd WE, Schiller AL, Goldring SR, Harris WH. Localized osteolysis in stable, non-septic total hip replacement. *J Bone Joint Surg Am.* 1986;68:912–919.
10. Johnston RC, Crowninshield RD. Roentgenographic results of total hip arthroplasty: a ten year follow-up study. *Clin Orthop.* 1983;181:92–98.
11. Hodgkinson JP, Shelley P, Wroblewski BM. The correlation between the radiographic appearance and operative findings at the bone–cement junction of the socket in Charnley low friction arthroplasties. *Clin Orthop.* 1988;228:105–109.
12. Schmalzreid TP, Kwong LM, Jasty MJ, Sedlacek RC, Haire TC, O'Connor DO, et al. The mechanism of loosening of cemented acetabular components in total hip arthroplasty: analysis of specimens retrieved at autopsy. *Clin Orthop.* 1992;274:60–78.
13. Engh CA, Griffin WL, Marx CL. Cementless acetabular components. *J Bone Joint Surg Br.* 1990;72:53–59.
14. Rorabeck CH, Bourne RB, Mulliken BD, et al. The Nicholas Andry award: comparative results of cemented and cementless total hip arthroplasty. *Clin Orthop.* 1996;325:330–344.
15. Barrack RL, Mulroy RD Jr, Harris WH. Improved cementing techniques and femoral component loosening in young patients with hip arthroplasty: a 12 year radiographic review. *J Bone Joint Surg Br.* 1992;74:385–389.
16. Alsema R, Deutman R, Mulder TJ. Stanmore total hip replacement: a 15 to 16 year clinical and radiographic follow-up. *J Bone Joint Surg Br.* 1994;76:240–244.
17. Capello WN, Salley PI, Feinberg JR. Omniflex modular femoral component: two to five year results. *Clin Orthop.* 1994;298:54–59.
18. Cox CV, Dorr LD. Five year results of proximal bone ingrowth fixation total hip replacement. *Orthop Trans.* 1992;16:748–749.
19. Beauchesne RP, Kukita Y, Knezevich S, Suthers K, Kukita Y. Roentgenographic evaluation of the AML porous coated acetabular component: a six year minimum follow-up study. *Orthop Trans.* 1992;16:834.
20. Engh CA, Hooten JP Jr, Zettl-Schaffer KR, Ghaffarpour M, McGovern TF, Macalino GE, et al. Porous coated total hip replacement. *Clin Orthop.* 1994;298:89–99.
21. Bettin D, Greitmann B, Polster J, Schulte-Eistrup S. Long term results of uncemented Judet hip endoprostheses. *Int Orthop.* 1995;19:144–150.
22. Goldberg VM, Ninomiya J, Kelly G, Kraay M. Hybrid total hip arthroplasty: a 7 to 11 year follow-up. *Clin Orthop.* 1996;333:147–154.
23. Woolson ST, Haber DF. Primary total hip replacement with insertion of an acetabular component without cement and a femoral component with cement: follow-up study at an average of 6 years. *J Bone Joint Surg Am.* 1996;78:698–705.
24. Goetz D, Smith EJ, Harris WH. The prevalence of femoral osteolysis associated with components inserted with and

without cement in total hip replacements. *J Bone Joint Surg Am.* 1994;76:1121–1129.
25. Mulroy RD Jr, Harris WH. The effect of improved cementing techniques on component loosening in total hip replacement: an 11 year radiographic review. *J Bone Joint Surg Br.* 1990;72:757–760.
26. Maloney WJ, Jasty M, Rosenberg A, Harris WH. Bone lysis in well-fixed cemented femoral components. *J Bone Joint Surg Br.* 1990;72:966–970.
27. Kim YH, Kim VE. Uncemented porous coated anatomic total hip prosthesis: results at six years in a consecutive series. *J Bone Joint Surg Br.* 1993;75:6–13.
28. Heekin RD, Callaghan JJ, Hopkinson WJ, Savory CG, Xenos JS. The porous-coated anatomic total hip prosthesis, inserted without cement: results after five to seven years in a prospective study. *J Bone Joint Surg Am.* 1993;75:77–91.
29. Woolson ST, Maloney WJ. Cementless total hip arthroplasty using a porous-coated prosthesis for bone ingrowth fixation: three and one half year follow-up. *J Arthroplasty.* 1992;7:381–388.
30. Martel JM, Pierson R III, Jacobs JJ, Rosenberg AG, Maley M, Galante JO. Primary total hip reconstruction with a titanium-fiber coated prosthesis inserted without cement. *J Bone Joint Surg Am.* 1993;75:554–571.
31. Tanzer M, Maloney WJ, Jasty M, Harris WH. The progression of femoral cortical osteolysis in association with total hip arthroplasty without cement. *J Bone Joint Surg Am.* 1992;74:404–410.
32. Santavirta S, Konttinen YT, Bergroth V, Eskola A, Tallroth K, Lindholm TS. Aggressive granulomatous lesions associated with hip arthroplasty: immunopathological studies. *J Bone Joint Surg Am.* 1990;72:252–258.
33. Charnley J. Tissue reactions to polytetrafluoroethylene. *Lancet.* 1963;1379.
34. Charnley J. The long term results of low-friction arthroplasty of the hip performed as a primary intervention. *J Bone Joint Surg Br.* 1972;54:61–76.
35. Charnley J, Cupic Z. The nine and ten year results of the low-friction arthroplasty of the hip. *Clin Orthop.* 1973;95:9–17.
36. Webb PJ, Wrught KWJ, Winter GD. The Monk "soft top" endoprosthesis: clinical, biomechanical, and histopathological observations. *J Bone Joint Surg Br.* 1980;62:174–177.
37. Willert HG, Bertram H, Buchhorn GH. Osteolysis in alloarthroplasty of the hip: the role of ultra-high molecular weight polyethylene wear particles. *Clin Orthop.* 1990;258:95–107.
38. Buechel F, Drucker D, Jasty M, Jiranek W, Harris WH. Osteolysis around uncemented acetabular components of cobalt-chrome surface replacement hip arthroplasty. *Clin Orthop.* 1994;298:202–211.
39. Lombardi AV, Mallory TM, Vaughn BK, Drouillard P. Aseptic loosening in total hip arthroplasty secondary to osteolysis induced by wear debris from titanium-alloy modular femoral heads. *J Bone Joint Surg Am.* 1988;71:1337–1342.
40. Buly RL, Huo MH, Salvati E, Brien W, Bansal M. Titanium wear debris in failed cemented total hip arthroplasty: an analysis of 71 cases. *J Arthroplasty.* 1992;7:315–323.
41. Schmalzreid TP, Jasty MJ, Harris WH. Periprosthetic bone loss in total hip arthroplasty: polyethylene wear debris and the concept of the effective joint space. *J Bone Joint Surg Am.* 1992;74:849–863.
42. Willert HG, Bertram H, Buchorn GH. Osteolysis in alloarthroplasty of the hip: the role of bone cement fragmentation. *Clin Orthop.* 1990;258:95–107.
43. Jasty M, Maloney WJ, Bragdon CR, Haire T, Harris WH. Histomorphological studies of the long term skeletal responses to well fixed cemented femoral components. *J Bone Joint Surg Am.* 1990;72:1220–1228.
44. Anthony PP, Gie GA, Howie CR, Ling RSM. Localised endosteal bone lysis in relation to the femoral components of cemented total hip arthroplasties. *J Bone Joint Surg Br.* 1990;72:971–979.
45. Willert HG, Semlitsch M. Reactions of the articular capsule to wear products of artificial joint prostheses. *J Biomed Mater Res.* 1977;11:157–164.
46. Harris W, Schiller AL, Scholler J-M, Freiberg RA, Scott R. Extensive localized bone resorption in the femur following total hip replacement. *J Bone Joint Surg Am.* 1976;58:612–618.
47. Maguire JK Jr, Coscia MF, Lynch MH. Foreign body reaction to polymeric debris following total hip arthroplasty. *Clin Orthop.* 1987;216:213–223.
48. Johanson NA, Bullough PG, Wilson PD, Salvati EA, Ranawat CS. The microscopic anatomy of the bone-cement interface in failed total hip arthroplasties. *Clin Orthop.* 1987;218:123–135.
49. Radin EL, Rubin CT, Thrasher EL, et al. Changes in the bone-cement interface after total hip arthroplasty. *J Bone Joint Surg Am.* 1982;64:1188–1200.
50. Goldring SR, Schiller AL, Roelke M, Rourke CM, O'Neil DA, Harris WH. The synovial-like membrane at the bone-cement interface in loose total hip replacements and its proposed role in bone lysis. *J Bone Joint Surg Am.* 1983;65:575–584.
51. Wang JT, Goldring SR. Biological mechanisms involved in the pathogenesis of aseptic loosening after total joint replacement. *Semin Arthroplasty.* 1993;4:215–222.
52. Jiranek WA, Machado M, Jasty M, Jevsevar D, Wolfe HJ, Goldring SR, et al. Production of cytokines around loosened cemented acetabular components: analysis with immunohistochemical techniques and in situ hybridization. *J Bone Joint Surg Am.* 1993;75:863–879.
53. Haynes DR, Rogers SD, Hay S, Pearcy M, Howie DW. The differences in toxicity and release of bone-resorbing mediators induced by titanium and cobalt-chromium-alloy wear particles. *J Bone Joint Surg Am.* 1993;75:825–834.
54. Horowitz SM, Doty SB, Lane JM, Burstein AH. Studies of the mechanism by which the mechanical failure of polymethylmethacrylate leads to bone resorption. *J Bone Joint Surg Am.* 1993;75:802–815.
55. Wang JT, Willis A, Jiranek B, Merritt K, Brown SA, Goldring SR. Metal particles of orthopaedic implant materials and their corrosion products stimulate release of PGE2 and interleukin 6, products implicated in pathological bone resorption. *Orthop Trans.* 1993;18:86.
56. Maloney WJ, Smith RL, Castro F, Schurman DJ. Fibroblast response to metallic debris in vitro: enzyme induction, cell proliferation, and toxicity. *J Bone Joint Surg Am.* 1993;75:835–844.

57. Goldring SR, Flannery MS, Petrison KK, Evins AE, Jasty MJ. Evaluation of connective tissue cell responses to orthopaedic implant materials. *Connect Tissue Res.* 1990;24:77–81.
58. Goldring SR, Bennett NE, Jasty MJ, Wang JT. In vitro activation of monocyte macrophages and fibroblasts by metal particles. In: St John KR, ed. *Particulate Debris from Medical Implants: Mechanisms of Formation and Biological Consequences.* Philadelphia, Pa: American Society for Materials Testing; 1992:136–142. ASTM STP 1144.
59. Athanasou NA, Quinn J. Immunophenotypic differences between osteoclasts and macrophage polykaryons: immunohistological distinction and implications for osteoclast ontogeny and function. *J Clin Pathol.* 1990;43:997–1003.
60. Jasty M, Bragdon CS, Jiranek WA, Chandler H, Maloney W, Harris WH. Etiology of osteolysis around porous coated cementless total hip arthroplasties. *Clin Orthop.* 1994;308:111–126.
61. Lalor PA, Revell PA, Gray AB, Wright S, Railton GT, Freeman MA. Sensitivity to titanium: a cause of implant failure? *J Bone Joint Surg Br.* 1991;73:25–28.
62. Jiranek WA, Jasty M, Wang JT, Bragdon C, Wolfe H, Goldberg M, et al. Tissue response to particulate polymethylmethacrylate in mice with various immune deficiencies. *J Bone Joint Surg Am.* 1995;77:1650–1661.
63. Goodman S, Wang JS, Regula D, Aspenberg P. T lymphocytes are not necessary for particulate polyethylene-induced macrophage recruitment. *Acta Orthop Scand.* 1994;65:157–160.
64. Gil-Albarova J, Lacleriga A, Barrios C, Canadell J. Lymphocyte response to polymethylmethacrylate in loose total hip prostheses. *J Bone Joint Surg Br.* 1992;74:825–830.
65. Goldring SR, Wojno WC, Schiller AL, et al. In patients with rheumatoid arthritis the tissue reaction associated with loosened total knee replacements exhibits features of a rheumatoid synovium. *J Orthop Rheum.* 1988;1:9–21.
66. Caplan A. Certain unusual radiological appearances in the chest of coal-miners suffering from rheumatoid arthritis. *Thorax.* 1953;8:29–35.
67. Tashjian AH, Hohman EL, Antoniades HN, Levine L. Platelet-derived growth factor stimulates bone resorption via a prostaglandin-mediated mechanism. *Endocrinology.* 1982;3:118–122.
68. Gilardetti RS, Chaibi MS, Strouinga J, et al. High affinity binding of PDGF-AA and PDGF-BB to normal human osteoblastic cells and modulation by interleukin 1. *Am J Physiol.* 1991;261:980–985.
69. Canalis E. Interleukin-1 has independent effects on deoxyribonucleic acid and collagen synthesis in cultures of rat calvariae. *Endocrinology.* 1986;118:74–81.
70. Thomson BM, Saklatvala J, Chambers TJ. Osteoblasts mediate interleukin 1 responsiveness of bone resorption by rat osteoclasts. *J Exp Med.* 1986;104:104–112.
71. Suda T, Takahashi N, Martin TJ. Modulation of osteoclast differentiation. *Endocr Rev.* 1992;13:66–80.
72. Quinn J, Joyner C, Triffit JT, Athanasou NA. Polymethylmethacrylate-induced inflammatory macrophages resorb bone. *J Bone Joint Surg Br.* 1992;74:652–658.
73. Murray DW, Rushton N. Macrophages stimulate bone resorption when they phagocytose particles. *J Bone Joint Surg Br.* 1990;72:988–992.
74. Solovieva SA, Ceponis A, Konttinen YT, Takagi M, Suda A, Eklund KK, et al. Mast cells in loosening of totally replaced hips. *Clin Orthop.* 1996;322:158–165.
75. Chiba J, Rubash HE, Kim KJ, Iwaki Y. The characterization of cytokines in the interface tissue obtained from failed cementless total hip arthoplasty with and without femoral osteolysis. *Clin Orthop.* 1994;300:304–312.
76. Kim KJ, Rubash HE, Wilson SC, D'Antonio JA, McClain EJ. A histologic and biochemical comparison of the interface tissues in cementless and cemented hip prostheses. *Clin Orthop.* 1993;287:142–151.
77. Goldring SR, Jasty M, Roelke MS, Rourke CM, Bringhurst FR, Harris WH. Formation of a synovial-like membrane at the bone–cement interface: its role in bone resorption and implant loosening after total hip replacement. *Arthritis Rheum.* 1986;29:836–842.
78. Konttinen YT, Xu J-W, Patiala H, Imai S, Waris V, Li T-F, et al. Cytokines in aseptic loosening of total hip replacement. *Curr Orthop.* 1997;40–47.
79. Goldring MB, Goldring SR. Skeletal tissue response to cytokines. *Clin Orthop.* 1990;258:245–278.
80. Goldring SR, Goldring MB. Cytokines and skeletal physiology. *Clin Orthop.* 1996;324:13–23.
81. Jiranek WA, Qiu JY, Yin C, Cardea JA. Differential cell populations and cytokine production by the different layers of the interface membrane around failing total joint arthroplasties. *Trans Orthop Res Soc.* 1996;21:21.
82. Herman JH, Sowder WG, Anderson D, Appel AM, Hopson CN. Polymethylmethacrylate-induced release of bone-resorbing factors. *J Bone Joint Surg Am.* 1989;71:1530–1541.
83. Shanbag AS, Jacobs JJ, Black J, Galante JO, Glant TT. Macrophage/particle interactions: effect of size, composition, and surface area. *J Biomed Mater Res.* 1994;2:81–90.
84. Pratten MK. Pinocytosis and phagocytosis: the effect of size of a particulate substrate on its mode of capture by rat peritoneal macrophages cultured in vitro. *Biochem Biophys Acta.* 1986;881:307–313.
85. Goodman SB, Fornasier VL, Kei J. The effects of bulk versus particulate polymethylmethacrylate on bone. *Clin Orthop.* 1988;232:255–262.
86. Goodman SB, Fornasier VL, Lee J, Kei J. The effects of bulk versus particulate titanium and chrome cobalt alloy implanted into the rabbit tibia. *J Biomed Mater Res.* 1990;24:1539–1549.
87. Goodman SB, Fornasier VL, Lee J, Kei J. The histological effects of the implantation of different sizes of polyethylene particles in the rabbit tibia. *J Biomed Mater Res.* 1990;24:517–524.
88. Gelb H, Schumacher HR, Cuckler J. In vivo inflammatory response to polymethylmethacrylate particulate debris: effect of size, morphology, and surface area. *J Orthop Res.* 1994;12:83–92.
89. Shanbhag AS, Jacobs JJ, Black J, Galante JO, Glant TT. Macrophage/particle interactions: effect of size, composition, and surface area. *J Biomed Mater Res.* 1994;28:81–90.

4
Dislocation Following Total Hip Arthroplasty

Douglas A. Dennis

Dislocation after total hip arthroplasty (THA) is a relatively infrequent, yet frustrating, complication of this operative procedure. After aseptic loosening, it is the second most common major complication of THA.[1-3] The reported incidence of postoperative dislocation varies widely from less than 1% to nearly 10%,[1,4,5] with most studies of primary THA reporting an incidence of 2% to 5%.[6-14] The incidence of dislocation following revision THA is substantially greater, with a rate as high as 26.6% (12 of 45) after multiple procedures.[15] This chapter reviews the mechanisms, timing, risk factors, and management of this complication.

Mechanisms

Postoperative dislocation in THA may occur in a posterior, anterior, or superior direction. Although the majority of dislocations occur posteriorly, the type of surgical approach directly influences the direction of dislocation. In a review of 10 500 THA, Woo and Morrey[3] observed that after a posterior surgical approach, 77% of dislocations occurred posteriorly; 20%, superiorly; and 3%, anteriorly. When an anterior approach was used, 46% of dislocations occurred anteriorly; 46%, posteriorly; and 8%, superiorly.

Posterior dislocations result from lower extremity positioning in excessive flexion, adduction, and internal rotation. This most commonly occurs when a patient transfers to or from a low sitting position or bends over. Limb placement in extension, adduction, and external rotation risks anterior dislocation.[1] Superior dislocation may result from excessive adduction, especially when associated with vertical acetabular component positioning.

Timing of Dislocation

The majority of initial dislocations occur early, with approximately 60% to 70% reported within the first 4 to 6 weeks following the operative procedure.[8,11,16] Patients suffering an initial dislocation after this early period are at greater risk of experiencing recurrent dislocation. The risk of recurrent dislocation is highly variable, with two large series showing an incidence of approximately 33%.[3,9]

Khan et al.[8] analyzed 142 patients with a dislocated THA who were part of a multicenter study of 6774 THA (2.1%). In 94 (66.2%) of these patients, the first dislocation occurred within the first 5 weeks postoperatively. Recurrent dislocation was experienced by 37 (39.3%) of these patients. In the remaining 48 patients, the initial dislocation occurred after the first 5 weeks postoperatively and in 28 (58.3%) of these cases, recurrence of dislocation was observed.

Lindberg et al.,[11] in a review of 1739 primary THAs, observed dislocation in 56 cases (3.3%). The initial dislocation occurred within the first postoperative month in 41 patients (73.2%) with 9 of these patients (21.9%) experiencing recurrent dislocation. In the remaining 15 patients in which the initial dislocation occurred beyond the first postoperative month, recurrence of dislocation was observed in 6 cases (40%).

Late dislocations, while uncommon, can occur. Coventry[7] analyzed the cases of 32 patients who dislocated for the first time between 5 and 10 years postoperatively. He compared this patient group with a control group of patients who had not dislocated postoperatively, and with a group who had experienced a dislocated THA earlier than 5 years after the primary operative procedure. He detected increased range of motion (especially flexion) and higher radiographic acetabular component loosening in patients encountering late dislocation. It was postulated that stretching of the hip pseudocapsule over time and extremes of motion may lessen soft tissue constraints and allow for late dislocation. The necessity of additional corrective surgery in this series was substantial with 44% of those suffering an initial late dislocation requiring additional operative procedures. Lachiewicz and Paterno[13] attributed late dislocation to extreme loss of body weight resulting in reduction of muscle mass and soft tissue laxity. Daly and Morrey[17] theorized that polyethylene wear and cold flow from prolonged use may allow increased range of motion and stretching of the hip pseudocapsule over time, enhancing the probability of late dislocation.

Risk Factors

Myriad risk factors for postoperative dislocation after THA have been reported. Woo and Morrey[3] have best classified these into preoperative, perioperative, and postoperative categories (Table 4.1).

Preoperative Factors

Numerous investigators have documented that one of the most predominant preoperative risk factors for dislocation is previous hip surgery.[1,3,4,8,11,12,18–21] In a review of 10 500 THA, Woo and Morrey[3] found a twofold increase in dislocation in those patients with previous hip surgery (158 of 3259, or 4.8%) compared with those who had not had previous hip surgery (173 of 7241, or 2.4%) ($p < 0.001$). Fackler and Poss[12] reported a 1.8% (22 of 1224) dislocation rate after primary THA versus a 5.5% (12 of 219) rate after revision THA. Patients who have undergone previous operations for femoral neck fracture or hip osteotomy were found by Lindberg et al.[11] to be at higher risk for dislocation.

Dislocation occurs more commonly in women in most series with a female-to-male ratio of approximately 2:1.[1,3,8,11,22] Even a greater female predominance (3:1, 24 of 32) was observed by Coventry[7] in his analysis of late dislocations. Various investigators have noted higher rates of dislocation in patients afflicted with mental health disorders,[8,12,23] neuromuscular disease,[8,11,12] or alcoholism.[11,12,24] Advanced age has been noted to be a risk factor for dislocation in some series.[13,25–26] Ekelund et al.[25] reported a dislocation rate of 9.2% in a group of 157 consecutive patients 80 years of age or older, whereas Newington et al.[26] noted 15.2% of patients (17 of 112) older than 80 years at the time of primary THA suffered a postoperative dislocation. The increased incidence of dislocation in octogenarians may be related in part to the fact that a higher percentage of patients in this age group require THA because of acute intracapsular hip fracture, which has been associated with a higher incidence of postoperative dislocation.[3] Lachiewicz and Paterno[13] postulated the reason for this association may be related to diminished proprioception, mental acuity, or muscle mass with increasing age.

Perioperative Factors

Intraoperative patient positioning can affect the incidence of dislocation by enhancing the probability of acetabular component malposition.[2,3,27–28] McCollum and Gray[2] performed a roentgenographic study comparing pelvic orientation of subjects in the standing, upright position versus the lateral decubitus position. A series of standing preoperative lateral roentgenograms was compared with intraoperative lateral roentgenograms obtained with the patient laterally positioned on the operating table. They found that the normal lumbar lordosis decreased from the standing position by as much as 20° to 35° with the patient in the lateral decubitus position, resulting in flexion of the pelvis by a similar amount. Therefore, if the acetabular component is oriented in 15° to 20° of forward flexion (anteversion) relative to the longitudinal axis of the body with the patient laterally positioned, when the patient stands and the normal lumbar lordosis is regained (pelvis extends) the acetabular component may be malpositioned in 10° to 15° of retroversion, an unstable orientation for THA. A series of anteroposterior pelvic roentgenograms was also obtained with patients laterally placed on the operating table. They found that the superior acetabulum was consistently adducted 10° to 15° toward the foot. If this change in pelvic orientation is not recognized and the acetabular component is positioned in 45° of horizontal abduction relative to the operating table, when the patient stands the acetabular component assumes an orientation of 55° to 60° of abduction, risking disloca-

Table 4.1. Reported risk factors in patients with dislocation after total hip arthroplasty.[3]

Preoperative	Perioperative	Postoperative
Previous hip surgery	Intraoperative patient positioning	Patient noncompliance
Gender (female)	Surgical approach	Incorrect limb positioning
Mental health disorders	Capsulectomy	Trochanteric nonunion/migration
Neuromuscular disorders	Component malposition	Retained foreign debris
Alcohol abuse	Decreased prosthetic offset	Entrapped soft tissues
Older age (octogenarians)	Decreased soft tissue tension	
	Femoral head–neck ratio	
	Retained periacetabular osteophytes/cementophytes	

tion. Finally, forward (anterior) tilting of the pelvis with the patient laterally positioned is not uncommon, and it may result in placement of the acetabular component in less anteversion than desired.[3]

Whereas some investigators have found no differences in the incidence of dislocation among the various surgical approaches,[8] most studies suggest a higher risk of dislocation with use of the posterolateral approach.[2,3,14,29] Robinson et al.[14] compared a consecutive series of THA performed through a lateral transtrochanteric approach with a closely matched group accomplished through a posterior approach. An alarming dislocation rate of 7.5% (12 of 160) was observed with the posterior approach, while no dislocations (0 of 156) were encountered when a lateral transtrochanteric approach was used. In their review of 3353 THA, Woo and Morrey[3] reported an incidence of dislocation of 2.3% (18 of 770) with use of an anterior approach; 3.1% (59 of 1898) with a lateral transtrochanteric approach; and 5.8% (40 of 685) with a posterior approach.

Charnley et al.[2,12,13,23,30–32] believe restoration of tissue tension is a critical factor in preventing dislocation after THA. Charnley routinely performed a transtrochanteric approach and advanced the greater trochanter 1 cm distally to increase abductor muscle tension. This concept is supported by a review of the literature, which demonstrates many of the lowest rates of dislocation have been reported in studies in which a lateral transtrochanteric approach was used.[4,30–32] In addition, Fackler and Poss[12] observed dislocation in 1.0% of 394 patients in whom THA was performed by using a lateral transtrochanteric approach versus 2.4% of 543 patients who did not have a transtrochanteric approach.

Duplication of anatomic soft tissue tension requires restoration of both vertical and horizontal soft tissue length.[23] Vertical length is determined by the level of femoral neck resection, length of the prosthetic neck selected, and position of the acetabular component in the vertical plane. The clinical importance of restoration of vertical length is controversial.[3,7,9,12,19,32] Woo and Morrey[3] found that patients with unstable THA actually had operative limb lengths that measured 1.6 mm longer than the nonoperative control lower extremity. Fackler and Poss[12] found no statistical correlation between postoperative limb length and the incidence of dislocation. In contrast, Carlsson and Gentz[19] reported a statistical correlation ($p < 0.05$) between the proximally placed acetabular component and dislocation. Similarly, Etienne et al.[32] observed a dislocation rate of 1.2% with proximal acetabular component placement, compared with 0.6% in patients in whom the acetabular component was accurately positioned.

Horizontal length is determined by the level of femoral neck resection and the geometry of the femoral component selected. Horizontal length (offset) may be increased by a more distal femoral neck resection and use of a femoral component with increased neck length. Conversely, offset can be reduced by resecting the femoral neck more proximally and use of a femoral component with a shorter neck length. This latter choice risks earlier impingement and dislocation by allowing the femur to be positioned closer to the pelvis. Certain prosthetic systems offer femoral components with multiple neck offsets for further adjustment of horizontal soft tissue tension. Fackler and Poss[12] reported a statistically higher incidence of dislocation when offset was reduced after THA ($p < 0.025$).

Component malposition has long been recognized as a critical risk factor in the dislocation of THA.[1,3,4,5,9,12,19,32] The position of the normal acetabulum has been reported to be 60° of abduction and 40° of anteversion,[33] which is considerably more abduction and anteversion than is recommended by most hip arthroplasty surgeons.[2,27–28] The normal hip is stable with this acetabular position because the femoral head is larger than the prosthetic femoral head and the supporting capsule and ligamentum teres have not been disrupted.[2] In an intraoperative, biomechanical study, McCollum and Gray[2] reported the most stable position of the acetabular component that would allow physiologic range of motion without impingement was 30° to 50° of abduction and 20° to 40° of anteversion. In another study, Lewinnek et al.[10] determined the safe zone of acetabular component position was 40° ± 10° of abduction and 15° ± 10° of anteversion. They reported a statistically lower incidence of dislocation (1.5%) when the acetabular component was positioned within the safe zone, compared with a 6% dislocation rate when the acetabular component was oriented outside this range ($p < 0.05$). Fackler and Poss[12] noted that 44% of their 34 patients suffering dislocation had malposition of one or both components versus only 6% of a control group who did not experience a dislocation.

Evaluation of component malposition requires determination of the acetabular component abduction angle, version of the acetabular component, and version of the femoral component. The abduction angle is measured on the anteroposterior roentgenogram as the angle formed by a line tangential to the face of the acetabular component and a line drawn tangential to the inferior margins of the ischial tuberosities.[3] Numerous methods, including direct measurement and mathematical calculations, have been developed to determine version of the acetabular component.[23,34–36] Although many investigators have observed error in determination of version of the acetabular component from a lateral cross-table roentgenogram,[3,12,34,35,37] this method remains in common use as a simple approximation of acetabular component version. The acetabular component version is measured as the angle formed by a line drawn tangential to the face of the acetabular component and a line perpendicular to the horizontal plane (Fig. 4.1). Femoral component version is difficult to mea-

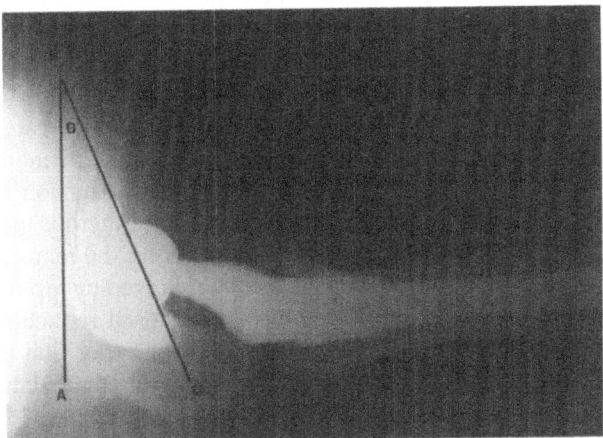

Figure 4.1. Lateral cross-table roentgenogram demonstrating measurement method to approximate acetabular component anteversion. Estimated acetabular anteversion is measured as the angle θ formed by a line drawn tangential to the face of the acetabular component (BC) and a line drawn perpendicular to the horizontal plane (AB).

sure on plain roentgenograms[1,3] and is best determined by using fluoroscopy,[12] computed tomography,[22] or mathematical calculations.[38] Rotational orientation of the femoral component appears less critical than acetabular component placement because femoral head coverage by the acetabular component changes only minimally with internal or external rotation of the femoral component except at the extremes of femoral component rotational malalignment.[2]

Prosthetic design features can play a role in the incidence of dislocation. As discussed previously, prosthetic designs that fail to restore horizontal soft tissue length (offset) are at greater risk for dislocation.[12] Amstutz et al.[39,40] have evaluated how the ratio of femoral head diameter to femoral neck diameter affects hip stability. Using a three dimensional protractor, they assessed the maximum in vitro range of motion of various femoral component designs before femoral neck–socket rim contact occurred. With the acetabular component positioned at 42° of abduction and 20° of anteversion, they observed femoral neck–socket rim impingement occurred at 80° of flexion with the Charnley femoral component (head-to-neck ratio of 1.74:1), compared with 114° of flexion with the Trapezoidal-28™ prosthesis (head-to-neck ratio of 1.97–2.97:1). Similar increases in rotation and abduction were recorded with prosthetic designs with higher head-to-neck ratios. These researchers proposed that femoral components with increased head-to-neck ratios should allow greater range of motion before neck–socket impingement occurs, lessening the chance of dislocation. Although logical in theory, numerous clinical studies[1,3,8,12,17,20] have failed to find a statistical correlation between femoral head size and prosthetic stability. In addition, a study with the use of femoral endoprostheses with normal femoral head diameter reported an incidence of hip instability of just over 2%, comparable to many analyses of THA in which femoral components with smaller femoral head diameters were used.[41]

Modular elevated-rim acetabular liners have been used commonly over the past decade with the purpose of improving hip stability by providing additional support in regions of compromised hip stability.[42,43] They provide the surgeon with the opportunity to place the augmented rim in a position that maximizes hip stability in each individual case. Cobb et al.[42] reviewed results of 5167 THA that included 2469 acetabular components with a 10° elevated-rim liner and 2698 cases in which a standard nonelevated liner was used. At 2 years postoperatively, dislocation occurred in 2.19% (48 of 2469) of hips with an elevated-rim liner versus 3.7% (101 of 2698) of those in which a standard liner was selected ($p = 0.001$). The advantage of elevated-rim liner use was greatest in cases of revision THA in which dislocation occurred in 4.4% (23 of 520) of hips with elevated-rim liners, compared with 9.6% (51 or 530) of hips with standard liners ($p = 0.005$). This contrasts with an incidence of dislocation of 1.3% (25 of 1949) of primary THA implanted with elevated-rim liners, compared with 2.35% (50 of 2168) with standard liners ($p = 0.04$). One must be aware of the potential of premature polyethylene wear and component loosening with the use of elevated-rim liners because of earlier neck–socket impingement.[42] In addition, the risk of anterior dislocation may be enhanced by premature impingement of the femoral neck on a posteriorly placed elevated rim, particularly if a skirted femoral head is used.[27] Similarly, femoral neck impingement on retained peripheral osteophytes has been reported to result in dislocation.[18,39,44]

The size and geometry of the proximal femoral neck have also been shown to affect hip range of motion before neck–socket impingement occurs. Krushell et al.[45] performed a prosthetic range of motion analysis of both modular and nonmodular femoral components by using an in vitro motion-testing apparatus. They observed reduced range of motion before neck-socket impingement occurred in modular versus nonmodular femoral components, theoretically increasing the risk of dislocation in these designs. They attributed the earlier impingement seen with modular designs to the larger cross-sectional diameter of their femoral necks, which typically have a round geometric shape as compared with many nonmodular femoral components in which the neck geometry is flattened (thinner) on the anterior and posterior surfaces. Anteroposterior neck diameter has the most substantial impact on the range of motion observed. The use of longer neck lengths with extended skirts resulted in dramatically reduced range of motion before impingement, secondary to the increased femoral neck diameter attributable to the extended skirt. Therefore, one must use femoral heads with extended skirts with caution to minimize the change of dislocation caused by neck–socket impingement.

Finally, retention and reconstruction of the capsule and supporting musculature may reduce the incidence of dislocation.[14,30,46,47] Robinson et al.[14] found a 7.5% incidence of hip dislocation with the use of posterior approach without attempted repair of either the posterior capsule or external rotator musculature. This resulted in a modification in their surgical technique to repair the capsule and external rotators. With reconstruction of these soft tissue structures, they incurred a dislocation rate of less than 1% in more than 1000 subsequent primary THA procedures.

Postoperative Factors

Noncompliance with postoperative instructions regarding limb positioning to maintain hip stability is probably the most frequent cause of early postoperative dislocation after THA.[13] Preoperative and continued postoperative education emphasizing the need to avoid lower limb positioning in excessive flexion, adduction, and internal rotation (posterior dislocation) or placement of the extended limb in marked external rotation (anterior dislocation) is imperative to minimize dislocation after THA.

Trochanteric nonunion after transtrochanteric surgical approach, especially if associated with proximal migration of the trochanteric fragment, has been observed by numerous investigators to increase the risk of postoperative dislocation.[1,3,22,27,28,30] Woo and Morrey[3] reported an incidence of dislocation of 2.8% (245 of 8750) in THA performed through a transtrochanteric approach in which an osseous or stable fibrous union of the greater trochanteric fragment was obtained. This contrasts with a 17.6% (34 of 194) rate of dislocation in THA with trochanteric nonunion and proximal migration of the osteotomized greater trochanter ($p < 0.0001$).

Entrapment of either soft tissue or foreign debris postoperatively may result in dislocation or prevent concentric reduction should dislocation occur.[48–52] Grigoris et al.[48] reported dislocation secondary to entrapment of the iliopsoas tendon posterior to the femoral neck, resulting in anterior dislocation. Others have found entrapment of interposed hip capsule, preventing concentric reduction after dislocation.[49] Entrapment of foreign materials, including suction drains,[50] fragmented trochanteric fixation wires,[51,52] and loose polymethylmethacrylate,[52] has been similarly noted.

Dislocation Management

Nonoperative Care

The best management of any medical complication is prevention. Dislocation of THA can be minimized by extensive preoperative and postoperative education to instruct patients on the mechanisms of dislocation and the importance of avoiding high-risk limb positions likely to cause dislocation (see Mechanism section).[1]

Should dislocation occur, the majority can be treated with closed reduction, usually facilitated by intravenous sedation or general anesthetic measures. Reduction of dislocated THA can be accomplished by numerous maneuvers, all of which use traction to bring the femoral head to the level of the acetabulum, followed by hip rotation.[23] Failure to achieve successful closed reduction can occur and is usually attributed to interposition of material, such as fragments of polymethylmethacrylate, broken wire, retained suction drains or soft tissues.[48–52]

After reduction, re-education of the patient on instructions to avoid recurrent dislocation is imperative. Additional external devices, such as knee immobilization splints, hip abduction braces, or hip spica casts, can be helpful to prevent patients from maneuvering the operative limb into a position in which dislocation may recur. Use of knee immobilization splints limits posterior dislocation by restricting hip flexion. These devices are of greatest value in obese patients who often tolerate hip braces or casting poorly.[53] The use of hip braces or casts has been reported by many[16,54–55] to reduce the incidence of recurrent dislocation. Clayton and Thirupathi[54] reported no recurrence of dislocation in 9 of 10 patients (90%) treated by hip abduction bracing after multiple dislocations. Mallory et al.[55] achieved hip stabilization in 92% of cases managed with a similar appliance. Williams et al.,[16] using a hip spica cast, were successful in preventing recurrent dislocation in 94% of patients.

The overall success of nonoperative management of dislocating THA varies among reported series, with 32% to 44% eventually requiring operative treatment.[3,7,20]

Operative Care

Approximately 1 of every 100 patients undergoing THA will require revision surgery for hip instability.[1] Operative treatment is considered when concentric reduction cannot be obtained by closed methods or in cases of recurrent episodes of dislocation despite extended periods of external bracing. Multiple operative procedures have been attempted (Table 4.2). The choice of operative method is based on the etiology of the dislocation and can be categorized on the basis of adequacy of component orientation.

In the author's experience, revision of the femoral component for rotational malalignment is infrequently required because acetabular component coverage of the femoral head changes only minimally with internal or external rotation of the femoral component except at the extremes of femoral component malrotation.[2] Because the preponderance of dislocations occur posteriorly, reorientation of the acetabular component often corrects the hip

Table 4.2. Operative options for recurrent hip instability.

> Component revision
> Extended lip liner
> Acetabular augmentation
> Trochanteric reattachment/advancement
> Constrained acetabular component
> Bipolar acetabular component
> Femoral head exchange
> Impingement correction

instability, particularly if the acetabular component is retroverted. Daly and Morrey,[17] in their review of 95 patients who experienced reoperation for chronic instability after THA, observed that correction of retroversion by acetabular component revision was the procedure most likely to produce a stable hip. Alternatively, insertion of a modular elevated-rim acetabular liner can reorient the peripheral boundaries of the acetabular component, providing additional support in regions of compromised hip stability,[4,42,43] although clear scientific data documenting the efficacy of this treatment method in recurrent dislocation cases is lacking. Also, the long-term durability of the unsupported polyethylene provided by the elevated rim is not yet known.

Others have attempted to gain hip stability by acetabular component augmentation.[56,57] In this technique, an additional section of a second polyethylene acetabular component is secured with screws to the previously implanted acetabular component. The augmentation section is positioned in the area in which dislocation is occurring. Bradbury and Milligan[57] reported on 16 patients managed with acetabular component augmentation. At an average follow-up period of 3 years, 14 patients (87.5%) had experienced no further dislocations, and there was no evidence of component loosening.

In cases in which soft tissue tension is believed to be inadequate, especially if component placement is satisfactory, distal advancement of the greater trochanter is to be considered to increase abductor muscle tension and function.[58,59] Kaplan et al.[58] reviewed 21 cases of trochanteric advancement in which no other cause of dislocation was apparent. In 76% (16 of 21) of these cases, no further dislocations occurred. Similarly, because of the increased incidence of dislocation with nonunion and proximal migration of the greater trochanter, reattachment of the avulsed greater trochanter is advised in these cases should dislocation recur.

In complex cases, often those in which the treatment modalities mentioned earlier have failed, additional treatment options include use of constrained acetabular components and insertion of bipolar acetabular devices. With constrained acetabular components, the femoral head is mechanically held within the acetabular liner, usually by a metal locking ring that grips the periphery of the acetabular liner. Indications for use of constrained acetabular components include extremity shortening, loss of musculature about the hip, weakening of the remaining hip musculature, altered kinesiology, placement in elderly and disoriented patients, and the multiply revised hip that continues to dislocate.[27,28,60] Disadvantages of these components include reduced range of motion and earlier impingement which theoretically may result in premature polyethylene wear and component loosening. Use of a 32 mm femoral head size that is nonskirted can improve motion and minimize the probability of impingement. Dislocation can still occur which usually necessitates open reduction and repositioning of the locking ring. Lombardi et al.[60] reviewed a series of 55 patients implanted with constrained acetabular components at an average follow-up of 30.2 months, obtaining hip stability in 91% (50 of 55).

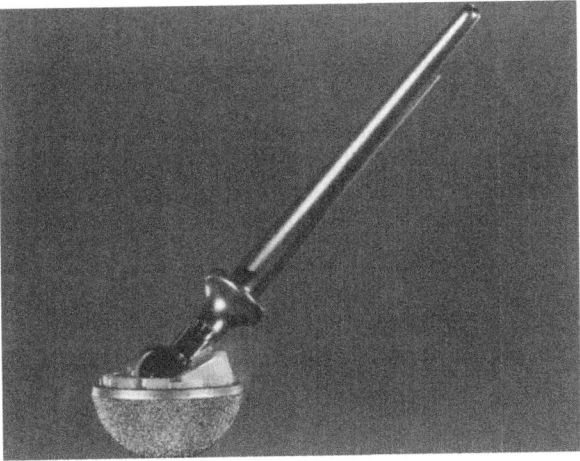

A

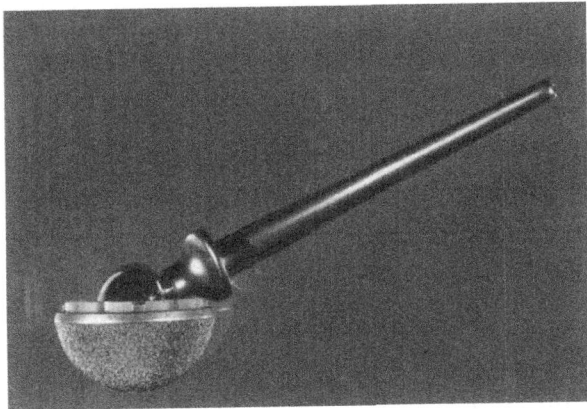

B

Figure 4.2. Photograph demonstrating reduction of motion due to premature neck–socket impingement from use of a skirted femoral head and elevated rim polyethylene liner (A) in comparison with use of a nonskirted femoral head with a nonelevated polyethylene liner (B).

Use of bipolar acetabular prostheses offers additional hip stability because motion can occur at two bearing surfaces and thus allow a greater range of motion before the femoral head dislodges from the acetabulum.[61,62] Ries and Wiedel[61] reported three cases of multiply revised THA complicated by recurrent dislocation, which was successfully managed with implantation of bipolar devices.

Finally, although rarely used as an isolated revision procedure, exchange of a modular femoral head for one with a larger diameter to increase motion before impingement occurs may be of benefit, especially when combined with other stabilization procedures. Also, selection of a modular femoral head with increased neck length can enhance hip stability by improving soft tissue tension. One must remain aware, however, that the longer neck lengths with skirted flanges may actually compromise hip stability by creating earlier neck–socket impingement, especially if used in conjunction with extended-rim acetabular liners (Fig. 4.2). Removal of any additional sources of impingement, such as osteophytes or cementophytes, is also critical to minimize the chance of recurrent dislocation.

Results of reoperation for hip instability are highly variable and are often related to both the type and the extent of the reoperative procedure. Woo and Morrey[3] reported on 91 patients who required reoperation for hip instability, obtaining stability in 69% (63 of 91) of cases. Daly and Morrey[17] analyzed reoperations for hip instability in 95 patients 7.6 years after the procedure. They reported 61% of patients had no further hip instability and concluded it was imperative to determine all etiologic factors preoperatively. In addition, all causative conditions must be confirmed and corrected at the time of reoperation. Failure to correct all factors contributing to dislocation intraoperatively was often associated with failure of the reoperation.

Conclusion

Dislocation after THA is a troublesome complication with a multifactorial etiology. A thorough understanding of all causative factors is required to minimize its occurrence. Prevention, through extensive preoperative and postoperative patient education and proper surgical technique, is the best form of management.

References

1. Morrey BF. Instability after total hip arthroplasty. *Orthop Clin North Am.* 1992;23:237–248.
2. McCollum DE, Gray WJ. Dislocation after total hip arthroplasty: causes and prevention. *Clin Orthop.* 1990;261:159–170.
3. Woo RYG, Morrey BF. Dislocations after total hip arthroplasty. *J Bone Joint Surg Am.* 1982;64:1295–1306.
4. Eftekhar NS. Dislocation and instability complicating low friction arthroplasty of the hip joint. *Clin Orthop.* 1976;121:120–125.
5. Ritter MA. Dislocation and subluxation of the total hip replacement. *Clin Orthop.* 1976;121:92–94.
6. Beckenbaugh BD, Ilstrup DM. Total hip arthroplasty: a review of three hundred and thirty-three cases with long follow-up. *J Bone Joint Surg Am.* 1978;60:306–313.
7. Coventry MB. Late dislocations in patients with Charnley total hip arthroplasty. *J Bone Joint Surg Am.* 1985;67:832–841.
8. Khan MAA, Brakenbury PH, Reynolds ISR. Dislocation following total hip replacement. *J Bone Joint Surg Br.* 1981;63:214–218.
9. Kristiansen B, Jorgensen L, Holmich P. Dislocation following total hip arthroplasty. *Arch Orthop Trauma Surg.* 1985;103:375–377.
10. Lewinnek GE, Lewis JL, Tarr R, Compere C, Zimmerman J. Dislocations after total hip replacement arthroplasties. *J Bone Joint Surg Am.* 1978;60:217–220.
11. Lindberg HO, Carlsson AS, Gentz CF, Pettersson H. Recurrent and non-recurrent dislocation following total hip arthroplasty. *Acta Orthop Scand.* 1982;53:947–952.
12. Fackler CD, Poss R. Dislocation in total hip arthroplasties. *Clin Orthop.* 1980;151:169–178.
13. Lachiewicz PF, Paterno SA. Dislocation of total hip replacements: causes, prevention, and outcome of treatment. *Complications Orthop.* 1996;3:14–18,30.
14. Robinson RP, Robinson HI Jr, Salvati EA. Comparison of the transtrochanteric and posterior approaches for total hip replacement. *Clin Orthop.* 1980;147:143–147.
15. Kavanagh BF, Fitzgerald RH Jr. Multiple revisions for failed total hip arthroplasty not associated with infection. *J Bone Joint Surg Am.* 1987;69:1144–1149.
16. Williams JF, Gottesman MJ, Mallory TH. Dislocation after total hip arthroplasty: treatment with an above-knee hip spica cast. *Clin Orthop.* 1982;171:53–58.
17. Daly PJ, Morrey BF. Operative correction of an unstable total hip arthroplasty. *J Bone Joint Surg Am.* 1992;74:1334–1343.
18. Grady-Benson JC. Instability after total hip arthroplasty. *Complications Orthop.* 1996;3:3–5.
19. Carlsson AS, Gentz CF. Postoperative dislocation in the Charnley and Brunswick total hip arthroplasty. *Clin Orthop.* 1977;125:177–182.
20. Dorr LD, Wolf AW, Chandler R, Conaty JP. Classification and treatment of dislocations of total hip arthroplasty. *Clin Orthop.* 1983;173:151–158.
21. Evanski PM, Waugh TR, Orofino CF. Total hip replacement with the Charnley prosthesis. *Clin Orthop.* 1973;95:69–72.
22. Turner RS. Postoperative total hip prosthetic femoral head dislocations: incidence, etiologic factors, and management. *Clin Orthop.* 1994;301:196–204.
23. Petty W, ed. Lower extremity replacement: the hip. In: *Total Joint Replacement.* Philadelphia, Pa: WB Saunders Co; 1991:304–314.
24. Hedlundh U, Fredin H. Patient characteristics in dislocations after primary total hip arthroplasty: 60 patients compared with a control group. *Acta Orthop Scand.* 1995;66:225–228.
25. Ekelund A, Rydell N, Nilsson OS. Total hip arthroplasty

in patients 80 years of age and older. *Clin Orthop.* 1992; 281:101–106.
26. Newington DP, Bannister GC, Fordyce M. Primary total hip replacement in patients over 80 years of age. *J Bone Joint Surg Br.* 1990;72:450–452.
27. Vaughn BK. Management of dislocation in total hip arthroplasty. *Oper Tech Orthop.* 1995;5:341–348.
28. Vaughn BK. Other complications of total hip arthroplasty. In: Callaghan JJ, Dennis DA, Paprosky WG, Rosenberg AG, eds. *Orthopaedic Knowledge Update: Hip and Knee Reconstruction.* Rosemont, Ill: American Academy of Orthopaedic Surgeons; 1995:163–170.
29. Vicar AJ, Coleman CR. A comparison of the anterolateral, transtrochanteric, and posterior surgical approaches in primary total hip arthroplasty. *Clin Orthop.* 1984;188: 152–159.
30. Charnley J. *Low Friction Arthroplasty of the Hip: Theory and Practice.* Berlin, Germany: Springer; 1979.
31. Pellici PM, Salvati EA, Robinson HJ. Mechanical failures in total hip replacement requiring reoperation. *J Bone Joint Surg Am.* 1979;61:28–36.
32. Etienne A, Cupic Z, Charnley J. Postoperative dislocation after Charnley low-friction arthroplasty. *Clin Orthop.* 1978;132:19–23.
33. Nordin M, Frankel BH. *Basic Biomechanics of the Musculoskeletal System.* 2nd ed. Philadelphia, Pa: Lea & Febiger; 1989.
34. Ackland MK, Bourne WB, Uhthoff HR. Anteversion of the acetabular cup: measurement of angle after total hip replacement. *J Bone Joint Surg Br.* 1986;68:409–413.
35. Goergen TG, Resnick D. Evaluation of acetabular anteversion following total hip arthroplasty: necessity of proper centering. *Br J Radiol.* 1975;48:259–260.
36. McLaren RH. Prosthetic hip angulation. *Radiology.* 1973; 107:705–706.
37. Herrlin K, Selvik G, Pettersson H, Kesek P, Onnerfalt R, Ohlin A. Position, orientation, and component interaction in dislocation of the total hip prosthesis. *Acta Radiol.* 1988; 29:441–444.
38. Magilligan DJ. Calculation of the angle of anteversion by means of horizontal lateral roentgenography. *J Bone Joint Surg Am.* 1956;38:1231–1246.
39. Amstutz HC, Lodwig RM, Schurman DJ, Hodgson AG. Range of motion studies for total hip replacements: a comparative study with a new experimental apparatus. *Clin Orthop.* 1975;111:124–130.
40. Amstutz HC, Markolf KL. Design features in total hip replacement. In: Harris WH, ed. *Proceedings of the Second Open Scientific Meeting of the Hip Society.* St Louis, Mo: CV Mosby; 1974.
41. Lowell JD. Complications of total hip replacement. *Instr Course Lect.* 1974;23:209–230.
42. Cobb TK, Morrey BF, Ilstrup DM. The elevated-rim acetabular liner in total hip arthroplasty: relationship to postoperative dislocation. *J Bone Joint Surg Am.* 1996;78:80–86.
43. Morrey BF, ed. Acetabulum. In: *Joint Replacement Arthroplasty.* New York, NY: Churchill Livingstone; 1991:569–572.
44. Coventry MB, Beckenbaugh RD, Nolan DR, Ilstrup DM. Two thousand twelve total hip arthroplasties: a study of postoperative course and early complications. *J Bone Joint Surg Am.* 1974;56:273–284.
45. Krushell RJ, Burke DW, Harris WH. Range of motion in contemporary total hip arthroplasty: the impact of modular head–neck components. *J Arthroplasty.* 1991;6:97–101.
46. Sculco TP, Moran MC. Posterior soft tissue reconstruction in primary total hip arthroplasty. Presented at 58th annual meeting of the American Academy of Orthopaedic Surgeons; March 11, 1991; Anaheim, Calif.
47. Potter HG, Montgomery KD, Padgett DE, Salvati EA, Helfet DL. Magnetic resonance imaging of the pelvis: new orthopaedic applications. *Clin Orthop.* 1995;319:223–231.
48. Grigoris P, Grecula MJ, Amstutz HC. Dislocation of a total hip arthroplasty caused by iliopsoas tendon displacement. *Clin Orthop.* 1994;306:132–135.
49. Soudry M, Juhn A, Mendes DG. Interposed soft tissue obstructing the reduction of a dislocated Charnley hip arthroplasty. *Orthopedics.* 1985;8:389–390.
50. Larson BJ, Zindrick M, Schwartz C, Demos TC. Postoperative dislocation of a total hip prosthesis due to a surgical drain. *AJR.* 1987;149:971–972.
51. Nordt W, Giangarra CE, Levy M, Habermann ET. Arthroscopic removal of entrapped debris following dislocation of a total hip arthroplasty. *Arthroscopy.* 1987;3: 196–198.
52. Vakili F, Salvati EA, Warren RF. Entrapped foreign body within the acetabular cup in total hip replacement. *Clin Orthop.* 1980;150:159–162.
53. Rao JP, Bronstein R. Dislocations following arthroplasties of the hip: incidence, prevention, and treatment. *Orthop Rev.* 1991;20:261–264.
54. Clayton ML, Thirupathi RG. Dislocation following total hip arthroplasty: management by special brace in selected patients. *Clin Orthop.* 1983;177:154–159.
55. Mallory TH, Vaughn BK, Lombardi AV Jr, Kraus TJ. Prophylactic use of a hip cast–brace following primary and revision total hip arthroplasty. *Orthop Rev.* 1988;17:178–183.
56. Olerud S, Karlstrom G. Recurrent dislocation after total hip replacement: treatment by fixing an additional sector to the acetabular component. *J Bone Joint Surg Br.* 1985;67: 402–405.
57. Bradbury N, Milligan GF. Acetabular augmentation for dislocation of the prosthetic hip: a 3 (1–6)-year follow-up of 16 patients. *Acta Orthop Scand.* 1994;65:424–426.
58. Kaplan SJ, Thomas WH, Poss R. Trochanteric advancement for recurrent dislocation after total hip arthroplasty. *J Arthroplasty.* 1987;2:119–124.
59. Fraser GA, Wroblewski BM. Revision of the Charnley low-friction arthroplasty for recurrent or irreducible dislocation. *J Bone Joint Surg Br.* 1981;63:552–555.
60. Lombardi AV Jr, Mallory TH, Kraus TJ, Vaughn BK. Preliminary report on the S-ROM constraining acetabular insert: a retrospective clinical experience. *Orthopedics.* 1991;14:297–303.
61. Ries MD, Wiedel JD. Bipolar hip arthroplasty for recurrent dislocation after total hip arthroplasty: a report of three cases. *Clin Orthop.* 1992;278:121–127.
62. Grigoris P, Grecula MJ, Amstutz HC. Maximum ball radius for total hip replacement dislocation. Presented at 58th annual meeting of the Western Orthopaedic Association; August 13–17, 1994; Long Beach, Calif.

5
Fracture

Mitchell Geiger, Merrill A. Ritter, and John B. Meding

A femur fracture in a patient with a total hip arthroplasty can be disastrous, but appropriate intervention with most fractures can lead to acceptable or good results. Many studies have examined the treatment of postoperative femur fractures associated with a hip arthroplasty.[1-10] However, little attention has been given to acetabular fractures in the postarthroplasty patient. This chapter examines the causes of bony fractures about total hip replacements in the postoperative situation, along with treatment options and results.

Incidence and Etiology

The incidence of postoperative femur fractures is higher in the revision total hip population (4.2%) than in the primary total hip population (0.1%).[11,12] Some periprosthetic fractures are clearly a result of high-energy trauma, as can occur in motor vehicle accidents and some falls. Often the fracture is comminuted. More commonly, a femur fracture adjacent to the site of a total hip replacement occurs in a patient with biomechanically weakened bone involved in a low-energy injury. Mechanical weakening can be due to stress risers (eg, screw holes), focal structural weakening (eg, polyethylene debris focal osteolysis), or diffuse structural weakening (eg, osteoporosis).[1,8,12,13-17] Table 5.1 lists some of the common causes of mechanical weakening of the femur after total hip surgery.

Brooks et al.[14] studied the effect of round cortical defects (eg, empty screw holes) on the torsional strength of the femur. They found that when round defects are less than 30% of the femur's cortical diameter, the stress concentration around the defect weakens the femur by 55% to torsional stress. Burstein et al.[18] demonstrated that in the dog model these defects fill in with bone and become structurally insignificant over an 8-week period. Larger defects, such as cortical windows or perforations due to eccentric reaming, may leave a large, long-lasting stress riser, particularly if cement fills the void. Some investigators advise filling all known bone defects with bone grafts.[15,17,19-21] Pellicci et al.[22] have recommended bypassing all such defects with a long-stem prosthesis by at least two or three times the shaft diameter to splint the weakened bone. Although some intramedullary devices provide excellent bending strength, they are not particularly strong in torsional support of a femur fracture because they are subject to slippage.[23,24] Although Larson et al.[25] found that a cemented long-stem prosthesis partially restored the torsional strength of a femur with a large defect, even with a long-stem prosthesis in place, weakened bone may fracture.[11,24] Therefore, in the treatment of a periprosthetic femoral fracture with a long-stem prosthesis, supplemental extramedullary fixation with cerclage wires and cortical allograft struts may be indicated to prevent mechanical failure.[20,24,26]

An unrecognized cortical fracture may occur with press-fitting in a total hip arthroplasty. With weight bearing the fracture may displace.[11,20,26-29] According to one study, use of an undersized broach resulted in a 20% intraoperative proximal femur fracture rate. Another study showed that use of a same-size broach resulted in a 2% intraoperative proximal femur fracture rate.[11] Schwartz et al.[29] noted that these fractures are identified half in the intraoperative and half in the postoperative period. Herzwurm et al.[30] demonstrated that, after placement of cerclage cables, the proximal femur can withstand two and one-half times larger hoop stresses before failing. Some surgeons routinely place cerclage wires about the proximal femur before press-fitting a femoral component.

Although acetabular fractures may occur during component press-fitting, true acetabular fractures sustained in the postoperative setting are rare. They have been seen after high-energy trauma such as motor vehicle accidents and after falls. Acetabular fractures frequently result in loosening of the prosthetic component.[21,25] Trochanteric fractures also can occur after falls. In our experience, however, they are rare in patients who have not had a previous trochanteric osteotomy.

5. Fracture

Table 5.1. Common causes of mechanical weakening of the femur after total hip surgery.

Stress Risers Seen about Total Hips
1. Empty screw holes
2. Cortical windows
3. Other bone defects filled with cement
4. Areas of eccentric reaming
5. Incomplete fractures from overzealous broaching or press-fitting
6. Focal lysis due to particulate wear debris
7. Osteotomy created during component revision
8. Cortical defects and thinnings due to drilling, burring, or use of cement osteotomies
9. Postinfection osteolysis
10. Stress-shielded bone after removal of femoral implant

Diffuse Bone Weakening: Metabolic Bone Diseases
1. Osteoporosis related to postmenopausal changes, senility, steroid use, calcium deficiency, etc.
2. Paget's disease
3. Calcium deficiency, malnutrition
4. Osteomalacia/renal osteodystrophy
5. Other: Endocrinopathy, Gaucher's disease, mucopolysaccharidosis

Diagnosis

Although displaced periprosthetic fractures are easy to diagnose, periprosthetic stress fractures may be difficult to confirm. A work-up may be required to rule out other painful periprosthetic conditions (eg, infection, loosening). Stress fractures about femoral prostheses may require bone scans or tomograms for visualization. The characteristic history of a femoral stress fracture includes gradually increasing thigh pain without recent trauma that begins weeks or months after surgery and decreases with restricted weight bearing. Likewise, stress fractures in the pubic ramus occurring in a patient with a hip prosthesis are characterized by insidious onset of groin pain, which resolves with a period of restricted weight bearing. The diagnosis is apparent when healing callus is seen on x-ray.[11,15,17,21,31,32]

Treatment Options and Results

Treatment options for periprosthetic femur fractures include nonoperative treatment, open reduction and internal fixation (ORIF), and revision. Nonoperative treatment consists of a period of bed rest with traction or a spica cast. This may be followed by a period of restricted

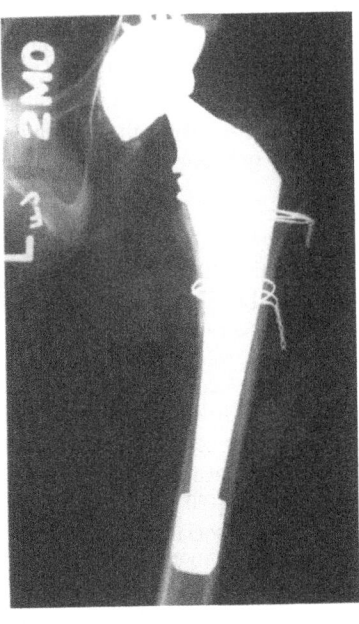 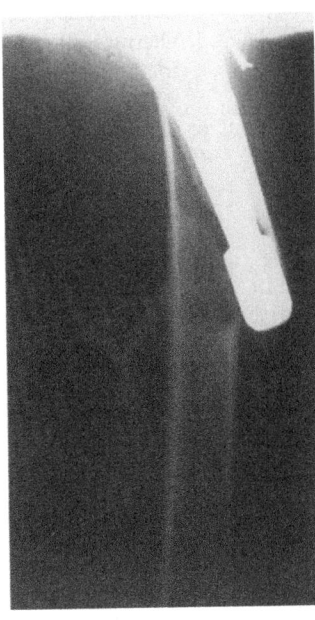 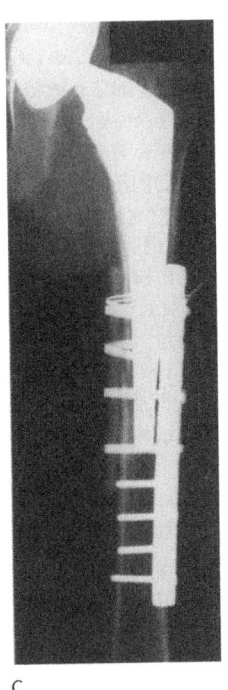 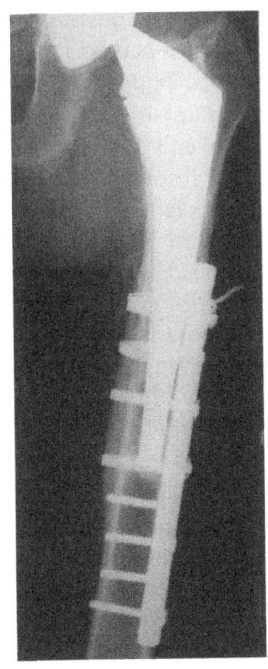

A B C D

Figure 5.1. This 28-year-old man underwent bilateral, primary, press-fit THRs for arthritis associated with ankylosing spondylitis. Cerclage wires were placed about the proximal femur prophylactically. The patient was ambulating independently at 2 months (A) and was painfree at 6 months follow-up. Eight months post-op, he twisted his leg while bowling and sustained an oblique femur fracture about the prosthesis (B). The fracture was stabilized by open reduction and internal fixation using an Ogden plate, allogenic tibial strut bone grafts, and screws and cerclage bands (C). After a period of restricted weight bearing, the fracture healed. At 3 years after surgery he was ambulating painfree. X-rays reveal graft incorporation (D).

weight bearing, often with a fracture brace. Although nonoperative treatment can lead to fracture healing, complications are common.[1,2,4,7,19,21,33,34] For example, Johansson et al.[33] noted healing of 9 of 10 periprosthetic femur fractures treated nonoperatively; however, only two had satisfactory results. Secondary procedures were needed because of malunion, nonunion, and prosthesis loosening.

In studies by Jensen et al.[4] and Beals and Tower[1] nonoperative treatment produced unsatisfactory functional results even though the fracture usually healed. Results of closed treatment for femur fractures associated with a loose prostheses are poor, whereas results of closed treatment for fractures associated with well-fixed prostheses vary with the level at which the fracture occurred. Specifically, distal femur fractures that occur well below a prosthesis have a satisfactory outcome with closed treatment, whereas proximal femur fractures that occur either at the level of the prosthetic stem or at the prosthetic stem tip have less predictable results.[1,4,13,19,33] Complications of proximal periprosthetic fractures treated with closed procedures include malunion, delayed union, late prosthesis loosening after fracture healing, bed sores, and death.

The results of open reduction and internal fixation of femur fractures associated with femoral hip prostheses are variable as well. Comparison of results from different studies is difficult because most studies reviewing ORIF include several surgical techniques. Techniques to correct these periprosthetic fractures include: AO plate and screws; Ogden plate with screws and cerclage; cerclage wires, cables, or bands; cortical bone graft struts and cerclage; and interfragmentary screw fixation.[1,2,4,8-10,33,35,36] Good results were noted with ORIF in some studies,[8-10] such as in the one by Wang et al.[9] who found satisfactory results in 5 of 6 cases. Other studies have revealed inferior results.[1,2,4] In general ORIF of periprosthetic femur fractures has an unacceptable success rate when a loose prosthesis is left in place.[1,2,4,9] The variable results seen in the literature with ORIF, even when the prosthesis is not loose, imply that adequate stabilization of the fracture is critical to obtain a satisfactory result (see Fig. 5.1).

Treatment of periprosthetic femur fractures by revision of the femoral component to a long-stem femoral component that bypasses the fracture has yielded the most consistent and satisfactory results. Of 78 cases of postoperative periprosthetic femur fractures treated with a long-stem revision that we have reviewed in the literature, only 15 demonstrated unsatisfactory results. The majority of the unsatisfactory long-stem femoral revisions involved cementing the femoral long-stem component.[1,4,9,33,37] A recent study by Beals and Tower[1] demonstrates that the best clinical results occur when a noncemented long-stem prosthesis is used to bypass the fracture site. Structural stability must be attained, however, with additional structural strut grafts, cerclage wires, or plate fixations. These techniques are discussed further in other sections of this book.

Conclusion

The incidence of postoperative femur fractures is higher after revision total hip arthroplasty, with the most common scenario being that of a low-energy fracture through biomechanically weak bone. When stress risers occur, prophylactic treatment with supplemental fixation with bone grafting is advised. When postoperative fractures occur, treatment options include nonoperative treatment, ORIF, and revision total hip replacement. When femoral prosthesis loosening is evident or rigid internal fixation cannot be achieved at the time of surgery, strong consideration should be given for treatment of a periprosthetic femur fracture with a long-stem prosthesis.

References

1. Beals RK, Tower SS. Periprosthetic fractures of the femur. *Clin Orthop.* 1996;327:238–246.
2. Bethea JS III, DeAndrade JR, Fleming LL, Lindenbaum SD, Welch RB. Proximal femoral fractures following total hip arthroplasty. *Clin Orthop.* 1982;170:95–106.
3. Fredin HO, Lindberg H, Carlsson AS. Femoral fracture following hip arthroplasty. *Acta Orthop Scand.* 1987;58:20–22.
4. Jenson JS, Barfod G, Hansen D, Larsen E, Linde F, Menck H, et al. Femoral shaft fracture after hip arthroplasty. *Acta Orthop Scand.* 1988;59:9–13.
5. Olerud S. Reconstruction of a fractured femur following total hip replacement. *J Bone Joint Surg Am.* 1979;61:937–938.
6. Olerud S, Karlstrom G. Hip arthroplasty with an extended femoral stem for salvage procedures. *Clin Orthop.* 1984;191:64–81.
7. Scott RD, Schilz JP. Femoral fracture and revision arthroplasty. In: Turner RH, Scheller AD, eds. *Revision Total Hip.* New York, NY: Grune & Stratton; 1982:133–145.
8. Serocki JH, Chandler RW, Dorr LD. Treatment of fractures about hip prostheses with compression plating. *J Arthroplasty.* 1992;7:129–135.
9. Wang GJ, Miller TO, Stamp WG. Femoral fracture following hip arthroplasty. *J Bone Joint Surg Am.* 1985;67:956–958.
10. Zenni EJ Jr, Pomeroy DL, Caudle RJ. Ogden plate and other fixations for fractures complicating femoral endoprostheses. *Clin Orthop.* 1988;231:83–90.
11. Kavanagh BF. Femoral fractures associated with total hip arthroplasty. *Orthop Clin North Am.* 1992;23:249–257.
12. Petty W. Total joint replacement. In: *Total Hip Arthroplasty: Complications.* Philadelphia, Pa: WB Saunders Co; 1991:291–299.
13. Booth RE, Balderston RA, Rothman RH. *Complications: Fractures about the Hip.* Philadelphia, Pa: WB Saunders, Co; 1988.
14. Brooks DB, Burstein AH, Frankel VA. The biomechanics of torsional fractures. *J Bone Joint Surg Am.* 1970;52:507–514.

15. Eschenroeder HC Jr, Krackow KA. Late onset femoral stress fracture associated with extruded cement following hip arthroplasty. *Clin Orthop.* 1988;236:210–213.
16. Fredin H. Late fracture of the femur following perforation during hip arthroplasty. *Acta Orthop Scand.* 1988;59:331–332.
17. Lotke PA, Wong RY. Stress fracture as a cause of chronic pain following revision total hip arthroplasty. *Clin Orthop.* 1986;206:147–150.
18. Burstein AH, Currey J, Frankel VH, Heiple KG, Lunseth P, Vessely JC. Bone strength. *J Bone Joint Surg Am.* 1972;54:1143–1156.
19. Cooke PH, Newman JH. Fractures of the femur in relation to cemented hip prostheses. *J Bone Joint Surg Br.* 1988;70:386–389.
20. Kavanagh BF, Ilstrup DM, Fitzgerald RH. Revision total hip arthroplasty. *J Bone Joint Surg Am.* 1985;76:517–526.
21. McElfresh EC, Coventry MB. Femoral and pelvic fractures after total hip arthroplasty. *J Bone Joint Surg Am.* 1974;56:483–492.
22. Pellicci PM, Wilson PD Jr, Sledge CB, Salvati FA, Ranawat CS, Poss R. Revision total hip arthroplasty. *Clin Orthop.* 1982;170:34–41.
23. Johnson KD, Tencher AF, Blumenthal S, August A, Johnston WC. Biomechanical performance of locked intramedullary nail systems in comminuted femoral shaft fractures. *Clin Orthop.* 1986;206:151–161.
24. Missakian JL, Rand JA. Fracture of the femoral shaft adjacent to long stem femoral components of total hip arthroplasty: report of seven cases. *Orthopedics.* 1993;16:149–152.
25. Larson JE, Chao EYS, Fitzgerald RH Jr, Kavanagh BF. Bypassing femoral cortical defects. *Orthop Trans.* 1988;12:414–415.
26. Kelley SS. Periprosthetic femoral fractures. *J Am Acad Orthop Surg.* 1994;2:164–172.
27. Christensen CM, Seger BM, Schultz RB. Management of intraoperative femur fractures associated with revision hip arthroplasty. *Clin Orthop.* 1989;248:177–180.
28. Mallory TH, Krauge TJ, Vollen BK. Intraoperative femoral fractures associated with cementless THA. *Orthopedics.* 1989;12:231–239.
29. Schwartz JT, Meyer JG, Engh CA. Femoral fracture during noncemented total hip arthroplasty. *J Bone Joint Surg Am.* 1989;71:1135–1142.
30. Herzwurm PJ, Walsh J, Pettine KA, Ebert F. Prophylactic cerclage: a method of preventing femur fracture in uncemented total hip arthroplasty. *Orthop Trans.* 1991;15:342–343.
31. Launder WJ, Hungerford DS. Stress fracture of the pubis after total hip arthroplasty. *Clin Orthop.* 1981;159:183–185.
32. OH I, Hardacre JA. Fatigue fracture of the inferior pubic ramus following total hip replacement for congenital hip dislocation. *Clin Orthop.* 1980;147:154–156.
33. Johansson JE, McBroom R, Barrington TW, Hunter GA. Fracture of the ipsilateral femur in patients with total hip replacement. *J Bone Joint Surg Am.* 1981;63:1435–1442.
34. Scott RD, Turner RH, Leitzes SM, Aufranc OE. Femoral fractures in conjunction with total hip replacement. *J Bone Joint Surg Am.* 1975;57:494–501.
35. Magerl F, Wyss A, Brunner C, Binder W. Plate osteosynthesis of femoral shaft fractures in adults. *Clin Orthop.* 1979;138:62–73.
36. Ruedi TP, Luscher JN. Results after internal fixation of comminuted fractures of the femoral shaft with DC plates. *Clin Orthop.* 1979;138:74–76.
37. Dohmae Y, Bechtold JE, Sherman RE, Puno RM, Gustilo RB. Reduction in cement–bone interface shear strength between primary and revision arthroplasty. *Clin Orthop.* 1988;236:214–220.

Part 2
Evaluation of the Painful Total Hip Arthroplasty

Thomas S. Thornhill

The most common complaint that brings the patient to the doctor is pain. By listening to the patient, we can frequently understand the process responsible for that pain. Is this nociceptive postoperative pain or is it a neuropathic pain? Is this a pain due to one of the common mechanisms of failure such as osteolysis and wear debris formation, mechanical loosening, infection, or another etiology amenable to surgical intervention? Is this a neuropathic pain such as reflex sympathetic dystrophy that should alert the surgeon to avoid further surgery? In the case of neuropathic pain, surgery should be avoided. The emphasis should be placed on management of that pain through use of pharmacologic agents such as Elavil™ and Tramadol™, which block re-uptake of serotonin and norepinephrine at the anterior horn cell and disrupt the painful reflex arc. Is this a pain on initiation of weightbearing that suggests loosening of the implant? Is this a pain that is inconsistent with radiographic findings, which might suggest infection? The experienced surgeon learns to listen to the patient, who is the best observer and can frequently lead the surgeon to the failure mechanism. This section deals with evaluation of the painful total hip as well as the radiographic studies most suitable to ascertaining the mechanism of failure and directing the surgeon onto the proper treatment path.

Radiographic evaluation of the painful total hip generally elucidates the failure mechanism. Consultation between the orthopedic surgeon and the orthopedic radiologist is essential to both direct and facilitate proper radiographic studies. In most cases plain radiographs including an AP and a Lowenstein or true lateral view are sufficient to determine the mechanism of failure.

Aseptic loosening can generally be differentiated from osteolysis by its position and the presence of endosteal focal erosion. Stress shielding is more likely to occur in cases of a distally fixed implant, and generally shows diffuse proximal osteopenia with distal sclerosis at the point where load is transferred from the implant to the bone. Scintigraphy using technetium is sensitive but not very specific. It can be very beneficial when the surgeon wants to determine whether the pain is due to the hip as a persistently hot bone scan one year after implantation. In some centers Indium-labeled white cell scans have been utilized in the evaluation of a potentially infected implant. Both CT and MRI have played limited roles because of metal artifact. More sophisticated techniques, however, have permitted subtraction of the metal artifact to the point where significant information can be gleaned.

In evaluating a painful total hip, the surgeon should have a low threshold for aspiration of the hip. This is best done under fluoroscopy with injection of a small amount of contrast to confirm the position of the needle. It is unclear whether aspiration should be performed routinely in evaluating the painful total hip, but it is agreed that any evidence of infection should be evaluated by an aspiration arthrogram and culture.

The ideal situation occurs when there is open communication between the orthopedist and the orthopedic radiologist and a systematic plan is developed for evaluation of the painful hip. In this era of managed care with limited resources, careful planning of radiographic procedures permits the most efficient use of radiology services necessary to confirm the mechanism of failure of the implant.

6
Evaluation of the Painful Total Hip Arthroplasty

Robert J. Carangelo and Arnold D. Scheller

There are many reasons for clinical failure of a total hip arthroplasty. The relationship between the arthroplasty and the surrounding tissues is complex. There are biologic, biomechanical, and structural factors that contribute to the success or failure of the arthroplasty composite. The composite structure consists of bone, cement, metal, and ultrahigh molecular weight polyethylene. A mechanism of failure could occur at any one or a combination of these materials that form the composite. The mode of failure may be as subtle and insidious as polyethylene wear particles inciting an inflammatory response leading to early or late osteolysis, or as obvious as component failure such as a femoral stem fracture. Failure mechanisms in hip arthroplasty may occur at the periarticular, articular, or extra-articular levels. (Table 6.1)

Many new developments have had an impact on the evaluation of the patient with a symptomatic total hip arthroplasty. Clinical entities have been described that can cause pain such as bone lysis with a stable implant. The interpretation of radiographs and some diagnostic tests has become more accurate. There are also methods of analyzing and differentiating an aseptic from a septic process. This has occurred in part because of the use of uncemented total hip arthroplasty. Conventional diagnostic tests used for cemented components had to be redefined to evaluate the patient with a symptomatic uncemented implant.

With an ever-increasing number of total hip revisions being performed currently and in the future, it is of paramount importance that the reconstructive surgeon understand the different types of failures that can occur, the diagnostic modalities available, and the treatment options. This chapter begins with the most important aspect of the evaluation: that is, the history and physical examination. It is followed by a description of the diagnostic tests available. Diagnostic algorithms are then presented to provide an organized approach to the management of the painful total hip arthroplasty.

Clinical Evaluation

History

The initial interview of a referred patient is crucial in establishing a productive patient–surgeon relationship. This is often complicated by the emotional state of the patient, who may be distrustful, depressed, and anxious about the situation. Special effort is necessary to understand such a patient. The rapport has hopefully been longstanding when the primary surgeon and revision surgeon are one and the same. Aufranc's admonitions never rang more true:

> Allow the patient to tell his story in his own way. Listen patiently until he has finished what he has to say. Do not interrupt the story until it is evident that some encouragement and direction are needed. Do not talk or try to explain conditions until all the essential facts of the patient's story, the preliminary examination, and any auxiliary studies that seem necessary have been evaluated. Ask more questions which will give a logical sequence of events in the development of the conditions and the past treatment.[1]

Although all patients being evaluated for a painful total hip arthroplasty will have pain, it is often nonspecific. Pain, being a subjective phenomenon, varies from person to person. The character of the pain, its location, radiation, duration, temporal patterns, exacerbating and ameliorating phenomena, and progression in its severity need to be clearly ascertained. It is common to have several different types of pain emanating from different sources. It is important to differentiate which is more debilitating.

The presence of a painfree interval after total hip arthroplasty suggests implant failure or indolent infection as the etiology. Failure to achieve pain relief may suggest an extrinsic source unrelated to the hip. Rest pain and night pain suggest a septic etiology. Pain on weight-bearing and a painful, restricted passive range

Table 6.1. Causes of hip pain.

Articular Mechanisms
- Aseptic loosening
- Septic loosening
- Dislocation
- Osteolysis
- Component failure

Periarticular Mechanisms
- Soft-tissue contracture
- Trochanteric nonunion
- Trochanteric bursitis
- Iliotibial band tendinitis
- Heterotopic ossification
- Periprosthetic fracture
- Limb length discrepancy

Extraarticular Mechanisms
- Lumbar disease
- Sacroiliac disease
- Ipsilateral degenerative joint disease of knee
- Vascular—aortoiliac disease
- Inguinal, femoral hernia
- Psychogenic factors

of motion are consistent findings in patients with a deep pyogenic infection. This may be of fulminant onset, but more characteristically progresses insidiously.

Pain that is aggravated with activity or weight-bearing and relieved with rest is often associated with aseptic loosening. Start-up pain after rising from a chair that improves after a few steps may be associated with a loose femoral component. Activity-related pain can also be associated with tendinitis or heterotopic ossification. Heterotopic ossification rarely causes significant pain, but it may mimic an inflammatory process with progressive pain and decreased range of motion within the first few months after total hip arthroplasty.

Acute and severe pain can be seen with component failure, such as stem or periprosthetic femur fracture, acetabular cup dissociation, and hip dislocation (see Fig. 6.1).

The location of the pain is also important in differentiating intrinsic from extrinsic pathology. Pain localized to the groin or buttock can be associated with acetabular pathology. Pain over the greater trochanter may be associated with trochanteric bursitis, iliotibial band tendinitis, nonunion of a trochanteric osteotomy or irritation from hardware used to secure the trochanteric osteotomy. Thigh pain with radiation to the anteromedial knee and leg is usually related to the femoral component. Thigh pain in patients with uncemented components is a new category. Persistent thigh pain in patients with porous ingrowth or press-fit components without radiographic evidence of loosening has been reported in 12% to 41% of patients at 2-year follow-up.[2-6] The etiology of this pain is unknown. Recalcitrant thigh pain leading to femoral stem revision has been described in components that were biologically ingrown and stable at surgery.[7,8] Fitzgerald[9] found that chronic pain in a cemented total hip arthroplasty was an indicator of an indolent infection. In the uncemented total hip arthroplasty, chronic thigh pain has been reported in most series to date.

In addition to the symptom of pain, the patient may describe a progressively worsening limp. This could be secondary to the pain or related to a leg length dis-

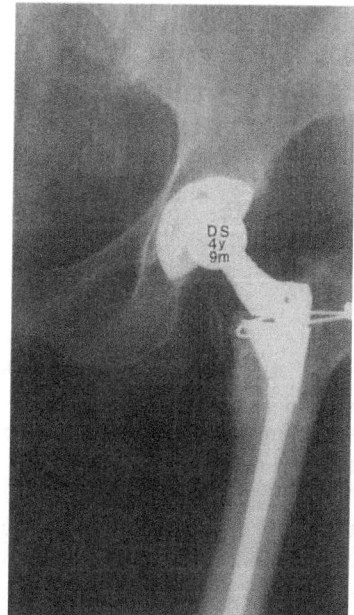 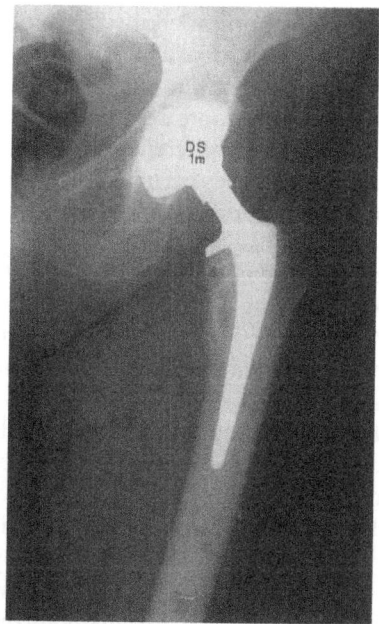

Figure 6.1. A. Radiograph of fractured stem. The fracture is located at the junction of the titanium SROM stem and ZTT sleeve. B. After extraction and revision to a cemented stem.

crepancy or abductor weakness, all of which could represent aseptic loosening with subsidence of the femoral implant or protrusion of the acetabular component. Decreasing range of motion may be the primary complaint. This may be associated with ectopic bone, soft tissue contracture, subsidence, protrusion or infection.

The patient may describe episodes of subluxation or dislocation. Questioning must be directed at defining which activities and in which positions the limb is in to initiate instability. Also, timing of the dislocation in relation to the index procedure is important to determine whether component malposition, bony impingement, or inadequate soft-tissue tension is the cause.

Systemic symptoms must also be investigated. Fever, chills, and night sweats may be associated with an indolent septic process. Contralateral hip, knee, or back pain could be related to primary disease or an altered gait pattern from a loose prosthesis.

After a thorough history is documented, a past medical and past surgical history is essential. Disorders that increase the risk of infection, such as diabetes, inflammatory arthritis, immune compromising disorders, history of prior hip infection, and multiple hip operations must be disclosed. Recent procedures such as dental work, colonoscopy, or cystoscopy must be documented in the face of a potential septic process.

Physical Examination

The physical exam of the patient with a painful total hip arthroplasty should proceed in a manner similar to that performed on all patients with hip pathology. Gait, with and without ambulatory aides, is observed for antalgia, limb length discrepancy, and Trendelenburg truncal sway. In a painful total hip arthroplasty there is often a shortened stance phase, a shortened length of stride, and abnormal pelvic rotation. The patient's stance is checked for pelvic obliquity, compensatory scoliosis, and contractures; a Trendelenburg test is performed. A positive Trendelenburg may indicate abductor weakness or trochanteric nonunion, an adduction deformity, a varus femoral component, ankylosis, or a loosened femoral component.

While the patient is standing, the back should be examined. Inspection may reveal scoliosis, excessive lumbar lordosis, or kyphosis. The lower back, sacroiliac joints, buttocks, and trochanters should be palpated to rule out pathology. Finally, range of motion is assessed. Range of motion should be painless throughout flexion, extension, and rotation. Pain signifies a potential extrinsic source for the hip pain. With the patient in the supine position, a passive straight-leg test is performed to observe for sciatic irritation.

While the patient is recumbent, active and passive range of motion of the hip is performed. Those positions that elicit pain or instability are recorded. Pain in the hip suggests mechanical dysfunction of one or both of the components. Patients with subluxation or a loose component may demonstrate a palpable and audible click or thud as the hip is brought into hyperflexion and adduction and then back into extension. Provocative tests, such as the Thomas test for hip flexion deformity and the Faber test (flexion, abduction, external rotation) to assess the sacroiliac joints, can also be performed.

With the patient on his or her side, abductor function is again observed as the patient attempts to elevate the limb against gravity and then against resistance. An Ober test can also be performed in this position to determine iliotibial band tension.

The true and apparent limb lengths are measured. If true progressive limb length inequality can be measured, this is highly suggestive of mechanical failure in fixation of the components. Apparent limb length discrepancies may give insight into abduction or adduction contractures, or into pelvic obliquity from scoliosis.

The skin around the hip is examined. Attention is directed at the type and number of incisions, excessive scar formation, abnormal healing, and sinus tracts. Palpation of the surrounding tissue may reveal swelling, a subcutaneous or subfascial mass, a fascial defect, or heterotopic ossification. New onset dermatitis in association with a loose implant may suggest a hypersensitivity reaction to the implant.

The exam is not complete until a thorough neurologic and vascular assessment are performed to rule out extrinsic etiology. Potential sources of infection should be sought, such as skin ulceration from venous stasis or arterial insufficiency, abscess formation, or skin breakdown. Occasionally, abdominal, rectal and pelvic exams may be necessary in complicated situations.

Extrinsic Disease

The pain associated with a total hip arthroplasty is commonly related to extrinsic disease. There are many causes of pain that may be confused with intrinsic pathology of the hip. Sciatic neuropathy in particular, be it primary or secondary, can present a confusing symptom complex. Protruding fourth or fifth lumbar discs are common causes of sciatica. Lumbar spondylosis, degenerative spondylolisthesis, and spinal stenosis frequently contribute to the array of symptoms seen in spinal pathology, all of which can refer pain to the hip region. Neurogenic claudication frequently refers pain to the hip and thigh region.

Neurologic complications from surgery are well documented. The reported incidence is 1%.[10-12] The majority of nerve injuries are neuropraxias due to retraction or limb lengthening and involve the sciatic nerve. These injuries are often transient and rarely last longer than a year.

Vascular claudication from chronic aortoiliac disease may also refer pain to the back, hips, thighs, and legs.[13,14] The characteristic symptoms of calf claudication may be absent secondary to collateral blood flow. Vascular injury during surgery has been reported.[15,16] Vascular claudication may occur after total hip arthroplasty because of the increased activity level.[17]

Other causes of pain in and around the hip include inguinal or femoral hernias, ectopic cement, pubic rami stress fractures, and metabolic neuropathies.

The final extrinsic mode of failure is seen in patients with emotional or psychologic problems who have high scores on the Minnesota Multiphasic Personality Inventory (MMPI). This test has indexes of depression, hysteria, and hypochondriasis. A finding of abnormalities in these areas is an unfortunate situation for both surgeon and patient. The surgeon should recognize, however, that operative intervention is not the solution to the patient's pain syndrome.

Diagnostic Evaluation

Laboratory Analysis

Once the extrinsic and periarticular modes of failure have been ruled out as a reason for the hip pain, the remaining etiologies are infection and aseptic loosening. Laboratory studies are the initial screening tests obtained to differentiate a septic from an aseptic process.

A standard profile should include CBC with differential, erythrocyte sedimentation rate (ESR), complete chemistries, and urinalysis. Additional tests may be performed if warranted by the history and physical exam. These include calcium, phosphorus, thyroid function studies, parathyroid hormone assay, alkaline phosphatase, serum electrophoresis, and C-reactive protein.

The WBC is generally of little value in the evaluation of the painful total hip. Leukocytosis is an uncommon manifestation unless there is fulminant sepsis. Despite the lack of absolute WBC elevation, however, a left shift may frequently be seen; therefore a differential should always be ordered.

The erythrocyte sedimentation rate (ESR) is a rough indicator of serum fibrinogen and immunoglobulin concentration and thereby a measurement of inflammation. There are disease and normal states that increase the ESR: pregnancy, connective tissue disorders, rheumatoid arthritis, neoplastic disease, and chronic infections.

After a total hip arthroplasty, the ESR remains elevated for 3 to 6 months and is therefore less reliable in predicting an infectious process.[18-20] The value should return to 30 mm/h approximately 6 months after surgery. A rate that remains elevated above 40 mm/h is highly suggestive of an infectious process. The ESR has a sensitivity of 73% to 100%, a specificity of 69% to 94%, and an accuracy of 73% to 88%.[18,21,22]

An alternative to the ESR is a test for the C-reactive protein (CRP). The CRP is an acute phase protein synthesized by hepatocytes. The significance of CRP in the assessment of acute infection and tissue destruction has been well documented.[23-25] A normal serum concentration appears to be 5 to 10 mg/l.[24] Several studies have demonstrated the efficacy of CRP in detecting infection in total hip arthroplasty.[19,26] The advantage of CRP is that it reaches maximum value usually 2 days postoperative and then returns to normal at 3 weeks.[19]

Radiographs

Plain radiographs should always be obtained in evaluation of the painful total hip arthroplasty. Examination of serial radiographs over time remains the most accurate method of determining component stability. The radiographs should be inspected for soft tissue abnormalities (heterotopic ossification), bony remodeling, radiolucencies, change in component position, and osteolysis.

There have been many radiographic criteria proposed for loosening of cemented femoral and acetabular components.[27-29] Most orthopaedists would agree, however, that loosening is definitely present if there is any migration of the components within the cement mantle, progressive complete radiolucency at the bone–cement interface of greater than 2 mm, and fracture of the cement mantle. Radiolucent lines on the femoral side have recently been thought to represent bone remodeling and not a decline in the bone–cement interface.[30,31]

On the acetabular side, however, Hodgkinson et al.[32] demonstrated that loosening was definite in 94% of Charnley cemented acetabular sockets if there was a continuous radiolucent line throughout all zones. If a radiolucent zone was found in zones 1 and 3 then only 7% of the components were loose.[32] Several studies have shown that determination of loosening of the femoral component is more accurate than for the acetabular component.[29,33]

In the absence of gross loosening, precise measurement of component migration is helpful to determine subtle changes in position of the implant. The Mueller template has been used to standardize measurements of component migration.[34] In addition, the hole-in-one technique uses the proximal extraction hole within the femoral implant and an implanted metal marker to measure femoral subsidence.[35]

The interpretation of radiographs of uncemented implants has been more clearly characterized by Engh et al.[36] They have defined the radiographic criteria to differentiate a stable from an unstable uncemented component. Again, the most reliable indicator of lack of osseointegration and instability of the femoral and acetabular implants was subsidence or migration. Measurement of this parameter is made more accurate by consistent positioning of the patient as described by Massin et al. to correct for pelvic rotation, and the use of Mueller templates.[37]

Even with the classification systems for stability of cemented and uncemented components, it is often not possible to differentiate aseptic from septic loosening solely on the basis of interpretation of plain radiographs.[38–40] There are specific radiographic signs, however, that suggest the presence of infection.[41] Lyon et al.[24] showed that endosteal scalloping and periosteal lamination were associated with infection in 90% of patients. Also, the rapid development of a continuous radiolucent line of greater than 2 mm or severe focal osteolysis within the first year is often associated with infection.[42,43]

Arthrogram and Aspiration

In addition to plain radiographs, arthrograms have been used to assess implant stability. They appear to be technique dependent with high-pressure or postambulation arthrograms having more accuracy. They have been used with less frequency because of the general lack of uniformity in the radiographic criteria for loosening in cemented components.[33,44,45] Maus et al.[40] have shown, however, a strong correlation between arthrography and component loosening at surgery. In the acetabulum, if contrast was present in all zones, zones I and II, or zones II and III, or there was a rim of contrast greater than 2 mm thick in any zone, there was greater than 90% of components loose at surgery. If the femoral criteria were satisfied, there was greater than 95% association with a loose femoral component. This study also demonstrated an improvement in the resolution of arthrography by using digital subtraction technique.

For uncemented implants there is even less consensus on the use of contrast arthrography. Barrack et al.[46] demonstrated a high incidence of false-positive (17%) and false-negative (25%) findings on the femoral side with sensitivity, specificity, and accuracy being only 60%. On the acetabular side, there were 31% false-negative findings and an accuracy of 62.5%. They concluded that there were significant limitations in using this procedure.

Nuclear arthrography has been used to improve the accuracy of diagnosis of a loose implant. Thus far it has been more useful on the femoral side with sensitivities ranging from 64% to 93% and specificities from 75% to 100% for both cemented and uncemented components.[47,48]

Aspiration

Aspiration of fluid from the hip joint has been touted as being the most important diagnostic procedure for differentiating a septic from an aseptic process. Whether it should be routinely used before all revisions is, however, controversial. Barrack et al.[49] reviewed a series of 270 total hip arthroplasties that were aspirated. Only 2% were determined to be infected, and in all 6 cases there was a clinical history and radiographic changes suggestive of infection. There were 32 (13%) false-positive aspirations. False-positive aspirations ranging from 16% to 30% have been reported in the literature.[33,50–52] They concluded from their study that selective aspiration should be performed in patients suspected of having an infection. In a similar study, Lachiewicz et al.,[53] found improved sensitivity (92%) and specificity (97%) of preoperative aspiration in prediction of infection, especially when combined with findings of an elevated ESR and implants that had been in place for less than 5 years.

Aspiration is performed under fluoroscopic guidance. The aspirate should be sent for cell count, gram stain, and aerobic and anaerobic cultures. The organisms cultured in the aspirate do not always correlate with those found at the time of surgery.[21] Skin flora are frequent isolates from the aspirate but could represent a contaminant or the true pathologic organism. Even though there are many confounding variables, aspiration remains a valuable diagnostic tool in the evaluation of the painful total hip arthroplasty.

Nuclear Medicine Evaluation

Nuclear medicine scans, which include technetium-99m-HDP, gallium citrate, WBC labeled with indium-111, and sulfur colloid bone marrow, have been used separately or in combination to diagnose the presence of infection in total hip arthroplasty. Because of variable sensitivity, specificity, and accuracy between studies the use of nuclear medicine scans is controversial.[31,38,54–57] Lieberman et al.[58] reviewed plain radiographs, bone scans, and hip aspirations in 54 patients with a painful cemented total hip and compared the results with operative findings. They concluded that technetium bone scan added little to the diagnosis of loosening or infection and is not necessary. Examination of serial plain radiographs was the most effective way to detect a loose component, and hip aspiration was shown to be very accurate in predicting infection.

In addition, it should be recognized that there will be variable uptake of these compounds in the bone surrounding normal cemented and uncemented implants. In fact, Utz et al.[59] demonstrated uptake in 20% of patients with cemented THA at 1 year. No patient had increased uptake beyond 1 year. For uncemented prostheses, Oswald et al.[60,61] observed stable or decreasing uptake of technetium-99m or indium-111 at 2 years. Because of the variable geometry of the uncemented prosthesis, bone remodeling will behave in different ways. Therefore interpretation of nuclear medicine scans may be of less value.

Technetium and gallium scans cannot be used to differentiate between septic and aseptic loosening. Combined, the studies are considered positive if uptake is incongruent or if gallium uptake is greater. There is a high specificity, but a low sensitivity, which means that a clearly positive scan suggests infection, whereas a negative scan provides little information.[29,38]

Indium-111-labeled WBC scans initially showed promise with high sensitivity, which increased further when combined with technetium-99m.[54] However, subsequent studies demonstrated variable results.[57] Palestro et al.[62] combined indium-111 and sulfur colloid bone marrow scans and found that incongruent uptake of the compounds had a sensitivity of 100%, specificity of 97%, and accuracy of 98% in predicting infection of a total hip arthroplasty.

Despite these data, the most useful result using either a technetium-99m or an indium-111 scan is as a negative test. A conservative approach can be followed when such tests are normal.

Intraoperative Evaluation

In some instances operative exploration is undertaken without a clear distinction of the etiology of hip pain. This should be approached cautiously especially if there is no objective evidence for loosening or infection.

The evaluation should proceed in an organized fashion. Range of motion should be ascertained before skin incision. The limits at which impingement, subluxation, or dislocation occur are noted. The soft tissue is examined for signs of inflammation. When the hip joint is exposed, a gram stain and culture of the fluid is obtained and numerous sections of capsule, synovium, and granulation tissue are obtained for permanent and frozen sections. There is some controversy as to the usefulness of these tissue samples. Results of the intraoperative gram stain have been relatively unpredictable.[49] Mirra et al.[63] reported that the presence of more than five polymorphonuclear leukocytes per high power field correlated with 95% of the total joint arthroplasties being infected. Using similar criteria, Feldman et al.[64] reported that the analysis of intraoperative frozen sections was a reliable predictor of infection. However, Fehring and McAlister[65] observed only 20% sensitivity for intraoperative frozen sections and 50% sensitivity for permanent sections.

The position of the implants needs to be checked, and the surgeon needs to make sure the version of the femoral stem and acetabulum are within acceptable range. Osteophytes surrounding the acetabulum or heterotopic ossification in the soft tissue is removed if it causes impingement.

Mechanical testing of the femoral stem with a torque wrench is necessary to demonstrate micromotion at the bone–implant or prosthesis–cement interface. The acetabular side is more difficult to test. If there is polyethylene wear, the liner should be removed. This will give access to the back of the socket, especially if there are screw holes. These should be cureted and checked for pockets of osteolysis that may need bone grafting.

Unfortunately if nothing is found on hip exploration to account for the patient's symptoms, revision of the component(s) may not be the solution.

Algorithms for the Painful Total Hip

Based on existing findings in the literature, algorithms have been developed for evaluation of the painful total hip arthroplasty. Harris and Barrack[66] provide several examples for uncemented and cemented total hips. They have been categorized as stable, loose, or lysis without looseness.

For stable cementless total hips, a distinction must be made between typical and atypical thigh pain. For typical thigh pain often a conservative treatment program is used unless the pain gets worse. At this stage an ESR and an aspiration with or without arthrogram are done. If the test findings are positive and there is clinical and radiographic correlation for infection, the component is removed. If the test results are negative, but there is progression of the pain, a technetium-99m/indium-111 scan is performed. If positive, the implant is either loose or infected. The surgeon can observe, repeat aspiration, or explore. For atypical pain the scenario is similar except a more aggressive approach is followed from the start (see Fig. 6.2).

For the loose cementless component, treatment depends on whether infection is present. With no indication of a septic process, revision depends on the degree of pain and instability. It is common over time for uncemented components to stabilize after migrating and then become osseointegrated (see Fig. 6.3).

Hip pain in a stable cemented component is much more ominous than in an uncemented component and warrants ESR and aspiration to rule out infection. If test results are definitely positive, resection and debridement is required. If a rare organism or contaminant is suspected, a second aspiration should be done. If the findings on aspiration are negative in the face of progressive pain, a technetium/indium scan, repeat aspiration, or exploration may be undertaken by the surgeon (see Fig. 6.4).

In a loose cemented total hip that has no clinical or radiographic sign of infection, revision of one or both components is warranted. If it is difficult to determine acetabular stability, a preoperative arthrogram may be of help. If there are signs of infection, an aspiration should be done, followed by resection if positive (see Fig. 6.5).

Much attention has been focused on the role of osteolysis in the painful total hip arthroplasty. Osteolysis is caused, in part, by particulate debris initiating an in-

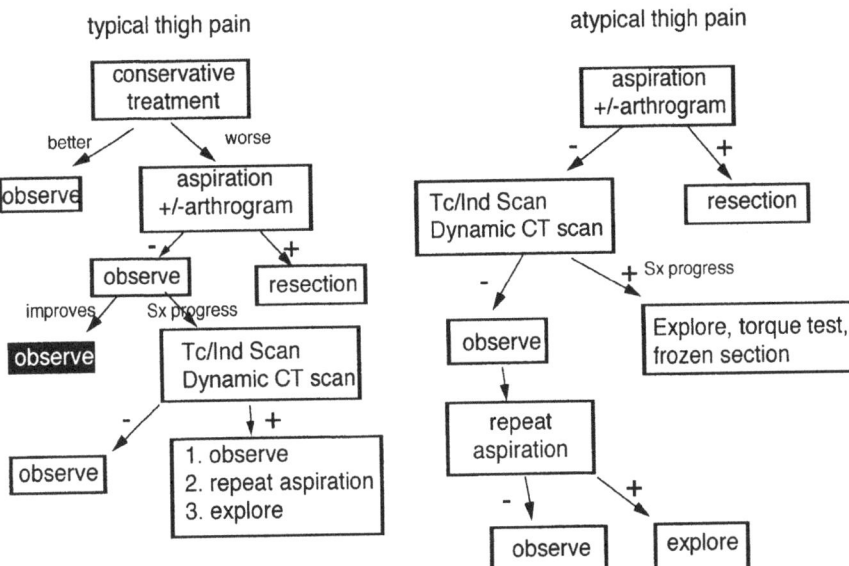

Figure 6.2. Algorithms for painful cementless total hip arthroplasty that appears stable radiographically.[66]

flammatory cascade that leads to periprosthetic bone loss.[67–71] It can be focal, diffuse, or linear and involve the entire effective joint space.[72] Osteolysis can occur in cemented and cementless implants, affecting the femoral and acetabular sides of the hip arthroplasty.[73–76] Its etiology appears to be multifactorial with the patient, type of implant, stability of the implant, and type of polyethylene all contributing to the severity of the osteolysis. The phenomenon of osteolysis without looseness of the components has been described by several investigators.[66,73,74] The concern is at what point does the surgeon intervene to halt the process of bone loss. Several questions about osteolysis are currently being investigated: How soon does the osteolytic process begin? How rapidly will the osteolytic lesions progress in size? In an asymptomatic patient when is surgery indicated? How extensive of a revision is necessary when there is just eccentric polyethylene wear?

Zhinian and Dorr[77] reported on the natural history of femoral focal osteolysis with a proximally ingrown stem. They found that if linear wear was greater than 0.2 mm/year or volumetric wear was greater than 150 mm^3/year focal osteolysis was seen on radiographs within the first 5 years. Seventy percent of the lytic defects presented within 6 months to 5 years. The size of

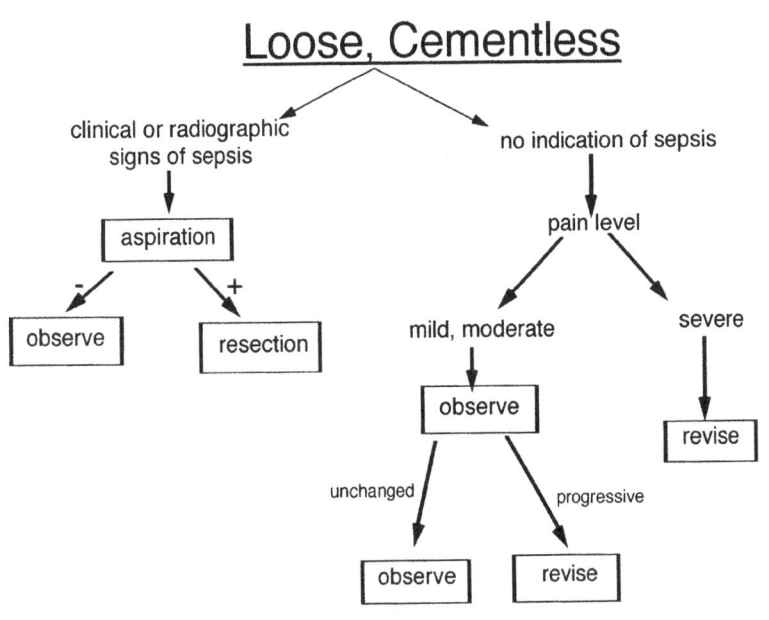

Figure 6.3. Algorithms for painful cementless total hip arthroplasty that appears loose radiographically.[66]

Figure 6.4. Algorithms for painful cemented total hip arthroplasty that appears stable radiographically.[66]

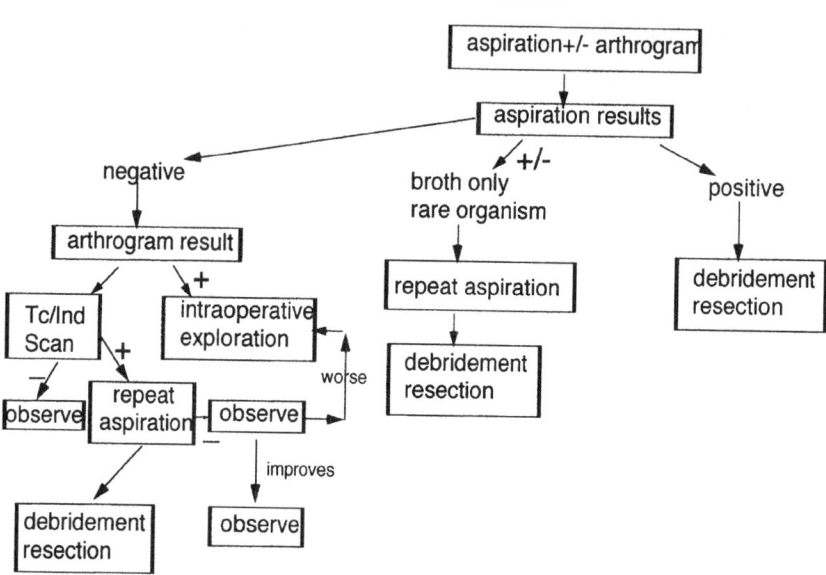

the defects increased at a slow rate of 0.9 mm/year, however the number of defects increased. If these defects involved six or more of the femoral zones defined by Gruen,[79] 56% of the stems were loose at revision. They concluded that revision should take place when linear and volumetric wear are excessive (>0.2 mm/year or >150 mm³/year) or if the patient is younger than 60 years with exchange of the femoral head and liner. Patients with small osteolytic defects that are asymptomatic should be monitored closely at 6-month intervals. If there is progression revision may be necessary.[72] Whether the revision entails just debridement and packing of the lytic defect with morcellized allograft or a proximal femoral allograft depends on the severity of the bone loss (see Fig. 6.6).

As for the acetabular side, Hozack et al.[78] recently reported on the relationship among polyethylene wear, pelvic osteolysis, and clinical symptoms in 54 patients with cementless acetabular components. From the findings, they developed an algorithm for treatment. They categorized patients into stages: I—radiographic polyethylene wear; IIa—wear and pain; IIb—wear, lysis, and no pain; and stage III—wear, lysis, and pain. The pain was often referred to the buttock or groin. In all cases there was evidence of polyethylene wear, and in 80% pelvic osteolysis was demonstrated. Patients in stages I and IIa were revised with particulate bone graft and cementless acetabular component. Patients in stage IIB or III required structural allograft in 79% of cases, and cemented components in 53%. They concluded that poly-

Figure 6.5. Algorithms for painful cemented total hip arthroplasty that appears loose radiographically.[66]

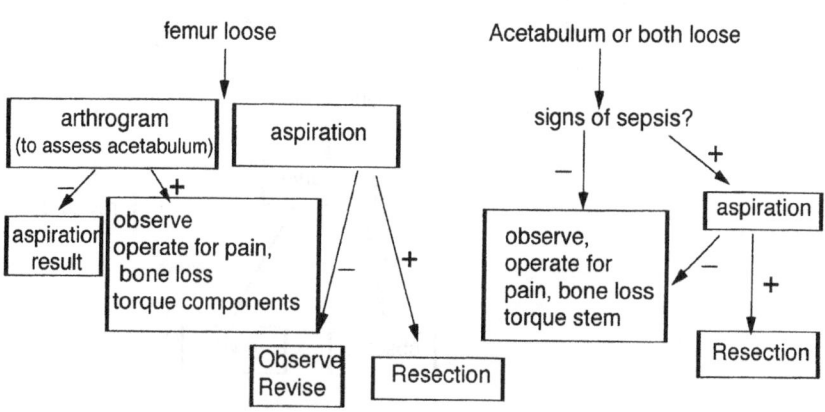

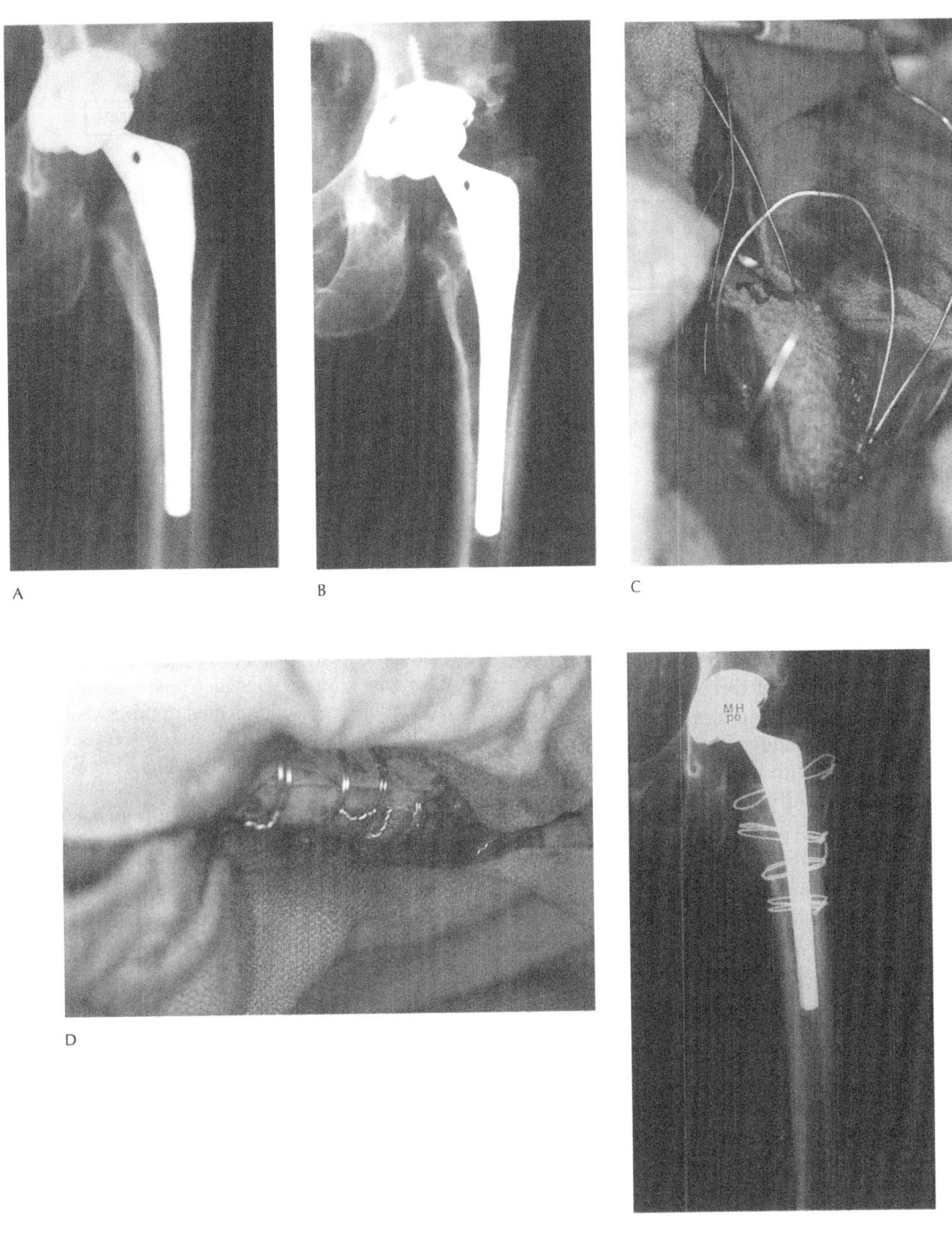

Figure 6.6. A. Radiograph of extensive femoral osteolysis in a stable stem B-E. Exposure requires extended trochanteric osteotomy, impaction of lytic defects with morcellized cancellous allograft, and fixation of the trochanteric osteotomy with wires.

ethylene wear in an asymptomatic patient foreshadows impending failure. The patient should be monitored closely and revised early. Revision is less complex with less bone loss.[78]

In the presence of a well-fixed ingrown acetabular component with eccentric polyethylene wear and focal osteolysis, often exchange of the liner and femoral head and impaction of the defect with morcellized allograft are all that is necessary. Removal of a ingrown component may cause additional bone loss. A CT scan of the pelvis preoperatively can depict the full extent of the lesion in most cases.

Figure 6.7. Algorithms.[66]

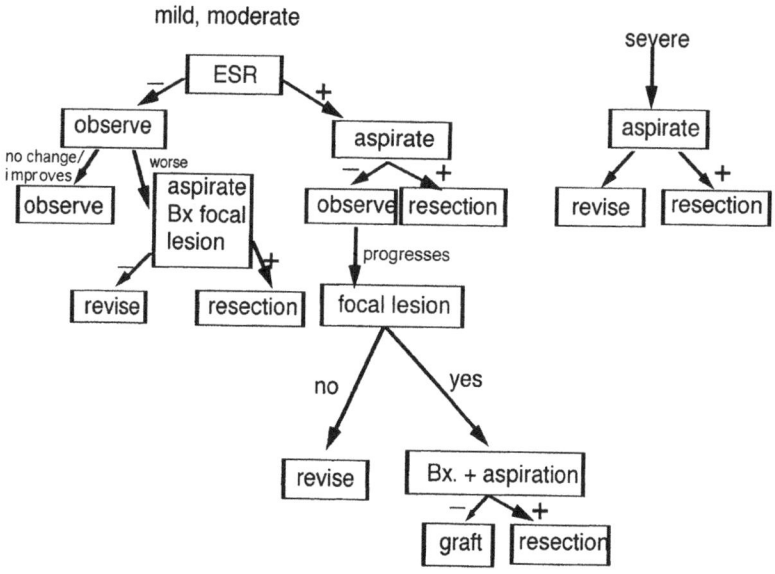

If a transtrochanteric or trochanteric slide had been used and the trochanter secured with a Dall-Miles Cable Grip™ system (Howmedica, Rutherford, NJ), close follow-up is warranted if the cable has broken or frayed. Metallic debris as a source of three-body wear can accelerate proximal femoral bone loss. If this occurs, removal of the cable grip is suggested. This phenomenon does not seem to occur with monofilament wire.

Early, severe, and rapidly developing osteolysis are signs of probable infection and therefore an ESR and aspiration should be obtained. If test results are positive, resection is indicated. However, if results are negative, the surgeon can proceed with a revision. The extent of revision will depend on the severity of bone loss (see Fig. 6.7).

Conclusion

The evaluation of the painful total hip arthroplasty can be quite complex and challenging. A thorough understanding of the patient's symptoms is the most important and often the limiting factor in the initial evaluation. One has to proceed in an orderly, systematic fashion beginning with the history and physical examination. In the current cost-conscious world the surgeon has to be selective in ordering diagnostic tests. New medical technologies on the horizon such as PCR amplification will, hopefully, improve the accuracy in differentiating septic from aseptic loosening.

References

1. Aufranc OE. *Constructive Surgery of the Hip.* St Louis, Mo: CV Mosby, Inc; 1962:18.
2. Callaghan JJ, Dysart SH, Savoy CG. The uncemented porous-coated anatomic total hip prosthesis: two year results of a prospective consecutive series. *J Bone Joint Surg Am.* 1988;70:337–346.
3. Haddad RJ Jr, Skalley TC, Cook SD, Brinkler MR, Cheramie J, Meyer R, et al. Clinical and roentenographic evaluation of noncemented porous-coated anatomic medullary locking (AML) and porous-coated anatomic (PCA) total hip arthroplasties. *Clin Orthop.* 1990;258:176–182.
4. Engh CA, Massin P, Suther KE. Roentgenographic assessment of the biologic fixation of porous-surfaced femoral components. *Clin Orthop.* 1990;257:107–128.
5. Peroutka RM, McCollum DE, Nunley JA. *Uncemented Primary Porous Coated Anatomic Total Hip Replacements: Preliminary Results.* Hot Springs, Va: American Academy of Orthopaedic Surgeons; 1988.
6. Vaughn BK, Mallory TH, Buchert PK, et al. *Porous Coated Anatomic Cementless Total Hip Replacement: Clinical and Roentgenographic Results with Minimum Two-Year Follow-up.* Atlanta, Ga: American Academy of Orthopaedic Surgeons; 1988.
7. Cook SD, Barrack RL, Thomas KA, Haddad RJ Jr. Quantitative analysis of tissue growth into human porous total hip components. *J Arthroplasty.* 1988;3:249–262.
8. Cook SD, Barrack RL, Thomas KA, Haddad RJ Jr. Tissue growth into porous primary and revision femoral stems. *J Arthroplasty.* 1991;6 Suppl:S37–S46.
9. Fitzgerald RH. Total hip arthroplasty sepsis: prevention and sepsis. *Orthop Clin North Am.* 1992;23:259–264.
10. Eftekhar NS, Stinchfield F. Total replacement of the hip joint by low friction arthroplasty. *Orthop Clin North Am.* 1973;2:483–501.
11. Weber ER, Daube JR, Coventry MB. Peripheral neuropathies associated with total hip arthroplasty. *J Bone Joint Surg Am.* 1976;58:66–69.
12. Schmalzried TP, Amstutz HC, Dorey FJ. Nerve palsy associated with total hip replacement: risk factors and prognosis. *J Bone Joint Surg Am.* 1991;73:1074–1080.

13. Dewolfe VG. Intermittent claudication of the hip and the syndrome of chronic aortoiliac thrombosis. *Circulation.* 1954;9:1–16.
14. Leriche R, Morel A. The syndrome of thromboembolic obliteration of the aortic bifurcation. *Ann Surg.* 1948;127:193–206.
15. Mallory TH. Rupture of the iliac vein from reaming the acetabulum during total hip replacement. *J Bone Joint Surg Am.* 1972;54:276–277.
16. Salama R, Stavorosky MM, Iellin A, Weissman SL. Femoral artery injury complicating total hip replacement. *Clin Orthop.* 1972;89:143–144.
17. Matos MA, Amstutz H, Machleder HI. Ischemia of the lower extremity after total hip replacement. *J Bone Joint Surg Am.* 1979;61:24–27.
18. Forster IW, Crawford R. Sedimentation rate in infected and uninfected total hip arthroplasty. *Clin Orthop.* 1982;168:48–52.
19. Aalto K, Osterman, K, Peltola H, Rasanen J. Changes in erythrocyte sedimentation rate and C-reactive protein after total hip arthroplasty. *Clin Orthop.* 1984;184:118–120.
20. Carlsson AS. Erythrocyte sedimentation rate in infected and unifected total hip arthroplasties. *Acta Orthop Scand.* 1978;49:287–290.
21. Manguson JE, Brown ML, Hauser MF, Berquist TH, Fitzgerald RH Jr, Klee GG. Indium-111-labeled leukocyte scintigraphy in suspected orthopaedic prosthesis infections: comparison with other imaging modalities. *Radiology.* 1988;168:235–239.
22. Patel D, Karchmer A, Harris WH. Role of preoperative aspiration of the hip prior to total hip replacement. *Hip* 1976;219.
23. Amos RS, Constable TJ, Crockson AP, Crockson AP, McConkey B. Rheumatoid arthritis: relation of serum C-reactive protein and erythrocyte sedimentation rates to radiographic changes. *Br Med J.* 1977;1:195–197.
24. Fisher CL, Gill C, Forrester MG, Nakamura R. Quantitation of "acute phase proteins" postoperatively: value in detection and monitoring of complications. *Am J Clin Pathol.* 1976;66:840–846.
25. Wilson PD, Aglietti P, Salvati EA. Subacute sepsis of the hip treated by antibiotics and cemented prosthesis. *J Bone Joint Surg Am.* 1974;56:879–898.
26. Sanzen L, Carlsson AS. The diagnostic value of C-reactive protein in infected total hip arthroplasties. *J Bone Joint Surg Br.* 1989;71:638–641.
27. Harris WH, McCarthy JC, O'Neill DA. Femoral component loosening using contemporary techniques of femoral cement fixation. *J Bone Joint Surg Am.* 1982;64:1063–1067.
28. Harris WH, Peneberg BL. Further follow-up on socket fixation using a metal packed acetabular component for total hip replacement. *J Bone Joint Surg Am.* 1987;69:1140–1143.
29. Lyons CW, Berquist TH, Lyons JC, Rand JA, Brown ML. Evaluation of radiographic findings in painful hip arthroplasties. *Clin Orthop.* 1985;195:239–251.
30. Jasty M, Maloney WJ, Bragdon CR, Haire T, Harris WH. Histomorphological studies of the long-term skeletal responses to well fixed cemented femoral components. *J Bone Joint Surg Am.* 1990;72:1220–1225.
31. Jacobs ME, Koeweiden EM, Slooff TJ. Plain radiographs inadequate for evaluation of the cement bone interface in the hip prosthesis: a cadaver study of femoral stems. *Acta Orthop Scand.* 1989;60:541–543.
32. Hodgkinson JP, Shelley P, Wroblewski BM. The correlation between the roentgenographic appearance and the operative findings at the bone cement junction of the socket in Charnley low friction arthroplasties. *Clin Orthop.* 1988;228:105–109.
33. O'Neill DA, Harris WH. Failed total hip replacement: assessment by plain radiographs, arthrograms, and aspiration of the hip joint. *J Bone Joint Surg Am.* 1984;66:540–546.
34. Wilson MG, Nikpoor N, Aliabadi P, Poss R, Weissman BN. The fate of acetabular allografts after bipolar revision arthroplasty of the hip: a radiographic review. *J Bone Joint Surg Am.* 1989;71:1469–1479.
35. Mulroy RD, Sedlacek RC, O'Connor DO, Estok DM 2d, Harris WH. A technique to detect migration of femoral components of total hip replacements on conventional radiographs. *J Arthroplasty.* 1991;6(suppl):S1–S4.
36. Engh CA, Bobyn JD, Glassman AH. Porous-coated hip replacement: the factors governing bone ingrowth, stress shielding, and clinical results. *J Bone Joint Surg Br.* 1987;69:45–55.
37. Massin P, Schmidt L, Engh CA. Evaluation of cementless acetabular component migration. *J Arthroplasty.* 1989;4:245–251.
38. Alibadii P, Tumeh SS, Weissman BN, McNeil BJ. Cemented total hip prosthesis: radiographic and scintigraphic evaluation. *Radiology.* 1989;173:203–206.
39. Cuckler JM, Star AM, Alivi A, Noto RB. Diagnosis and management of the infected total joint arthroplasty. *Orthop Clin North Am.* 1991;22:523–530.
40. Maus TP, Berquist TH, Bender CE, Rand JA. Arthrographic study of the painful total hip arthroplasty: refined criteria. *Radiology.* 1987;162:721–727.
41. Evans BG, Cuckler JM. Evaluation of the painful total hip arthroplasty. *Orthop Clin North Am.* 1992;23:303–311.
42. Bergstrom B, Lidgren L, Lindberg L. Radiographic abnormalities caused by postoperative infection following total hip arthroplasty. *Clin Orthop.* 1974;99:95–102.
43. Wetzner SM, Newberg AH, McKenzie JD. Radiographic evaluation of the symptomatic hip arthroplasty. In: Turner RH, Scheller AD, eds. *Revision Total Hip Arthroplasty.* New York, NY: Grune & Stratton; 1982:25–48.
44. Hendrix RW, Wixson RL, Rana NA, Rogers LF. Arthrography after total hip arthroplasty: a modified technique used in the diagnosis of pain. *Radiology.* 1983;148:647–652.
45. Hardy DC, Reinus WR, Totty WG, Keyser CK. Arthrography after total hip arthroplasty: utility of postambulation radiographs. *Skeletal Radiol.* 1988;17:20–23.
46. Barrack RL, Tanzer M, Kattapuram SV, Harris WH. The value of contrast arthrography in assessing loosening of symptomatic uncemented total hip components. *Skeletal Radiol.* 1994;23:37–41.
47. Maxon HR, Schneider HJ, Hopson CN, Miller EH, Von Stein DE, Kereiakes JG, et al. A comparative study of indium-111 DTPA radionuclide and iothalamate meglumine roentgenographic arthrography in evaluation of the painful total hip arthroplasty. *Clin Orthop.* 1989;245:156–159.
48. Resnik CS, Fratkin MJ, Cardea JA. Arthroscintigraphic evaluation of the painful total hip prosthesis. *Clin Nucl Med.* 1986;11:242–244.

49. Barrack RL, Harris WH. The value of aspiration of the hip joint before revision total hip arthroplasty. *J Bone Joint Surg Am.* 1993;75:66–76.
50. Fitzgerald RH Jr, Peterson LF, Washington JA 2d, Van Scoy RE, Coventry MB. Bacterial colonization of wounds and sepsis in total hip arthroplasty. *J Bone Joint Surg Am.* 1973;55:1242–1250.
51. Murray WR. Results in patients with total hip replacement arthroplasty. *Clin Orthop.* 1973;95:80–90.
52. Phillips WC, Kattapuram SV. Efficacy of preoperative hip aspiration performed in the radiology department. *Clin Orthop.* 1983;179:141–146.
53. Lachiewicz PF, Rodger GD, Thomason HC. Aspiration of the hip joint before revision total hip arthroplasty: clinical and laboratory factors influencing attainment of a positive culture. *J Bone Joint Surg Am.* 1996;78:749–754.
54. Johnson JA, Christie MJ, Sandler MP, Parks PF Jr, Homra L, Kaye JJ. Detection of occult infection following total hip arthroplasty using sequential technetium-99m HDP bone scintigraphy and indium-111 WBC imaging. *J Nucl Med.* 1988;29:1347–1353.
55. Merkel KD, Brown ML, Dewanagee MK, Fitzgerald RH Jr. Comparison of indium labeled leukocyte imaging with sequential technetium gallium scanning in the detection of low grade musculoskeletal sepsis. *J Bone Joint Surg Am.* 1985;67:465–476.
56. McKillop JH, McKay I, Cuthbert GF, Fogelman I, Gray HW, Sturrock RD. Scintigraphic evaluation of the painful prosthetic joint: a comparison of gallium-67 citrate and indium-111 labeled leukocyte imaging. *Clin Radiol.* 1984;35:239–241.
57. Wukich DK, Abrue SH, Callaghan JJ, Van Nostrand D, Savory CG, Eggli DF, et al. Diagnosis of infection by preoperative scintigraphy with indium labeled white blood cells. *J Bone Joint Surg Am.* 1987;69:1353–1360.
58. Lieberman JR, Huo MH, Schneider R, Salvati EA. Evaluation of painful hip arthroplasties: are technetium bone scans necessary? *J Bone Joint Surg Br.* 1993;75:475–478.
59. Utz JA, Lull RJ, Galvin EG. Asymptomatic total hip prosthesis: natural history determined using Tc-99m MDP bone scans. *Radiology.* 1986;161:509–512.
60. Oswald SG, Van Nostrand D, Savory CG, Callaghan JJ. Three phase bone scan and indium labeled white blood cell scintigraphy following porous coated hip arthroplasty: a prospective study of the prosthesis tip. *J Nucl Med.* 1989;30:1321–1331.
61. Oswald SG, Van Nostrand D, Savory CG, Anderson JH, Callaghan JJ. The acetabulum: a prospective study of three-phase bone and indium white blood cell scintigraphy following porous coated hip arthroplasty. *J Nucl Med.* 1990;31:274–280.
62. Palestro CJ, Kim CK, Swyer AJ, Capozzi JD, Solomon RW, Goldsmith SJ. Total hip arthroplasty: periprosthetic indium-111–labeled leukocyte activity and complementary technetium-99m-sulfur colloid imaging in suspected infection. *J Nucl Med.* 1990;31:1950–1955.
63. Mirra JM, Marder RA, Amstutz HC. The pathology of failed total joint arthroplasty. *Clin Orthop.* 1982;170:175–183.
64. Feldman DS, Lonner JH, Desal P, Zuckerman JD. The role of intraoperative frozen sections in revision total joint arthroplasty. *J Bone Joint Surg Am.* 1995;75:1807–1813.
65. Fehring TK, McAlister JA. Frozen histologic section as a guide to sepsis in total joint arthroplasty. Presented at 58th meeting of the American Academy of Orthopaedic Surgeons, 1991.
66. Harris WH, Barrack RL. Contemporary algorithms for evaluation of the painful total hip replacement. *Orthop Rev.* 1993;22:303–311.
67. Maloney WJ, Smith RL, Schmalzried TP, et al. Isolation and characterization of wear particles in patients who have had failure of a hip arthroplasty without cement. *J Bone Joint Surg Am.* 1995;75:1301–1309.
68. Maloney WJ, Smith RL. Periprosthetic osteolysis in total hip arthroplasty: role of particulate wear debris. *Instr Course Lec.* 1996;45:171–182.
69. Goldring SR, Schiller AL, Roelke M, Rourke CM, O'Neil DA, Harris WH. The synovial-like membrane at the bone cement interface in loose total hip replacements and its proposed role in bone lysis. *J Bone Joint Surg Am.* 1983;65:575–584.
70. Athanasou NA, Quinn J, Bulstrode CJK. Resorption of bone by inflammatory cells derived from the joint capsule of hip arthroplasties. *J Bone Joint Surg Br.* 1992;74:57–62.
71. Murray DW, Rushton N. Macrophages stimulate bone resorption when they phagocytose particles. *J Bone Joint Surg Br.* 1990;72:988–992.
72. Schmalzried TP, Jasty M, Harris WH. Periprosthetic bone loss in total hip arthroplasty: polyethylene wear debris and the concept of the effective joint space. *J Bone Joint Surg Am.* 1992;74:849–863.
73. Jasty MJ, Floyd WE 3d, Schiller AL, Goldring SR, Harris WH. Localized osteolysis in stable, nonseptic total hip replacement. *J Bone Joint Surg Am.* 1986;68:912–919.
74. Maloney WJ, Jasty MJ, Rosenberg A, Harris WH. Bone lysis in well fixed cemented femoral components. *J Bone Joint Surg Br.* 1990;72:966–970.
75. Maloney WJ, Peters P, Engh CA, Chandler H. Severe osteolysis of the pelvis in association with acetabular replacement without cement. *J Bone Joint Surg Am.* 1993;75:1627–1635.
76. Maloney WJ, Jasty M, Harris WH, Galante JO, Callaghan JJ. Endosteal erosion in association with stable uncemented femoral components. *J Bone Joint Surg Am.* 1990;72:1025–1034.
77. Zhinian W, Dorr LD. Natural history of femoral focal osteoylsis with proximal ingrowth smooth stem implant. *J Arthroplasty.* 1996;11:718–725.
78. Hozak WJ, Mesa JL, Carey C, Rothman RH. Relationship between polyethylene wear, pelvic osteolysis, and clinical symptomatology in patients with cementless acetabular components: a framework for decision making. *J Arthroplasty.* 1996;11:769–772.
79. Gruen TA, McNeice GM, Amstutz HC. Modes of failure of cemented stem type femoral components–A radiographic analysis of loosening. *Clin Orthrop and Rel Rsch.* 1979;141:17–27.

7
Radiographic Evaluation of the Painful Total Hip Arthroplasty

Arthur H. Newberg, Steven M. Wetzner, and John M. Ellis

The successful development of reliable total hip arthroplasty for the treatment of severely diseased hips has led to its increasing application, with more than 200,000 implants placed in the United States each year. As with any mode of therapy, the more frequent its use, the greater the chance of complications or failure.

Ten percent of total hip arthroplasties will require revision after 10 years because of loosening. Component failure in the total hip arthroplasty is a complex mechanism, involving mechanical, biologic, and structural factors that affect the integrity of the component as a whole. The most frequent of these complications are component loosening[1] and osteolysis secondary to particle disease related to the shedding of the high molecular weight polyethylene in the acetabular component.

Differentiation of aseptic loosening from infection can be a clinical and diagnostic dilemma. The presenting symptom in both loosening and infection is most often a painful arthroplasty.[2] The clinician must use information derived from sequential plain films, radionuclide studies, and aspiration with or without arthrography of the affected joint. Plain radiographs of septic hip prostheses often show normal findings but can show focal bone loss that mimics aggressive granulomatosis. In the end, no matter how methodical the work-up, clinical judgment may be the deciding factor in dictating the appropriate treatment option. The following discussion attempts to integrate the various imaging modalities and how they can be used to help sort out the difficult problems of the hip arthroplasty patient.

Radiography

The radiographic evaluation of the total hip arthroplasty allows analysis of the components' interactive environment among the bone, acrylic cement, metal, and high-density polyethylene. Routine radiographs remain the most important diagnostic imaging modality in the evaluation of a painful total hip arthroplasty. The availability of sequential films that are obtained in a reproducible fashion will be sufficient in most cases to assess whether or not the implant and its host bone have undergone a change over time (Fig. 7.1).

In addition to an anteroposterior radiograph of the pelvis including both hips, a true lateral view of the postoperative hip will give the best assessment of the anteversion or retroversion of the acetabular component. The acetabular component ideally is placed in slight anteversion or forward flexion. The actual degree of acetabular anteversion can be measured only on the true lateral radiograph. The degree of apparent anteversion seems to vary considerably with the accuracy in centering the film over the acetabulum.[3] In addition, we have used the modified Lowenstein as part of the routine radiographic film series. This view is a modified frog lateral view of the affected hip. The knee is flexed on the affected side, and the thigh is drawn up to at least a 45° angle. The patient is rotated so that the affected thigh touches the top of the radiographic table. This view optimizes assessment of the acetabulum and femoral shaft. The proximal half of the femur should be included on the radiograph as well[4] (Fig. 7.2). One final point must be emphasized. It is imperative that the entire prosthesis, including the area below the tip of the femoral component, be included on the radiographs. Position change, component fracture, motion, or infection can easily be missed if the information is not visible.

Another recently described plain film view is the caudal oblique view, which may be useful in assessing preoperatively whether there is a large posterior bony defect in the acetabulum that may require bone grafting.[5] It has been demonstrated that routine views, even including Judet obliques (45° anterior and posterior radiographs), may underestimate these posterior defects. These defects are often discovered at the time of acetabular revision surgery. If these defects can be evalu-

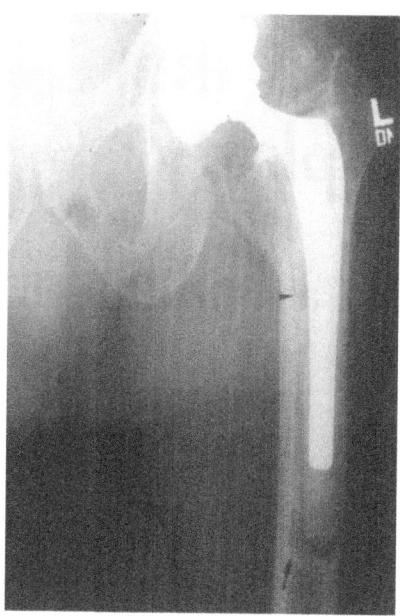

Figure 7.1. Anteroposterior (AP) radiograph of the left hip demonstrating femoral component loosening. There is a cement fracture (arrowhead) and osteolysis distal to the cement mantle (arrow).

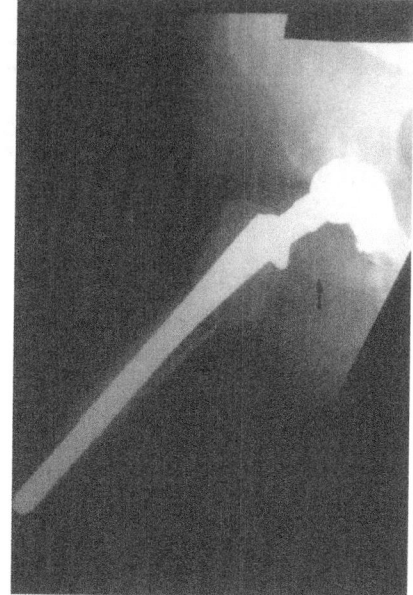

Figure 7.2. Example of the modified Lowenstein view of the hip. Note the polyethylene wear in the cup resulting in marked femoral head asymmetry within the acetabulum. There is also evidence of metal synovitis characterized by increased density in the periarticular soft tissues (arrow).

ated preoperatively, better preop planning will be possible for the type of graft and materials that will be needed at the time of surgery. This view is obtained by rotating the affected hip anteriorly about 30°, a position similar to that used in the obturator Judet oblique. Next the central x-ray beam is oriented by angling the tube 30° to the feet (caudad) (Fig. 7.3).

Some investigators have advocated the use of computed tomography (CT) in the assessment of total hip arthroplasties.[6] This technique is limited to date because of the metal artifact. We have used CT, however, to look for periprosthetic abscess or intraabdominal or pelvic fluid collections. In addition, 3D CT software programs have been developed to allow the design of custom total hip implants in patients with extremely narrow medullary cavities, as is often seen in juvenile chronic arthritis (JRA) or hip dysplasia.

Plain Film Radiography

The plain film diagnosis of loosening of cemented prosthetic components has been defined radiographically by the presence of radiolucent lines at cement–bone or metal–cement interfaces. Various factors are thought to contribute to loosening, including insufficient cement or uneven cement distribution; presence of less than 1 cm of cement between the calcar and the stem; insufficient removal of cancellous bone lateral to the stem; insufficient cement beyond the stem tip; and positioning of the femoral component in alignment other than slight valgus.[7] Loosening of a cemented stem is usually identified by change in position of the stem, cement fracture, prosthesis fracture, or development of progressive radiolucent lines (Fig. 7.4). Lucent lines that measure 1 to 2 mm and are nonprogressive are probably not signifi-

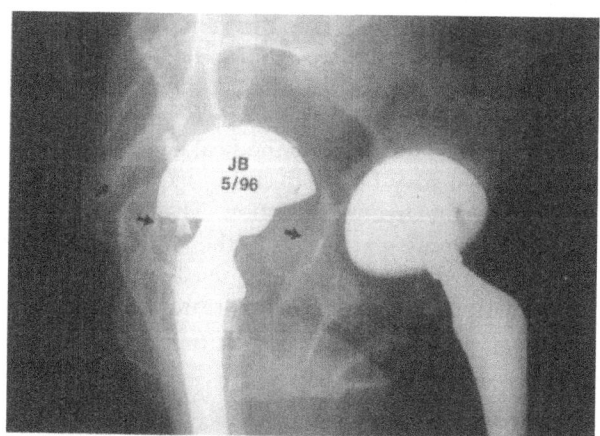

Figure 7.3. The caudal oblique view is helpful in detecting bony deficiencies. This failed revision arthroplasty demonstrates both anterior and posterior bony defects (arrows), suggestive of pelvic discontinuity that was indeed found at the time of surgery.

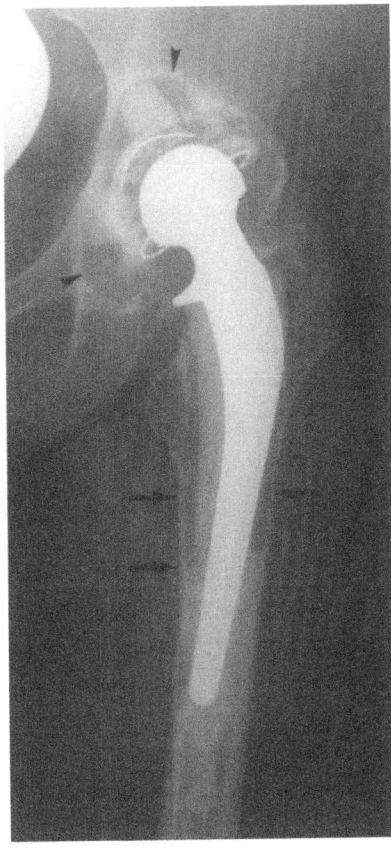

Figure 7.4. AP radiograph demonstrating loose cemented acetabular and femoral components. Note the thinning of the femoral cortex secondary to osteolysis (arrows). The polyethylene cup shows increased radiolucencies at the cement–bone interface (arrowheads).

patient did the radiographic findings change the clinical management. Some investigators have recommended postoperative radiographs at 6 weeks, 3 months, 6 months, and then every 6 to 12 months thereafter. The time intervals at which to perform radiography in asymptomatic patients are less straightforward. To our knowledge, the only potentially asymptomatic complications of hip arthroplasty are stress shielding and aggressive granulomatosis[11] (Fig. 7.5).

Mechanical friction between the components during movement wears small (1–4 μm) particles away from the polyethylene surface. This debris incites a foreign body granulomatous reaction that induces localized bone resorption. Migration of this debris and its accompanying reaction along cement–bone or metal–bone interfaces may lead to loosening.[12] Wear debris has evolved as the major player in mechanical loosening of cemented as well as uncemented arthroplasties. Osteolysis results from particle debris formation and this has been most commonly reported secondary to polyethylene wear debris.[13,14] The radiographs in these patients

cant. On the other hand, if lucencies are greater than 2 mm and progressive on sequential films, this picture probably represents true loosening.[8] Aliabadi and coworkers[9] found that a complete radiolucent line of 2 mm or wider along the femoral interface on conventional radiographs proved to be 54% sensitive and 96% specific for loosening.

Ectopic cement distribution should be noted. Rarely, cement in the pelvis has eroded the bladder and/or femoral vessels, with resultant sepsis and hemorrhage or hematuria.[10] In addition, the extension of cement through breaks in the femoral shaft cortex should be noted. Such breaks may be potential sites of component failure. Examination of the AP pelvis film may yield information with regard to the postoperative presence of protrusio acetabuli or stress fractures of the ischium.

It is difficult to know exactly how often patients should have follow-up radiographic studies. Certainly, clinical findings are more important in determining clinical management than are the results of radiography. In one study[11] of 148 postoperative patients, in only one

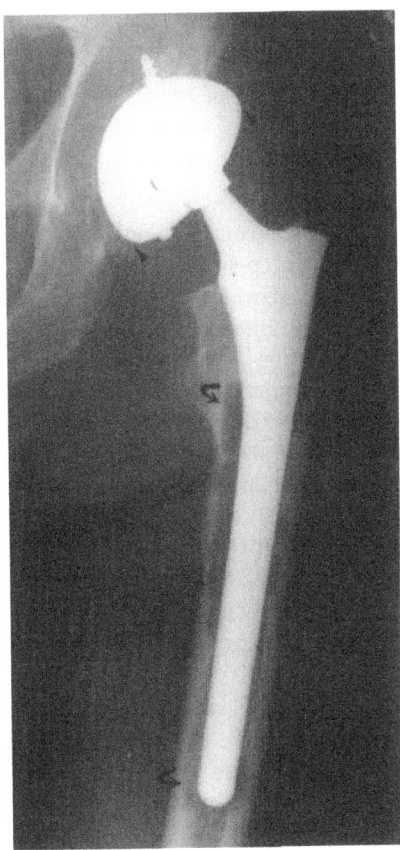

Figure 7.5. Radiograph of the hip demonstrating aggressive granulomatosis (curved arrows) of the femur in an uncemented total hip replacement. Note the asymmetry of the cup due to polyethylene wear (arrowheads).

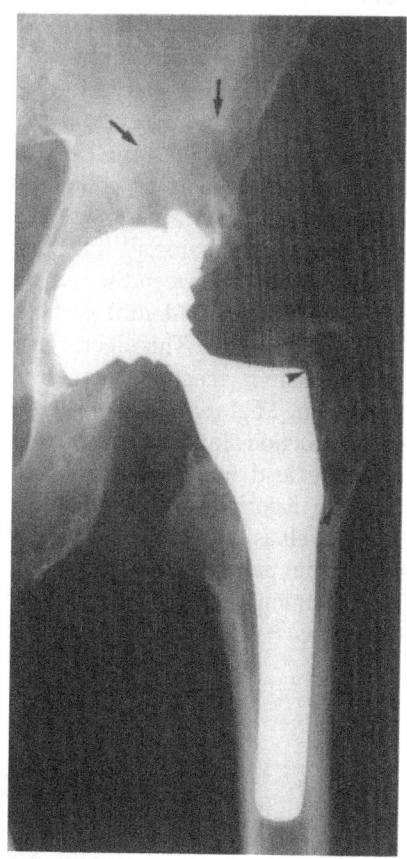

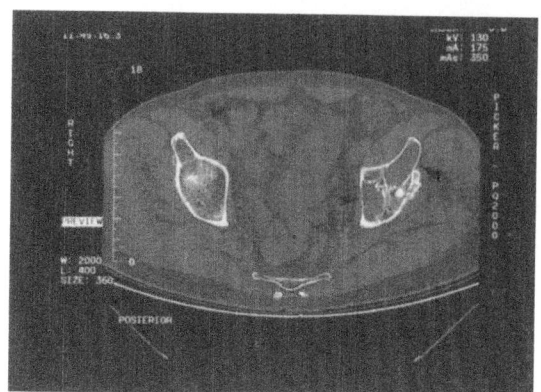

Figure 7.6. (A) Radiograph demonstrating acetabular osteolysis mimicking a bone tumor (arrows). There is also asymmetry of the femoral component in the cup due to wear as well as proximal femoral osteolysis (arrowheads). (B) Image from an axial CT scan through the supra-acetabular area demonstrating the pseudotumor appearance created by aggressive granulomatosis (arrowheads).

will show areas of bone destruction[15] (Fig. 7.6). Because of this phenomenon, pelvic osteolysis is becoming a more frequent indication for revision, and its incidence will most likely continue to increase, as documented with long-term studies.[16] Osteolysis secondary to wear debris on the acetabular side may produce large areas of bone destruction, so destructive that they may in fact mimic tumor in older patients. On the femoral side, one may see variable focal areas of osteolysis presenting as focal areas of endosteal cortical bone erosion. The plain film differentiation between particle debris osteolysis and sepsis can be difficult and sometimes impossible.

We also evaluate sequential plain radiographs for the development of cup asymmetry to help decide whether there is cup wear (Fig. 7.7). Because in most acetabular components the polyethylene liner is of equal diameter, if on follow-up radiographs asymmetry is seen between the femoral prosthetic head and the cup one can conclude there has been poly wear. As a secondary phenomenon, if the polyethylene liner wears through, one may see increased density in the joint representing metal synovitis. Separation of the polyethylene from the metal also allows metal-on-metal friction, which sheds metal fragments into the joint. Metal deposition is seen radiographically as dense, sometimes curvilinear, deposits in a periarticular distribution.[17] Usually the plain films show superolateral displacement of the femoral component within the acetabulum as a manifestation of the wear of the cup (Fig. 7.8). Histologically, one sees the

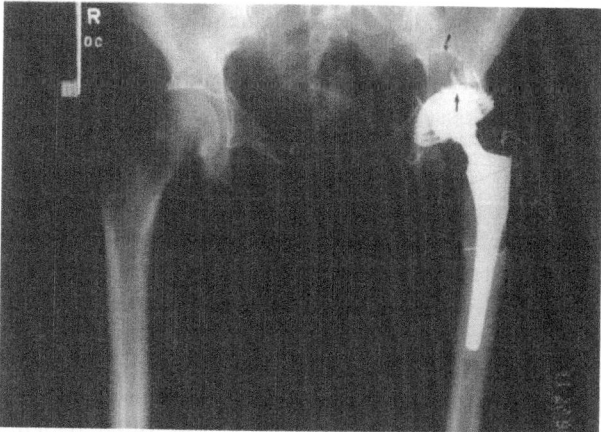

Figure 7.7. AP radiograph demonstrating polyethylene wear of the cup. There has been superior migration of the femoral component (arrow), and there is osteolysis in the acetabulum (curved arrow).

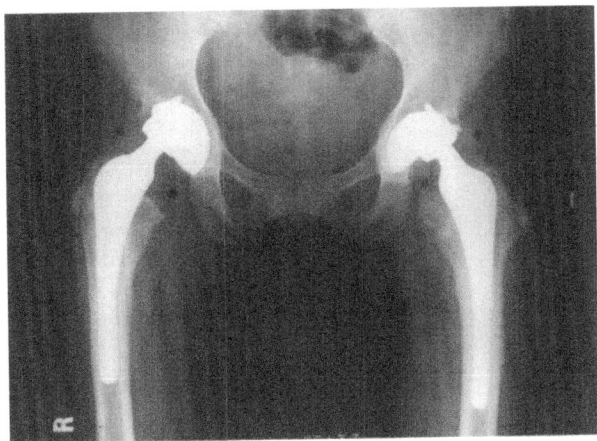

Figure 7.8. Radiograph illustrating bilateral metal synovitis characterized by increased density around the acetabular soft tissues (arrows). Note the marked wear of the acetabular components resulting in metal-to-metal contact.

off of the medial femoral neck (calcar area), and an overall decrease in proximal femoral bone density.

Loosening of these uncemented stems is suggested by lucent zones of 2 mm or more, shedding of implant surface beads, or well-defined areas of osteolysis representing the granulomatous response to polyethylene debris. A study by Kattapuram et al.[18] revealed that subsidence was the most important indicator of clinical outcome. Subsidence is said to occur when the medullary cavity is too wide relative to the stem, which allows the prosthesis to settle. Subsidence was measured as the distance from the superomedial extent of the porous coating to the most superomedial point of the calcar (Fig. 7.10). If subsidence stabilized without progressing to more than 5 mm, the hips in this series had excellent clinical results.

Focal cortical thickening may be seen and is most likely the result of localized increase in stress transfer from the prosthesis to bone. This finding may occur when there is motion or poor fixation of the prosthesis

metallic materials imbedded in the periarticular cells and interstitium.

Therefore, even in the aymptomatic patient, radiographic follow-up is indicated to screen for aggressive osteolysis accompanying arthroplasty failure. Aggressive foreign body osteolysis usually begins 3 years or more postoperatively and therefore asymptomatic patients should be screened beginning 3 years postop.

Evaluation of Uncemented Stems

According to some surgeons and in some institutions, advances in technology point to the use of a reverse hybrid hip. In these cases an uncemented stem, which allows for bone ingrowth, is combined with a cemented cup. With the use of porous-coated implants, the surgeon hopes to achieve a cancellous metaphyseal bond by using the distal stem merely as a keel to counteract bending stresses. These stems must be evaluated over time for changes that may indicate loosening. In these bone ingrowth stems, one may see "spot welds" representing focal areas of new bone growing to the surface of the ingrowth material. Sclerotic lines are often noted about the smooth portions of femoral components, and they represent a reaction to fibrous tissue. When sclerotic lines completely outline the bone ingrowth area, fibrous ingrowth rather than bone ingrowth has taken place. A bony pedestal at the distal tip of a bone ingrowth component suggests loosening particularly when the component has long areas for bone ingrowth (Fig. 7.9). Bone resorption in areas of the femur that are relatively unstressed (termed stress-shielding) indicates that bone ingrowth fixation has occurred. This bone loss is seen proximally as thinning of the cortex, rounding

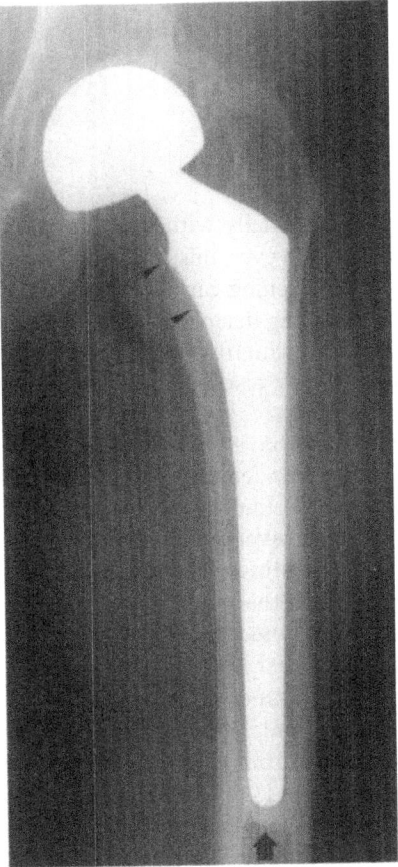

Figure 7.9. Radiograph demonstrating a loose, subsided bipolar arthroplasty. Note the bead-shedding proximally (arrowheads). There is pedestal formation adjacent to the distal tip of the femoral component (arrow).

Figure 7.10. (A and B) AP radiographs of the right hip 4 years apart. There is progression of the subsidence. Note the relationship of the proximal medial femoral stem to the calcar femoris (arrowheads).

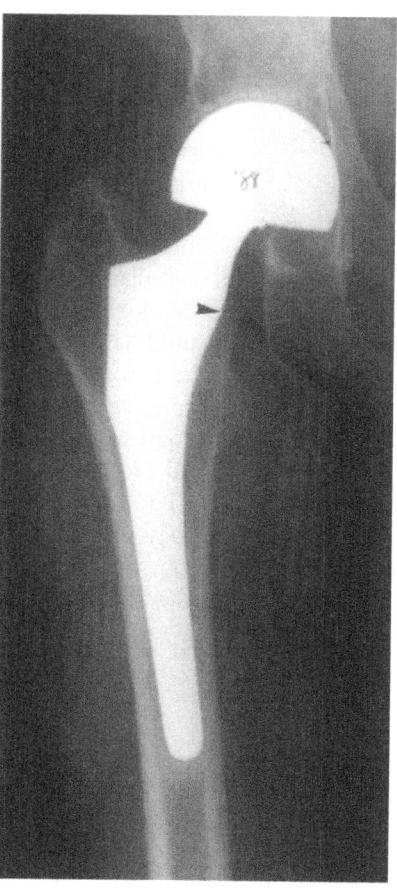
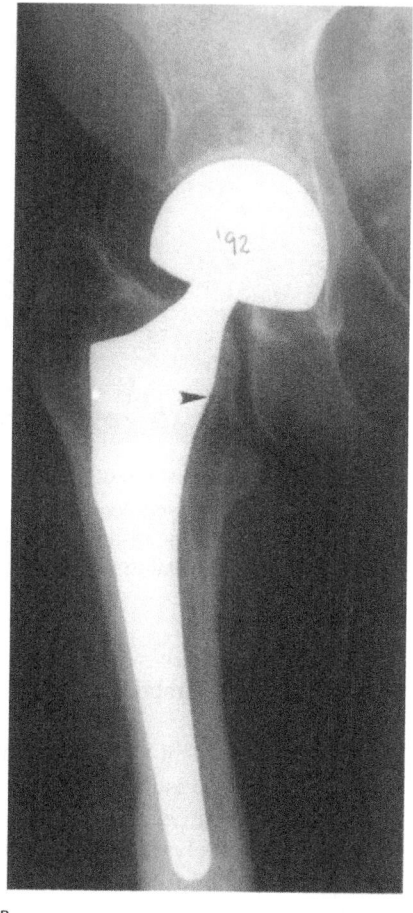

A

B

proximally and medially with lateral migration of the distal stem tip. However, this finding is nonspecific because cortical thickening can also represent an accommodative remodeling that occurs when the femur flexes relative to the firmly ingrown rigid prosthesis. Thus cortical thickening may also indicate a successful arthroplasty.[19]

In patients who have undergone high-pressure cement techniques for femoral component insertion, a rare postoperative finding is the identification on postop films of intravenous methyl methacrylate.[20,21] With current cementing techniques, methylmethacrylate is packed into the medullary cavity under high pressure with a cement gun. This intravascular cement will appear as a linear line of increased density in the medial thigh soft tissues originating from the medial cortex of the proximal femur and extending proximally toward the groin (Fig. 7.11). This intravenous cement may extend for a variable distance. Intravascular cement is not associated with any postoperative complications and is merely a radiographic curiosity not to be misinterpreted as a foreign body. Rarely, drain fragments can be left behind; in one reported case they are alleged to have contributed to postop dislocation.[22]

Evaluation for Heterotopic Ossification

Postoperative heterotopic bone (HO) is another complication that occurs in patients who have undergone multiple hip operations. It is also associated with ankylos-

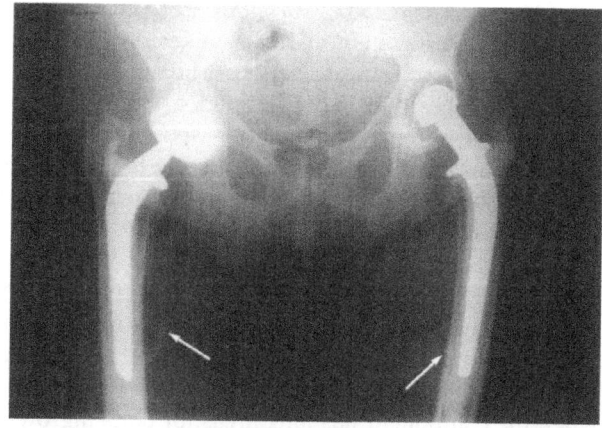

Figure 7.11. Pelvis radiograph demonstrating intravenously injected methylmethacrylate in medial thigh soft tissue bilaterally characterized by a density that is somewhat linear in shape (arrows).

ing spondylitis, possibly diffuse idiopathic skeletal hyperosotosis (DISH), extensive intraoperative trauma, hypertrophic osteoarthritis, and posttraumatic arthritis.[23] The most common clinical signs are pain and decreased range of motion. Up to 30% of patients presenting with radiographic signs of peri-implant HO will develop typical clinical symptoms, which include increasing pain and restricted hip motion leading to complete ankylosis of the hip. Hip aspiration in the patient with HO can be difficult because it may be difficult to gain access into the joint capsule from an anterolateral route. In some cases, the hip aspiration might be better performed under CT guidance, wherein the needle can be placed into the joint where the CT scan demonstrates there is a small area devoid of HO. This will make access into the joint easier than that accomplished with ordinary fluoroscopic guidance.[24] Patients who undergo resection of HO are treated with perioperative radiotherapy.[23,25] Prophylactic perioperative radiotherapy has successfully prevented progression of HO in more than 90% of all high-risk patients.

Evaluation of Dislocation

In addition to the radiographic observations relating to the integrity of the components and their relation to the host bone, other radiographic observations regarding the configuration and position of the prosthesis are notable. Dislocation of the components most commonly occurs in the immediate postoperative period and relates to either improper positioning of the patient's leg during that time or improper positioning of the components. When dislocation occurs later than 3 months postoperatively, it is usually indicative of malposition of components, overzealous rehabilitation, or possibly subsidence of the components. The position of the greater trochanter relative to the lateral acetabular rim is of importance. A high trochanter at this level can act as a lever to facilitate dislocation as it abuts the acetabular rim during abduction. In addition, excessive anteversion or retroversion of the acetabular component potentiates the chance for dislocation.

The need to relocate a dislocated hip necessitates some degree of urgency. In the past, these relocations were performed in the radiology department on the radiographic fluoroscopy table. Patients undergoing this procedure in the x-ray department with mild intravenous sedation often experienced increased pain and morbidity. In addition, the procedure required a number of assistants to help with the relocation. Currently, we recommend prompt reduction of the dislocated hip in the operating room under anesthesia. This has resulted in increased patient satisfaction and less chance for femoral fracture during the attempted relocation.

Aspiration and Arthrography

Contrast arthrography is a common procedure used for evaluating prosthetic hip complications, especially loosening and infection. There is some controversy, however, as to the utility of this procedure. Some investigators have reported that arthrography is not uniformly effective in detecting loosening of the components.[26] As a result, some radiology departments use arthrography only as far as is necessary to place the needle into the prosthetic hip joint for aspiration in those patients in whom there is suspicion of sepsis.

A number of methods have been suggested to improve resolution, including subtraction arthrography, color subtraction, and digital subtraction arthrography.[27-29] Of more importance than the choice of method, however, seems to be the technique of performing the arthrogram. Use of high injection pressures and/or postambulation arthrograms have increased diagnostic accuracy.[30,31] By using improved techniques and refined criteria for interpretation, some investigators have reported an accuracy of 96% for both acetabular and femoral component loosening.[32]

The technique of placing a needle into the prosthetic hip joint requires careful attention to detail. Under fluoroscopic guidance we place an opaque marker over the anterolateral aspect of the hip joint that will be studied. We recommend that the skin be marked in an area corresponding to the upper edge of the greater trochanter. This anterolateral approach avoids all vessels and provides a direct route into the joint. This anterolateral position of the needle also allows it to be fluoroscopically discerned from the underlying prosthesis without any overlap. If a direct anterior approach is used, the needle may be obscured by the prosthesis. With the use of a standard commercially available arthrogram tray, the radiologist—who is gloved and masked—prepares the patient's skin. Local anesthetic is instilled into the skin and subcutaneous tissues. We have recently started adding about 2 mL of an 8.4% solution of sodium bicarbonate to 8 mL of 1% lidocaine. This combination of local anesthetic and bicarbonate apparently neutralizes the acidity of the local anesthetic agent and has resulted in a marked decrease in patient pain and discomfort, leading to better patient acceptance during the anesthetizing process. Care should be taken not to introduce anesthetic into the hip joint because it is a bacteriostatic solution.

Next, a 20-gauge, 3-inch needle is advanced into the hip joint. The patient may experience some discomfort as the capsule is perforated. The needle placement is constantly checked fluoroscopically. We attempt to place the needle on the prosthetic femoral neck. One can actually feel the metal scraping the needle tip if it is in the correct place. Almost all hips do have some joint fluid. The fluid is gently aspirated, and all air is removed from the syringe before the specimen is sent to the laboratory for gram stain as well as aerobic and anaerobic cultures. The necessary laboratory forms should be correctly filled out. If the patient was receiving antibiotics for an infected hip, these should have been discontinued 3 weeks before the procedure, if possible. If there is sufficient fluid aspirated, one can also consider sending a separate specimen to be analyzed for cell count, differential, and polyethylene wear debris analysis under polarized light. However, the physician must be sure that the laboratory is equipped to perform the latter test. If the only procedure to be performed is an aspiration, the needle is withdrawn, and the procedure is complete.

If no fluid can be obtained, several additional maneuvers can be tried. First, the needle position can be changed. This should be done below the skin surface. Every attempt should be made to avoid violating the skin surface more than once. If the needle is removed we will often use a new needle for the second stick. One can introduce 5 mL of nonbacteriostatic saline. If the saline cannot be reaspirated, one can be almost certain that the needle is not intraarticular. An alternative measure is to inject a small amount of radiographic contrast material. This will serve two purposes: first, it will confirm whether the needle is indeed intraarticular (if the contrast flows quickly away from the tip of the needle); second, the contrast material can be reaspirated and sent to the laboratory for culture and sensitivities as well as gram stain. Radiographic contrast material is not bacteriostatic. If the injected contrast streaks diagonally across the femoral neck, the needle is extraarticular and most likely in the psoas sheath despite the tactile feeling that the needle is touching the prosthetic femoral neck.

Not all patients who are about to undergo a revision hip arthroplasty need to have a preoperative aspiration or arthrogram. Gould et al.[33] prospectively studied 78 patients undergoing revision arthroplasty. In their series, they found no cases of infection in patients with a low suspicion of infection. They concluded that routine percutaneous hip aspirations do not need to be performed when a revision is contemplated if the clinical suspicion for infection is low. Hip aspiration and arthrography should not be eliminated, however, when the clinical suspicion is equivocal or high or there is no apparent cause for the patient's pain. It should be remembered that septic loosening is much less common than aseptic loosening, with less than 1% of loose hip prostheses being infected. Tigges et al.[34] have noted that hip aspiration is an accurate and cost-effective method of evaluating the potentially infected hip prosthesis. In their study, they were able to diagnose infection accurately in 13 of 14 infected hips and to rule out infection in 122 of 133 cases. Fitzgerald[35] reserves aspiration and arthrogram for evaluation of patients with non-inflammatory arthritis and a painful total hip arthroplasty who have an elevated ESR or an elevated C-reactive protein concentration.

If the radiologist is also performing an arthrogram, we connect the dye to the needle via a syringe filled with about 25 mL of contrast material and the extension tubing that is included with the arthrogram tray. First, under fluoroscopic guidance the prosthesis is positioned in the center of the fluoroscopic field. A 14" × 14" film is used, and the film is split on the control panel to obtain two separate fluoroscopic spot films. A scout film is obtained after the needle and tubing are connected and the injection is ready to begin. The second spot radiograph is obtained with the patient in the same position after about 10 mL of contrast has been injected. The film is then exchanged for another 14" × 14" cassette. This film is divided into three sections and an exposure is obtained centering on the femoral component. Contrast is constantly injected during this time. The end point of the injection is the point at which the patient experiences pain or when about 20 to 25 mL has been injected. We then perform push-and-pull films with the remaining two exposures. After the procedure is completed, because the needle has been left in place during the entire procedure, the contrast is withdrawn to decrease postprocedure patient discomfort. In rare cases we need to instill 2% lidocaine along with the contrast. This is occasionally done to evaluate the troublesome arthroplasty that shows no abnormalities on sequential plain films. In these cases, the contrast is obviously not withdrawn but the needle is removed.

A recent report by Braunstein and coworkers[36] described the instillation of bupivacaine along with the contrast material to assess for pain relief. The investigators suggest that this technique may be valuable to assess whether the pain is coming from an intracapsular source. They added 7 mL of bupivacaine to about 10 to 15 mL of radiographic contrast material. We do not ambulate our patients with contrast in the hip joint. This technique has been advocated by Hardy and coworkers[30] in an attempt to increase the accuracy of detecting loosening after hip arthrography. In their study, they had improved detection of prosthetic loosening by using postexercise arthrography. Nearly half of their study group had improved visualization of the pertinent findings on postambulation radiographs.

Arthrography in uncemented stems may be more difficult to assess. Barrack et al.[37] found that uncemented femoral component loosening had a sensitivity of 57%, specificity of 60%, and accuracy of 58%. In their study, there were relatively high incidences of both false-negatives and false-positives. The investigators believe that arthrography has distinct limitations in identifying the fixation status of uncemented total hip components. They postulate that extensive ingrowth can coexist with enough empty space in the porous surface to allow contrast penetration and tracking, resulting in a false-positive result.

To improve visualization of the contrast–bone and contrast–metal interface, conventional subtraction arthrography can also be used. In this technique, however, it is imperative that the patient not move between radiographic exposures. The inability to hold still in these often difficult patients may be a limiting factor. Also the technique requires time, extra darkroom manipulation of the images, and patient cooperation.

We[28] and others[29] have used digital subtraction arthrography in the assessment of prosthetic hip components (Fig. 7.12). This technique may be better than others in assessing loosening because it does allow real time visualization of the contrast material.[29] Walker et al.[27] demonstrated that digital subtraction arthrography of the femoral component demonstrated a 96% sensitivity and 100% specificity for loosening. Sensitivity and specificity for acetabular loosening were 83% and 80%, respectively. In addition, digital images were superior in demonstrating lymphatic or vascular opacification.

Another arthrographic technique that has not met with widespread acceptance is nuclear arthrography.[38] This technique advocates combining radiographic contrast material with the isotope and injecting both into the hip joint. It is suggested that the advantage of nuclear arthrography is that the viscosity of the saline vehicle in which the isotope has been dissolved is less than that of contrast material. Therefore, the radionuclide is better able to penetrate small areas of loosening at bone–

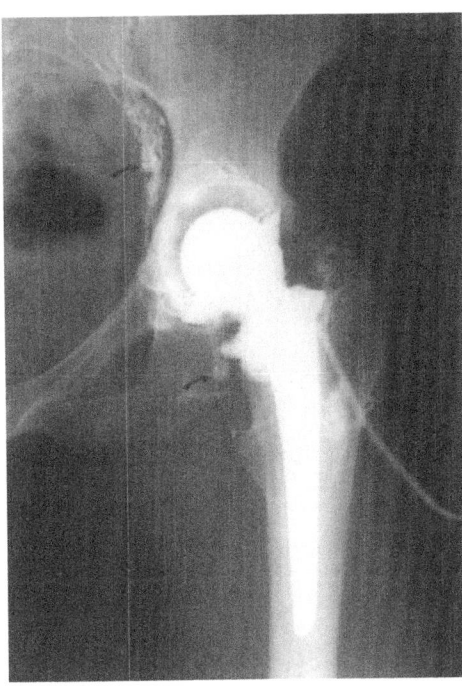

Figure 7.13. Radiograph obtained during a hip aspiration–arthrogram. Both components are loose, and there is marked lymphatic opacification (arrows).

cement or bone–metal interfaces. Contrast plus nuclear arthrography together are better than either alone in making a diagnosis of loosening.

Some of the false-negative results of arthrography can be explained on the basis of interposition soft tissue (such as granulation tissue, fibrous tissue, or pus) blocking passage of contrast into the metal–cement or cement–bone interface. Another reason for false-negative results can be large bursae or cavities around the prosthesis, which may hinder filling of the interfaces because of reduced injection pressure.[29]

Lymphatic opacification during hip arthrography is usually related to one of three etiologies: pressure of injection, overdistention of the joint capsule, or an inflammatory process in the synovium (Fig. 7.13). There is no correlation between lymphatic opacification during a hip arthrogram and prosthetic loosening with or without infection.[39,40] On the other hand, filling of venous structures is usually seen in loosening of components (Fig. 7.14). In patients with recurrent dislocation we have often noted the filling of a large posterior hip pseudobursa, which may represent a chronically distended joint capsule from the repeated dislocations (Fig. 7.15). This large bursal cavity probably needs to be resected at the time of revision surgery. Berquist et al.[41] reported on the appearance of bursae around the hip in arthroplasty patients. These bursae can be a source of pain especially with those occurring around

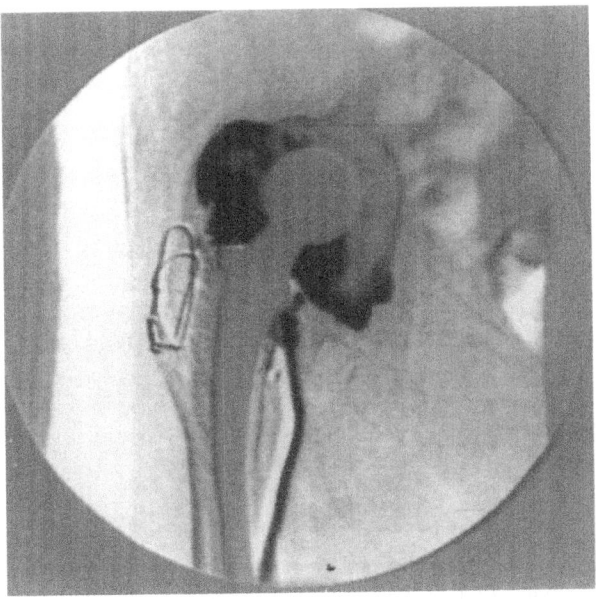

Figure 7.12. Image from a digital subtraction arthrogram showing loosening of both the femoral and acetabular components of this cemented hip arthroplasty.

Part 2. Evaluation of the Painful Total Hip Arthroplasty

the acetabulum and those located over the greater trochanter.

The patient who has had the total hip arthroplasty removed because of infection (ie, the resected hip arthroplasty patient or the Girdlestone arthroplasty patient), may require frequent or follow-up joint aspiration to assess the results of antibiotic treatment and possibly help determine the proper time for a new reimplanted hip. These patients require a modified technique for hip aspiration. Obtaining fluid for culture is particularly challenging in these patients; therefore we fluoroscopically localize a point midway between the medial and lateral edges of the proximal femur.[42] This corresponds to a point bisecting the greater and lesser trochanters (Fig. 7.16). The skin overlying this area is then prepped and the needle advanced straight down into the pseudojoint in an attempt to aspirate fluid for culture. This area is more likely to yield joint fluid than the area of the patient's true acetabulum, which in most cases will not yield a successful joint aspiration.

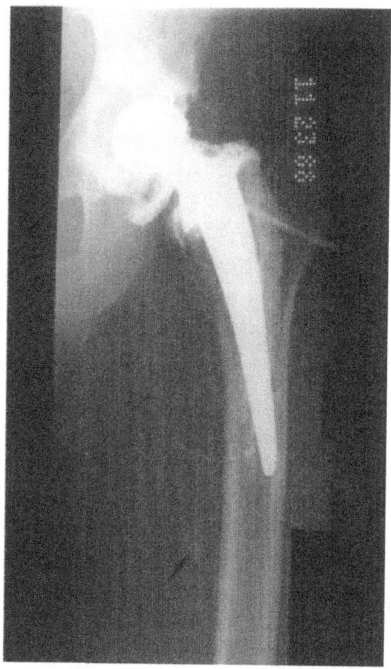

Figure 7.14. A representatve fluoroscopic spot film obtained during an aspiration and arthrogram. The femoral component is loose, and there is both venous (arrow) and lymphatic (open arrows) opacification in the medial thigh. These findings are supportive evidence of component loosening.

Evaluation of Infection

Sepsis in the total hip arthroplasty patient has decreased markedly since this surgical procedure was first introduced. Deep postoperative infections occur in less than

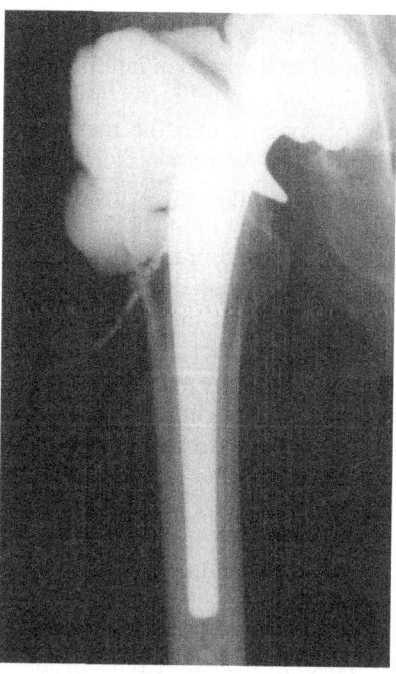

Figure 7.15. Fluoroscopic spot film demonstrating a large collection of injected contrast material filling a prominent pseudobursa posterior to the hip joint. The patient had a history of recurrent dislocations.

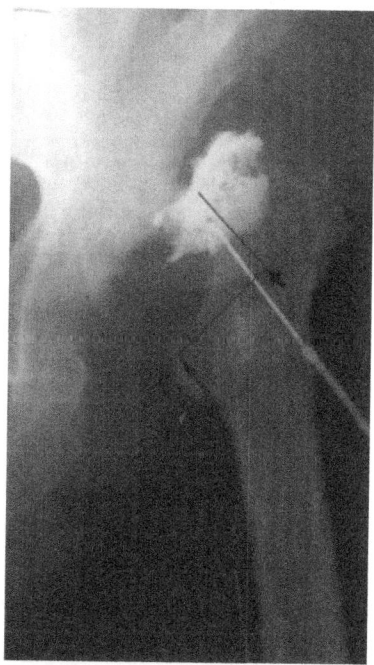

Figure 7.16. Spot radiograph demonstrating the technique for performing a hip aspiration in the Girdlestone arthroplasty patient. The needle has been placed midway between the trochanters and confirmed to be within the pseudocapsule with a small amount of injected contrast material.

0.5% of arthroplasty patients.[35] The diagnosis of deep sepsis around a total hip replacement can be made on the basis of the clinical history and physical examination in approximately 25% of patients.[35] In 50% of patients, the diagnosis of infection may require the use of laboratory investigation, including radiography, culture of joint aspirates, nuclear imaging, and blood tests (white count and sedimentation rate).

There is no apparent set timeframe for the occurrence of postoperative infection in the hip arthroplasty patient. The incidence of delayed sepsis appears to increase as the postoperative interval lengthens. Early infections tend to be fulminant in character, whereas late infections may either be fulminant or indolent (Fig. 7.17). Patients undergoing reoperations have an increased incidence of infection, twice that associated with the virgin hip. Prosthetic loosening is a severe complication of joint space infection, accounting for 7% to 56% of the total number of loose prostheses. Delay in treatment of an infected joint promotes increased bone destruction with resultant loosening of components.

It is usually difficult to distinguish between loosening secondary to infection versus mechanical factors on the basis of either plain radiographs or arthrography. The diagnosis usually rests on the results of culture of the joint aspirate. There are, however, some radiographic findings that indicate infection. Plain radiographs in sepsis often show normal findings but can show focal bone loss that mimics aggressive granulomatosis.[43] Rapid bone resorption and widening of the radiolucent zone at the bone–cement interface greater than 2 mm both suggest the possibility of infection. Similarly, the presence of periosteal new bone adjacent to the proximal femur is suggestive of infection (Fig. 7.18). During an arthrogram, filling of adjacent abscess cavities or communication with periarticular cavities may suggest an infected joint. Dussault et al.[44] found five patients in whom there was contrast filling of such communicating cavities; these patients were subsequently proven to have infected hip replacements.[44]

Lymphatic opacification during arthrography may be minimally suggestive of infection; more likely, it represents synovial inflammation. This finding must be considered nonspecific and may relate to the volume of contrast injected during arthrography, as well as to the force of the injection. Unfortunately, plain film radiographic abnormal findings are present in only 1% to 2% of patients with infected arthroplasties. In spite of radiographic evaluation, in the end surgical exploration alone may be the definitive method for diagnosing infection of prosthetic joints, because hips with negative culture results may have confirmed infection at surgery. This is most likely due to the surgeon's ability to obtain specimens from the actual joint space during surgery, as op-

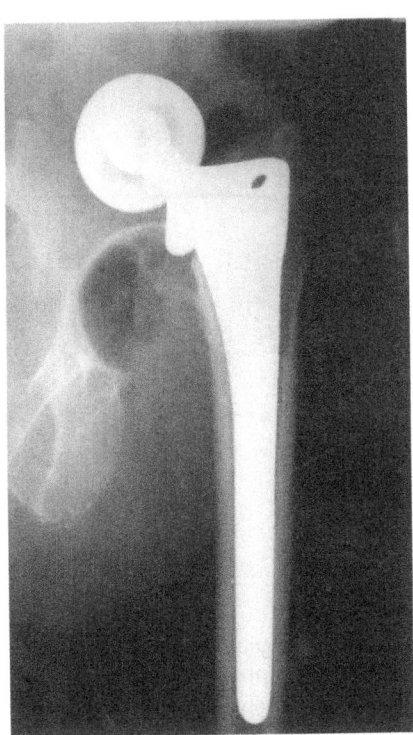

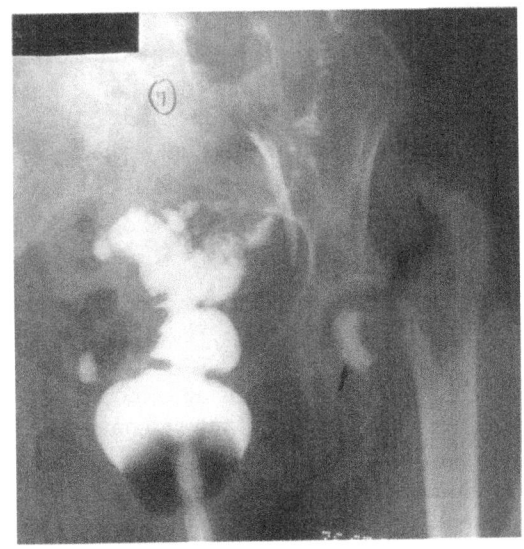

Figure 7.17. (A) Postoperative radiograph of the left hip demonstrating a septic dislocation of a left hip bipolar arthroplasty. There is air in the joint space. The arthroplasty was inserted 3 weeks earlier for a hip fracture. (B) Radiograph taken after a barium enema demonstrating diverticulae in the sigmoid colon. There is an extraluminal streak of barium, and there is barium in the left hip (arrow). The septic hip was caused by diverticulitis with abscess formation.

and diagnose complications of arthroplasty.

The initial application of bone scintigraphy has been the diagnosis of component infection or loosening. The practical difficulty with this imaging technique is that it exhibits high degrees of sensitivity but relatively low degrees of specificity.[46,49] Therefore, radionuclide evaluation of complications of arthroplasty surgery has been studied extensively over the past two decades in order to refine specificity. Some investigators believe that bone scintigraphy is most useful when the images reveal normal findings, because increased uptake may reflect not only postoperative changes but also infection or component loosening[50] (Fig. 7.19). In attempting to improve specificity, we have routinely used three-phase bone scintigraphy as our initial imaging procedure.[51]

Twenty microcuries of ^{99m}Tc methylene diphosphonate (MDP), an agent that localizes in areas of increased blood flow and bone turnover, is injected, and the patient is scanned dynamically to evaluate initial vascular distribution of isotope. After this, the patient remains under the gamma camera, and an early phase distribution image is obtained approximately 20 minutes after injection. Finally, after patient hydration and a delay of 3 to 4 hours, a scan of the affected area is obtained. Some investigators believe this sequential approach to bone

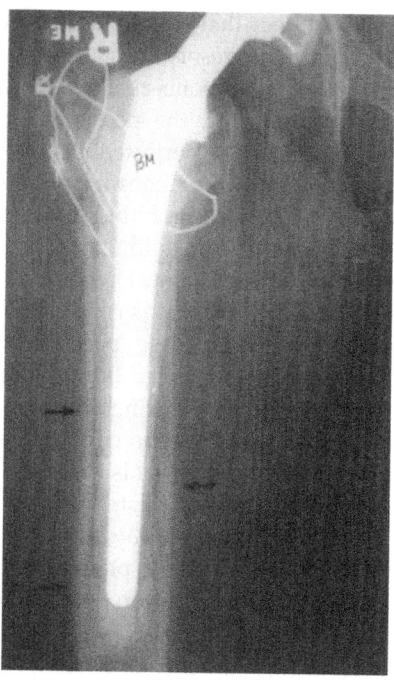

Figure 7.18. Radiograph of the right hip demonstrating the plain film findings of osteomyelitis in a total hip patient. There is diffuse periosteal reaction along the femoral shaft (arrows).

posed to a potential peripheral location during arthrography.

Ultrasound, as a noninvasive diagnostic modality, has been used to detect infection.[45] Ultrasound was used in 33 patients who had hip pain after arthroplasty. All patients who had an intraarticular effusion with extraarticular extension seen on sonograms proved to have infection.

Radionuclide Imaging of the Revision Hip Arthroplasty

Radionuclide imaging has been used as an important diagnostic adjunct in the evaluation of the outcome of various interventions involving total joint replacement surgery. These techniques have been applied to the evaluation of the painful prosthesis, heterotopic bone formation, component failure, component loosening, vascular viability (including that of allografts), and infection.[46,47] Of these indications, loosening and infection are the most common problems that initiate the request for these imaging procedures.[47] The use of newer imaging modalities, such as CT and MRI, is particularly limited with regard to revision arthroplasties because of extensive metallic artifacts that arise from the orthopedic hardware.[48] Therefore the burden of proof, as it were, has fallen to nuclear imaging techniques to define

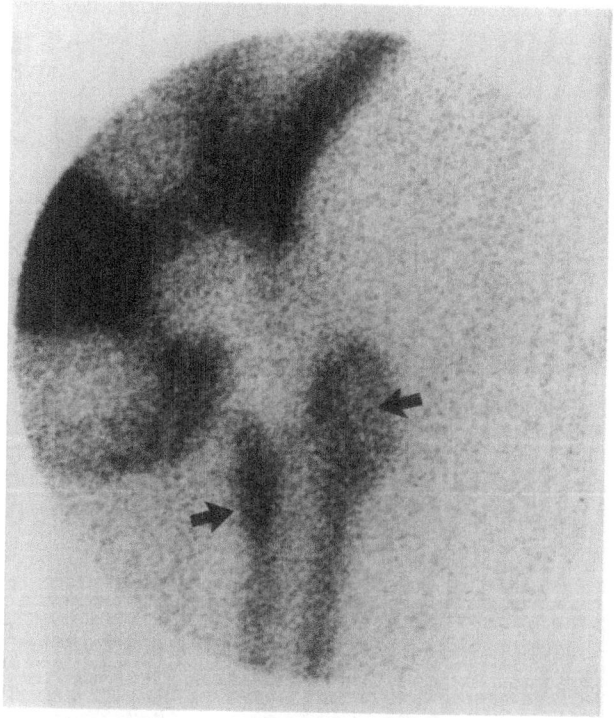

Figure 7.19. Conventional bone scintigraphy with use of ^{99m}Tc MDP has nonspecific increased affinity for any area of increased bone activity. In this AP view of the left hip, increased uptake is noted surrounding medial and lateral aspects of this loose femoral component (arrows).

scintigraphy, coupled with an analysis of the patterns of uptake, significantly increases exam specificity[51] (Fig. 7.20). Tehranzadeh et al.[49] have shown that focal uptake, especially surrounding the prosthesis stem tip or trochanters, is specific for loosening, whereas diffuse periprosthetic uptake is specific for infection. There is normally increased periprosthetic uptake in the cemented prosthesis for approximately 1 year postsurgery, and 10% of these patients will have persistent increased uptake indefinitely.[52,53] This obviously limits

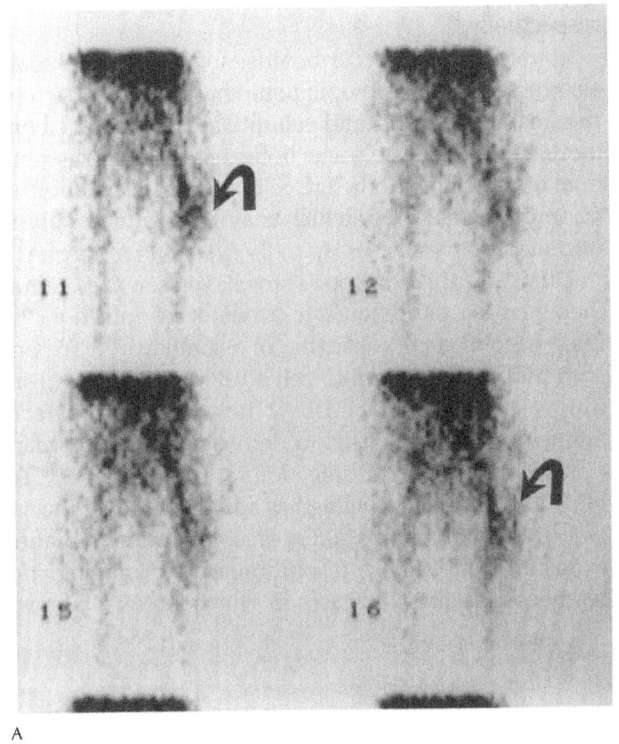

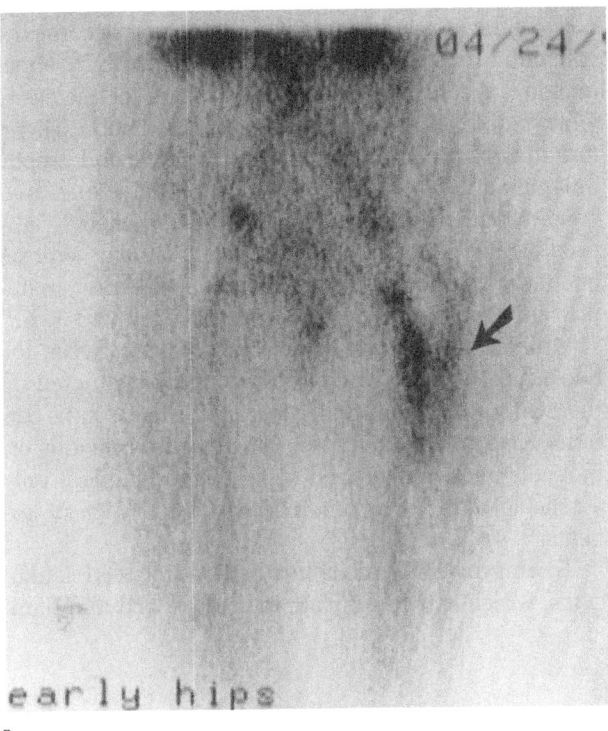

Figure 7.20. Three-phase bone scintigraphy improves discrimination of component loosening related to infection. (A) In the initial flow study, increased vascular distribution of isotope (^{99m}Tc MDP) is noted in both the region of the left femur and the soft tissues surrounding the femoral component (curved arrows). (B) In the early distribution phase, there is increasing intensity of both periprosthetic and soft tissue uptake (arrow). (C) Delayed imaging 4 hours postinjection shows intense uptake surrounding all aspects of the femoral component as well as the lateral region of the acetabular component (arrows). This sequential progression of uptake is pathognomonic of infection.

early detection of complications, especially loosening. Newer porous-coated prostheses that allow bone and fibrous tissue ingrowth into the prosthesis may have different patterns of uptake than originally described and have been reported to have increased activity for at least 2 years. Therefore, conventional bone imaging may have limited value during this period.[51-53]

Dual-tracer studies, focusing primarily on the diagnosis of the infected joint replacement, have become the convention. Gallium (^{67}Ga citrate), originally a bone-imaging agent, is also localized in areas of increased white blood cell accumulation and inflammation. Therefore there is accumulation in areas of septic and aseptic inflammation, as well as in any other region of increased bone turnover resulting in low specificity when ^{67}Ga is used alone.[50] The use of dual-isotopic scanning with sequential ^{99m}Tc/^{67}Ga scintigraphy has been shown to improve diagnostic accuracy of infection to 60% to 80%.[54] The diagnosis relies on discordant uptake between the two scans, with increased asymmetric uptake noted on the ^{67}Ga scan indicating infection. Equivalent uptake patterns occur in 46% to 72% of patients with previous orthopedic interventions, and hence this technique is only a reliable indicator of infection in 25% to 33% of patients.[55]

To improve specificity further, radiolabeled leukocytes, which can accumulate in areas of active inflammation, have been used to detect infection complicating revision arthroplasties (Fig. 7.21). Because these agents theoretically do not accumulate in areas of nonspecific bone turnover, loosening would not be expected to cause false-positive results. However, the results obtained by using labeled leukocytes alone have been somewhat disappointing with sensitivity and specificity ranging from 50% to 100% and 23% to 100%, respectively.[50]

Sources of error occur because increased uptake can also be seen in heterotopic bone that contains marrow, rheumatoid arthritis, and cellulitis. Periprosthetic bone localization may also occur because of altered distribution of reticuloendothelial cells and accumulation of tracer at the stem tip, which may be seen normally in uncemented prostheses up to 3½ years after surgery.[56]

Dual- and triple-isotope scans have been used to further increase the diagnostic accuracy of infection.[54,55] Dual-isotope scans consisting of a standard ^{99m}Tc bone scan and a labeled white cell scan with either 111-indium (^{111}In) or ^{99m}Tc-HMPAO (hexamethyl propylene-amine-oxine) can be used to define areas of discordant uptake suggestive of infection.[57] The use of ^{99m}Tc-HMPAO white cell labeling has advantages over the use of ^{111}In scanning in that there is lower patient radiation exposure, better image resolution, earlier imaging, and ready availability.[48] In cases in which a clear diagnosis

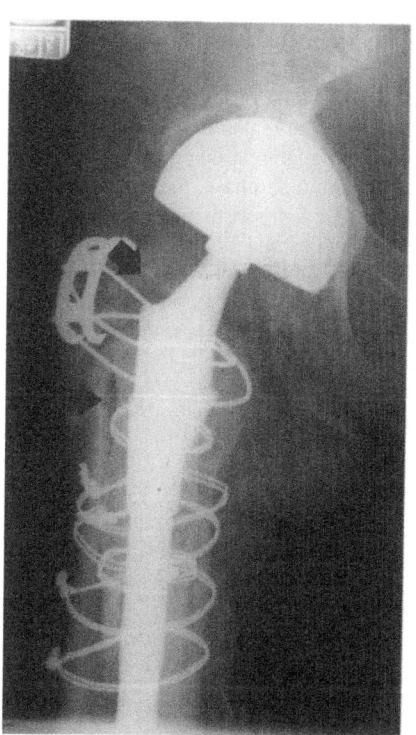

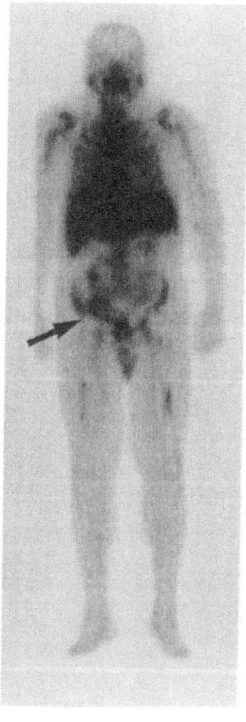

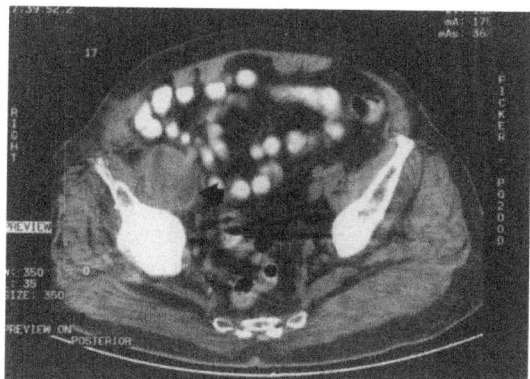

Figure 7.21. Labeled leukocyte scans improve the reliability of diagnosis of occult sepsis in patients after revision surgery. (A) In an AP radiograph of a symptomatic revision arthroplasty, resorption is noted surrounding the bone cement interface of the femoral component and the greater trochanter (arrowheads). (B) A whole-body ^{99m}Tc HMPAO-labeled leukocyte scan shows normal distribution of isotope to the liver and spleen and focally intense uptake (arrow) in the region of the acetabular component and proximal femur of the right hip indicative of sepsis. (C) Axial CT image of the pelvis in the same patient reveals an abscess adjacent to the right iliac bone (arrowheads) in the region of the abnormal uptake.

of infection cannot be reached by using the dual-isotope approach, a third tracer, ^{99m}Tc sulfur colloid, may be used to differentiate further increased uptake defined on the white cell scan. Although both sulfur colloid and labeled white cells accumulate in the marrow, only leukocytes accumulate in areas of infection. Thus, this technique facilitates the differentiation of labeled leukocyte uptake in aberrant, but not abnormal marrow from uptake indicative of active infection. The reported accuracy of this technique exceeds 90%.[54]

The current diagnostic scheme for the evaluation of a potentially infected arthroplasty should therefore begin with the use of a three phase bone scan as a screening exam because of its high sensitivity, low cost, and ready availability. If the scan results are positive, but inconclusive with regard to active infection, a labeled leukocyte scan can then be performed; finally, if needed, a ^{99m}Tc sulfur colloid scan can be performed to resolve any diagnostic uncertainty.[54]

Just as new radionuclide techniques have been developed to facilitate the diagnosis of the infected prosthesis, new techniques involving radionuclide arthrography have been used to better define component loosening.[58] Radionuclide arthrography is performed contemporaneously with radiographic arthrography in that both iodinated contrast and ^{111}In colloid are injected into the joint under fluoroscopic guidance. Oyen et al.[58] found that nuclear arthrography performed better than or equal to radiographic arthrography regarding component failure and had a higher diagnostic accuracy than conventional bone scans with the use of ^{99m}Tc-MDP images alone. They believed that nuclear arthrography added value over radiographic arthrography and bone scanning alone in the detection of prosthetic loosening, especially for the evaluation of the femoral component.

Thus, in the past two decades there has been continued evolution of nuclear imaging from primarily examinations of high sensitivities but of limited true diagnostic value. Through the use of newer isotopes, labeling, and imaging techniques nuclear imaging is now capable of providing accurate and meaningful diagnostic information regarding clinical outcomes of revision hip arthroplasties.

Advanced Imaging Techniques

In addition to conventional radiography and radionuclide examination, newer imaging modalities have been used to aid in the evaluation of the revision total hip arthroplasty. These include angiography, ultrasound, CT, MRI, and three-dimensional imaging techniques such as digital holography.

Angiography has been used in preoperative evaluation of arterial and venous anatomy before complex revision total hip arthroplasty. Angiography allows the depiction of a vascular road map, which defines the relationship of vascular structures to the acetabulum and femoral head, particularly in patients with protrusio, chronic dislocation, longstanding Girdlestone, or severe CDH before corrective reduction. In addition, in elderly patients distal arterial run-off can be evaluated, so that postoperative limb viability will not be jeopardized (Fig. 7.22).

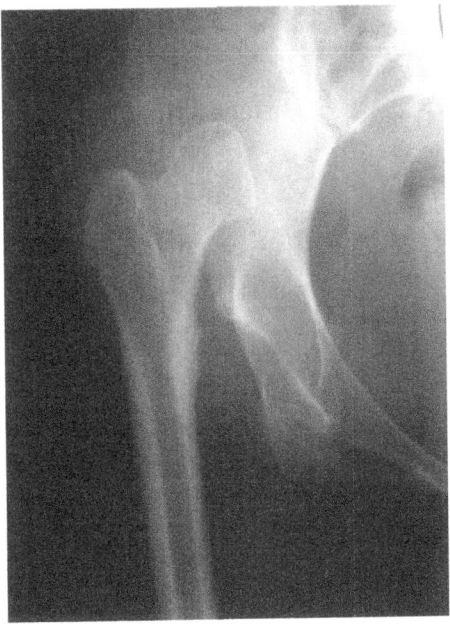

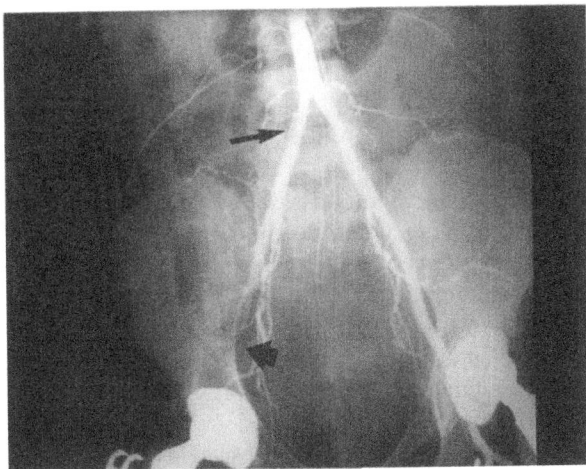

Figure 7.22. (A) AP radiograph showing longstanding hip dislocation secondary to CDH. Following corrective surgery, the patient had symptoms of vascular occlusion. (B) Arteriogram demonstrating a tear in the right iliac artery (arrow) and an embolic occlusion of the right external iliac artery (arrowhead) resulting from the stretching trauma of relocating the femur in anatomic position.

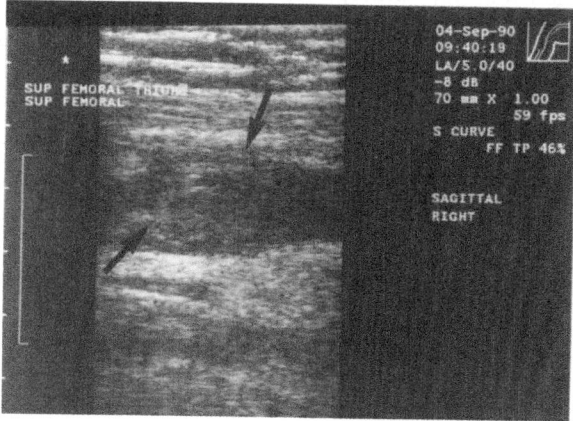

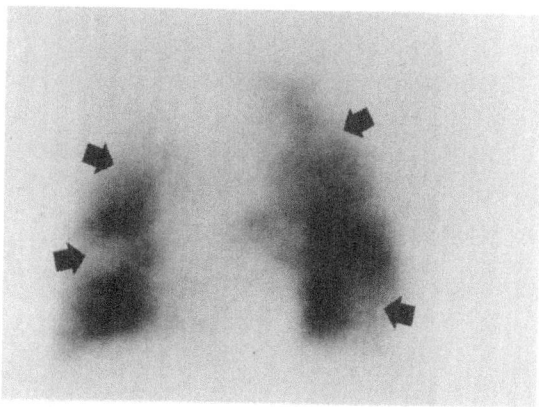

Figure 7.23. (A) Compression ultrasound of the right femoral vein in a postoperative patient demonstrates the vein to be noncompressible and filled with echogenic thrombus (arrows). (B) Perfusion lung scan subsequently performed in the same patient shows multiple perfusion defects (arrowheads) consistent with pulmonary emboli.

technology, duplex ultrasound affords a complete vascular evaluation of symptomatic vascular segments. Similarly, duplex ultrasound allows the differentiation of venous thrombosis from arterial stenosis or occlusion as a cause of a painful lower extremity.

More importantly, many investigators have suggested the routine use of duplex ultrasound pre- and postoperatively to evaluate for the presence of either symptomatic or asymptomatic venous thrombosis.[59-61] Compression ultrasound of venous structures, coupled with augmented pulsed Doppler and color Doppler imaging, has resulted in a diagnostic accuracy of greater than 90% in detection of clinically significant deep venous thrombosis above the level of the popliteal trifurcation.[60-62] Although the detection of DVT in the calf has a lower accuracy rate of 81%, many investigators believe that these distal DVTs have no clinical significance.[60] Detection and diagnosis of DVT in the perioperative revision arthroplasty patient, the occurrence of which is usually not an insurmountable therapeutic

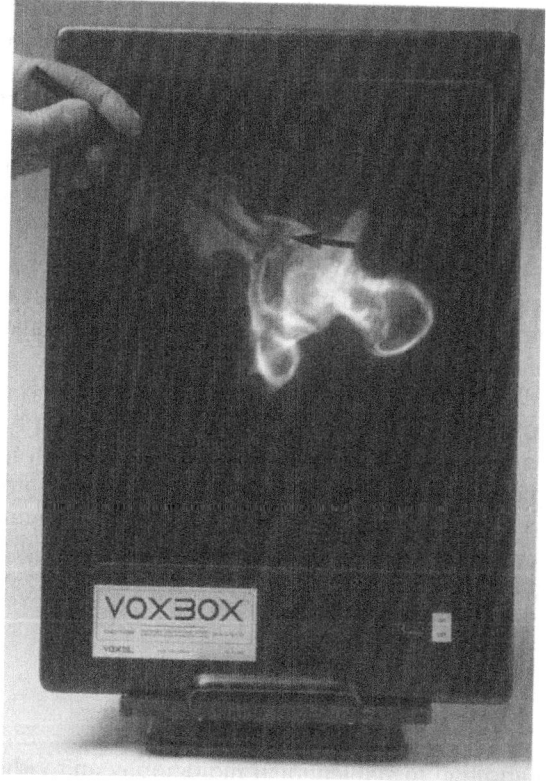

Figure 7.24. Digital hologram derived from a high-resolution CT scan is displayed on a specialized light box. Although the three-dimensional image cannot be effectively reproduced on the printed page, the true displayed image provides a depiction of anatomic relationships of the fragments of this fractured pelvis (arrow) captured on the scan and allows viewer interaction. In using such a display, a surgeon may plan a surgical procedure preoperatively.

Similarly, ultrasound has been used to evaluate arterial and venous patency before surgery. Such vascular disease can affect overall tissue perfusion and influence the likelihood of appropriate tissue healing. With this information in hand, an informed clinical decision can be made before surgery regarding the need for vascular therapeutic interventions to preserve limb viability and improve wound healing.

The evaluation can be accomplished in two ways. First, the competency of the arterial run-off can be screened by using noninvasive pulse volume recording and segmental pressure analysis. Once an area of abnormality is identified, duplex ultrasound can be used to evaluate the vascular anatomy surrounding the abnormal segment. Duplex ultrasound is capable of not only defining the intimal geography of the vascular lumen but simultaneously demonstrating the physiologic flow characteristics of blood within the lumen. Coupled with color Doppler dilemma, is focused on preventing the occurrence of significant related unsuspected complications, such as pulmonary emboli or extension of venous thrombi beyond the lower extremities[63] (Fig. 7.23).

Computed tomography and MRI have limited use in the evaluation of revision hip arthroplasty patients primarily because of extensive artifacts originating from the patient's existing implant. Computed tomography can be used to evaluate surrounding soft tissue structures and the quality of existing bone stock. High-resolution CT scans have been used as the source for pseudo-three-dimensional displays of complex anatomy. These techniques often require the use of complex software and dedicated workstations. The resultant output, usually viewed at a workstation console, has been used to allow the creation of custom prostheses or plan an operative approach.

In addition, we have used a new three-dimensional imaging technique, digital holography (DH), to provide hard copy spatial imaging.[64,65] Digital holography is capable of displaying on a single film, in true three-dimension, the intricate anatomic relationships captured sequentially on the slices of a scan. The DH is viewed on a special portable viewbox, allowing the surgeon a clear appreciation of spatial relationships in complex cases and therefore allowing appropriate preoperative planning. Our experience with DH is that it provides the surgeon with a form of tactile evaluation before surgery, as well as promotes the communication of a proposed therapy to the patient, affording better understanding of planned corrective surgery and therefore enabling a more accurate informed consent[64,65] (Fig. 7.24).

Conclusion

The evolution of therapeutic approaches to total hip arthroplasty has moved the radiologist to develop new imaging techniques to provide useful diagnostic clinical information. Although many of the procedures performed have not changed significantly in the past 15 years, the way their results are interpreted and applied has changed. More advanced and more specific nuclear studies are providing needed clinical information regarding sepsis and component loosening. Future understanding of the causes of component failure may result in the development of more precise imaging techniques that can improve patient satisfaction and clinical outcome.

References

1. Amstutz HC. Complications of total hip replacement. *Clin Orthop.* 1970;72:123–137.
2. Beabout JW. Radiology of total hip arthroplasty. *Radiol Clin North Am.* 1975;13:3–19.
3. Goergen TG, Resnick D. Evaluation of acetabular anteversion following total hip arthroplasty: necessity of proper centering. *Br J Radiol.* 1975;48:259–263.
4. Bontrager K. *Textbook of Radiographic Positioning and Related Anatomy.* 3rd ed. St Louis, Mo: Mosby-Year Book; 1993: 231.
5. Mason B, Wardell SR, Stamos VP, et al. Radiographic assessment of posterolateral acetabular defects in revision total hip arthroplasty: a cadaveric study. Presented at annual meeting of the American Academy of Orthopaedic Surgeons; March 19–23, 1997. San Francisco.
6. Egund N, Pettersson H, Frost S, Lidgren L. The potential of computed tomography in visualizing structures inside the metal cup in surface replacement total hip arthroplasty. *Skeletal Radiol.* 1987;16:201–204.
7. Beckenbaugh RD, Ilstrup DM. Total hip arthroplasty. *J Bone Joint Surg Am.* 1978;60:306–313.
8. Griffiths HJ, Priest DR, Kushner D. Total hip replacement and other orthopedic hip procedures. *Radiol Clin North Am.* 1995;33:267–287.
9. Aliabadi P, Tumeh SS, Weissman BN, McNeil BJ. Cemented total hip prosthesis: radiographic and scintigraphic evaluation. *Radiology.* 1989;173:203–206.
10. Weissman BN. Radiographic evaluation of total joint replacement. In: Kelley WN, Harris ED, Ruddy S, et al, eds. *Textbook of Rheumatology.* Philadelphia, Pa: WB Saunders Co; 1980:2020–2054.
11. Tigges S, Roberson JR, Cohen DE. Hip arthroplasty: the role of plain radiographs in outpatient management. *Radiology.* 1995;194:73–75.
12. Chew FS, Lev MH. Polyethylene osteolysis. *AJR.* 1992;159: 1254.
13. Huo MH, Betts F, Bogumill GP, Kenmore PI, Hayek RJ, Martinelli TJ. Metallic wear debris in acetabular osteolysis in a mechanically stable cementless total hip replacement: report of a case. *Orthopedics.* 1993;16:1277–1281.
14. Reinus WR, Gilula LA, Kyriakos M, Kuhlman RE. Histiocytic reaction to hip arthroplasty. *Radiology.* 1985;155:315–318.
15. Scott WW Jr, Riley LH Jr, Dorfman HD. Focal lytic lesions associated with femoral stem loosening in total hip prosthesis. *AJR.* 1985;144:977–982.
16. Petrera P, Rubash HE. Revision total hip arthroplasty: the acetabular component. *J Am Acad Orthop Surg.* 1995;3:15–21.
17. Quale JL, Murphey MD, Huntrakoon M, Reckling FW, Neff JR. Titanium-induced arthropathy associated with polyethylene–metal separation after total joint replacement. *Radiology.* 1992;182:855–858.
18. Kattapuram SV, Lodwick GS, Chandler H, Khurana JS, Ehara S, Rosenthal DI. Porous coated anatomic hip prostheses: radiographic analysis and clinical correlation. *Radiology.* 1990;174:861–864.
19. Kaplan PA, Montesi SA, Jardon OM, Gregory PR. Bone ingrowth hip prostheses in asymptomatic patients: radiographic features. *Radiology.* 1988;169:221–227.
20. Weissman BN, Sosman JL, Braunstein EM, Dadkhahipoor H, Kandarpa K, Thornhill TS, et al. Intravenous methylmethacrylate after total hip replacement. *J Bone Joint Surg Am.* 1984;66:443–450.
21. Brandser E, El-Khoury G, Riley M, Callaghan J. Intravenous methylmethacrylate following cemented total hip arthroplasty. *Skeletal Radiol.* 1995;24:493–494.

22. Larson BJ, Zindrick M, Schwartz C, Demos TC. Postoperative dislocation of a total hip prosthesis due to a surgical drain. *AJR*. 1987;149:971–972.
23. Seegenschmiedt MH, Goldmann AR, Martus P, Wolfel R, Hohmann D, Sauer R. Prophylactic radiation therapy for prevention of heterotopic ossification after hip arthroplasty: results in 141 high-risk hips. *Radiology*. 1993;188:257–264.
24. Chew FS, Brown JH, Palmer WE, Kattapuram SV. CT-guided aspiration in potentially infected total hip replacements complicated by heterotopic bone. *Eur J Radiol*. 1995;20:72–74.
25. DeFlitch CJ, Stryker JA. Postoperative hip irradiation in prevention of heterotopic ossification: causes of treatment failure. *Radiology*. 1993;188:265–270.
26. O'Neill DA, Harris WH. Failed total hip replacement: assessment by plain radiographs, arthrograms, and aspiration of the hip joint. *J Bone Joint Surg Am*. 1984;66:540–546.
27. Walker CW, FitzRandolph RL, Collins DN, Dalrymple GV. Arthrography of painful hips following arthroplasty: digital versus plain film subtraction. *Skeletal Radiol*. 1991;20:403–407.
28. Newberg AH, Wetzner SM, Digital subtraction arthrography. *Radiology*. 1985;154:238–239.
29. Ginai AZ, van Biezen FC, Kint PA, Oei HY, Hop WC. Digital subtraction arthrography in preoperative evaluation of painful total hip arthroplasty. *Skeletal Radiol*. 1996;25:357–363.
30. Hardy DC, Reinus WR, Totty WG, Keyser CK. Arthrography after total hip arthroplasty: utility of post ambulation radiographs. *Skeletal Radiol*. 1988;17:20–23.
31. Cone RO, Yaru N, Resnick D, Gershuni D, Guerra J Jr. Intracapsular pressure monitoring during arthrographic evaluation of painful hip prostheses. *AJR*. 1983;141:885–889.
32. Maus TP, Berquist TH, Bender CE, Rand JA. Arthrographic study of painful total hip arthroplasty: Refined criteria. *Radiology*. 1987;162:721–727.
33. Gould ES, Potter HG, Bober SE. Role of routine percutaneous hip aspirations prior to prosthesis revision. *Skeletal Radiol*. 1990;19:427–430.
34. Tigges S, Stiles RG, Meli RJ, Roberson JR. Hip aspiration: a cost-effective and accurate method of evaluating the potentially infected hip prosthesis. *Radiology*. 1993;189:485–488.
35. Fitzgerald RH Jr. Infected total hip arthroplasty: diagnosis and treatment. *J Am Acad Orthop Surg*. 1995;3:249–262.
36. Braunstein EM, Cardinal E, Buckwalter KA, Capello W. Bupivicaine arthrography of the post-arthroplasty hip. *Skeletal Radiol*. 1995;24:519–521.
37. Barrack RL, Tanzer M, Kattapuram SV, Harris WH. The value of contrast arthrography in assessing loosening of symptomatic uncemented total hip components. *Skeletal Radiol*. 1994;23:37–41.
38. Swan JS, Braunstein EM, Wellman HN, Capello W. Contrast and nuclear arthrography in loosening of the uncemented hip prosthesis. *Skeletal Radiol*. 1991;20:15–19.
39. Heenan SD, Chirambasukwa W, Stoker DJ. Lymphatic filling in arthrography following total hip replacement. *Clin Radiol*. 1995;50:90–94.
40. Bloom RA, Gheorghiu D, Krausz Y. Lymphatic opacification in the prosthetic hip. *Skeletal Radiol*. 1991;20:43–45.
41. Berquist TH, Bender CE, Maus TP, Ward EM, Rand JA. Pseudobursae: a useful finding in patients with painful hip arthroplasty. *AJR*. 1987;148:103–106.
42. Swan JS, Braunstein EM, Capello W. Aspiration of the hip in patients treated with Girdlestone arthroplasty. *AJR*. 1991;156:545–546.
43. Tigges S, Stiles RG, Roberson JR. Appearance of septic hip prostheses on plain radiographs. *AJR*. 1994;163:377–380.
44. Dussault RH, Goldman AB, Ghelman B. Radiologic diagnosis of loosening and infection in hip prostheses. *J Can Assoc Radiol*. 1977;28:119–127.
45. vanHolsbeeck MT, Eyler WR, Sherman LS, Lombardi TJ, Mezger E, Verner JJ, et al. Detection of infection in loosened hip prostheses: efficacy of sonography. *AJR*. 1994;163:381–384.
46. Wellman HN, Schauwecker DS, Capello WN. Evaluation of metallic osseous implants with nuclear medicine. *Semin Nucl Med*. 1988;18:126–136.
47. Aliabadi P, Tumeh SS, Weissman BN, McNeil BJ. Cemented total hip prosthesis: radiographic and scintigraphic evaluation. *Radiology*. 1989;173:203–206.
48. Copping C, Dalgliesh SM, Dudley NJ, Griffiths PA, Harrington M, Potter R, et al. The role of ^{99m}TC-HMPAO white cell imaging in suspected orthopedic infection. *Br J Radiol*. 1992;65:309–312.
49. Tehranzadeh J, Gubernick I, Blaha D. Prospective study of sequential technetium ^{99m} phosphate and gallium imaging in painful hip prostheses (comparison of diagnostic modalities). *Clin Nucl Med*. 1988;13:229–236.
50. Palestro CJ. Radionuclide imaging after skeletal interventional procedures. *Semin Nucl Med*. 1995;25:3–14.
51. Rubello D, Borsulo N, Chierichetti F, Zanco P, Ferlin G. Three phase bone scintigraphy by pattern of loosening in uncemented prostheses. *Eur J Nucl Med*. 1995;22:299–301.
52. Utz JA, Lull RJ, Galvin EG. Asymptomatic total hip prosthesis: natural history determined using Tc99m MDP bone scans. *Radiology*. 1986;161:509–512.
53. Li DJ, Miles KA, Wraight EP. Bone scintigraphy of hip prostheses: can analysis of patterns of abnormality improve accuracy? *Clin Nucl Med*. 1994;49:112–115.
54. Palestro CJ, Kim CK, Swyer AJ, Capozzi JD, Solomon RW, Goldsmith SJ, et al. Total hip arthroplasty: periprosthetic indium 111 labeled leukocyte activity and complementary technetium 99m sulfur colloid imaging in suspected infection. *J Nucl Med*. 1990;31:1950–1957.
55. Seabold JE, Nepola JV, Marsh JL, Hawes DR, Justin EP, Ponto JA, et al. Postoperative bone marrow alterations: potential pitfalls in the diagnosis of osteomyelitis with In-111 labeled leukocyte scintigraphy. *Radiology*. 1991;180:741–747.
56. Johnson JA, Christie MJ, Sandler MP, Parks PF Jr, Horma L, Kaye JJ. Detection of occult infection following total joint arthroplasty using sequential technetium 99m HDP bone scintigraphy and indium 111 WBC imaging. *J Nucl Med*. 1988;29:1347–1353.
57. Glithero PR, Grigori P, Harding LK, Hesslewood SR, McMinn DJ. White cell scans and infected joint replacements. *J Bone Joint Surg Br*. 1993;75:371–374.
58. Oyen WJ, Lemmens JA, Claessens RA, van Horn JR, Sloof TJ, Corstens FH. Nuclear arthrography: combined scintigraphic and radiographic procedure for diagnosis

of total hip prosthesis loosening. *J Nucl Med.* 1996;37:62–70.
59. Weinman EE, Salzman EW. Deep-vein thrombosis. *N Engl J Med.* 1994;331:1630–1641.
60. Cronan JJ. Venous thromboembolic disease: the role of US. *Radiology.* 1993;186:619–630.
61. Barnes RW, Nix ML, Barnes CL, Lavender RC, Golden WE, Harmon BH, et al. Perioperative asymptomatic venous thrombosis: role of duplex scanning versus venography. *J Vasc Surg.* 1989;9:251–260.
62. Lewis BD, James EM, Welch TJ, Joyce JW, Hallett JW, Weaver AL. Diagnosis of acute deep venous thrombosis of the lower extremities: prospective evaluation of color Doppler flow imaging versus venography. *Radiology.* 1994;192:651–655.
63. Kalodiki E, Domjan J, Nicolaides AN, Cunningham DA, Al-Kutoubi A, Birch R, et al. V/Q defects and deep venous thrombosis following total hip replacement. *Clin Radiol.* 1995;50:400–403.
64. Robertson DD, Sutherland CS, Chan BW, Hodge JC, Scott WW, Fishman EK. Depiction of pelvic fractures using 3D volumetric holography: comparison of plain x-ray and CT. *J Comput Assist Tomogr.* 1995;19:967–974.
65. Wetzner SM, Newberg AH, Bierbaum BE, Terrono AL, Robbins AH. Multiple exposure volumetric holography of orthopedic injuries. *Orthop Trans.* 1995;19:431–432.

8
Pain Syndromes in Revision Total Hip Arthroplasty

Ross J. Muscomeci

This chapter addresses pain medication issues. The anatomy and physiology of pain, and the mechanism of pain relief with many types of treatment are not yet well understood. Furthermore, the theories currently proposed to explain how pain is transmitted and modified suggest that the process is far more complex than that of a single pain–single nerve system. Although it is not necessary for readers to have a detailed knowledge of pain theory and anatomy, it is helpful to have an understanding of some basic concepts in this area. Differential diagnosis of pain in the hip or lower extremity is best approached by trying to define the type of pain present and then attempting to ascertain the possible causes. The chapter begins with a brief overview of the different types of pain, and then moves to evaluation of the painful hip, specific pain syndromes related to total hip arthroplasty, and treatment options.

Overview

For practical purposes, pain is commonly classified as acute or chronic pain, and is then further defined by its mechanism and location. *Acute pain* after hip surgery is *usually* associated with a well-understood condition and has limited duration. Generally, acute pain in this situation has an important biologic function and causes a stress response that includes hormonal and emotional aspects. This pain is predominantly a physical phenomenon, and rarely is it primarily due to psychologic factors.[1]

Chronic pain has been defined as pain lasting at least 1 month beyond the time that would normally be expected for a painful condition to heal, pain that is associated with a chronic pathologic process that causes continuous pain, or pain that recurs at intervals for months or years.[1] In contrast to acute pain, chronic pain never has a biologic function and is an illness itself in that it has a negative impact on the physical, emotional, economic, and social condition of a patient. There is no stress response as in acute pain. There is usually a significant contribution to the pain condition made by psychologic and emotional factors, and in some cases the pain may be caused by these factors.[1]

Pain is divided, on the basis of its source, into *visceral* and *somatic* pain. Each has markedly different characteristics. Pain related to total hip arthroplasty will invariably be somatic in origin, so the discussion here is limited to types of somatic pain. Somatic pain can be divided into pain of musculoskeletal or neuropathic origin. Musculoskeletal pain is undoubtedly the type of pain with which readers are most familiar. It is predominantly mechanical in origin, and the quality of pain is usually described as aching, pressure, throbbing, crushing, or stabbing. Acutely, this type of pain usually responds well to a combination of opioids and nonsteroidal anti-inflammatory agents. Chronic pain syndromes within this category respond variably to medications and include arthritis, skeletal pain, myofascial pain and fibromyalgia.

Neuropathic pain is generally defined as pain resulting from injury to or a primary disorder of a portion of the nervous system. Although there are many variations of neuropathic pain and considerable overlap with the symptoms of other types of pain, pain that is predominantly of neuropathic origin has characteristic features that help identify it. Unlike sensations described with musculoskeletal pain, neuropathic pain is usually described as shooting, electrical, pins and needles, or burning. It is also frequently associated with allodynia, hyperalgesia, and hyperpathia. It is important to identify this type of pain because it is characteristically resistant to many analgesics and responds much better to nonopioid adjunctive medications. Neuropathic pain can be divided further into categories determined by the location of the insult with peripheral, central, and autonomic types being the most common.

Of the three types of neuropathic pain, *peripheral mononeuropathies* are commonly encountered after total hip arthroplasty. Entrapment and trauma are the most frequent causes of mononeuropathy. Other causes include postherpetic neuralgia from shingles, diabetes, carcinomatous neuropathy, systemic lupus erythematosus, rheumatoid arthritis, and tumor invasion.[2] Mononeuropathies are identified by pain that is limited to the distribution of one nerve. The pain is described as a burning or throbbing, and it is usually associated with sharp, lancinating exacerbations; paresthesias; and motor or sensory abnormalities. It is not unusual to see vasomotor changes in the distribution of the injured nerve, and hyperalgesia is a common finding.

Central pain results from interruption of central somatosensory pathways at the level of the spinal cord or brain.[3] The pain is frequently delayed in onset, and the distribution coincides with all or part of the lesion created by an insult to the central nervous system. The quality of the pain is similar to that associated with peripheral nerve lesions, and it is easily exacerbated by multiple causes. This type of pain is notoriously difficult to treat; because it is rarely limited to areas around the hip, it will not be discussed further here.

Pain secondary to *autonomic dysfunction* is also rarely, if ever, limited to the hip or associated regions, but it may occur after total hip arthroplasty. There are many names for this type of pain, the most common of which are reflex sympathetic dystrophy (RSD) and causalgia. The nomenclature that is currently being used for this syndrome is complex regional pain syndrome, with type I (previously called RSD) resulting from many different types of injury and type II (previously called causalgia) resulting from major nerve injury. The inciting injury can range from avulsion of a major nerve trunk to something so minor that the patient cannot even remember being injured. Pain from this source is characteristically burning in nature. Although it may be described with other terms as well, burning will usually be at least part of the description. Another hallmark of the syndrome is that the pain is out of proportion to any injury present or physical findings on exam. It is associated with allodynia, vasomotor, and sudomotor abnormalities, and it occurs in one or more extremities. It is usually diffuse, and it tends to be more distal than proximal. Although history and physical exam findings suggest the diagnosis of sympathetically mediated pain, a more definitive diagnosis requires sympathetic nerve blockade, and treatment usually involves a series of such blocks.[4] Other treatment modalities are discussed later in the chapter.

Differential Diagnosis of Hip Pain

Intra-Articular Sources

Pain of intra-articular origin in the nonoperative hip is likely to result from injury or arthritis. The arthritides include both acute and chronic forms. Acute arthritides may be related to infection or hemarthrosis. Chronic arthritides include rheumatoid arthritis, gouty or psoriatic arthrosis, degenerative osteoarthritis, and, in younger patients, pigmented villonodular synovitis.[5] Pain is usually experienced in the groin, over the greater trochanter, in the buttock, or down the anterior and inner thigh, but may be referred to the distal thigh or knee because of overlapping innervation by the obturator nerve.[6] If it is difficult to distinguish between intra- and extra-articular sources, an arthrogram with the use of a local anesthetic should be helpful.

Treatment of arthritis beyond the use of mild analgesics and nonsteroidal anti-inflammatory medications or aspirin is covered in texts on rheumatology. Intraarticular pain in the postoperative hip is covered briefly in later sections of this chapter, and more extensively elsewhere in this book.

Extra-Articular Sources of Musculoskeletal Origin

Some extra-articular disorders may cause pain in the hip as well. Trochanteric bursitis causes pain over the greater trochanter and lateral thigh. Iliopectineal bursitis causes pain in the lateral portion of Scarpa's triangle, with anterior thigh pain from femoral nerve irritation in some cases. Finally, ischiogluteal bursitis causes pain in the area of the ischial tuberosity, and the pain worsens with sitting.[5,7]

Abnormalities in the femoral shaft, pelvic bones, and spine may also elicit pain in the area of the hip. Lumbar facet syndrome has back pain as its chief complaint, but the pain frequently radiates to the hip, buttocks, thigh, or knee.[8] Sacroiliac joint dysfunction also causes pain that radiates to the same locations.[9] Nerves have been identified in the marrow, periosteum, and cortex of long bones, and some fibers from the periosteum are known to penetrate the cortex by way of Volkmann's canals.[10] Bone is capable of producing pain in response to internal or external pressure, physical distortion, inflammation, or periosteal injury.[11]

Myofascial pain can also cause pain in the region of the hip. Myofascial pain is either primary, in which case it is caused by a traumatic disease of the muscle, or secondary, in which case a disorder outside the muscle is causing painful foci within the muscle. The hallmark of both is the "trigger point." Trigger points are exquisitely tender sites within muscle, bone–tendon junction, or associated fascia, and they feel like a firm nodule or band. They are anatomically constant in that they are always found in the same part of the muscle, and palpation can refer pain to distant sites in a pattern that is not radicular.[11] The proposed mechanisms for the formation of trigger points include damage to the sarcoplasmic reticulum with calcium ion release and local uncontrolled hypermetabolism, and injury causing release of local mediators of pain with subsequent sensitization.[12]

Myofascial pain syndromes that are known to cause pain in the region of the hip include those with trigger points in the following muscles: gluteus medius, gluteus minimus, piriformis, tensor fascia lata, and iliopsoas. The gluteus medius syndrome consists of trigger points along the posterior portion of the iliac crest that radiate in a pattern covering the gluteal region and posterior thigh. Diagnosis can be made by palpating trigger points along the iliac crest and recreating the pattern of pain that the patient has experienced before the exam. The gluteus minimus syndrome is similar but with trigger points located more inferiorly in the gluteal region.

Piriformis syndrome is frequently misdiagnosed as lumbar nerve root compression because in severe cases the muscle compresses the sciatic nerve, producing an entrapment syndrome. Spasm in the piriformis muscle will cause external rotation of the thigh at rest and limit adduction and internal rotation on exam. Pain is localized to the gluteal and greater trochanteric areas, and the trigger point is best palpated with the patient lying on the unaffected side with hip and knee flexed. Pain due to trigger points in the tensor fascia lata can extend along the entire length of the lateral aspect of the leg from thigh to ankle, but trigger points in the proximal portion of the muscle just below the anterior superior iliac spine cause pain localized to the hip area.

The iliopsoas syndrome is a result of trigger points in the iliacus and psoas muscles and above the femoral attachment of the iliopsoas tendon. Pain is produced in an area extending along the ipsilateral lumbosacral spine and extends downward to the sacroiliac, inguinal, and upper anterior thigh regions. The diagnosis can be made by observing that the involved muscles are shortened, causing external rotation and flexion at the thigh with flattening of the normal lumbar lordosis. Tenderness is found over the lesser trochanter at the medial aspect of the femoral triangle, in the iliacus muscle at the midpoint of the iliac crest just medial to the brim of the pelvis, and in the psoas muscle palpated with deep abdominal pressure just inferior to the umbilicus and just lateral to the rectus abdominus.[13] The treatment for myofascial pain includes local infiltration of a local anesthetic and corticosteroid in conjunction with physical therapy as the mainstay. It may also include electrical muscle stimulation therapy, acupuncture, and biofeedback training.[14-17]

Fibromyalgia is a syndrome of chronic musculoskeletal pain, but by definition it is diffuse and not difficult to distinguish from disorders localized to the hip or lower extremity. Painful areas are specific and constant, and are distinguished from trigger points in that there is no palpable band or nodule, and only focal tenderness is present. To make the diagnosis of fibromyalgia, tenderness must be found in at least 11 of 18 specific locations, of which the greater trochanter and gluteal region are included. The remaining locations are remote from the hip, so this topic will not be covered further in this chapter.[11]

Extra-Articular Sources of Neuropathic Origin

Mononeuropathies that are likely to cause pain in the region of the hip, groin, or thigh include lumbar plexitis; femoral, sciatic, or obturator neuralgia; meralgia paresthetica; and postherpetic neuralgia. Lumbar plexitis is a poorly understood condition caused by an inherited autosomal dominant trait, viral infection, radiation therapy, or nonspecific inflammation. The initial complaint is of pain in the hip associated with the onset of paresis. Proximal muscles are involved more than distal, and motor changes are more pronounced than sensory ones. Meralgia paresthetica is the name given to lateral femoral cutaneous neuralgia. It is associated with pain on the anterolateral surface of the thigh made worse by standing or walking and has no associated motor abnormalities. Femoral, sciatic, or obturator neuropathies are associated with pain and motor abnormalities in the distribution of these nerves and should not present diagnostic difficulty.[2] Postherpetic neuralgia in the T12 or L1 nerve root causes radicular pain in the region of the hip and groin, but there is usually a history of a preceding vesicular rash.

Spinal cord abnormalities may also cause unilateral or bilateral pain of a radicular nature, including spinal stenosis, arachnoiditis, and herniated nucleus pulposus. These should be considered in the differential diagnosis of hip or thigh pain.[18]

Postoperative Hip Pain

Spinal stenosis has been implicated in both continued postoperative hip pain and postoperative footdrop after total hip arthroplasty. These patients present some diagnostic difficulty, but once correctly diagnosed and treated the majority experience resolution of symptoms.[19,20] Herniated nucleus pulposus has also presented diagnostic difficulty after hip arthroplasty. Mallory and Halley[21] described a case in which a patient experienced postoperative buttock pain without radicular symptoms. They postulated that stress placed on the lumbosacral spine during surgery may have contributed to the disc herniation. Postoperative pubic ramus fractures have been discussed in at least two case reports as presenting confusing clinical pictures with unexplained groin pain. This pain could easily be confused with late infection or loosening of a hip prosthesis. In both cases, conservative management was successful.[22,23]

Postoperative mononeuropathies of the lower extremity occur with increased frequency in revision hip arthroplasty. The reported incidence in primary hip replacement is 0.09% to 5.9%, and in revision surgery it ranges from 2.0% to 7.6%. The nerve most commonly involved is the peroneal nerve, but sciatic, femoral, obturator, and upper extremity nerve injuries have also been reported.[24] Mononeuropathy and its treatment are discussed in more detail later.

Evaluation and Treatment of the Painful Hip and Lower Extremity

It is assumed that readers are well acquainted with physical examination of the hip and lower extremity, so the focus of this discussion is on physical findings and diagnostic modalities specific to the symptomatic hip arthroplasty and related pain syndromes. In general, when obtaining history for a complaint of pain, the important aspects to consider are: time and character of onset, location, duration, exacerbating or ameliorating phenomena, temporal relationships, radiation, associated physiologic abnormalities, and—perhaps most important—the character or quality of the pain. If a careful and detailed history is obtained, the differential diagnosis can be considerably narrowed in most cases.

Evaluation of Postoperative Hip Pain

Evaluation of the painful total hip arthroplasty has been discussed by many investigators.[25–28] Evans and Cuckler[26] make the point that a painfree interval after total hip arthroplasty suggests either fixation or implant failure or sepsis as the etiology of the pain, while failure to achieve pain relief suggests sources extrinsic to the joint. Rest pain and nocturnal pain suggest possible infectious etiology, and pain that is increased with activity is commonly associated with aseptic loosening. They also discuss the importance of noting location. Thigh and leg pain can indicate a problem with the femoral component, but are a common complaint in porous ingrowth and press-fit devices that have no evidence of loosening. Pain resulting from acetabular pathology causes symptoms in the groin and buttock.[26] Horne et al.[27] divided postoperative pain for total hip arthroplasty into pain that occurs either earlier or later than 6 months postoperatively. Their reason for approaching the problem in this fashion is that standard methods for investigating painful hip arthroplasty, including erythrocyte sedimentation rate and technetium polyphosphate bone scans, do not return to baseline levels until 6 months after primary total hip arthroplasty. For pain that occurs earlier than 6 months postoperatively they suggest that fracture or dislocation of the prosthesis or surrounding bone and infection should be considered, along with the possibility that the hip was not the original source of the pain. They mention five disorders that may mimic the pain of an arthritic hip: (1) spinal stenosis; (2) neoplasm of the pelvis or lumbosacral spine; (3) meralgia paresthetica; (4) Paget's disease of the pelvis, femur, or lumbosacral spine; and (5) other joint diseases such as rheumatoid arthritis, ankylosing spondylitis, or septic arthritis of the lumbosacral spine or sacroiliac joints. For pain that occurs later than 6 months postoperatively, they believe that greatest attention should be paid to the cement–bone or cement–prosthesis interface.[27]

Aspects of the physical exam that may be helpful include observation of the gait, relationship to passive motion, and leg length. Pain with a normal gait suggests that sources other than the prosthesis are more likely to be the source of the pain. Pain with passive motion or progressive limb length inequality suggests mechanical dysfunction or failure in fixation. When the source of the pain is not clear, it is important to include abdominal, pelvic, and rectal examinations as part of the evaluation.[26]

Laboratory studies used in evaluation of the symptomatic hip arthroplasty include white blood cell count (WBC), erythrocyte sedimentation rate (ESR), and C-reactive protein (CRP). The WBC is of little value in the absence of fulminant sepsis. The ESR may be helpful, but it does not return to baseline values for up to 6 months postoperatively, and it may be elevated in a number of conditions. In a patient who is more than 6 months past the date of operation and has no other identifiable causes for an elevated ESR, infection should be suspected. This test has a sensitivity of 73%–100%, a specificity of 69%–94%, and an accuracy of 73%–88%.[39] The CRP has been studied as a marker of infection in postoperative total hip replacements. In one study,[27] CRP levels increased in the early postoperative period but returned to normal in all patients by 3 weeks. Although there are no available data regarding sensitivity, specificity, or accuracy, it seems that CRP may be of some value in helping to differentiate between septic and aseptic loosening of hip prostheses.[26,27]

Plain radiographs, arthrograms, joint aspiration, nuclear medicine scans, CT scans, and intraoperative tests may all play a role in evaluation of the painful total hip arthroplasty. These are discussed in detail elsewhere in this book and will not be discussed further here.

Related Pain Syndromes and Their Treatment

Reflex Sympathetic Dystrophy

The patient with unusual or unexplained postoperative lower extremity pain should be evaluated for sympathetically mediated factors as the cause. As previously stated, this syndrome has many names, and the correct terminology currently is complex regional pain syndrome (CRPS) type I. Because the most widely recognized term is reflex sympathetic dystrophy, that term will be used in this chapter.

Reflex sympathetic dystrophy may be produced by any type of trauma, and the incidence, severity, and course of the symptoms are not related to the severity of injury or extent of surgery that caused them. The pain is typically severe, burning, lancinating, easily exacerbated, and unrelieved by rest. Symptoms usually start distally and move proximally over time. Allodynia, hyperalgesia, hyperesthesia, and both vasomotor and sudomotor abnormalities are all characteristic.[29]

In the early stages, the limb is frequently red and warm or cool and pale and painful. The typical patient with early RSD will present with a painful extremity and usually a negative work-up for other causes. The limb is frequently not symmetric with regard to color, temperature, or both, and in severe cases the patient will guard the extremity. The history will be suggestive of allodynia in that even the slightest stimulation will create pain. Patients will frequently sleep with the affected extremity uncovered because even sheets on top of the skin or wind blowing over the skin will cause discomfort. Pain and physical signs do not conform to known patterns of peripheral nerve distribution.

In later stages of the disorder, severe disability occurs with weakness, atrophy, and trophic changes of the skin becoming prominent and leaving the patient with a contracted cold, pale, painful limb with waxy or brawny skin, coarse hair, and brittle nails. The severity of symptoms varies. Although all cases will show similar pathology, one sign or symptom will frequently be out of proportion to the others.[29] In my experience, RSD of the lower extremity is particularly prone to varied symptoms, and that pain, which is not characteristic of sympathetically mediated pain but remains unexplained, will sometimes respond to treatment for RSD.

If history and examination are suggestive of RSD, a number of diagnostic methods may be used. In established cases of RSD plain radiographs will reveal diffuse and periarticular soft tissue swelling, osteopenia, and endosteal and intracortical bone resorption 75% to 100% of the time.[30] Delayed images of three-phase bone scans have a characteristic pattern in RSD and are very sensitive and specific with high negative predictive value in patients with diagnostic uncertainty.[31]

Response to sympathetic blockade remains the mainstay of diagnosis, and its efficacy was first established in trauma victims in World War II.[29] During World War II, patients with high-velocity missile injuries to major nerve trunks would occasionally develop the syndrome of sympathetically maintained pain, which has been called causalgia in the presence of major nerve injury. Doup et al.[32] suggested that the pain relief produced by sympathetic block in these patients was prompt, complete, and so dramatic that this pain relief should be considered diagnostic for the syndrome. The lumbar sympathetic chain supplies the lower extremity and is located anterolateral to the lumbar vertebral bodies and immediately adjacent to the inferior vena cava and aorta. The sympathetic chain is separated from somatic nerve trunks by the psoas muscle and fascia, so sympathetic blockade should not create loss of sensation unless spread of the medication is atypical. The expected spread is both superior and inferior. If adequate volume is administered, the longitudinal spread is usually adequate to create full sympathetic blockade of the extremity. Bupivacaine 0.25% to 0.5% is usually used with a volume of 15 to 30 mL. The injection can be done under CT or fluoroscopic guidance, as well as without radiologic assistance by using anatomic landmarks only. If radiologic guidance is used, a small amount of contrast material mixed with a local anesthetic is frequently used as a method of checking placement before injection of the full volume of local anesthetic.[33] The patient is usually placed in the prone position. An intravenous catheter is inserted, and the injection is placed at the anterolateral aspect of the L2 or L3 vertebral body. The intravenous phentolamine test has also been used to diagnose RSD, but it has limited application and is not used in our pain clinics.[34]

Treatment of RSD usually consists of a combination of sympathetic blocks in a series combined with physical therapy and oral medications as needed. If the diagnostic sympathetic block is successful, a series of blocks is performed, with the frequency being determined by the duration of the patient's response. Initially the blocks may be performed as frequently as every day, but intervals are usually not more than 2 weeks apart.[35] Pain relief obtained from these blocks usually lasts far longer than the duration of the block itself, and successive blocks are expected to give progressively longer duration of pain relief. Physical therapy sessions are recommended as closely after the blocks as possible, so that patients can participate aggressively in therapy without being limited by the pain associated with RSD. I believe that physical therapy and use of the extremity are at least as important as sympathetic blocks in treatment of this syndrome, and they should be used in conjunction whenever possible. Sympathetic blocks are continued until pain has resolved or no progressive benefit is seen, in which case other treatment options are considered. Intravenous regional blockade is frequently used as a second step in treatment. Medications that have been used as part of the block mixture for therapeutic effect include reserpine, guanethidine, nifedipine, and others.[35] The medication most frequently used for this purpose in our clinic is bretylium. For RSD that is resistant to traditional forms of therapy, more invasive treatments are available. These include radiofrequency thermocoagulation of the sympathetic chain, surgical or chemical sympathectomy, and implantation of a dorsal column stimulator. (Further discussion of these treatment options is beyond the scope of this book.) Oral medications, such as narcotic analgesics, tricyclic antidepressants, and other adjunctive medications, are also used when needed, and they will be discussed later.

The response to treatment is highly variable and has not been well documented. In one study of 125 cases involving pain in the upper extremity, almost 60% of patients had residual symptoms despite adequate treatment.[36] In my experience, most patients will experience at least some improvement in both symptoms and level of functional ability.

Peripheral Neuropathies

As previously discussed, lower extremity mononeuropathies occur with increased frequency as a complication of revision hip arthroplasty. The nerve most commonly affected is the peroneal nerve, but sciatic, obturator and femoral nerves may also be injured, along with upper extremity nerves secondary to patient positioning during the longer revision surgeries. In a retrospective study Nercessian et al.[24] reviewed 7133 consecutive total hip arthroplasties and noted a 0.15% incidence of upper extremity nerve injury, with the ulnar nerve being involved most often. Risk factors for nerve injury were not limited to revision surgery and included female gender, a diagnosis of congenital dislocation of the hip, and having a resident as the primary surgeon. These investigators also found a higher incidence of permanent nerve injury in revision surgery, suggesting that the injuries are not only more frequent in revisions, but also more severe. Finally, although leg lengthening has frequently been cited in orthopedic literature as a cause of nerve injury,[37–39] the study by Nercessian et al.[24] did not support that finding. In another study, Nercessian et al.[40] found that postoperative alterations in the center of rotation of the hip did not correlate with an increased incidence of nerve injury. In a prospective study, Navarro, et al.[41] examined the effect of surgical approach on the incidence of postoperative nerve palsy. Although previous studies have indicated a decreased incidence with use of the transtrochanteric approach,[24] this study found no relationship between surgical approach and the incidence of nerve palsy in either primary or revision surgery.

The cause of postoperative nerve palsy is unknown in most cases.[42] Previously reported etiologies other than leg lengthening include intraoperative trauma,[43] thermal injury from polymerization of cement,[44] paralysis as a complication of bleeding,[45] entrapment of the sciatic nerve by wire,[46] and migration of trochanteric wires.[47] Proper evaluation for these potential causes of nerve injury should include a careful review of the operative course, and serious consideration should be given to reexploration if there is any question about trauma to the involved nerve because surgical intervention can improve the prognosis in some cases.[47,48]

Peripheral mononeuropathy will create symptoms that are predominantly in the distribution of the affected nerve. Local tenderness and sensitivity to movement, radiating or lancinating pain, and altered sensation are all characteristic.[2] Weakness, muscle atrophy, fasciculations, cramps, and loss of tendon reflexes are also frequently seen. Paresthesias, hyperesthesia, hyperpathia, and autonomic disturbances may be seen. Descriptors commonly used in peripheral mononeuropathy include aching, burning, lancinating or shooting, and throbbing. It is sometimes difficult to differentiate sympathetically mediated pain from a sympathetic-independent peripheral mononeuropathy if symptoms are not well localized. In addition, sensory changes may be selective for only certain types of sensation.[49] Sympathetic blockade is useful in making this distinction. If a sympathetic block creates only partial pain relief in suspected RSD, I reexamine the patient carefully to check specifically for a dermatomal distribution on the assumption that there may be a peripheral nerve injury with an overlying sympathetic dysfunction.

Although there are many similarities in the treatment of sympathetically mediated (RSD) and sympathetic-independent neuropathic pain, there are also important differences. It is useful, therefore, to distinguish between the two. The treatment of sympathetic-independent neuropathic pain includes the use of intermittent peripheral nerve blocks with local anesthetic and corticosteroid and a variable combination of tricyclic antidepressants, phenothiazines, membrane-stabilizing agents, and clonidine. Afferent stimulation, TENS and topical capsaicin are also used. Capsaicin acts by depleting substance P at nerve terminals, and TENS presumably works by reducing the transmission of pain impulses at the level of the spinal cord. Intravenous lidocaine may be infused to test the responsiveness to that class of medications. If the test infusion is successful, oral mexiletine may be used.[50] There is evidence that some patients with this type of pain may respond to GABA receptor agents such as baclofen or NMDA–receptor antagonists such as ketamine or dextromethorphan. For particularly resistant cases of mononeuropathy, implantable peripheral nerve stimulators have been used with fairly good success.

Sympathetic-independent neuropathic pain is notoriously unresponsive to narcotic analgesics and usually one of the more difficult types of pain to treat. Although it is tempting to treat a suffering patient with the more familiar pain relievers, this type of pain responds best to a combination of drugs, use of narcotics alone or as the primary agent is likely to be disappointing for both the clinician and the patient.

Medications Used in the Treatment of Pain

Nonsteroidal Anti-Inflammatory Medications (NSAIDs)

It is assumed that nonsteroidal anti-inflammatory medications (NSAIDs) are familiar to the reader, so they will not be discussed in detail here. It is worth mentioning that the World Health Organization has published guidelines on the treatment of pain that uses the concept of an analgesic ladder. The idea behind the analgesic ladder is that the treatment of pain should begin with the simplest dosage schedules and least invasive pain management modalities first. Mild to moderate pain is treated with NSAIDs, aspirin, or acetaminophen first with or without adjunctive medications. If response to these agents is not adequate, a mild opioid analgesic is added, followed by a potent opioid if necessary. These different classes of medications are considered to be complementary, not mutually exclusive, so the addition of an opioid should not prompt the discontinuation of an NSAID or adjunctive medication.

Some aspects of NSAIDs that are worth mentioning include the fact that despite extensive literature on the myriad drugs available in this category, none has been shown to be superior to the others for the purposes of analgesia. It is also important to read the literature on this subject carefully because the measured variable in many studies is the anti-inflammatory effect and not necessarily analgesia. This is important because there is a documented lack of association between the analgesia and anti-inflammatory effects of these medications.[51]

It is common to see a difference in the way an individual will respond to different NSAIDs, although this is not a predictable finding. If a patient is not achieving the desired degree of analgesia, it is frequently possible to switch to another category of NSAID and get better results. Categories of commonly used NSAIDs are salicylates, paraaminophenol, acetic acid derivatives, propionic acid derivatives, oxicam derivatives, and naphthylalkanones. Salicylates include aspirin, choline magnesium trisalicylate (Trilisate), and diflunisal (Dolobid). Acetaminophen is a paraaminophenol derivative and is the lone NSAID in this category. Acetic acid derivatives include diclofenac (Voltaren), indomethacin (Indocin), sulindac (Clinoril), tolmetin (Tolectin), etodolac (Lodine), and ketorolac (Toradol). Propionic acid derivatives include ibuprofen (Motrin), fenoprofen (Nalfon), ketoprofen (Orudis), flurbiprofen (Ansaid), oxaprozin (Daypro), and naproxen (Naprosyn, Anaprox, Naprelan). Daypro and Naprelan have the advantage of once daily dosing. The only oxicam derivative in clinical use is piroxicam (Feldene). Naphthyl-alkanones are a new class of NSAID, and the only clinically available drug in this class currently is nabumetone (Relafen). Nabumetone has been shown to result in fewer gastric lesions than aspirin, naproxen, or ibuprofen, and at a dosage of 1 g/day for 7 days resulted in no change in bleeding time.[52]

Opioids

Although most readers are familiar with the use of opioid analgesics for acute pain in the postoperative period, there are important differences in how they are used for chronic pain states. The first important difference concerns the pharmacokinetics (what the body does to the drug) and pharmacodynamics (what the drug does to the body) of the agents that are selected. Most agents that are used for acute pain, such as oxycodone or hydrocodone, are in an immediate-release form and have a clinical effectiveness of 3 to 4 hours. When the medication is administered the serum level rises rapidly, creating a rapid peak level, and then falls just as rapidly. Because these medications are usually prescribed on a pro re nata (PRN) basis, the patient moves in and out of a therapeutic serum level as though being on an analgesic rollercoaster. Although this may work adequately for acute pain syndromes, it does not work as well in chronic pain syndromes. Maintaining a more stable serum level over a longer period of time seems to create a better analgesic effect with a lower total dosage. Several agents are available for this purpose, including MS Contin and Oramorph; both use morphine as their active ingredient. Oxycontin is a newer medication that has oxycodone as the active ingredient and has the same slow release properties of MS Contin. We also find methadone to be a very useful agent. Although it is known for its use in heroin detoxification clinics, it is also an excellent analgesic. The biggest advantage is that it is inexpensive compared with the other long-acting opioid analgesics. The disadvantages of methadone are related to the stigma associated with its use and its variable half-life. Fentanyl is available in a transdermal release system called Duragesic, which needs to be replaced only once every 72 hours. Because the system creates a reservoir of fentanyl in subcutaneous adipose tissue, users should expect a 12- to 18-hour delay in both onset and termination of effect once the patch is placed or removed. It is also likely to be less effective in extremely thin individuals.

One of the main concerns with the use of opioid analgesics over long periods is the development of addiction. Portenoy[53] has defined *addiction* in a manner relevant to the chronic pain patient as being characterized by (1) intense desire for the drug and overwhelming concern about its continued availability; (2) compulsive, unsanctioned, or inappropriate drug use; and (3) manipulative behavior, hoarding, or obtaining medication from multiple sources. This is distinct from drug *depen-*

dence, which is a pharmacologic property of opioids that causes a withdrawal syndrome if the drug is withheld. Although dependence is usually present in addiction, addiction is not necessarily present in dependence. *Pseudoaddiction* describes behavior that mimics addiction in a patient who has severe pain that is being inadequately treated. Use of the term pseudoaddiction implies that the patient is seeking medication for the appropriate reasons but is doing so in an inappropriate fashion because he or she is desperate to get relief. Good literature on this subject is scarce. However, the risk of addictive behavior developing in a patient who has a chronic pain syndrome and is to receive narcotics long term is probably 1% if the patient has no previous history of addictive behavior. In individuals who do have a history of addictive behavior, chronic narcotic use is relatively contraindicated.

Tolerance is also a characteristic of opioids; it manifests itself as an increasing dose requirement to achieve the same therapeutic effect that evolves over long-term use. The rate and degree to which tolerance develops will vary from patient to patient. Although its existence does not indicate a failure of opioid therapy, in extremes it may prompt either a drug holiday or use of an alternative opioid. Although high doses of opioids are alarming to most health care professionals, many chronic pain patients require extremely high doses to achieve the desired effect. A good analogy is to consider titration of an opioid for pain control as being similar to titration of insulin for control of blood glucose level. The medication must be carefully increased in an incremental fashion, but a high dose, although unfamiliar, is not inherently dangerous. Opioids are titrated to effect and should not be withheld at an arbitrary ceiling level. The one exception is meperidine because of the potential toxicity from its metabolite normeperidine. Meperidine is not considered to be appropriate for chronic use.

Adjunctive Medications

Adjunctive medications are so named because they are usually used as adjuncts to narcotic analgesics or some other primary method of treatment. In some cases this may be a misnomer because they are sometimes used as primary analgesics.

Tricyclic antidepressants are one of the most frequently used adjunctive medications. Chronic pain syndromes have been linked to decreased levels of the neurotransmitters serotonin and norepinephrine, and these medications are presumed to have an analgesic capability based on their ability to alter the levels of these neurotransmitters.[54] Interestingly, their analgesic effect is unrelated to and precedes their antidepressant effect. There is currently some debate as to how long it takes for these medications to achieve their analgesic effect, so a trial period of 2 to 3 weeks is indicated before discontinuing them.[55] When taken at bedtime, they improve the patient's ability to have uninterrupted sleep, thereby decreasing the stress level and making them better able to deal with the pain they are experiencing. Although the dose used for pain management is far below that used for depression, it is common to see some mood-enhancing effect. These drugs are particularly effective in the treatment of pain that is described as either burning or tingling and is constant rather than episodic.

Although they are helpful in chronic pain syndromes, tricyclic antidepressants do not appear to be as effective in acute pain. Kerrick et al.[56] performed a randomized, placebo-controlled, double-blind study of 28 patients who underwent elective hip or knee arthroplasty. These patients received morphine or meperidine patient-controlled analgesia and received either amitriptyline or placebo for 3 days postoperatively. They found no opioid sparing effect or improvement in general well-being in the study group compared to the placebo group.

Anticonvulsants are also used to treat certain types of pain, and they are particularly useful in peripheral neuropathies that have lancinating or shooting pain with an electrical quality to it. Phenytoin, valproic acid, carbamazepine, and clonazepam are the drugs most frequently used. I have recently begun prescribing the agent gabapentin, and it is currently the agent I prescribe most frequently. These medications exert their anticonvulsant action by reducing spontaneous neuronal firing in the brain. Although it is not clear whether they have the same effect on peripheral nerves, the success seen in treating trigeminal neuralgia has prompted their use in other peripheral neuropathies.[57]

Phenothiazines may also be used in chronic pain syndromes, although I do not frequently prescribe them. Chlorpromazine and fluphenazine are two frequently used agents in this class of medication. Butyrophenones have a high affinity for opiate receptors and may be direct opiate agonists as well as having potent antiemetic effects. Both phenothiazines and butyrophenones are frequently used in combination with narcotics for these reasons.[57]

Alpha receptor agents are also frequently used to treat neuropathic pain of all types. Clonidine, a selective alpha$_2$ receptor agonist, has known analgesic properties and is being used more widely in the treatment of pain as evidence accumulates for its effectiveness.[58,59] It is also useful for mitigating the symptoms associated with narcotic withdrawal.[60] Phenoxybenzamine, a nonselective alpha receptor antagonist, has been used successfully in diseases with a large component of vasoconstriction. It is useful in neuropathic pain states that exhibit this characteristic as well.[61]

Treatment Challanges in the Patient with Pain

Psychologic Issues

When treating a patient in pain, and particularly a patient in chronic pain, it is important to remember that pain is a complex entity that is made up of both physiologic and psychologic components. An afferent stimulus may reach the brain by way of Aδ and C fibers, but once there it is subject to modification by the emotional state of the individual, and the response to that impulse is determined to a large extent by the learned behavior of the individual. Learned behavior is a result of past experiences as well as ethnic, religious, and cultural factors. It may be altered by the context of the situation. Social influences may also play a large role. Secondary gain is a term used to describe the benefit an individual might derive from pain, such as affection, attention, monetary gain, or distraction from other unpleasant issues, and it can sometimes play a large role in symptom magnification. This is not meant to suggest that these individuals deliberately mislead others regarding the extent of their pain, which is malingering but, rather, that these nonphysiologic factors play a role in altering people's perception of their painful stimulus.

Because psychologic factors play a significant role in the experience of pain, it follows that the treatment of chronic pain states should include treatment of this aspect of pain. Most patients who experience pain on a daily basis for extended periods will be depressed, fatigued, and in need of psychologic support. Failure to address this aspect of care will limit the success of treatment. The treatment of pain has developed into a multidisciplinary specialty with psychologists or psychiatrists playing a significant and important role.

In addition to counseling, psychologists routinely administer various tests designed to give a relatively objective evaluation of the patient's psychologic state, emotional state, and ability to cope with the situation. The tests combined with the psychologist's evaluation during interviews, will frequently yield information that is very useful in treatment.

Psychologic tests have proved to be particularly useful before implantation of dorsal column (spinal cord) stimulators and intrathecal morphine pumps. Patients who are considered candidates for the implantation of these expensive and relatively invasive devices are subjected to a battery of tests as part of the preparation process. In the event that the tests reveal previously unrecognized aspects of the patient's psychologic or emotional state that have been found to correlate with poor outcome, the patient is referred for psychologic rehabilitation before implantation proceeds. Although the psychologic impact of primary total hip arthroplasty has been very positive,[62] the situation in a patient undergoing revision surgery may be somewhat different. Thus the concept of preoperative psychologic evaluation—and intervention, where indicated—may warrant consideration in patients who do not present a straightforward clinical picture. It is far more effective to identify important psychologic issues and address them in an aggressive fashion preoperatively rather than postoperatively.

Chronic Opioid Therapy

Many patients who have been receiving relatively high doses of opioids for extended periods, such as cancer patients, will need surgery. It is important to realize that these patients will have developed tolerance to opioids and require elevated doses of medication to achieve pain relief. The way that I approach this problem is to consider the patient's chronic and acute postoperative pain as separate entities for the purposes of treatment. The opioid dose that the patient was receiving preoperatively is continued throughout the perioperative period, with equivalent conversions made to parenteral or transdermal drugs if the patient is unable to take oral medications. An additional quantity of opioid is then added to treat the acute postoperative pain, which is superimposed on the chronic pain syndrome. This additional dose of opioid should be proportional to the dose of medication the patient was receiving preoperatively, so that it reflects the tolerance the patient has developed.

As mentioned earlier, it is also important to approach these patients in a multidisciplinary fashion. For individuals who are not familiar or comfortable with long-acting opioids, and conversion between opioids, or for the purpose of facilitating a multidisciplinary approach, a consultation with a pain specialist is appropriate. If a consultation is planned, it is best to involve the consultant preoperatively.

History of Substance Abuse

The need for a multidisciplinary approach to managing pain is probably greatest in the patient with a previous or ongoing history of substance abuse. The problem is that there is no way to determine definitively whether a patient's complaint of pain is real, or whether he or she is attempting to obtain opioids for alternative reasons. My approach to this situation is to assume that every patient is truthful and treat postoperative pain based on the patient's description of its severity. Nonopioid medications and neural blockade are used whenever possible to minimize the use of opioids, but opioids are used when needed. Doses are elevated in response to complaints of pain, and dose escalation is limited only by side effects or the achievement of pain relief.

During the immediate postoperative period, a relationship is established with the patient in which pain complaints are aggressively treated, but limits are also set if inappropriate behavior, such as harassment or manipulation of medical staff, is exhibited. Once an adequate period has passed for wound healing and pain reduction to have occurred in the average patient, opioid doses are slowly reduced. If the patient complains of continued pain, the cause is aggressively sought. If none is found and no physiologic evidence of pain is seen, opioid weaning is continued. During this time, all available nonopioid methods of pain control are used, and psychologic support is advisable. I do not attempt to detoxify active substance abusers in the postoperative period. If they express a desire to undergo detoxification, I refer them to an appropriate center. In my experience, the more structure and support these patients are provided with the better they tend to do. Referral to a pain specialist and psychologist is definitely appropriate in this setting.

References

1. Bonica JJ. Definitions and taxonomy of pain. In: Bonica J, ed. *The Management of Pain*. 2nd ed. Philadelphia, Pa: Lea & Febiger; 1990:18–27.
2. Loeser JD. Peripheral nerve disorders. In: Bonica JJ, ed. *The Management of Pain*. 2nd ed. Philadelphia, Pa: Lea & Febiger; 1990:211–219.
3. Tasker RR. Pain resulting from central nervous system pathology (central pain). In: Bonica JJ, ed. *The Management of Pain*. 2nd ed. Philadelphia, Pa: Lea & Febiger; 1990: 264–283.
4. Warfield CA. Sympathetic dystrophy. In: Warfield CA, ed. *Manual of Pain Management*. Philadelphia, Pa: JB Lippincott; 1991:154–157.
5. Bonica JJ. General considerations of pain in the low back, hips, and lower extremities. In: Bonica J, ed. *The Management of Pain*. 2nd ed. Philadelphia, Pa: Lea & Febiger; 1990:1395–1447.
6. Gilliland BC. Arthritis and periarthritic disorders. In: Bonica J, ed. *The Management of Pain*. 2nd ed. Philadelphia, Pa: Lea & Febiger; 1990:329–351.
7. Bonica JJ, Spengler DM. Painful disorders of the hip region. In: Bonica J, ed. *The Management of Pain*. 2nd ed. Philadelphia, Pa: Lea & Febiger; 1990:1530–1556.
8. Raj PP, Neumann MN. Facet blocks. In: Raj PP, ed. *Pain Medicine: A Comprehensive Review*. St Louis, Mo: CV Mosby, Inc; 1996:266–270.
9. Calder TM, Rowlingson JC. Low back pain. In: Raj PP, ed. *Pain Medicine: A Comprehensive Review*. St Louis, Mo: CV Mosby, Inc; 1996:406–416.
10. Bjurholm A. Substance P and CGRP immunoreactive nerves in bone. *Peptides*. 1988;9:165–171.
11. Burton RJ Jr. Musculoskeletal pain. In: Raj PP, ed. *Pain Medicine: A Comprehensive Review*. St Louis, Mo: CV Mosby, Inc; 1996:418–428.
12. Perl ER. Pain and nociception. In: Smith D, ed. *Handbook of Physiology, Section I: The Nervous System*. vol 3. Bethesda, Md: American Physiology Society; 1984.
13. Bonica JJ, Sola SE. Other painful disorders of the low back. In: Bonica JJ, ed. *The Management of Pain*. 2nd ed. Philadelphia, Pa: Lea & Febiger; 1990:1484–1514.
14. Simons DG. Myofascial pain syndromes of head, neck and low back. In: Dubner R, Gebhart GF, Bond MR, eds. *Pain Research and Clinical Management*. vol. 3. Proceedings of the Fifth World Congress on Pain. New York, NY: Elsevier; 1988:186–200.
15. Lee MH, Itoh M, Yang GW, Eason AL. Physical therapy and rehabilitation medicine. In: Bonica JJ, ed. *The Management of Pain*. 2nd ed. Philadelphia, Pa: Lea & Febiger; 1990:1769–1788.
16. Chapman CR, Gunn CC. Acupuncture. In: Bonica JJ, ed. *The Management of Pain*. 2nd ed. Philadelphia, Pa: Lea & Febiger; 1990:1805–1821.
17. Fischer AA. Documentation of muscle pain in soft tissue pathology. In: Kraus H, ed. *Diagnosis and Treatment of Muscle Pain*. Chicago, Ill. Quintessence Publishing; 1988:55–65.
18. Loeser JD. Pain of neurologic origin in the hips and lower extremities. In: Bonica JJ, ed. *The Management of Pain*. 2nd ed. Philadelphia, Pa: Lea & Febiger, 1990: 1515–1529.
19. Bohl WR, Steffee AD. Lumbar spinal stenosis: a cause of continued pain and disability in patients after total hip arthroplasty. *Spine*. 1979;4:168–173.
20. Pritchett JW. Lumbar decompression to treat foot drop after hip arthroplasty. *Clin Orthop*. 1994;303:173–177.
21. Mallory TH, Halley D. Posterior buttock pain following total hip replacement: a case report. *Clin Orthop*. 1973;90: 104–106.
22. Laudner WJ, Hungerford DS. Stress fracture of the pubis after total hip arthroplasty. *Clin Orthop*. 1981;159:183–185.
23. Cracchiolo A. Stress fractures of the pelvis as a cause of hip pain following total hip and knee arthroplasty. *Arthritis Rheum*. 1981;24:740–742.
24. Nercessian OA, Macaulay W, Stinchfield FE. Peripheral neuropathies following total hip arthroplasty. *J Arthroplasty*. 1994;9:645–651.
25. Barrack RL. Assessment of the symptomatic total hip. *Orthopedics*. 1994;17:793–795.
26. Evans BG, Cuckler JM. Evaluation of the painful total hip arthroplasty. *Orthop Clin North Am*. 1992;23:303–311.
27. Horne G, Rutherford A, Schemitsch E. Evaluation of hip pain following cemented total hip arthroplasty. *Orthopedics*. 1990;13:415–419.
28. Nakahara M. An objective examination for painful hip after total hip arthroplasty. *Acta Orthop Scand*. 1982;53: 591–596.
29. Bonica JJ. Causalgia and other reflex sympathetic dystrophies. In: Bonica JJ, ed. *The Management of Pain*. 2nd ed. Philadelphia, Pa: Lea & Febiger; 1990:220–243.
30. Genant HK, Kozin F, Bekerman C, McCarty DJ, Sims J. A comprehensive analysis using fine-detail radiography, photon absorptiometry, and bone and joint scintigraphy. The reflex sympathetic dystrophy syndrome. *Radiology*. 1975;117:21–32.
31. Holder LE, MacKinnon SE. Reflex sympathetic dystrophy in the hands: clinical and scintigraphic criteria. *Radiology*. 1984;152:517–522.
32. Doupe J, Cullen CH, Chance GQ. Post-traumatic pain and the causalgic syndrome. *J Neurol Neurosurg Psychiatry*. 1944;7:33–48.
33. Lofstrom JB, Cousins MJ. Sympathetic neural blockade of

upper and lower extremity. In: Cousins MJ, Bridenbaugh PO, eds. *Neural Blockade in Clinical Anesthesia and Management of Pain.* 2nd ed. Philadelphia, Pa: JB Lippincott; 1988:461–500.
34. Nehme AE, Warfield CA. Diagnostic measures. In: Warfield CA, ed. *Principles and Practice of Pain Management.* New York, NY: McGraw-Hill International Book Co; 1993:53–61.
35. McLeskey CH, Balestrieri FJ, Weeks DB. Sympathetic dystrophies. In: Warfield CA, ed. *Principles and Practice of Pain Management.* New York, NY: McGraw-Hill International Book Co; 1993:219–234.
36. Subbarao J, Stillwell GK. Reflex sympathetic dystrophy syndrome of the upper extremity: analysis of total outcome of management of 125 cases. *Arch Phys Med Rehabil.* 1981;62:549–554.
37. Edwards BN, Tullos HS, Nobel PC. Contributory factors and etiology of sciatic nerve palsy in total hip arthroplasty. *Clin Orthop.* 1987;218:136–141.
38. Lazansky MG. Complications revisited: the debit side of total hip replacement. *Clin Orthop.* 1973;95:96–103.
39. Johansen NA, Pellicci PM, Tsairis P, Salvati EA: Nerve injury in total hip arthroplasty. *Clin Orthop.* 1983;179:214–222.
40. Nercessian OA, Piccoluga F, Eftekhar NS. Postoperative sciatic and femoral nerve palsy with reference to leg lengthening and medialization/lateralization of the hip joint following total hip arthroplasty. *Clin Orthop.* 1994;304:165–171.
41. Navarro RA, Schmalzried TP, Amstutz HC, Dorey FJ. Surgical approach and nerve palsy in total hip arthroplasty. *J Arthroplasty.* 1995;10:1–5.
42. Nercessian OA, Piccoluga F, Eftekhar NS. Postoperative sciatic and femoral nerve palsy with reference to leg lengthening and medialization/lateralization of the hip joint following total hip arthroplasty. *Clin Orthop.* 1994; 304:165–171.
43. Mclean M. Total hip replacement and sciatic nerve trauma. *Orthopedics.* 1986;9:1121–1127.
44. Poss GM, Lusskin R, Waugh TR, Battista AE. Femoral neuropathy secondary to pressurized cement in total hip replacement treatment by decompression and neurolysis: a case report. *J Bone Joint Surg Am.* 1987;69:623–625.
45. Fleming RE Jr, Michelsen CB, Stinchfield FE. Sciatic paralysis: a complication of bleeding following hip surgery. *J Bone Joint Surg Am.* 1979;61:37–39.
46. Mallory TH. Sciatic nerve entrapment secondary to trochanteric wiring following total hip arthroplasty: a case report. *Clin Orthop.* 1983;180:198–200.
47. Asnis SE, Hanley S, Shelton PD. Sciatic neuropathy secondary to migration of trochanteric wire following total hip arthroplasty. *Clin Orthop.* 1985;196:226–228.
48. Kim DH, Kline DG. Surgical outcome for intra- and extrapelvic femoral nerve lesions. *J Neurosurg.* 1995;83:783–790.
49. Armstrong PJ, Murphy TM. Peripheral neuropathies and neuralgias. In: Warfield CA, ed. *Principles and Practice of Pain Management.* New York, NY: McGraw-Hill International Book Co; 1993:295–300.
50. Paggioli JJ, Racz GB: Intravenous and oral anesthetics in pain management: reflections on intravenous lidocaine and mexiletine. *Pain Digest.* 1995;5:69–72.
51. McCormack K, Brune K. Dissociation between the antinociceptive and anti-inflammatory effects of the nonsteroidal anti-inflammatory drugs: a survey of their analgesic efficacy. *Drugs.* 1991;41:533–547.
52. Katz JA. Opioids and nonsteroidal antiinflammatory analgesics. In: Raj PP, ed. *Pain Medicine. A Comprehensive Review.* St Louis, Mo: Mosby-Year Book, Inc; 1996:126–140.
53. Portenoy RK. Chronic opioid therapy in nonmalignant pain. *J Pain Symptom Manage.* 1990;5(suppl):S46–S62.
54. Stein JM, Warfield CA. Systemic analgesics. In: Warfield CA, ed. *Manual of Pain Management.* Philadelphia, Pa: JB Lippincott; 1991:233–237.
55. Haddox JD. Coanalgesic agents. In: Raj PP, ed. *Pain Medicine: A Comprehensive Review.* St Louis, Mo: Mosby-Year Book, Inc; 1996:142–153.
56. Kerrick JM, Fine PG, Lipman AG, Love G. Low-dose amitriptyline as an adjunct to opioids for postoperative orthopedic pain: a placebo-controlled trial. *Pain.* 1993;52: 325–330.
57. Warfield CA. Psychotropic drugs. In: Warfield CA, ed. *Manual of Pain Management.* Philadelphia, Pa: JB Lippincott; 1991:238–240.
58. De Kock M, Crochet B, Morimont C, Scholtes JL. Intravenous or epidural clonidine for intra- and postoperative analgesia. *Anesthesiology.* 1993;79:525–531.
59. Eisenach J, Detweiler D, Hood D. Hemodynamic and analgesic actions of epidurally administered clonidine. *Anesthesiology.* 1993;78:277–287.
60. Stoelting RK. Antihypertensive drugs. In: *Pharmacology and Physiology in Anesthetic Practice.* 2nd ed. Philadelphia, Pa: JB Lippincott; 1991:311–323.
61. Stoelting RK. Alpha- and beta-adrenergic receptor antagonists. In: *Pharmacology and Physiology in Anesthetic Practice.* 2nd ed. Philadelphia, Pa: JB Lippincott; 1991:295–310.
62. Petrie K, Chamberlain K, Azariah R. The psychological impact of hip arthroplasty. *Aust N Z J Surg.* 1994;64:115–117.

Part 3
Preoperative Planning

James V. Bono and Joseph C. McCarthy

The importance of preoperative planning in revision total hip surgery cannot be overemphasized. This cognitive exercise should not be overlooked or left until the last minute. There are many surgical pitfalls that can be avoided by thorough planning of the surgical approach, removal of existing implants and cement, and placement of revision components. Although the focus of the following discussion is the technical aspects of the revision surgical procedure, preoperative planning must address broader issues regarding the patient's general health status and living conditions. A thorough medical evaluation should be performed on all patients undergoing revision hip surgery. Adequate time is allowed for optimization of the patient's medical condition before the elective surgery procedure. Anticipation of blood loss and the length of surgery is important in choosing the method of blood conservation and anesthetic to be used.

Preoperative planning begins in the office setting and includes a thorough history and physical examination of the patient and evaluation of adequate preoperative x-rays. A thorough knowledge of previous surgical procedures is mandatory. Although tedious, obtaining hospital records, including implant stickers, is often necessary in order to identify the patient's existing components.

A complete orthopedic examination of the patient is essential. An assessment of motor and sensory function should be well documented and repeated the morning of surgery. Limb length is routinely assessed in the office and measured by using blocks placed under the shortened extremity. Any discrepancy between apparent and actual limb length needs to be investigated. Often, the hemipelvis is elevated because of an adduction contracture of the hip. Over time, this may create a fixed pelvic obliquity with or without a lumbar scoliosis. An AP radiograph of the pelvis with the patient sitting can sometimes differentiate a fixed from a flexible pelvic obliquity. A limb length discrepancy resulting from a fixed pelvic obliquity can create an apparent limb length discrepancy when in actuality the limb lengths are equal. If the pelvic obliquity is fixed, limb length will not be restored by soft tissue release alone. This condition often requires lengthening of the operative extremity based on the measured discrepancy.

The goals of revision surgery are to restore limb length and offset while maximizing abductor muscle function. The acetabular and femoral implants must provide initial as well as long-term stability. The femoral component should be of adequate length and sized appropriately to the proximal and distal geometry of the femur. The acetabular component must have structural support which is often compromised by bony erosion. The condition and amount of host bone that is in contact with the prosthesis determines the biologic character of the reconstruction. If there is sufficient host bone to allow porous ingrowth, a cementless component may be considered. However, if there is insufficient host bone or the host bone appears biologically unsatisfactory, the prospect of cementless fixation is poor. Alternative methods of fixation need to be considered in this setting, including the use of cement or a bipolar hemiarthroplasty.

An assessment of existing bone stock as well as a prediction of soft tissue integrity are fundamental. An AP radiograph of the pelvis is used to determine the interteardrop axis. This is the most accurate radiographic reference to measure preoperative limb length discrepancy. In cases of an aplastic hemipelvis or posttraumatic deformity, the axis along the inferior aspect of the SI joints is used. These references are the most reproducible when accounting for differences in radiographic technique and pelvic tilt. Lateral and oblique views of the pelvis can be used to assess the integrity of anterior and posterior columns. The use of three-dimensional imaging can help in assessing extent and location of preoperative bone loss. Assessment of acetabular bone loss is useful in predicting requirements for bone graft, prosthesis selection, and implant fixation. Cavitary lesions are usually managed with the use of morsellized allograft. For massive medial cavitary lesions with protrusio, reconstructive options include hanging the cup on the existing rim with backgrafting of the lesion with particulate or solid allograft.

Alternatively, a deep profile component can be used, which makes up the defect by virtue of a thicker metal shell. Identification of a large segmental peripheral defect implies the lack of structural support for the implant and generally precludes a press-fit or rim-fit of the acetabular component. This finding should alert the surgeon to the potential need for a bulk structural allograft. A femoral head, distal femoral, or whole acetabular allograft is prepared and contoured to the size of the defect. Appropriate fixation devices (eg, screws, plates) need to be available. Alternatively, an oblong acetabular component or reinforcement ring, if considered, should be on hand. Preoperative identification of a pelvic discontinuity requires additional surgical exposure and equipment to attach the top of the pelvis to the bottom. This may be done in several ways, including through the use of a pelvic reconstruction plate, acetabular cage, or anti-protrusio device. With massive cavitary and segmental deficiencies, the editors of this book have used a replicating device made by Midas Rex, which uses an intraoperative mold of the defect as a template to contour the allograft.

Preoperative planning for femoral component revision is usually simpler than for the acetabulum. Limb length discrepancies are measured radiographically and correlated to the clinical discrepancy with the use of blocks. The clinical measurement often supersedes the radiographic measurement if there is a disparity between the two. To achieve limb length equalization, the surgeon must first determine the center of the acetabular reconstruction by templating the acetabular component in appropriate position, given the existing bone, or in the position anticipated after structural grafting. Once this point is known, the position of the femoral implant is measured. If the limb is to be intentionally lengthened, the center of the head of the femoral component is placed superior to the center of the acetabular component. Consequently, when the hip is reduced the leg will be lengthened by the measured amount. Similarly, femoral component offset may be adjusted by varying the neck length of the prosthesis and resection level of the bone. Often, increased offset requires use of a longer neck prosthesis with deeper seating of the femoral component. Templates are used to choose the appropriate diameter of the femoral stem both proximally and distally, and to anticipate the anterior bow of the femur. The AP radiograph is used to assess any lateral bowing of the femur, angular deformity, and any cortical defects, whether complete or partial. Typically, the revision stem bypasses existing defects by two femoral diameters.

Incomplete or cavitary femoral deficiencies may be ignored or filled in with graft material. Segmental proximal deficiencies, however, may preclude proximal fixation. These deficiencies are occasionally not identified on the preoperative radiograph. The inability to visualize a continuous anterior and posterior cortex, often attributed to poor radiographic technique, identifies a proximal segmental femoral deficiency. The use of a proximal femoral allograft, long-stem cemented implant, or fully porous-coated stem should be anticipated. Allograft onlay strut grafts should always be available to reinforce pre-existing or iatrogenic distal femoral perforations.

Frequently, few anatomic landmarks remain on the proximal femur in the revision setting. The lesser trochanter may be poorly visualized or obscured by heterotopic bone. Often, the only landmark that remains is the collar of the existing prosthesis. The location of the existing prosthesis serves as an intraoperative landmark to reference subsequent component position, and it should be carefully marked before removal.

The AP radiographs must be scrutinized for trochanteric overhang. With the femoral stem aligned within the canal, a line is drawn proximally to predict the path of femoral component insertion. If an excessive amount of trochanter overhangs, several potential complications can occur. First, if the trochanteric bone is not resected, the new femoral stem will be placed in varus, with or without lateral femoral perforation. Second, if too great a lateral force is placed on the trochanter during canal preparation or stem insertion, a trochanteric fracture can result. Finally, the trochanteric bed may be excessively thinned to introduce the femoral stem, resulting in trochanteric fracture or abductor avulsion.

Preoperative planning must address not only the particular implant that is to be used, but also the expected surgical exposure required. On the acetabular side, adequate exposure requires translation of the femur either anteriorly or posteriorly. Surgical scarring in the revision situation can make this quite difficult. A complete capsulectomy is often required to allow sufficient translation of the femur. A psoas tenotomy is infrequently required, but it should be performed if necessary. Superior acetabular exposure is often limited, particularly when a superior segmental defect is to be reconstructed. In this setting, conventional trochanteric osteotomy yields the greatest exposure. The trochanteric remnant can be retracted superiorly and the abductor musculature can be subperiosteally elevated from the iliac wing. A trochanteric slide or extended trochanteric osteotomy, in which the abductor mechanism is left in continuity, allows greater anterior retraction of the abductor mechanism but is not as extensile as a conventional osteotomy. The use of a pre-existing skin excision is often adequate. However, with the requirement for major structural acetabular grafting, the surgeon cannot compensate for a poorly placed initial incision. Therefore a proximal extension should be considered.

On the femoral side, surgical exposure must anticipate removal of both the existing prosthesis and all hardware and cement. Cement removal may be facilitated by making a bony window or by using a trochanteric slide or extended trochanteric osteotomy. This decision is based on the location and extent of the cement column, and an assessment of whether the cement is loose. The extent and location of the osteotomy is determined pre-operatively to provide adequate exposure. Occasionally, a transverse osteotomy may be required to compensate for angular deformity and may allow for expedient removal of cement.

A template of the selected implant should be placed over the AP radiograph. The presence of trochanteric overhang, as mentioned previously, should alert the surgeon to potential problems. The temptation to preserve the trochanter can result in excessive thinning of the bone or inadvertent detachment of the abductor tendon. A trochanteric slide, extended trochanteric osteotomy, or transverse femoral osteotomy should be considered in these situations. Although the concept of femoral osteotomy may seem somewhat radical, it prevents the potential pitfalls of trochanteric fracture or abductor injury and may actually be a more conservative option.

In summary, preoperative planning must anticipate the required surgical exposure, removal of existing implants, and safe and accurate placement of revision components. There is never a single preoperative plan. Rather, several plans need to be considered in the event of intraoperative complication or unexpected finding. It is far better to be overprepared than underprepared.

9
Bone Stock Loss and Allografting: Acetabulum

Wayne G. Paprosky, Michael S. Bradford, and Todd D. Sekundiak

Reconstructive surgery of the failed acetabulum in revision arthroplasty is increasingly difficult to perform because of the increased bone loss as compared with that in a primary procedure. Being able to predict the bony defect preoperatively allows the surgeon to create the appropriate armamentarium for successful reconstruction. As the number of joint replacements and the time they remain in vivo increase, bony defects also increase.[1-7] A historical and clinical perspective of the patient must be combined with a radiographic assessment to determine a protocol for the appropriate reconstructive procedure.

Causes of Acetabular Bony Defects

Acetabular bony defects occur from multiple etiologies. The patient can have either structural bone loss from the index disease process or defects created iatrogenically from previous operative procedures. Early operative failures that occur aseptically tend to be a result of poor technique, and the acetabular defect should not have progressed from the time of the previous procedure. Unfortunately most failures that occur late and are related to aseptic loosening tend to be a result of progressive osteolysis. With osteolysis being relatively painfree, bone loss can progress and be extensive.[8-15] It is therefore essential to accurately classify the defects radiographically so the joint can be reconstructed. The final caveat in assessing the preoperative defect is to ensure one accounts for the bone loss that may occur with removal of in situ components. Stable components that require removal because of incompatibility, poor design, or recurrent dislocation can lead to further significant bone loss.

Correlation of Acetabular Bony Defects with Reconstruction

The acetabulum is in the shape of an inverted horseshoe, with the limbs of the horseshoe being formed by the anterior and posterior walls and columns. The apex of these limbs forms the superior dome, with the horns at the open end forming the cotyloid fossa with the transverse acetabular ligament. The cotyloid fossa is the medial portion of the anterior and posterior wall and determines the medial extent of the acetabular fossa. The anterior and posterior columns unite at the apex of the acetabulum to form an inverted Y. This Y needs to be in continuity to support the acetabular component or provide a buttress for structural allografts. The radiographic assessment will determine the degree of alteration that has occurred to this anatomy, which will affect the reconstruction chosen.

When evaluating the acetabulum and classifying the defect, one must correlate the defect to the type of reconstruction chosen.[6,15] For example, a porous acetabular cup requires approximately 50% host contact to obtain a stable fit and eventual ingrowth. Larger defects will not support a press-fit cup and require custom cups, particulate graft techniques, or bulk structural allografts.[16] Therefore the classification system should correlate reconstruction with the type of defect. Further, the classification system needs to be clinically and radiographically reproducible, so that it can be used in the clinical setting.

We have concerns with the AAOS acetabular defect classification in that it provides only a descriptive explanation of the defects without giving options for the problems present.[17] Further, it is a classification system that can be used only intraoperatively because it provides no determinants radiographically for preoperative assessment. For instance, the use of structural allografts can be indicated in segmental, combined segmental and cavitary, pelvic dissociation, and even arthrodesed classifications.

Classification System for Acetabular Reconstruction

We use a classification that is simple, reproducible, and predictive for the acetabular reconstruction required. It uses the bony landmarks on an anterioposterior radiograph to reconstruct the three-dimensional acetabulum. By assessing the degree and direction of migration of the hip center, the amount of ischial osteolysis, the destruction of the acetabular teardrop, and the breach in Kohler's line, the surgeon can reconstruct the acetabular rim, columns, and medial wall. Once the degree of bone loss has been determined, the surgeon can determine the intraoperative needs.

Migration of Hip Center and Breach in Kohler's Line

The method of Gore et al.[18] can be used to determine the extent and direction of hip center migration if there is a normal contralateral hip. Otherwise, the method of Ranawat et al.[19] can be used. We determine the amount of superior migration by constructing a horizontal line through the most superior extent of each obturator foramen and measuring the distance to the failed hip center.[16] Migration greater than 2 cm above the normal hip center or 3 cm above the obturator foramen reference line is classified as significant. It is important to factor in the amount of superior cement or metal augmentation that has been used to fill preexisting superior acetabular defects. It has previously been determined that the average normal hip center is 10.9 mm above the obturator line.[16] With the greater amount of superior migration, more destruction of the columns occurs.

Direction of migration also determines degree of bone destruction. Superior migration that also occurs in a lateral direction tends to cause more posterior column damage. It also tends to occur more rapidly. This may be secondary to the loads, which are highest when the hip center is displaced in a superior, lateral, and posterior direction. Supermedial migration signifies destruction of the anterior column. Although this migration tends to be less progressive than the superolateral migration or break-out pattern, one must be aware of the extreme difficulty in reconstructing the anterior column and therefore forewarned of severe break-in patterns.

The final migration pattern may be mostly medial or protrusio. Obviously, this signifies medial wall destruction and some degree of anterior column involvement. The degree of medial migration can be determined by assessing the integrity of Kohler's line. This can then be used to assess the amount of anterior column bone loss. Migration that is still lateral to Kohler's line is grade I. Migration to but not through Kohler's line is grade II. Migration that occurs into the pelvis but with medial expansion of the pelvic wall is grade II+. Disruption of Kohler's line with migration into the pelvis signifies grade III, whereas marked medial migration of the component into the pelvis is grade III+. By combining this sign with the assessment of the acetabular teardrop destruction and ischial lysis, the amount of antero- and posteroinferior wall and column destruction, respectively, can be determined.

Acetabular Teardrop Destruction

The acetabular teardrop is a radiographic representation formed by the cotyloid fossa and the inner table of the pelvis. The cotyloid fossa represents the medial aspect of the acetabulum. With destruction of the lateral aspect of the teardrop, only the inferior portion of the acetabular wall tends to be involved, with preservation of the antero- and posteroinferior columns. When destruction of the teardrop also includes its medial side, inferior column involvement must be suspected. This finding is then correlated with the degree of ischial lysis to determine whether destruction is more anterior or posterior.

Ischial Osteolysis

Ischial osteolysis represents damage to the inferior aspects of the posterior wall and column. As determined by previous studies, the millimeters of involvement of the ischium determines the degree of posterior wall and column involvement. This measurement is taken from the superior transverse obturator reference line, as discussed for hip center migration. Mild lysis of 0 to 7 mm tends to have little effect on the wall or column. Seven to 14 mm of involvement leads to greater wall destruction and is moderate in classification. Greater involvement is severe and indicates structural loss of the posteroinferior wall and column.

By combining these radiographic criteria and including the obvious historical and clinical caveats, one can determine the ability of the acetabulum to support a prosthesis or the augmentation required to ensure long-term fixation and survivability.

Reconstructive Approach by Type of Bony Defect

Type I

A Type I acetabular defect resembles a primary acetabulum (Fig. 9.1). There is no superior migration of the failed head center. The teardrop and ischium are intact and medial migration is at most grade I. There will be greater than

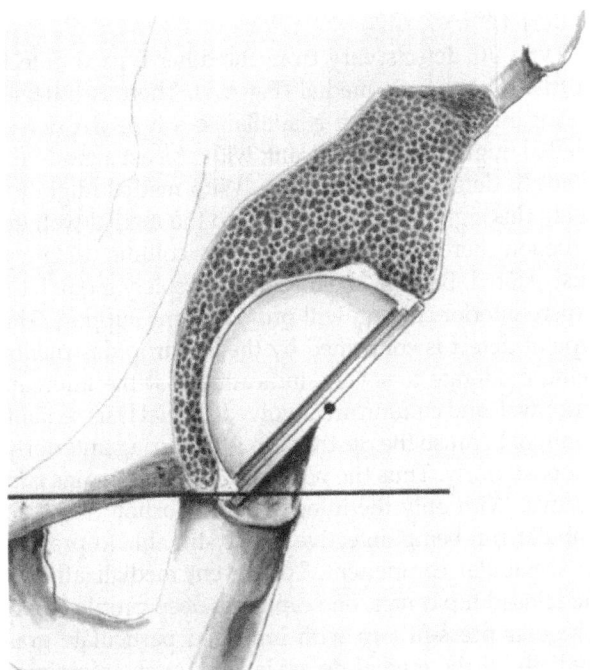

Figure 9.1. Type I acetabular defect. Teardrop Lysis: None. Ischial Lysis: None. Kohler's Line: Grade I. Migration: None. (See color insert.)

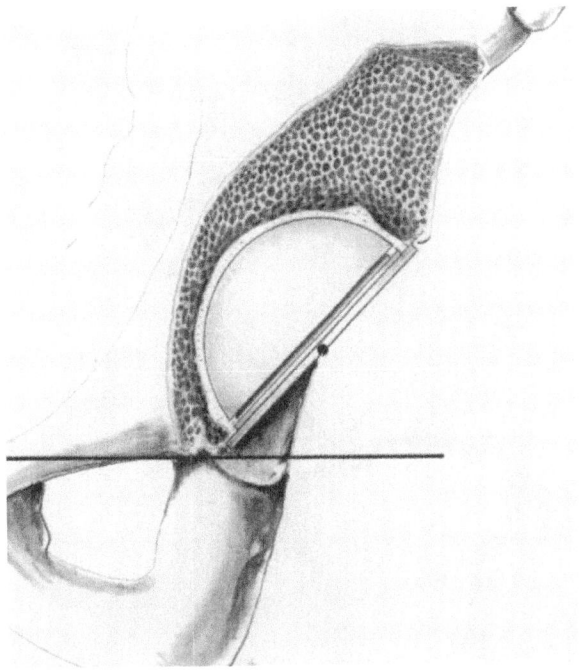

Figure 9.2. Type IIA acetabular defect. Teardrop Lysis: Mild. Ischial Lysis: Mild. Kohler's Line: Grade I. Migration: <3.0 cm. (See color insert.)

90% host bone contact with the component, which will allow acceptance of a press-fit or cemented component. There is minimal bone loss, and the only graft proposed would be particulate bone to fill previous cement lug holes or small, contained defects from localized osteolysis.

Type II

Type II defects are the most commonly seen defects in the revision setting (Figs. 9.2, 9.3, 9.4). Migration of the hip center is present, with increasing loss of the teardrop and destruction of the ischium. Kohler's line integrity can be variable, but in all cases the anterior and posterior columns are intact and supportive. These defects inherently have a minimum of 70% of the host bone contacting a press-fit acetabular component. Bone grafts with these types of defects are performed to restore bone stock, but they are not required to support component fixation. The same cannot be said for attempts to place a cemented component. Cementing components with type II defects can be fraught with hazards and this approach should be used only when combined with impaction graft techniques.[20]

Type IIA defects are similar to type I defects, with slightly increased bone loss (Fig. 9.2). Migration is well below the significant level of 3 cm from the superior transverse obturator line. Kohler's line disruption is grade I. Teardrop lysis is minimal with only a portion of the lateral border of the teardrop being involved. Ischial lysis is well below the mild limit of 7 mm. Reconstruction can proceed in a manner similar to that in type I defects, with the realization that slightly greater amounts of particulate bone may be required to fill defects. If one is contemplating cementing an acetabular

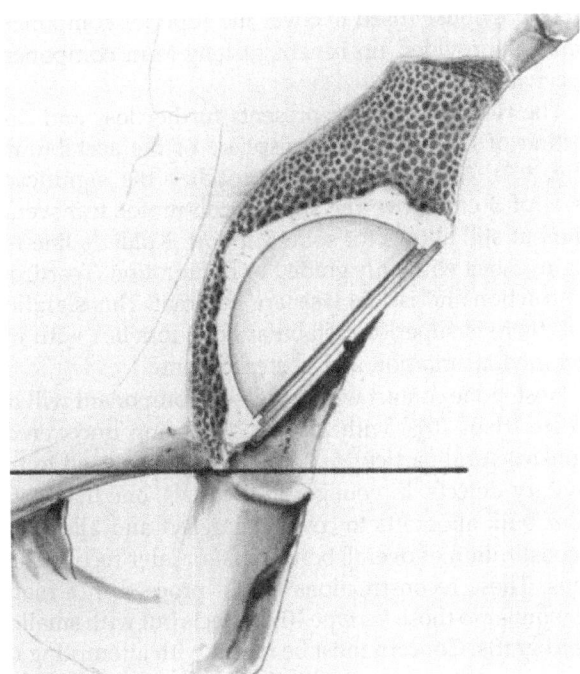

Figure 9.3. Type IIB acetabular defect. Teardrop Lysis: Mild. Ischial Lysis: Mild. Kohler's Line: Grade I–II. Migration: <3.0 cm. (See color insert.)

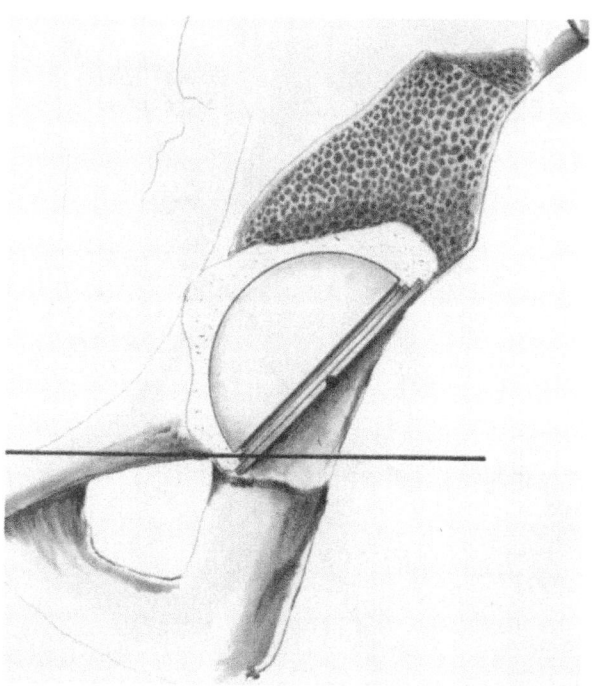

Figure 9.4. Type IIC acetabular defect. Teardrop Lysis: Moderate/Severe. Ischial Lysis: Mild. Kohler's Line: Grade III. Migration: <3.0 cm. (See color insert.)

component, one must ensure the bone graft is impacted and that only 85% host bone contact may be available for obtaining cement penetration. This amount of contact is more than adequate to support a press-fit component. Loss of the 10% to 15% contact tends to occur superiorly. Small bulk allografts (ie, femoral heads) were previously used to cover the superior component rim but provided no benefit to long-term component survivability.

The type IIB defect represents further loss and distortion of the superior hemisphere of the acetabulum (Fig. 9.3). Migration now approaches the significant level of 3 cm above the superior obturator transverse line but still allows for some support. Kohler's line remains intact with only grade I or II migration. Teardrop destruction and ischial lysis are minimal. This signifies that there is superior acetabular bone loss but with intact medial, anterior, and posterior bone.

Host–bone contact with a press-fit component will be greater than 70%, with 20% to 30% being uncovered. Nonstructural particulate bone can again be used to fill cavitary defects. In younger individuals, one may consider bulk allografts to cover the defect and allow for reconstitution of overall bone mass for later reconstructions. These reconstructions would proceed in a manner similar to those for type IIIA defects but with smaller sized grafts. Concern must be raised with attempting to cement a component into this defect.[1–3,5,6,7,10–12,20–25] An impaction acetabular graft is an option, but we personally have no experience with this type of defect and cannot correlate the findings in the literature with this type of defect.[19]

Type IIC defects vary from the other type II defects in that migration is medial (Fig. 9.4). There is little superior migration, which is similar to a type IIA defect. Medial migration is significant, with at least a grade II+ if not III defect in Kohler's line. With medial migration being this significant, in addition to the medial wall destruction there is loss in the anterior column, as previously stated. Because the migration is solely medial, the superoanterior column will provide some support. This type of defect is confirmed by the teardrop destruction being moderate to severe, indicating that the inferoanterior wall and column are involved. Ischial lysis remains minimal because the destruction is occurring anteriorly, not posteriorly. Thus the posterior column remains supportive. With only the inferoanterior portion of the acetabular rim being defective one is still able to press-fit an acetabular component. To prevent medialization of the revised hip center, one can use a deep profile cup or a regular press-fit cup with impacted particulate graft medially. If the medial defect is large or the remaining membrane is nonsupportive to the particulate graft, a napkin-ring type of femoral head graft can be impacted in place. This can be grouted with particulate graft for further stability and shaped with the acetabular reamers. If cement is an option, one would consider an impaction graft technique after making the defect contained with mesh or block allograft. Cement-ing a component directly into this defect would not be advisable.

Type III

Type III defects have progressed to a significant level of structural acetabular bone loss. The superior dome is nonsupportive. With defects extending into the anterior and posterior columns, they also lose their ability to support a prosthesis. Defects are large enough that less than 70% of the press-fit component will be in contact with the host bone. Press-fit components will obtain some initial, although minimal, stability and still require augmentation or structural allograft to allow for bony ingrowth. In cases in which defects are so large that only 50% of host bone would be contacting a hemispheric press-fit implant, ingrowth cannot be obtained. Therefore one must consider an acetabular transplant. The type III defects have been subcategorized on the basis of criteria to support a hemispheric cup.

The type IIIA defect has migrated 3 cm above the superior obturator transverse line, signifying severe superior bone loss with no supportive superior dome (Fig. 9.5). Kohler's line may still be intact or expanded into the pelvis (grade II or II+). Thus migration is more superior than medial, signifying that a portion of the anterior column is supportive. A portion of the posterior column is also supportive unless migration is massive. Teardrop lysis remains mild to moderate, indicating some inferoanterior column support. This can be correlated with the degree of Kohler's line involvement to assess the superanterior column. Ischial lysis also remains mild to moderate, with lysis being less than 15 mm below the superior obturator transverse line. Thus the inferior portion of the posterior column will also provide for some support.

"Double-bubble cups" may provide initial stability to obtain biologic fixation, although follow-up is not available and technique is critical because increased bone loss is produced with further reaming. The use of jumbo press-fit cups can result in some initial stability in these defects.[26] Fifty to 70% of host bone contact is required. Fixation is augmented with a structural bulk allograft, which improves the initial stability and allows for eventual bone ingrowth of the acetabular shell. Incorporation of the bone graft also reconstitutes bone which can lessen the size of defect and possibly make future revisions easier.[27-31] The size, type, and technique of bulk structural allografting is described elsewhere.[31-34] The graft chosen must be large enough to span the defect and of adequate structural integrity to accept load and resist resorption. Routinely, we use a distal femoral allograft with proximal tibias or femurs as an alternative. Rarely is a femoral head used because of its small size and weak structure. A viable alternative to bulk structural allografts, as reported by Berry and Muller,[36] is to use impaction bone grafts within the defects. A metal

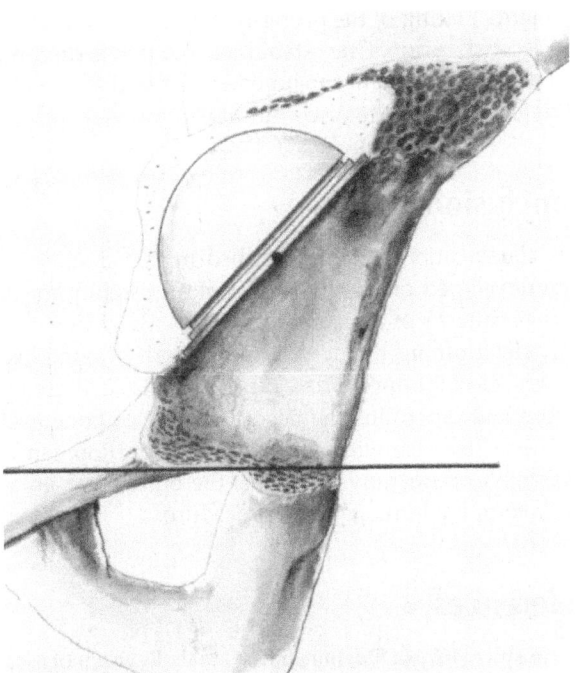

Figure 9.6. Type IIIB acetabular defect. Teardrop Lysis: Severe. Ischial Lysis: Severe. Kohler's Line: Grade III+. Migration: <3.0 cm. (See color insert.)

cage is then used to contain the graft, with the cage being supported by the remaining rim and fixation occurring in the ischium and ilium. Failure rates are moderate, but the technique restores bone stock and allows for easier re-revisions.[35-37]

The most severe acetabular defects are the Type IIIB (Fig. 9.6). The entire acetabulum is nonsupportive. Migration is significant and more than 3 cm from the superior obturator line, again signifying significant superior dome involvement. Kohler's line destruction has now progressed to grade III or III+, thus signifying both medial wall and anterior column involvement. The teardrop is obliterated, signifying extension of the anterior column loss to the inferior portion of the acetabulum. Further ischial lysis is severe with greater than 15 mm of involvement. If superior migration is massive, both superior and inferior portions of the posterior column will be nonsupportive. One can hope at best for 50% of host–bone contact with a press-fit cup and usually less than 40%. Attempts at obtaining fixation of a press-fit cup with bulk structural allograft are fraught with hazard and associated with a reported failure rate of 63%.[39] Reconstruction with a total acetabular transplant graft and a cemented all-polyethylene cup is recommended.[40] Reconstruction with an acetabular cage is also recommended, although fixation and support for the cage can be tenuous.[35-38]

A final caveat is given for all severe defects. Before any reconstruction proposed earlier is attempted, pelvic discontinuity must be ruled out. The discontinuity may

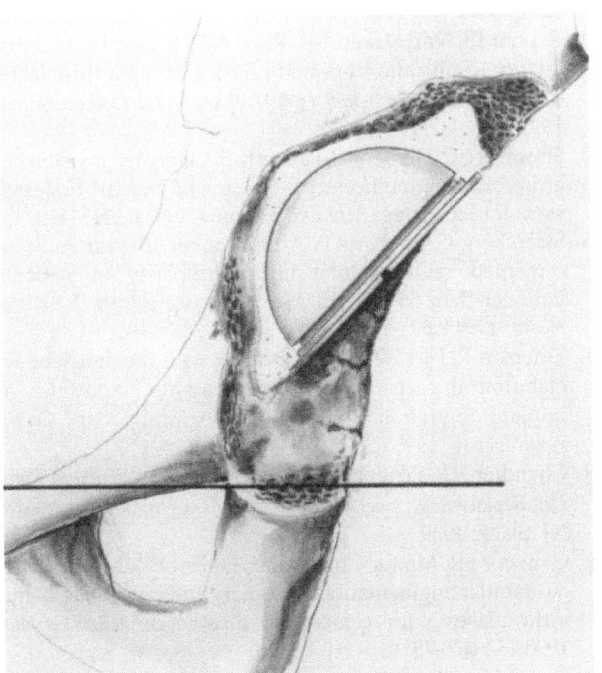

Figure 9.5. Type IIIA acetabular defect. Teardrop Lysis: Moderate. Ischial Lysis: Mild/Moderate. Kohler's Line: Grade II–II+. Migration: <3.0 cm. (See color insert.)

be occult and must be assessed by adequate, generous exposure. Plating of the posterior column must precede any reconstruction. Once stabilized, the pelvic discontinuity can be treated in a manner similar to that used for its defect without the discontinuity.

Conclusion

This classification system described in this chapter has been developed on the basis of clinically significant recurrent patterns of acetabular bone loss. By radiographically determining the degree and pattern of bone loss, one can select the appropriate type of reconstructive component and determine the need and type of bone graft required. The ease with which the classification can be performed preoperatively lessens the burden for an already complex intraoperative procedure.

References

1. Amstutz HC, Ma SM, Jinnah RH, Mai L. Revision of aseptic loose total hip arthroplasties. *Clin Orthop*. 1982;170: 21–33.
2. Cameron HU, Bhimji S. Design rationale in early clinical trials with a hemispherical threaded acetabular component. *J Arthroplasty*. 1988;3:299–304.
3. Lachiewicz PF, Hussamy OD. Revision of the acetabulum without cement with use of the Harris-Galante porous coated implant. *J Bone Joint Surg Am*. 1994;76:1834–1839.
4. Mallory TH, Vaughn BK, Lombardi V Jr., Reynolds HM Jr., Koenig JA. Threaded acetabular components: design rationale and preliminary clinical experience. *Orthop Rev*. 1988;17:305–314.
5. Marti RK, Schuller HM, Besselaar PP, Vanfrank Haasnoot EL. Results of revision hip arthroplasty with cement. *J Bone Joint Surg Am*. 1990;72:346–354.
6. Paprosky WG, Magnus RE. Principles of bone grafting in revision total hip arthroplasty. *Clin Orthop*. 1994;298:147–155.
7. Pellicci PM, Wilson PD Jr, Sledge CB, Salvati EA, Ranawat CS, Poss R. Revision total hip arthroplasty. *Clin Orthop*. 1982;170:34–41.
8. Pellicci PM, Wilson PD Jr, Sledge CB, Salvati EA, Ranawat CS, Poss R, et al. Long-term results of revision total hip replacement: a follow-up report. *J Bone Joint Surg Am*. 1985;67:513–516.
9. Cameron HU, Jung YB. Acetabular revision with a bipolar prosthesis. *Clin Orthop*. 1990;251:100–103.
10. Hunter GA, Welsh RP, Cameron HU, Bailey WH. The results of revision of total hip arthroplasty. *J Bone Joint Surg Br*. 1979;61:419–421.
11. Kavanaugh BF, Ilstrup DM, Fitzgerald RH Jr. Revision total hip arthroplasty. *J Bone Joint Surg Am*. 1985;67:517–526.
12. Kavanaugh BF, Fitzgerald RH. Multiple revisions for failed total hip arthroplasty not associated with infection. *J Bone Joint Surg Am*. 1987;69:1144–1149.
13. Murray WR. Acetabular salvage in revision total hip arthroplasty using a bipolar prosthesis. *Clin Orthop*. 1990; 251:92–99.
14. Oakeshott RD, Morgan DAF, Zukor DJ, Rudan JF, Brooks PJ, Gross AE. Revision total hip arthroplasty with osseous allograft reconstruction: a clinical and roentgenographic analysis. *Clin Orthop*. 1987;225:37–61.
15. Pollock FH, Whiteside LA. The fate of massive allografts in total hip acetabular revision surgery. *J Arthroplasty*. 1992;7:271–276.
16. Paprosky WG, Perona PG, Lawrence JM. Acetabular defect classification and surgical reconstruction in revision arthroplasty: a 6 year follow-up evaluation. *J Arthroplasty*. 1994;9:33–44.
17. D'Antonio J, Capello WN, Borden LS, Barger WL, Bierbaum BF, Boettcher WG, et al. Classification and management of acetabular abnormalities in total hip arthroplasty. *Clin Orthop*. 1989;243:126–137.
18. Gore DR, Murray MP, Gardner GM, Mollinger LA. Comparison of function two years after revision of failed total hip arthroplasty and primary hip arthroplasty. *Clin Orthop*. 1986;208:168–173.
19. Ranawat CS, Dorr LD, Inglis AE. Total hip arthroplasty in protrusio acetabuli of rheumatoid arthritis. *J Bone Joint Surg Am*. 1980;62:1059–1065.
20. Azuma T, Yasuda H, Okagaki K, Sakai K. Compressed allograft chips for acetabular reconstruction in revision hip arthroplasty. *J Bone Joint Surg Br*. 1994;76:740–744.
21. Callaghan JJ. Total hip arthroplasty: clinical perspective. *Clin Orthop*. 1992;276:33–40.
22. Callaghan JJ, Salvati EA, Pellicci PM, Wilson PD Jr, Ranawat CS. Results of revision for mechanical failure after cemented total hip replacement, 1979 to 1982: a two to five year follow-up. *J Bone Joint Surg Am*. 1985;67:1074–1085.
23. Mulroy RD, Harris WH. The effect of improved cementing techniques on component loosening in total hip replacement: an 11-year radiographic study. *J Bone Joint Surg Br*. 1990;72:757–760.
24. Repten JB, Varmarken J-E, Rock ND, Jensen JS. Unsatisfactory results after repeated revision of hip arthroplasty: 61 cases followed for 5 (1–10) years. *Acta Orthop Scand*. 1992;63:120–127.
25. Stromberg C, Herberts P, Palmertz B. Cemented revision hip arthroplasty: a multicenter 5–9 year study of 204 first revisions for loosening. *Acta Orthop Scand*. 1992;63:111–119.
26. Stromberg C, Herberts P. A multicenter 10–year study of cemented revision total hip arthroplasty in patients younger than 55 years old: a follow-up report. *J Arthroplasty*. 1994;9:595–601.
27. Emerson RH Jr, Head WC. Dealing with the deficient acetabulum in revision hip arthroplasty: the importance of implant migration and use of the jumbo cup. *Semin Arthroplasty*. 1995;6:96–102.
28. Chandler HP, Penenberg BL. *Bone Stock Deficiency in Total Hip Replacement: Classification and Management*. Thorofare, NJ: Slack; 1989.
29. Convery FR, Minter-Convery M, Devine SD, Meyers MH. Acetabular augmentation in primary and revision total hip arthroplasty with cementless prostheses. *Clin Orthop*. 1990;252:167–75.
30. Gross AE, Allan DG, Catre M, Garbuz DS, Stockley I. Bone grafts in hip replacement surgery: the pelvic side. *Orthop Clin North Am*. 1993;24:679–695.
31. Knight JL, Fujii K, Atwater R, Grothaus L. Bone-grafting

for acetabular deficiency during primary and revision total hip arthroplasty: a radiographic and clinical analysis. *J Arthroplasty*. 1993;8:371–382.

32. Paprosky WG, Bradford MS, Jablonsky WS. Acetabular reconstruction with massive acetabular allografts. *Instr Course Lect*. 1996;45:149–159.

33. McAllister CM, Borden LS. Allograft reconstruction of the acetabulum in revision hip surgery. *Semin Arthroplasty*. 1993;4:80–86.

34. Patch DA, Lewallen DG. Reconstruction of deficient acetabula using bone graft and a fixed porous ingrowth cup: a 5 year roentgenographic study. *Orthop Trans*. 1993;17:151.

35. Silverton CD, Rosenberg AG, Sheinkop MB, Kull LR, Galante JO. Revision total hip arthroplasty using cementless acetabular component: technique and results. *Clin Orthop*. 1995;319:201–208.

36. Berry DJ, Muller ME. Revision arthroplasty using an anti-protrusio cage for massive acetabular bone deficiency. *J Bone Joint Surg Br*. 1992;74:711–715.

37. Peters CL, Curtain M, Samuelson KM. Acetabular revision with the Burch-Schneider anti-protrusio cage and cancellous allograft bone. *J Arthroplasty*. 1995;10:307–312.

38. Rosson J, Schatzker J. The use of reinforcement rings to reconstruct deficient acetabulae. *J Bone Joint Surg Br*. 1992;74:716–720.

39. Paprosky WG, Bradford MS, Jablonsky WS. Acetabular reconstruction with massive acetabular grafts. *Instr Course Lect*. 1996;45:149–159.

40. Bradford MS, Paprosky WG. Total acetabular transplant allograft reconstruction of the severely deficient acetabulum. *Semin Arthroplasty*. 1995;6:86–95.

10
Bone Stock Loss and Allografting: Femur

Donald B. Longjohn and Lawrence D. Dorr

Significant loss of femoral bone stock in total hip revision presents a challenge to the joint replacement surgeon. There are several mechanisms that can result in the periprosthetic loss of bone stock in the femur. These include infection, mechanical loosening, stress-shielding due to large diameter stiff stems with distal fixation, and osteolysis secondary to particulate debris such as polyethylene. Loss of femoral bone stock causes difficulty in obtaining support for the femoral component at the time of revision surgery. Several reports of the early experience with revision total joint replacement describe worse results when bone loss was severe.[1-4] This has led to the development of different techniques and prosthetic designs to address this problem.

Careful preoperative planning is essential before revision total joint arthroplasty is undertaken in the hip with extensive femoral bone loss. The surgeon must have an accurate estimation of the pattern of bone loss in the femur. This is necessary to determine what inventory of materials will be required to complete the operation. In centers for hip joint replacement a large inventory of prostheses, instruments, and bone graft is available on site. At such centers, nearly any defect can be defined and dealt with at the time of surgery by an experienced revision surgeon, because all required resources are at his or her disposal. At hospitals where complex hip revisions are not performed on a routine basis, this inventory of supplies and instruments will not be available. Special implants, instruments, and supplies will have to be ordered in advance to have them available at the time of surgery. This is a significant cost to the hospital, particularly when large structural allografts are contemplated or custom implants may be required. Therefore it is important that the appropriate types and sizes be obtained. Even more unfortunate for a surgeon and the patient is to unexpectedly encounter a problem at surgery requiring a structural allograft or a different type of implant that is not available. Consequently, thorough preoperative planning in revision hip surgery not only benefits the patient but can help control costs.

Classification Systems

Several classification systems for femoral bone loss have been described in the literature. These were presented in conjunction with reports on reconstructive techniques in revision and served as a way of categorizing results. Chandler and Penenberg,[5] Dorr et al.,[6] Engh and Glassman,[7] Gross et al.,[8] Mallory,[9] and Paprosky[10] have all proposed classification systems that have differed in their complexity and in their descriptive terms. All have proved useful for their given purposes, but none has been universally accepted and used as a way to compare reconstructive efforts and report results among investigators. In 1993, D'Antonio et al.[11] published a comprehensive classification system for femoral deficiencies in total hip arthroplasty that represents the recommendations of the American Academy of Orthopedic Surgeons (AAOS) Committee on the Hip. This system uses the same descriptive terms as those in the AAOS classification system for acetabular deficiencies.[12] This classification system is presented in Table 10.1.

AAOS Classification System

In the AAOS classification system femoral deficiencies are described as segmental or cavitary. A segmental defect is any loss of bone in the femoral cortical shell (Fig. 10.1A). A cavitary defect is a loss of cancellous bone and/or endosteal cortical erosion without violation of the outer cortical shell (Fig. 10.1B).

Segmental defects are subdivided into proximal, intercalary, and those involving the greater trochanter. Proximal segmental defects can be either partial or complete. The partial defects are described as being anterior, medial, or posterior, and they can extend from the proximal femur to any level distally in the femur.

10. Bone Stock Loss and Allografting: Femur

Table 10.1. AAOS Classification of femoral bone loss.[11]

I. Segmental deficiencies
  A. Proximal
    1. Partial
      (a) Anterior
      (b) Medial
      (c) Posterior
    2. Complete
  B. Intercalary
  C. Greater trochanter
II. Cavitary deficiencies
  A. Cancellous
  B. Cortical
  C. Ectasia
III. Combined segmental and cavitary deficiencies
IV. Malalignment
  A. Rotational
  B. Angular
V. Femoral stenosis
VI. Femoral discontinuity

Circumferential loss of bone of the proximal femur is considered a complete proximal segmental defect. Intercalary defects are defects in the cortical tube that have intact bone above and below (ie, cortical windows and perforations). The greater trochanter is considered separately because of the unique problems that its loss causes.

Cavitary defects are subdivided according to the degree of bone loss in the involved femur. Cancellous cavitary defects involve loss of the cancellous medullary bone, whereas cortical cavitary defects have endosteal erosion of cortical bone as well. Ectasia is a situation in which there is complete loss of the cancellous bone with severe endosteal erosion of cortical bone with expansion of the femoral canal (Fig. 10.1B).

Frequently, segmental and cavitary defects coexist in the revision situation and are designated as combined segmental and cavitary defects in the AAOS classification (Fig. 10.1C). In our experience, most femoral revisions have combined deformities with segmental and cavitary defects, each being present to some degree. An example of a combined deformity would be a femur with endosteal erosion due to osteolysis with perforation of the cortex by the tip of a stem that has migrated into varus.

Because the AAOS classification system was designed to apply in both primary and revision situations, it also includes categories for malalignment, stenosis, and discontinuity of the femur. Malalignment can be either angular or rotational (Fig. 10.1D). Stenosis is relative or absolute and can be caused by an old fracture site or a distal pedestal of neocortical bone at the tip of a loose uncemented stem (Fig. 10.1E). Femoral discontinuity can be the result of a fracture or nonunion in the primary or revision setting (Fig. 10.1F).

With the use of the AAOS classification system, femoral defects are also described according to the level of bone loss. Level I includes bone proximal to the inferior portion of the lesser trochanter. Level II is an area below the inferior lesser trochanter and within 10 cm distal to it. Level III is bone greater than 10 cm distal to the lesser trochanter.

The AAOS grading system attempts to grade the femoral reconstruction (Table 10.2). Grade I reconstructions demonstrate complete contact between the prosthesis and the host bone. No graft is required, and the implant is stable. In grade II reconstructions, there is incomplete contact between the prosthesis and the host bone, but the implant is stable and no structural graft is required. Nonstructural graft may be used to fill gaps. In our practice this represents the most common situation. Grade III reconstructions require structural grafts to stabilize the prosthesis. Such grafts could be cortical strut grafts or en bloc grafts such as proximal femoral allografts.

The AAOS classification system for femoral bony abnormalities has emerged as the most comprehensive

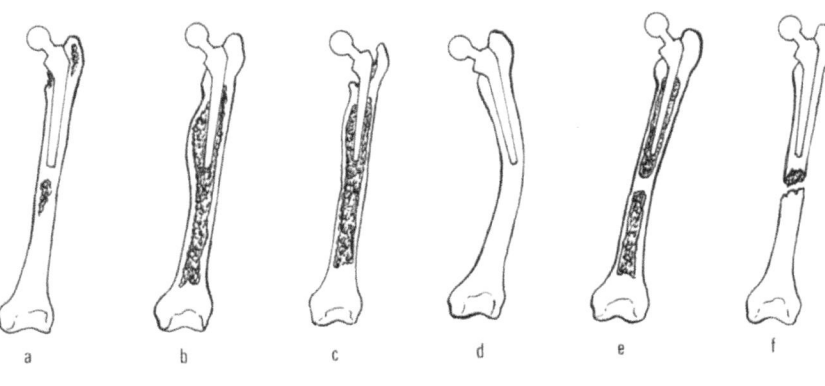

Figure 10.1. A. Segmental defect: Any loss of bone in the femoral cortical shell. B. Cavitary defect: Cancellous bone loss and/or endosteal cortical erosion with intact cortical shell. Ectasia is severe endosteal erosion of cortical bone with expansion of the femoral canal. C. Combined segmental and cavitary defects. D. Malalignment: Can be either angular or rotational. E. Stenosis: Relative or absolute, often caused by an old fracture or pedestal. F. Femoral discontinuity: Result of fracture or nonunion in primary or revision setting.

Table 10.2. AAOS grading system of femoral reconstructions[11]

Grade I	Complete prosthesis–host bone contact
	No graft required
Grade II	Incomplete host bone contact
	Prosthesis stable in host bone
	Filler graft may be required
Grade III	Incomplete prosthesis–host bone contact
	Prosthesis not stable in host bone
	Structural allograft required to stabilize prosthesis

system yet devised. It is useful for classifying bone loss in both the revision situation and primary total hip arthroplasties in which there are femoral bony abnormalities. It is a fairly complex system to use. However, a simplified system would not be as comprehensive, nor would it adequately classify the varying patterns of femoral bone defects. A large advantage is that the descriptive language used is the same as that used in the AAOS classification system for acetabular abnormalities. This provides for a common language for discussion and reporting of hip reconstructions.[13]

Organization of Femoral Revisions

At our institution, we divide femoral reconstructions into five categories on the basis of difficulty, involvement for the patient, and cost (Table 10.3). Although not actually a new classification system in itself, our system helps us organize our thoughts and resources in a practical manner.

Revision with Primary Stem

The simplest, least involved reconstruction for the patient, and the most cost-effective femoral revision, is a procedure in which the femur can be revised with another primary stem. This can be either cemented or uncemented; however, the technique of cementing into a bed of impacted cancellous graft is considered separately.

Revision with a primary uncemented stem is usually performed in a relatively young patient with good remaining bone stock including the proximal femoral neck, which is important for rotational stability with the proximally porous-coated anatomic stems that we use. Significant segmental or cavitary bone loss would preclude the use of this technique. This would be an example of an AAOS grade I femoral reconstruction.

Cemented revision with a primary stem is more often performed in older less active patients who have a reasonable amount of remaining bone. Third-generation cementing techniques are used as in primary cemented cases. Occasionally, a cortical strut graft may be required to cover a cortical defect such as a perforation and to protect stress risers and prevent fracture. With level I segmental defects the stem may occasionally need to be cemented "proud" to maintain proper hip length. Many cavitary and minor segmental defects can be reconstructed in this manner. The important thing to remember is that the final construct must be judged to be sufficiently durable to support the patient's given level of activity. If not, another more involved technique may need to be used.

Revision with Longer "Revision" Stem with Proximal and Distal Fixation

The next most involved reconstruction is revision with a long "revision" stem (Fig. 10.2). These stems are designed to be implanted into a femur with some degree of bone loss. They are designed to be stabilized and fixed in the diaphysis and they may have an anterior bow to match the anterior bow of the femur. The increased stem length allows extension past proximal areas of bone loss, which occur with shorter primary stems. These revision stems vary as widely in their design as do primary stems. The revision stem that we have used is made of titanium to decrease the modulus of elasticity, and in larger diameter sizes the distal end is split to decrease stiffness further.[6,14] This stem has a large proximal cross section designed to maximize fit in the proximal femur at the level of the lesser trochanter. The proximal portion of the stem is porous-coated, and the middle portion of the stem is grit blasted. The neck-shaft angle of the stem is increased (140°) to maintain length of the hip, given the lower level of placement of the stem in the femur, while not disproportionately increasing offset. Other stem designs have similar features in that they are designed to be placed into the distal femur and bypass missing or deficient proximal femoral bone.

This category constitutes AAOS grade I and II reconstructions because the stem achieves a stable fit in the femur. Varying degrees of cavitary and segmental bone loss from the proximal femur and upper diaphysis can be reconstructed in this manner, including partial and complete segmental loss in level 1 and intercalary segmental and cavitary defects in level 2. Because the stem is long, it can bridge areas of partial intercalary

Table 10.3. Organization of femoral revisions based on complexity of the reconstruction

I. Revision with primary stem
   A. Uncemented
   B. Cemented
II. Revision with longer "revision" stem—proximal and distal fixation
III. Revision with longer "revision" stem—diaphyseal fixation only
   A. Proximal nonstructural bone graft
   B. Proximal cement
   C. Proximal bulk allograft—load sharing
IV. Revision with long stem and reduction osteotomy
V. Revision with impaction grafting and cemented fixation

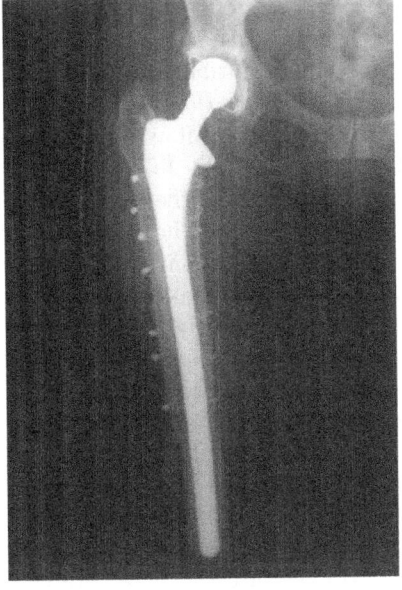
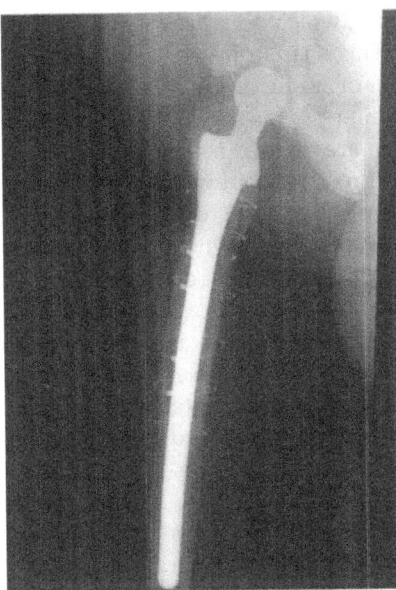

Figure 10.2. A. Anteroposterior radiograph of a femur that has been revised with the APR revision stem. The length of the stem allows it to be inserted past areas of proximal bone loss into intact distal host bone. The stem is designed to be seated at a lower level, anticipating loss of the femoral neck. The increased neck–shaft angle with the increased neck length restore hip length without disproportionately increasing the offset. Proximal segmental defects have been successfully repaired with cortical strip grafts and cerclage cables. B. Lateral radiograph demonstrating the anterior bow of the revision stem that matches the anatomic bow of the femur. This allows insertion of the long stem into the diaphysis without perforation of the anterior cortex. The proximal geometry of the stem is designed to maximize fit in the proximal femur at the level of the calcar.

bone loss and protect the femur from fracture through stress risers. Supplemental filler graft material may be required to fill cavitary defects, and occasionally, cortical strip grafts may be used to patch cortical defects. In these reconstructions we still attempt to achieve proximal bone ingrowth into the porous-coated area of the stem. The middle portion of the stem is grit blasted to obtain additional mechanical grip in the diaphysis and also to obtain biologic fixation through appositional bone ongrowth onto the grit-blasted surface.[15–17] Other stem designs have extensively porous coated surfaces and attempt to achieve ingrowth in the diaphysis.[3]

Revision with Longer "Revision" Stem— Diaphyseal Fixation Only

The third most involved reconstruction is revision with a long revision stem, obtaining diaphyseal fixation. These procedures represent AAOS grade II and III reconstructions. Extensive segmental and/or cavitary bone loss is present in levels 1, 2, and 3 (above and below the lesser trochanter; Fig. 10.3). In these femurs it is not possible to obtain adequate fixation in the remaining proximal bone, and a proximally porous-coated stem could not achieve fixation. Fixation must be obtained in the diaphysis. For these revisions we use a long titanium stem, which is entirely grit blasted with proximal hydroxylapatite coating and has eight longitudinal sharp-edged flutes. The presence of the flutes serves two purposes. First, by cutting into the endosteal cortical bone, they provide immediate rotational stability. Second, they increase the surface area of the stem in

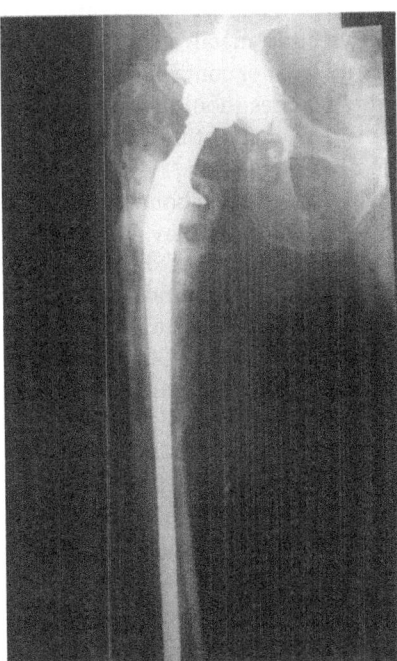

Figure 10.3. Anteroposterior radiograph showing extensive segmental and cavitary bone loss of the proximal femur that extends into the diaphysis. In such situations there is inadequate bone remaining in the proximal femur to achieve fixation with a proximally porous-coated stem. Fixation will need to be achieved in the diaphysis. The proximal femur can be reconstructed with allograft or, in patients with low activity levels, with a modular endoprosthetic system.

direct contact with the bone to increase the area of biologic fixation. The stem is also tapered, which decreases the diameter of the stem distally. This shape plus the use of titanium decrease the modulus of elasticity which helps prevent proximal stress-shielding.

In grade II reconstructions, which are defined as incomplete host bone contact with the prosthesis but with the prosthesis being stable in the host bone, structural allograft will not be required. In these cases in which the stem has axial and rotational stability in the host diaphysis, an attempt can be made to restore the proximal femoral bone loss with nonstructural graft, such as cancellous filler graft material with or without supplemental cortical strip grafts. This is a good option for younger patients with a longer life expectancy and higher activity level. In older, sedentary patients or patients whose activity level is otherwise limited, the proximal femoral bone loss can be replaced by cement. This is an acceptable alternative in these patients if the stem has adequate fixation in the diaphysis. Cement provides additional and immediate stability and fills proximal defects.

If a trochanteric slide has been performed and the trochanter has to be reattached to the remainder of the femur, fixation wires or cables should not be placed directly against the metal of the stem. If this should happen, the wires or cables will abrade against the stem and may create grooves in the stem, weakening its structural integrity and creating metal debris particles that can cause third-body wear or contribute to lysis. To prevent this, the cables or wires should be placed against bone medially or even around or through cement in cases in which this is used proximally.

In cases with catastrophic bone loss from the proximal femur (see Fig. 10.3), we may elect to use solid bulk allograft to reconstruct the proximal femur. The allograft provides proximal structural support for the stem, is load sharing, and can assist in rotational stability as well. These procedures are AAOS grade III reconstructions. In these cases there is complete segmental loss of the proximal femur and often disruption of the greater trochanter. We prefer proximal femoral allograft; however proximal tibial allograft is preferred by some surgeons. Because of an early high failure rate associated with stems press-fit into allografts, we currently recommend cemented fixation of the stem into the allograft and uncemented fixation in the host bone.[18] We use a long stem that will obtain diaphyseal fixation in the host bone. Diaphyseal fixation is important and the design of the stem used must provide for this. The stem should be long enough to allow fixation in the diaphysis and should be textured distally in some manner to allow biologic fixation by bone ingrowth or ongrowth.

Long, extensively porous-coated titanium or CoCr stems have been used with success by a number of investigators. We favor a long grit-blasted titanium stem with eight longitudinal cutting fins to obtain a press-fit into the remaining, often sclerotic bone of the host femoral diaphysis.[19] The proximal stem should not be large and stiff because these attributes can cause resorption of the allograft with time (Fig. 10.4). Often the intramedullary canal of the allograft will have to be reamed up to obtain an adequate 2- to 3-mm cement mantle for the cemented fixation of the stem that will have a press-fit in the often widened host diaphysis. If possible, we make matching step cuts in the distal portion of the allograft and the proximal end of the host bone to fit them together. Alternatively, 45° oblique cuts can be used. If there is remaining expanded host bone proximally in the upper diaphysis or lower metaphysis of the host femur, we may press-fit the stem distally into the diaphysis and press-fit the allograft proximally into the expanded area of host bone. If at all possible, remaining thin nonsupportive host bone with attached soft tissue can be bivalved and wrapped around the graft–host junction to serve as a vascularized autograft (Figs. 10.4, 10.5).[8] The graft–host junction can be fixed with dynamic compression plates, or with cortical strip grafts and cerclage wires or cables. There are often remaining areas of thin or deficient bone that would benefit from the addition of cortical strip grafts.

We attempt to preserve the greater trochanter with as much attached lateral cortex as possible and with the gluteus medius insertion and vastus lateralis origins intact. This facilitates reattachment. Maintenance of the greater trochanter promotes hip stability and strength and provides protection against postoperative dislocation. In our experience, the trochanter usually achieves fibrous union to allograft bone, but this still provides hip support.[18] The use of allografts will be discussed in more detail later in the chapter.

In elderly patients with very low activity levels we may elect to reconstruct this amount of femoral bone loss with a modular endoprosthetic system as may be used in oncologic reconstructive procedures (Fig. 10.6). This approach can simplify the surgery, but it increases the cost, and the long-term durability of such reconstructions is not known.

Revision with Long Stem and Reduction Osteotomy of Femoral Shaft

Perhaps the most difficult revision situation is the femur with extensive segmental loss proximally and extensive cavitary loss involving the entire diaphysis (levels I to III). In these bones with extensive ectasia of the diaphysis, a press-fit cannot be obtained because the canal has become too expanded. In these cases, we will reconstruct the femur with a proximal femoral allograft and perform a reduction osteotomy in the diaphysis. The reduction osteotomy is performed by removing a longitudinal strip of bone from the lateral cortex. The

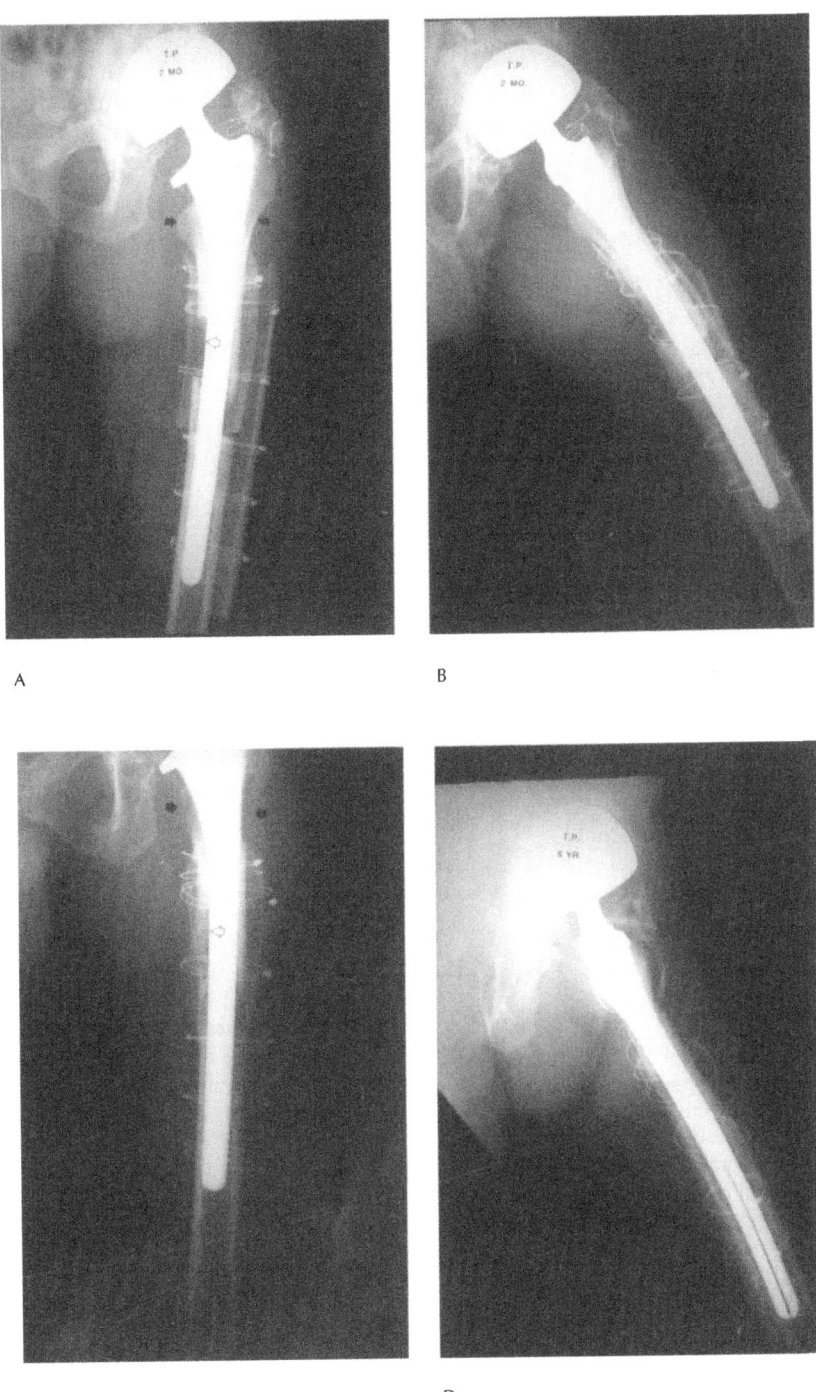

Figure 10.4. A. Anteroposterior radiograph taken 2 months postoperatively after reconstruction of a femur with severe proximal bone defects. A long stem has been cemented into a proximal femoral allograft (heavy solid arrows) and the distal portion of the stem then press-fit into the host diaphysis. Remaining proximal host bone has been wrapped around the graft-host junction and an additional allograft strut has been placed laterally. Note the gap medially between the graft and the host diaphysis (open arrow). The trochanter was not able to be successfully reattached. B. Lateral radiograph taken 2 months postoperatively. Note the gap between the graft and the host bone seen posteriorly (open arrow). Note also the remaining section of host femur anteriorly at the graft-host junction and the strut graft overlying it. C. Anteroposterior radiograph of same hip 5 years postoperatively showing significant resorption of portions of the proximal femoral allograft, believed to be related to stress-shielding because of the large stiff stem proximally (heavy solid arrows). The gap seen medially at the graft-host junction has now filled in with bone (open arrow). The proximal 1/3 of the lateral strut allograft has been resorbed (small arrow). D. Lateral radiograph taken 5 years postoperatively showing healing at the graft-host junction and ossification of the previous posterior gap (open arrow). Incorporation of the strut allograft is seen but with resorption of the proximal 1/3 (small arrow).

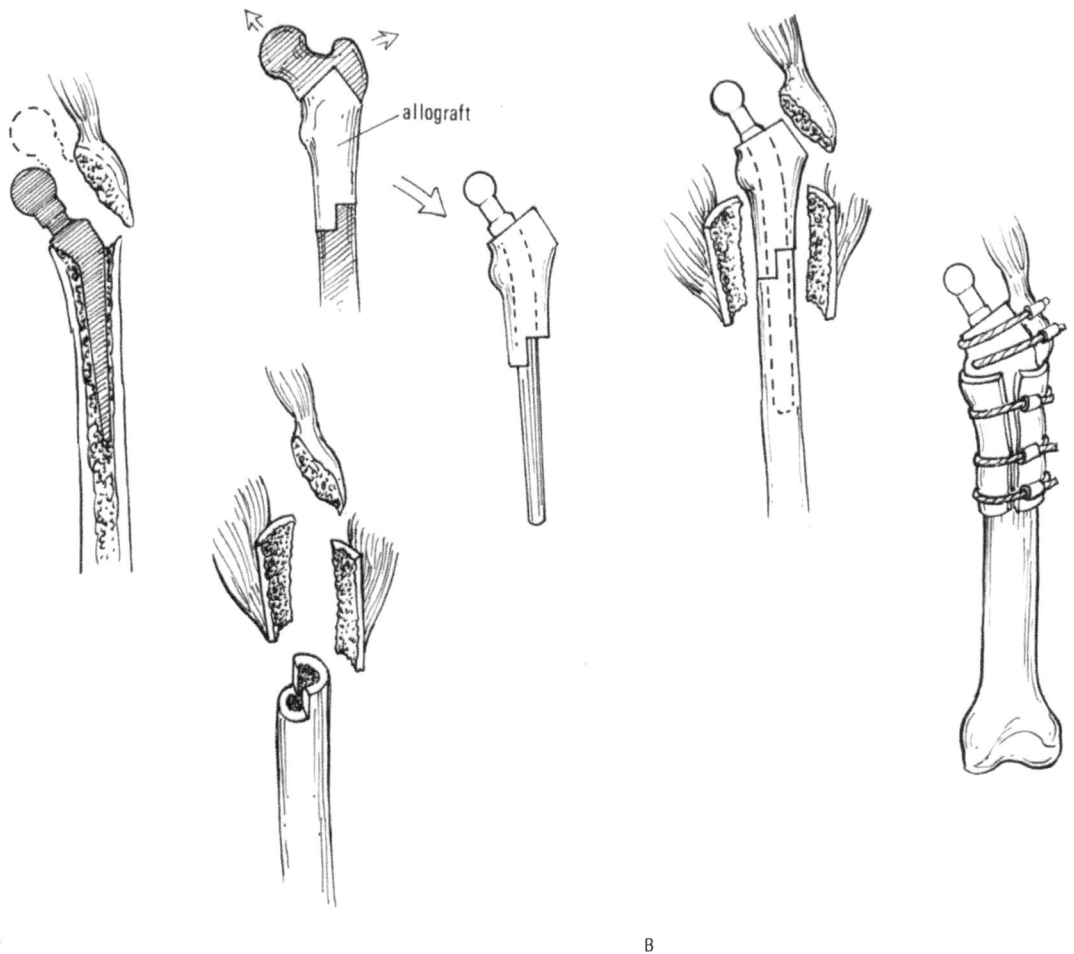

Figure 10.5. A: Severe segmental proximal femoral bone loss with a subsided stem and detached greater trochanter. After removal of the stem a step cut is made in the diaphysis. Any thin remaining segments of proximal cortical bone are left with their attached soft tissues. A matching step cut is made in a proximal femoral allograft and the head and greater trochanter are removed. After appropriate reaming, a long stem is cemented into the allograft. B: The distal portion of the long stem is press-fit into the remaining host diaphysis until the allograft contacts the host bone. The trochanter is then cabled to the allograft and the remaining portions of proximal host cortex with their soft tissue attachments are wrapped around the graft-host junction as vascularized autografts. Careful planning and preparation is required to determine the correct length of allograft that will result in the appropriate femur length to stabilize the hip.

width of the strip of bone depends on how much the diameter needs to be reduced. The strip of bone is retained and used as autograft material. The host bone is reduced around the stem and tightened with cerclage cables or wires, which brings the endosteal cortex into intimate contact with the textured surface of the stem. Biologic fixation can then replace the immediate mechanical fixation. The cortical bone of the host diaphysis is often thin and needs to be supplemented with cortical strip grafts (Fig. 10.7). In these patients we use a hip cast–brace postoperatively for 3 months to facilitate bone healing.

In elderly patients with low activity levels and this pattern of severe femoral bone loss, we may choose to reconstruct with a modular endoprosthetic system, which is cemented into the expanded femoral diaphysis. The durability of such reconstructions is not optimal, but it may suffice in an elderly person with a low activity level. It also decreases operative time and morbidity and allows easier rehabilitation.

Revision with Impaction Grafting and Cemented Fixation

Although believed to be primarily useful for proximal cavitary defects, proponents of this method feel that many defects can be addressed with this technique.[20] Segmental defects can be repaired with cortical strip grafts and cerclage wiring, and cavitary defects can be filled with impacted particulate graft. This technique is described in more detail elsewhere in this book.

Use of Structural Allograft for Femoral Bone Deficiencies

The first large series of allograft transplantations was reported in 1908 by Lexer who performed 23 whole knee transplants and 11 hemijoint knee transplants. He reviewed the progress of these patients 12 years later in 1923 and reported 50% successful results.[21] Reports of several large series did not appear in the literature again until the 1960s. This renewed interest was stimulated by the discovery that the immunogenicity of grafts could be reduced by freezing.[20]

Structural allograft bone is used as either cortical strip grafts or entire segmental grafts, such as proximal or distal femurs.

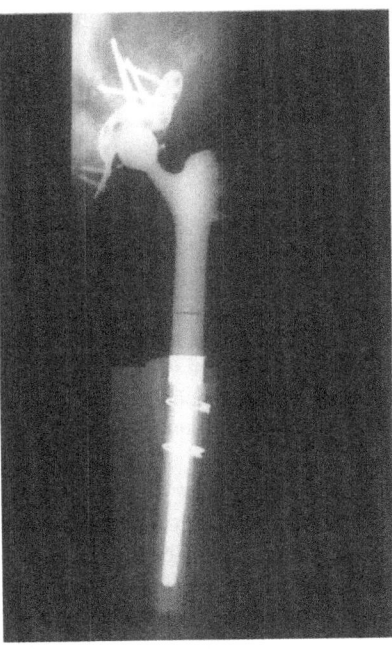

Figure 10.6. Anteroposterior radiograph of a severely bone-deficient proximal femur reconstructed with a modular oncologic-type endoprosthesis. This revision was performed in an elderly man with severe pulmonary disease who had a low activity level. This was the second stage of a two stage revision for an infected, loose total hip with a periprosthetic femur fracture. A remaining shell of the greater trochanter with attached abductors was attached to the "trochanter" on the prosthesis by pronged washers and bolts. Because of significantly osteoporotic bone in the remaining diaphysis, fixation with a press-fit stem would only have been possible with reduction osteotomy followed by protected weight-bearing for an extended period of time. Therefore cemented fixation of the stem was performed to allow earlier weight-bearing.

Cortical Strip Grafts

Cortical strip grafts can be used to augment lost femoral bone stock and restore structural integrity to the femur (see Fig. 10.4). Cortical strip grafts do become biologically active and achieve union to host bone in a matter of months if properly applied. They incorporate faster and more completely than do segmental allografts. Cortical strip grafts go though a predictable series of radiographic changes during the healing process: round-off, scalloping, partial bridging, complete bridging, and remodeling of host bone and graft.[22,23]

In a canine model, Emerson et al.[22] demonstrated formation of a callus-like structure at 8 weeks that had 60% to 80% of the strength of that in controls. The edges and portions of the graft not opposed to host bone underwent osteoclastic resorption. Complete bridging to host bone was evident at 12 weeks, and the biomechanical strength was equal to that in controls. At 24 weeks, the struts were radiographically indistinguishable and grossly were entirely blended into host bone. Major portions of the grafts had remodeled to new cortical bone. There is general agreement between the canine model and the human clinical experience. The time sequence of healing differs in that human graft repair occurs six to eight times more slowly than in the dog.

Patient series of revision total hips using cortical strip grafts demonstrate a 96% to 98% incidence of graft union with an average time to union of 7.3 to 8.4 months.[22,23] In one large series,[22] there was an overall subsidence rate of 7%. Revisions in this series that included the use of a calcar replacement stem had a subsidence rate of 2.7%. In both series there was a higher incidence of failure when the prosthesis was supported by graft. Therefore the prosthesis should always be supported by host bone and not by the strut graft alone.[22,23]

Buoncristiani et al.[14] reported 32 revision total hip arthroplasties in which partially demineralized microperforated cortical strut grafts were used. Demineralization imparts osteoinductive properties to the graft by activating bone matrix proteins. The microperforations become centers for ossification early in graft incorporation. The grafts are partially demineralized to allow more active ossification while retaining adequate rigidity. The grafts healed at an average of 9.3 months. Remodeling, defined as complete incorporation into the femoral cortex was seen at an average of 19.3 months. One graft completely resorbed, and 12 grafts partially resorbed. Of these 12 grafts, 11 resorbed proximally only, and 6 resorbed to the distal level of fixation on the medial side of the stem, indicating that the partial resorption was due to stress shielding and not to a failure of incorporation. The study revealed that the demineralized strut grafts were frequently united to frozen proximal femoral allografts. This phenomenon was attributed to the dynamic osteogenesis induced by demineralization.

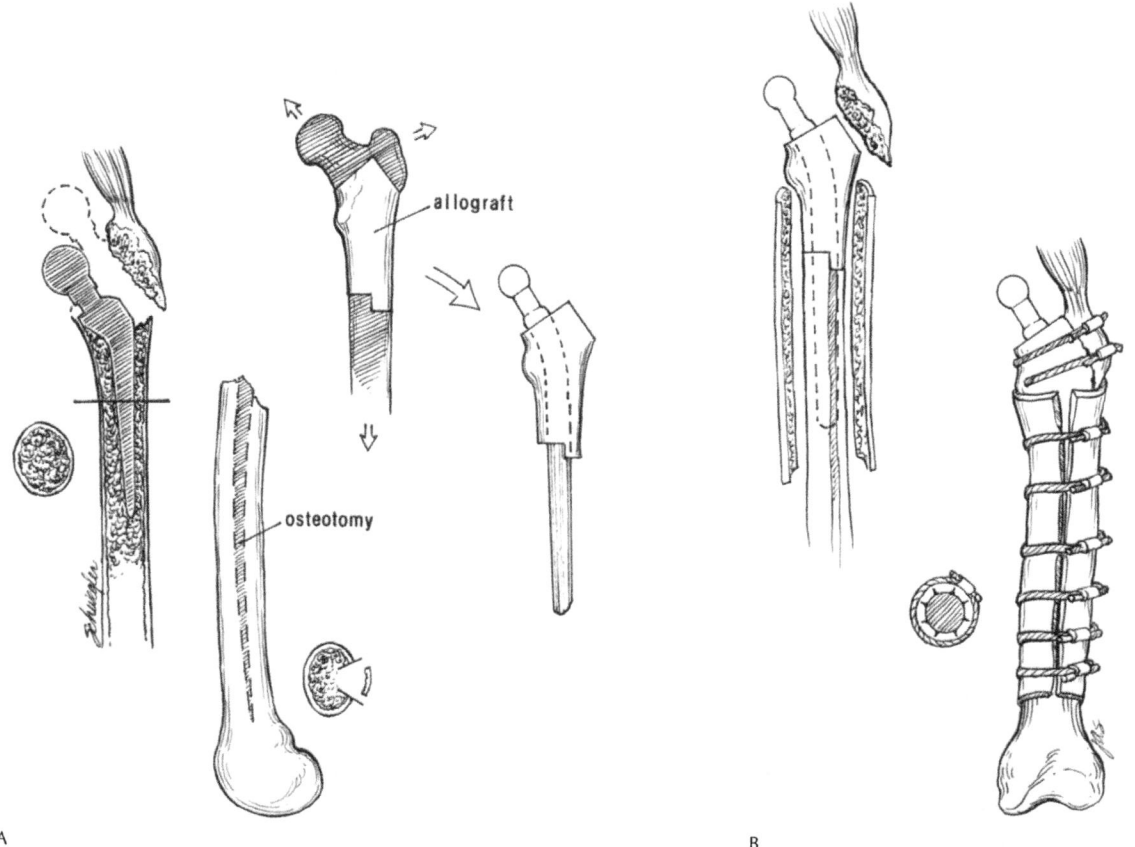

Figure 10.7. A. Severe segmental and cavitary bone loss of the proximal femur with subsidence of the stem and significant cavitary bone loss in the diaphysis with an expanded canal (ectasia). A press-fit will not be possible in this enlarged diaphyseal canal. The inner diameter of the widened diaphysis is decreased with a reduction osteotomy. A proximal femoral allograft is prepared by shaping it appropriately and creating a distal step-cut. A long stem is then cemented into the segmental allograft. B. The stem–allograft composite is then inserted into the host bone, which has been prepared with a matching stem-cut at the graft–host junction. The reduction osteotomy can first be closed down and fixed with cerclage wires or cables, and then the stem can be press-fit into the diaphysis. Alternatively the stem can be inserted into the host bone, and then the reduction osteotomy can be closed down over the stem. The graft–host junction and the thin diaphyseal bone are buttressed with cortical strip grafts. The host trochanter is reattached to the segmental allograft with cerclage cables.

These studies support the use of cortical strip grafts to help restore areas of segmental bone loss in revision total hip arthroplasty. In addition to replacement for segmental defects, cortical strip grafts may also be used to increase the cortical width of the femoral shaft. This may be helpful in cases of diaphyseal cortical thinning and the use of a large diameter stiff stem. In such cases, thigh pain may result from the poor stem:cortical stiffness ratio. Cortical strip grafts can buttress femoral bone stock, increasing the relative stiffness of the cortical bone and thus favorably affecting the stem:cortical stiffness ratio.

Bulk Solid Allografts

An option for reconstruction of substantial segmental bone loss from the proximal femur is segmental replacement with an implant that replaces the proximal femur. These implants are often used for reconstruction after neoplastic diseases, but their use has been expanded to include reconstruction in nonneoplastic diseases as well.[24] Although this technique is simple to perform, there are disadvantages associated with this method in patients with normal life expectancies and activity levels. Extensive loss of the lateral femoral cortex eliminates the ability to obtain secure reattachment of the greater trochanter and abductor muscles, so that significant limp, dislocation, or both may result. If the lateral cortex can be preserved for trochanteric reattachment, these components can offer a more reliable and simple reconstruction for elderly patients with severe periprosthetic bone loss.

In younger, more active patients with extensive segmental bone loss of the proximal femur, segmental allograft replacement of bone offers advantages. The use of allograft replacement of large segmental femoral defects allows the possibility of replacing lost bone stock and restoring the mechanical integrity of the femur. Solid allograft is usually used in segmental or combined segmental and cavitary deficiencies (AAOS grades II or III). Although the bulk of the cortical bone in these grafts usually remains necrotic long after implantation, union at the graft–host junction is seen in most patients in whom stable fixation is achieved.[8,18,23,25–28] After healing at the graft–host junction occurs, the graft can become load bearing and enhance the ability of the prosthesis to resist rotational and axial forces. This ability to restore bone support from the proximal femur and the ability to use a common revision stem, as opposed to a more expensive custom or modular proximal femoral replacement stem, are distinct advantages.

The use of bulk solid allograft bone in reconstruction of femoral bone loss is not without disadvantages. These include the risk of disease transmission,[29] providing a nidus for infection in the nonvascularized allograft, resorption of the graft, and fracture or fragmentation of the allograft. Perhaps the greatest disadvantage of bulk cortical allografts is the unpredictability of incorporation which is related to antigenicity, immune response, and processing (eg, freezing) of the graft.[25,28]

Stevenson et al.[28] studied the antigenicity and effects of freezing on incorporation of segmental cortical allografts. They found that syngeneic grafts were incorporated more readily than grafts with a minor histocompatibility mismatch, and these grafts, in turn, were incorporated more readily than grafts with a major histocompatibility mismatch. Freezing had two main effects on incorporation: (1) It muted the effects of histocompatibility mismatching, and (2) it reduced the biologic activity of the graft. Histocompatibility matching was the critical functional determinant of incorporation of fresh grafts, but among the frozen grafts, the effects of freezing were dominant. Overall, they found that *fresh* syngeneic grafts incorporated quickly; frozen syngeneic and fresh frozen grafts with a minor histocompatibility mismatch incorporated, but more slowly; *frozen* grafts with a major histocompatibility mismatch (which is representative of most grafts used in joint reconstruction) had the least predictable process of incorporation, which was slow and variable; fresh grafts with a major mismatch underwent rapid failure.

Mankin et al.[21] have one of the largest series of massive allograft reconstructions. Seventy percent of 91 patients who underwent allograft reconstruction after tumor resection had good to excellent results at 2-year follow-up. Failures were associated with infection, graft fracture, and nonunion, and they usually occurred within 2 years. If early major complications did not occur, the clinical results remained stable at 8 to 10 years.

Head et al.[30] used freeze-dried allografts to reconstruct massive bone loss associated with failed cemented total hip arthroplasties in 22 patients and reported similar good results. Function was improved in 73% of hips. They reported one nonunion and six dislocations in five patients.

Gross et al.[8] reported an 85% success rate in a series of 40 large proximal femoral allografts (average length, 10.4 cm.). They reported primary osseous healing in 75% of patients; bridging union with persistent junction in 7.5%; stable nonunion in 2.5%; and unstable nonunion in 7.5%. Eleven percent of grafts subsided. The trochanter united to the graft in 38%, 42% obtained a stable fibrous union, and there was trochanteric nonunion escape with greater than 1 cm of proximal migration in 21%. No large allografts were resorbed, and none were revised for mechanical failure. Four grafts required resection: three for infection and one for recurrent dislocation.

In contrast, when calcar allografts (defined by Gross et al.[8] as less than or equal to 3 cm in length) were used there was significant resorption. In 40% there was resorption of greater than half the initial allograft, with an additional 10% with a third to half the graft resorbed. Subsidence was seen in 43% with an average of 1.1 cm. With cementing of the graft, the incidence of resorption and fracture decreased. Resorption of greater than one third of the graft was seen in 79% of grafts without cement and in only 10% of grafts with cement.

Zmolek and Dorr[18] reported an 82% incidence of radiographic union at 4-year follow-up in 11 patients who underwent segmental replacement of the proximal femur with large proximal femoral allografts during revision total hip arthroplasty. Radiographic union occurred at an average of 12 months. They also reported subsidence of an average of 7 mm in 64% of the hips. This was believed to be the result of press-fitting the stems into the allografts. Five hips subsequently underwent revision with the femoral component cemented into the allograft. No subsidence has been seen in these hips at 2-year follow-up. Implant retrieval in one patient and reoperation in three patients revealed no muscular attachments to the allograft. Biopsy of the allograft revealed no evidence of revascularization at an average of 12 months after implantation, even when union had occurred. Six of 11 patients experienced at least one postoperative dislocation.

Oakeshott et al.[26] reported on 112 frozen allografts used in 72 patients. They reported that clinical objectives were achieved in 85% of patients at 6 to 72 months follow-up. Twenty-six of these grafts were calcar allografts and did not extend below the inferior edge of the lesser trochanter. Nineteen were proximal femurs, and 7 were proximal tibias. Five of 7 tibial grafts united, and 8 of 19 femoral grafts united. One required resection for infection. Two resorbed completely; one, partially. Twelve subsided, with 11 subsiding 1 cm or more. Only 4 of the 12 subsided grafts were cemented into the allograft. These 4 migrated as a single unit into the host bone. Two allografts fractured, and these were associated with nonunion at the graft–host junction. Oakeshott et al. also reported that 14 of 23 trochanteric osteotomies healed by stable fibrous union; two of 23 escaped; and seven of 23 healed by bony union.

Robertson[27] used 20 large proximal femoral allografts and four distal femoral allografts to reconstruct femoral bone deficiency in 24 revision total hip arthroplasties. He reported 22 of 24 hips demonstrated evidence of incorporation at the graft–host junction, and 18 of 24 hips united at the graft–trochanter junction at a mean follow-up of 44 months. In 22 of 24 patients, the operation was successful in decreasing pain and increasing mobility. Significant graft resorption was seen in two patients, but there were no graft fractures. Other complications included one dislocation, two leg length discrepancies, two shaft nonunions, six trochanteric nonunions, and two infections.

From the reports described above, it can be seen that severe femoral bone defects can be reconstructed with solid allograft with acceptable results. To maximize the chance for success several guidelines, based on the results of these clinical studies, should be followed. Bone ingrowth cannot be expected from dead bone. To prevent subsidence of the stem and resorption of the graft the stem should be cemented into the allograft. Smaller calcar allografts (<3 cm) have a high incidence of resorption and failure and should not be used. In general, defects small enough to be reconstructed with such a small allograft can be reconstructed with other methods, such as use of a stem that replaces the calcar bone or cortical strut grafts. Fixation of the stem in host bone is necessary for success. Stems with a smooth distal surface will not achieve biologic fixation into the host diaphysis. A long stem with a distal textured surface, such as a porous-coated or a grit-blasted surface, should be used. By using a stem that extends past the allograft, biologic fixation in the host diaphysis is achieved. By following these recommendations, the surgeon will improve the chance for a successful outcome in reconstruction with a segmental allograft.

Conclusion

Revision total hip arthroplasty can be a challenging undertaking. The importance of proper preoperative planning cannot be overemphasized. Frequently, periprosthetic bone loss from the femur requires some form of grafting to restore lost bone stock. In some cases the filling of limited cavitary defects with particulate autograft, allograft, or bone graft substitute material is all that is required. In more severe cases of segmental or combined segmental and cavitary defects, structural graft may be required as well. Often, cortical strip grafts can be used to restore lost bone stock and structural integrity to the femur. In such cases it is important that adequate fixation of the prosthesis in host bone be achieved to optimize results. In severe cases of proximal bone loss, segmental replacement of the proximal femur may be required with either a custom or modular stem, or with a bulk allograft and a long stem. If allograft is to be used, it is important to cement the stem into the allograft even if the stem is to be press-fit into the host bone. In elderly, less active patients, a modular segmental femoral replacement stem may be a good choice, but in a young, more active patient with a normal life expectancy, the chance of restoring lost bone stock warrants consideration of the use of an allograft. Unfortunately, the most commonly used allograft in orthopedics is the frozen unmatched graft. This is the least predictable with regard to incorporation. Although it is unlikely that tissue typing, as is done for other organ transplants, could feasibly be expanded to bone allografts, it is possible that the process of graft incorporation could one day be pharmacologically manipulated, making the use of allograft bone a more attractive option.

References

1. Callaghan JJ, Salvati EA, Pellici PM, Wilson PD, Ranawat CS. Results of revision for mechanical failure after cemented total hip replacement, 1979 to 1982: a two to five-year follow-up. *J Bone Joint Surg Am.* 1985;67:1074–1085.
2. Kavanagh BF, Ilstrup DM, Fitzgerald RH. Revision total hip arthroplasty. *J Bone Joint Surg Am.* 1985;67:517–526.
3. Engh CA, Glassman AH, Griffin WL, Mayer JG. Results of cementless revision for failed cemented total hip arthroplasty. *Clin Orthop.* 1988;235:91–110.
4. Marti RK, Schuller HM, Besselaar PP, Vanfrank Haasnoot EL. Results of revision of hip arthroplasty with cement: a five to fourteen-year follow-up study. *J Bone Joint Surg Am.* 1990;72:346–354.
5. Chandler HP, Penenberg BL, eds. *Bone Stock Deficiency in Total Hip Replacement: Classification and Management.* Thorofare, NJ: Slack; 1989:19–164.
6. Dorr LD, Dierdorf D, Carn RM. Principles of cementless total hip revision and use of the APR revision hip. *Tech Orthop.* 1987;2:20–33.
7. Engh CA, Glassman AH. Cementless revision of failed total hip replacement. *Orthop Rev.* 1990;14(suppl):23–28.
8. Gross AE, Allen DG, Lavoie GJ, Oakeshott RD. Revision arthroplasty of the proximal femur using allograft bone. *Orthop Clin North Am.* 1993;24:705–715.
9. Mallory TH. Preparation of the proximal femur in cementless total hip revision. *Clin Orthop.* 1988;235:47–60.
10. Paprosky WG. Femoral defect classification: clinical application. *Orthop Rev.* 1990;14(suppl):9–15.
11. D'Antonio J, McCarthy JC, Barger WL, Borden LS, Cappelo WN, Collis DK, et al. Classification of femoral abnormalities in total hip arthroplasty. *Clin Orthop.* 1993;296:133–139.
12. D'Antonio J, Capello WN, Borden LS, Barger WL, Bierbaum BF, Boettcher WG, et al. Classification and man-

agement of acetabular abnormalities in total hip arthroplasty. *Clin Orthop.* 1989;243:126–137.
13. Masri BA, Duncan CP. Classification of bone loss in total hip arthroplasty. In: Pritchard DJ, ed. *Instructional Course Lectures.* vol 45. Rosemont, Ill: American Academy of Orthopaedic Surgeons; 1996:199–208.
14. Buoncristiani AM, Dorr LD, Johnson C, Wan Z. Cementless revision of total hip arthroplasty using the anatomic porous replacement revision prosthesis. *J Arthroplasty.* 1997;12:403–415.
15. Zweymuller KA, Lintner FK, Semlitsch MF. Biologic fixation of a press-fit titanium hip joint endoprosthesis. *Clin Orthop.* 1988;235:195–206.
16. Feighan JE, Goldberg VM, Davy D, Parr JA, Stevenson S. The influence of surface-blasting on the incorporation of titanium-alloy implants in a rabbit intramedullary model. *J Bone Joint Surg Am.* 1995;77:1380–1395.
17. Lester DK, Campbell P. 100-year-old patient with press-fit prosthesis: a postmortem retrieval study. *Am J Orthop.* 1996;25:30–34.
18. Zmolek JC, Dorr LD. Revision total hip arthroplasty: the use of solid allograft. *J Arthroplasty.* 1993;8:361–370.
19. Wehrli U. [Wagner revision of prosthesis stem]. *Z Unfallchir Versicherungsmed.* 1991;84:216–224.
20. Gie GA, Linder L, Ling RSM, Sim J-P, Slooft TJJH, Timperley AJ. Impacted cancellous allograft and cement for revision total hip arthroplasty. *J Bone Joint Surg Br.* 1993;75:14–21.
21. Lexer E. cited by: Mankin HJ, Doppelt S, Tomford W. Clinical experience with allograft implantation. *Clin Orthop.* 1983;174:69–86.
22. Emerson RH Jr, Malinin TI, Cuellar AD, Head WC, Peters PC Jr. Cortical strut allografts in the reconstruction of the femur in revision total hip arthroplasty: a basic science and clinical study. *Clin Orthop.* 1992;285:35–44.
23. Head CH, Wagner RA, Emerson RH, Malinin TI. Restoration of femoral bone stock in revision total hip arthroplasty. *Orthop Clin North Am.* 1993;24:697–703.
24. Freedman EL, Eckardt JJ. A modular endoprosthetic system for tumor and nontumor reconstruction: preliminary experience. *Orthopedics.* 1997;20:27–36.
25. Goldberg VM, Stevenson S. Natural history of autografts and allografts. *Clin Orthop.* 1987;225:7–16.
26. Oakeshott RD, Morgan DAF, Zukor DJ, Rudan JF, Brooks PJ, Gross AE. Revision total hip arthroplasty with osseous allograft reconstruction. *Clin Orthop.* 1987;225:37–61.
27. Robertson RJ. Proximal femoral bone loss after total hip arthroplasty. *Orthop Clin North Am.* 1992;23:291–302.
28. Stevenson S, Li XQ, Davy DT, Klein L, Goldberg VM. Critical biological determinants of incorporation of nonvascularized cortical bone grafts. *J Bone Joint Surg Am.* 1997;79:1–16.
29. Tomford WW. Transmission of disease through transplantation of musculoskeletal allografts. *J Bone Joint Surg Am.* 1995;77:1742–1754.
30. Head WC, Berklacich FM, Malinin TI, Emerson RH Jr. Proximal femoral allografts in revision total hip arthroplasty. *Clin Orthop.* 1987;225:22–36.

11
Bone Stock Loss and Allografting: Trochanter

Geoffrey H. Westrich

Complex deformities of the femur are becoming increasingly common in revision total hip arthroplasty. In preparing for such cases, the surgeon must assess not only the acetabulum and femur shaft, but also the proximal femur.[1-5] Preoperative planning is essential for a successful outcome, and routine assessment of the status of the trochanter is mandatory. An overall evaluation of the quality and quantity of proximal femoral bone stock, as well as of the amount of osteopenia is a prerequisite to surgical intervention. Although many etiologies for proximal femoral bone loss exist, osteolysis secondary to particulate debris from polyethylene, bone cement, or metal particles is the most common.[6] With the bearing surface of metal on polyethylene that is used in current total hip arthroplasty designs, such wear debris is unfortunately prevalent. Secondary causes of proximal femoral bone loss that involves the trochanteric region include advanced age, stress-shielding, osteolysis from infection, and abrasive loss from loose or migrating femoral stems.[4,6,7] In addition, iatrogenic bone loss may occur from the revision surgery itself. The preoperative assessment of osteolysis involving the greater trochanter is important, and as a result may reduce the risk of intraoperative fractures. In addition, osteolysis may necessitate the restoration of trochanteric bone stock.

Other problems with the greater trochanter are observed in patients who had previous hip surgery. In patients with a trochanteric osteotomy performed during a previous operation, nonunion of the trochanter may occur.[1,8-13] Thus the surgeon must fully evaluate the interface between the greater trochanter and the proximal femur. The recognition of a trochanteric nonunion is important not only for exposure, but also for subsequent reconstruction. A final category of trochanteric problems is in patients who have previous hardware. It is necessary to evaluate the type of hardware used and also recognize that old hardware may add difficulty to the revision procedure.

Classification

Classification of femoral bony abnormalities is useful for preoperative planning in revision total hip arthroplasty. A classification for femoral bone loss was developed by the American Association of Orthopedic Surgeons Committee on the Hip. (Table 11.1).[14,15] This classification system was adopted from a similar classification of acetabular lesions.

There are two basic categories of bone loss: segmental and cavitary. Segmental defects are noncontained lesions involving loss of the supporting cortical bone from the femoral shell. Cavitary defects are contained lesions that represent an excavation of cancellous and/or endosteal cortical bone from within, and they have an intact cortical shell.

Segmental defects are divided into three subcategories: proximal, intercalary, and greater trochanter lesions. Proximal segmental defects can be either partial or complete, with partial defects involving the anterior, medial, or posterior aspect of the femur. Segmental intercalary defects are denoted by an area of cortical bone loss with intact bone above and below the lesion. Because of the unique and difficult problems associated with a greater trochanter segmental defect, a separate category for greater trochanter involvement was established.

Cavitary defects involve a contained lesion with erosion of cancellous bone or loss of endosteal cortical bone from within the femur. Thus the outer cortical shell remains intact. Cavitary lesions have a wide spectrum of bony deficiency from simple loss of cancellous medullary bone to an ectatic form, with severe dilation of the femoral canal. It is noteworthy that a patient may have a combination of segmental and cavitary defects, and this frequently exists in the setting of revision hip surgery.

Other categories of femoral bone abnormalities include malalignment, stenosis, and discontinuity. Malalignment

Table 11.1 AAOS classification of femoral abnormalities.[10]

I. Segmental
   A. Proximal
      1. Partial
      2. Complete
   B. Intercalary
   C. Greater trochanter
II. Cavitary
III. Combined segmental and cavitary
IV. Malalignment
   A. Rotational
   B. Angular
V. Stenosis
VI. Discontinuity

can be either rotational or angular and noted at any level of the femur. Stenosis is observed with a relative or absolute narrowing of the femoral canal. The final category, discontinuity, involves the absence of bony integrity of the femoral shaft seen with femoral fractures.

Another useful grading system involves the level of bone loss within the femur (Table 11.2). Level I is defined as bone loss proximal to the level of the inferior lesser trochanter, whereas level II is localized from the level of the inferior lesser trochanter to a point 10 cm distal. Level III includes any femoral bone loss distal to level II. In using this system, any bone loss that involves the greater trochanter would be classified as level I.

Grading of the type of femoral reconstruction (Table 11.3) is also helpful and recommended by some investigators.[16] A grade I reconstruction involves complete stability of the femoral prosthesis without the need for bone grafting. A grade II reconstruction depicts incomplete contact of the host bone with the prosthesis. Although the prosthesis is stable, bone grafting may be used to address the defects. The last category, grade III, denotes incomplete host bone contact with the prosthesis and an unstable situation. As such, structural bone graft is necessary to stabilize the prosthesis.

Nonunion

Historically, osteotomy of the greater trochanter was used routinely for exposure during primary total hip arthroplasty.[8,11,13] Charnley popularized the transtrochanteric approach; however, he and a colleague (Ferreira) noted several complications with its use.[17] Problems related to trochanteric osteotomy included increased blood loss and operative time, trochanteric bursitis, and trochanteric nonunion resulting in pain, a limp, and dislocation.[18] Unfortunately, nonunion of the greater trochanter was a well-recognized complication after trochanteric osteotomy.

Most primary and revision total hip arthroplasties are performed without osteotomy of the greater trochanter. Therefore, several advantages are achieved and include decreased blood loss, absence of nonunion, and lack of hardware.[5] In selected cases, however, osteotomy of the greater trochanter is mandatory. Femoral shortening during total hip arthroplasty will produce laxity in the abductor muscles, and as such, osteotomy of the greater trochanter with advancement is indicated to prevent limp and dislocation.[5] In addition, some difficult primary and revision total hip arthroplasties require wide exposure. Therefore osteotomy of the greater trochanter is necessary to prevent technical errors.[5]

Although trochanteric osteotomy is no longer performed for the routine primary total hip arthroplasty, the reported incidence of nonunion varies considerably from 1% to 17.5% depending on the series.[8,13] In evaluating a cohort of 728 total hip arthroplasty patients treated with a transtrochanteric approach, Amstutz and Maki[19] noted a 4.8% (35 of 728) incidence of trochanteric nonunion. Nonunion of the greater trochanter is also associated with weakness in the abductor muscle group, a limp, and pain. In the study by Amstutz and Maki, the amount of weakness was correlated with the amount of separation, with greater than 2 cm resulting in profound abductor weakness. Although some patients with a stable fibrous nonunion of the greater trochanter may not experience pain, many patients complained of lateral hip pain with ambulation. Jenson and Harris,[16] in a study of 804 total hip arthroplasties (725 primary and 79 revision) with standard trochanteric osteotomy, noted only a 1% nonunion rate. Furthermore, they noted that delayed union (>6 months) occurred in 2.3% of the primary cases and 7.6% of the revision cases.

In preoperative planning for a revision total hip arthroplasty, a nonunion of the greater trochanter should be addressed. Although the nonunion may provide for easier exposure during the revision surgery, proper reduction and fixation of the greater trochanter

Table 11.2. Level of femoral bone loss.

I. Proximal to inferior lesser trochanter
II. Inferior lesser trochanter to 10 cm below
III. Bone distal to level II

Table 11.3. Grading femoral reconstruction.

I. Complete prosthesis–host bone contact
   A. No bone graft required
II. Incomplete prosthesis–host bone contact
   A. Prosthesis stable in host bone
   B. Bone graft may be added
III. Incomplete prosthesis–host bone contact
   A. Prosthesis is not stable in host bone
   B. Structural bone graft required to stabilize prosthesis

From *American Academy of Orthopaedic Surgeons Committee on the Hip* is necessary for a successful outcome. The long lever arm created by the greater trochanter not only assists the abductor muscles, but also decreases the joint reactive force in the hip.[20–22] Restoration of the greater trochanter in revision hip surgery is essential to reestablish normal hip biomechanics.[1] Improper repositioning and fixing of the greater trochanter on the proximal femur may lead to repeated nonunion with pain, limp, and dislocation.[1]

Certain criteria have been elucidated that predispose to nonunion of the greater trochanter. In a series by Jenson and Harris,[16] osteoporotic bone, inadequately tightened vertical wires, and placement of the trochanter on cement were associated with nonunion. Amstutz and Maki[19] identified several other factors that contribute to nonunion of the greater trochanter, including osteoporosis, excessive body weight, intraoperative trochanteric fracture, inability of the patient to protect the hip after surgery, inadvertent scoring or kinking of the wire, and poor fixation of the greater trochanter in a tilted position.

Several options are currently available to reattach the greater trochanter to the proximal femur. These include wire, cable, clamps, screws, or a combination of such items and techniques. In patients with intact proximal femoral bone stock, fixation to the patient's bone may be achieved with drill holes through the femoral shaft and/or lesser trochanter. However, with proximal segmental bony defects, fixation to the prosthesis is more prudent. As such, several revision femoral stems are designed to allow fixation of wires or screws to aid in reattaching the greater trochanter.

Osteolysis

It is essential to recognize osteolysis of the greater trochanter before revision total hip arthroplasty. Many etiologies for osteolysis of the greater trochanter exist, however the most common include bone loss secondary to particulate debris from polyethylene, bone cement, or metal particles.[23] Bearing surfaces in current arthroplasty designs include metal on polyethylene, ceramic on polyethylene, and metal on metal. With such bearing surfaces, production of wear debris and the subsequent inflammatory response, are unfortunately prevalent.[4] Secondary causes of proximal femoral bone loss involving the greater trochanter include osteolysis from infection and abrasive loss from loose or migrating femoral stems. In addition, iatrogenic bone loss may occur from the revision surgery itself.

Preoperative assessment of osteolysis involving the greater trochanter may reduce the risk of intraoperative fracture. If the surgeon appreciates the extent of osteolysis of the greater trochanter, adequate preoperative planning may be performed. Unintentional fracture of the greater trochanter can have a devastating effect on a patient's outcome, as well as prolong postoperative rehabilitation.

Osteolysis of the proximal femur may necessitate restoration of trochanteric bone stock, depending on the degree of destruction. As such, the surgeon should be prepared to excise an osteolytic lesion and graft the cavitary or segmental lesion involving the greater trochanter with bone.[6,15] Bone grafting should be considered, provided the bone graft will be contained by the prosthesis and not be free to migrate within the hip joint.

Osteopenia

Osteopenia of the proximal femur can exist both in patients without previous hip surgery and in patients after primary total hip arthroplasty.[7,17] Potential deleterious effects of osteopenia involving the proximal femur are the possibility of intraoperative fracture of the greater trochanter and nonunion of a trochanteric osteotomy.[2] Fracture may occur at several stages of the revision arthroplasty, including with exposure of the acetabulum with retraction of the greater trochanter, removal of the femoral prosthesis, or reinsertion of a new femoral component. Therefore in preoperative planning for a revision total hip arthroplasty, the surgeon needs to assess the bone density of the greater trochanter carefully to determine whether potential weakness of the bony architecture exists.

Although the most common cause of osteopenia may be advanced patient age, other etiologies, such as stress-shielding, can occur. Bone remodeling around hip implants can be explained as an effect of mechanical adaptation consistent with Wolff's law. As the load to the proximal femur is rerouted through the prosthesis and away from this area, osteopenia of the greater trochanter ensues. The bone is greatly weakened and at subsequent risk for fracture. Several investigators have suggested that bone resorption is more extensive around cementless as compared with cemented femoral stems.[17,18] Most likely this is due to material properties and flexibility of the implant. Therefore, a more rigid femoral implant will create more stress-shielding. Both the geometry of the implant and the extent of porous coating are responsible for the amount of stress-shielding and resultant osteopenia.

Several investigators have noted that osteopenia of the greater trochanter is associated with nonunion of a trochanteric osteotomy. In 1978, Amstutz and Maki[19] reported that decreased bone density was associated with nonunion after trochanteric osteotomy in both primary and revision total hip arthroplasties. Subsequently, in 1986 Jenson and Harris[16] identified poor bone quality as a predisposing factor in the development of trochanteric nonunion. Therefore, the surgeon must carefully inspect the bone quality of the greater trochanter before performing a revision total hip arthroplasty. This may prevent inadvertent fracture of the trochanter as well as ascertain in the preoperative plan whether reinforcement of the greater trochanter (ie, with wire mesh) will be required.

Hardware

Several techniques have been described for performing an osteotomy of the greater trochanter. Depending on the type of osteotomy, the fixation and hardware used vary greatly. Six different modifications in the type of trochanteric osteotomy exist:[5]

1. the standard trochanteric osteotomy
2. anterior trochanteric slide
3. oblique trochanteric osteotomy
4. horizontal trochanteric osteotomy
5. vertical trochanteric osteotomy
6. extended trochanteric osteotomy.

It is essential that the surgeon appreciate the indications for using these techniques. Application of the different trochanteric osteotomies varies with primary and revision total hip arthroplasties.

The standard trochanteric osteotomy is used in primary cases that require a complex acetabular exposure, such as in severe development dysplasia, and in cases of a high hip center with a lax abductor.[5] The trochanter is repaired with a simple four-wire technique by using two horizontal wires and two vertical wires.[8,10,13,24] If the trochanter is to be advanced distally, the transverse holes in the femoral shaft should be placed more distally. In a study of 804 total hip arthroplasties (725 primary and 79 revision) with a standard trochanteric osteotomy, Jenson and Harris[16] noted a 99% union rate. Furthermore, they noted that delayed union (>6 months) occurred in 2.3% of the primary cases and 7.6% of the revision cases. Investigators have identified certain criteria that predispose to nonunion of the greater trochanter, and these include osteoporotic bone, inadequately tightened vertical wires, and placement of part of the trochanter on cement.[5,13]

The anterior trochanteric slide technique was first reported by Glassman et al.[21] in 1987. However, variations of the technique were described previously by others.[5,25] Indications for the technique are similar to those for the standard trochanteric osteotomy, but several advantages are proposed. With this type of osteotomy, the distal attachment of the vastus lateralis muscle is left intact as a sleeve. This provides continuity to the abductor–lateralis myofascial sleeve and prevents proximal migration of the greater trochanter. Reattachment of the greater trochanter is usually performed with two wires passed through drill holes in the medial femoral cortex. In using this technique for 90 cases (1 primary, 89 revision), Glassman et al.[21] noted that nonunion occurred in 10% (9 of 90) of cases at a mean follow-up of 21 months.

The oblique trochanteric osteotomy was created to increase exposure during the direct lateral approach in primary total hip arthroplasty, and it is rarely used for revision total hip arthroplasty.[5] The horizontal trochanteric osteotomy is used in revision hip surgery when the proximal femoral anatomy is such that a standard trochanteric osteotomy would not allow a cancellous bony bed to reattach the greater trochanter fragment.[5] As such, a horizontal or short oblique osteotomy of the greater trochanter is performed, thus requiring advancement of the abductor mechanism with reattachment of the greater trochanter fragment onto a cancellous bed. Two vertical and two horizontal wires are used to reattach the osteotomized fragment to the lateral cancellous bed. If the greater trochanter fragment is of poor bone quality, augmentation with wire mesh may be performed to assist in evenly distributing the forces. In a study of 28 revision hip cases in which a horizontal osteotomy was used, nonunion occurred in 11% (3 of 28).[1] The vertical trochanteric osteotomy is indicated only after a previous osteotomy in which the greater trochanter was advanced to the lateral cortex (ie, previous horizontal osteotomy). Therefore, this type of osteotomy is rarely required in revision hip surgery. To reattach the trochanter fragment after a vertical osteotomy, three cerclage wires are used and occasionally reinforced with wire mesh.

Finally, the extended trochanteric osteotomy is indicated for the removal of well-fixed cemented or uncemented femoral components.[2,4,5] In addition, this technique is used for removal of a well-fixed cement mantle in a patient with a loose femoral component. Although it is rare to remove a well-fixed component, infection, osteolysis without loosening, and recurrent dislocation may necessitate that this be done.[5] The extended trochanteric osteotomy is a useful adjunct to the techniques of the arthroplasty surgeon. The extended trochanteric osteotomy is performed with an osteotome, a saw, or a high-speed drill.[1,2,4,5] The posterior limb of the osteotomy is made just anterior to the linea aspera, whereas the other part is fashioned anteriorly one third the circumference of the femur under the vastus lateralis and intermedius and parallel to the posterior cut. In an attempt not to devascularize the osteotomy fragment, the muscle may be left attached to the fragment with the anterior part of the osteotomy performed with multiple drill holes or a narrow osteotome through the vastus muscle. The distal part of the osteotomy is transverse to the long axis of the femur and may be oblique or dove-tailed to assist in locking the distal fragment into the host bone during reattachment. After the bone is cut, the osteotomy fragment is lifted off the prosthesis or cement mantle with a combination of straight and curved osteotomes. The femoral stem is then removed, and the remaining femur debrided thoroughly in preparation for reimplanting a new prosthesis. In the reinsertion of an uncemented femoral component, the extended trochanteric osteotomy may be repaired after the insertion of the prosthesis. However, use of a cemented femoral component necessitates reattachment of the osteotomy before cementing. If cement is to be used, gelatin foam can serve as a gasket between the osteotomy fragment and the femur to prevent cement from extruding into the osteotomy site.[5] This foam does not interfere with bone healing.[26] Monofilament cerclage wires or cable may be used to reattach the extended trochanteric osteotomy. If the trochanter requires advancement, the distal aspect of the osteotomy fragment can be shortened and advanced distally before fixation to the femur.

In studying 20 cases of uncemented revision total hip arthroplasty incorporating an extended trochanteric osteotomy, Younger et al.[27] noted that all patients healed at an average of 3 months. In addition, trochanteric migration greater than 2 mm was not observed.[5]

Although the above trochanteric osteotomies were all described with the classical hardware configurations, cables are now used in place of wire by some surgeons. In addition, trochanteric grips are currently manufactured to be used with cable for certain applications. Although cable appears to be more user friendly to some individuals, concerns about fraying and wear debris are common. The choice as to the use of a particular type of hardware is left to the discretion of the surgeon.

Postoperative Care

After trochanteric osteotomy, patients are allowed to bear partial weight with the use of a walker or two crutches until the osteotomy heals. Although this may require up to 3 months of restriction, the radiographic appearance of union is the preferred guide to reestablishing full weight bearing.[5] During postoperative exercise active hip abduction against gravity and passive hip adduction should be avoided until union of the trochanter occurs. Assistive device support is slowly advanced to one crutch or a cane, which can be eliminated when the patient can ambulate without a limp.

Conclusion

In most patients, routine total hip arthroplasty is a successful operation with highly predictable pain relief and restoration of normal function. Revision total hip arthroplasty, however, is more complicated with less predictable results. To afford the patient the greatest likelihood of success, careful preoperative planning is essential. A thorough assessment of the greater trochanter is necessary to plan for the appropriate procedure, prevent intraoperative complications, expedite the revision surgery, and determine the postoperative rehabilitation protocol.

References

1. Bobyn JD, Tanzer M, Dujovne AR, Brooks CE. Risk factors for stress shielding and bone resorption after cementless total hip arthroplasty. In: Galante JO, Rosenberg AG, Callaghan JJ, eds. *Total Hip Revision Surgery.* New York, NY: Raven Press; 1995:141–149.
2. Clarke RP Jr, Shea WD, Bierbaum BE. Trochanteric osteotomy: analysis of pattern of wire fixation failure and complications. *Clin Orthop.* 1979;141:102–110.
3. Harris WH, Jones WN. The use of wire mesh in total hip replacement surgery. *Clin Orthop.* 1975;106:117–121.
4. McGrory BJ, Bal BS, Harris WH. Trochanteric osteotomy for total hip arthroplasty: six variations and indications for their use. *J Am Acad Orthop Surg.* 1996;4:258–267.
5. Sumner DR, Turner TM. Stress shielding. In: Galante JO, Rosenberg AG, Callaghan JJ, eds. *Total Hip Revision Surgery.* New York, NY: Raven Press; 1995:151–158.
6. Fulkerson JP, Crelin ES, Keggi KJ. Anatomy and osteotomy of the greater trochanter. *Arch Surg.* 1979;114:19–21.
7. Markolf KL, Hirschowitz DL, Amstutz HC. Mechanical stability of the greater trochanter following osteotomy and reattachment by wiring. *Clin Orthop.* 1979;141:111–121.
8. Berry DJ, Muller ME. Chevron osteotomy and single wire reattachment of the greater trochanter in primary and revision total hip arthroplasty. *Clin Orthop.* 1993;294:155–161.
9. Cameron HU. Use of a distal trochanteric osteotomy in hip revision. *Contemp Orthop.* 1991;23:235–238.
10. D'Antonio J, McCarthy JC, Barger WL, Borden LS, Cappelo WN, Collis DK, et al. Classification of femoral abnormalities in total hip arthroplasty. *Clin Orthop.* 1993;296:133–139.
11. Hungerford DS, Krackow KA, Lennox DW. The PCA primary and revision hip systems. In: Fitzgerald R, ed. *Noncemented Total Hip Arthroplasty.* New York, NY: Raven Press; 1988:433–450.
12. Jacobs JJ, Urban RM, Glant TT, Galante JO. Clinical implications of osteolysis. In: Galante JO, Rosenberg AG, Callaghan JJ, eds. *Total Hip Revision Surgery.* New York, NY: Raven Press; 1995:81–90.
13. Learmonth ID, Hussell JG, Grobler GP. Unpredictable progression of osteolysis following cementless hip arthroplasty. *Acta Orthop Scand.* 1996;67:245–248.
14. Bal BS, Maurer BT, Harris WH. Trochanteric union following revision total hip arthroplasty. *J Arthroplasty.* 1998;13:29–33.
15. Free SA, Delp SL. Trochanteric transfer in total hip replacement: effects on the moment arms and force-generating capacities of the hip abductors. *J Orthop Res.* 1996;14:245–250.
16. Jensen NF, Harris WH. A system for trochanteric osteotomy and reattachment for total hip arthroplasty with a ninety-nine percent union rate. *Clin Orthop.* 1986;208:174–181.
17. Charnley J, Ferreira SD. Transplantation of the greater

trochanter in arthroplasty of the hip. *J Bone Joint Surg Br.* 1964;46:191–197.
18. Peters PC Jr, Head WC, Emerson RH Jr. An extended trochanteric osteotomy for revision total hip replacement. *J Bone Joint Surg Br.* 1993;75:158–159.
19. Amstutz HC, Maki S. Complications of trochanteric osteotomy in total hip replacement. *J Bone Joint Surg Am.* 1978;60:214–216.
20. Cobden RH, Thrasher EL, Harris WH. Topical hemostatic agents to reduce bleeding from cancellous bone: a comparison of microcrystalline collagen, thrombin, and thrombin-soaked gelatin foam. *J Bone Joint Surg Am.* 1976;58:70–73.
21. Glassman AH, Engh CA, Bobyn JD. A technique of extensile exposure for total hip arthroplasty. *J Arthroplasty.* 1987;2:11–21.
22. Gottschalk FA, Morein G, Weber F. Effect of the position of the greater trochanteric osteotomy for total hip arthroplasty. *J Arthroplasty.* 1988;3:235–240.
23. Kadoya Y, Revell PA, al-Saffar N, Kobayashi A, Scott G, Freeman MA. Bone formation and bone resorption in failed total joint arthroplasties: histomorphometric analysis with histochemical and immunohistochemical technique. *J Orthop Res.* 1996;14:473–482.
24. Harris WH, Crothers OD. Reattachment of the greater trochanter in total hip replacement arthroplasty. *J Bone Joint Surg Am.* 1978;60:211–213.
25. Haantejens P, DeBoeck H, Opdecam P. Proximal femoral replacement prosthesis for salvage of failed hip arthroplasty. *Acta Orthop Scand.* 1996;67:37–42.
26. D'Antonio JA. Classification of femoral bony abnormalities. In: Galante JO, Rosenberg AG, Callaghan JJ, eds. *Total Hip Revision Surgery.* New York, NY: Raven Press; 1995:351–358.
27. Younger TI, Bradford MS, Magnus RE, Paprosky WG. Extended proximal femoral osteotomy: a new technique for femoral revision arthroplasty. *J Arthroplasty.* 1995;10:329–338.

12
Blood Management in Revision Total Hip Arthroplasty

Thomas P. Sculco and David E. Tate

The goals of blood management in revision total hip replacement are to avoid the use of allogeneic (homologous) blood and to utilize all other methods of augmentation or retrieval of autogenous blood appropriate for each patient. Because of the nature of orthopedic surgery and revision total hip replacement in particular, blood loss tends to be significant. The surgical exposures in revision total hip replacement often require ample dissections about the hip through fibrotic tissue. These tissues may be quite vascular, and hemostasis is difficult to achieve because of their friable nature. Often there are diffuse sites of bleeding as well. Wide tissue flaps often need to be dissected, and therefore oozing for prolonged periods during revision procedures is encountered. This significantly increases the amount of blood loss.

The actual techniques of implant removal during revision total hip replacement require extensive manipulation of bone and soft tissue, and with these techniques, there is significant blood loss. This blood loss from exposure and implant removal is further compounded by the continued blood loss as the revision component is inserted. These revision procedures are often performed on elderly patients in whom vessels are fragile and bony bleeding from the exposed surfaces is unsuitable for conventional cautery or ligature hemostasis. Therefore, it is not unreasonable that reports of revision total hip replacement document intraoperative blood loss in the 1000 to 2000 mL range.[1,2]

The blood management options available to the orthopedic surgeon include reduction of the intraoperative blood loss and use of blood retrieval and augmentation methods. Measures to lessen intraoperative blood loss include careful hemostasis, atraumatic technique, and improved anesthetic management. In 1975, Sculco and Ranawat[3] reported significantly reduced total operative blood loss in total hip replacement with spinal anesthesia. Currently, all joint replacement procedures, including revision total hip replacement, at the Hospital for Special Surgery are performed under hypotensive epidural anesthesia. This has led to significantly reduced blood loss, improved bony surfaces for implant fixation, and shorter surgical time.[4] Average total blood loss for routine total hip replacement has been documented as less than 600 mL. Intraoperative blood loss averaged under 250 mL in a series of 250 consecutive hip replacements.[5] Experience with revision total hip replacement has been similar (see Chapter 13).

From a surgeon's viewpoint, patients tolerate the use of hypotensive epidural anesthesia well, and there has been no increased perioperative morbidity associated with it. The adjunctive use of hypotension in the revision total hip replacement patient has not produced an increase in cardiovascular or cerebral morbidity.[4] The added benefit in revision total hip replacement of the patient having the ability to control postoperative pain by maintaining the epidural catheter for analgesia has also facilitated recovery from these complex procedures.

Aside from anesthesia management being important in reducing blood loss, there are other perioperative measures that should be taken in preparing the patient for revision hip surgery. Patients should be advised to refrain from taking antiplatelet medication before surgery. Nonsteroidal anti-inflammatory (NSAID) medications have the ability to increase intraoperative bleeding by affecting platelet function. If at all possible, these should be discontinued 5 to 7 days before surgery. Robinson et al.[6] documented a statistically significant increase in intraoperative blood loss and postoperative transfusion needs in primary total hip arthroplasty with long-term (6 months or longer) NSAID users compared to a control group not using NSAIDS. The relationship between blood loss and NSAID therapy held true with both general and spinal anesthesia. All operations were performed by the same surgeon by means of the posterior approach, and all anesthetics were administered by the same anesthesia consultant.

Careful attention should be paid to patients' coagulation profile. Prothrombin time and partial thromboplastin time are useful in identifying a patient who may have an occult bleeding dyscrasia.

Techniques for Blood Salvage

Aside from intraoperative anesthesia management, which is important in reducing blood loss, all methods of autogenous blood retrieval and augmentation should be used when appropriate. These include preoperative autologous blood deposit, hemodilution, intraoperative blood retrieval, postoperative blood retrieval, and the preoperative use of recombinant erythropoietin to increase red blood cell mass.

Preoperative Autologous Blood Donation

Because of the significant risks associated with allogeneic red blood cell transfusion, preoperative autologous blood donation is used routinely in most elective orthopedic procedures in which anticipated blood loss is great. Although many patients are aware of the risks associated with transfusion of homologous blood, only about 5% of the blood transfused in the United States is autologous.[7] Orthopedic surgery, because of the elective nature of many of its nontraumatic procedures, is ideally suited for the use of predeposited autologous programs. At the Hospital for Special Surgery, where most surgical procedures are elective, about 80% of the blood transfused is autologous. Autologous blood is usually drawn at weekly intervals before surgery, and the amount obtained varies depending on expected blood loss. For routine hip and knee replacement, one unit is obtained. For complex revision joint replacement and spine surgery, in which blood loss is greater, two to four units may be obtained. Iron must be administered during the time of blood donation.[2,8,9]

In comparison with allogeneic blood, autologous blood has numerous advantages for the patient. Certainly one of the greatest benefits is the absence of risk of disease transmission with autologous blood. This includes infection with diseases such as HIV, hepatitis, cytomegalovirus, and, less commonly, malaria. Although HIV is the most feared consequence of transfusion-related infection, its transmission risk is estimated at 1 in 225 000 units, whereas for hepatitis C, the risk is about 1 in 3300 units. About half of patients who develop hepatitis C develop chronic liver disease, and in about 10% of these patients, the disease progresses to cirrhosis.[10,11]

Predeposited autologous blood has additional benefits aside from safety from disease transmission. The bone marrow is primed when autologous blood is taken, and reticulocytosis is underway before the bone marrow is stimulated by surgical blood loss. The lag effect is not present for the production of mature red cells, as is the case in nonpredonating patients. In addition, red cell mass is reduced by the removal of autologous blood, and this reduces the loss of red cells at the time of surgery.[9]

Although the benefits of autologous blood are significant, it is not without problems. Simpson et al.[12] documented their experience with a pediatric autologous blood program with 175 patients and noted a series of clinical and clerical errors. They describe a group of nine patients in whom autologous blood could not be used because of delays in the operating room schedule and expiration of the autologous blood; three of these patients subsequently required allogeneic blood. Even more serious was a series of clerical errors. Three patients received homologous blood before all their autologous units were given. One patient's autologous blood was misplaced, resulting in allogeneic transfusion, and one patient received a unit of autologous and allogeneic blood when only the autologous unit was ordered.

An additional issue is that of cost of autologous blood and its underuse. An average unit of autologous blood costs between $200 and 400.[1,13] It is therefore the responsibility of the surgeon to estimate carefully the patient's transfusion needs and order only that amount of blood preoperatively. Biesma et al.[14] studied preoperative autologous blood collection for primary total hip arthroplasty. They compared allogeneic blood exposure in patients who had predonated 4 units ($n = 50$) to that in patients who had predonated 2 units ($n = 50$). There was no significant difference in allogeneic blood exposure between the two groups. For the group that donated two units, eighteen units were discarded, whereas for the group that donated four units, 51 were discarded. Iron stores were also significantly lower in the group that predonated four units.[14] Iron is the rate-limiting factor in hematopoiesis after phlebotomy.[15]

The preoperative hemoglobin level should be considered when determining the need for autologous units of blood. In patients in whom hemoglobin levels are 14 gm (2.17 mmol/L) or greater, one unit is generally adequate; often no blood may be needed if hemoglobin levels are greater than 15 gm (2.32 mmol/L). In a 1994 study from the Hospital for Special Surgery, patients who underwent simultaneous bilateral total knee replacements required an average of 2.6 units of blood.[16] This is similar to the amount required for patients undergoing simultaneous bilateral hip replacements. Patients undergoing revision joint replacement procedures may require three or more units.[1]

Another possible complication related to autologous blood programs is adverse patient reactions. Syncopal episodes may produce traumatic injury to elderly patients.[8] Although uncommon, cardiovascular events may also occur.[9]

Hemodilution

Hemodilution has been used successfully in prostate surgery.[17] It involves drawing blood just before or during the surgical procedure and reinfusing the blood postoperatively. By using this technique, there is a reduction in red cell mass immediately and this consequently effects a reduction in red cell loss intraoperatively. The blood retrieved is fresh whole blood, and it is also rich in platelets and coagulation factors, products not present in processed units of packed autologous red cells. As detailed in Chapter 13, this method requires an anesthesia team familiar with its application because it can be quite labor intensive. Hemodilution may not be suitable for many elderly patients with profound cardiac and pulmonary comorbidities who are revision total hip arthroplasty candidates. Hemodilution in the setting of revision total hip arthroplasty may be best for the special circumstance of a complex revision in a young, otherwise healthy patient for whom blood loss of 2000 mL is anticipated.

Intraoperative Blood Salvage

Blood shed during orthopedic surgical procedures may be salvaged and reinfused into patients. Blood is collected by a suction technique, which anticoagulates the blood immediately with heparin sodium as it is retrieved. These red cells are then washed and packed by centrifugation. The effluent, which contains heparin as well as cellular and tissue debris, is removed as part of the washing and centrifugation process, and packed red cells can then be reinfused into the patient either intraoperatively or postoperatively. About 55% of the red cells shed can be collected for reinfusion.[18]

Intraoperative blood salvage is cost effective when expected blood loss is 1000 mL or greater. Guerra and Cuckler[13] found that in patients undergoing primary total hip arthroplasty with no predonated blood, the cell saver reduced both the risk of allogeneic blood exposure by 40% and the mean transfusion requirement from 2.6 to 1.5 units per patient ($p < 0.05$). These findings are reinforced by a study from Law and Weidel,[1] who reported that on patients undergoing revision THA, an average of 7.6 units of red blood cells were salvaged when bone grafts of both femur and acetabulum were needed. In revisions that required no bone grafts, however, an average of only 2.1 units per patient were required. Revisions that required grafts of either the femur or the acetabulum yielded a need for an average of 3.0 and 3.2 units, respectively. These investigators found that, overall, autologous blood with intraoperative salvage accounted for 72% of the perioperative blood needs in their patients, but that use of the cell saver device became cost effective at their institution when four or more units were salvaged.

An additional benefit of using blood salvaged during surgery, as in using blood from hemodilution, is that 2,3-diphosphoglycerate is preserved. This compound enhances the ability of red blood cells to deliver oxygen to tissues.[18] Ray et al.[19] also studied radiolabeled, reinfused red blood cells and radiolabeled allogeneic and autologous red cells. They found the 30-day survival was the same for all three groups, confirming that the viability of these cells is maintained despite the trauma of processing and reinfusion.

Postoperative Blood Reinfusion

Postoperative reinfusion of shed blood was initially studied by thoracic surgeons in an attempt to reinfuse blood lost from mediastinal drainage. In 1978 and in a larger study in 1979, Schaff et al.[20,21] demonstrated that the need for allogeneic blood replacement was reduced by 50% when a mediastinal reinfusion drain was used. Recognizing that this technique might have application to reinfusing postoperative drainage, in the mid-1980s Sculco[22] investigated the retrieval and reinfusion mediastinal device and studied the quality and quantity of blood present in the collected postoperative drainage. Additional filters for bone debris and fat were added to the mediastinal system. Postoperative drainage from arthroplasty wounds was studied to determine whether an adequate volume was available and whether red cells maintained their viability. The drainage averaged about 350 mL per patient. Plasma hemoglobin level was measured and found to be low, demonstrating adequate red cell survival similar to that with intraoperative retrieval. The hematocrit of the shed blood was 0.22, also affirming that the reinfusion would provide a significant number of red blood cells.

Two randomized cohorts undergoing postoperative retrieval and infusion of shed blood were studied to determine the need for cell washing. Acid-citrate-dextrose solution was added to the blood to prevent clotting. Group 1 ($n = 19$) underwent collection of postoperative drainage. The drainage was washed, centrifuged, and reinfused with the modified mediastinal drainage system. In group 2 (n = 16), drainage was collected in a similar fashion and reinfusion was performed without washing of the cells. There were no complications or untoward events noted in the reinfusion of the washed shed blood in group 1. In group 2, however, two patients had severe hypotension during the reinfusion process, with the systemic pressure returning to baseline levels with termination of the transfusion.[23] The explanation for these hypotensive events was unclear but may have been related to the release of cytokines or other vasoactive substances as a response to this drainage being reinfused. Arnested et al.[24] found elevated levels of cytokines in collected unwashed wound drainage and in the sera of patients to whom unwashed blood was administered. Filtration did not decrease the levels of these cytokines. Cytokine levels were not evaluated in washed drainage as a part of this study. Of note is that cytokines are implicated in severe allergic and anaphylactic reactions.[24]

Healy et al.[25] found that the relative risk of transfusion was 2.5 times greater in patients who did not receive reinfused blood than in those who did. The study group was a set of patients undergoing either hip or knee arthroplasty or spinal fusion. No untoward events (febrile episodes, clotting abnormalities, thromboembolic events, or transfusion reactions) were noted. No polymethylmethacrylate monomer was detected on analysis of blood obtained from arthroplasty patients.

Faris et al.[26] found hyperthermia in 16 of 154 patients receiving reinfusion of unwashed blood. There was a direct correlation between hyperthermia and time to reinfusion. When the extracorporeal time was limited to 4 hours or less, the incidence decreased to 2 in 99 patients.

The usefulness of postoperative reinfusion was questioned by Ritter et al.,[27] from the same institution as Faris et al., when they reported that there was no significant difference in the need for postoperative transfusion whether or not drains were used. They reported no significant difference in the groups in terms of either wound problems or hematoma. There were no infections in either group of total hips, and there was one infection each in the total knee groups. There were equivalent numbers of patients in each group who required brief immobilization because of excessive wound drainage. The investigators concluded that postoperative drains were not necessary and therefore postoperative reinfusion of drainage is not feasible if no drain is used.

There appears to be a role for postoperative drainage reinfusion in patients in whom there is significant blood loss postoperatively. This bloody drainage is collected and available for reinfusion. The data seem to indicate that the safest method of reinfusion of these red cells is by washing the cells. There is expense involved in this process, and this must be considered in its implementation. Only in bilateral arthroplasty procedures and revision procedures such as hip revision does reinfusion seem to be indicated because of the tendency for the drainage to be copious in these patient groups. If the technique is used, patients must be monitored carefully to identify untoward hyperthermic or hypotensive reactions. The technique is useful but has the potential for systemic reactions during blood reinfusion.

Preoperative Use of Recombinant Human Erythropoietin

Recombinant human erythropoietin (epoetin alfa) has a role in patients undergoing orthopedic procedures with anticipated substantial blood loss. Erythropoietin is normally produced primarily in the kidney, and its level in serum is increased in response to reduced hemoglobin in the circulating blood as it passes through the kidney. Erythropoietin has a direct effect on the bone marrow by acting on precursor cells to red blood cell production. There is a lag effect, therefore, when erythropoietin acts on the bone marrow until fully mature red cells appear. This lag time is 5 to 7 days. As red cell mass is increased, the stimulus to produce erythropoietin is reduced, and a steady state is established.

Recombinant human erythropoietin has been shown to produce the same effect on erythropoiesis as human erythropoietin.[28] Recombinant erythropoietin must be administered parenterally. According to the manufacturer,[28] patients with a hematocrit in excess of 0.36 to 0.39 presently are not candidates for epoetin alfa. Adequate iron stores should be present for recombinant erythropoietin to be effective. The serum transferrin saturation should be at least 20% and serum ferritin level should be at least 100 μg/L.

Levine et al.,[29] using three groups of baboons, investigated the efficacy of different dosing regimens for recombinant human erythropoietin. Group 1 received no medication; Group 2 received 1000 U/kg daily for 5 days preoperatively; and Group 3 received 5 daily preoperative doses of 1000 U/kg along with 14 daily doses postoperatively. All animals underwent laparotomy, followed by exchange transfusion to reduce the hematocrit to 0.15. Group 3 returned to baseline hematocrit significantly faster than the control group (12.6 days versus 28.2 days, $p < 0.01$). The return to baseline in Group 2 was also faster than that in the control group, but not significantly so.

Goodnough et al.[8] used a regimen of 300 U/kg of erythropoietin twice weekly versus placebo in surgical patients preparing to predonate blood before surgery for orthopedic procedures associated with high blood loss. Preoperative donations were significantly higher in the medicated patients, with 5.4 units per patient versus 4.1 units per patient in the placebo group.

In a multicenter trial, Faris et al.[30] used daily epoetin alfa regimen in patients who were unable to predonate blood. The patients were divided into three groups. Group 1 received epoetin alfa 300 U/day subcutaneously for 10 days preoperatively, on the day of surgery, and 4 days postoperatively. Group 2 received 100 U/day subcutaneously for 10 days preoperatively, on the day of surgery, and 4 days postoperatively. Group 3 received a placebo for 10 days preoperatively, on the day of surgery, and 4 days postoperatively. Allogeneic blood use was significantly less in the groups receiving recombinant human erythropoietin. Transfusions with allogeneic blood were required by 16.7% of patients in group 1; 25% of patients in group 2; and 53.7% of patients in group 3.

Goldberg et al.[31] documented equal efficacy between a weekly and daily dosing regimen. The study randomized primary hip or knee arthroplasty patients older than 18 years of age who had pretreatment hemoglobin levels of 10–13 mg/dl (1.55 to 2.02 mmol/L) into two groups. Group 1 received 600 U/kg of epoetin alfa once a week for 3 weeks before surgery and 600 U/kg on the day of surgery. Group 2 received 300 U/kg daily for 10 days before surgery, on the day of surgery, and for 4 days after the procedure. Mean increase in hemoglobin level was higher in patients in the weekly dosing group. Overall, 84% of patients in the weekly dosing group and 80% of patients in the daily dosing group did not need allogeneic blood. In primary joint arthroplasty, therefore, weekly dosing appears equally efficacious to daily dosing in helping reduce the need for allogeneic banked blood. In addition, weekly dosing should be more convenient for patients, and it requires less medication (3000 U/kg total for weekly dosing versus 4500 U/kg total for daily dosing) as presented in this study.

Use of recombinant human erythropoietin has also been reported in Jehovah's Witnesses, a religious group that will not accept blood that has been extracorporeal. Its use was first presented in a case report in 1991. The patient in question suffered a decrease in hematocrit to 0.13 after an automobile accident. The patient was given erythropoietin 300 U/kg daily for 3 days, followed by 150 U/kg three times a week for 2 weeks. Her hematocrit increased to 0.20 8 days after starting therapy and peaked at 0.37 3 weeks after treatment began.[32] Of note is that, although erythropoietin is a recombinant product, each milliliter contains 2.5 mg of human albumin. As McGraw pointed out in correspondence, some Jehovah's Witnesses may refuse the product on that basis.[33] In most cases, however, these patients will accept erythropoietin.

Nelson and Fontenot[2] have reported on the use of erythropoietin in a Jehovah's Witness patient undergoing revision total hip arthroplasty. The red blood cell mass in this patient was augmented with the use of recombinant human erythropoietin. Because both the femoral and the acetabular components were believed to be loose, the predicted blood loss for revision with a preoperative hematocrit of 0.33 was believed to be unacceptable without additional intervention. The patient received 100 U/kg of recombinant human erythropoietin for 10 weeks preoperatively, along with iron, folate, and vitamin C supplementation. Her hematocrit increased to 0.43. Blood loss was 1350 mL at revision, with 750 mL reinfusion from a cell saver device. Her lowest recorded hematocrit was 0.32, and she made an uneventful recovery. While some Jehovah's Witnesses will not accept the use of a cell saver device, it has considerable utility in those who will permit its use, as this case demonstrated.

Complications related to the use of recombinant human erythropoietin have been uncommon. Hypertension in response to erythropoietin therapy is encountered in renal dialysis patients but this has been infrequent in orthopedic patients. However, all patients receiving erythropoietin therapy need regular blood pressure monitoring. An excessive rise in blood pressure may necessitate stopping the drug.[8,28] An additional potential side effect from the drug is increased viscosity of the blood which might increase the incidence of deep venous thrombosis. There has been no increase in DVT, however, in the studies published on orthopedic patients, when compared to findings in the control cohort of patients.

Recombinant human erythropoietin before surgery is an additional method that is useful for revision total hip replacement patients. With dosing regimens at weekly levels demonstrating similar efficacy to daily dosing, the inconvenience to the patient has been reduced. The FDA has approved the use of the drug in patients with hemoglobin levels of 10–13 gm/dl (1.55 to 2.02 mmol/L). Therefore reimbursement for this drug is possible. This approval has facilitated the use of recombinant erythropoietin in indicated patients because the cost of the drug has been a major deterrent to its use previously.

Conclusion

Techniques of blood management in revision total hip replacement surgery should be used routinely. The total approach to blood management for these patients should include consideration for preoperative autologous blood donation, intraoperative use of the cell saver and postoperative blood reinfusion in a carefully monitored environment. Erythropoietin should also be considered in patients who have low hemoglobin levels, because this drug can promote additional autologous blood for predonation as well as increase the hematocrit at the time of surgery. Patients who can predonate blood should do so. Intraoperative reinfusion has been useful for procedures with blood loss in excess of 1000 mL. Postoperative reinfusion is controversial. If used, washing the blood before reinfusion and performing the reinfusion within 4 hours are probably the safest measures to observe. Recombinant human erythropoietin has shown promise in boosting red blood cell mass, but its use must be planned for because it cannot be administered acutely. By carefully evaluating the blood requirement needs of each patient preoperatively and using these methods, the revision hip surgeon can minimize patient exposure to allogeneic blood and use the available blood management resources in an efficient and safe manner.

References

1. Law JK, Weidel JD. Autotransfusion in revision total hip arthroplasties using uncemented prostheses. *Clin Orthop.* 1989;245:145–149.
2. Nelson CL, Fontenot HJ. Ten strategies to reduce blood loss in orthopaedic surgery. *Am J Surg.* 1995;170(suppl): 64S–68S.
3. Sculco TP, Ranawat C. The use of spinal anesthesia for total hip replacement. *J Bone Joint Surg Am.* 1975;57:173–177.
4. Sharrock NE, Mineo R, Urquhart B, Salvati EA. The effect of two levels of hypotension on intraoperative blood loss during total hip arthroplasty performed under lumbar epidural anesthesia. *Anesth Analg.* 1993;76:580–584.
5. Lieberman JR, Huo MM, Hanaway J, Salvati EA, Sculco TP, Sharrock NE. The prevalence of deep venous thrombosis after total hip arthroplasty with hypotensive epidural anesthesia. *J Bone Joint Surg Am.* 1994;76:341–348.
6. Robinson CM, Christie J, Malcolm-Smith N. Nonsteroidal antiinflammatory drugs, perioperative blood loss, and transfusion requirements in elective hip arthroplasty. *J Arthroplasty.* 1993;8:607–610.
7. Keeling MM. Blood transfusion medicine 1993. In: *Orthopaedic Knowledge Update 4.* American Academy of Orthopaedic Surgeons; 1993:215.
8. Goodnough LT, Rudnick S, Price TH, Ballas SK, Collins ML, Crowley JP, et al. Increased preoperative collection of autologous blood with recombinant human erythropoietin therapy. *N Engl J Med.* 1989;321:1163–1168.
9. Stanisavljevic S, Walker RH, Bartman CR. Autologous blood transfusion in total joint arthroplasty. *J Arthroplasty.* 1986;1:207–209.
10. Dodd RY. The risk of transfusion-transmitted infection. *N Engl J Med.* 1992;327:419–421.
11. Walker RH. Special report: transfusion risks. *Am J Clin Pathol.* 1987;88:374–378.
12. Simpson MB, Georgopoulos G, Orsini E, Eilert RE. Autologous transfusions for orthopaedic procedures at a children's hospital. *J Bone Joint Surg Am.* 1992;74:652–658.
13. Guerra JJ, Cuckler JM. Cost-effectiveness of intra-operative autotransfusion in total hip arthroplasty surgery. *Clin Orthop.* 1995;315:212–222.
14. Biesma DH, Marx JJM, van de Wiel A. Collection of autologous blood before elective total hip replacement. *J Bone Joint Surg Am.* 1994;76:1471–1475.
15. Finch S, Haskins D, Finch CA. Iron metabolism: hematopoiesis following phlebotomy—iron as a limiting factor. *J Clin Invest.* 1950;28:1078–1086.
16. Jankiewicz JJ, Sculco TP, Ranawat CS, Behr C, Tarrentino S. One-stage versus 2-stage bilateral total knee arthroplasty. *Clin Orthop.* 1994;309:94–101.
17. Ness PM, Bourke DL, Walsh PC. A randomized trial of perioperative hemodilution versus transfusion of preoperatively deposited autologous blood in elective surgery. *Transfusion.* 1992;32:226–230.
18. Flynn JC, Metzger CR, Csencitz TA. Intraoperative autotransfusion (IAT) in spinal surgery. *Spine* 1982;7:432–435.
19. Ray JM, Flynn JC, Bierman AH. Erythrocyte survival following intraoperative autotransfusion in spinal surgery: an in-vivo comparative study and 5-year update. *Spine.* 1986;11:879–882.
20. Schaff HV, Hauer JM, Bell WR, Gardner TJ, Donahoo JS, Gott VL, et al. Autotransfusion of shed mediastinal blood after cardiac surgery. *J Thorac Cardiovasc Surg.* 1978;75:632–641.
21. Schaff HV, Hauer JM, Gardner TJ, Donahoo JS, Watkins L Jr, Gott VL, et al. Routine use of autotransfusion following cardiac surgery: experience in 700 patients. *Ann Thorac Surg.* 1979;27:493–499.
22. Sculco (data on file)
23. Clements DH, Sculco TP, Burke SW, Mayer K, Levine DB. Salvage and reinfusion of postoperative sanguineous wound drainage. *J Bone Joint Surg Am.* 1992;74:646–651.
24. Arnested JP, Bengtson A, Bengtson JP, Tylman M, Redl H, Schlag G. Formation of cytokines by retransfusion of shed whole blood. *Br J Anaesth.* 1994;72:422–425.
25. Healy WL, Pfeifer BA, Kurtz SR, Johnson C, Johnson W, Johnston R, et al. Evaluation of autologous shed blood for autotransfusion after orthopaedic surgery. *Clin Orthop.* 1994;299:53–59.
26. Faris PM, Ritter MA, Keating EM, Valeri CR. Unwashed filtered shed blood collected after hip and knee arthroplasties. *J Bone Joint Surg Am.* 1991;73:1169–1178.
27. Ritter MA, Keating EM, Faris PM. Closed wound drainage in total hip or total knee replacement. *J Bone Joint Surg Am.* 1994;76:35–38.
28. Amgen, Inc. Procrit/epoetin alfa product description; 1995.
29. Levine E, Gould S, Rosen A, Sehgal LR, Egrie JC, Sehgal HL, et al. Perioperative recombinant human erythropoietin. *Surgery.* 1989;106:432–438.
30. Faris PM, Ritter MA, Abels RA. The effects of recombinant human erythropoietin on perioperative transfusion requirements in patients undergoing major orthopaedic surgery. *J Bone Joint Surg Am.* 1996;78:62–72.
31. Goldberg MA, McCutchen JW, Jove M, D. Cesare P, Friedman RJ, Poss R, et al. A safety and efficacy comparison study of two dosing regimens of epoetin alfa in patients undergoing major orthopaedic surgery. *Am J Orthop.* 1996;25:544–552.
32. Koester JA, Nelson LD, Morris JA, Safcsak K. Use of recombinant human erythropoietin in a Jehovah's Witness refusing transfusion of blood products: case report. *J Trauma.* 1990;30:1406–1408.
33. Mc Graw JP. Use of recombinant human erythropoietin in a Jehovah's Witness [letter; comment]. *J Trauma.* 1991;31: 1017–1018.

13
Anesthesia Considerations: Hypotension and Hemodilution

Nigel E. Sharrock

There has been an ever-increasing interest in avoiding allogeneic blood transfusion. This began with the recognition of the risk of both hepatitis B virus transmission and transfusion reactions. Currently, concerns have focused on transmission of HIV, hepatitis C or *Yersinia*. In addition, there are immunologic consequences to transfusion, and an increased risk of infection in patients who are transfused.[1] Finally, cost has become an issue. These multiple concerns have brought patients, surgeons, physicians, anesthesiologists, hematologists, and hospital administration personnel together (for a change) in a concerted effort to reduce the use of allogeneic transfusions.[2] This chapter deals with three techniques that can have a major impact on transfusion requirements after total hip arthroplasty (THA).

Hemodilution

Hemodilution involves infusing a large volume of fluid (crystalloid or colloid) into a patient immediately preoperatively as blood is withdrawn from the patient.[2-4] The volume of crystalloid infused is three to four times the volume of blood withdrawn. If colloid is infused rather than crystalloid, lesser volumes may be used but the procedure is more expensive.[5] The goal is to withdraw 2 to 4 units of blood preoperatively—blood that can be reinfused toward the end of surgery or in the immediate postoperative period. The combination of crystalloid infused and concurrent withdrawal of blood dilutes the patients' hemoglobin level intraoperatively but preserves the circulating blood volume.

Rationale

The basis of hemodilution assumes that patients will bleed a similar amount during surgery. Rather than losing blood with a hematocrit of 0.40, the blood loss will have a hematocrit of perhaps 0.20 to 0.25, thereby conserving red blood cell mass. The withdrawn blood is then reinfused when the blood loss slows at the end of surgery. By using these basic concepts, it follows that hemodilution will be more efficacious if the intraoperative hematocrit is lower (ie, more blood is withdrawn, resulting in greater hemodilution); the preoperative hematocrit is higher (enabling more hemodilution to be safely performed); and the intraoperative blood loss is greater (ie, if blood loss is low, the benefit is negligible).[6]

How Is It Done?

Typically, blood is withdrawn passively from an arterial line and stored in a blood transfusion bag (containing acid-citrate-dextrose solution). It is important that as the blood is withdrawn, it is slowly agitated to prevent clotting. By using a system of stopcocks, 1 to 5 units of blood can be withdrawn. The blood is kept in close proximity to the patient and the patient's name should be attached to each bag. Because the blood is kept at room temperature, it must be reinfused within 6 hours.

Concurrently, the patient receives crystalloid or colloid intravenously. To preserve volume status, it is important to monitor central venous pressure and, ideally, cardiac output if larger volumes are to be withdrawn. It is mandatory that volume status be preserved because volume depletion from losing blood leads to low cardiac output, especially when the patient is under general anesthesia. This can lead to shock with adverse consequences.

During surgery, the hematocrit should be checked if there is significant blood loss because it is probably unwise to allow the hematocrit to fall below 0.20 to 0.25 in most patients undergoing THA. Lower levels of hemodilution can be tolerated in young patients, provided that cardiac output is increased, because this enables the oxygen transport to be maintained.[7] The withdrawn blood can be reinfused if the hematocrit begins to fall. The remaining blood should be transfused toward the end of surgery or in the immediate postoperative period.

The reinfusion of blood can lead to fluid overload. Increases in central venous pressure (CVP) or pulmonary artery pressure (PAP) should be normalized with the use of diuretics or vasodilation. On emergence from general anesthesia, increases in CVP or PAP are common because of vasoconstriction. Thus patients who have received additional fluid are at an increased risk of pulmonary edema. In higher risk cases, it may be advisable to maintain patients on a ventilator until central venous pressure and oxygenation are stabilized. Aggressive diuresis can also lead to hypokalemia. Therefore, serum potassium levels should be monitored and abnormalities should be corrected. It is important to warm all fluids and blood to prevent hypothermia in these patients. Customarily included are monitoring of heart rate and rhythm by electrocardiogram, oxygen saturation by pulse oximetry, temperature, blood pressure by radial artery catheter, and central venous or pulmonary artery pressure. In addition, serial hematocrits, arterial blood gas values, and serum electrolyte levels are evaluated.

It is clear from this description that aggressive hemodilution (withdrawal of 4 to 5 units of blood or 2 L) is a labor-intensive process, with added complexity involving additional costs.

Physiologic Effects

The safety of hemodilution is based on the fact that the normal physiologic response to acute anemia is to preserve oxygen transport by increasing cardiac output. In addition, tissues can extract additional oxygen. Finally, patients are usually administered hyperoxic concentrations of anesthetic gases, so that they will have additional oxygen dissolved in blood. These combined mechanisms act to preserve oxygen delivery.

The increase in cardiac output is partly compensatory and partly due to the decreased viscosity of blood. The circulatory response involves a decrease in peripheral vascular resistance and an increase in heart rate and cardiac output. If filling pressures are preserved (as they need to be), stroke volumes are normal or enhanced (due to decreased end systolic volume). These adaptive changes (especially increased heart rate) are well tolerated by young patients. However, elderly patients or those with heart disease may not be able to increase their heart rate safely, limiting the use of this technique in many patients undergoing THA. In addition, the myocardium maximally extracts oxygen under normal circumstances. Therefore, reduced oxygen delivery to the coronary arteries, because of a low hemoglobin level, may lead to coronary ischemia in patients with cardiac disease. For these reasons, the technique is not normally recommended in higher risk patients (who represent most patients undergoing revision THA).

Hemodilution leads to several other physiologic changes, which may limit its utility. Hemodilution leads to a decline in serum protein, which reduces oncotic pressure, leading to significant sequestration of fluid into tissues. Tissue edema may have an impact on gastrointestinal function, wound healing, or oxygen uptake by the lung. The hemodilution also dilutes the clotting factors. With minor degrees of hemodilution, this is well tolerated because both coagulant and anticoagulant factors are diluted out. However, more extreme hemodilution leads to an increase in activated partial thromboplastin time, (aPTT), marked dilution of coagulation factors, and a propensity to bleed intraoperatively. The disturbances may lead to postoperative coagulation disturbances as well.[3] It is also possible that if the anticoagulants (antithrombin III, proteins C and S) are too diluted, a postoperative procoagulant state could ensue, favoring genesis of venous thrombosis.

Efficacy

A number of investigators have analyzed the utility of hemodilution on the basis of theoretical consideration.[6] It appears that the minor degrees of hemodilution (withdrawal of 1 to 2 units of blood) have minimal, if any, beneficial effect on preventing homologous transfusions because the hemoglobin mass saved is so small. It is also clear that the technique has limited use if the preoperative hematocrit is less than 0.36 or the intraoperative blood loss is less than 1 L. This basically means that the technique has little, if any, role in primary THA.[5]

Theoretic studies have also demonstrated that to save 2 units of homologous blood, patients must have a preoperative hematocrit of 0.40, be diluted to 0.20 intraoperatively and have an intraoperative blood loss of at least 2 L.[6] This means that the only clinical setting in which this technique may be helpful would be for one-stage bilateral or complex revision THA. Furthermore, significant hemodilution is not well tolerated in elderly patients or in those with underlying cardiac disease. For these reasons, I believe hemodilution has limited applications in THA except in complex or bilateral one-stage procedures in healthy patients.

Earlier studies that claimed that hemodilution was beneficial often allowed patients to have lower hematocrits than their historic controls. As will be discussed shortly, toleration of lower hematocrits leads to a dramatic lowering of transfusion requirements. For these reasons, it is conceivable that much of the presumed benefit assumed to be due to hemodilution was merely due to accepting lower postoperative hematocrits.

Hypotensive Anesthesia

Blood loss is related to the mean arterial pressure (MAP) during surgery: the higher the pressure, the greater the blood loss. Conversely, lower blood pressures reduce bleeding. The relationship is quite steep such that for every 10 mmHg increase in pressure, bleeding increases by about 50%. From this, it is apparent that keeping MAP at about 50 mmHg results in about one-third to one-fifth the blood loss that is noted with normotension (MAP of 80 to 100 mmHg). The typical intraoperative blood loss (IBL) with a MAP of 50 mmHg is 150 to 250 mL, whereas that in normotension ranges from 500 to 1000 mL for a primary THA.[8,9] This reduction in intraoperative IBL results in a reduction in homologous transfusion.[9]

Bleeding during surgery is not related to cardiac output, only MAP.[10] Thus bleeding is related to the pressure within, not the flow through, the vessels. During THA performed in the lateral decubitus position, the surgical wound is above the level of the heart so it is not surprising that IBL is not related to central venous pressure. At the end of surgery, when the MAP increases, wound drainage is not increased. Thus, the reduction in bleeding results in a net saving in blood loss and a reduction in transfusion requirements.

Techniques

Induced hypotension can be produced with several techniques by using general or regional anesthesia.[11] By using general anesthesia, MAP can be reduced by arterial vasodilation or cardiac depression. In practice, a combination of techniques is often used by infusing vasodilators (eg, sodium nitroprusside, nitroglycerin), in combination with beta-blockers or inhalation agents. Alternatively, agents such as labetalol (both a beta-blocker and an alpha-blocker) or deep inhalation anesthesia may be used. All these techniques reduce MAP, thereby reducing intraoperative bleeding. Hemodynamically, these techniques are characterized by a reduction in stroke volume and cardiac output (unless heart rate increases). If filling pressures are not maintained, significant reductions in cardiac output can occur. It is not possible to monitor brain function effectively because patients are asleep.

With regional anesthesia, intraoperative blood loss is less than that with general anesthesia.[12–15] This is almost certainly due to the lower MAP associated with spinal or epidural anesthesia. In studies in which MAP has been maintained within the normotensive range with spinal or epidural anesthesia, intraoperative blood loss is greater than 1 L.

With hypotensive epidural anesthesia (HEA), MAP is maintained at 45 to 55 mmHg while maintaining a stable heart rate, filling pressure, stroke volume, and cardiac output.[16] This is achieved by producing an extensive epidural blockade and infusing epinephrine at 1 to 5 µg/min to maintain circulatory stability.[9] This technique has the physiologic advantage of preserving cardiac output with a normal heart rate and being able to monitor the patient's neurologic function by keeping him or her awake, if required. For these reasons, this technique has proved to be safe in elderly, high-risk patients who constitute most patients undergoing THA.[17] Intraoperative blood loss for primary THA is 100 to 250 mL with this technique.[18]

Results

All studies of THA have demonstrated a reduction in intraoperative blood loss with hypotensive anesthesia, compared to normotensive anesthesia. Intraoperative blood loss is reduced by 60% to 70%. There is no increase in postoperative wound drainage, so transfusion requirements are reduced by at least 50% (Table 13.1).[19,20,21]

The experience at the Hospital for Special Surgery is similar. With the introduction of spinal anesthesia in the 1970s, Sculco and Ranawat[12] noted that IBL and transfusion requirements were halved when compared to general anesthesia. When HEA was introduced in 1986 to 1987, a retrospective review revealed that blood loss fell 50% and transfusion requirements fell significantly. In patients who did not predonate autologous blood, the average patient received 1.2 units of homologous blood and 70% were transfused by using normotensive anesthesia. After introduction of HEA, the mean number of homologous units transfused was 0.7 liters; 38% of patients received homologous blood. In a series of high-risk patients in a controlled trial of hypotensive epidural

Table 13.1. Intraoperative blood loss and inhospital transfusion with hypotensive anesthesia.

	Intraoperative blood loss (mL)		Inhospital transfusion (units)	
	Normotension	Hypotension	Normotension	Hypotension
Thompson and colleagues[19]	1183	326	1.3	0.5
Vazeery and Lunde[20]	1638	212	3.2	1.6
Rosberg and colleagues[21]	1780	660	2.2	1.1

anesthesia, only 5% of patients received homologous blood.[27] This ultimate success in avoiding transfusion is due to a combination of predonation of autologous blood, hypotensive epidural anesthesia, and toleration of lower hematocrits. This is in stark contrast to current experience from other centers in which the average blood replacement is 1 to 2 units of blood with intraoperative blood loss of 500 to 1500 mL.[4,8,9]

Other Benefits

Hypotensive anesthesia may have additional benefits other than avoiding transfusion. It may result in a shorter operative time. The reduction in intraoperative blood loss means that less crystalloid is needed, which reduces cost, risk of hypothermia, postoperative pulmonary edema, and the likelihood of dilutional disturbances in coagulation.[3] Rates of deep venous thrombosis are low when hypotensive epidural anesthesia is used.[22] This may be due to enhanced blood flow in the patient's legs with this technique or a more specific response to hypotensive anesthesia by not losing blood during surgery.[22,23] Finally, hypotensive anesthesia provides a dry bone interface, which enables better cement penetration into the cancellous bone.[24] Hypotensive anesthesia has been shown to improve the radiographic results of cemented acetabular fixation. Presumably, the fixation of femoral components is also improved. These data were collected in primary THA and whether they apply to revision THA is unknown.

Safety Issues in High-Risk Cases

Unlike primary THA, revision THA is typically performed in elderly patients. The surgery is longer, more complex, and often associated with significant blood loss. Thus the potential benefits of hypotensive anesthesia are greater in revision THA than in primary THA. The question is, How safe is hypotensive anesthesia in high-risk cases?

Hypotensive epidural anesthesia has been used in thousands of high-risk cases at the Hospital for Special Surgery.[17] The technique is used in patients with hypertension, chronic obstructive pulmonary disease (COPD), and ischemic heart disease, as well as in elderly patients. With appropriate monitoring, patients with mitral regurgitation and minor degrees of aortic stenosis can be safely managed. The duration of hypotension is not a limiting factor. Patients undergoing revision THA should be monitored with central venous or pulmonary artery catheters. With hypotensive anesthesia, preservation of filling pressures is vital to ensure a stable cardiac output.

Induced hypotension by using general anesthesia can be used for revision THA in more healthy patients, but the safety of these techniques for longer revisions cases in the elderly high-risk cases is yet to be demonstrated in large series.

Toleration of Low Hematocrit

Perhaps the cheapest and most effective way to avoid homologous transfusion after revision THA is to lower the so-called transfusion trigger.[2] This is the hematocrit at which one transfuses blood. Traditionally, this was a hematocrit of 0.30; but in recent years, experience has shown that this can be lowered to 0.20 in healthy patients.[2] Patients with COPD or ischemic heart disease may not tolerate a hematocrit of less than 0.30. If these patients become at all symptomatic, hypotensive, or tachycardic, it is better to transfuse at a hematocrit of 0.30. On the other hand, hematocrits of less than 0.30 are usually well tolerated even in the elderly.

Outcome data suggest that postoperative hematocrits of less than 0.30 do not adversely affect outcome. For these reasons, most centers are re-evaluating transfusion criteria and restricting elective transfusion unless the hematocrit is less than 0.25 or 0.26. Reasons to transfuse at higher hematocrits are usually reserved for symptomatic patients with medical comorbidities.

In a person who weighs 70 kg and has a preoperative hematocrit of 0.40, simple calculations can demonstrate that if one reduces the transfusion trigger from 0.30 to 0.24, this will save 2 units of blood. From this, it is clear how much of an impact such a policy may have on transfusion requirements.

Conclusion

Lowering of the transfusion trigger is a simple, cheap, and effective measure of reducing the need for allogeneic transfusion. It must be used selectively, but quite low hematocrits (≈ 0.20) can be tolerated in young, fit patients. Higher values of 0.25 to 0.26 are tolerated in otherwise well elderly patients and in many with compensated cardiopulmonary diseases. Hypotensive anesthesia, especially HEA, can reduce intraoperative blood loss by 60% to 70%. Intraoperative blood loss in a complex revision THA may be 2 L with normotensive anesthesia, but 600 to 700 mL is typical with HEA. This may save up to 3 to 4 units of blood, making the use of cell savers unnecessary. When HEA is used in conjunction with an autologous blood program, allogeneic blood is not usually needed. Hemodilution has a role in young healthy patients for complex THA in which anticipated blood losses approach 2 L.

The best approach to avoid homologous transfusion is to use several modalities at once (eg, lowering of the transfusion trigger, HEA, cell saver, and autologous predonation. Cost issues, anesthesia staffing, and practice patterns may determine what combination of strategies is best in each institution.

References

1. Landers DF, Hill GE, Wong KC, Fox IJ. Blood transfusion–induced immunomodulation. *Anesth Analg.* 1996;82:187–204.
2. Weiskopf RB. More on the changing indications for transfusion of blood and blood components during anesthesia: editorial views. *Anesthesiology.* 1996;84:498–501.
3. McLoughlin TM Jr, Fontana JL, Alving B, Mongan PD, Bunger R. Profound normovolemic hemodilution: hemostatic effects in patients and in a porcine model. *Anesth Analg.* 1996;83:459–465.
4. Habler OP, Kleen MS, Podtschaske AH, Hutter JW, Tiede M, Kemming GI, et al. The effect of acute normovolemic hemodilution (ANH) on myocardial contractility in anesthetized dogs. *Anesth Analg.* 1996;83:451–458.
5. Mielke LL, Entholzner EK, Kling M, Breinbauer BE, Burgkart R, Hargasser SR, et al. Preoperative acute hypervolemic hemodilution with hydroxyethylstarch: an alternative to acute normovolemic hemodilution? *Anesth Analg.* 1997;84:26–30.
6. Weiskopf RB. Mathematical analysis of isovolemic hemodilution indicates that it can decrease the need for allogeneic blood transfusion. *Transfusion.* 1995;35:37–41.
7. van Iterson M, van der Waart FJM, Erdmann W, Trouwborst A. Systemic haemodynamics and oxygenation during haemodilution in children. *Lancet.* 1995;346:1127–1129.
8. Sharrock NE, Mineo R, Urquhart B, Salvati EA. The effect of two levels of hypotension on intraoperative blood loss during total hip arthroplasty. *Anesth Analg.* 1993;76:580–584.
9. Sharrock NE, Salvati EA. Hypotensive epidural anesthesia for total hip arthroplasty. *Acta Orthop Scand.* 1996;67:91–107.
10. Sharrock NE, Mineo R, Go G. The effect of cardiac output on intraoperative blood loss during total hip arthroplasty. *Reg Anaesth.* 1993;18:24–29.
11. Van Aken H, Miller ED Jr. Deliberate hypotension. In: Miller RD, ed. *Anesthesia.* New York, NY: Churchill Livingstone; 1994:1481–1503.
12. Sculco TP, Ranawat C. The use of spinal anesthesia for total hip replacement arthroplasty. *J Bone Joint Surg Am.* 1975;57:173–177.
13. Modig J. Beneficial effects on intraoperative and postoperative blood loss in total hip replacement when performed under lumbar epidural anesthesia: an explanatory study. *Acta Chir Scand Suppl.* 1988;550:95–103.
14. Modig J. Regional anaesthesia and blood loss. *Acta Anaesthesiol Scand Suppl.* 1988;32:44–48.
15. Keith I. Anaesthesia and blood loss in total hip replacement. *Anaesthesia.* 1977;32:444–450.
16. Sharrock NE, Mineo R, Urquhart B. Haemodynamic effects and outcome analysis of hypotensive extradural anaesthesia in controlled hypertensive patients undergoing total hip arthroplasty. *Br J Anaesth.* 1991;67:17–25.
17. Sharrock NE, Cazan MG, Hargett MJ, Williams-Russo P, Wilson PD Jr. Changes in mortality after total hip and knee arthroplasty over a ten-year period. *Anesth Analg.* 1995;80:242–248.
18. Sharrock NE, Ranawat CS, Urquhart B, Peterson M. Factors influencing deep vein thrombosis following total hip arthroplasty. *Anesth Analg.* 1993;76:765–771.
19. Thompson GE, Miller RD, Stevens WC, Murray WR. Hypotensive anesthesia for total hip arthroplasty: a study of blood loss and organ function (brain, heart, liver, and kidney). *Anesthesiology.* 1978;48:91–96.
20. Vazeery AK, Lunde O. Controlled hypotension in hip joint surgery: an assessment of surgical haemorrhage during sodium nitroprusside infusion. *Acta Orthop Scand.* 1979;50:433–441.
21. Rosberg B, Fredin H, Gustafson C. Anesthetic techniques and surgical blood loss in total hip arthroplasty. *Acta Anaesthesiol Scand.* 1982;26:189–193.
22. Lieberman JR, Huo MM, Hanway J, Salvati EA, Sculco TP, Sharrock NE. The prevalence of deep venous thrombosis after total hip arthroplasty with hypotensive epidural anesthesia. *J Bone Joint Surg Am.* 1994;76:341–348.
23. Bading B, Blank S, Sculco TP, Pickering TG, Sharrock NE. Augmentation of calf blood flow by epinephrine infusion during lumbar epidural anesthesia. *Anesth Analg.* 1994;78:1119–1124.
24. Ranawat CS, Beaver WB, Sharrock NE, Maynard MJ, Urquhart B, Schneider R. Effect of hypotensive epidural anaesthesia on acetabular cement–bone fixation in total hip arthroplasty. *J Bone Joint Surg Br.* 1991;73:779–782.

14
Preoperative Templating in Revision Total Hip Arthroplasty

Kenneth B. Mathis, Philip C. Noble, and Hugh S. Tullos

The goals of preoperative templating for total hip replacement are to provide: (1) an estimate of the size of the femoral and acetabular components needed at surgery; (2) the appropriate level of femoral osteotomy; (3) the assurance that the medial offset of the femoral head can be reproduced without excessive lengthening of the extremity; and (4) the assurance that a corresponding modular neck is available to achieve this goal.

Templating in revision total hip arthroplasty is challenging in that reproducing limb length, achieving stable press-fit of the implant, and restoring offset are complex issues. The need for special equipment (ie, high-speed drills, cables, ultrasonic cement removal tools, allograft bone, somatosensory evoked potentials, and modular custom prostheses) can be ascertained by templating. In addition, shortened operative time, decreased complications, and the need for fewer implants and implant systems in the operating room can be expected. Failure to template adequately before surgery will most likely lead to less than optimal results and may occasionally prevent completion of the planned procedure.

The first step in preoperative templating is preparation of adequate radiographs of the hip, pelvis, and femur. An anteroposterior (AP) radiograph of the pelvis, an AP radiograph of the proximal two thirds of the femur, and a Lowenstein lateral are the minimum views needed. The AP radiograph should show the femur in 15° to 20° of internal rotation to present the head and neck in a true AP view and reveal the head and neck offset accurately. However, in the arthritic hip it is not always possible to rotate the limb internally 15° to 20°. Consequently, the contralateral uninvolved hip may be used as a guide to the offset of the affected femur. If both hips are involved and cannot be rotated, an alternative positioning will be needed. By having a posterior radiograph made with the patient prone and the foot externally rotated 15° to 20° with the opposite hip elevated, the femoral neck can be presented in a true AP plane for templating purposes.[1] It is also important to determine the correct magnification of each radiograph to ensure the accuracy of templating. The magnification of standard radiographs can be checked by use of markers placed at the same distance from the radiographic cassette as the shaft of the femur. Alternatively, a device can be used to measure the diameter of the femoral head on the radiograph. Comparison with the known head diameter then gives the percent magnification of the image. It is recommended that radiographs of the entire involved femur be prepared, especially in the presence of an ipsilateral total knee arthroplasty or previous trauma to the distal femur.

The first step in radiographic templating is to measure the difference in limb length of the affected and contralateral extremities on the AP pelvic radiograph. A line is first drawn connecting the most inferior aspects of the ischial tuberosities (Fig. 14.1). The vertical distance from this line to the center of the lesser trochanter is measured for the ipsilateral and contralateral femora. The difference between these measurements is usually an accurate indication of limb length inequality, and it is marked on the radiograph for later reference. However, to be precise this measurement needs to be performed by using radiographs with the same amount of abduction and rotation bilaterally. In addition, one should not rely on this measurement alone, but should check a clinical estimate of limb length against the x-ray measurement because limb length inequality that is not due to the hip disease will not be detected with this method. If polio, a distal femoral epiphyseal disorder, an old fracture, or a congenital disorder is present, scanograms will be necessary to determine accurately the limb length and amount of correction to be obtained. If contractions are present, a computer tomographic scanogram may be necessary.

In cases in which the contralateral femur is abnormal so that it cannot be used as a reference for determining head offset, an alternative method must be used to lo-

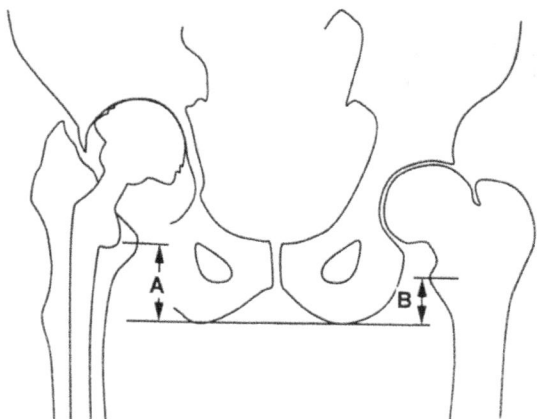

Figure 14.1. Inferior ischial line measurement of limb length inequality. A − B = Limb length discrepancy.

cate the head center. In a recent anatomic study performed by Sugano and coworkers,[2] correlations between the position of standard radiographic landmarks and the height and medial offset of the femoral head center were calculated for a group of 32 cadaveric femora with neck-shaft angles ranging from 115° to 146°. This study showed that the height of the head center could not be predicted from the height of the greater trochanter with any accuracy. Although the tip of the trochanter was located 10.3 mm proximal to the femoral head center of the average femur, the relative distance between these two points varied by more than 20 mm.

The strongest correlations were found between the position of the head center and the point along the neck axis where the neck was narrowest (Fig. 14.2). As a rule of thumb, it was found that the height of the head center could be predicted to ±5.1 mm by adding 10 mm to the height of the midpoint of the neck isthmus above the lesser trochanter. Similarly, the medial offset of the head center was predicted to ±4.6 mm by adding 15 mm to the offset of the midpoint of the neck isthmus from the medullary axis. These rules form a useful basis for defining normal femoral anatomy in situations in which the normal anatomy is not readily available.

Acetabulum

Preoperative templating is also essential for planning the correct position of the acetabular component. The failed acetabular component has usually migrated superiorly and possibly medially. The resulting acetabular defects are generally categorized as segmental or cavitary according to the American Academy of Orthopedic Surgeons classification.[3] Type I (segmental) defects are characterized by loss of bone from the supporting rim of the acetabular margin or the medial wall. Type II defects are contained, cavitary lesions in the presence of an intact acetabular rim, and they are subdivided by location (superior, medial, anterior, and posterior). If segmental and cavitary bone loss is present, the defect is classified as type III, whereas type IV defects include a pelvic discontinuity with disruption of both the anterior and posterior columns. In type I and III defects, the percentage of the cup that would be uncovered or unsupported needs to be estimated. Porous, hemispheric shells can span these defects most of the time.

Landi et al.[4] examined the capacity of the acetabulum to accommodate acetabular cups of increased diameter (megacups) as a means of filling bony defects at revision. They found that the average acetabulum can be enlarged by 11% (6 mm) without loss of adequate coverage or a gross reduction in implant stability. In this process, the surface of the shell was displaced an average of 6.5 mm posteriorly and 7.7 mm superiorly, indicating the theoretic limits of this method of filling bony defects.

Occasionally, a structural allograft or autograft will be required. However, the long-term success of bulk structural allograft is poor, with failure rates of 44% to 70% reported at 2- to 5-year follow up.[5–7] Nonetheless, in the young patient the use of bulk allograft may still be favored, considering the potential for restoration of bone stock. If it is necessary to ream up more than 10 mm from the diameter of the original shell to fill the acetabulum, a reinforcement ring may be needed for ad-

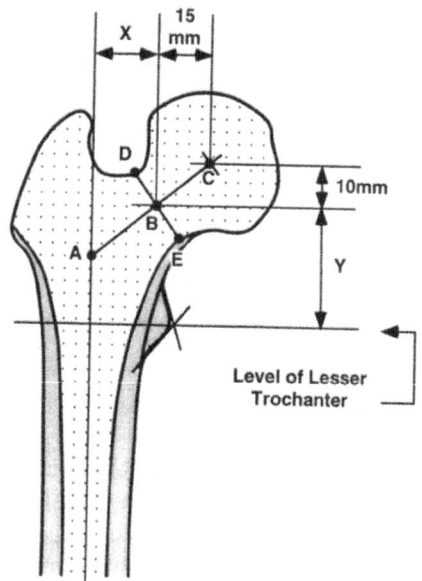

Figure 14.2. The femoral head center (C) may be predicted from the coordinates (X, Y) of the center of the isthmus of the femoral neck (point B). This point is defined by the intersection of the neck axis (AC) and the line perpendicular to AC where the line crossing the femoral neck (DE) is shortest.

equate reconstruction. This is because the rigid screw fixation provided by the ring allows the cup to span defects and helps shield allograft from forces until it can incorporate. Success rates up to 76% have been reported with this method.[8]

Type II defects that are relatively small are managed well by grafting. In addition, if the hip center has migrated proximally, an uncemented shell placed high with good bone contact is preferable to the use of a structural allograft despite the increased mechanical stresses placed on the higher hip center.

Another promising option is to use cups of an oblong or double-cup design. These components allow an intimate fit of the uncemented shell to the distorted acetabulum and restoration of the hip center without the use of structural grafts (Fig. 14.3). However, long-term follow-up is not yet available on these devices, and their use in the younger population may be contraindicated. This is because they do not rebuild lost bone stock and may make the next revision even more challenging. In cases of pelvic discontinuity (Type IV defects), it is necessary to plan for fixation of the pelvis with plates and

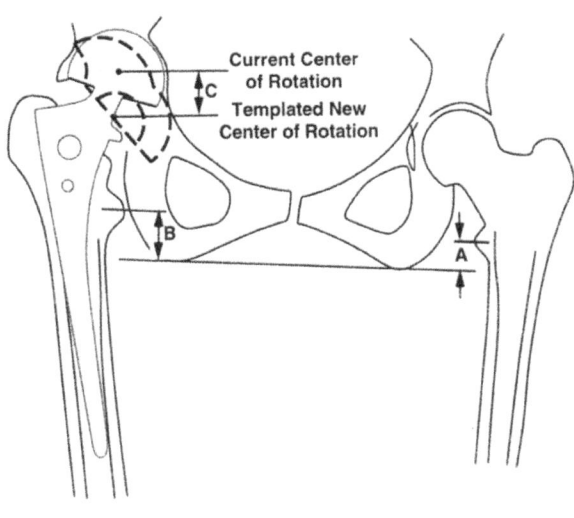

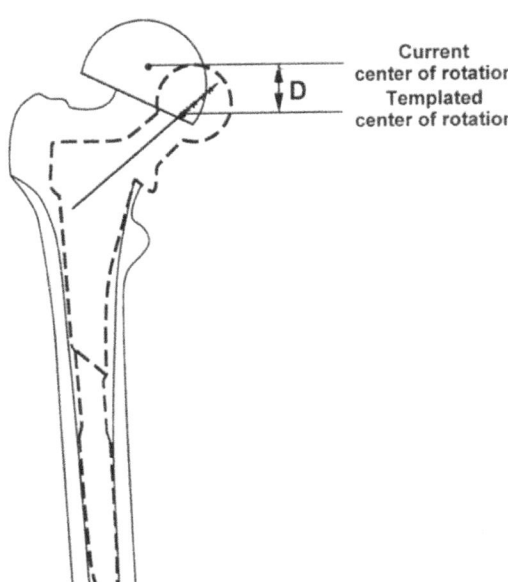

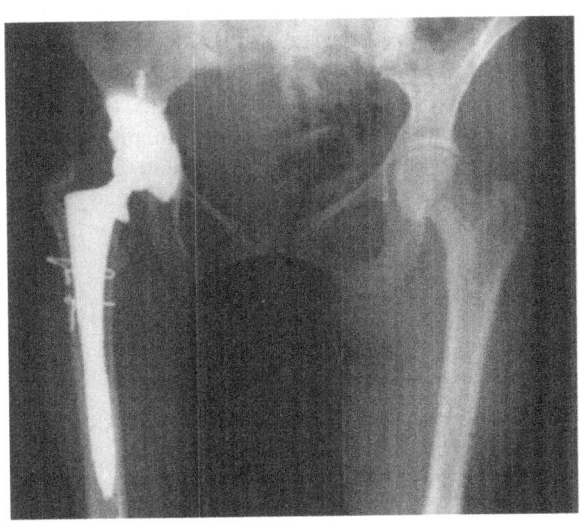

Figure 14.3. A. Type II defect. Bringing the center of rotation back down to original position will overlengthen the patient's leg. B − A = Amount of shortening present; C = Amount of length gained by restoring acetabular centers of rotation. Because C > B − A, the femoral neck length will need to be shortened. B. Template of prosthesis planned. D = Amount of shortening that can be obtained. C. Oblong cup filling acetabular defect with restoration of limb length.

screws in addition to the acetabular socket reconstruction.

To template the acetabulum preoperatively for simpler reconstructions, the AP radiograph may be used to select the cup size that appears to contact the remaining bone superiorly and inferiorly and the teardrop medially. This template is then placed beneath the x-ray film, and an x-ray pencil is used to outline the cup to 45° of lateral tilt. The new planned center of rotation is also marked. The vertical distance from the current center of rotation is measured and compared with the limb length discrepancy. If the value is less, additional length will need to be restored through higher placement of the femoral prosthesis within the femur or selection of a modular head of increased neck length (Fig. 14.4).

Femur

The next step in templating involves evaluating the femur. If the quality of the metaphyseal bone stock is good to excellent, the templating is performed with the goals of maximum fit and fill of the metaphysis. In this situation, either a distally fixed or a proximally fixed stem is appropriate, although distal fixation is probably more reliable. However, it is important to note that for distally fixed implants to perform satisfactorily, a close fit must be achieved through the canal isthmus with contact between the distal stem and at least two opposite cortices. Although the appropriate size prosthesis may be estimated from conventional AP radiographs, several studies have shown that conventional templating only predicts the appropriate size of cementless stems in 42% to 60% of cases because of variations in femoral rotation and radiographic magnification.[9]

Therefore, we have developed a routine CT scan protocol for accurately sizing the femur in preoperative planning for revision total hip replacement. This proto-

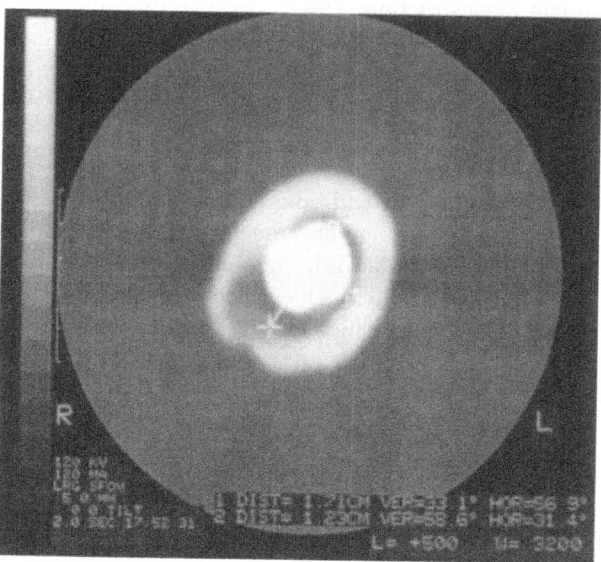

Figure 14.5. CT scan for canal templating. Note oblique, oval shape of canal (17 × 12 mm).

col consists of only five slices through the femur, starting at the lesser trochanter and extending distally at intervals of 2 cm. By prior arrangement with the radiologist, measurements of the major and minor diameters of the canal are measured at each level (Fig. 14.5). Note that the medullary canal averages 35% larger on anteroposterior than on mediolateral direction. This oval is generally rotated slightly out of the direct AP plane.

Consequently, to get increased diaphyseal contact and enhanced rotational stability of the implant, it is usually necessary to ream away some of the medial and lateral cortical bone. Less bone reaming is necessary when a fluted prosthesis is used because of the enhanced rotational stability afforded by this mode of distal fixation. In addition, because the scan requires no interpretation and few slices, the scan at our institution is relatively inexpensive. With these data, the amount of reaming is calculated preoperatively, and errors caused by sizing of implants on the basis of the "feel" of reamers are eliminated. Relying on perception of contact by reaming can lead to erroneous undersizing, especially if retained cement is present within the canal.

Attention is next directed to the selection of the optimum neck length. The center of rotation of each available modular head is examined with the x-ray template placed in the position of maximum filling of the metaphysis. The options for head position are marked on the film and compared with the existing center of rotation of the hip (Fig. 14.6). The vertical differences can be measured and added to the value obtained for the shift in position of the acetabulum.

Attention is also paid to offset. If the contralateral hip is normal, this value can be measured on the normal hip

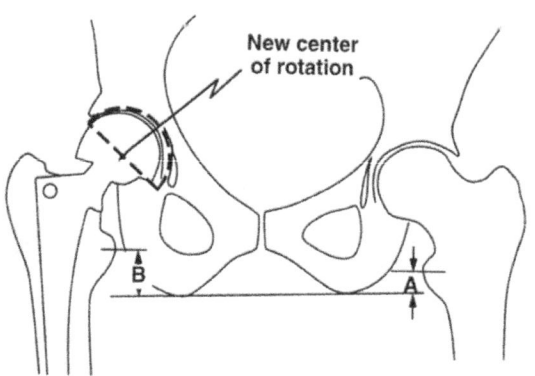

Figure 14.4. Template of acetabular component with new centers of rotation. A + B measure distance between lesser trochanter and trans-ischial line. A − B = limb length discrepancy.

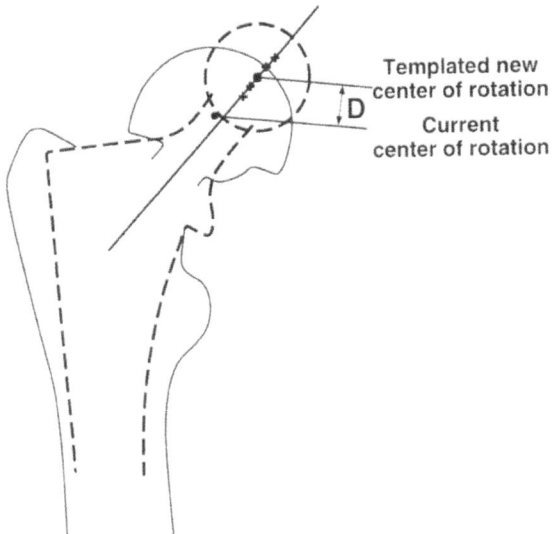

Figure 14.6. Templating new center of rotation. D = Increase in limb length obtained by this prosthesis.

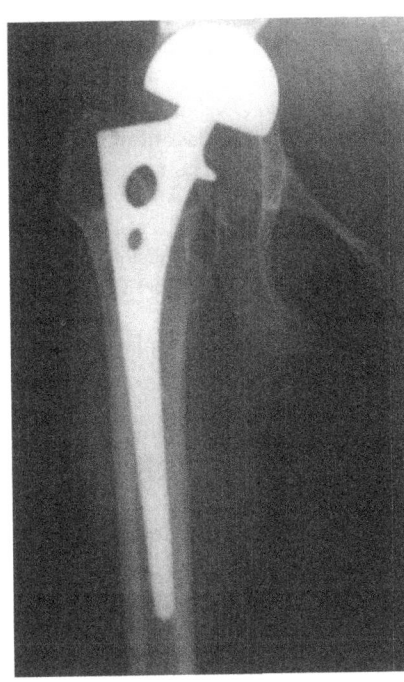

Figure 14.7. Lateral endosteal line demonstrating lateral margin of a proposed new prosthesis. A trochanteric osteotomy will be required in this example.

and restored by templating the proposed implant on the normal hip and placing the template at the same neck resection level seen on the affected side. If significant lengthening is planned on the revision side, exact restoration of medial offset is less critical because tightening of the myofascial envelope will occur as the extremity is lengthened. If lengthening of greater than 2.5 cm is needed, either somatosensory evoked potentials (SSEP) or a wake-up test may be needed to minimize the risk of sciatic nerve palsy.

It is also important to assess the AP radiograph to check for a varus deformity of the proximal femur. This can be performed by drawing a line along the lateral endosteal surface of the femur up to the greater trochanter (Fig. 14.7). This line corresponds to the position of the lateral edge of a rigid canal reamer and the surface of the prosthesis when it is implanted in neutral alignment within the medullary canal. If the line passes through the lateral cortex of the femur below the level of the greater trochanter, a varus deformity is present. This should be corrected with an osteotomy before the femur is prepared for implantation of the prosthetic component.

Once an implant has been selected on the basis of the AP radiograph, the corresponding lateral template is placed on the Lowenstein lateral views of the femur. This is done to ensure that the implant will fit the metaphyseal portion of the bone and not impinge on the anterior cortex distally because of the curvature of the canal.

Even greater preoperative planning is required for more complicated revisions that involve extensive loss of proximal bone stock. In these cases, preoperative scanograms for limb length are routinely recommended because of the lack of an identifiable lesser trochanter. If there is inadequate metaphyseal bone for stable proximal fixation, a distally fixed implant will be required. For this to be successful, direct contact between the distal stem of the prosthesis and the medullary canal must be achieved over a length of at least 5 cm. In cases in which the bone loss extends distally past the isthmus or there is insufficient contact between the distal stem and the cortical bone, distally fixed cementless stems will not provide adequate stability. Either impaction grafting or cement fixation are necessary in these cases.

For proximal femoral defects that are contained, we recommend use of morselized autograft or allograft as long as stability of the implant does not depend on the graft. Segmental defects in the calcar of less than 3 cm are best treated with use of a prosthesis of a calcar-replacing design. Use of standard prostheses in this situation with extra long neck lengths and femoral heads with a "skirt" is generally to be avoided. The extra width of the neck from the skirt restricts range of motion, especially when combined with a hooded polyethylene liner. This leads to impingement and increased risk of dislocation.

References

1. Engh C. Recent advances in cementless total hip arthroplasty using the AML prosthesis. *Tech Orthop.* 1991;6:3.

2. Sugano N, Noble P, Kamaric E, et al. Predicting the position of the femoral head. In: Proceedings of the American Association of Hip and Knee Surgeons meeting; November 8–10, 1996; Dallas, Tex.
3. D'Antonio J, Capello WN, Borden LS, Bargar WL, Bierbaum BF, Boettcher WG, et al. Classification and management of acetabular abnormalities in total hip arthroplasty. *Clin Orthop.* 1989;243:126–137.
4. Landi S, Noble P, Kamaric E, et al. Anatomic constraints on the use of mega-cups in revision THR. In: Proceedings of the ISTA meeting; September 24–27, 1997; San Diego, Calif.
5. Paprosky W, Magnus R. Principles of bone grafting in revision total hip arthroplasty: acetabular technique. *Clin Orthop.* 1994;298:147–155.
6. Hooten J Jr, Engh C. Failure of structural acetabular allografts in cementless revision hip arthroplasty. *J Bone Joint Surg Br.* 1994;76:419–422.
7. Kwong L, Jasty M, Harris W. High failure rate of bulk femoral head allografts in total hip acetabular reconstructions at 10 years. *J Arthroplasty.* 1993;8:341–346.
8. Berry D, Miller M. Revision arthroplasty using an anti-protrusion cage for massive acetabular bone deficiency. *J Bone Joint Surg Br.* 1992;74:711–715.
9. Knight J, Atwater R. Pre-operative planning for total hip arthroplasty. *J Arthroplasty.* 1992;7:403–409.

15
Biomechanics of Revision Hip Replacement

Philip C. Noble

In revision total hip replacement, biomechanical challenges confront the surgeon in restoring the normal mechanics of the hip joint while achieving stable, long-term fixation of the prosthetic components in host bone. In this chapter, we will briefly review the biomechanics of the hip joint and the effect of variables describing the design of the femoral component on load-sharing and fixation within the revision femur. Because the fundamental goal of joint replacement is to restore the physiologic motion of the hip joint, we will also discuss challenges confronting the revision surgeon in recreating the normal anatomic relationship between the pelvis and femur.

Forces Acting on the Hip Joint

Large forces and moments are developed within the hip joint during normal activities, including walking, running, stair-climbing, and rising from a chair. Using instrumented hip prostheses, several investigators have reported in vivo measurements of hip joint forces for periods of up to 3 years after implantation.[1-5] These studies show that during normal gait, the peak force developed across the hip ranges from 2.6 to 4.1 times body weight (typically, 390–620 lb), whereas the torque acting on the hip prosthesis ranges from 74 to 189 in-lb, with peak values of up to 291 in-lb. The in vivo readings show that joint forces increase with walking speed, body weight, and stride length, with forces of up to eight times the body weight during strenuous activities.

The effect of individual parameters on loading of the hip joint can be appreciated from a simplified mechanical model of the hip joint during one-legged stance (Fig. 15.1).[6] In this model, the forces acting across the hip are represented in the sagittal plane. The weight of the body supported by the hip joint is represented by a single force (W^1) passing through the center of gravity of the body. Typically, the hip joint supports five-sixths of the total body weight (BW) (ie, $W^1 = 5/6$ BW). This force is balanced by muscle contraction, which stabilizes the pelvis by counteracting the leverage developed by the weight of the body. In this model, the sum of these muscle forces is represented by a net abductor muscle force (F_A), which acts in the direction of the glutei muscles.

A stable mechanical equilibrium is reached when the abducting effect of the forces equals the adducting effect of the body weight acting around the hip joint fulcrum. This balance is expressed mathematically by the equation

$$F_A \cdot r = \frac{5}{6} W \cdot L$$

where: r = the minimum distance from the abductor muscles to the joint center
W = body weight
L = horizontal distance from the center of gravity of the body to the joint center

This equation can be rearranged to solve for the net abductor force:

$$F_A = \frac{5}{6} W(L/r)$$

This indicates that the abductor force necessary to maintain hip joint stability is proportional to the ratio between L and r. For a typical value of this ratio (eg, $L/r = 2.5$), the estimated value of the abductor force is 2.1 times body weight. From this expression it can be seen that the abductor force (and thus the total joint force) may be decreased by either leaning over the hip joint (decreasing L) or maximizing the distance of the abductor insertion from the center of the femoral head (increasing r). Moreover, the more valgus the femoral neck, the larger the ratio L/r and, thus, the greater the abductor force necessary to balance body weight.

It is also possible to calculate the total force (F_R) acting on the hip joint by adding the vertical and horizon-

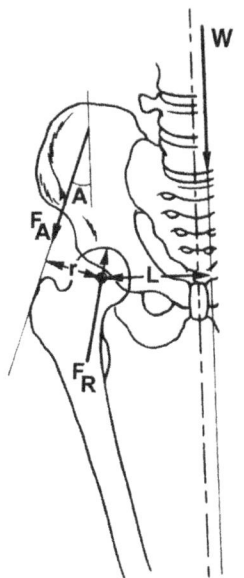

Figure 15.1. Diagrammatic representation of the forces acting on the hip joint during single-legged stance (coronal plane projection) (Noble et al,[6] with permission)

tal components of the joint reactive force. If the ratio $L/r = 2.5$, this leads to the expression

$$F_R = \frac{5}{6}W(725 + 5 \cos A)^{1/2}$$

For a typical value of the angle A (20°), the predicted value of F_R is 2.88 times body weight. Thus the total force supported by the hip joint is almost equal to the algebraic sum of the abductor force (2.1 BW) and the weight of the supported body (0.83 BW).

This analysis demonstrates that the joint reaction force is primarily determined by the magnitude of the muscle forces controlling joint motion. Because muscles normally act closer to the joint than to the center of gravity of the rest of the body, the force developed by muscle contraction must be several times larger than the weight of the body to balance the forces causing joint motion. With activities necessitating greater joint motion (eg, walking, running, stair-climbing), the center of gravity of the body moves even further from the joint, leading to greatly increased muscle and joint reaction forces.

Load Transmission Across the Implant–Bone Interface

The response of the femur and the femoral prosthesis to loading significantly influences the clinical success of total hip replacement. Long-term, asymptomatic performance of hip replacements depends on direct attachment of bone to the surface of the prosthesis. For this to occur, relative motion between the bone and the implant must be limited to 50 to 100 μm through the mechanical fixation achieved intraoperatively. Once biologic incorporation occurs, changes in the stresses developed within the femur initiate remodeling of the bone, leading to restoration of missing bone stock or atrophy of existing bone as a new equilibrium is reached within the skeleton.

In this section, we examine the loading response of the implant–bone construct after revision hip total replacement.

Intramedullary Fixation of Cementless Femoral Prostheses

Rigid fixation of the implant–bone interface is an important prerequisite for successful clinical performance of cementless prostheses. Numerous factors affect the relative motion of the prosthesis and the femur under physiologic loads.[7,8] Factors presented by the patient include intracortical geometry; quality of the bone stock; and weight, height, and activity of the individual. Factors that come under the control of the surgeon include fit of the implant to the endosteal contours of the femur, area of contact between the surface of the prosthesis and the implant site, and position of implantation of the prosthesis within the bone (including the level of the femoral neck osteotomy).

In primary hip replacement, stable fixation of the cementless interface can be achieved through an accurate fit between the prosthesis and the strong cancellous and cortical bone of the femoral metaphysis.[9] However, in revision arthroplasty, the cancellous bone of the proximal femur is often compromised and incapable of stabilizing the prosthesis. This has led to the widespread use of prostheses that provide distal fixation with the cortical walls of the medullary canal.

Kendrick, et al.[10] investigated the contribution of the cross-sectional configuration of the distal stem to stability of the bone–implant interface. By testing several stem designs implanted in cadaveric bone, these investigators examined the ability of cementless designs to provide torsional resistance comparable with that of cemented stems. Four cross-sectional designs were investigated: fluted stem, finned stem, porous-coated stem, and slotted fluted stem (Fig. 15.2). A knurled stem was also cemented into each specimen at the conclusion of testing to act as a control.

Large differences were observed in the rigidity of fixation of the five designs. The torque required to cause 100 μm of displacement at the bone–stem interface ranged from 13.7 ± 0.8 N-m with the porous-coated component to 30.1 ± 3.7 N-m with the fluted design ($p < .0001$) (Fig. 15.3). Intermediate values of 19.5 ± 1.4 and 19.9 ± 2.3 N-m were observed with finned and slotted fluted designs, respectively, compared with 34.0 ±

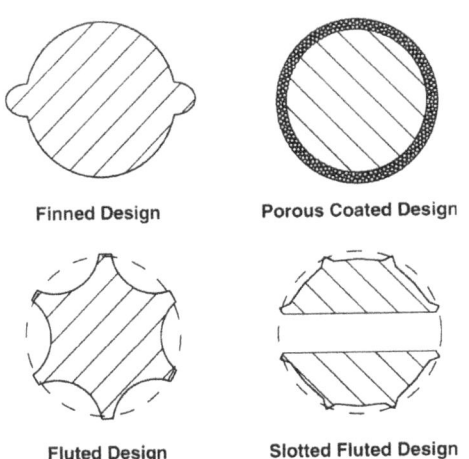

Figure 15.2. Cross-sectional designs of four cementless stems tested by Kendrick and colleagues.[10] (Reproduced with permission.)

3.0 N-m resisted by cemented controls. Statistical analysis demonstrated that the porous-coated, finned, and slotted fluted designs were all significantly weaker in torsion than the cemented component. There was no statistically significant difference in torsional resistance between the solid fluted (unslotted) and cemented stems.

In view of the large forces developed in torsion during loading of the hip joint, it is recommended that surgeons attempt to gain proximal and distal support of implants within the femur. In cases of severe metaphyseal deficiency in which proximal support is unavailable, it is often necessary to provide fixation over 70 mm of the distal stem of the prosthesis to gain adequate stability for normal activities.

Effect of Implants on Cortical Loading

During weight-bearing, loads imposed on the head of the hip prosthesis are passed back to the femur at points of fixation between the implant and bone. This pattern of load transfer is strongly influenced by several factors, including distribution and rigidity of the points of fixation and relative stiffness of the implant and the femur. If the implant surface is uniformly bonded to the bone, large stress concentrations occur within the femur at the junction of the implant and the femoral neck osteotomy proximally, and adjacent to the tip of the prosthesis distally.[11] Because the implant shares some of the load normally borne by the femur, average cortical stresses are often 30% to 60% lower than physiologic levels. This effect is termed stress-shielding of the bone by the prosthesis.

To understand the mechanical basis of stress-shielding, it is instructive to review the factors affecting the mechanical stiffness of femoral prostheses relative to the femur. This subject was studied by Dujovne et al.,[12] with the use of CT scans of a collection of 65 femora and the geometric profiles to two contemporary designs of cementless prostheses. For standard cobalt–chromium components, they determined that the bending stiffness of the distal stem matches that of the average femur with a canal diameter of approximately 13.5 mm. In smaller canals, the femur is stiffer than the corresponding prosthesis. However, in larger canals the stiffness of the implant exceeds the original femur by a factor of 1.5 at 15 mm and 2.5 at 18 mm (Fig. 15.4). In all cases, they found that in bending, the proximal third of the femoral stem was more stiff than the femur by a factor ranging from 4× at 12 mm to 10× at 18 mm. Compared with CoCr, fabrication of the prosthesis from titanium 6 aluminum 4 vanadium (Ti6Al4V) alloy led to a twofold reduction in bending stiffness, independent of prosthesis size.

As the bending stiffness of the femur increases with canal diameter and cortical thickness, the relative load-sharing between a bone and a rigidly fixed prosthesis depends on the intra- and extramedullary dimensions of the femur.[13] In theoretic terms, the reduction in normal physiologic stresses borne by the femur after implantation of the prosthesis is given by the expression

$$\frac{\text{Bone Stress (with Implant)}}{\text{Bone Stress (without Implant)}} = \frac{[(D/d)^4 - 1]}{[(D/d)^4 + (n - 1)]}$$

where d = Distal diameter of the prosthesis
D = External diameter of the femoral shaft
n = Ratio of the elastic moduli of the implant and cortical bone

For cobalt–chromium alloys, the value of n is approximately 10. In primary cementless hip replacement, the external diameter of the femur within the isthmus is typically 2.1 ± 0.3 times the diameter of the medullary canal. Once such a canal is filled with a CoCr stem, the corresponding reduction in cortical stresses is approximately 35%.

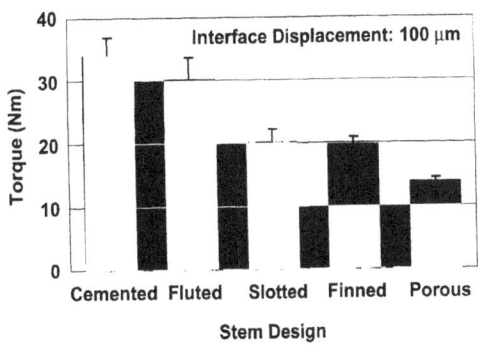

Figure 15.3. Torque required to cause 100 μm of interface displacement of five modes of diaphyseal fixation (Kendrick et al,[10] with permission.)

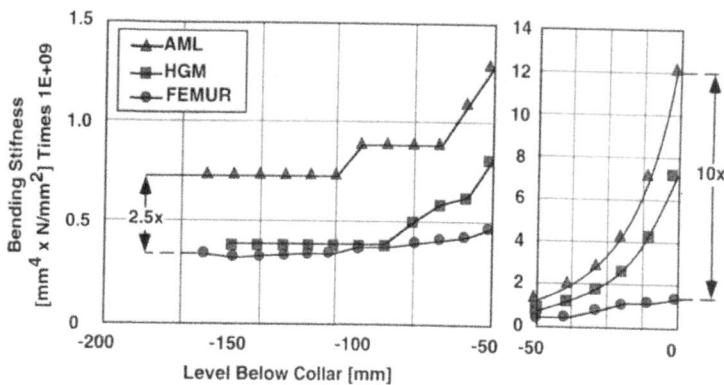

Figure 15.4. Average values of the bending stiffness of a femur with an 18 mm canal, compared with corresponding cementless prosthesis fabricated from CoCr (AML) and Ti6Al4V (HGM). Values are plotted as a function of position of each section along the axis of the femur. The CoCr prosthesis is seen to be 2.5 times stiffer than the femur in the isthmus and 10 times stiffer at the level of the proximal osteotomy (from Dujovne et al,[12] with permission)

At revision THR, some thinning of the cortices is generally present with expansion of the medullary canal. Typically, the canal of the revision femur is 1 to 3 mm larger than the corresponding primary femur. This can dramatically change the mechanics of load transfer between the femur and the prosthesis as the ratio of femoral and stem diameters is reduced, leading to a significant increase in the proportion of the applied load borne by the prosthesis. Typically, enlargement of the medullary canal by 2 mm leads to a 15% reduction in cortical stresses (50% versus 35%) if there is no change in the external diameter of the diaphysis.

Response of the Femur to Stress-Shielding

Because remodeling is determined by the stress level within the bone, stress shielding can lead to dramatic bone loss after total hip replacement. The relationship between design factors and periprosthetic remodeling was studied by Engh and Bobyn[13] in a review of 411 cases of primary cementless total hip replacement performed with one design of porous-coated CoCr prosthesis. The effect of variations in the extent of porous coating and the diameter of the distal stem on the severity of bone loss was examined at 2-year follow-up. In 72% of cases, some degree of bone loss was present on anteroposterior and lateral radiographs, including an 18% incidence of pronounced cortical resorption (bone loss at five or more of 16 sites). In keeping with the predictions of engineering analysis, the severity of bone loss increased dramatically with the diameter of the femoral stem. With small stems (≤12 mm), the overall incidence was 5.6%, compared with 28% in cases performed by using implants of larger distal diameter (≥13.5 mm, $p < 0.05$).

This conclusion has been further confirmed by the experimental studies of Bobyn et al.[14] who performed bilateral cementless hip replacements in dogs by using two designs of femoral prostheses of the same external geometry. One design consisted of a solid Co-Cr stem with extensive porous coating, whereas the second design was fabricated from Ti6Al4V alloy and was hollow distally. This led to a fourfold difference in bending and torsional stiffness. Both designs were implanted bilaterally in the femora of each experimental animal. At 6 and 12 months postoperatively, gross differences were observed in the remodeling patterns of the right and left femora directly correlating with the stiffness of the prosthesis. Severe bone resorption was observed around most of the stiffer CoCr prostheses, but around none of the more flexible titanium components. Moreover, quantitative analysis of histologic sections revealed that the area of cortical bone surrounding the prostheses was 25% to 35% greater in the flexible components, compared with components of greater stiffness.

Although bone loss secondary to stress-shielding is frequently observed in cementless hip replacement, especially after implantation of femoral stems with extensive porous coating, adverse clinical sequelae have rarely been reported. Nonetheless, some surgeons are concerned that, in the long term, adverse remodeling will increase access of particulate debris generated within the joint space, leading to a greater incidence of osteolysis. Evidence supporting this hypothesis is lacking, but many surgeons remain interested in practical measures to reduce bone loss within the femur secondary to stress-shielding. One strategy is to provide points of rigid implant fixation as proximal as possible within the femur, thereby increasing proximal load transfer. Another strategy is to apply a bioactive coating to the proximal stem to maximize the chances of bony attachment. Research is also underway to develop femoral stems fabricated from lower modulus materials (eg, fiber-reinforced composites and new titanium alloys) to reduce their bending stiffness, thereby minimizing adverse bony remodeling.

Thigh Pain

Another significant complication of cementless hip arthroplasty is anterior thigh pain. This symptom varies in severity and frequency but has been reported in 1% to 45% of patients in different cementless series.[15] Although this phenomenon is multifactorial, bone scans confirm that patients reporting thigh pain after cementless THR do have increased uptake of technetium-99m-medronate methylene diphosphate (a bone-imaging agent) within the femur adjacent to the tip of the prosthesis.[16] Although few of these patients have prostheses that could be classified as loose in the traditional sense, evidence from many cementless series suggests that thigh pain is often indicative of inadequate proximal fixation, leading to increased distal loading of the femur.[17] This suggests that excessive micromotion localized within discrete areas of the implant–bone interface may lead to discomfort. This view is supported by a review of 175 cases of cementless femoral revisions performed with extensively porous-coated stems in which the overall incidence of significant thigh pain was only 4.2% in cases with bone-ingrown interfaces, compared with 18.5% in cases with stable fibrous fixation.[18] This dramatic difference suggests that thigh pain and interface micromotion are directly related.

An additional factor is the pattern of load-sharing developed between the implant and the femur. Thigh pain occurs most frequently in patients with large medullary canals, especially when a mismatch is present between the bending stiffness of the distal stem and the femur. In these cases, there is an abrupt transition in stiffness from the implant to the femur at the distal tip of the prosthesis. This generates a local stress concentration adjacent to the distal tip that may be reduced with time through local thickening of the cortices. This hypothesis is consistent with the observation that the incidence of thigh pain can be dramatically reduced by increasing the flexibility of the distal tip of the prosthesis, most commonly through the addition of a longitudinal slot within the coronal plane.

Biomechanics of the Hip Joint Articulation

Considerations related to the global motion of the hip joint have a fundamental bearing on the successful function of joint replacements. To restore normal joint function, it is necessary to recreate the geometric relationship between the pelvis and the femur while preventing impingement at the extremes of joint motion.

Restoration of the Joint Center

One of the most important factors influencing the stability of an artificial hip joint is the accuracy of restoration of normal joint anatomy. At the extremes of joint motion, the mechanical stability of the joint is critically affected by the tone of the abductor muscles. The force of contraction of these muscles is determined by their operating length and cross-sectional area. Any change in the relative position of the femur and the pelvis will cause a change in the moment arm of each muscle and thus the force of contraction needed to stabilize the hip joint. This, in turn, will alter the compressive force acting across the hip joint. For example, if the femur is displaced medially, the mechanical advantage of the abductor mechanism is reduced, so that a larger force must be generated by muscle contraction to balance the weight of the body. Larger muscle forces will directly increase the joint reaction force and the loading of the acetabular component, leading to accelerated wear of the articulating surfaces.

This subject is of considerable practical significance in revision total hip replacement. In cases of superior migration of the acetabular component, the surgeon must often decide whether to accept displacement of the hip center, primarily through use of an oversized cup, or to strive to restore the joint center to its original location, possibly through use of an allograft. Similar considerations confront reconstruction of dislocated hips secondary to congenital dislocation of the hip. In a computer study, Delp and Maloney[19] examined the effect of superoinferior, anteroposterior, and mediolateral displacement of the hip center on the moment-generating capacity of four groups of hip muscles. Displacements of 20 mm in each direction caused changes of 20% to 50% in the moment developed by each muscle group acting across the hip joint. This confirmed the importance of restoration of normal joint anatomy, given the sensitivity of muscle forces to changes in the location of the hip joint.

A common radiographic observation after revision THR is medial displacement of the femur with respect to the pelvis. In this situation, the tone of the abductors and the normal stability of the prosthetic joint may be restored by lengthening the extremity or by changing the position of the trochanter on the femur. However, because few patients will accept lengthening of the leg and most surgeons do not favor a trochanteric osteotomy, a better solution is to select a prosthesis that allows the medial offset of the prosthesis to replicate the original offset of the femur with additional allowance for the effects of any deformity and medialization of the acetabulum.

For this to work in practice, the femoral prosthesis must provide sufficient variation in neck length to restore the original head position without excessive limb lengthening. This is a difficult task, because the medial head offset of the normal femur varies from approximately 29 to 58 mm (95% confidence limits) because of the combined effect of variations in the length and inclination of the femoral neck (Fig. 15.5).[21] Even within

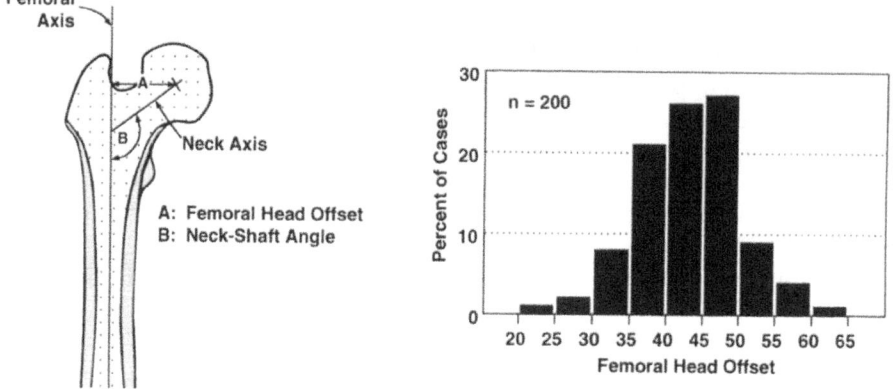

Figure 15.5. Anatomic distribution of the medial offset of the femur (from Noble,[21] with permission)

femora of the same canal size, the range of medial head offset is approximately 20 mm. This means that a 28-mm range in prosthetic neck length is required to restore the original offset of the femur, compared with a range of only 15 to 20 mm that is generally available through the use of modular femoral heads.[21]

A similar problem is presented by the variable position of the femoral head in the sagittal plane. Across the anatomic range, the anteversion of the femoral neck with respect to the distal condyles varies by approximately 35° (95% confidence limits). Conventional, monolithic stems only restore normal anteversion to within ±10°, because the rotational position of the prosthesis within the femur is dictated by its fit within the canal.[22]

Because many cementless femoral stems are stable in only one rotational position within the femur, variations in the anatomic relationship between the femoral neck and the medullary canal lead to errors in restoration of the anterior offset. In some instances, the shape of the canal and/or the femoral neck can cause posterior displacement of the head center of up to 10 mm, leading to a potentially unstable joint. In cases in which the femoral metaphysis remains intact, the risk of placement of the femoral head in a retroverted position may be reduced through use of modular prostheses, because these implants allow the distal stem to be rotated with respect to the metaphyseal segment of the prosthesis. Alternatively, asymmetric components can be selected that have been designed to sit within the neck of the femur, thereby restoring the original head position.

In the revision femur, these considerations are often less of a problem because the rotational orientation of distally fixed prostheses can be varied, provided that the proximal body of the prosthesis does not impinge on the metaphysis. If the normal anatomic features of the proximal femur are absent or distorted, the rotational position of the implant must be determined by external landmarks, including the overall alignment of the extremity if retroversion or excessive anteversion is to be prevented. Thus, the final rotational position must be established before seating the prosthesis, because additional adjustment of implant position is impossible once the distal stem is engaged within the medullary canal.

Impingement and Dislocation

The range of stable motion of the prosthetic hip is influenced by many variables, including the design of the prosthetic components. In general, dislocation occurs after impingement of the neck of the femoral stem on the edge of the acetabular liner, so that any measures that

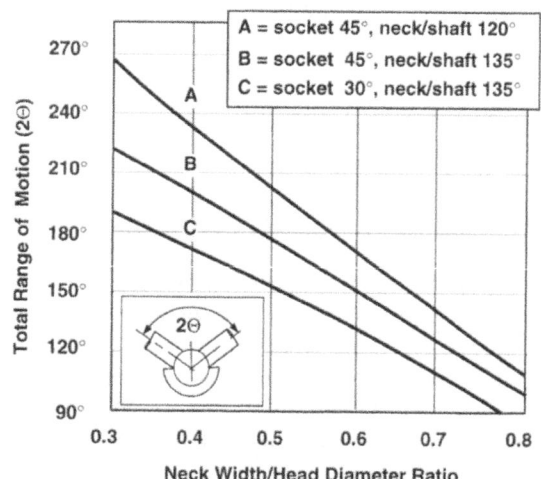

Figure 15.6. Range of motion of the prosthetic hip joint as a function of the ratio between the neck width and head diameter. (From Walker, Courtesy of Charles C Thomas, Publisher, Ltd, Springfield, Illinois.[24])

increase the allowable motion of the joint before impingement will reduce the risk of dislocation.[23] These measures include adequate lateralization of the femur to increase tissue tension, placement of acetabular cup in sufficient anteversion to prevent anterior impingement, and selection of the largest possible femoral head. Because prosthetic wear increases with the size of the head of the prosthesis, selection of femoral heads larger than 28 mm is generally avoided. Consequently, prostheses with the narrowest possible neck should be selected to maximize the ratio of the head and neck diameter and, thus, the range of motion of the artificial joint (Fig. 15.6).[24]

A common factor in dislocation of prostheses is the use of modular heads with skirts to extend the length of the femoral neck. Potentially, this modification allows the surgeon to compensate for an unusually low femoral neck osteotomy or superior placement of the acetabular cup while still restoring the original position of the joint center. However, because the skirt covers the neck of the prosthesis, increasing its outer diameter by 4 to 5 mm, the ratio of the head-to-neck diameter is dramatically reduced. This severely limits the range of motion of the joint. In view of this complication, calcar replacement prostheses are strongly recommended in cases of medial bone-stock loss because these components are designed to be placed at a lower resection level and do not necessitate the use of skirted femoral heads to restore the normal head center.

References

1. Bergmann G, Graichen F, Rohlmann A. Load directions at hip prostheses measured in-vivo. *J Biomech*. 1989;22:986.
2. Bergmann G, Graichen F, Rohlmann A. Hip joint loading during walking and running, measured in two patients. *J Biomech*. 1993;26:969–990.
3. Davy DT, Kotzar GM, Brown RH, Heiple KG, Goldberg VM, Heiple KG Jr, et al. Telemetric force measurements across the hip after total arthroplasty. *J Bone Joint Surg Am*. 1988;70:45–50.
4. English TA, Kilvington M. In vivo records of hip loads using a femoral implant with telemetric output. *J Biomed Eng*. 1979;1:111–115.
5. Rydell NW. Forces acting on the femoral head prosthesis. *Acta Orthop Scand Suppl*. 1966;88:139–145.
6. Noble P, Scheller A Jr, Tullos H, Levy RN, Turner RH. Design and selection of prosthetic components in total hip replacement. In: Stillwell W, ed. *The Art of Total Hip Arthroplasty*. New York, NY: Grune & Stratton; 1986:51–67.
7. Capello W. Technical aspects of cementless total hip arthroplasty. *Clin Orthop*. 1990;261:102–106.
8. Noble P. Biomechanical advances in total hip replacement. In: Niwa S, Perren SM, Hattori T, eds. *Biomechanics in Orthopedics*. Tokyo, Japan: Springer-Verlag; 1992:46–75.
9. Poss R, Walker P, Spector M, Reilly DT, Robertson DD, Sledge CB. Strategies for improving fixation of femoral components in total hip arthroplasty. *Clin Orthop*. 1988;235:181–194.
10. Kendrick J, Noble P, Tullos H. Distal stem design and the torsional stability of cementless femoral stems. *J Arthroplasty*. 1995;10:463–469.
11. Huiskes R. Some fundamental aspects of human joint replacements: analysis of stresses and heat conduction in bone–prosthesis structures. *Acta Orthop Scand*. 1980;185:109–200.
12. Dujovne A, Bobyn J, Krygier J, Miller JE, Brooks CE. Mechanical compatibility of noncemented hip prostheses with the human femur. *J Arthroplasty*. 1993;8:7–22.
13. Engh C, Bobyn J. The influence of stem size and extent of porous coating on femoral bone resorption after primary cementless hip arthroplasty. *Clin Orthop*. 1988;231:7–28.
14. Bobyn J, Glassman A, Goto H, Krygier JJ, Miller JE, Brooks CE. The effect of stem stiffness on femoral bone resorption after canine porous-coated total hip arthroplasty. *Clin Orthop*. 1990;261:196–213.
15. Glassman A. Cementless primary total hip replacement. In: Callaghan J, Dennis D, Paprosky W, Rosenberg AG, eds. *Orthopaedic Knowledge Update: Hip and Knee Reconstruction*. Rosemont, Ill: American Academy of Orthopaedic Surgeons; 1995;23:191–206.
16. Pohlemann T, Steinmetz M, Ehrenheim C, Hundeshagen H, Tscherne H. The importance of roentgenological and scinitigraphic studies in patients with and without thigh pain following cementless PCA hip endoprosthesis. *Z Orthop Ihre Grenzgeb*. 1995;133:25–33.
17. Campbell A, Rorabeck C, Bourme R, Chess D, Nott L. Thigh pain after cementless hip arthroplasty: annoyance or ill omen. *J Bone Joint Surg Br*. 1992;74:63–66.
18. Moreland J, Bernstein M. Femoral revision hip arthroplasty with uncemented, porous-coated stems. *Clin Orthop*. 1995;319:141–150.
19. Delp SL, Maloney W. Effects of hip center location on the moment-generating capacity of the muscles. *J Biomech*. 1993;26(4–5):485–499.
20. Noble P. Contributions of basic applied sciences to hip replacement in older persons. In: Schafer M, ed. *Instr Course Lect*. Chicago, Ill: American Academy of Orthopaedic Surgeons; 1994;43:382–392.
21. Noble P, Alexander J, Lindahl L, et al. The anatomic basis of femoral component design. *Clin Orthop*. 1988;235:145–165.
22. Noble PC, Lucas MJ. Femoral anteversion following cementless total hip replacement. *Orthop Trans*. 1989;13:391–392.
23. Daly P, Morrey B. Operative correction of an unstable total hip arthroplasty. *J Bone Joint Surg Am*. 1992;74:1334–1343.
24. Walker PS. Human joints and their artificial replacements. Springfield, Ill: Charles C Thomas Publisher; 1977.

16
Equipment Overview

James C. Slater

A learning curve exists with every surgical procedure, and revision total hip arthroplasty is no exception. Successful mastery of this art requires focused attention to numerous details before, during, and after the operative intervention. This includes preoperative planning and preparation. Technologic advances continually occur and provide surgeons with new materials and equipment of ever increasing precision and complexity. However, technology alone is not enough to yield consistently successful results. Judgment, ability, and adherence to fundamental biologic and surgical principles are mandatory and have been emphasized by Aufranc and others.[1-3]

Preparation for surgery of this complexity includes optimizing the operating theater and the surgical team. Various aspects of preoperative planning are covered to maximize efficiency and sterile technique in the operating room environment and to ensure the availability of necessary equipment and tools for exposure and removal of cement and/or implants. Bone graft selection and instruments for preparation are also discussed. Finally, implant options and equipment for managing unique situations will be considered. Preoperative planning and preparation are mandatory to allow surgery of this magnitude and complexity to proceed expeditiously while successfully addressing many different surgical contingencies.

The relative importance of these considerations cannot be overstated. A well-known caveat reads, "Preoperative planning facilitates intraoperative decision making" (written communication, R.H. Turner and B.E. Bierbaum, January, 1993). Most complications can be prevented at this point—before the surgeon enters the operating room.

Operating Room Environment

Many factors are considered in assessing the operating room environment. Basic concerns include the adequacy of size and use of space, lighting for visualization, patient positioning, methods of equipment sterilization and use, barrier systems, air quality, and sterile technique.

Postoperative infections are often multifactorial, and relative incidences increase with various risk factors.[4,5] The primary focus of this segment of preoperative planning is the consideration of operating room factors influencing potential bacterial contamination. This should increase the likelihood of aseptic technique, but it remains controversial whether these methods will actually reduce postoperative infection rates. In the operating room, bacterial sources are considered endogenous if they originate from the patient. Examples would include organisms from local skin and tissue or a hematogenous source. Exogenous sources include the OR personnel, equipment, implants, and the surrounding air. Airborne contaminants are carried on moisture droplets and particles. Much effort has been directed toward developing techniques to decrease the size, quantity, and concentration of foreign material and exogenous sources of bacterial contamination during operative procedures. Significant success has resulted. However, no clinically significant level of maximum allowable wound inoculum or number of bacteria at clean air supply terminals has been established. Ultraclean air standards have been set at a maximum 10 colony forming units per cubic meter.[6] Despite the inherent limitations, postoperative infection rates remain the standard of comparison as we consider these various methods to control them. Many of these methods are controversial and serve as recommendations only.

Direct bacterial contamination occurs with a break in sterile technique. Proper draping is critical in maintaining the sterile field. Modern draping typically includes the use of adherent drapes as a skin barrier adjacent to the incision. Antibiotic-impregnated drapes are also available. Disposable nonwoven barriers are much less porous than woven materials and should isolate the field more effectively.[7] Recommendations also include double gloving, together with outer glove changes after draping, before handling cement or implants, and at appointed time intervals during the procedure. Sanders et al.[8] showed undetected holes in latex gloves are frequent and correlate with the duration the glove is in use. The efficacy of periodic antibiotic wound irrigation after intraoperative cultures are obtained is not known, but this measure is routinely performed in our institution.

Indirect contamination occurs with airborne particles and bacteria. Many will recall Charnley's "clean room within the operating room" used in an early effort to further isolate both surgeon and patient or even patient appendage from potential contaminants.[9] Techniques to decrease potential indirect contamination currently in widespread use include laminar flow clean air rooms, positive pressure, and minimization of OR traffic. In some centers, isolation body exhaust suits are also used. Laminar flow clean air rooms have high-efficiency particulate air filters that remove 99.97% of particles at or greater than 0.3 μm, and significantly reduce numbers of airborne bacteria entering the OR. The laminar flow of air can be vertical or horizontal. It is responsible for removing particles generated exogenously within the OR as the air leaves through exhaust vents during the multiple room air turnovers per hour. Minimization of air flow obstruction and turbulence is necessary, making patient, equipment, personnel, and overhead lighting positions important considerations.

In considering all these technologic advances, it should be noted that perioperative antibiotic prophylaxis is generally credited with the greatest decline in infection rates in total joint arthroplasty.[10] Lidwell et al.[6] showed that the use of laminar flow ultraclean air rooms and body exhaust suits significantly reduced infection rates both with and without the prophylactic use of antibiotics. A small, but nonetheless further, reduction in infection rates was seen with the combination of ultraclean air, body exhaust suits, and antibiotics. However, data were not randomized and the results were not statistically significant. In series of prospective randomized and blinded cases at the Mayo Clinic, Fitzgerald[10] found no significant difference in infection rates for antibiotic prophylaxis cases with and without horizontal clean air. Body exhaust suits were not used. Isolation body exhaust suit systems, together with additional measures that include antibiotics and laminar flow clean air, have been reported in a retrospective study to decrease potential bacterial contamination and infection rates.[11] This has been attributed to presumed diminished bacterial contamination from personnel in the area of the sterile field. The relative contribution from the isolation system has been difficult to quantify. Using a specific filtered exhaust helmet system, investigators measured air samples over the sterile field in an ultraclean nonlaminar flow air exchange system and found no increased protection over that provided by conventional paper hoods and masks.[12] Advantages of modern body exhaust systems include increased convenience resulting from battery-powered individual units. Protection of the surgeon from splatter and airborne particles is also increased.

Disadvantages include the bulkiness of the isolation suits and attachment hoses in older less portable systems, potential communication difficulties with surgical assistants, and cost. Ultraviolet light has been shown to be effective in decreasing live bacterial contamination counts.[13] Proper protective gear is mandatory to decrease skin exposure and possible cornea damage. These factors are also likely to decrease traffic flow of personnel.

Use of battery-powered or electric drills, saws, and reamers can potentially decrease contamination, in comparison with pneumatic-powered instruments. Gas leakage occurs, making adequate equipment sterilization imperative. However, the relatively decreased torque pressures and duration of battery cell charge have kept battery-powered instruments from more widespread use. Current developments with electric instruments appear promising, but long-term durability remains an issue.

Component Removal

The first task in revision surgery is safe exposure and removal of the failed construct. Optimal exposure is mandatory, and this subject is covered in Part 4. After the removal of failed components, bone deficits are invariably present. Also, the residual bone is of poorer quality for replantation. Available bone may be thin and sclerotic, osteolytic and/or osteoporotic. This remaining bone significantly affects the reconstructive options, and preservation of host bone throughout the extraction process remains of vital importance.

Preoperative Planning

Preoperative planning will influence the types of equipment necessary and the techniques used. Available instruments should include hand-held straight and curved osteotomes, narrow flexible osteotomes, extended-length cement extraction tools and gouges, straight and angled curets, impactors and bone tamps, standard and high-speed burrs, drills, and a screwdriver set matching the implants and any internal fixation devices in place. A modular screwdriver system that matches the screwheads of multiple implants is now available. Implant extraction devices (either universal or component specific) should be readily available. Cerclage wires or cables, trochanteric reattachment devices, screws, and pelvic reconstruction plates are often needed. Flexible fiberoptic lighting, extended-length suction devices, a radiolucent operating table, and flouroscopic image intensifier will all facilitate work in the distal femur. Additional equipment considerations will be covered later as they pertain to the specific implant removed. Intraoperative and postoperative blood reinfusion techniques are discussed in Chapter 12.

Removal of Acetabular Components

Preoperative x-rays are helpful in planning acetabular exposure and removal. The cemented socket should be assessed for the relative stability of fixation, as well as for the quality, quantity, and position of methylmethacrylate. The relative position and extent of radiolucencies, bone loss, osteolysis, stress-shielding, migration patterns (subsidence), or protrusio must also be considered. Often this is difficult to determine on radiographic studies. Radiographs should include anteroposterior (AP) pelvis and AP and Lowenstein lateral x-rays of the hip. Magnification markers are placed along the lateral aspect of the trochanter and femoral shaft for preoperative templating. In addition, 45° internal and external Judet views and inlet view of the pelvis may be helpful. CT scans can yield additional information with all-polyethylene components. However, metal-backed components typically cause significant artifact, making CT scanning less useful.

Assessment of the cementless socket should proceed in the same manner with additional attention to the stability of fixation, relative socket position, modularity of the insert, and presence of additional stabilization methods (eg, screws, pegs, spikes, or threads). Exposure proceeds with disarticulation of the femoral and acetabular components. A bone hook is helpful in applying a distraction force without excessive torque on the potentially weakened femoral shaft. After disarticulation, removal of the modular femoral head, when present, facilitates acetabular exposure. If acetabular revision alone is planned, removal of the modular femoral head should be accomplished without trauma to the Morse taper or to the implant interfaces. We prefer to use a graduated U-shaped wedge driven between the head and a flat U-shaped base resting on the femoral neck or collar. Use of a simple bone punch will often score the taper, either directly or indirectly, as the taper is asymmetrically disrupted. Others have described a relatively atraumatic method of removal by selectively heating the cobalt–chromium head relative to the cooler titanium stem.[14] We have no experience with this technique.

The femoral component Morse taper or the nonmodular head should be protected, and we accomplish this with a surgical sponge with radiopaque x-ray marker. With posterolateral approaches, the neck is placed anterior and superior to the socket to aid exposure. Soft tissue elevation from the anterior inferior iliac spine or anterior capsulectomy facilitates this and can be performed through the psoas sheath with the psoas tendon protecting the anterior neurovascular structures. If lateral or anterolateral approaches are used, the femoral component can be placed posterior to the socket if the leg is maintained in flexion and external rotation. The posterior pseudocapsule can be released by using periosteal dissection or electrocautery with particular care to prevent injury to the sciatic nerve. The leg should also be supported to prevent traction injury to the sciatic nerve.

If acetabular exposure is still compromised, we prefer to use a trochanteric slide osteotomy as described by Glassman and Engh[15] and outlined in Part 4. Trochanteric reattachment equipment is needed and options include cerclage wires, cables, claw grip, or femoral component-specific attachment devices.[16,17] Other options for exposure would include a formal trochanteric osteotomy or, in certain cemented smooth stems, the tap out-tap in technique originated by Smith-Peterson and reported by Nabors et al.[18] and Lieberman et al.[19]

When both femoral and acetabular components are being revised, the femoral component is removed first to facilitate acetabular exposure. Recommended techniques are discussed in a subsequent section of this chapter. The acetabular component should be widely exposed with complete 360° access to the peripheral margins.

Removal of Cemented Socket

In removing the cemented all-polyethylene socket, the cement–socket interface should be addressed initially. The interval is usually easily identified, and unless the socket and adherent cement are grossly loose, removal should proceed in this manner. Straight osteotomes are used to disrupt the peripheral margins. Curved osteotomes are then advanced to further loosen the cement–socket interval. Long curved Moreland (Smith-Peterson) acetabular gouges then follow the contour of the cup to the dome to disrupt the interface completely and extract the cup from the cement bed. The shape of these gouges decreases the likelihood of bone or pelvic penetration. Prying should never be attempted because fracture and bone loss can result. Instead, a side-to-side motion should be used.

Another technique involves the use of a high-speed burr to remove a triangular-shaped section of the socket. The cup can then be imploded on itself and removed, or additional sections can be cut and removed with curved gouges. Large amounts of polyethylene debris are generated with this technique, and soft tissue protection and complete debris removal can be very difficult. A pneumatic impact wrench (Cup-Out®) has been developed to remove well-fixed cemented or cementless sockets, and Lachiewicz and Anspach have reported their early experience with this technique.[20] Another method for cemented socket removal involves an acetabular extractor that obtains purchase by threading into a hole previously drilled in the polyethylene.[21] Insertion of the threaded portion brings a platform in contact with the socket rim to allow a back-and-forth rocking motion as a distraction force is applied. Concern exists for potential fracture or bone loss because of the large forces and torque generated with this technique.

After socket removal, the cement can be excised under direct visualization. Osteotomes or high-speed burrs can be used to fractionate the cement, and curets are used to remove cement fragments and underlying fibrous and inflammatory tissue. The amount of intrapelvic cement is often larger than the exposed tunnel and should be left in situ; exceptions would be if the cement caused symptoms or in cases of sepsis when all foreign material must be excised. When intrapelvic cement or severely protrused components must be removed, potential exists for injury to vascular or neural structures, as well as to the ureter, bladder wall, or bowel. In this setting, preoperative arteriogram and intravenous pyelogram are helpful to define the abnormal anatomy, and a retroperitoneal approach and exposure should be considered, as outlined in Part 4.[22,23]

Removal of a cemented metal-backed socket that is not grossly loose begins with removal of the polyethylene insert. This can be quickly and easily accomplished with the drill-and-tap technique, wherein the liner is initially drilled with a 3.2-mm drill bit. A 6.5-mm screw is then introduced and tightened to separate the liner from the metal cup. Other methods include the use of osteotomes or high-speed burrs to fragment the liner and disrupt the locking mechanism.

Once the polyethylene liner is removed, the cement–metal interface is addressed. Again, curved acetabular gouges can be used to disrupt the cement–metal interval circumferentially from the periphery to the dome, following the contour of the cup while protecting the cement bed and host bone. The pneumatic impact wrench technique (Cup-Out®) can also be considered. Any technique of disruption is more difficult if the metal has a textured or porous surface with interdigitated cement. Care should be taken as the curved gouges are passed because all or part of the cement may come out with the metal socket, and significant bone loss may result. In rare circumstances, sectioning of the metal cup is necessary for safe extraction. Carbide-tipped bits are available for high-speed drills to accomplish this. The amount of metal debris generated is significant, and meticulous tissue protection and debris removal are recommended.

After the metal shell is loosened from the cement bed, it is driven out with an offset impactor placed on the superior lateral rim and directed caudally. As the component leaves the cement bed, the impactor is moved sequentially higher on the dome until extraction is complete. Remaining cement is then removed under direct visualization as outlined previously.

Removal of Cementless Socket

Removal of the stable cementless socket also begins with removal of the polyethylene insert. Most components are modular, and new implants may have locking mechanisms that facilitate liner removal. Other techniques for removal were described earlier. Screws, if present, are removed at this point. Scar tissue should be completely excised from the screwhead to allow complete seating of the screwdriver. If stripped, the heads are removed with the high-speed burr, and the shafts are excised later with small trephines, pliers, or a commercially available broken screw removal set. Curved gouges are then used to follow the contour of the implant as the bone–implant interface is disrupted. This proceeds circumferentially from the periphery to the dome, with the surgeon taking into consideration any pegs, spikes, threads, or altered geometry. Threaded sockets have extraction devices designed to grasp and rotate out stable components, though these have not worked well. Concern exists for potential fracture with the forces generated. Curved osteotomes and long curved gouges are again preferred. Screw or dome holes, when present, can also yield access for curets, small osteotomes, or burrs to disrupt fixation.

With bone graft placement at original surgery, bone may actually protrude through the holes and bone may need to be removed. After the metal shell is circumferentially loosened to the polar region, we prefer to drive it out with an offset impactor placed on the superior lateral rim with the force directed caudally to further protect any weakened bone in the acetabular columns or dome. As the socket exits the bony bed, the impactor is moved higher on the dome until removal is complete. Traction, if needed, can be applied simultaneously with any grasping tool, such as pliers or clamps. Other traction devices include special cup extractors that obtain purchase on ledges or screw holes and allow distraction forces. Socket designs with threaded dome holes allow extractors to be screwed securely to the cup for additional traction.

The technique of bipolar socket removal from the femoral component is determined by the locking mechanism present. Various modern designs can be disarticulated by inserting a disassembly key, dislodging a polyethylene locking ring with osteotomes, or with disassembly instruments that spread metal locking rings. Unfortunately, removal of some older models can be more difficult and is typically accomplished with osteotomes disrupting a segment of the polyethylene locking assembly on the inferior aspect. Another technique involves drilling through the polyethylene from the inferior aspect with the surgeon taking care to prevent drill contact with the femoral head if femoral revision is not planned. A screw is then advanced until it contacts the inner surface of the metal dislodging it from the polyethylene liner. The liner is then levered off the femoral component.[24]

Removal of Femoral Component

Preoperative x-rays are particularly helpful in planning femoral component removal. Both AP and Lowenstein lateral views are reviewed. Considerations include evaluating for femoral deformity and determining whether the implant is modular and has a collar, as well as whether it is a cemented or cementless device. With cemented implants, the surgeon should assess the relative stability of fixation; location and extent of bone loss; amount of cement present; and quality of the mantel. The proximal and distal cement thickness should be determined, together with the presence or absence of a distal cement plug. Radiolucencies at the cement–prosthesis junction or cement–bone interface will influence ease of removal. Areas of weakened bone are identified, and prophylactic circumferential wiring may be used to prevent fracture or perforation during implant or cement removal. Implant surface texturing or cement precoating will determine the degree of difficulty in disrupting the prosthesis–cement junction for removal. Collars vary in size and shape and can block access to parts of the implant–cement interface in the femoral metaphysis. The surgeon should also note whether the stem is straight or curved, and whether any extraction holes or threaded insertion sites are present. Finally, if any extraction equipment exists that is unique to the implant, it should be made available from preoperative identification of the component.

Exposure of the entire proximal margin of the femur and the femoral component should be completed with osteotomes and rongeurs. Scar tissue frequently builds up and is easily removed. Assessment is made of the stability of the implant and the status of surrounding bone and cement. At times, manual traction will remove a grossly loose femoral component from the cement mantel. More commonly, attention should be directed first to the lateral shoulder of the prosthesis. Any cement, bone overgrowth, or scar tissue present can hinder component removal and predispose to metaphyseal fracture during extraction. Osteotomes, wide and narrow rongeurs, or high speed-burrs can be used to accomplish component removal. Exposure in this area allows a direct line of sight down the shaft for tools used later during distal cement removal. This also seems to lessen the likelihood of reaming the canal in a varus position or perforating through the lateral femur distally. If lateral exposure is still not optimal, we prefer the trochanteric slide described by Glassman and Engh.[15] The method is described in Part 4 of this book. This technique allows exposure for cement and implant removal, as well as for subsequent adjustment of abductor tension and joint stabilization.

After complete exposure proximally, most loose, smooth, cemented stems can be safely and easily removed with an extractor. Components with nonmodular heads are typically removed with a loop extractor with sliding hammer mechanism passed over the head and held against the neck while distraction forces are directed in line with the femur. Offline forces should be avoided because they may fracture or weaken bone already damaged by osteolysis, stress shielding, and/or disuse osteoporosis. Components with modular heads cannot be removed with loop extractors because the Morse taper provides no ledge. Extraction may be accomplished with hooks passed through extraction holes when present in the component. If a collar is present, it can be used as a ledge or platform for an impactor driven in a retrograde manner. Most manufacturers of modular head components have extraction devices available for their implants. Preoperative identification of the stem will allow availability at the time of surgery. A universal modular stem extractor is available, and it fits a wide array of implants.[25] Individual sleeves match the implant manufacturer's taper and lock on the stem and the extractor. Another relatively universal extractor is also available and attaches by means of a locking mechanism on the neck just below the Morse taper.[21] If no ledge or indentation is present, a carbide-tipped burr is used to fashion one.

Cemented components with irregular surfaces, texturing, porous coating, or cement precoating will be more difficult to remove. The cement–prosthesis interface must be disrupted first. Thin flexible osteotomes or small high-speed burrs are recommended in the metaphyseal areas. Thin high-speed burrs have the advantage of creating a working space in the cement as it is removed. In contrast, rigid osteotomes do not create a space for their thickness, and their wedging effect may exceed the absorbing capacity of the bone and cause fracture. Trochanteric osteotomy may improve exposure and implant/cement removal. When indicated, we prefer the trochanteric slide osteotomy previously discussed. Some surgeons recommend routine use of extended osteotomies or oval windows to facilitate exposure and extraction of the prosthesis and for subsequent cement removal.[26,27] We consider these methods only when other techniques have failed or when preoperative planning includes a corrective osteotomy for deformity. The area of porosity or precoating is cleared of cement with hand instruments or high-speed burrs. The implant is then driven out from below with carbide-tipped punches or extracted from above as previously described. Circumferential wires or cables are used to further stabilize the osteotomy or cortical windows before the revision component is inserted. Bone grafting of these areas follows. Long-stem components are necessary to bypass any cortical deficiencies by at least 1.5 to 2 femoral diameters measured at the level of the stress riser. Recent work with laser technology for implant removal has been reported with favorable results.[28] Issues and concerns include the vaporization products generated, amount of heat transferred, the learning curve, and the relative expense.[29] Removal of stable cementless components requires significant preoperative assessment. Clinical history and exam together with radiographic studies, yield information regarding the relative stability of fixation and design characteristics unique to the implant. The location and extent of any surface treatment such as areas of macrotexturing, porous coating, or biologic fixation such as hydroxylapatite, should be determined. The likelihood of bony or fibrous ingrowth or bone ongrowth should be assessed.

Collars, when present, may serve as a ledge for impactors during extraction, but they can hinder access to the proximal bone–implant interface. Carbide-tipped burrs may be necessary for partial removal to allow disruption of the medial bone–implant surface. Proximal and distal stem geometry and relative canal filling will influence access for extraction tools. Presence of extraction holes or threaded insertion or extraction sites should be noted. Again, any extraction equipment unique to the implant should be made available from preoperative identification of the component. The location and extent of any radiolucencies or bone loss will identify potential areas of fibrous ingrowth or prosthesis loosening to aid extraction or bone weakness requiring additional support during component removal.

Complete proximal femoral exposure is necessary with circumferential exposure of the implant. As with cemented stems, particular attention should be directed to exposure of the lateral shoulder of the implant to remove any barrier to extraction and to lessen the likelihood of metaphyseal fracture. Narrow straight or flexible osteotomes or a thin high-speed burr is used to disrupt the bone–prosthesis interface in the metaphyseal area. A thin flexible gouge is also available to fit along the rounded lateral shoulder of several implant types. Broad or curved rigid osteotomes are again avoided because their wedging effect may exceed the absorbing capacity of bone and cause fracture. Bone preservation and structural integrity of the femur remain high priorities at all times as the instruments are passed around all margins of the implant. When the interface is disrupted, extraction devices (as previously described) are used to remove the stem from the canal. If the stem still cannot be extracted because of more extensive porous coating in the diaphyseal femur or unique stem geometry, more aggressive measures must be considered. These include creating small oval windows or an extended osteotomy.[30,31] An anterior oval window strategically placed to allow access to further disrupt the interface can then allow the prosthesis to be driven out with punches in a retrograde manner. A step-cut, extended trochanteric osteotomy made with a high-speed burr can provide wide exposure to the prosthesis–bone interface. The trochanteric bed of bone is preserved as possible for reattachment and cerclage wires are used for increased proximal femoral stability.

Removal of stable, bone-ingrown, extensively porous-coated stems can be particularly challenging. At this time, the best technique includes proceeding as previously outlined for the proximal aspect of the stem. The implant is then exposed at the junction of the proximal flare with the distal cylindric portion through a small anterior oval window. The stem is sectioned with a small carbide-tipped high-speed burr. The proximal stem is extracted, and the distal stem is removed with hollow trephines.[32] Broken stems have become less common with advances in biomaterials and metallurgy. Predisposing risk factors are discussed in Part 4. The technique of extraction depends on the level of implant failure and the relative access to the retained portion. Stem geometry, method of fixation, and relative stability are also influencing factors.

References

1. Aufranc OE. Arthroplasty. In: Crenshaw AH, ed. *Campbell's Operative Orthopaedics.* 5th ed. St. Louis, Mo: CV Mosby; 1971:1244–1285.
2. Aufranc OE. Evaluation of the patient with an arthritic hip. In: Stillwell WT, ed. *The Art of Total Hip Arthroplasty.* New York, NY: Grune & Stratton; 1987:15.
3. Calandruccio RA. Arthroplasty of hip. In: Crenshaw AH, ed. *Campbell's Operative Orthopaedics.* 7th ed. St Louis, Mo: CV Mosby; 1987:1460–1491.
4. Poss R, Thornhill TS, Ewald FC, Thomas WH, Batte NJ, Sledge CB, et al. Factors influencing the incidence and outcome of infection following total joint arthroplasty. *Clin Orthop.* 1984;182:117–126.
5. Maderazo EG, Judson S, Pasternak H. Late infections of total joint prostheses. *Clin Orthop.* 1988;229:131–142.
6. Lidwell O, Lowbury EJL, Whyte W, Blowers R, Stanley SJ, Lowe D. Effect of ultraclean air in operating rooms on deep sepsis in the joint after total hip or knee replacement: a randomized study. *Br Med J.* (Clin Res Ed) 1982;285:10–14.
7. Dorsey R. The operating room environment. In: Stillwell WT, ed. *The Art of Total Hip Arthroplasty.* New York, NY: Grune & Stratton; 1987:179–191.
8. Sanders R, Fortin P, Ross E, Helfet D. Outer gloves in orthopaedic procedures. *J Bone Joint Surg Am.* 1990;72:914–917.
9. Charnley J. Low friction arthroplasty of the hip. Berlin, Germany: Springer; 1979:152–168.
10. Fitzgerald RH. Treatment of infected total hip arthroplasty. Presented at 8th annual Orthopaedics Research Symposium; November 1993; Chicago, Ill.
11. Schutzer SF, Harris WH. Deep wound infection after total hip replacement under contemporary aseptic conditions. *J Bone Joint Surg Am.* 1988;70:724–727.
12. Shaw JA, Bordner MA, Hamory BH. Efficacy of the

Sterishield filtered exhaust helmet in limiting bacterial counts in the operating room during total joint arthroplasty. *J Arthroplasty.* 1996;11:469–473.
13. Goldner JL. Ultraviolet light in orthopaedic operating rooms at Duke University. *Clin Orthop.* 1978;96:195–205.
14. Robinson RA, Simonian PT. Thermal expansion modular femoral head extractor for revision total hip arthroplasty. *J Arthroplasty.* 1995;10:476–479.
15. Glassman AH, Engh CA, Bobyn JD. Proximal femoral osteotomy as an adjunct in cementless revision total hip arthroplasty. *J Arthroplasty.* 1987;2:47–63.
16. Dall DM, Miles AW. Reattachment of the greater trochanter: the use of the cable grip system. *J Bone Joint Surg Am.* 1983;65:55–59.
17. Scher MA, Jakim I. Trochanteric reattachment in revision total hip arthroplasty. *J Bone Joint Surg Am.* 1990;72:435–438.
18. Nabors ED, Liebelt RA, Mattingly DA, Bierbaum BE. Removal and reinsertion of cemented femoral components during acetabular revision. *J Arthroplasty.* 1996;11:146–152.
19. Lieberman JR, Moeckel BH, Evans BG, Salvati EA, Ranawat CS. Cement-within-cement revision hip arthroplasty. *J Bone Joint Surg Br.* 1993;75:869–871.
20. Lachiewicz P, Anspach W. Removal of a well fixed acetabular component. *J Bone Joint Surg Am.* 1991;73:1355–1356.
21. Moreland JR. Techniques for removal of the prosthesis and cement in hip revision arthroplasty. In: Tullos H, ed. *Instr Course Lect.* Park Ridge, Ill: American Academy of Orthopaedic Surgeons; 1991:163–170.
22. Eftakar NS, Nercessian O. Intrapelvic migration of total hip prostheses. *J Bone Joint Surg Am.* 1989;71:1480–1486.
23. Kremchek TE, McCarthy JC, Turner RH. Retroperitoneal approach to the hip for the removal of intrapelvic cement. Presented at AAOS 60th annual meeting; 1993; San Francisco, Calif.
24. Harkess JW. *Arthroplasty of Hip.* In: Crenshaw AH, ed. *Campbell's Operative Orthopaedics.* 8th ed. St Louis, Mo: CV Mosby; 1992:441–626.
25. Bohn W. Modular femoral stem removal during total hip arthroplasty using a universal modular stem extractor. *Clin Orthop.* 1992;285:155–157.
26. Cameron HU. Femoral windows for easy cement removal in hip revision surgery. *Orthop Rev.* 1990;19:909–912.
27. Sydney SV, Mallory TH. Controlled perforation: a safe method of cement removal from the femoral canal. *Clin Orthop.* 1990;253:168–172.
28. Sherk HH, Kollmer C. Revision arthroplasty using a CO_2 laser. In: Sherk HH, ed. *Lasers in Orthopaedics.* Philadelphia, Pa: JB Lippencott; 1990:75–103.
29. Moreland JR, Sherk HH, et al. Symposium: techniques for removal of prosthesis and cement in total hip revision surgery. *Contemp Orthop.* 1990;601.
30. Cameron HU. Proximal femoral osteotomy in difficult revision hip surgery: how to revise the unrevisable. *Contemp Orthop.* 1989;28:565.
31. Younger TI, Bradford MS, Jablonsky WS, Paprosky WG. Extended proximal femoral osteotomy: a new technique for femoral revision arthroplasty. *J Arthroplasty.* 1995;10:329–338.
32. Glasman AH, Engh CA. The removal of porous-coated femoral stems. *Clin Orthop.* 1992;285:164–180.

17
Use of the Cup-Out® Device for Difficult Acetabular Revisions

Paul F. Lachiewicz

Loose cemented acetabular components are usually easy to remove at the time of revision arthroplasty. However, cemented metal-backed components and metal porous-coated acetabular components may be extremely difficult to remove, without substantial damage to the adjacent acetabulum and pelvis. Secure porous-coated acetabular components may require removal for polyethylene wear or dissociation (if they are nonmodular), malposition with recurrent dislocations, and infection. The Cup-Out® pneumatic impact wrench was developed and tested at the University of North Carolina at Chapel Hill in 1988 and is available on a rental basis from Anspach® (Palm Beach Gardens, FL). A previous study on torque testing of cemented and porous-coated acetabular components to determine the strength of the fixation provided the idea for the instruments.[1] The pneumatic impact wrench delivers repetitive rotatory loads to the acetabular component (Fig. 17.1). Shear stresses develop at the implant–cement or implant–bone interface to loosen the component.

Wide exposure of the acetabulum is achieved either by trochanteric osteotomy or a posterior approach with anterior capsulectomy. The polyethylene insert of the modular or nonmodular metal-backed acetabular component is removed. A driver of the appropriate size is then selected, and the metal component is marked for placement of the studs of the driver. Grooves approximating the size of the studs (6 mm wide and 6 mm deep) are cut into the component with a high-speed burr with use of a carbide cutter. The driver is then fitted into the component, and the impact wrench is engaged. A similar technique for removal of a nonmodular polyethylene component can be used, except that three grooves are made instead of two to help prevent the driver from cutting out. The peak torque delivered is controlled by the pressure of the nitrogen applied to the impact wrench, which ranges from 276 to 1379 kPa (40–200 psi). The driver is designed to pass through an arc of only 15° to prevent fracture of the acetabulum. The surgeon should begin at mid-range (828 kPa or 120 psi) and reverse direction before increasing the torque. The pressure is applied by the impact wrench for 15 to 30 seconds before direction is reversed.

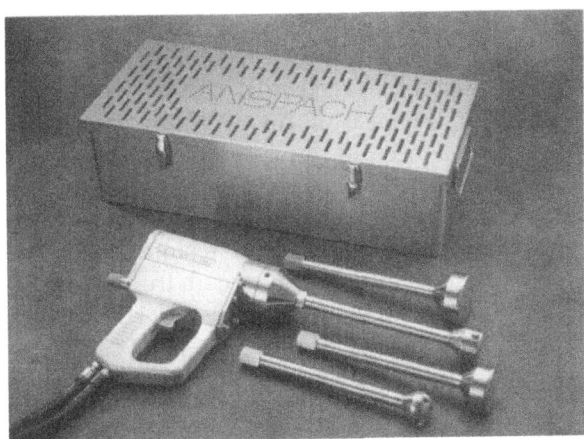

Figure 17.1. The Cup-Out® device comes with a pneumatic impact wrench and several sizes of drivers. (Courtesy of Dr. Paul F. Lachiewicz.)

This instrument has been used successfully by me and many surgeons throughout the country during the past 7 years. I have used the device to remove six well-fixed porous-coated acetabular components for infection or recurrent dislocation. Other surgeons reported successful use of the device to remove eight well-fixed cementless acetabular components. The Cup-Out® is a valuable and extremely helpful device for removal of well-fixed acetabular components in difficult revision operations.

Reference

1. Lachiewicz P, Anspach W. Removal of a well fixed acetabular component. *J Bone Joint Surg Am.* 1991;73:1355–1356.

18
Hand Tools

James V. Bono

The removal of implants and cement can be exhaustive without proper instruments. A complete set of hand tools is an absolute requirement when preparing for revision surgery. The instruments are designed to facilitate the removal of implants, cement, and cement plugs. Several special instruments are required to remove most femoral components on the market. A hook extractor is designed for removal of Austin Moore type stems, whereas a one-piece universal stem extractor will effectively remove stems with a fixed head of up to a 38 mm diameter. A multipiece universal stem extractor is designed for removal of modular femoral stems with stepped trunions. A universal smooth trunion stem extractor is used with various size inserts designed to fit varying neck tapers to create a three-point contact that securely holds the trunion during stem extraction (Fig. 18.1).

Stem extractors attach to a universal handle that can be used with a slotted hammer. A femoral head extractor, consisting of a holder and wedges, allows for quick removal of most modular heads. A femoral stem punch may be utilized in cases where the stem has fractured within the femur and the metal component is difficult to retrieve.

Special instruments are required for the removal of cementless acetabular components. Removal of acetabular screws is facilitated by several different style screwdrivers, from solid shafts to flexible shafts and a screw trephine for extraction of stripped or broken screws. Acetabular osteotomes are used with a curvature that will conform to the outer diameter of the acetabular implant. A unique instrument in the industry, the TreBay™ "bear claw" acetabular cup and liner extractor, will remove poly liners or metal acetabular cups (Fig. 18.2). An acetabular cup liner chisel is utilized for separation of the liner from the shell and should be used in conjunction with the acetabular "bear claw." The "poly claws" are designed with sharp tips for extraction of plastic acetabular components only.

Cement removal tools are designed to preserve valuable bone during the most challenging cement removal procedures. Cement removal tools include sharp cement extraction hooks that are utilized to remove cement in the femoral canal, blunt extraction hooks that may be used as feelers to locate defects in the canal wall, and cement extraction curettes with extended shafts for easy access to deep cavities. A thumb guide on the handle

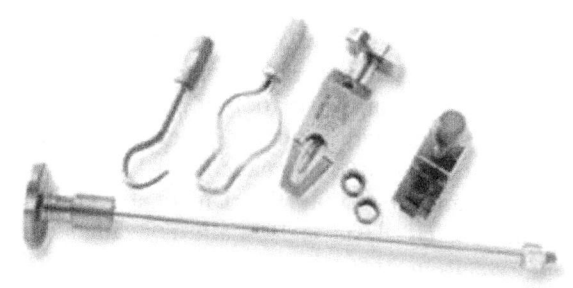

Figure 18.1. Femoral stem removal instruments of the Trebay™ system designed for easy extraction of Austin Moore stems, monolithic stems, modular stepped, or smooth trunion style implants.

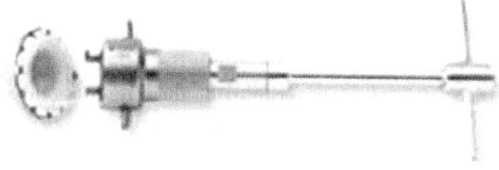

Figure 18.2. The "bear claw" acetabular cup and liner extractor of the Trebay™ system.

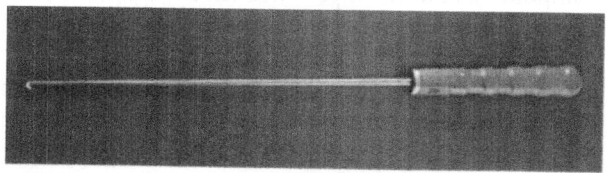

Figure 18.3. Cement removal tool of the Trebay system. (See color insert.)

18. Hand Tools

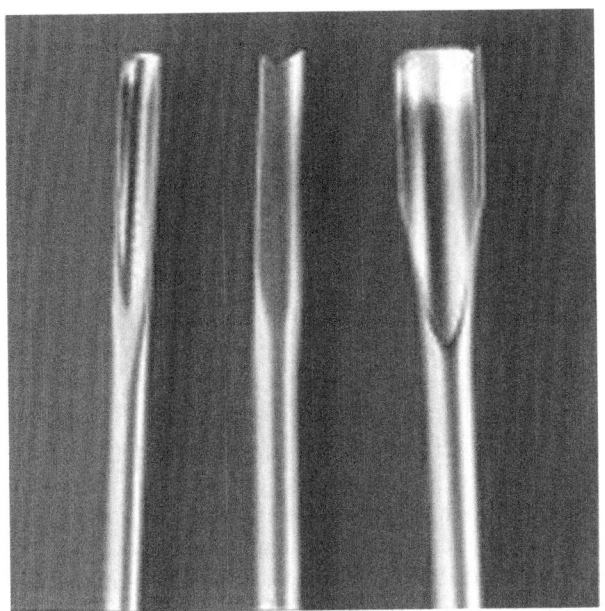

Figure 18.4. Circular cement chisel of the Trebay system. (See color insert.)

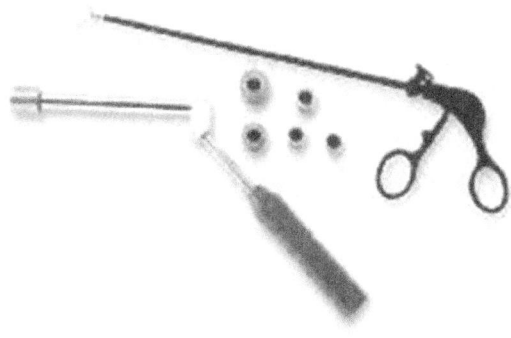

Figure 18.5. Extraction of the femoral plug and distal cement can be accomplished using a drill with the Trebay system centering handle. Grasping forceps extract cement debris from the distal canal. (See color insert.)

helps to orient the working tip of the instrument (Fig. 18.3). A metal strike plate at the top of the shaft provides a solid base for use with a slotted or slide hammer. A cement-splitting chisel will efficiently split the cement mantle. Circular chisels are used to disrupt the cement–bone interface (Fig. 18.4).

For removal of the cement plug and cement distal to the stem, a drill guide may be used with various size centering cones, which will properly align the drill in preparation for removing the femoral plug and any remaining distal cement. A variety of tap extractors may then allow for removal of the cement plug and distal cement (Fig. 18.5). Grasping forceps are used to remove cement fragments and debris.

Both hard tools and power tools should be available if the cement removal to be undertaken is extensive. Visualization of the medullary canal is assisted considerably by the use of a head-mounted fiberoptic light source.

The task of cement removal can be divided into two parts: first, the proximal cement that is accessible; and second, the distal cement that is relatively inaccessible. The proximal cement can be fragmented using the hand instrument as described above.

The farther distal (and less accessible) the cement, the more important it is to revert to the "gold standard" for distal cement removal: the Midas Rex™ drill under precise biplane fluoroscopic control. This technique has been described in great detail by Turner and Emerson[1] and will not be repeated here.

Reference

1. Turner RH, Emerson RH. Femoral revision arthroplasty. In: RH Turner and AD Scheller, Ed. *Revision Total Hip Arthroplasty*. New York: Grune & Stratton, 1982:75–106.

19
Ultrasonic Cement Removal

Richard L. Wixson

With revision of failed cemented total hip replacements, removal of bone cement can vary from simple pulling out of loose pieces to extraction of well-fixed components completely encased in cement, which extends well down the femoral diaphysis. Traditional methods of cement removal have involved fragmentation with osteotomes and manual instruments, reamers and high-speed burrs (Midas Rex or Anspach) or the use of extended trochanteric osteotomies or creation of cortical windows. All these methods either involve or carry the risk of violation of the femoral cortex with fracture or perforations.

An alternative approach was developed by Klapper et al. and Caillouette[1–4] using ultrasonic energy for cement removal. Ultrasonic devices have a long history of use in dentistry to break up dental plaque without injury to underlying hard structures or adjacent soft tissues. Other applications have involved devices to fragment cataracts for removal in ophthalmic procedures and tumor destruction in neurosurgery. For bone cement removal, rather than fragmenting the cement, the ultrasonic tool softens the material, allowing its removal. The system does not send ultrasonic waves into the bone or cement. A power source sends electrical energy to a crystal, which pulsates because of the Piezo electric effect. The crystal is housed in an ultrasonic transducer, which converts the electrical energy into mechanical energy. This mechanical energy causes tool tips, attached to the handpiece, to vibrate at high rates. Polymethylmethacrylate (PMMA), or bone cement, transmits heat poorly, but it has a high capacity for energy absorption. When the tool tips come in contact with the PMMA, the surrounding cement softens, which allows its removal.

Although the vibration of the tool tip does not produce heat, the cement softening results in significant heat release. Because bone necrosis can occur at temperatures of 47°C for more than a minute,[5] there is potential for thermal damage. Using thermal transducers in bone and at the bone cement interface, Caillouette et al.[2,3] found a maximum temperature of 40°C during ultrasonic prosthesis removal. Brooks et al.[6] found higher temperatures of up to 50°C, which were, however, transitory in very small areas and could be reduced by irrigation. They concluded that with the use of irrigation, the temperature produced would not exceed the threshold for bone viability. Both histologic bone analysis and torsional strength testing of canine femurs after ultra-

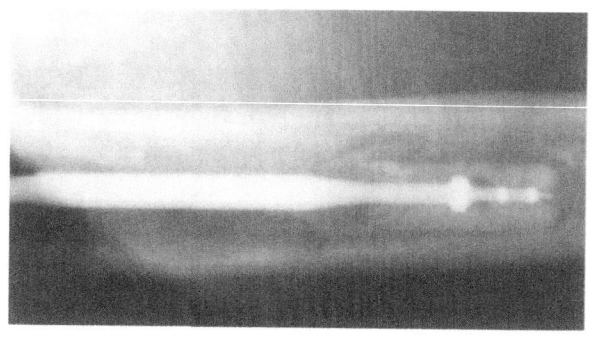
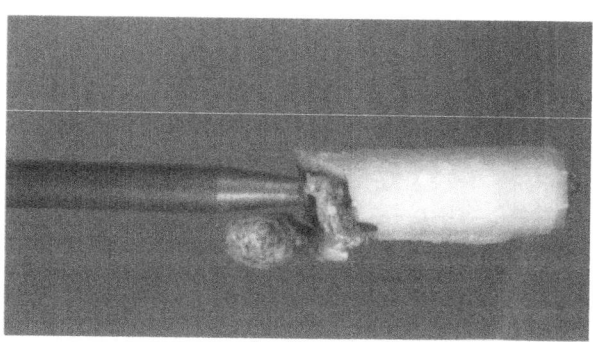

A   B

Figure 19.1. A. Intraoperative radiograph of ultrasonic plug puller tip inside distal cement plug. B. Photograph of the extracted plug.

sonic cement removal showed no deleterious effect.[2,4] Additional studies by Cautilli and Hozack[7] established that there was no danger from any fumes generated during ultrasonic cement removal.

A major advantage of the ultrasonic system is the ability of the surgeon to sense or feel the difference between cutting through the bone cement and coming into contact with cortical bone. Except for very thin cortical bone, there is much less likelihood of perforation, compared with the use of manual osteotomes or high-speed burrs.[8] In 90 reported revision cases with ultrasonic tools, the new perforation rate was 1%.[9] In addition, unlike the use of high-speed burrs, intraoperative fluoroscopy or x-rays are rarely needed.

If the femoral implant is well fixed, several thin osteotome-like ultrasonic tips can be used to separate the prosthesis from the metal–cement interface until the prosthesis can be extracted. Large masses of cement or thick cement mantles can then be removed with other tips, which function like gauges or curets to scoop out softened PMMA. The remaining cement mantle can then be cut into quarters longitudinally with thin ultrasonic tips down to the bone, at which point the cut sections can be removed more easily with manual instruments. It is important that large amounts of irrigation be used to reduce any temperature elevation in the cement being cut near the bone.[6] Once the cement mantel has been removed, the biggest problem is often an intact cement plug in the cortical diaphysis below where the prosthesis ended. A plug-puller tip can be used to penetrate the cement plug with the ultrasonic tool activated. Once the power is turned off, the cement then hardens around the tip, which can then be extracted. (See Fig. 19.1). For tight plugs or large extensions of cement, a central canal can be made down the shaft of the femur with a disc drill tip. Usually, either additional ultrasonic instruments or manual instruments can be used to pull out the remaining cement. On the acetabular side, the device is useful for both cutting up the cement mass for removal and using the plug puller to remove intrapelvic cement masses.

Compared with other methods, ultrasonic cement removal is a reliable technique for cement removal with much less risk or the requirement of femoral disruption or damage.

References

1. Klapper RC, Caillouette JT. The use of ultrasonic tools in revision arthroplasty procedures. *Contemp Orthop.* 1990;20:273–279.
2. Caillouette J, Gorab R, Klapper RC, Anzel S. Revision arthroplasty facilitated by ultrasonic tool cement removal: histologic analysis of endosteal bone after cement removal. *Orthop Rev.* 1991;20:435–440.
3. Caillouette J, Gorab R, Klapper RC, Anzel S. Revision arthroplasty facilitated by ultrasonic tool cement removal: in vitro evaluation. *Orthop Rev.* 1991;20:353–357.
4. Klapper RC, Caillouette JT, Callaghan JJ, Hozack WJ. Ultrasonic technology in revision joint arthroplasty. *Clin Orthop.* 1992;285:147–154.
5. Eriksson AR, Albrektsson T. Temperature threshold levels for heat-induced bone tissue injury: a vital microscopic study in the rabbit. *J Prosthet Dent.* 1983;50:101–107.
6. Brooks AT, Nelson CL, Stewart CL, Skinner RA, Siems ML. Effect of ultrasonic device on temperatures generated in bone and on bone–cement structure. *J Arthroplasty.* 1993;8:413–418.
7. Cautilli GP, Hozack WJ. Analysis of fume emission from ultrasonic removal of methyl methacrylate cement in revision hip surgery. *J Arthroplasty.* 1994;9:305–306.
8. Brooks AT, Nelson CL, Hofmann O. Minimal femoral cortical thickness necessary to prevent perforation by ultrasonic tools in revision joint surgery. *J Arthroplasty.* 1995;10:359–362.
9. Gardiner R, Hozack WJ, Nelson C, Keating EM. Revision total hip arthroplasty using ultrasonically driven tools. *J Arthroplasty.* 1993;8:517–521.

20
Drill and Excavation

Frank B. Gray

Among the many techniques available for femoral cement removal, one of the most consistently reliable and safe has been the use of cannulated end mills. End mills are used in two separate and distinct ways, each complementing the other in the extraction of femoral cement.[1]

Router Technique

The first technique involves the use of the instrument as a router, clearing cement from the proximal femoral sidewalls. This is performed with a gentle brushing motion. Because the end mill only rotates at about 300 rpm, there is less heat build-up and less risk of femoral perforation than with high-speed burrs. A step-cut technique often is used in the proximal canal during this stage of the procedure to redefine the proximal ledge of the cement mantle, facilitating subsequent splitting with hand tools. This technique is continued into the canal to the distal extent of the femoral stem recess. As the solid distal wall of cement is encountered, the second end mill technique is used.

Cannulated End Mill Technique

A long 10 × 1/8 inch drill bit, designed to drill cement, is directed into the distal cement. If the cement column is not extensive, the drill is passed through to the far side of the cement, and a 2.0-mm guide pin is inserted through the drill hole. Gentle probing with the guide pin confirms intramedullary location. Over this is passed a cannulated end mill. This technique is possible because the end mills are end cutting as well as side cutting. On the other hand, if the cement column is extensive, the drill may be progressed in millimeter increments, left embedded in the cement, and used as the guide over which the end mill is passed (see Fig. 20.1).

Conclusion

The major advantages of the use of cannulated end mills are controlled access to the distal femoral cement, safer removal of proximal cement, and overall cost effectiveness. Inadvertent femoral cortical perforation, if such should occur, involves little more than a 1/8-inch drill hole, which is readily recognized before further cortical damage occurs. This technique appears to offer certain advantages, in particular to lower volume total hip revision surgeons, because of better control and a shorter learning curve than with some of the other current techniques available.

Reference

1. Gray F. Prosthesis and cement removal techniques. *Orthop Clin North Am* 1992;23:313–319.

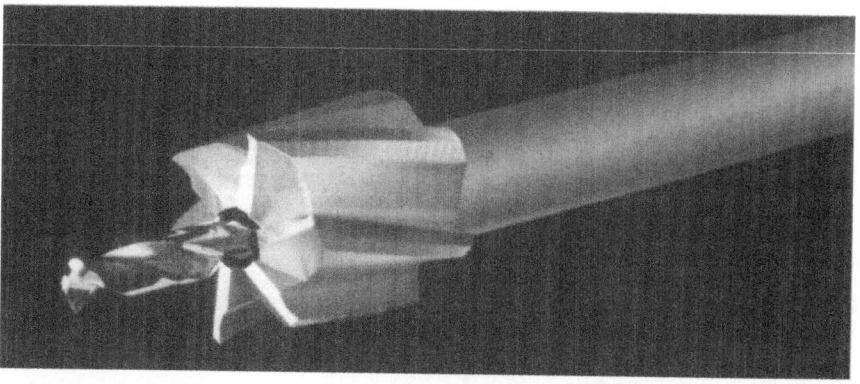

Figure 20.1. The end mill is passed over a 10-inch cement drill. (Courtesy of Howmedica, Inc, Rutherford, NJ.)

21
Bone Bank/Bone Graft

James C. Slater

After the removal of failed components or cement, bone deficits are invariably present. This results from the components themselves and any motion or subsidence that occurs. Other contributing factors include osteolysis, stress-shielding, disuse osteoporosis, and additional loss occurring during removal of the failed implants. As previously noted in Chapters 9 to 11, the residual bone may be thin and sclerotic with deficits being cavitary, segmental, combined, or with discontinuity. The remaining bone significantly affects the reconstructive options, and preservation of host bone is vital.

Various classification systems address bone deficits on both the femoral and acetabular sides and help guide the reconstruction.[1-4] (See Chapters 9 to 11.) Reconstructive options include bone replacement with metallic implants, custom components, or bone graft–implant constructs from autologous and/or allogeneic sources. Use of bone grafting to address deficits has several advantages, including more normal transfer of implant forces to host bone,[5] potential restoration of bone stock for future surgery, and possible soft tissue attachment and fixation. In addition, it allows for the use of more conventional noncustom implants. Various grafts are available, and they are often used in combination in revision total hip arthroplasty. Factors in selection include the availability of graft types, biomechanical forces the graft will receive, metabolic and nutritional status of the patient, and characteristics of the graft–host–implant construct.[6] Donor age, anatomic site and graft geometry affect strength and mechanical properties. Once bone grafting has been selected, biologic and biomechanical concerns must be addressed together with the relative adequacy of fixation methods to host bone.

Bone graft incorporation is dynamic and proceeds through various stages, depending on the type of graft used. The desired goal is a source of osteogenesis that becomes a physiologicically stable and biomechanically supportive structure.[7] To achieve this end point, the surgeon must have a working knowledge of the biology of graft incorporation.

Primary Osteogenesis

Primary osteogenesis is the synthesis of new bone by transplanted cells that remain viable. This occurs only with autografts because processed allografts contain no live cells. Fresh, unprocessed allografts are no longer used because of the intense immunologic response evoked through both humoral and cell-mediated pathways.[8] Processing of allografts destroys primary osteogenesis capability but also reduces the immune response.[9] Commonly used processing techniques include fresh-freezing, and the response can be further reduced with freeze-drying.[10] These two processes maintain the osteoinductive and osteoconductive properties of the grafts.[11]

Osteoinduction and Osteoconduction

Osteoinduction involves the migration of host osteoprogenitor stem cells into the graft, which then differentiate into osteoblasts. This begins with host blood vessels invading the graft as cutting cones, with osteoclasts and osteoblasts simultaneously resorbing and laying down bone in a process called creeping substitution. This process is mediated in part by bone morphogenic proteins (BMPs) that are low molecular weight peptides. These proteins participate in the recruitment and differentiation of stem cells.[12,13] They remain active in fresh-frozen, freeze-dried, and decalcified allografts but are destroyed by autoclaving.[11] *Osteoconduction* is the process whereby the graft serves as a scaffolding for ingrowth from the host with a new blood supply and new cells for bone formation.

Autologous Bone Graft

Autologous bone graft remains the gold standard and should be used whenever possible. Its advantages include an absence of immunologic rejection and more complete incorporation. Disadvantages include the relatively small supply available, donor site morbidity, and difficulty in reconstructing large segmental defects. Cancellous autograft has primary osteogenesis capability. Revascularization is rapid because of the large surface area, and osteoblasts and osteoclasts proliferate early. Apposition of new viable bone occurs before resorption of old necrotic bone.[14] Complete replacement by new bone is often accomplished by one year after placement.[11]

Cortical autografts differ in that they can provide early partial structural support. However, revascularization is slower than with cancellous bone because of the density and smaller available surface area. Osteoclastic resorption must occur before extensive revascularization and new appositional bone formation. This process weakens the graft and typically peaks around 6 months after implantation.[6] Some investigators estimate maximal weakening at 60% of original strength by 12 weeks, with this level remaining until 1 year and gradually increasing to the original strength by 2 years after implantation.[14] With proper technique, physiologic loading, and implant-host bone stability, complete resorption probably never occurs, and the bone remains a mixture of graft and new bone.[6] Concerns include nonunion, infection, late fracture, or graft failure.

Allograft Bone

Advantages of allograft bone include the wide selection of available shapes and sizes and the absence of any donor site morbidity. With graft maturation, the desired end point is a biologic reconstruction that may partially revascularize and regain some capability of biologic self-repair.[15] Potential allograft disadvantages include the immunologic response, with possible rejection or resorption. Other concerns include systemic disease transmission and increased rate of deep wound infections.[16] Delayed complications include nonunion of graft–host junctions or late graft fracture or failure.[15]

Processing and Procurement

Allograft bone must be processed to decrease the host immunologic response. Techniques include freezing, freeze-drying, decalcifying, or irradiating the bone or exposing it to chemical agents or cryopreservatives. Another primary concern is preventing disease transmission, and procurement and bone-banking protocols and guidelines must be stringently enforced. Standards are published and made available by the American Association of Tissue Banks (AATB). Commercial bone banks provide service regionally or nationally, and some hospitals provide bone locally or through limited networks.

Graft procurement, storage, and use must be accomplished while the risk of disease transmission is minimized. This begins with comprehensive donor screening.[17] Past medical history and circumstances surrounding death are monitored for any potential systemic source of infection. Any evidence of bacterial, fungal, or viral organisms on appropriate cultures makes harvest unacceptable. Blood and body fluids are cultured, and serologic tests are performed to assess for hepatitis viruses and HIV. Live donors (eg, femoral heads) are retested 3 to 6 months later to exclude potential HIV(+) patients who have not seroconverted at the time of harvest.[18] The time between infection and seropositive conversion is referred to as the negative window. It should be noted, however, that negative windows up to 3 years and possibly longer have been reported.[19] Patients with metabolic and neoplastic diseases, exposure to toxic substances, diseases of unknown origin, or conditions predisposing to osteomyelitis are also excluded.

Deep-freezing and storage of bone at $-70°C$ or $-80°C$ is standard protocol.[20,21] Cell necrosis occurs while osteoconductive and osteoinductive properties are maintained. Mild immunogenesis remains, and disease transmission can still occur. Because freezing alone does not sterilize the allograft, procurement must be by aseptic means. Cultures are obtained at harvest and we recommend repeating them when bone is thawed for use. In contrast, freeze-drying to a residual moisture of 3% to 5% allows storage at room temperature in sterile vacuum sealed containers.[22] This measure further diminishes the immune reaction and may also decrease the potential for disease transmission.[23] Unfortunately, mechanical properties are changed, resulting in a weaker structure. This factor should be considered in the final construct. Compression strength is maintained, but bending and torsional strengths are significantly diminished.[24,25]

Another method of preparation involves decalcifying the allograft. This removes all rigidity and strength, but osteoinduction continues. Several new products have become available, and clinical investigation continues. Use typically occurs in conjunction with structurally supportive materials.

Harvest and storage of allograft occurs with sterile technique, or with clean technique and subsequent sterilization. Sterilization of allografts occurs with irradiation or use of chemicals, such as ethylene oxide, acids, alcohol, or thimerosal. Irradiation has been reported to inactivate HIV, but considerable controversy exists regarding the amount required. Inactivation of HIV is dose dependent making the initial HIV bioburden the most important factor.[26] Additional variables include whether the bone is cortical or cancellous and dried or frozen. Doses from 1.5–2.5 Mrads (0.015 to 0.025 mGy) have been used in tissue banks.[27] Graft strength has been reported to be diminished with doses greater than 2.5 Mrads (0.025 mGy).[28] Other investigators have shown no significant alteration of mechanical properties up to 3.0 Mrads (0.03 mGy).[29] Osteoinductive properties are also diminished at varying levels of irradiation.[30] Much work is still required to determine optimal radiation levels for sterilization of various tissue types while maintaining strength and osteoinductive ability and minimizing risk of HIV transmission.

Use

Allograft can be used in cancellous or cortical structure. Cancellous sources include femoral heads or freeze-dried chips. One method involves sectioning femoral heads with an oscillating saw and then morsellizing the bone with rongeurs or hand-driven or pneumatic bone mills. The powered mills have a tendency to jam with cortical pieces against the blade. Another method involves hemisectioning the femoral head and then using small modular "cheese-grater" acetabular reamers. As each reamer fills with morsellized graft, larger sizes are used. The morsellized bone is densely packed and easily removed with a wide curet from the locking orifice in the same manner as that used to remove autograft during acetabular reaming. Osteogenesis is then enhanced by mixing the allograft with host bone marrow or any available autograft reamings from the pelvis. Contained acetabular defects are packed with graft and impacted with acetabular reamers in reverse. Femoral defects are grafted, as are any bone junctions, windows, or osteotomies. Impaction grafting technique for cemented stems requires a more coarse morsellized graft with fragments of 3 to 5 mm, and bone milling is recommended in this case.[31]

Cortical allografts or autografts can be used for femoral reinforcement or, in severe cases, structural deficiencies when no other options exist. Success is very technique dependent, and correct biomechanical principles must be observed.[32,33] First, do not sacrifice or devascularize any host bone and do not rely on the graft for primary structural support if cementless constructs are used. The importance of precise shaping and accurate rigid graft fixation, together with a stable joint construct, cannot be overstated. Finally, the graft must be stressed (Wolff's law) to prevent resorption, but it should not be relied on for stability except in salvage cases.

Preparation

Allograft preparation is facilitated by having extra tables for sterile working space. A second surgeon or surgical team expedites completion so that graft preparation occurs while the component or bone cement is being removed. This decreases operative time and potential blood loss. We prefer fresh-frozen grafts, and these are thawed in warm triple-antibiotic saline solution after cultures are obtained. An alternative method is to thaw the allograft in warm Betadine solution.[5] A table vise is preferred, but bone holders or towel clamps can also secure the graft while shaping and contouring are completed. An oscillating saw is used to cut grafts into segments or for hemisectioning of whole allografts. Wedges of varying size, shape, or diameter can be cut from femoral heads, and the saw is also useful in removing cartilage or shaving off bone. All soft tissue and cartilage are removed before implantation.

High-speed burrs are used to shape structural grafts. In the acetabulum, some surgeons may prefer to use female reamers of varying sizes to shape large allografts. Trabeculae and screw fixation are aligned along the anatomic weight-bearing axis. K-wires are used for provisional fixation, and partially threaded cancellous screws with washers impact and secure the graft after morsellized graft is placed at the interface. Fixation of the graft to host bone is obtained independent from the acetabular component. Transverse bolts are not used. Reaming of the graft is minimized, so that strong subchondral bone is left intact. Cancellous surfaces are not exposed except to host bone. Early and mid-range results suggest that greater than 50% of the socket should be supported by host bone if cementless techniques are used.[2,33–35] Host bone contact in the anterior and posterior columns is vital[33] and some investigators recommend significant socket medialization to obtain this.[36] Also, good fit and apposition of the graft to the host without gaps are particularly important. Pelvic reconstruction plates and screws are used to secure graft for major column deficiencies or pelvic discontinuity. At times, whole anatomic acetabular allografts are needed to salvage these severe deficits. Posterior plating, obtaining intraoperative x-rays, and cementing the socket are recommended. Cement is kept out of the graft–host junctions. Use of reinforcement rings or cages attached to host bone and bridging the graft may be indicated, and these should be made available on the basis of preoperative planning, as will be discussed in the next chapter.

Preparation of onlay cortical strut allografts for femoral reinforcement should be done in a manner to maximize graft-host bone contact. The proximal and distal femur and the proximal tibia are excellent sources. Endosteal contouring with the Midas Rex™ high-speed burr yields an inner diameter of the graft that closely matches the outer diameter of the host femur. The graft is then placed over femoral deficiencies, fractures, perforations, osteotomies, femoral windows, or massive graft–host bone junctions. The interfaces are grafted with morselized bone before the onlay graft is positioned, and the margins of the onlay allograft are also grafted. To avoid weakening the allograft, screws and plates are not used, and holes are not drilled except for trochanteric reattachment, if needed. Cerclage wires or cables are used for fixation, and cable passers facilitate passage without injury to neural or vascular structures. The surgeon should watch for injury to perforating branches from the profunda femoris artery, which can retract and bleed significantly.

Proximal Femoral Reconstruction Allografts

Circumferential proximal femoral deficiency can occur with either a thin diaphyseal shell remaining or with total bone absence. Options for approach to this extremely complex scenario are outlined in Chapter 26. If a whole proximal femoral allograft technique[37] is selected, strong fresh-frozen ipsilateral femur bone from a young donor is recommended. Standardized preoperative x-rays of the graft should be inspected for size, shape, and bone quality.[38] A radiographic scoring system has been developed in an attempt to correlate morphologic features with probable in vivo mechanical properties on the basis of the Singh index, cortical shaft index, calcar width, and isthmus-to-canal ratio.[39]

Graft preparation is completed on the back table. High speed drills are used to prepare the intramedullary portion of the graft, with care to avoid excessive bone removal because this will weaken the graft. Coarse reamers are avoided because they may torque and split the bone. The proximal aspect of the long-stem or modular metaphyseal sleeve is cemented into the graft but not into host bone. Sterile methylene blue dye can be used to mark the graft and host–bone junction for proper rotation and version. If step-cuts in the graft are planned for rotational control, they are marked and completed with a high-speed burr, rather than with an oscillating saw. Cement is not used at the junction or distally with this technique. Morsellized autograft and allograft are used at the interface. Extended-length cortical onlay grafts then reinforce the junction medially and laterally, and they are secured with No. 16 Luque cerclage wires or cables.

If a thin ectatic diaphyseal shell of bone is present, it can be collapsed around the implant with a reduction osteotomy by using cerclage wires or cables. Alternatively, if whole proximal femoral allografting is used, the bone is split (maintaining its vascularity) and collapsed around the graft junction externally and secured with cerclage wires or cables.

References

1. D'Antonio JA, Capello WN, Borden LS, Barger WL, Bierbaum BF, Boettcher WG, et al. Classification and management of acetabular abnormalities in total hip arthroplasty. *Clin Orthop.* 1989;243:126–137.
2. Paprosky WG, Perona PG, Lawrence JM. Acetabular defect classification and surgical reconstruction in revision arthroplasty. *J Arthroplasty.* 1994;9:33–44.
3. D'Antonio JA, McCarthy JC, Barger WL, Borden LS, Cappelo WN, Collis DK, et al. Classification of femoral abnormalities in total hip arthroplasty. *Clin Orthop.* 1993;296:133–139.
4. Masri BA, Duncan CP. Classification of bone loss in total hip arthroplasty. In: Pritchard DJ, ed. *Instr Course Lect 45.* Park Ridge, Ill: American Academy of Orthopaedic Surgeons; 1996:199–208.
5. Gross AE, Allan DG, Leitch KK, Hutchison CR. Proximal femoral allografts for reconstruction of bone stock in revision arthroplasty of the hip. In: Pritchard DJ, ed. *Instr Course Lect 45.* Park Ridge, Ill: American Academy of Orthopaedic Surgeons; 1996:143–147.
6. Goldberg V. Bone grafting in revision total hip arthroplasty. In: Tullos HS, ed. *Instr Course Lect XL.* Park Ridge, Ill: American Academy of Orthopaedic Surgeons; 1991:177–184.
7. Friedlaender GE, Goldberg VM, eds. *Bone and Cartilage Allografts: Biology and Clinical Applications.* Park Ridge, Ill: American Academy of Orthopaedic Surgeons; 1991:xiii.
8. Horowitz MC, Friedlaender GE. The immune response to bone grafts. In: Friedlaender GE, Goldberg VM, eds. *Bone and Cartilage Allografts: Biology and Clinical Applications.* Park Ridge, Ill: American Academy of Orthopaedic Surgeons; 1991:85–101.
9. Curtiss PH, Powell AE, Herndon CH. Immunological factors in homogenous bone transplantation, III: the inability of homogenous rabbit bone to induce circulating antibodies in rabbits. *J Bone Joint Surg Am.* 1959;41:1482–1488.
10. Friedlaender GE, Strong DM, Sell KW. Studies of the antigenicity of bone, II: donor specific anti-HLA antibodies in human recipients of freeze dried allografts. *J Bone Joint Surg Am.* 1984;66:107–116.
11. Goldberg VM, Stevenson S, Shaffer JW. Biology of autografts and allografts. In: Friedlaender GE, Goldberg VM, eds. *Bone and Cartilage Allografts: Biology and Clinical Applications.* Park Ridge, Ill: American Academy of Orthopaedic Surgeons; 1991:3–12.
12. Urist MR, Strates BS. Bone morphogenic protein. *J Dent Res.* 1971;50:1392–1406.
13. Mitzutani H, Urist MR. The nature of bone morphogenetic protein (BMP) fractions derived from bovine bone matrix gelatin. *Clin Orthop.* 1982;171:213–223.
14. Springfield DS. Massive autogenous bone grafts. *Orthop Clin North Am.* 1987;18:249–257.
15. Berry BH, Lord CF, Gebhardt MC, Mankin HJ. Fractures of allografts. *J Bone Joint Surg Am.* 1990;72:825–833.
16. Lord CF, Gebhardt MC, Tomford WW, Mankin HJ. Infection in bone allografts. *J Bone Joint Surg Am.* 1988;70:369–376.
17. Doppelt SH, Tomford WW, Lucas AD, Mankin HG. Operational and financial aspects of a hospital bone bank. *J Bone Joint Surg Am.* 1981;63:1472–1481.
18. American Association of Tissue Banks. 180-Day quarantine for HCV and HIV for living donors effective April 1, 1991. *Am Assoc Tissue Banks Newsl.* 1990;13:1.
19. Imagoua DT, Lee MH, Wolinsky SM, Sano K, Morales F, Kwok S, et al. Human immunodeficiency virus type 1 infection in homosexual men who remain seronegative for prolonged periods. *N Engl J Med.* 1989;320:1458–1462.
20. Ehrlich MG, Lorenz J, Tomford WW, et al. Collagenase activity in banked bone. *Trans Orthop Res Soc.* 1983;8:166.
21. Pelker RR, Friedlaender GE. Biomechanical considerations in osteochondral grafts. In: Friedlaender GE, Goldberg VM, eds. *Bone and Cartilage Allografts: Biology and Clinical*

Applications. Park Ridge, Ill: American Academy of Orthopaedic Surgeons; 1991:155–162.
22. Malinin JI, Wu NM, Flores A. Freeze drying of bone for allotransportation. In: Friedlaender GE, Mankin HJ, Sell KW, eds. *Osteochondral Allografts: Biology, Banking, and Clinical Applications*. Boston, Mass: Little Brown; 1983: 181–192.
23. Bottomfield S. HIV transmission incident. *Am Assoc Tissue Banks Newsl*. 1991;14:1.
24. Triantafyllou N, Sotiropoulos E, Triantafyllou JN. The mechanical properties of the lyophilized and irradiated bone grafts. *Acta Orthop Belg*. 1975;41(suppl):35–44.
25. Pelker RR, Friedlaender GE, Markham TC. Biomechanical properties of bone allografts. *Clin Orthop*. 1983;174:54–57.
26. Czitrom AA. Principles and techniques of tissue banking. In: Heckman JD, ed. *Instr Course Lect*. Park Ridge, Ill: American Academy of Orthopaedic Surgeons; 1993;42: 359–362.
27. Strong DM, Sayers MH, Conrad EU. Screening tissue donors for infectious markers. In: Friedlaender GE, Goldberg VM, eds. *Bone and Cartilage Allografts: Biology and Clinical Applications*. Park Ridge, Ill: American Academy of Orthopaedic Surgeons; 1991:193–209.
28. Bright RW, Smarsh JD, Gambill VM. Sterilization of human bone by irradiation. In: Friedlaender GE, Mankin HJ, Sell KW, eds. *Osteochondral Allografts: Biology, Banking, and Clinical Applications*. Boston, Mass: Little Brown; 1983: 223–232.
29. Komender J, Komender A, Dziedzic-Goclawska A, Ostrowski K. Radiation sterilized bone grafts evaluated by electron spin resonance technique and mechanical tests. *Transplant Proc*. 1976;8:25–37.
30. Lane JM, Kopman C, Newman JC, Burstein A, Boskey A, Einhorn TA. The effect of storage and radiosterilization on the osteoinductive properties of demineralized bone matrix. *Orthop Trans*. 1984;8:227–228.
31. Nelissen RG, Bauer TW, Weidenhielm LR, LeGolvan DP, Mikhail WE. Revision hip arthroplasty with the use of cement and impaction grafting. *J Bone Joint Surg Am*. 1995;77: 412–422.
32. Chandler HP. Management of the bone deficient hip-structural grafting of the acetabulum. *Orthopedics*. 1995;18: 863–864.
33. Young SK, Dorr LD, Kaufman RL, Gruen TA. Factors related to failure of structural bone grafts in acetabular reconstruction of total hip arthroplasty. *J Arthroplasty*. 1991; 6:S73–S82.
34. Paprosky WG, Bradford MS, Jablonsky WS. Acetabular reconstruction with massive acetabular allografts. In: Pritchard DJ, ed. *Instr Course Lect 45*. Park Ridge, Ill: American Academy of Orthopaedic Surgeons; 1996:149–159.
35. Zmolek JC, Dorr LD. Solid allograft in revision total hip arthroplasty. *J Arthroplasty*. 1993;8:361–370.
36. Dorr LD. Ten years experience with non-cemented sockets. Presented at Symposium IV Acetabular Revision, 23rd open meeting of The Hip Society; February 1995; Orlando, Fla.
37. Chandler HP, Penenberg BL. Femoral reconstruction. In: Chandler HP, Penenberg BL, eds. *Bone Stock Deficiency in Total Hip Replacement*. Thorofare, NJ: Slack, Inc; 1989: 137–164.
38. Tomford WW, Mankin HJ. Principles and practical applications of bone banking. In: Chandler HP, Penenberg BL, eds. *Bone Stock Deficiency in Total Hip Replacement*. Thorofare, NJ: Slack, Inc; 1989:13–17.
39. Bloebaum RD, Lauritzen RS, Skedros JG, Smith EF, Thomas KA, Bennett JT, et al. Roentgenographic procedure for selecting proximal femur allograft for use in revision arthroplasty. *J Arthroplasty*. 1993;8:347–360.

22
Implant Inventory

Geoffry Van Flandern

A pivotal ingredient in preoperative planning is implant selection. All revision total hip cases are not performed in centers supplying massive implant inventories. In modern health care, it is difficult for hospitals to justify a large selection of specialized revision components in permanent inventory. As hospital implant inventories shrink, preoperative planning for predicted intraoperative problems becomes critical. The surgeon must fully investigate each revision scenario and plan for a sufficient inventory of equipment to meet all predicted needs.

In the following discussion, component selection is divided according to component type: acetabulum, femur, and greater trochanter. Examples of implant inventory options are provided. Before a discussion of individual defects and components is begun, it is important to emphasize that the surgeon needs to be comfortable with the revision case. That surgeon must be familiar with the bone defects to be addressed, so that the plan will include an inventory of all necessary implants and as little extra equipment as possible.

Acetabulum

Defects in the acetabulum are as individual as patients themselves. For simplification of implant discussion, we have divided acetabular defects into those identified by D'Antonio et al., but in the following order: cavitary defects, segmental defects (noncontained cavitary including medial defects), and pelvic discontinuity.[1] Each acetabular revision may include any number of these deficiencies, even in the same case. For the purposes of discussion, we will attempt to make implant suggestions on the basis of these more general categories.

Contained cavitary defects represent the majority of acetabular problems encountered in revision hip surgery. An inventory of cementless cups with peripheral and/or dome screws will provide a solution for most problems.[2] Screwless acetabular implants are an option, but revision bone anatomy and quality may leave initial fixation inadequate (Fig. 22.1A). All but the most straightforward revision situations will require screw fixation for metal-backed acetabular components (Fig. 22.1B). Large or jumbo sizes are an important inventory consideration. Even contained defects may involve large areas of bone loss or inconsistency that will need to be reconstructed. The contained cavitary lesion assumes a stabilizing rim, which may provide support for a large or even jumbo component (Fig. 22.1C, D).[1]

As mentioned earlier, screw fixation can be pivotal to early acetabular interface stability. Because cavitary defects will tend to involve the cancellous bone of the iliac wing, ischium, and pubis, dome screw fixation alone may prove inadequate. Acetabular revision components such as those manufactured by Joint Medical Products (now Johnson & Johnson) or De Puy include peripheral screws as a fixation option. Peripheral screws add screw fixation in alternate directions to dome screws. The peripheral screws are directed toward the cortical bone of the medial iliac wall. This may provide better or alternative purchase in the case of cavitary defects surrounding the acetabulum (Fig. 22.1C, D).

Acetabular components that provide lateralization may be helpful with large defects. As deficiencies increase in size, even large or jumbo cups may leave the center rotation of the hip too medial. An acetabular component providing medial bulk with lateralization can better restore the center of rotation and abductor tension. Preoperative planning for acetabular inventory should take into account a possible need for lateralized acetabular components (Fig. 22.1E).

Cemented revision acetabular components may be in the preoperative plan for the very limited deficiency or in the low-activity patient. This option may require filling some surrounding deficiencies with cement. The surgeon should assume a difficult bone–cement interface with cemented acetabular revision.[3,4] Cemented acetabular components will be an inventory consideration for revision hip surgery only in very specific and isolated situations (Fig. 22.1F).

Allograft bone should be considered an inventory item, as it would be for any other component. In treatment of contained cavitary defects, morselized allograft

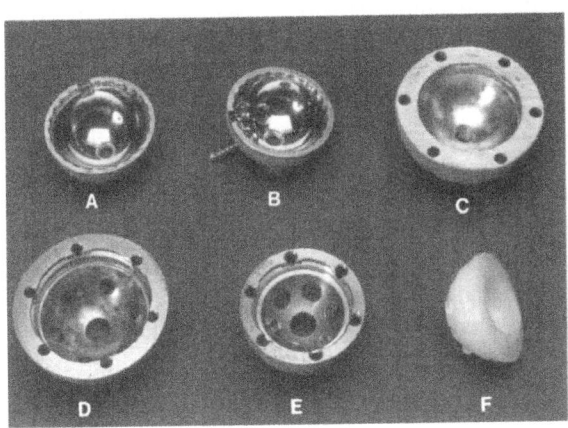

Figure 22.1. A. Reflection screwless acetabular component. (Smith Nephew Richards, Memphis, Tennessee.) B. Reflection acetabular component with cluster screw holes. (Smith Nephew Richards, Memphis, Tennessee.) C. Jumbo size acetabular component with peripheral screws. (De Puy, Warsaw, Indiana.) D. Jumbo size acetabular component with peripheral screw and dome screw capability. (Johnson & Johnson, Raynham, Massachusetts.) E. Deep profile +6-mm lateral acetabular component with peripheral screw and dome screw capability. (Johnson & Johnson, Raynham, Massachusetts.) F. Cemented acetabular component. (Smith Nephew Richards, Memphis, Tennessee.)

or autograft will complete the preoperative inventory needs.[1,5] Morselized allograft can be used to fill cavitary deficiencies in the contained cavitary defect. Allograft request and preparation should be considered critical to the preoperative planning and inventory organization.

Segmental or noncontained cavitary defects are significantly more technically involved. Segmental defects include those with superior and/or posterior and/or medial deficiencies sizable enough to preclude stability of a hemispheric implant without structural graft or additional implant support.[1,5]

In the segmental defect, bone graft must be considered in a bulk or structural type. Allograft should be ordered and preoperatively planned, as it would be for any other revision component. Availability of femoral head or especially distal femoral allografts must be considered in the preoperative plan.[6] Screw fixation of the allograft is necessary. An inventory of large-fragment, partially threaded screws with washers will be necessary. If allograft is used and host bone involves more than 50% of the bed, cementless hemispheric components may be the implant of choice.[6] If allograft provides more than 50% of the bed for reconstruction, cemented acetabular components may be the implant of choice.[6] An inventory of small to moderate sizes of cemented acetabular components may be necessary when the bed consists of more than half allograft bone.

Attempts to avoid the use of structural allograft have included use of oval- or oblong-type acetabular components. The oblong cup by Johnson & Johnson provides superior as well as anterior/posterior fill with a second or bilobed section (Fig. 22.2A). The bilobed configuration allows a posterosuperior defect to be filled with metal ingrowth surface and then anchored through multiple screw holes in the oblong cup.

The bilobed or second section of the oblong cup provides multiple screw hole options in different orientations for fixation. The inventory of bilobed cups includes different primary acetabular sizes combined with two different second lobe or bilobed sizes for each primary size. This size flexibility can accommodate many superior and posterior defects.

A final inventory option for segmental defects would include ring-stabilized components. The Birch–Schneider ring, the Walderman Link partial pelvis replacement ring (with and without caudal flange), and the Mueller O ring can be used to span large areas of deficiency (Fig. 22.2B, C, D, E). After fixation of the ring to the bone, a cemented acetabular component is fixed to the ring itself. Ring supports generally span areas of deficiency and are fixed to bone with large screws and surrounded by morselized graft. An inventory of large-fragment screws and allograft is necessary.

Deficiencies involving the medial wall, or protrusio, may need additional inventory considerations. In simple deepened medial defects, a metal-backed hemispheric component may be adequate. Rim fit by a metal-backed or a jumbo metal-backed component can be

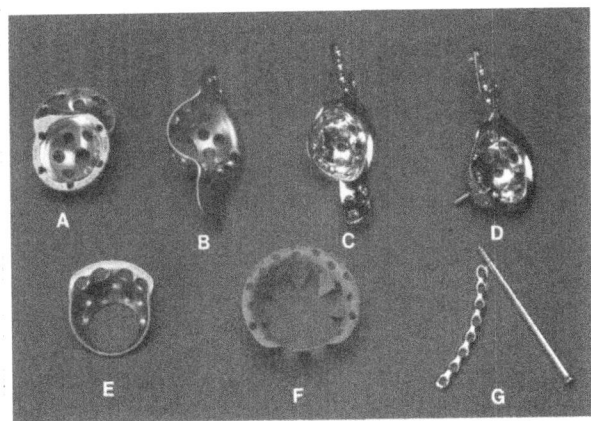

Figure 22.2. A. Oblong acetabular component. Note bilobed section. (Johnson & Johnson, Raynham, Massachusetts.) B. Birch–Schneider acetabular ring. (Distributed by Intermedics Corp, Austin, Texas.) C. Partial pelvis replacement with additional caudal flange. (Waldemar Link Corp, Hamburg, Germany.) D. Partial pelvis replacement ring. (Waldemar Link Corp, Hamburg, Germany.) E. Mueller O ring. (Distributed by Intermedics Corp, Austin, Texas.) F. Protrusio ring. (De Puy, Warsaw, Indiana.) G. Pelvic reconstruction plate and partially threaded lag screw. (Synthes Corp.)

supplemented by medial morselized graft (see Fig. 22.1C, D). A lateralized hemispheric component may be useful in restoring the center of rotation of the hip and abductor anatomy (Fig. 22.1E). In more advanced medial deficiencies, a cage or protrusio ring with bone graft may be the solution. De Puy's protrusio ring provides a great deal of medial support with adequate space for morselized bone graft (Fig. 22.2F).

Larger medial deficiencies, especially when combined with other areas of bone loss, may best be addressed with ring-support systems, as briefly noted earlier. The Link America partial pelvis replacement provides ring support with fixation to the iliac wing, as well as optional fixation through use of a caudal flange (Fig. 22.2C, D). The Birch–Schneider ring allows screw fixation into the ilium and ischium (Fig. 22.2B). Supplemental morselized bone is quite useful in reconstructions using these two ring implants. A small cemented all-polyethylene acetabular component completes the reconstruction inventory needs when ring fixation is considered.

Pelvic discontinuity proposes a major challenge to the revision hip surgeon. Both pelvic stability and bone–implant interface fixation must be addressed. Inventory sufficient to accomplish both may be addressed separately or together. If addressed separately, pelvic fixation is addressed first. A selection of pelvic reconstruction plates, screws, and lag screws will prove necessary to provide adequate pelvic fixation (Fig. 22.2G). Plate fixation will adequately stabilize the pelvis to permit predictable interface fixation of a metal-backed cup with multiple screw augmentation.[1]

Pelvic discontinuity can also be bridged with a single implant. Birch–Schneider or Walderman Link rings provide fixation into the ilium as well as the ischial–pubic region (Fig. 22.2B, C, D). Again morselized graft can be used to complete the reconstruction. Small cemented acetabular components are a necessary inventory consideration for the use of the ring fixation systems.

A final inventory option for reconstructions involving massive bone loss would be the total allograft acetabulum. This allograft segment is bolted to the ilium and possibly to the ischial or pubic structures.[6] Reconstruction plates, dynamic compression (DCP) plates, or lag screws will be necessary in multiple lengths and dimensions (Fig. 22.2G). The allograft acetabulum will need to be reamed. Because of the bone type involved, an inventory of cemented components will be necessary as the final reconstructive implant.[6]

Femur

Femoral reconstruction can be addressed in many different ways. A brief discussion of cemented femoral revision options is followed by more involved suggestions for cementless revision femoral stems on the basis of femoral deficiency.

Cemented femoral components are considered an option for revision surgery in the hip with fresh femoral

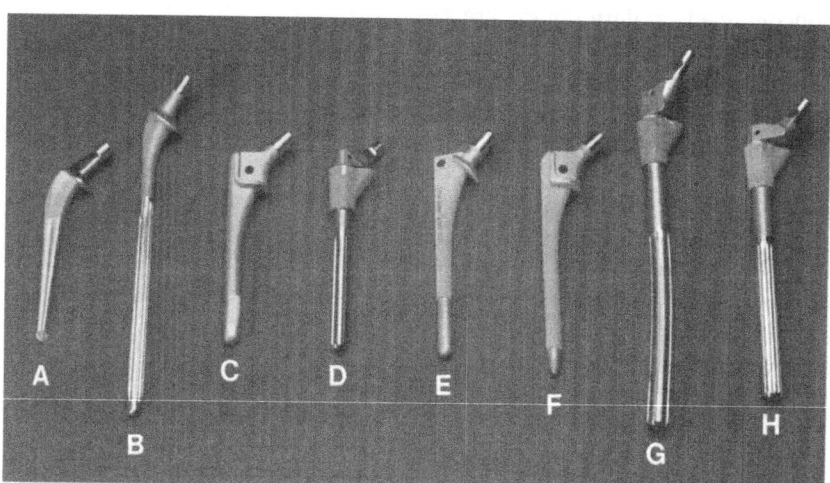

Figure 22.3. A. Spectrum primary cemented femoral component. (Smith Nephew Richards, Memphis, Tennessee.) B. Long-stem cemented femoral component. (Howmedica Corp, Rutherford, New Jersey.) C. Cemented calcar-replacing AML prosthesis. (De Puy, Warsaw, Indiana.) D. S-ROM standard length cementless modular femoral component. (Johnson & Johnson, Raynham, Massachusetts.) E. 5/8 coated cementless AML femoral cementless prosthesis. (De Puy, Warsaw, Indiana.) F. Calcar-replacing 7/8 coated AML cementless femoral component. (De Puy, Warsaw, Indiana.) G. S-ROM long-bowed stem cementless femoral component with modular proximal metaphyseal section and calcar-replacing femoral neck. (Johnson & Johnson, Raynham, Massachusetts.) H. S-ROM long-stem straight femoral component with proximal metaphyseal modularity and standard neck. (Johnson & Johnson, Raynham, Massachusetts.)

bone stock available or in the patient with limited predicted demand (Fig. 22.3A). Cemented components, as with cementless counterparts, must include options for longer stems and calcar replacement (Fig. 22.3B, C). Femoral bone stock must be rather optimal for cemented revision to be considered.[3]

For most revision settings, proximal metaphyseal bone is the likely area of deficiency. Proximal femoral bone loss must be assessed to make an accurate prediction of preoperative inventory demands. Femoral bone deficiencies can be difficult to predict, making inventory for femoral revisions challenging to organize. For implant suggestion purposes, we have divided femoral deficiencies into three categories: mild proximal metaphyseal deficiency, moderate proximal metaphyseal deficiency, and severe proximal metaphyseal deficiency including intercalary shaft deficiencies.[7] A discussion of neck length and offset closes this section on femoral revision implant inventory.

In the femur with minimal proximal bone deficiency, an inventory of unibody or primary modular cementless stems may be all that is necessary (Fig. 22.3D, E). With limited proximal deficiency, the metaphysis will provide bone for ingrowth, rotational stability, and adequate femoral length.

Moderate proximal bone deficiencies require intraoperative flexibility from implants. An inventory of distal diaphyseal ingrowth components such as the anatomic medullary locking (AML), fully coated component can be used (Fig. 22.3F).[7] Proximally coated modular revision components such as the S-ROM can use remaining metaphyseal bone for support and still gain rotational stability through fluted longer stems.[8] Bowed stems are a necessary inventory item in situations in which the stem will extend into the middle section of the diaphysis in an anatomically correct femur (Fig. 22.3G). Straight long stems are an inventory consideration for osteotomized femurs or those with distortion of the normal femoral bow (Fig. 22.3H). If deficiency extends to or below the lesser trochanter, neck length must be addressed preoperatively to have calcar replacing components amongst the revision inventory.

In the most severe proximal bone loss situations, the more distally coated, fixed components may be necessary. A fully coated device with diaphyseal fixation such as the AML revision system may be quite adequate for more severe proximal bone loss (Fig. 22.3F).[7] In the most severe situations of proximal bone loss, the inventory may include a proximal femoral allograft. A total proximal femoral allograft will need to be combined with a component suitable for cement fixation into the allograft as well as diaphyseal fixation of the host femur either with or without cement. A selection of long-stem components such as the S-ROM will permit cement fixation to the proximal allograft with press-fit rotational purchase of the host diaphysis distally (Fig. 22.3G).[9] A long-stem cemented component can offer cement fixation to both proximal allograft and host bone (Fig. 22.3B).

Intercalary defects in the femur must be considered preoperatively. Defects must be bridged by a distance of two and one half canal diameters to protect intercalary deficiencies.[10] Predicted defects can be those already existing or those that may be necessary for existing implant or cement removal. A long-stem prosthesis can be bowed or straight as noted earlier (Fig. 22.3G, H). Unless there is an osteotomy performed or abnormal femoral anatomy, an inventory of bowed stems will be necessary when length past the proximal third of the diaphysis is desired.

Long stems such as the S-ROM can provide proximal modularity, flute rotational stability, and tuning fork construction for distal flexibility. When intercalary defects are suspected preoperatively or intraoperatively, fresh-frozen strut allograft might also be considered in the prosthetic inventory.[11] Wires (16 or 18 gauge) will be necessary to fix strut allografts or longitudinal splits that may be discovered during or caused by revision prosthesis placement (Fig. 22.4A). A single fixed cable system (eg, Dall-Miles cable system) can be used but cannot be retightened after being crimp-fixed (Fig. 22.4B).

Femoral reconstruction inventory in deficiencies to or below the lesser trochanter must include a calcar-replacing neck prosthesis. As has been touched on earlier, implant inventory should include a selection of calcar-replacing prostheses (Fig. 22.4C, D, E). With these, lateralized necks and additional offset should be considered in the inventory as well. Lateralized neck components such as the S-ROM +8 lateral prosthesis can re-

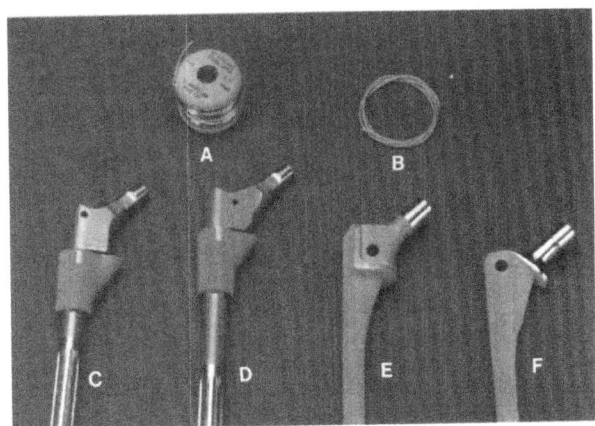

Figure 22.4. A. 18-gauge stainless steel wire. (V Mueller & Co.) B. Dall–Miles cable. (Howmedica Corp, Rutherford, New Jersey.) C. S-ROM calcar-replacing femoral neck. (Johnson & Johnson, Raynham, Massachusetts.) D. S-ROM calcar-replacing neck +8-mm lateralized component. (Johnson & Johnson, Raynham, Massachusetts.) E. AML calcar-replacing femoral neck. (De Puy, Warsaw, Indiana.) F. Lateralized cementless femoral AML component. (De Puy, Warsaw, Indiana.)

store substantial abductor tension and stability without distorting length (Fig. 22.4D, E, F).[10]

Greater Trochanter

Many reconstructive hip surgeries will necessitate fixation of the trochanter at the end of the procedure. Trochanteric fixation can be necessary in the insufficiency fracture of revision proximal bone or after elective trochanteric or extended trochanteric osteotomies.

The insufficiency fracture can occur in any hip revision setting. Inventory for revision hip surgery must include some type of possible fixation. A 16- or 18-gauge wire can be cut in length adequate for wire trochanteric fixation (Fig. 22.5A). Prepackaged clamps (eg, Dall-Miles cable clamps) provide predictable purchase of the trochanter and secure fixation around the proximal femur (Fig. 22.5B). Dall-Miles trochanteric clamps are available in three sizes and can fit most revision bone needs.

Trochanteric bolts are also available. This fixation alternative involves bolt fixation through the trochanter into the hip revision prosthesis. This option is available in the S-ROM revision prosthesis. The bolt fixes the trochanteric clamp directly to the shoulder of the prosthesis (Fig. 22.5C). An inventory of trochanteric fixation devices is critical to complete the revision total hip surgical inventory.

Conclusion

Hospital implant inventories are rapidly shrinking to cut costs. For specialized cases, the surgeon and hospitals are forced to import implants. The surgical team must attempt to accurately predict the intraoperative needs for the revision total hip arthroplasty. Preoperative planning must be done early enough to have specialized equipment available, completely enough to have implant flexibility for all possible problems, but efficiently enough not to have large volumes of unnecessary equipment on hand.

References

1. D'Antonio J, Capello W, Borden L, Barger WL, Bierbaum BF, Boettcher WG, et al. Classification and management of acetabular abnormalities in total hip arthroplasty. *Clin Orthop.* 1989;243:126–137.
2. Padgett D, Kuff L, Rosenburg A, Sumner DR, Galante JO. Revision of the acetabular component without cement after total hip arthroplasty: 3–6 year follow-up. *J Bone Joint Surg Am.* 1993;75:663–673.
3. Callaghan J, Salvati E, Pellicci P, Wilson PD Jr, Ranawat CS. Results of revision for mechanical failure after cemented total hip replacement, 1979–1982: a 2–5 year follow-up. *J Bone Joint Surg Am.* 1985;67:1074–1085.
4. Estok D, Harris W. Long term results of cemented femoral revision surgery using second-generation techniques: an average 11.7 year follow-up evaluation. *Clin Orthop.* 1994;299:190–202.
5. Gross A, Allan D, Catre M, Garbuz DS, Stockley I. Bone grafts and hip replacement surgery: the pelvic side. *Orthop Clin North Am.* 1993;24:679–695.
6. Paprosky W, Magnus R. Principles of bone grafting in revision total hip arthroplasty: acetabular technique. *Clin Orthop.* 1994;298:147–155.
7. Lawrence J, Engh C, Macalino G. Revision total hip arthroplasty: long term results without cement. *Clin Orthop.* 1993;24:635–644.
8. Cameron H. The two to six year results with a proximally modular noncemented total hip replacement used in hip revisions. *Clin Orthop.* 1994;298:47–53.
9. Chandler HP, Clark J, Murphy S, McCarthy J, Penenberg B, Danylchuk K, et al. Reconstruction of major segmental loss of the proximal femur in revision total hip arthroplasty. *Clin Orthop.* 1994;298:67–74.
10. D'Antonio J, McCarthy J, Bargar W, Borden LS, Cappelo WN, Collis DK, et al. Classification of femoral abnormalities in total hip arthroplasty. *Clin Orthop.* 1993;296:133–139.
11. Pak J, Paprosky W, Jablonsky W, Lawrence JM. Femoral strut allografts in cementless revision total hip arthroplasty. *Clin Orthop.* 1993;295:172–178.

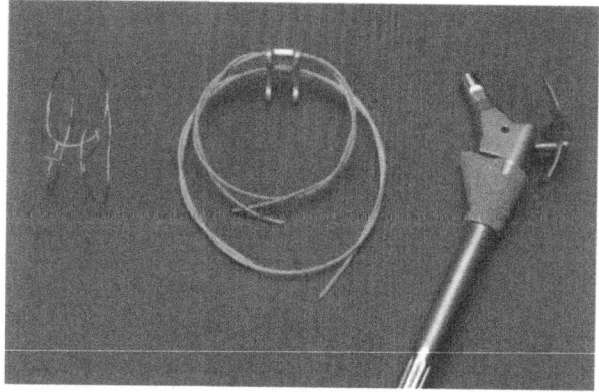

Figure 22.5. A. 18-gauge stainless steel wire for trochanteric fixation. (V Mueller Co.) B. Dall–Miles Cable Grip™ system. (Howmedica Corp., Rutherford, New Jersey.) C. S-ROM revision femoral stem with trochanteric bolt. (Johnson & Johnson, Raynham, Massachusetts.)

Part 4
Surgical Techniques in Revision Total Hip Arthroplasty

Section 1
Femur

Joseph C. McCarthy and James V. Bono

Although acetabular component reconstruction is a common occurrence in revision total hip surgery, it is femoral component reconstruction that presents the most formidable challenge to the surgeon. Failure of the femoral prosthesis may be the result of cemented or cementless loosening, malposition, component and/or bony fracture, infection, instability, leg length discrepancy, or osteolysis. (See Part 1.) Component failure is often accompanied by remarkable segmental or cavitary bone loss or stress-shielding. Implant extraction is considerably more difficult in this environment. Prophylactic cerclage femoral wiring may be necessary to avoid shattering the femur.

In addition, the femur may contain a long cement column or distal plug that is adherent to the cortex. It may be difficult to distinguish the methylcrylate from endosteal bone, especially about the isthmus. Careful cement removal methods are necessary or bone stock will be further compromised. A well ingrown but malpositioned or infected femoral prosthesis is a special challenge. An extensile surgical approach (see Part 4.2) and designated tools, such as flexible high-speed bits or diamond wheels to disrupt the porous bond and/or cut the implant are often required.

After component extraction has been accomplished, femoral bone stock needs to be reassessed and provisions made for the new implant. In this part, we examine the rationale and specific techniques of bone graft augmentation and implant reconstruction. All authors detail their methods, surgical decision making, and tips for obtaining a successful outcome. After implant fixation is addressed, trochanteric reattachment is discussed.

Part 4
Surgical Techniques in Radical Tumor Surgery

23
Reconstruction of Cavitary Defects: Bone Grafting

James P. Jamison

Femoral cavitary defects present a true challenge to the reconstructive hip surgeon. As described by D'Antonio et al., cavitary defects are contained lesions. The cortical shell remains intact while cancellous and endosteal cortical bone are eroded through several different mechanisms.[1] The surgeon is faced with a sclerotic, irregular endosteal surface, which may provide neither osseous apposition nor stability for the revision implant.[2] Discussion of treatment for this difficult problem focuses on the state of the revision femur, classification of femoral deficiencies, philosophies in revision, preoperative planning, component choices, and grafting options. Despite variations in systems of classification, approach, and management of this difficult problem, the goals of pain relief, bone loss arrest, bone stock restoration,[3] and long-term mechanical stability are constants throughout the literature.[4]

State of the Revision Femur

Loss of femoral bone stock in the revision setting is the result of a multifactorial process. Osteolysis is a frequent culprit in failure because of bone erosion and loosening, producing great potential for femoral destruction and creating difficult problems in revision. Osteolysis is initiated by wear particles of polyethylene, cement, and metal, and it may present with either isolated or generalized bone loss. The membrane within these osteolytic lesions contains wear particle debris and secretes enzymes responsible for bony destruction.[5] Areas of osteolysis may be separated by areas of solid fixation of bone, cement, and prosthesis. As a result, stress risers are formed at the points of osteolytic defects, necessitating early intervention to prevent further bone loss or fracture of bone or prosthesis. In such situations, the bone is usually fragile, exposure and cement removal are difficult, and blood loss is large.[6]

The deficient femur can result from other sources as well. Mechanical instability caused by osteolysis compounds the problem.[7] Aging causes decreased bone mass by means of endosteal resorption and poor periosteal bone formation.[8] The resultant widened canal diameter compensates for decreased cortical thickness, in an attempt to protect the femur against torsional and bending stresses. This process may or may not compromise component fixation.[9,10] Iatrogenic bone loss in revision surgery with component and cement removal is often unavoidable. Stress-shielding promotes cortical hypertrophy at the point of fixation of a stiff metal stem, with atrophy more proximally in the less stiff, unstressed femur. The surgeon must also be suspicious of infection as a source of osteolysis in the revision setting.[11] The avascular state of the bone and of the scarred, contracted, and indurated soft tissues, heightens the risk of infection.[12,13]

Other possible pitfalls must also be recognized. Cortical defects may result purposefully by the creation of cortical windows for component and cement removal or inadvertently with the use of power tools. A longer stem is then required to bypass the defect and prevent fracture. The smooth sclerotic endosteal surface encountered when revising a cemented stem makes cemented revision more difficult, with poor cement interdigitation into bone and reduced shear strength at the bone–cement interface, as compared with findings in primary arthroplasties.[14] Suboptimal quality of the soft tissues and potential for leg shortening can lead to instability and dislocation.[15]

Classification of Femoral Deficiencies

Classification systems are meant to assist the surgeon in determining the best treatment options for a given problem, to aid in uniform evaluation and reporting of cases, and to be easy to remember and apply. Several systems have been described for evaluation and management of femoral cavitary defects, although no one system has received universal acceptance.[16]

Engh, Glassman, et al.[4,17] reported a relatively simple guide to this problem, categorizing defects as mild, moderate, or severe bone loss. Cases in which the neck and isthmus remain intact, bone loss is minimal, and no grafting is required are described as mild. Moderate damage describes those cases in which the isthmus remains intact, but the femoral neck and intertrochanteric area are deficient such as in a failed cemented stem collapsed into varus. In this category, diaphyseal bone stock remains intact. There are no cortical perforations, but there is proximal thinning and calcar destruction. Severe bone loss refers to damage in both the femoral neck and the isthmus.

Paprosky[18] categorized femoral deficiency relative to the femur's ability to support an extensively porous-coated femoral component. Type I femurs have partial calcar, anterior and posterior loss and an intact metaphysis and diaphysis. They require no bone graft. Type II femurs have major anteroposterior bone loss and a deficient calcar, but the diaphysis is intact. Subgroups a to c describe degrees of metaphyseal loss. Type III refers to those femurs that have progressed to loss of diaphyseal as well as metaphyseal bone with deficiency of the entire proximal femur.

Two other simple methods of describing femoral defects have been devised. Mallory[6] used a grading system for the revision femur in which type I indicates an essentially intact femoral cortex and medullary canal, and type II refers to loss of medullary bone only with an intact cortex. Progression is seen in type III to involve the cortex. Subgroups of type III describe the level of cortical involvement. Gustillo and Pasternak[15] divided component loosening and bone loss into four types. In type I minimal endosteal or inner cortical bone is lost, whereas in type II the proximal canal may be enlarged by 50% or more, possibly with a small lateral wall defect. Type III indicates gross instability with a posteromedial wall defect involving the lesser trochanter, whereas in type IV there is total proximal circumferential loss.

Chandler and Penenberg[19] based their classification system of femoral defects on femoral anatomy. Type I involves calcar deficiency, either intramedullary or total, whereas type II concerns the deficient trochanter. Types III and IV describe cortical thinning and perforation, respectively. Type V includes fracture about or below the implant, and type VI involves circumferential deficiency of the metaphysis and proximal diaphysis.

D'Antonio et al. and the American Academy of Orthopedic Surgeons (AAOS) Committee on the Hip developed a classification of femoral abnormalities in a collaborative effort to standardize nomenclature for assistance in preoperative planning and reporting of cases. This system resembles the AAOS classification for acetabular defects reported in 1989.[20] Type I describes segmental defects, or lesions in the supporting shell, further categorized as proximal, intercalary, or involving the greater trochanter. Cavitary defects, the focus of this chapter, constitute type II. Subgroups are referred to as cancellous (mild), cortical (moderate), and ectatic (medullary expansion). Type III involves combined segmental and cavitary lesions, whereas type IV describes malalignment. Type V indicates femoral stenosis, and type VI involves femoral discontinuity or fracture. Each category is further assigned a level of involvement. Level I lies proximal to the inferior border of the lesser trochanter. Level II extends 10 cm below level I. Level III is distal to level II. Bone loss is also graded in this system. Grade I indicates minimal bone loss with maintenance of host–prosthesis contact and no requirement for bone grafting. Grade II describes some loss of host–prosthesis contact, but sustained prosthesis support. Morselized grafting is not required for stability in revision in these cases, but it may be beneficial to fill voids. Grade III is most severe with great loss of host–prosthesis contact such that successful revision relies on the use of structural grafting.[1] Although somewhat involved, this system is believed to be the most comprehensive and widely accepted.[16]

Philosophies in Revision

Several investigators have outlined their approach to revision of femoral components. Although specific preferences may vary, many of the basic principles run current through their management of these difficult cases.

Hozack et al.[3] list the goals of revision hip surgery as pain relief, bone loss arrest, and bone stock restoration. A primary tenet in realizing these ends is achieving initial stability of the implant on host bone to reduce the chance of failure and further bone loss.[2,4,6,21,22] To prevent catastrophic implant failure from progressive defects, early intervention is recommended once progressive bone loss is identified on serial radiographs.[6,11] At times intervention may be indicated before the hip becomes symptomatic.[6]

Cemented revision is advocated by some investigators in specific situations. However, cementless implants are favored by most investigators. Two schools of thought predominate: (1) proximal fixation and restoration of proximal femoral bone stock loss through grafting, which may pose a risk to immediate implant stability,[15,21] or (2) immediate fixation and stability in distal healthier bone, which risks the effects of proximal stress-shielding[4,11] and possible worsening of bone loss. Bone grafting is considered to be an integral step in bone stock restoration by most investigators, but it is avoided by others. Ideas on management with respect to preoperative planning, implant choice, and bone grafting are discussed next.

Preoperative Planning

Management of cavitary femoral defects in revision total hip surgery begins, as always, with proper preoperative evaluation and planning. Radiographs in the anteroposterior and lateral planes that reveal the entire length of the existing implant and cement column are critical. Oblique views may show areas of cortical thinning not seen on routine films. The addition of magnification markers is beneficial in determining implant sizes. Such analysis will allow classification of femoral defects and evaluation of bone grafting or special implant requirements.[1,16,19]

A reflex thought in evaluation of the painful total hip replacement should be suspicion of infection. As noted earlier, infection may cause osteolysis and cavitary defects.[11] Work-up for possible infection usually consists of laboratory tests (sedimentation rate, white blood cell count, and C-reactive protein), aspiration, and/or bone scans.[1,6,16]

Identification of the existing implants from the patient's old records is quite helpful, and templating in both the AP and lateral planes is a key step to a successful revision. The proper width and length of stem to fill the canal and bypass defects can be estimated, as can appropriate neck length and offset to restore leg length, abductor function, and femoral head center of rotation.[1,6]

Component Options

Cemented Femoral Components

Pierson and Harris[23] described a series of 29 cemented revisions of cemented femoral components, all with moderate or extensive cortical osteolysis. No bone graft was used. At an average follow-up of 8.5 years, recurrence of osteolysis was seen in two cases (6.9%). Subsidence was seen in one, and 25 components (86%) remained well fixed radiographically. Mean Harris hip scores improved from 53 preoperatively to 81 after revision. These results illustrate success with cemented revision in femurs with large cavitary defects without osteolytic progression.

In their report on 106 cemented revisions without bone graft for severe femoral osteolytic cavitary defects, Raut et al.[24] found 95.3% to be well fixed at a mean follow-up of 6.3 years. New endosteal cavitations were seen in 16%, but they were defined as large in only 1.9%. These investigators cited the work by Gie et al. and their success in reconstitution of bone stock with allografting,[7] but Raut et al. found their own results without bone grafting to be encouraging.[24]

Turner et al.[25] reviewed their series of 165 long-stem cemented revision stems inserted without bone graft for aseptic loosening of cemented primary arthroplasties. Clinical follow-up of 139 hips revealed failure in 17 cases (12%), with 11 cases of aseptic loosening, two component fractures, one shaft fracture, and three infections. Radiographic analysis showed 24% with progressive femoral lucencies at average follow-up of 6 to 7 years. Twenty-one percent of femurs demonstrated lucencies involving greater than 50% of the bone-cement interface. Three serious complications (myocardial infarction, prolonged hypotension, and death) occurred during cementing. An advantage of the cemented long stem was seen in the ability to bypass deficiencies in the proximal femur to obtain rigid bone–cement fixation in distal bony trabeculae. Stability obtained with isthmus fixation was believed to prevent motion, which could lead to further bone resorption and component loosening. Disadvantages included cement intrusion into distal normal bone, increased technical difficulty, and potential stress-shielding of the previously pathologic proximal femur.[25,26] The investigators reviewed the work of Pellicci et al.[27,28] and Callaghan et al.,[29] showing significant postoperative and progressive radiolucencies after cemented femoral revision and the overall inferior quality of cemented fixation in revision surgery, as compared with findings in primary arthroplasty. They found a high correlation of loosening with proximal bone stock deficiencies and radiolucent lines on initial postoperative radiographs. In light of these findings, Turner et al.[30] narrowed their indications for cemented revisions to older patients with a shorter life expectancy and poorer rehabilitation potential, previously septic cases to allow use of antibiotic-impregnated cement, and cases demonstrating long-term tolerance to cement (no significant osteolysis or bone defects). A move toward cementless revision was preferred in younger patients and cases with fracture or bone stock deficiencies requiring bone grafting.

Wilson[31] outlined his criterion for cemented versus cementless femoral revision. He found the degree of bone stock compromise to be far more important than gender, age, weight, or diagnosis for determining implant selection. Cemented stems were selected in cases with good preservation of bone stock or in which sound bone–cement fixation could be obtained with larger and/or longer stems. Examples included fractured femoral components with a healthy bone–cement interface and aseptic loosening when revision was addressed before much bone stock damage had occurred. Cementless fixation was preferred in cases with large cavitary bone stock deficiencies requiring grafting, including those with femoral subsidence, and autograft was favored over allograft (see later discussion).

Wirta et al.[32] described a series of 16 hips revised with cemented stems for aggressive granulomatosis or cavitary defects. Twelve were multifocal, and four were solitary. Three were located distally. Two patients developed recurrence of aggressive granulomatous lesions at their original sites. Because of this 12.5% recurrence, the investigators noted their move to revision with cementless femoral components and bone grafting of defects.

In cases with an essentially intact cortex and medullary contents after component removal, Mallory[6] advocated use of either cemented or cementless stems. Cemented revision was preferred in the elderly patient (older than 60 years), and cementless was preferred in patients younger than 60 years with a greater potential for bone ingrowth. In all other revision situations Mallory opted for cementless components. Hedley et al.[33] also supported cemented components for first-time revisions in elderly patients, but they preferred cementless revision with bone grafting in most cases.

Cementless Femoral Components

Bargar et al.[21] reported on a series of 47 revisions with the use of porous-ingrowth femoral prostheses custom designed from plain findings on radiographs and computer tomography scans. The choice of the custom stem was not based on the presence of a particular bone defect pattern or location. Thirty-four percent required structural grafting to restore bone stock, not for prosthesis stability. Particulate grafting was used in all cases. All defects were bypassed by 3 canal diameters with stems extending at least 3 canal diameters into the isthmus. Nineteen percent had intraoperative proximal femur fractures with seating of the prosthesis, and 15% subsided greater than 3 mm. These investigators favored the custom prosthesis to reduce the amount of bone graft required to fill defects, thereby encouraging more successful ingrowth for fixation and possibly reducing graft donor site morbidity. They also believed that the custom implant may provide more uniform implant loading and stress transfer, preventing stress-shielding or fracture. Any failure of ingrowth was attributed to the relatively small surface area of the porous surfaces placed anteriorly, posteriorly, and medially. Defects were classified according to AAOS criteria.[1] Proximal cancellous cavitary defects were present in nearly every case. Cortical defects were usually in levels I and II, and they were present in 70% of cases. The custom canal-filling metaphyseal portion of the stem addresses the proximal cavitary defects because it was designed to contact remaining cortical bone circumferentially. Cortical cavitary defects at level III were treated as stress risers, bone grafted, and bypassed by the stem.[21]

Engh et al.[4,17] cited reports[27,34] of cemented femoral component instability ranging from 25% to 51%, as the stimulus for their investigation of cementless femoral revision. They reported a series of 127 such cases. Immediate implant stability was noted as an absolute necessity. In cases of significant bone loss the osteogenic potential of the thin, sclerotic, hypovascular bone was believed to be minimal. They favored obtaining initial implant stability by press-fitting an extensively porous coated stem into the healthy bone distal to the defects. Bone grafting was not believed to be beneficial (see discussion later). Fixation was graded as optimal in 86% of cases and as fibrous stable in 13%. One percent of failures of fixation were with a cylindric stem. Using this technique they found no correlation between the extent of femoral bone stock loss and final radiographic stability.[4] A minimum 3-year follow-up of this same group of patients, now with 202 femoral revisions, 81% were classified as stable with bone ingrowth; 12%, as stable with fibrous encapsulation; and 7%, as mechanical failures, half of which were re-revised. Mechanical failure was somewhat more likely in the face of severe bone stock damage, but the ability to maintain stability—bony or fibrous—did not differ.[17]

A long-stem, extensively porous-coated prosthesis was also favored by Roberson[11] when revising femurs with extensive proximal cavitary deficiencies. He noted that the component must be of large diameter to fit the canal and long enough to bypass deficiencies and reach the isthmus for stability, facilitating ingrowth.

In their evaluation of 57 cementless revisions with a proximal porous ingrowth stem and bone grafting, Gustillo and Pasternak[15,35] documented reconstitution of cortical bone with increased density and thickness in many cases. Subsidence was noted in 11 patients and was progressive in 5, 4 of whom underwent re-revision. They preferred this technique, with collar contact at the calcar, proper neck length and anteversion, and a long, curved stem being essential for stability and enhancement of ingrowth.

Hedley et al.[33] showed a preference for cementless revision, usually with a standard length stem. Fifty-four femoral revisions were reported, all with bone graft in the form of slurry placed within the canal to fill defects. Clinical results were excellent or good in 90% of cases. New radiolucencies covering more than 50% of the stem–bone interface were seen in 10% of cases, whereas new radiolucencies covering less than 50% of the interface were seen in 60%. Overall, more radiolucencies were noted distally over the smooth portion of the stem. A positive response of proximal cancellous bone was seen with hypertrophic densification in one third of cases. Cortical hypertrophy was seen distally. Despite substantial proximal bone stock destruction, maximum subsidence was 5 mm.

Contrary to Engh et al.,[4,17] Peters and co-authors[36] found a trend toward decreased stability with increased severity of bone loss in cementless revision. Forty-nine cases with a proximal ingrowth stem were evaluated at an average follow-up of more than 5 years. At revision, 84% had cortical or ectatic cavitary metaphyseal bone loss. All cases involved particulate grafting of the femur. Analysis demonstrated 96% chance of survival at 6 years with revision as the end point, but only 37% chance of survival at 6 years with subsidence added as an indicator of failure. Forty-five percent of cases had progressive subsidence or definite loosening. No statistical significance was reached, but a definite trend was seen toward decreased component stability with increased preoperative loss of femoral bone stock. Both a qualitative and a quantitative increase in proximal bone stock was noted in the most deficient femurs. Their findings demonstrated enhancement of bone stock in the more severely deficient femurs and preservation of bone stock even in the face of subsidence. Despite good clinical results, the rate of subsidence and loosening was unacceptably high. They concluded that a noncircumferentially porous-coated, long-stem, titanium femoral component is not appropriate for revision with moderate or severe metaphyseal bone loss.

Grafting Options

Opinions vary on both the necessity of bone graft and the optimal grafting substance in treatment of cavitary lesions at the time of femoral revision. Greis and co-authors[37] and Kang et al.[38] outlined characteristics of the ideal graft material in hip surgery. It should be readily available, aid in providing initial support to the prosthesis despite the defect, and promote both rapid defect healing and bone ingrowth at the adjacent porous-coated implant surface to provide biologic fixation and enhance stability. The following review examines the use of bone graft and the effectiveness of different regimens in achieving these ends.

Revision without Bone Graft

In reports of revision with a fully porous-coated femoral component, Engh et al.[4,17] maintain that morselized bone graft is of no benefit in providing immediate stability, facilitating proximal ingrowth, or augmenting viable bone stock. The ability of their straight, cylindric, canal-filling stem to gain direct contact with viable bone distal to any proximal defects seemed to preclude the use of graft.

Meding and co-authors[39] reviewed 32 long-stem revision procedures performed without bone grafting. Maximal proximal and distal canal fill was observed. Proximal osteopenia (stress-shielding) progressed with time up to 2 years. Cortical hypertrophy at the tip of the stem was present in 41% of cases at final evaluation, and endosteal new bone formation was noted in 25%. Prosthetic subsidence greater than or equal to 2 mm was found in 9% of cases, and 53% of cases formed pedestals. Distal pedestal formation and distal cortical hypertrophy correlated with proximal osteopenia. All 32 had excellent function and 26 were painfree at final evaluation. Despite the proximal osteopenia, the investigators believed that a proximally coated, uncemented, long-stem femoral component provided good clinical outcome and adequate early fixation without bone grafting.

The success of cemented revision without bone grafting in the face of moderate or extensive osteolysis, as described by Raut et al.[24] and Pierson and Harris,[23] was discussed earlier. However, no mention was made, nor does it seem likely, that bone stock reconstitution can result from this technique.

At New England Baptist Hospital, the majority of femoral cavitary defects are currently managed by revision with a proximally porous-coated, distally fluted modular implant without bone grafting. In developing this technique, recognition was given to the difficulty in placing particulate bone graft accurately within canal defects. In addition, the risk of fracture with insertion of a canal-filling stem into a medullary cavity packed with bone graft was also recognized. Success with this approach is illustrated in Fig. 23.1. The physiologic response of bone to early postoperative weight-bearing is believed to assist in bone stock reconstitution (J. Bono, unpublished data, 1997).

Revision with Bone Graft

In a review of 59 cementless femoral revisions in patients with focal femoral cavitary defects, Hozack et al.[3] used cancellous allograft bone paste in 28 cases, noting that their technique did not guarantee complete filling of all defects. No components migrated and all were observed to be stable by using Engh criteria.[40] At minimum 2-year follow-up, no cavitary lesions had progressed, and 56% had healed completely. No difference was found in healing potential with respect to proximity to porous or smooth zones of the stem. Interestingly, no difference was noted in healing potential when comparing grafted to nongrafted defects. They identified surgical debridement of defects to be the key to stabilizing defect progression. Although no real benefit was found with grafting, the investigators recognized that a more meticulous technique of graft application may demonstrate a positive effect.[3]

Bargar et al.[21] support the use of particulate autogenous bone graft to fill defects whenever possible. Their custom cementless stem was designed to contact remaining cortical bone, serving a theoretic dual purpose. First, it gave greater stability to the implant without reliance on bone graft. Second, it decreased the amount of autograft required to fill the defects, so as to save the creation of a donor site in many cases, avoiding the morbidity inherent therein. They found ingrowth in at least one of three proximal mesh pads in 74% of cases. Subsidence of greater than 3 mm was noted in seven cases, five of which stabilized. They believed that bone graft in small quantities was beneficial. However, it was believed to hinder fixation when required for implant support or when placed in large quantities between host bone and the ingrowth surface.

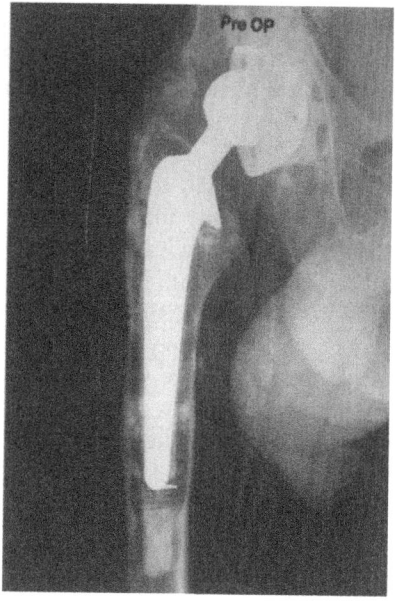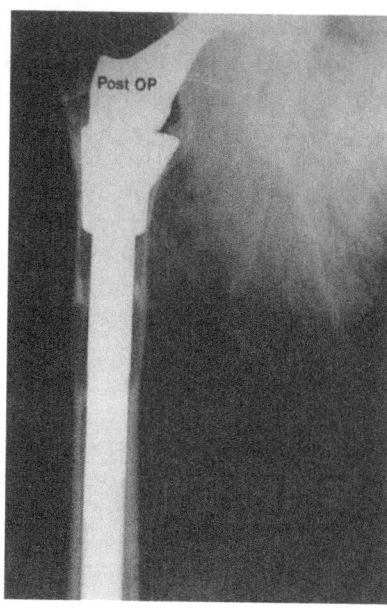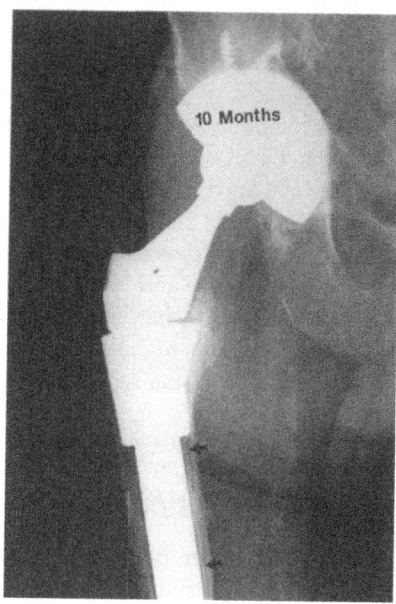

Figure 23.1. Use of a proximally porous-coated, distally fluted modular implant without bone grafting.

Eskola et al.[41] described cementless femoral revision for aggressive granulomatous lesions in 16 cases, 9 of which involved cancellous bone grafting of cavities. Consolidation of the cavitary defects was noted by an average of 16 months with grafting and 14 to 19 months without grafting. No criterion for grafting versus no grafting was stated, nor was the type of graft used. No components subsided. The investigators noted their previous success in treating such cases with cemented revision, but they cited the risk of possibly catastrophic recurrence of cavitary defects as cause for concern. Results with cementless revision and bone grafting were favored.

Wilson[31] stated his preference for cementless revision and autografting for revision femurs with bony deficiencies. Eight cases showed significant femoral bone loss, all of which were revised with a porous ingrowth stem supplemented by autograft. Defect size required the addition of allograft in two of these cases, but Wilson took care to place autograft only in contact with the porous ingrowth plates. No report of outcome was given, but Wilson's preferences were clear.

Gustillo and Pasternak[15] used autograft, allograft, or both to fill defects, along with a porous ingrowth prosthesis. They observed increased thickness and density of cortical bone at 12 to 24 months postoperatively. The four re-revisions for loose femoral components in their 57-case series were attributed to component undersizing, not to prevention of ingrowth from the presence of a mass of bone graft.

In a canine model, McDonald et al.[2] evaluated the effect of autograft and allograft in enhancing ingrowth fixation in femoral revision. Much greater ingrowth was seen in grafted specimens versus those without graft, with no significant difference being observed between autograft and allograft groups. The autograft group showed greater ultimate shear strength than the control group, with a positive correlation to ingrowth. Radiographic evaluation demonstrated more frequent radiolucencies and subsidence in the nongrafted control group, with significantly less ingrowth and strength of fixation. The investigators preferred autograft as the material of choice to repair bony defects, but they recognized allograft bone as a viable alternative.

Autograft and freeze-dried allograft enhancement of ingrowth into porous coated implants in dog humeri was investigated by Kienapfel et al.[42] They found that across a 3-mm gap packed with graft, autograft specimens showed new bone formation at 2 weeks with some ingrowth. By 8 weeks, they resembled normal bone with extensive areas of ingrowth. Allograft specimens showed some new bone formation, although less than autograft specimens; no ingrowth at 2 weeks; and only occasional ingrowth at 8 weeks. In mechanical testing autograft implants had much greater strengths of fixation than implants in the control group at 4 weeks. Allograft strength of fixation was greater, but not significantly so. By 8 weeks fixation, strength in autografts was double that of controls, but not with statistical significance. There was no difference between allografts and controls at 8 weeks. These authors concluded that autograft enhances new bone formation, bone ingrowth, and strength of fixation. By comparison, freeze-dried allograft did not improve new bone formation or ingrowth, with only a small increase in strength of fixation being observed. Autograft was clearly superior, whereas allograft was recognized as being of some benefit in facilitating new bone formation across the defect. These results would imply that, although autograft is better overall, freeze-dried allograft is useful in filling defects around implant surfaces in which there is no porous coating and no expectation for ingrowth.

In their review of 49 cementless revisions, Peters et al.[36] reported using particulate allograft bone, autograft bone, or both to fill defects in the femoral canal in each case. They believed that cancellous endosteal bone graft, whether autograft or allograft, enhances bone stock in severely deficient femora.

Nelson et al.[43] reported three cases in which cemented femoral components were revised with uncemented stems and cancellous particulate allograft. Their technique involved packing the medullary canal with graft to ensure complete filling of defects, then milling a fresh canal through the graft to seat the prosthesis. They noted adequate allograft incorporation in each case.

In their study of cementless femoral revision, Hedley and associates[33] used allograft bone to supplement defects. Although subsidence was noted, they considered a maximum of 5 mm in this series to be small, considering the substantial proximal bone stock destruction in many cases. Often the proximal porous surface of the stem was nearly surrounded by allograft bone slivers or paste. No evidence of late bone ingrowth from consolidated allograft was noted, and fixation in these cases was assumed to be primarily fibrous. Overall, these investigators noted a remarkable reconstitution of cortex with the use of bone graft and a noncemented stem.

Fitzgerald et al.[22] evaluated the performance of autograft, allograft, and hydroxylapatite-tricalcium phosphate (HA/TCP) crystals in filling defects and enhancing ingrowth. In a revision setting in dogs, ingrowth was much greater with the use of autograft or allograft, when compared with no grafting, with no statistically significant difference between the grafting groups. Greater stability was seen with autograft, because vertical subsidence was more common without grafting and with allograft. Radiolucencies were noted in each of the nongrafted specimens (three of three), two of which subsided. In the autograft group radiolucencies were apparent in three of six specimens, with one subsidence. The allograft group demonstrated radiolucencies in only one of five cases, with no subsidence. Histologic evaluation demonstrated equal incorporation of autograft and allograft at 12 weeks in this canine model. They concluded that autograft and allograft incorporated equally well and provided comparable fixation and mechanical strength.

Kang et al.[38] conducted an evaluation of femoral and acetabular defect response to no grafting, grafting with autologous bone, and grafting with a 50:50 mixture of autologous bone and HA/TCP in dogs. Implants were fiber–metal porous ingrowth prostheses. Focusing on the femoral results, no radiographic evidence of lucencies or subsidence was noted. The least amount of new bone formation was demonstrated in the ungrafted control group, in which bone was found only on the fiber–metal side of the defect. In contrast, both grafted groups demonstrated complete defect filling with mature trabecular bone at 6 and 12 weeks. With regard to porous ingrowth, no significant differences were found among the three groups on the femoral side, but trends paralleled the interesting findings in the acetabulum. At 6 weeks, the control and graft mixture groups demonstrated much greater ingrowth, compared with the autograft group. At 12 weeks, the graft mixture group showed much greater ingrowth than that in the autograft group, which had predominantly fibrous ingrowth. This finding was believed to be due in part to the resorptive process required for autograft before new bone formation can occur. The authors concluded that autograft incorporates well but that bone ingrowth in regions of autografting during revision arthroplasty appears to be unlikely.

Greis et al.[37] investigated in dogs the response of 4.5-mm cortical femoral defects to use of a fiber–metal component with and without a coating of HA/TCP. Defects were treated with no graft in controls, autograft, a 50:50 mixture of autograft and HA/TCP, and a collagen–HA/TCP–bone marrow mixture. Analysis of defect healing and ingrowth was conducted at 6, 12, and 24 weeks. Defect healing was better in all grafted groups at 6 and 12 weeks, as compared with controls, but grafting had no statistically significant effect on ingrowth, which maximized at 12 weeks. The HA/TCP coating did not enhance ingrowth in the femur. All femoral components were stable, with no porous surface radiolucencies.

Lewis et al.[44] investigated the efficacy of autograft, fresh-frozen allograft, and beta-tricalcium/phosphate (TCP) in filling a 2-mm gap between bone and a porous surface, providing bony ingrowth, and enhancing stability. These groups were compared with a press-fit control group with no gap and a nongrafted gap control group. Biomechanical push-out testing showed the nongrafted gap group had much lower values than all other groups at 4, 8, and 16 weeks. No statistically significant difference in push-out strength was noted among the press-fit control, autograft, fresh-frozen allograft, or beta-TCP groups. Histologic evaluation showed full-thickness circumferential ingrowth in the press-fit control group by 8 weeks. The nongrafted control group had no ingrowth at 8 weeks and only minimal ingrowth at 16 weeks in one specimen. Autografted specimens demonstrated full-thickness circumferential ingrowth by 8 weeks. The fresh-frozen allograft and beta-TCP groups did reveal ingrowth at 8 and 16 weeks, though less than that found in the autograft specimens. No statistically significant quantitative differences could be demonstrated among the three grafted groups. Qualitatively, the greatest new bone formation was seen in the autograft group, followed by the TCP and the allograft specimens. A similar pattern was noted for bone ingrowth. They concluded that, without grafting, bone has a limited ability to cross a void or provide effective stabilization of the implant.

Conclusion

As can be seen from this discussion, no consensus exists in the management of cavitary defects of the revision femur. Strong differences of opinion continue with respect to the preferred implant and bone grafting options. However, experience and adherence to the general principles of revision will point the surgeon toward success in management of even the most difficult cases of femoral cavitary defects.

References

1. D'Antonio J, McCarthy JC, Bargar WL, Borden LS, Cappelo WN, Collis WK, et al. Classification of femoral abnormalities in total hip arthroplasty. *Clin Orthop.* 1993;296:133–139.
2. McDonald D, Fitzgerald R, Chao E. The enhancement of fixation of a porous-coated femoral component by autograft and allograft in the dog. *J Bone Joint Surg Am.* 1988;70:728–737.
3. Hozack W, Bicalho P, Eng K. Treatment of femoral osteolysis with cementless total hip revision. *J Arthroplasty.* 1996;11:668–672.
4. Engh CA, Glassman AH, Griffin WL, Mayer JG. Results of cementless revision for failed cemented total hip arthroplasty. *Clin Orthop.* 1988;235:91–110.
5. Jasty MJ, Floyd WE 3d, Schiller AL, Goldring SR, Harris WH. Localized osteolysis in stable, non-septic total hip replacement. *J Bone Joint Surg Am.* 1986;68:912–919.
6. Mallory T. Preparation of the proximal femur in cementless total hip revision. *Clin Orthop.* 1988;235:47–60.
7. Gie GA, Linder L, Ling RS, Simon JP, Slooff TJ, Timperley AJ. Impacted cancellous allografts and cement for revision total hip arthroplasty. *J Bone Joint Surg Br.* 1993;75:14–21.
8. Ruff C, Hayes W. Subperiosteal expansion and cortical remodeling of the human femur and tibia with aging. *Science* 1982;217:945–948.
9. Comadoll J, Sherman R, Gustillo R, Bechtold JE. Radiographic changes in bone dimensions in asymptomatic cemented total hip arthroplasties: results of nine to thirteen-year follow-up. *J Bone Joint Surg Am.* 1988;70:433–438.
10. Jasty M, Maloney W, Bragdon C, Haire T, Harris WH. Histomorphological studies of the long-term responses to well fixed cemented femoral components. *J Bone Joint Surg Am.* 1990;72:1220–1229.
11. Roberson J. Proximal femoral bone loss after total hip arthroplasty. *Orthop Clin North Am.* 1992;23:291–302.
12. Dennis D, Dingman C, Meglan D, O'Leary JF, Mallory TH, Berme N. Femoral cement removal in revision total hip arthroplasty: a biomechanical analysis. *Clin Orthop.* 1987;220:142–147.
13. Eftekhar N. Rechannelization of cemented femur using a guide and drill system. *Clin Orthop.* 1977;123:29–31.
14. Dohmae Y, Bechtold J, Sherman R, Puno RM, Gustilo RB. Reduction in cement–bone interface shear strength between primary and revision arthroplasty. *Clin Orthop.* 1988;236:214–220.
15. Gustillo R, Pasternak H. Revision total hip arthroplasty with titanium ingrowth prosthesis and bone grafting for failed cemented femoral component loosening. *Clin Orthop.* 1988;235:111–119.
16. Masri B, Duncan C. Classification of bone loss in total hip arthroplasty. In: Pritchard D, ed. *Instr Course Lect.* Rosemont, Ill: American Academy of Orthopaedic Surgeons; 1996;45:199–208.
17. Engh C, Glassman A. Cementless revision of a failed total hip replacement: an update. In Tullos H, ed. *Instr Course Lect.* Park Ridge, Ill: American Academy of Orthopaedic Surgeons; 1991;40:189–197.
18. Paprosky W. Femoral defect classification: clinical application. *Orthop Rev.* 1990;14S:9–15.
19. Chandler H, Penenberg B. Femoral reconstruction. In: Chandler H, Penenberg B, eds. *Bone Stock Deficiency in Total Hip Arthroplasty. Classification and Management.* Thorofare, NJ: Slack, Inc; 1989:103–164.
20. D'Antonio JA, Capello WN, Borden LS, Barger WL, Bierbaum BF, Boettcher WG, et al. Classification and management of acetabular abnormalities in total hip arthroplasty. *Clin Orthop.* 1989;243:126–137.
21. Bargar WL, Murzic WJ, Taylor JK, Newman MA, Paul HA. Management of bone loss in revision total hip arthroplasty using custom cementless femoral components. *J Arthroplasty.* 1993;8:245–252.
22. Fitzgerald R, Chao E, McDonald D, et al. A comparison of autografts, allografts, and tricalcium phosphate hydroxyapatite crystals. In: Fitzgerald R, ed. *Non-cemented Total Hip Arthroplasty.* New York, NY: Raven Press; 1988:159–174.
23. Pierson J, Harris W. Cemented revision for femoral osteolysis in cemented arthroplasties: results in 29 hips after a mean 8.5 year follow-up. *J Bone Joint Surg Br.* 1994;76:40–44.
24. Raut V, Siney P, Wroblewski B. Cemented Charnley revision arthroplasty for severe femoral osteolysis. *J Bone Joint Surg Br.* 1995;77:362–365.
25. Turner R, Emerson R. Femoral revision total hip arthroplasty. In: Turner R, Scheller A, eds. *Revision Total Hip Arthroplasty.* New York, NY: Grune & Stratton; 1982:75–106.
26. Scheller A, D'Errico J. Hip biomechanics and prosthetic design and selection in revision total hip arthroplasty. In: Turner R, Scheller A, eds. *Revision Total Hip Arthroplasty.* New York, NY: Grune & Stratton; 1982:49–73.
27. Pellicci PM, Wilson PD Jr, Sledge CB, Salvati EA, Ranawat CS, Poss R. Revision total hip arthroplasty. *Clin Orthop.* 1982;170:34–41.

28. Pellicci PM, Wilson PD Jr, Sledge CB, Salvati EA, Ranawat CS, Poss R, et al. Long-term results of revision total hip replacement: a follow-up report. *J Bone Joint Surg Am.* 1985; 67:513–516.
29. Callaghan J, Salvati E, Pellicci P, et al. Two to five year results of revision total hip replacement. Presented at American Academy of Orthopaedic Surgeons 52nd annual conference meeting; January 1985; Las Vegas, Nev.
30. Turner R, Mattingly D, Scheller A. Femoral revision total hip arthroplasty using a long-stem femoral component. *J Arthroplasty.* 1987;2:247–258.
31. Wilson P. Revision total hip arthroplasty: current role of polymethylmethacrylate. *Clin Orthop.* 1987;225:218–228.
32. Wirta J, Eskola A, Santavirta S, Tallroth K, Konttinen YT, Lindholm S. Revision of aggressive granulomatous lesions in hip arthroplasty. *J Arthroplasty.* 1990;5(suppl):S47–S52.
33. Hedley A, Gruen T, Ruoff D. Revision of failed total hip arthroplasties with uncemented porous-coated anatomic components. *Clin Orthop.* 1988;235:75–90.
34. Kavanagh B, Ilstrup D, Fitzgerald R. Revision total hip arthroplasty. *J Bone Joint Surg Am.* 1985;67:517–526.
35. Gustillo R. Revision of femoral component loosening with titanium ingrowth prosthesis and bone grafting. *Instr Course Lect.* 1986;35: 161–163.
36. Peters CL, Rivero DP, Kull LR, Jacobs JJ, Rosenberg AG, Galante JO. Revision total hip arthroplasty without cement: subsidence of proximally porous-coated femoral components. *J Bone Joint Surg Am.* 1995;77:1217–1226.
37. Greis PE, Kang JD, Silvaggio V, Rubash HE. A long-term study on defect filling and bone ingrowth using a canine fiber metal total hip model. *Clin Orthop.* 1992;274:47–59.
38. Kang JD, McKernan DJ, Kruger M, Mutschler T, Thompson WH, Rubash HE. Ingrowth and formation of bone in defects in an uncemented fiber–metal total hip-replacement model in dogs. *J Bone Joint Surg Am.* 1991;73:93–104.
39. Meding JB, Ritter MA, Keating EM, Faris PM. Clinical and radiographic evaluation of long-stem femoral components following revision total hip arthroplasty. *J Arthroplasty.* 1994;9:399–408.
40. Engh C, Massin P, Suthers K. Roentgenographic assessment of biologic fixation of porous-surfaced femoral components. *Clin Orthop.* 1990;257:107–128.
41. Eskola A, Santavirta S, Konttinen YT, Hoikka V, Tallroth K, Lindholm TS. Cementless revision of aggressive granulomatous lesions in hip replacements. *J Bone Joint Surg Br.* 1990;72:212–216.
42. Kienapfel H, Sumner DR, Turner TM, Urban RM, Galante JO. Efficacy of autograft and freeze-dried allograft to enhance fixation of porous coated implants in the presence of interface gaps. *J Orthop Res.* 1992;10:423–433.
43. Nelson I, Bulstrode C, Mowat A. Femoral allografts in the revision of hip replacement. *J Bone Joint Surg Br.* 1990;72: 151–152.
44. Lewis C, Jones L, Hungerford D. Effects of grafting on porous metal ingrowth: a canine model. *J Arthroplasty.* 1997;12:451–460.

24
Reconstruction of Cavitary Defects: Endosteal Grafting

James J. Elting

After 25 years of experience with total hip arthroplasty, aseptic loosening of the femoral component continues to be the most frequent mode of failure and thus the primary reason for revision surgery. Typically, the failure manifests at the bone–cement or bone–implant interface. The femora to be revised by definition have cavitary and segmental defects, as classified by the American Academy of Orthopedic Surgeons[1] or Endo–Klinik[2] grading systems. Most importantly, in each case the endosteal scaffold has been destroyed, regardless of the design or mode of fixation of the unstable stem to be exchanged.[2-4]

This chapter deals with approaches to reconstruction of cavitary defects, which may range in severity from a small cystic area of endosteal bone lysis to an expansible circumferential lesion enveloping much of the proximal femur and rendering it structurally incompetent—the so-called ballooning femur. It is essential that the surgeon appreciate the location and extent of these cavitations when planning for revision surgery.

The challenge facing the orthopedic surgeon at the time of any revision arthroplasty is to provide not only an immediately stable construct for the deficient proximal femur, but a construct that will endure. Many techniques for femoral exchange arthroplasty have been advocated over the years, and indeed the debate has intensified as greater numbers of patients require exchange of painful loose components and the process of osteolysis is better understood. Likewise, the discussion in the literature has broadened to include considerations of the mechanics and biology of bone grafting as well as of implant design, mode of fixation, and surgical technique.[2-18]

Many investigators have reported on several approaches to femoral revision arthroplasty. Cementless stems with distal fixation, cemented constructs, revision and custom prostheses, modular implants, segmental allografts, and femoral strut grafts are all described elsewhere in this book. Cavitary defects are bypassed to obtain solid distal fixation in both cemented and cementless techniques with the use of long stems. Morselized bone or polymethylmethacrylate can be used to fill the lesions, or cortical strut grafts can be onlayed to bridge or reinforce areas of weakness. In addition, segmental allograft can be used to replace femur that has been rendered incompetent by massive osteolysis. An alternative approach, whereby these cleaned and constrained cavitations provide the substrate for a biologic reconstitution of the proximal femur, is the innovation of Gie et al.[2] Results of midterm experience have demonstrated that impaction grafting can provide both immediate stability of the femoral revision construct and a favorable environment for osteoconduction and ultimate rebuilding of femoral bone stock.[2,13,15-18]

McCollum et al.[19] in 1980 and Gates et al.[20] in 1990 described a technique for compacting morsellized cancellous allograft in protrusio acetabuli defects and stabilizing the construct with a cemented cup. Slooff et al.[21] extended and adapted this pelvic impaction grafting for use in femoral revision arthroplasty. Credit must be given to Gie, Ling, et al., who in 1988 first achieved immediate stability of a revision component in a deficient femur by using impacted morselized cancellous allograft and a cemented, collarless, polished taper stem. In 1993, they reported on their very favorable early results with this method.[2] Other reviews have followed, and the midterm experience lends encouragement to further investigation and development of impaction grafting for femoral revision arthroplasty.[15-18]

Technique

The surgical technique for femoral revision arthroplasty involves six distinct steps, which are described next in operative sequence, followed by a description of aftercare and patient follow-up.

Preparation of Canal

Complete removal of all foreign material from the proximal femur is carried out. This includes implant, polymethylmethacrylate (PMMA), osteolytic debris, granulomata, fibrous membrane, and spacers. If there is a stable polyethylene or polymethylmethacrylate plug or a bony pedestal below the region of implant loosening and osteolysis, this may be left intact. Extended trochanteric osteotomy may be a surgical necessity and is well suited to impaction grafting techniques. In the course of dissection and debridement, new and more severe endosteal defects may be appreciated and/or created. This should not be looked on as a surgical complication, although it will lead to moments of despair. What often remains to build on, then, is a patulous, translucent, incompetent, and deficient femoral envelope, complete with fenestration, fracture, or discontinuity.

Occlusion of the Canal

The canal is occluded 3 cm distal to either the most inferior region of osteolysis or the point at which the tip of the new prosthesis will lie. The bony pedestal, old plug, or residual polymethylmethacrylate (PMMA) may be useful in this regard. A calibrated guide wire is threaded into a stiff medullary plug of appropriate diameter. The guide wire, in turn, is threaded through the cannula of the largest cylindric packer that can be accommodated by the femoral canal (Fig. 24.1A). The plug is driven to the area of proper seating, and the next smaller packer is introduced to confirm seating (Fig. 24.1B). If a pedestal, old cement restrictor, or residual PMMA remains to occlude the canal, the cannulated packer or tamp is used to guide the threaded-tip calibrated guide wire for central fixation. It is critical that the guide wire be fixed in the center of the femoral tube, regardless of the mode of occlusion. This will facilitate solid circumferential packing of the allograft chips. If an extremely long stem has been removed, it may be necessary to fill the distal part of the canal with packed cancellous chips and then insert a plug more proximally.

Circumferential Restraint

The circumferential integrity of the proximal femoral envelope is addressed next. Visual and manual examination are carried out, both within the canal by means of a flexible light and along the surface exposed by a generous dissection. If the femoral cortical shell is intact, no further reinforcement is indicated. Fenestrations, fractures, and areas of weakened cortex are reinforced with fine cobalt–chromium screening secured by cables or cerclage wires. This is done by introducing the largest taper tamp that can be accommodated within the bony vault, taking care to achieve proper version (neutral to 10° anteversion) and use this as a mold for the screening, cerclage wires, and cables. In some cases of extreme bone loss, the screening may wrap completely around the upper femur, and there may be gaps (measurable in centimeters) in the cortex (Fig. 24.2). The object is to create a "basket," which will be filled by tightly compacted morsellized cancellous allograft. Infractions distal to the length of the new stem may be fixed with a long lateral

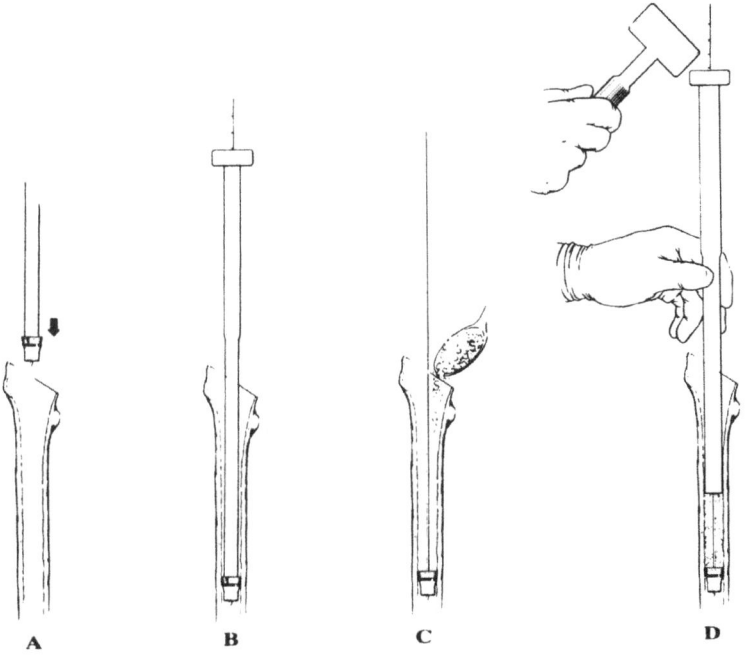

Figure 24.1. (From Nelissen, Bauer, Weidenhielm, et al[15] by permission of *The Journal of Bone and Joint Surgery*.) A. The femoral canal cement restrictor is introduced with the calibrated guide wire screwed in. B. Appropriate depth and seating are gauged by the cylindric packer. C. Morselized allograft is introduced. D. The allograft is packed distally in the cleaned femoral vault.

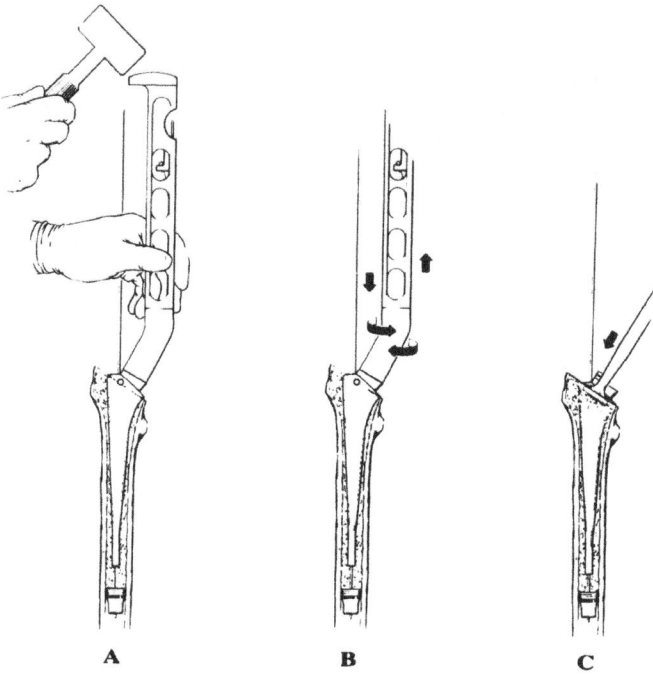

Figure 24.2. (From Nelissen, Bauer, Weidenhielm, et al[15] by permission of *The Journal of Bone and Joint Surgery*.) A. The smooth taper tamp repeatedly compacts the bone cereal as forceful hammer blows are struck. B. Impaction is complete when the tamp resists manual attempts at torsion and extraction. C. Proximal packing is essential to fill all cavitary defects adequately and ensure good implant and polymethylmethacrylate seating.

side plate or cortical strut grafts. Of special importance are those weakened or thinned areas of lateral cortex at the level of the tip of a stem that has failed in varus.

Impaction of Morselized Allograft

The morselized graft (3–8 mm in dimension; greater than 75% cancellous, less than 25% cortical, allograft) is delivered into the plugged canal, packed distally, and tamped vigorously. This is done over the calibrated centralized guide wire that has been screwed into the center of the canal plug. The chips are introduced by using a spoon (Fig. 24.1C) and packed with the cylindric device used to introduce the plug. Filling and packing are repeated several times until approximately the distal third of the cavity is tightly filled (Fig. 24.1D). More bone cereal is spooned in, and the largest smooth taper tamp used in step three (described earlier) is impacted until it is seated at an acceptable level. If the distal packing is too dense to allow the taper tamp to find an appropriate depth, it may be necessary to use a cannulated reamer to remove some of the allograft. The tamp is a smooth taper oversized in each dimension to the comparable stem to allow for a cement mantle 2 mm in circumference and 5 mm medially at the upper end, as well as 1.5 cm distally. Iterative filling and tamping are carried out with sequentially smaller tamps until the appropriate size is seated (Fig. 24.3A). This is judged at the operating table with the preoperative templating in mind. It cannot be emphasized too strongly how much force must be delivered to impact the graft properly. When the seated tamp is immovable to manual twist-ing and extraction attempts (Fig. 24.3B), a trial reduction may then be done with a head–neck assembly, which attaches to the now torsionally stable tamp. Additional proximal packing completes the impaction to the level of the shoulder of the tamp (Fig. 24.3C). Rectangular tamps are best suited for this step, which completes the construction of a neomedullary canal constrained within the proximal femoral envelope (Fig. 24.4A).

Introduction of Cement and Pressurization

After removal of the guide wire, polymethylmethacrylate is delivered in a retrograde fashion by means of a small bore or tapered nozzle and cement gun, so that this neomedullary canal fashioned from allograft is filled (Fig. 24.4A). To protect the graft, the acrylic is introduced somewhat earlier than in a primary arthroplasty, yet in a doughy state. Pressurization is maintained by a proximal seal, which surrounds the junction of barrel and nozzle of the gun (Fig. 24.4C). While pressurizing the PMMA, the surgeon will appreciate extravasation of blood and fluid from canal and allograft, often bubbling through thin cortex and/or screening.

Introduction of Femoral Component

A collarless, polished taper stem is introduced as the polymethylmethacrylate is curing. Again, a seal is used to prevent acrylic extrusion and maintain pressurization (Fig. 24.4D). Moderate force must be applied both to insert the stem in the doughy cement and to maintain its

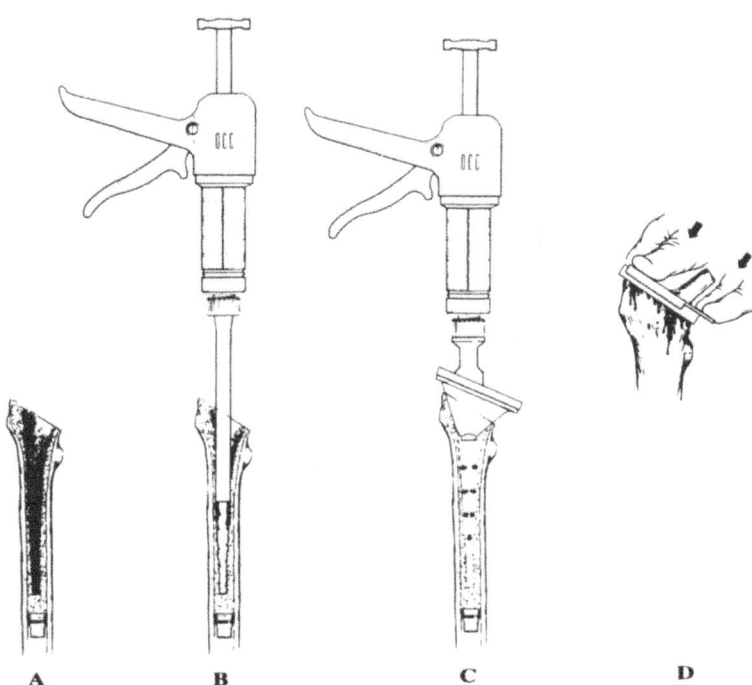

Figure 24.3. (From Nelissen, Bauer, Weidenhielm et al[15] by permission of *The Journal of Bone and Joint Surgery*.) A. The neomedullary canal has been shaped, formed by impacted allograft contained circumferentially by the upper femur. B. The polymethylmethacrylate is introduced by means of cement gun and modified nozzle. C. The PMMA is pressurized with proximal seal firmly in place. D. With the acrylic in a doughy state, the collarless polished taper stem is introduced with a proximal seal maintained to prevent extension of PMMA.

depth as the composite stiffens, recalling that the extrusion force will equal intrusion pressure with a double taper wedge. The intrusion pressure of polymethylmethacrylate must also be greater than the blood pressure in bone to prevent lamination of acrylic. For this reason, we insist on the use of hypotensive anesthesia for both primary and revision arthroplasty surgery.

Aftercare

Postoperatively, patients are mobilized rapidly, discharged from the hospital within a week, and encouraged to bear weight lightly with double support for 6 weeks. Those at risk for dislocation are in a brace, as proposed by Lima et al.[22] Use of a single cane is sug-

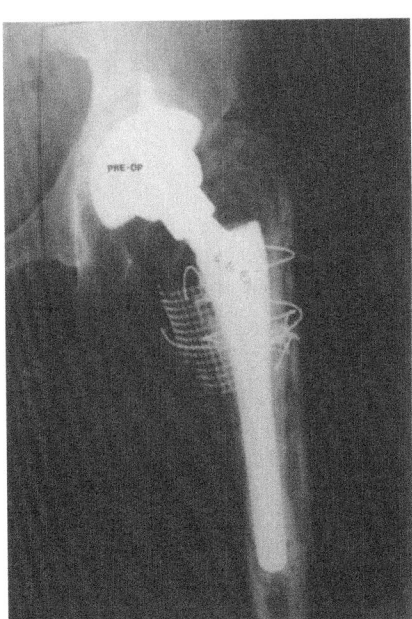
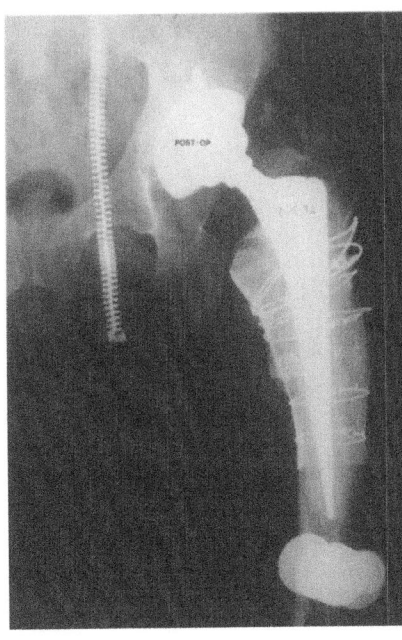

Figure 24.4. Preoperative and 3-month postoperative radiographs of a 42-year-old man with a loose stem in an incompetent proximal femur. Circumferential screening was necessary to create a "basket" into which morselized allograft could be impacted.

gested for the second 6 weeks. Thereafter the patient is systematically evaluated, with annual clinical and radiographic evaluations commencing 2 years postsurgery.

Early and Mid-Term Results

Several investigators have reported their early and midterm results in patients who have had impaction grafting femoral exchange arthroplasty.[2,13,15–18] Gie and colleagues[2] reported in 1993 on 56 hips with a mean followup of 30 months (range, 18–48 months) and our review[18] of our initial 56 hips with a mean follow-up of 31 months (range, 24–64 months) published in 1995 yielded virtually identical results. The average Harris hip score was 90, with 80% of patients reporting no pain referable to the revised hip. Seventy-eight percent of patients used no support in ambulation, 17% took a cane on long walks, 11% preferred a single cane full time, and 4% used a walker. As in any series of patients with hip revision surgery, age, infirmity and systemic disease had an impact on the lowest scores. However, no individual in either series showed a decrease in clinical rating over the time studied; in fact, several individuals scored slightly higher at a longer-term review point.

Serial radiographs are examined for (1) stem subsidence, (2) mantle subsidence, and (3) radiolucent lines between both stem and cement and cement and bone, as described by Gruen et al.[23] We also perform a subjective evaluation of graft incorporation by grading the serial x-rays for cortical new bone formation, trabecular lines, cortical or trabecular incorporation (or incorporation of both resorptive areas), or any other changes in appearance. This has proved to be a difficult and controversial exercise because there are no published criteria, and these collarless, polished taper stems in the PMMA–allograft composite may behave in a manner that cannot be quantified by methods applicable to collared textured stems. Also the hardware used to constrain the upper femur will obscure the roentgenographic image of the area that has been grafted (Fig. 24.5). Subsidence of stem within PMMA that was measurable on plain radiographs was seen in 48% of our cases[18] and in 80% of those reviewed by Gie et al.[2] Only 7% and 14% in the respective series of femurs x-rayed showed settling of the entire composite. The average distal migration of stem within acrylic in our early group[18] was 2.8 mm, with 17% showing greater than 2 mm. All except one had stabilized at 2 years, and we have revised that one case with progressive subsidence at 6 years.

Lucent lines between stem and mantle or mantle and bone were infrequently seen on radiographic review (2% and 4%, respectively, of possible zones at each interface). Ninety-three percent of x-rays showed progressive radiographic evidence of impacted graft incorporation; only one individual had what appeared to be an area of graft resorption. With that one exception there had been no x-ray evidence of deterioration of graft incorporation over time. There appears to be no correlation between the nature and severity of preoperative bone loss and ultimate radiographic appearance. Likewise, the clinical scores did not reflect a relationship between degree of pre-revision cavitary and/or segmental bone loss and ultimate clinical score.

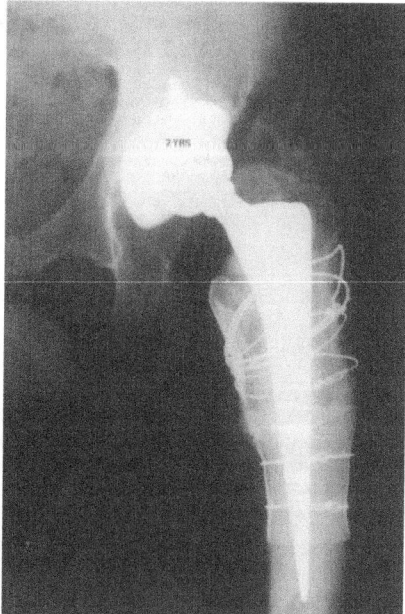 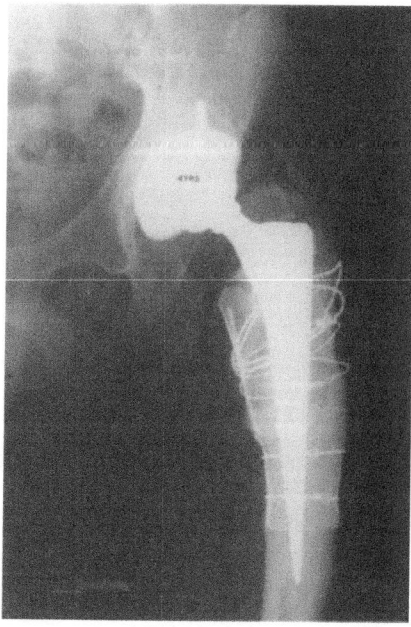

Figure 24.5. X-Rays at 2 and 4 years postimpaction grafting reflect the maintenance of stable geometry, absence of subsidence, and difficulty visualizing the grafted area because of the screening. Functional result is excellent.

Our latest review, after 7 years experience in 150 cases (average age 65 years at revision femoral arthroplasty) has yielded 112 hips that have been monitored for more than 2 years. Of these, 103 were evaluated at an average of 46 months after surgery. The Harris hip score average remains 90, with 81% reporting no pain, and the same number reporting no use support in ambulation. Review of radiographs reflected less than 2 mm average measurable subsidence of stem within mantle in fewer than 50% of cases. Sinkage of the entire construct occurred in 5%, to a depth of less than 2 mm on average. Radiolucent lines, either at implant–PMMA interface or between composite and bone, were rare (2% and 4% of zones, respectively). One individual's revised hip has failed, with subsidence progressing over 6 years, disappearance of graft on x-ray, and increase in pain. This patient, a large woman who has insulin-dependent diabetes and intermittently receives high doses of steroids for rheumatoid disease, was recently re-impacted.

Ten patients have had further surgery related to revised hip or femur: five for femur fractures (4 shaft, 1 supracondylar), 3 for cup revisions, 1 for cerclage wire removal, and one late aseptic loosening. All four shaft fractures occurred at or just distal to the tip of prosthesis. Two early breaks were through compromised cortex; two late breaks were the result of considerable trauma. In none of the fractured femurs was the implant changed or the impaction redone. The fracture was stabilized in each case with a lateral side plate without supplemental bone graft and without opening the hip joint. Each has healed solidly. We have not seen this complication since 1994, possibly because we have been more likely to use a lateral plate or cortical strut graft to reinforce compromised distal cortex. Also, we have had the advantages of being able to use the cannulated instrumentation (unavailable for the first 2 years of our experience) and time on the learning curve.

Reoperation has provided us with a wealth of histologic evidence as to the fate of the impacted cancellous allograft. Nelissen et al.[15] in 1995 published a histologic analysis of four cases of impaction grafting. Biopsy specimens were obtained from the proximal femur at the time of removal of symptomatic trochanteric wires in four patients at 11 to 27 months post-revision hip arthroplasty. These investigators described three zones as they interpreted sections microscopically: an inner zone consisting of bone cement, fibrous tissue, and partially necrotic trabeculae with evidence of bone remodeling; a middle zone consisting of viable trabecular bone and probable formation of so-called neocortex with few particles of bone cement; and an outer zone of viable cortex. In one case of cup exchange in our series,[17] we took sections of lateral femoral cortex in an area in which there had been full-thickness bone loss secondary to osteolysis before impaction grafting 30 months earlier. The pathologist's interpretation was "living lamellar bone" in this tissue from the outer zone. Likewise, Ling and coworkers[24] have reported the results of histologic examinations of one femur biopsied at reoperation and another retrieved at autopsy. Analysis of postmortem tissue from the proximal femur 3½ years after impaction grafting revealed three zones, described as "regenerated cortical bone," an "interface zone," and a deep layer, with findings similar to those of Nelissen et al.[15]

One important finding in these reports lies in the discovery of areas of creeping substitution, in which necrotic trabecular bone is being replaced by viable new bone. The small size of the trabecular fragments and their location and appearance suggested to the authors that these pieces of bone undergoing osteoconduction are allograft. We have biopsied full-thickness calcar in a femur impacted 56 months before exchange of the previously unrevised acetabular prosthesis. In this instance, we could identify very little necrotic trabecular bone in the inner zone, but there appeared to be good interdigitation of polymethylmethacrylate with viable endosteal spicules and no fibrous membrane. On gross examination, the stem and mantle were solidly fixed at surgery.

Synthesis of Findings

As has been described, impaction grafting—the innovation of Gie, Ling, and associates—represents an abrupt departure from methods of femoral revision athroplasty advocated previously. Most significantly, no attempt is made to bridge or fill the areas of cavitary endosteal bone lysis with either a long or bulky revision prosthesis or a large quantity of PMMA. Instead, the circumferentially restrained proximal femoral envelope is packed tightly with morselized cancellous allograft, thus constructing a neomedullary canal. Polymethylmethacrylate inserted under pressure provides the initial stability for the collarless, polished taper stem–cement–graft composite. The clinical results in the mid-term are most encouraging, and both radiographic and histologic evidence supports the fact that osteoconduction does indeed proceed in this environment.

Controversy has been sparked, however, by the radiographic appearance of early subsidence of stem within mantle of these polished stems in a percentage (50%,[18] 80%[2]) of cases reported. Although this subsidence is on average at the lower limits of detection on x-ray and its progression typically ends less than 24 months after surgery, some observers have cited this phenomenon as evidence for instability of the proximal femoral reconstruction. Radiographic criteria for femoral stability in cemented arthroplasty may not apply to those cases in which a collarless, polished, double taper stem is implanted, whether it be in the primary or revision operation. Review of intermediate and long-term clinical results with these polished stems suggests that they may behave quite differently within the cement mantle than do stems with textured surfaces and collared design.[25] Bench testing of the stem–acrylic composite, finite element analysis, as well as basic engineering research into the properties of PMMA under load in physiologic conditions have contributed to current understanding.

The collarless, polished, double taper stem exerts radial compressive forces on the cement mantle as it engages, while the hip is subjected to loading forces.[25] These forces are transmitted through PMMA to the morselized graft and femoral tube, thus loading the allograft–PMMA composite in compression. This polished, double taper design will actually become more tightly fixed with subsidence within the mantle. Verdonschot and Huiskes[26] have confirmed the early work of Lee and Ling, who demonstrated that polymethylmethacrylate cured and loaded in a physiologic milieu will behave as a viscoelastic solid and exhibit the property of creep. Further, these experiments showed that because of creep, the prosthesis could subside in the cement mantle without the development of cracks in the acrylic. Radiographically, the symmetric appearance of trabecular incorporation with maturation of the impacted graft implies continued cyclic loading by means of the radial compressive forces generated during gait.[2]

It must be remembered that PMMA exhibits its strength when loaded in compression, and it will fail in tension or shear.[27] Fowler et al.[28] report bench testing, which has been used to investigate the forces developed at the stem–cement interface of both the polished taper and rough surface designs. Whereas the textured surface yielded shear stresses in proportion to the surface roughness, the polished stem loaded the acrylic mantle in more compression with proportional reduction of shear. Verdonschot and Huiskes[27] have investigated stem–cement interface characteristics by using three-dimensional finite element techniques. In this model, they found that the failure index of the cement–bone interface was reduced when friction at the stem–cement interface was reduced. Their conclusions, derived from the simulated loading conditions described, were that a polished taper stem design may be desirable for the cement–bone interface mechanics. The Morse taper, used to lock head on neck in all modular femoral prosthetic designs, is another example of the stability of the taper once engaged.

Bevrins et al.[29] have conducted in vitro studies of mechanical stability and effects of cement pressurization in the impacted allograft construct for femoral revision arthroplasty. Their model, utilizing fresh-frozen human cadaveric femurs, was carried out with a collared, precoated femoral stem. Those specimens undergoing impaction grafting were compared for stability against cemented and uncemented constructs. Initial migration and micromotion were measured. The impacted morselized allograft composite behaved more like the cemented than the cementless implant. Increased pressurization of PMMA increased the penetration into the bone cereal, but it did not increase the stability of the construct. The authors hypothesized that the stability provided with the combination of allograft and cemented reconstruction is adequate for graft incorporation. Similarly, Smith and coworkers[30] have tested synthetic femora subjected to impaction grafting with collarless, polished taper stems and found a high degree of strength and stability in the composite.

Having considered the physical environment in impaction grafting, we must relate those characteristics to the biologic processes that must evolve so that the upper femur can be reconstituted. For the ultimate success of bone grafting (ie, stable new bone formation), several physiologic and biomechanical criteria must be fulfilled. Cells that will form bone are a prerequisite, as are a scaffold for osteoconduction, a bony bed, a blood supply, stability, and bone morphogenic and growth factors.[31–33] Morselized, fresh-frozen, cancellous allograft provides an appropriate scaffold for creeping substitution and bony reconstitution.[34] The cleaned and constrained upper femoral vault is a bony bed enveloped in a well-vascularized musculature. As has been discussed, polymethylmethacrylate, appropriately introduced and pressurized, acts to stabilize the bone cereal immediately in the interzone between taper stem and femoral cortex.[29,30]

Cancellous bone for impaction grafting has come from a number of sources and has been prepared in a variety of ways. Safety is of paramount concern. Therefore, whatever the source, the allograft must be screened bacteriologically, and donors must be tested for human immunodeficiency virus and hepatitis A, B, and C viruses. Early applications for impaction grafting were with fresh-frozen femoral heads obtained from hospital bone banks. These were morselized in a commercially available bone mill in the operating room. Femoral heads are currently available from bone banks, as are distal femurs or prepackaged cubed cancellous bone or a cortical–cancellous mix of chips. Studies of aggregate mechanics have shown maximum compression with an array of sizes of allograft pieces, ranging from 3 to 10 mm. It is unclear whether freeze-dried and/or irradiated bone is appropriate for use in impaction grafting. Most surgeons advocating this technique have continued to use the fresh-frozen allograft. Mechanical testing of impacted specimens would indicate that heparinized blood should be avoided,[30] and our clinical data would suggest that high-dose steroid therapy may have a negative effect on the ultimate formation of new bone in the impacted area. Likewise, exactly how much weight bearing in ambulation is beneficial early postsurgery is not clear. Compressive forces must be applied by cyclic axial loading, but not to the detriment of the structural integrity of stem–cement–allograft–cortex construct.[30]

We do know that at the time of surgery the impacted allograft must impart stability in resisting torsional and axial forces. Our choice of material at this time is an aggregate mix, 3 to 8 mm in dimension, of approximately 75% cortical and 25% cancellous chips. Proper compaction demands that it have the texture of a dry cereal and in no way resemble a mush.

Conclusion

Impaction grafting imparts in femoral reconstruction those conditions necessary for a biologic rebuilding of compromised or lost structural bone. They are (1) appropriate size allograft to provide a lattice work for osteoconduction, (2) well-vascularized bony bed, (3) immediate stabilization by PMMA of the compacted stem–acrylic–allograft cereal–cortical composite, and (4) appropriate cyclic compressive load over time with axial forces converted to compression by means of collarless, polished taper stem.

The clinical experience over 8 years confirms satisfactory results with this method. Patients' lack of pain and high degree of function are most encouraging. Exciting work is being carried out at a number of centers, which may determine (1) the optimum allograft material; (2) whether impaction grafting can be successful with stems other than the collarless, polished, double taper design; and (3) the precise nature of femoral stem–cement interface. We continue to monitor these patients closely and will continue to use impaction grafting, the innovation of Gie, Ling, and coworkers, for all femoral exchange arthroplasty.

References

1. D'Antonio J, McCarthy JC, Bargar WL, Borden LS, Cappelo WN, Collis WK, et al. Classification of femoral abnormalities in total hip arthroplasty. *Clin Orthop.* 1993;296:133–139.
2. Gie GA, Linder L, Ling RS, Simon JP, Slooff TJ, Timperley AJ. Impacted cancellous allografts and cement revision total hip arthroplasty. *J Bone Joint Surg Br.* 1993;75:14–21.
3. Mulroy WF, Harris WH. Revision of the total hip arthroplasty with use of so-called second-generation cementing techniques for aseptic loosening of the femoral component. *J Bone Joint Surg Am.* 1996;78:325–330.
4. McLaughlin JR, Harris WH. Revision of the femoral component of a total hip arthroplasty with the calcar-replacement femoral component. *J Bone Joint Surg Am.* 1996;78:331–339.
5. Engh CA, Glassman AH, Griffin WL, Mayer JG. Results of cementless revision for failed cemented total hip arthroplasty. *Clin Orthop.* 1988;235:91–110.
6. Goldberg V, Stevenson S. Bone graft options: fact and fancy. *Orthopedics.* 1994;17:809–810, 821.
7. Head WC, Emerson RH, Peters PC Jr, Hillyard JM. Second generation of proximal femoral allografts in total hip arthroplasty revision. *Orthop Trans.* 1993;16:650.
8. Emerson RH, Malinin TI, Cueller AD. Cortical strut allografts in the reconstruction of the femur in revision total hip arthroplasty. *Clin Orthop.* 1992;285:35–44.
9. Hussamy O, Lachiewicz PF. Revision total hip arthroplasty with the BIAS femoral component: three to six year results. *J Bone Joint Surg Am.* 1994;76:1137–1148.
10. Kershaw CJ, Atkins RM, Dodd CA, Bulstrode CJ. Revision total hip arthroplasty for aseptic failure: a review of 276 cases. *J Bone Joint Surg Br.* 1991;73:564–568.
11. Rubash HE, Harris WH. Revision of nonseptic, loose, cemented femoral components using modern cementing techniques. *J Arthroplasty.* 1988;3:241–248.
12. Schüller HM, Marti RK, Besselaar PP. Aseptic failure in revision hip replacement. *Acta Orthop Scand.* 1988;59: 34–35.
13. Simon JP, Fowler JL, Gie GA, Ling RS, Timperley AJ. Impaction cancellous grafting of the femur in cemented total hip revision arthroplasty. *J Bone Joint Surg Br.* 1991; 73(Suppl I):73.
14. Strömberg CN, Herberts P, Ahnfelt L. Revision total hip arthroplasty in patients younger than 55 years old: clinical and radiologic results after 4 years. *J Arthroplasty.* 1988; 3:47–59.
15. Nelissen RG, Bauer TW, Weidenhielm LR, LeGolvan DP, Mikhail WE. Cemented revision hip arthroplasty with impaction grafting: histology of four cases. *J Bone Joint Surg Am.* 1995;77:412–422.
16. Weidenhielm LR, Mikhail WE, Nelissen RG, et al. Surgical technique and early results in revision of a total hip arthroplasty with a cemented, collarless, tapered, polished stem and contained morselized allograft. *J Orthop Tech.* 1994;2: 113–121.
17. Elting JJ, Zicat BA, Mikhail WE, Hubbell JC, House BS. Impaction grafting: preliminary report of a new method for exchange femoral arthroplasty. *Orthopedics.* 1995;18: 107–112.
18. Elting JJ, Mikhail WE, Zicat BA, Hubbell JC, Lane LE, House B. Preliminary report of impaction grafting for exchange femoral arthroplasty. *Clin Orthop.* 1995;319:159–167.
19. McCollum DE, Nunley JA, Harrelson JM. Bone-grafting in total hip replacement for acetabular protrusion. *J Bone Joint Surg Am.* 1980;62:1065–1073.
20. Gates HS, McCollum DE, Poletti SC, Nunley JA. Bone-grafting in total hip arthroplasty for protrusio acetabuli. *J Bone Joint Surg Am.* 1990;72:248–251.
21. Slooff TJ, Huiskes R, van Horn J, Lemmens AJ. Bone grafting in total hip replacement for acetabular protrusion. *Acta Orthop Scand.* 1984;55:593–596.
22. Lima D, Magnus R, Paprosky WG. Team management of hip revision patients using a post-op hip orthosis. *J Prostl Orthop.* 1994;6:20–24.
23. Gruen TA, McNeice GM, Amstutz HC. "Modes of failure" of cemented stem-type femoral components: a radiographic analysis of loosening. *Clin Orthop.* 1979;141:17–27.
24. Ling RSM, Timperley AJ, Linder L. Histological findings in a case of cemented femoral revision treated by endosteal impaction grafting. *Acta Orthop Scand.* 1992;63(suppl 248):29.
25. Gie GA, Fowler JL, Lee AJC, Ling RS. The long-term behaviour of a totally collarless, polished femoral component in cemented total hip arthroplasty. *J Bone Joint Surg Br.* 1990;72:935.
26. Verdonschot N, Huiskes R. Creep behavior of hand-mixed

Simplex P bone cement under cyclic tensile loading. *J Appl Biomater.* 1994;5:235–243.
27. Verdonschot N, Huiskes R. Mechanical effects of stem cement interface characteristics in total hip replacement. *Clin Orthop.* 1996;329:326–336.
28. Fowler JL, Gie GA, Lee AJ. Experience with the Exeter total hip replacement since 1970. *Orthop Clin North Am.* 1988;19:477–489.
29. Bevzins A, Sumner DR, Wasielewski RC. Impacted particulate allograft for femoral revision total hip arthroplasty. *J Arthroplasty.* 1996;11:500–506.
30. Smith EJ, Richardson JB, Evans P, Nelson K, Lee RJ. The initial stability of femoral impaction grafting. *Orthop Trans.* 1995;19:369.
31. Goldberg V, Stevenson S. Natural history of autografts and allografts. *Clin Orthop.* 1987;225:7–16.
32. Lance EM. Some observations on bone graft technology. *Clin Orthop.* 1985;200:114–124.
33. Urist M, O'Connor B, Burwell G. *Bone Grafts, Derivatives and Substitutes.* Oxford, England: Butterworth-Heinemann, Ltd; 1994.
34. McLaren A, Stamp G. Morselized cancellous bone graft for bone defects: autograft vs. allograft. *J Bone Joint Surg Br.* 1991;73(suppl I):46.

25
Reconstruction of Segmental Defects: Onlay Allografting

Roger H. Emerson, Jr. and William C. Head

Successive total hip revisions are associated with loss of bone stock, and revision for loosening of one hip component is associated with an increased rate of subsequent loosening of that same component.[1-4] Stromberg and Herberts[4] attributed the poor results they found in a 10-year follow-up study of revision total hip arthroplasty in young patients (ie, younger than 55 years of age) to poor bone quality at the time of revision. Callaghan et al.[1] also found that mechanical failure and progressive radiolucencies in revision hip arthroplasties correlated significantly with poor-quality bone stock of the preoperative femur. Femoral bone loss—in the form of osteolytic defects, cortical windows, and perforations—has been associated with stem breakage,[5] femoral fracture,[6,7] femoral subsidence,[8] and femoral loosening.[9] At the extreme, loss of femoral bone stock can preclude prosthesis reimplantation,[3,10] but any loss of bone means some loss of implant bone support.

The logical conclusion is that loss of bony structural support from the femur is one factor leading to failure of a femoral revision arthroplasty. Accordingly, appropriate restoration of femoral bone stock is an important part of the revision operation. Onlay cortical strut allografts have several advantages over other allograft options, morsellized allograft and bulk whole-bone allografts. Struts can provide some structural support in situations in which bone chips cannot. Because struts are on the periosteal surface of the femur, they allow for a viable endosteal bone–implant interface, with the prospect of bony ingrowth of the femoral component in the setting of cementless revision surgery. Allograft struts follow the same biologic fundamentals as those of whole-bone segments; namely, that union depends on rigid fixation and incorporation depends on union of the allograft–host junction. The very nature of strut grafts takes advantage of this biology, because they are easily rigidly fixed and have an extensive junction with the host for union, with little depth of bone to be incorporated. Animal and human studies have shown that struts are metabolically very active and incorporate and remodel very quickly.[11]

Biology of Onlay Strut Allografts

The original research on the biology of onlay struts was done by Kreutz et al.[12] in a fracture model using freeze-dried bone, although without the use of stable fixation. Malinin et al.[13] have described a series of radius fractures in a dog model, comparing a metal plate with a bone allograft plate, both fixed with screws. The allograft series healed more quickly with more strength. In this dog model by 12 weeks, the allograft strut could no longer be separated from the host, with trabecular bridging seen spanning the interface between the graft and host cortex with remodeling of the graft edges. At this stage, the biomechanical strength of the grafted radius is equal to that of the normal contralateral limb, with new fractures occurring with mechanical testing of the specimens through the screw holes, rather than through the osteotomy site. Histologic evaluation at 12 weeks shows that the strut has been completely transformed into a callus-like structure. The host–graft junction has formed trabecular spaces with bone marrow elements. The underlying host radius has also undergone revascularization. In 24-week specimens, the strut is distinguishable radiologically, but grossly it has blended entirely with the host bone. Although cancellous bone and dense mesenchymal tissue are still present, the major portion of the graft has remodeled to new cortical bone. Not only has the graft remodeled, but the host bone under the struts has undergone similar histologic remodeling.[11]

Radiographic study of human struts used for femoral reconstruction at the time of total hip revision has shown the same radiologic sequence as that in the dog model, although it occurred more slowly.[11] The average length of grafts in this study was 12.6 cm (range, 4.8–21.0

cm). Strut union was seen on average by 8.4 months. (SD = 3.2 months), defining union as at least 50% bridging between the host cortex and graft. The average time of onset of cortical round-off of the strut edges was 7.0 months; partial bridging between the graft and host, 8.3 months; and complete bridging, 12.5 months. The overall rate of graft union was 96.6%. Although several grafts demonstrated some surface scalloping (especially between fixation wires) and other struts demonstrated even more extensive resorption, many struts showed periosteal new bone forming over the graft or extending down the periosteal cortex of the host at the ends of the strut. By 27 months, radiographs revealed that the grafts had completed the healing process.[11] Further observation of these struts reveals that they ultimately take on the same appearance as that of the underlying host bone, apparently responding to the same local mechanical environment as the host bone. Biopsy of human strut grafts and retrievals show a similar histology to the animal model (written communication, Malanin TI, March, 1995).

Clinical Experience

The best means of accomplishing bone augmentation of the femur at revision total hip arthroplasty has not been established. Callaghan et al.[1] recommended aggressive grafting of bone defects and all fractures, but they did not specify a method to use. Engh et al.[14] found that morsellized bone graft does not significantly restore lost bone stock. Gustillo and Pasternak[15] found that postoperative Harris clinical scores diminished with increasing pre-revision bone loss, despite use of both morselized autograft to fill cavitary defects and a long-stem revision femoral component. Those revisions with the best bone averaged scores of 93 points, whereas those with the worst bone averaged 78 points. Gie et al.[16] have shown that impacted cancellous allografting can restore bone to the proximal femur, but this technique is very new with no long-term studies of the fate of the femoral component or the bone graft. The extent to which impacted cancellous bone can provide reliable structural support remains to be established.

Cortical onlay struts have proved to be more reliable clinically than whole-bone allografts. It must be pointed out that the extent of the bone loss that can be reconstructed with a strut is much less, and it follows that strut cases are generally less complicated than cases requiring bulk grafting. Allan et al.[17] noted no nonunions and an average improvement of 42 points in the Harris hip score with struts, compared with 35 points for the whole-bone grafts. Emerson et al.[11] described a large series of femoral strut grafts: 146 grafts in 115 patients with 34 months average follow-up. In this series, clinical outcome was independent of the original femoral bone deficiency, whereas historic controls[14] have shown that clinical outcome is best in those femurs with the best starting bone stock. The average Harris score for this group of strut revisions was 79, compared with 70 for a series of bulk allograft patients as reported by Head et al.[18] Chandler and Penenberg[19] have described a series of twelve patients with cortical thinning in which the investigators used a cortical onlay allograft to reconstruct the femur with good results. Chandler et al.[20] have also presented a series of fractures below a femoral hip component treated with allograft struts, with an 89% fracture union rate.

Operative Technique

Regional femoral cortical bone loss is ideal for strut reconstruction. The best strut is made from freeze-dried bone because this is the least antigenic of allograft bone.[21] It is a weaker material compared with fresh-frozen bone. However, in the setting of regional bone loss in total hip revision strength is not as important as it is in the setting of segmental loss in which the allograft will need to provide substantial if not complete

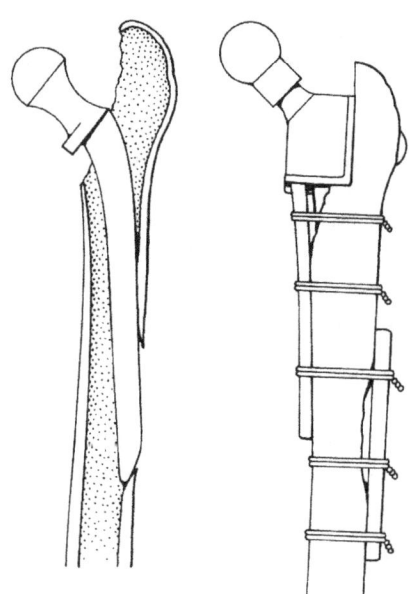

Figure 25.1. A. Varus drift of a loose femoral component with bone loss in the calcar region medially and the lateral cortex below the metaphysis. This common type of bone loss significantly compromises the structural support of the native femur for a revision implant. B. A proximal platform–loading calcar–deficient revision femoral component with cortical strut augmentation of medial and lateral bone loss. The medial strut does not provide full implant support, but it does contribute to implant stability. The host femoral tube must still provide the majority of the implant support.

support for the implant. The strut should be long enough to span the area of deficiency and provide significant mechanical support to the adjacent femur.

The most common and important regional bone loss related to a failed implant occurs in the medial femoral calcar. It is caused by osteolysis or stress-shielding,[22] and it is frequently complicated by varus collapse of the failed prosthesis. The combination of a calcar deficient prosthesis and a medial strut makes a very strong construct for this bone loss pattern. This is because this implant design puts axial load on the top of the strut, and the strut in turn can provide some rotational support to the implant. (See Fig. 25.1.) The strut, however, cannot provide full axial support of the implant. Windows made for cement removal are best done anteriorly or laterally in the femur to prevent dangerous weakening of the femur from the bone defect created. Cortical windows placed near the tip of the revision prosthesis are especially significant. (See Fig. 25.2.) A long strut over the window area will protect the femur from fracture. Struts that are placed on the medial femur require more soft tissue stripping, but they are well tolerated, whereas struts on the anterior or lateral femur may make it difficult to repair the quadriceps. When positioned distal to the bow of the femur, the strut can be a source of local discomfort with knee range of motion because of the added bulk of the graft impinging on the femur. In the latter setting, the graft should be trimmed and contoured to prevent extensor mechanism irritation.

Simple cerclage wires are sufficient fixation for most grafts. The fixation must be absolutely rigid. One advantage of wires over a cable system is that the wires can be successively tightened in a back-and-forth manner along the graft, as the graft is brought down onto the surface of the host cortex.

References

1. Callaghan JJ, Salvati EA, Pellicci PM, Wilson PD Jr, Ranawat CS. Result of revision for mechanical failure after cemented total hip replacement. *J Bone Joint Surg Am.* 1985;67:1074–1085.
2. Hunter GA, Welsh RP, Cameron HU, Bailey WH. The results of revision of total hip arthroplasty. *J Bone Joint Surg Br.* 1979;61:419–421.
3. Kavanagh BF, Fitzgerald RH. Multiple revisions for failed total hip arthroplasty not associated with infection. *J Bone Joint Surg Am.* 1987;69:1144–1149.
4. Stromberg CN, Herberts P. A multicenter 10-year study of cemented revision total hip arthroplasty in patients younger than 55 years old: a follow-up report. *J Arthroplasty.* 1994;9:595–601.
5. Gruen TA, McNeice GM, Amstutz HC. "Modes of failure" of cemented stem–type femoral components: a radiographic analysis of loosening. *Clin Orthop.* 1979;141:17–27.
6. Maloney WJ, Jasty M, Rosenberg A, Harris WH. Bone lysis in well-fixed cemented femoral components. *J Bone Joint Surg Br.* 1990;72:966–970.
7. Scott RD. Femoral fractures in conjunction with total hip replacement. *J Bone Joint Surg Am.* 1975;57:494–501.
8. Kavanagh BF, Ilstrup DM, Fitzgerald RH. Revision total hip arthroplasty. *J Bone Joint Surg Am.* 1985;67:517–526.
9. Huddleston HD. Femoral lysis after cemented hip arthroplasty. *J Arthroplasty.* 1988;3:285–297.
10. Pazzaglia UE, Ghisellini F, Ceffa R, Riccardi C, Ceciliani L. Evaluation of reimplant total hip prostheses and resection arthroplasty. *Orthopedics.* 1988;11:1141–1145.
11. Emerson RH Jr, Malinin TI, Cuellar AD, Head WC, Peters PC. Cortical strut allografts in the reconstruction of the femur in revision total hip arthroplasty: a basic science and clinical study. *Clin Orthop.* 1992;285:35–44.
12. Kreutz FP, Hyatt GW, Basset AL. The preservation and clinical use of freeze-dried bone. *J Bone Joint Surg Am.* 1951;33:863–872.
13. Malinin T, Latta LL, Wagner JL, Brown MD. Healing of fractures with freeze-dried cortical bone plates. *Clin Orthop.* 1984;190:281–286.
14. Engh CA, Glassman AH, Griffin WL, Mayer JG. Results of cementless revision for failed cemented total hip arthroplasty. *Clin Orthop.* 1988;235:91–110.
15. Gustillo RB, Pasternak HS. Revision total hip arthroplasty with titanium ingrowth prosthesis and bone grafting for failed cemented component loosening. *Clin Orthop.* 1988;235:111–119.
16. Gie GA, Linder L, Ling RS, Simon JP, Slooff TJ, Timperley

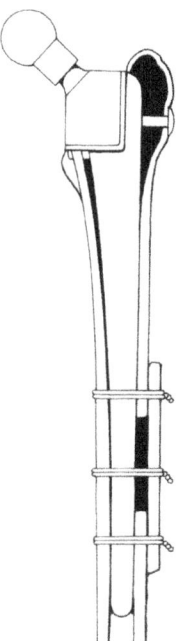

Figure 25.2. A distal cortical window for cement removal restored with a cortical strut, which goes above and below the defect to provide support to the deficient femur.

AJ. Impacted cancellous allografts and cement for revision total hip arthroplasty. *J Bone Joint Surg Br.* 1993;75:14–21.

17. Allan DG, Lavoie GJ, McDonald S, Oakeshott R, Gross AE. Proximal femoral allografts in revision hip arthroplasty. *J Bone Joint Surg Br.* 1991;73:235–240.

18. Head WC, Hillyard JM, Emerson RH Jr, et al. Proximal femoral allografts in revision total hip arthroplasty. *Semin Arthroplasty.* 1993;4:92–98.

19. Chandler HP, Penenberg BL. Femoral reconstruction. In: Chandler HP, Penenberg BL, eds. *Bone Deficiency in Total Hip Replacement.* Thorofare, NJ: Slack, Inc; 1989:103–164.

20. Chandler HP, King D, McCarthy J, et al. The treatment of femoral fractures following total hip arthroplasty. Presented as a scientific exhibit, American Academy of Orthopaedic Surgeons annual meeting: 1991; Anaheim, Calif.

21. Friedlaender GE, Strong DM, Sells KW. Studies on the antigenicity of bone. *J Bone Joint Surg Am.* 1976;58:854–858.

22. Salvati EA, Wilson PD Jr, Jolley MN, Vakili F, Aglietti P, Brown GC. A ten-year follow-up study of our first one hundred consecutive Charnley total hip replacements. *J Bone Joint Surg Am.* 1981;63:753–767.

26
Use of Femoral Allografts in Reconstruction of Major Segmental Defects

Hugh P. Chandler and Robert J. Carangelo

Major segmental bone loss of the proximal femur in revision total hip surgery presents a formidable challenge to the reconstructive surgeon. Resection arthroplasty is not an option because it results in a very short and unstable extremity.[1,2] Cemented proximal femoral replacement components have been used extensively in tumor surgery, but in our experience they have not done well in revision total hip replacement. The femoral endosteal canal is smooth and sclerotic from the previous stem, and cement intrusion is not optimal.[3,4,5,6] Unlike some tumor patients, the patient with a femoral revision may live for many years and place high demands on the fixation of the femoral component. Distally sintered components achieve distal fixation, but may compromise proximal bone quality even further because of stress shielding.[7,8,9,10,11] In rare instances of severe bone deficiency, it may be necessary to add intramedullary bone graft to expanded femoral canals.[12]

We have used a proximal femoral allograft combined with an S-ROM modular stem™ (Johnson & Johnson) in 44 hips in 42 patients since July of 1989. The average age of the patient was 62 (range 35–84). The problems were formidable. The average patient had undergone five previous hip operations (range 1–16). Eight had experienced septic event that required resection arthroplasty, although none had positive cultures at the time of their reconstruction with the allograft. The preoperative defects within the proximal femur ranged from 10–25 cm. All patients required two crutches or a walker.

Technique for Reconstruction of Proximal Femoral Deficiency

Surgical Approach

The trochanteric slide is the appropriate exposure because the trochanter (or the sleeve of the abductors and quadriceps if the trochanter is absent) will be resting against a nonviable allograft bed and union may not occur. The quadriceps tethers the trochanter and, even if union does not occur, this muscle prevents the trochanter from migrating proximally (Fig. 26.1). If bone is available for an extended trochanteric osteotomy, this technique should be used because it increases the surface area of viable bone that is in contact with the allograft, providing a better chance of union, and it allows for better fixation of the trochanter to the graft (Fig. 26.2, 26.16, and 26.17).

Choice of Graft Material

The surgeon should select an ipsilateral allograft femur that is the same size or slightly larger than the host bone. A smaller graft is contraindicated because it is necessary to prepare the metaphysis and the medullary canal of the allograft 2 mm larger than the host canal. We have not attempted to match tissue types of the allograft and the host.

Choice of Stem

The S-ROM modular stem (Johnson and Johnson, Raynham, MA) has proven to be the most satisfactory of all the stems we have tried in conjunction with a proximal femoral allograft (Fig. 26.3). Because this stem is modular, the proximal ZT sleeve can be selectively cemented to the allograft and the stem can be press-fit to the host. The distal portion of this stem is a constant diameter and resists bending forces. The flutes provide rotational control, even in an eburnated canal. Because of these features, a simple butt joint can be used between the allograft and the host bone. The uncemented distal portion of the stem that is within the host bone permits early impaction of the graft to the host through the transverse butt joint. The diameter of the stem is deter-

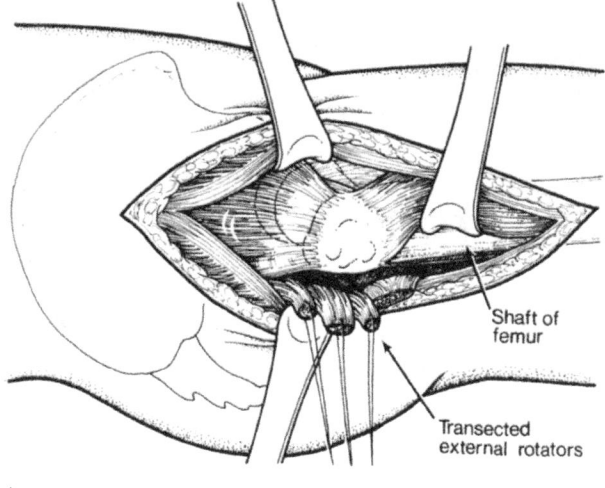

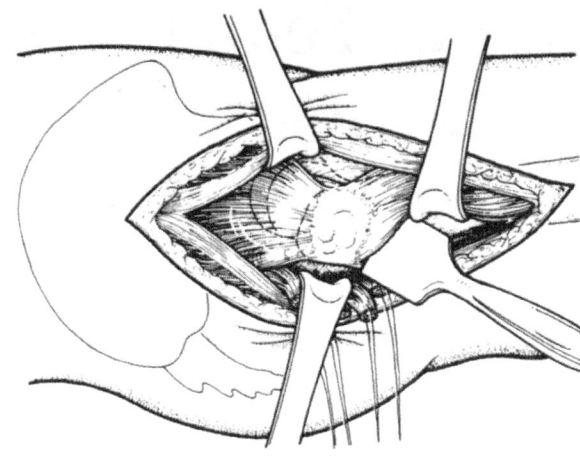

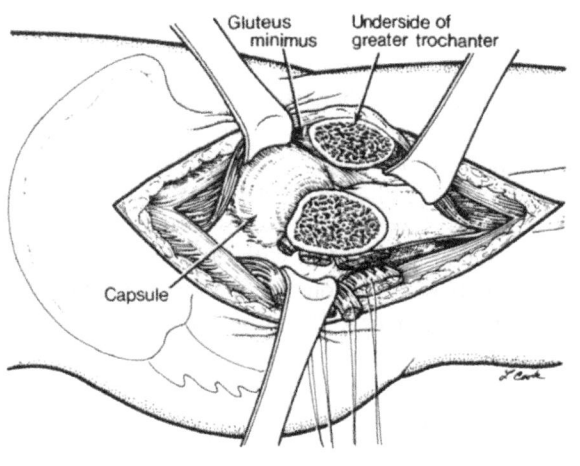

Figure 26.1. With the trochanteric slide, the short external rotators and the posterior capsule are divided from the greater trochanter and tagged for later reconstruction. B. An osteotomy of the greater trochanter is performed. C. The abductors and the quadriceps are kept in continuity with the greater trochanter.

mined by the diameter of the host medullary canal. A variety of curved and straight stem lengths are available. The stem should extend at least 8 cm within the host femur.

Preparation of the Host

Proximal host bone that is not structurally strong should be removed with a saw, leaving a transverse surface that can support the graft. Fragments of host bone that are divided from the distal shaft should be saved for later autogenous grafting at the host–graft junction. If possible, these fragments should be left attached to the quadriceps so they receive a blood supply. The distal medullary canal is prepared with flexible reamers that are the same diameter as the inner diameter of the selected stem (Fig. 26.4). The fact that the flutes are 1.2 mm larger than the stem ensures that rotational control of the stem will be achieved within the host femur. The rare exception could be the situation in which the allograft segment is very short and the majority of the curved portion of the stem will be in the host bone. In this circumstance, the host canal should be prepared 1 mm larger than the stem to ensure that the femur will not be fractured as the stem is inserted. If the host canal is too tight, the stem can potentially jam within it and become difficult to advance or remove.

Preparation of the Graft

The graft is prepared with standard S-ROM milling tools to a size that is 2 mm larger than the final stem to be used (Fig. 26.5). This provides space for a cement mantle around the sleeve and ensures that the bowed stem will pass through the allograft easily without risk of allograft fracture.

A trial ZT sleeve 2 mm larger than the stem that will eventually be used is placed in the femoral allograft. A trial stem of the same diameter as the selected stem is attached to the trial proximal stem body. The shortest neck lengths and the shortest head lengths are assembled on the trial component. With the trial prosthesis inserted within the allograft and the trial head reduced into the acetabular component, maximum traction is ap-

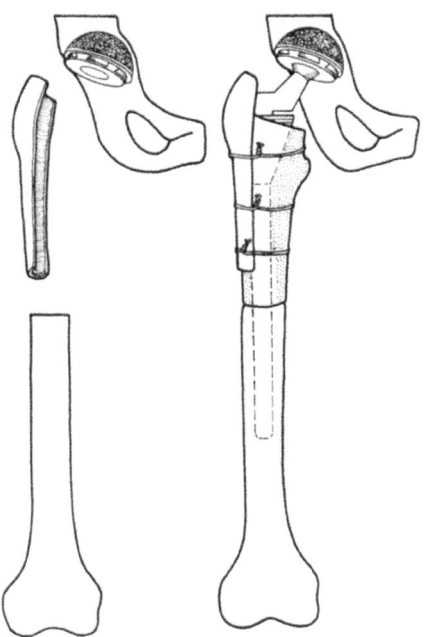

Figure 26.2. The extended trochanteric osteotomy is useful because it increases the surface area of viable bone in contact with the allograft, providing a better chance of union. B. The extended trochanteric fragment is reattached to host bone with cerclage wires.

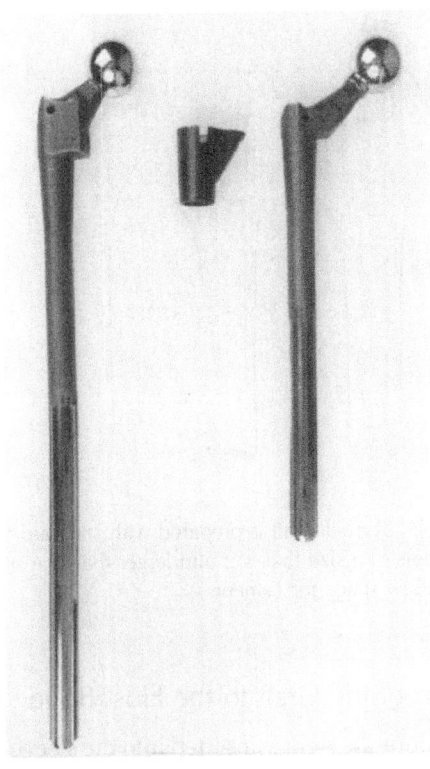

Figure 26.3. The S-ROM stem is modular. The proximal sleeve (ZT) can be selectively cemented to the allograft, and the stem can be press-fit to the host. The distal portion of the stem is a constant diameter and resists bending forces. The flutes resist rotation.

plied to the distal host femur and the resection line is marked using methylene blue (Fig. 26.6). A transverse cut through the allograft is made with an oscillating saw. If too much bone is resected from the allograft, longer neck and/or head lengths can be used to make up the discrepancy. Since most patients who require proximal femoral allografts are very short preoperatively, it may be difficult to reestablish normal length at the index grafting procedure; recurrent dislocation can potentially occur postoperatively when the soft tissues have stretched out. In this situation, revision is accomplished easily: a stem with a longer neck or head length is chosen, and the sleeve is left cemented to the allograft.

The anteversion of the allograft in relation to the host bone is marked with methylene blue (Fig. 26.6). The oversize trial sleeve is removed and the appropriate ZT (2 mm smaller than the trial) is selected. The graft is cleaned with pulsatile lavage and dried with sponges. Half a package of liquid cement is forced into the open trabeculae of the prepared allograft using finger pressure, and thicker cement is later placed around the ZT sleeve (Fig. 26.7). Alignment instruments ensure proper positioning of the sleeve as it is cemented to the proximal femoral allograft. Care should be taken to avoid inserting the sleeve too far distally into the allograft because this could prevent the maintenance of a circumferential cement mantle.

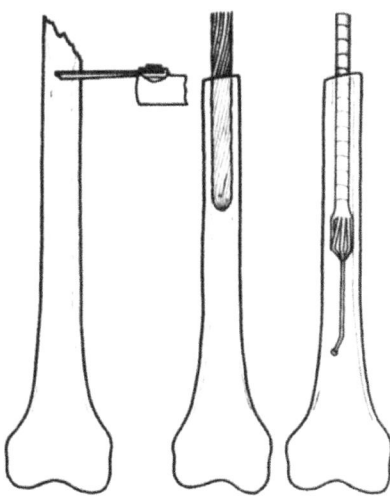

Figure 26.4. Proximal host bone that is not structurally strong is removed with a saw, leaving a flat transverse surface that can support the graft. The medullary canal is prepared with flexible reamers that are the same diameter as the selected stem.

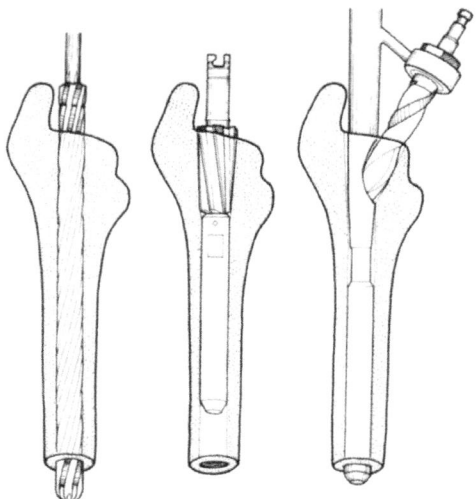

Figure 26.5. The allograft is prepared with standard S-ROM milling tools to a size that is 2 mm larger than the selected stem to allow space for cement.

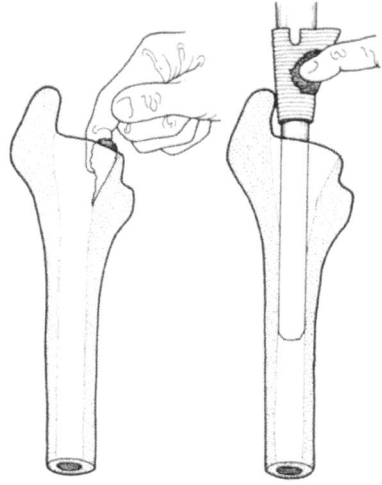

Figure 26.7. Half a package of cement is used to cement the sleeve to the allograft. Liquid cement is forced into the open trabeculae by using a gloved finger, and thicker cement is later placed around the sleeve. Care should be taken not to insert the sleeve too deeply into the allograft to ensure that there will be an adequate cement mantle.

Fixation of the Graft to the Host Bone

The appropriate stem is inserted into the sleeve (already cemented to the allograft) and the Morse taper between the sleeve and the stem is engaged and locked by impaction. Reaming the diaphysis of the graft 2 mm larger than the stem permits a bowed stem to pass through the allograft easily without risk of fracture. If there is any concern that the stem is tight within the allograft, the allograft should be protected with temporary cerclage wires, cables, or hose clamps. We prefer to use hose clamps because they are very strong and very inexpensive, and they can be removed after the stem has been inserted (Fig. 26.8).

A high risk of fracture of the host bone exists as the fluted stem is introduced within the medullary canal because the canal has been reamed to match the inner diameter of the stem. Therefore, the host bone should be protected by double No. 16 twisted wires, crimped cables, or hose clamps. It is safer to insert protective cerclage devices proximally just below the junction of the graft and the host and distally about 5 or 6 cm (Fig. 26.9). The stem is inserted into the host canal, matching the previously marked anteversion. Care should be taken to start the stem in the appropriate anteversion because

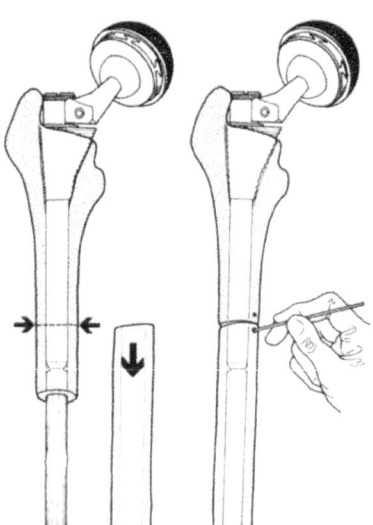

Figure 26.6. The trial prosthesis with the shortest neck and head length is inserted within the allograft and reduced into the acetabular component. Maximum traction is applied to the distal host femur and the resection line is marked with the allograft. A transverse cut through the allograft is made with an oscillating saw.

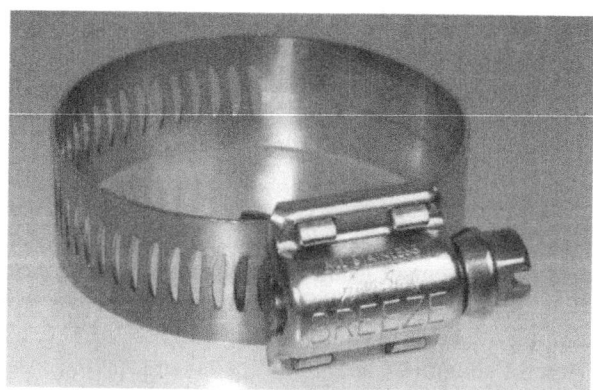

Figure 26.8. Hose clamps can be used to protect the graft and the host temporarily.

26. Use of Femoral Allografts in Reconstruction of Major Segmental Defects

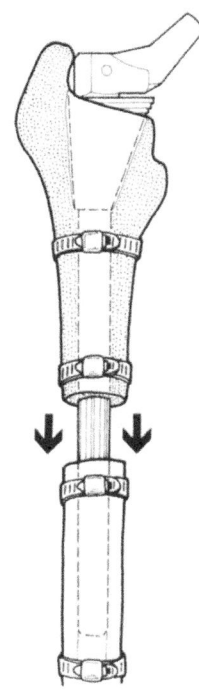

Figure 26.9. Cerclage wires, cables, or hose clamps are placed around the allograft and the host bone as the stem is inserted to prevent potential fracture.

this location cannot be changed once the flutes have engaged the host bone. Impaction should be steady and frequent without excessive hard blows. The stem will slowly advance into the host bone. When the allograft impacts against the host bone, the butt joint may not fit perfectly. A thin oscillating saw may be used to trim away high points. The graft is then impacted again and the process is repeated until the contact area is optimal (Fig. 26.10). Care should be taken not to scratch the stem with the oscillating saw because a fracture of the stem could result.

It is quite easy to obtain a perfect butt joint, and a step-cut is not necessary because rotational stability is almost always maintained by the fluted distal portion of the S-ROM stem. However, it is very important to ensure that the graft is stable in rotation. If instability can be proven intraoperatively, the strut graft or a fracture plate should be placed on the lateral cortex. We prefer to use a fracture plate because such plates are cheaper and stronger than strut grafts. The plate is held in place with temporary hose clamps, which provide extraordinary compressive strength, slightly deforming the plate outside the femur and the stem within it. Double No. 16 stainless steel twisted wires are placed at 2½-cm intervals between the hose clamps, and then the hose clamps are removed (see Fig. 26.14D). Autologous bone that has been removed from the proximal femur should be placed around the junction of the graft and the host.

Cerclage wires or sutures may be used to hold the bone in place.

Trochanteric Reattachment

In cases of a healthy host trochanter, the greater trochanter of the allograft should be resected to provide a bed for the host trochanter. The greater trochanter can be attached to the allograft with either wires or the Dall Miles Cable Grip System™ (Howmedica, Rutherford, N.J.). In cases of extended trochanteric osteotomy, fixation of the distal cortical strut is easily achieved by cerclage wires (Fig. 26.2, 26.16, 26.17). In the absence of a host trochanter, the soft tissue sleeve of the abductors and the quadriceps should be sutured to the posterior capsule and to the posterior fascia of the quadriceps. We prefer not to drill holes in the allograft itself to suture the abductor sleeve to the bone.

Postoperative Management

Because the allograft femur is obtained from healthy young donors, it is very strong. The stem protects the allograft and the host bone from fracture. Early weight-bearing is helpful in impacting the allograft to the host bone, ensuring early union and later remodeling. Usually, patients can be mobilized by the first or second day, depending on comfort, and they are encour-

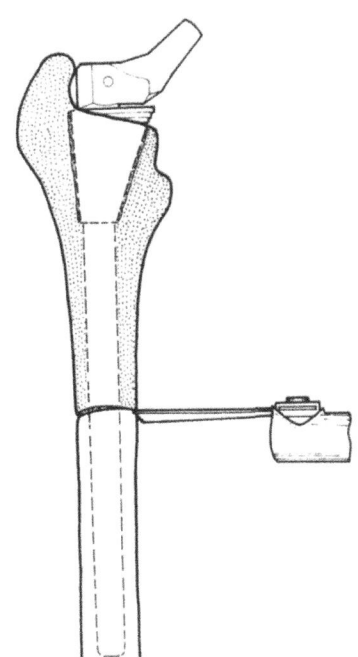

Figure 26.10. After the allograft is impacted against the host bone, a thin oscillating saw is used to trim away any high points. Further impaction of the allograft provides a perfect fit at the allograft–host junction.

aged to put at least 60 to 80 pounds of weight on the extremity. The only reason that immediate full weight-bearing is not permitted is to ensure that the trochanter stays in apposition to the proximal allograft. At 6 weeks, all patients are encouraged to bear full weight; the only stipulations are that they should avoid pain and should not limp. Many patients can walk without support or limp at 6 to 8 weeks.

Dealing with the Patulous Host Canal

In a host medullary canal larger than 19 mm, it is very difficult to obtain a proximal femoral allograft large enough to permit preparation of the allograft 2 mm larger than the component to be used. Stems larger than 19 mm can also cause distal thigh pain.

On three occasions, we have used a tibial allograft, milled to a cylindrical shape with an outer diameter of 21 mm[16] (Fig. 26.11). The patulous host canal is gently drilled with a 21-mm drill to ensure that it is of a constant diameter. The medullary canal of the tibial graft is prepared with 13-mm reamers to accept an 18/13 stem. The allograft proximal femur is prepared as described earlier, with milling tools 2 mm larger than the planned stem. If an intramedullary tibial graft is used in the host bone, it is preferable to assemble the sleeve and the stem first, engaging the Morse taper, and then cementing the sleeve and the proximal portion of the stem together into the allograft (Fig. 26.12). The reason for cementing both the sleeve and the proximal stem to the allograft,

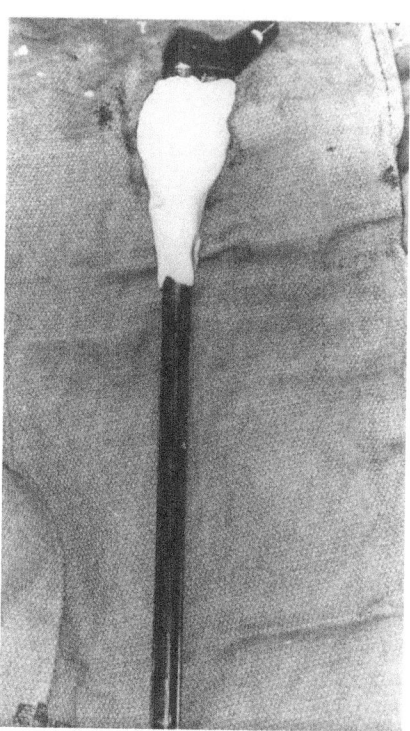

Figure 26.12. If an intramedullary tibial graft is used, it is probably better to assemble the sleeve and the stem first and then to cement both to the allograft.

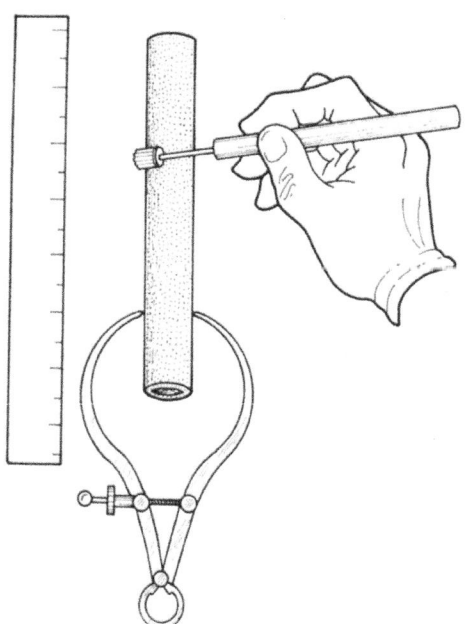

Figure 26.11. A tibial diaphyseal allograft is milled with a high-powered burr to a cylindric shape with an outer diameter to match the inner diameter of the host femur.

rather than cementing only the sleeve, is that a distal pedestal cannot form within the tibial graft. On one occasion in our experience, the stem subsided, fracturing the proximal allograft (Fig. 26.13F, G, H). Cementing of the sleeve and the proximal stem provides a larger area of cement fixation.

On one occasion we inserted the allograft tibia within the host canal and held it with distal transverse screws to provide rotational stability (Fig. 26.13C). On two other occasions, we assembled the distal allograft on the stem prior to insertion into the host bone (Fig. 26.14A–G). The latter technique is preferable; however, a lateral strut or, preferably, a fracture plate must be added to control rotation because the tibial graft is cylindrical and could theoretically twist within the canal.

Results

The average preoperative Harris hip score was 33, and the postoperative rating was 81, including the failures. All patients required a walker or crutches preoperatively. At last follow-up, 25 walked without support; 12 used a cane; 4 used crutches; and 2 elderly patients continue to use a walker for balance only. Radiographic union of the graft to the host occurred in 42 of 44 hips (97%). There was only one proven nonunion.

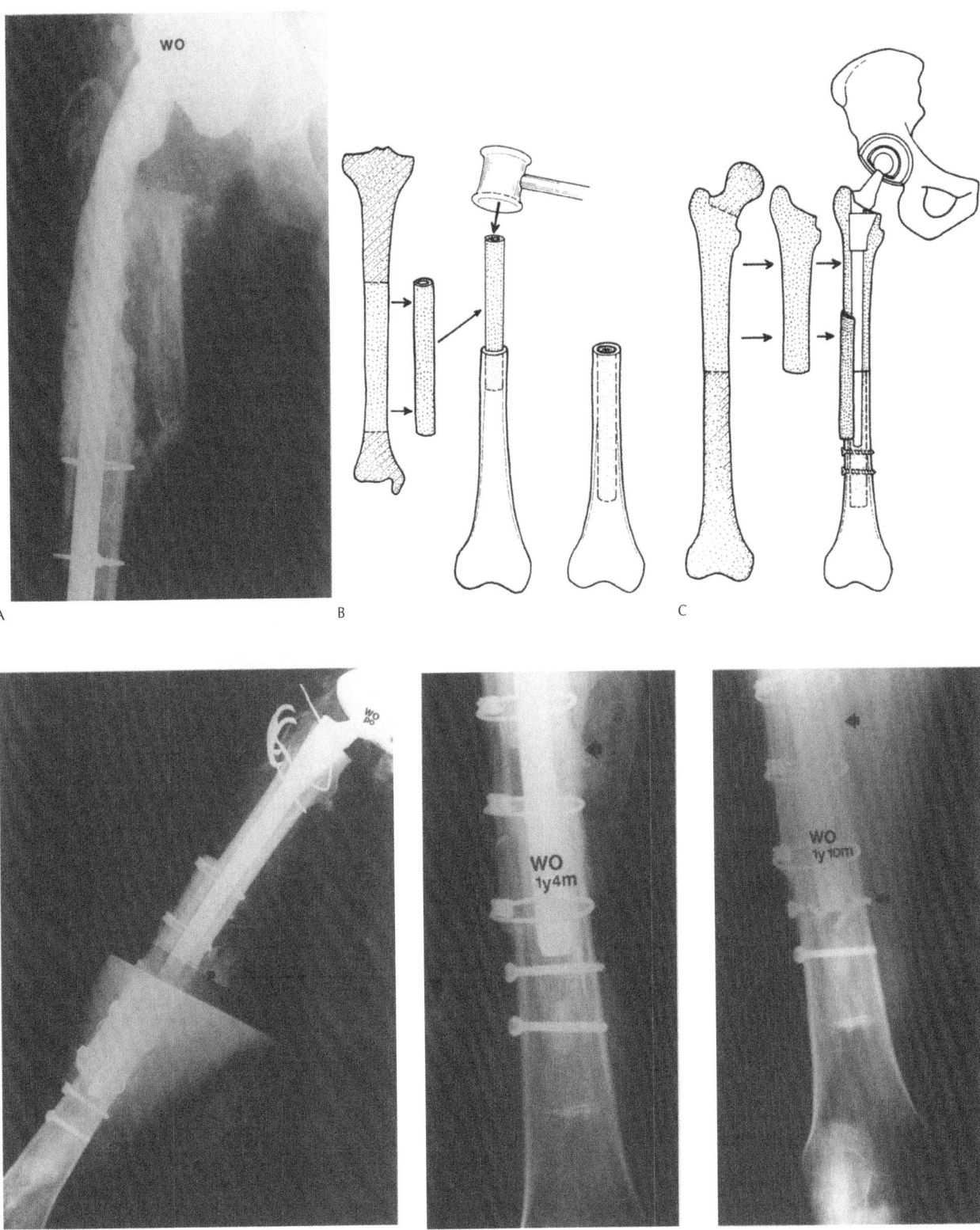

Figure 26.13. A. This 36-year-old man had undergone nine previous hip operations. A. He presented with a septic hip. The organism was *Staphylococcus aureus*. After debridement, a spacer coated with antibiotic-impregnated cement was used. Systemic antibiotics were discontinued at 6 weeks. An aspiration 10 days later was negative for infection. The hip was reconstructed 7 days after the aspiration. B. A tibial allograft was then impacted within the medullary canal. C. A proximal femoral allograft was used with the standard technique except that a smaller stem was placed within the medullary canal of the tibia. Rotation was controlled with two distal screws and a lateral onlay strut. D. The junction of the femoral allograft and the host bone is obvious on the postoperative radiograph (arrow). At 6 weeks after surgery, the patient began using a cane. E. At 1 year 4 months, the proximal femoral allograft and the host bone have united (arrow). The patient used a cane only for long walks. F. At 1 year 10 months, the patient had thigh pain and (subjectively reported) shortening of the extremity. Radiographs showed distal subsidence of the stem with fracture of the proximal screw.

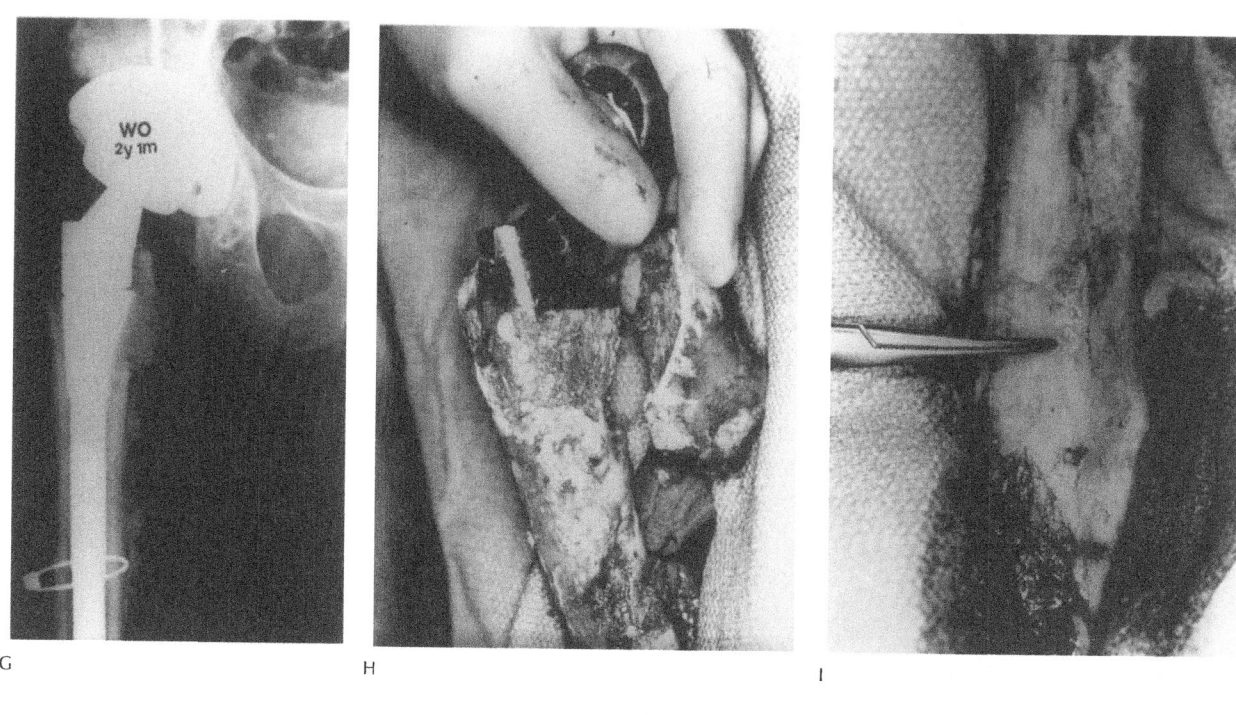
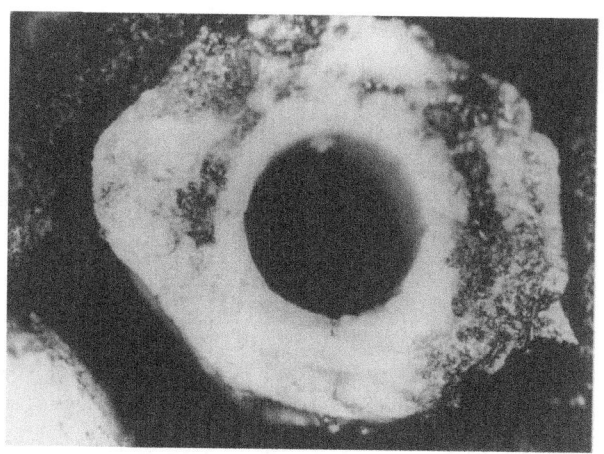
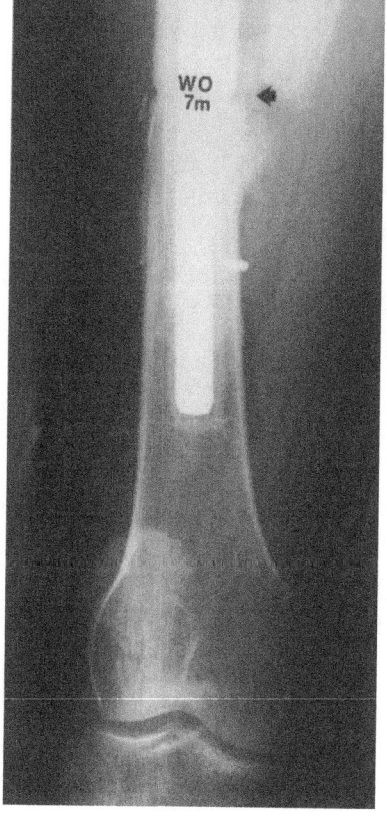

Figure 26.13. Continued. G. X-ray at 2 years 1 month shows subsidence of the proximal portion of the prosthesis. H. The proximal portion of the allograft had fractured as the stem subsided. I. The graft–host junction was solidly united. The onlay allograft strut had united to the host, but not entirely to the proximal femoral allograft. J. The intramedullary tibial graft had united to the host femur. Note the grooves made by the flutes. K. A new proximal femoral allograft was used, but the proximal stem and sleeve were cemented as one unit (see Fig. 26.12). The new stem was placed within in the previous tibial graft, and the flutes engaged the grooves made by the original stem. At 7 months, the junction of the proximal femoral allograft and the host bone appear to have united. The patient uses a cane for long walks.

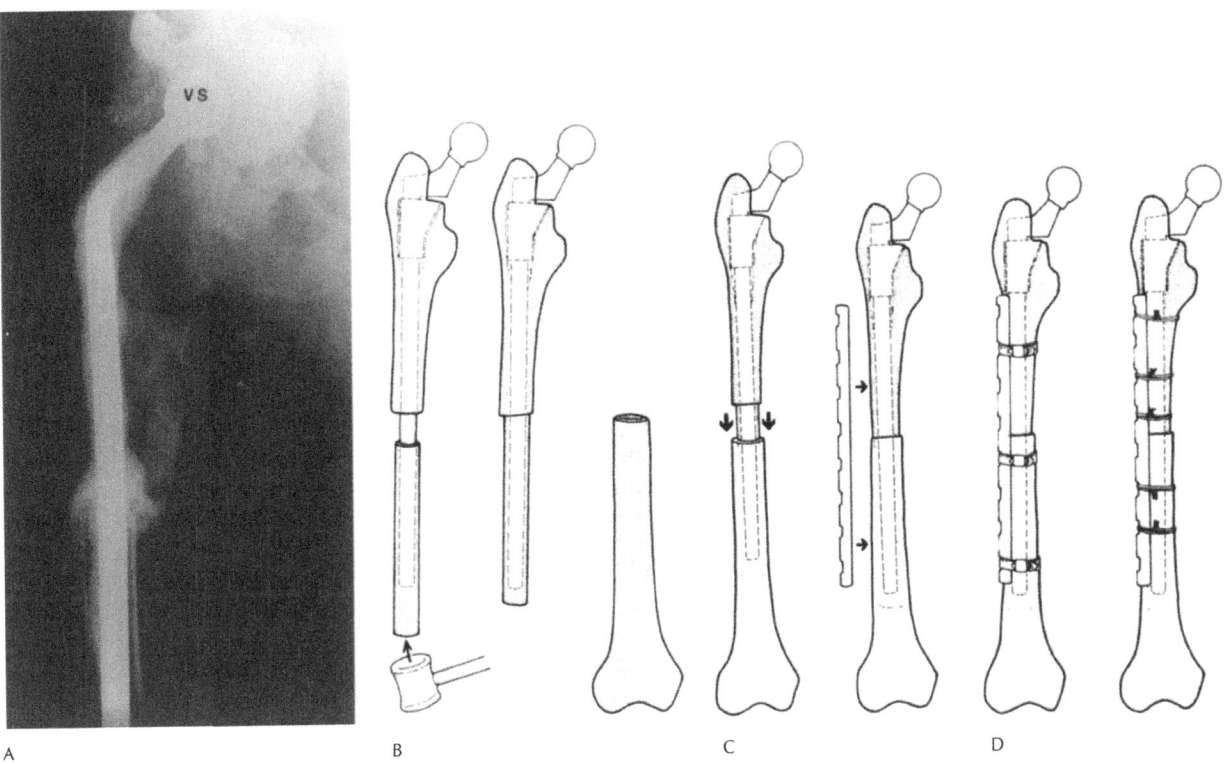

Figure 26.14. This 79-year-old woman had undergone nine previous hip operations. A. She presented with a *Staph epidermidis* infection. Debridement of grossly infected proximal femoral bone left a major defect. A temporary articulating spacer with antibiotic-impregnated cement was used for 6 weeks. Ten days after a negative aspiration, the hip was reconstructed. A tibial allograft was milled to an outside diameter of 21 mms. The medullary canal of the tibial allograft was prepared with 13-mm reamers. The standard technique of proximal femoral allograft reconstruction was used proximally, except that the sleeve and the proximal stem were cemented together (see Fig. 26.12). B. The tibial graft was protected temporarily with hose clamps and impacted onto the distal portion of the stem. The host canal was prepared with a 21-mm reamer. The host femur was temporarily protected with hose clamps. C. The distal tibial graft was impacted within the medullary canal of the host femur until the proximal femoral allograft contacted the host femur. D. A fracture plate was used to control rotation. Hose clamps were used initially, and they slightly deformed the stem and the plate. The hose clamps were replaced by double No. 16 wires.

One patient had a resection arthroplasty for sepsis 3 weeks after a proximal femoral allograft (Fig. 26.15A–E). Ten weeks later, she underwent a reconstruction with a new allograft. At 8 months, the graft is united to the host femur. None of the patients who had previously experienced sepsis had recurrence of their initial infection. One patient with no previous infections developed a *Staph aureus* infection.

In many patients it was difficult to determine whether or not the greater trochanter had united. The greater trochanter migrated proximally by over 1 cm (range 1.2–2 cm) in five patients. However, because the quadriceps tethered the trochanter from more proximal migration, a limp was seldom present, even if the trochanter had obviously not united.

The most common serious complication was dislocation, which occurred in nine cases, five of which required revision because of recurrent dislocation.

There were four graft failures. One patient, who had undergone seven previous total hip replacements but no prior sepsis, developed a *Staph aureous* infection that required resection arthroplasty with removal of the graft and the components. An antibiotic-impregnated spacer was used, and the patient was treated with intravenous antibiotics for 6 weeks. After a negative aspiration 10 days after cessation of antibiotics, another allograft prosthesis reconstruction was performed 8 weeks after the initial debridement. That patient remains infection-free with a united graft at 7 years (Fig. 26.15A–E).

There was one nonunion at the graft–host junction because the initial stem was undersized. At revision a larger stem, combined with a fracture plate and autogenous bone, was used. Union occurred. One patient, who had undergone an intramedullary distal tibial graft, sustained a fracture of the proximal allograft when the stem and sleeve subsided (Fig. 26.13A–K). One patient experienced major resorption of the femoral allograft, but currently functions well because a distal pedestal was formed in the host bone. We believe this

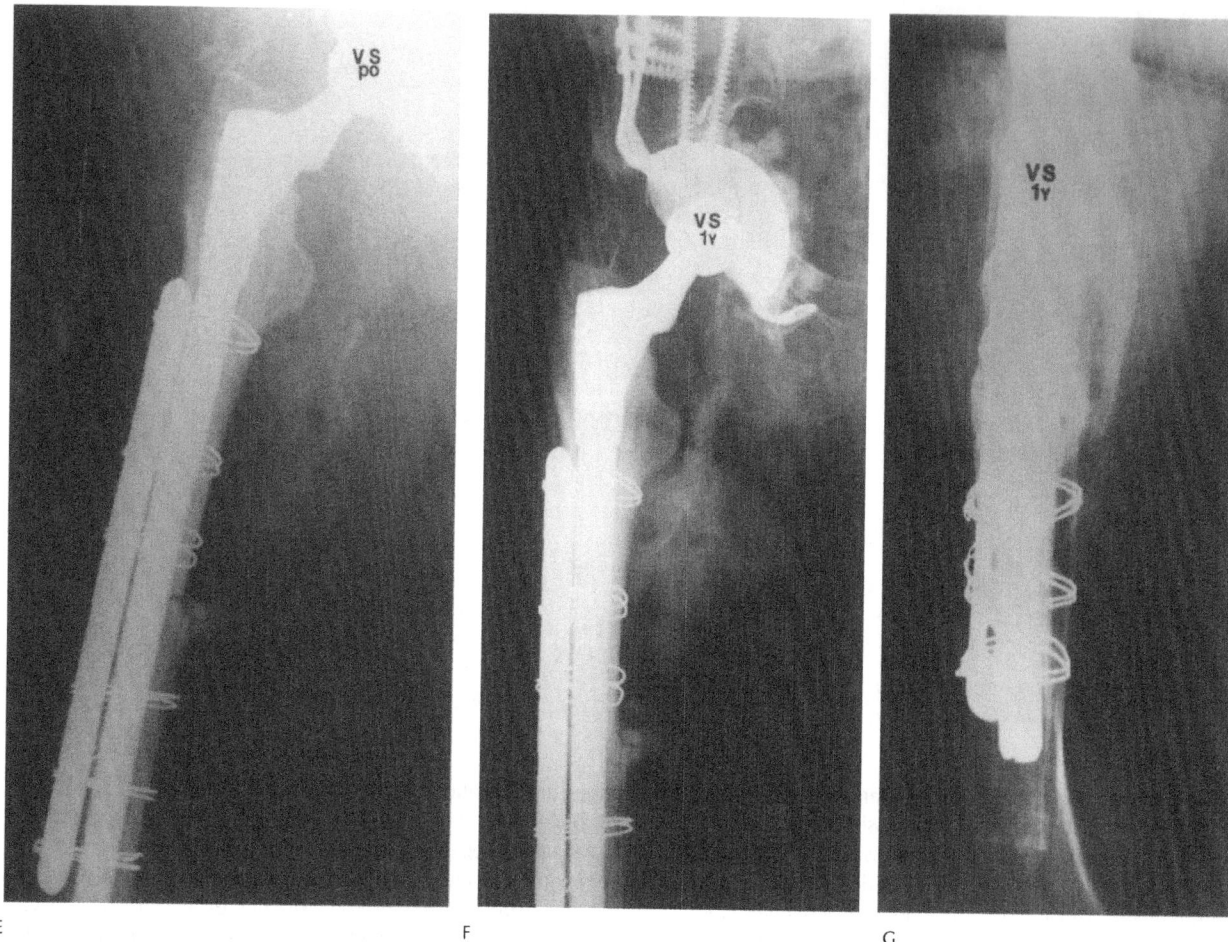

E F G

Figure 26.14. Continued. E. AP postoperative radiograph of proximal femoral allograft reconstruction. F. The patient at 1 year postoperative is comfortable and infection free. She uses a walker for balance. AP x-ray demonstrates union at the host–allograft junction. G. The lateral view also demonstrates union at the host–allograft junction and the intramedullary graft.

resorption was probably an antigenic response to the allograft, because the patient had undergone two previous acetabular allografts and two previous proximal femoral allografts (using other techniques) and had received multiple homologous transfusions. This patient is considering revision because of moderate shortening. If proximal femoral graft is used in a second revision, we plan to employ appropriate tissue typing to prevent future antigenic response.

Questions

Several technical questions arise concerning the use of a proximal femoral allograft combined with a revision component used to reconstruct major femoral deficiency in revision total hip replacement.

The first question is whether fresh-frozen or freeze-dried allograft bone should be used. Our experience has been only with fresh-frozen bone, but Head et al.[13] have reported positive results using freeze-dried allografts, with union at the graft host junction occurring at an average of 36 weeks. Provided that the graft is protected by a stem, either fresh-frozen or freeze-dried grafts can be used with equal success.

The second question is whether the femoral component should be cemented to the allograft. Initially we used uncemented components within a proximal femoral allograft, but these components had a high failure rate because they prevent ingrowth. Subsidence of uncemented collarless components occurred routinely and, on one occasion, a collared, uncemented prosthesis failed very quickly because the collar split the allograft as it subsided. Zmolek and Dorr[14] also noted subsidence in 7 of 11 uncemented femoral components used with structural proximal allografts. They recommend cementing the femoral component to the allograft. Head et al.[15] reported no subsidence in 22 patients with cemented femoral components used with structural

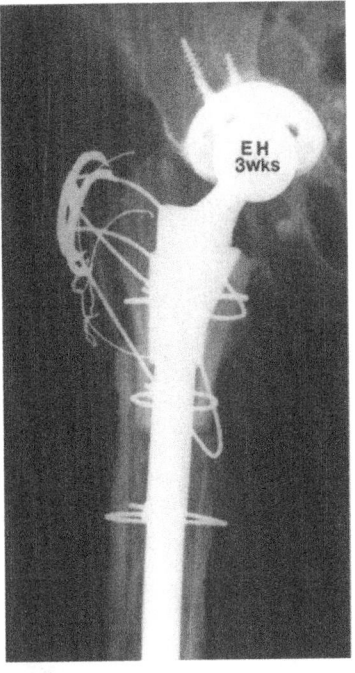

A

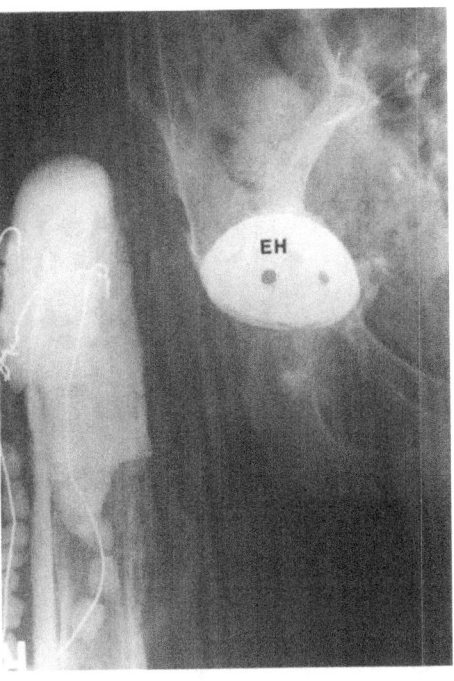

B

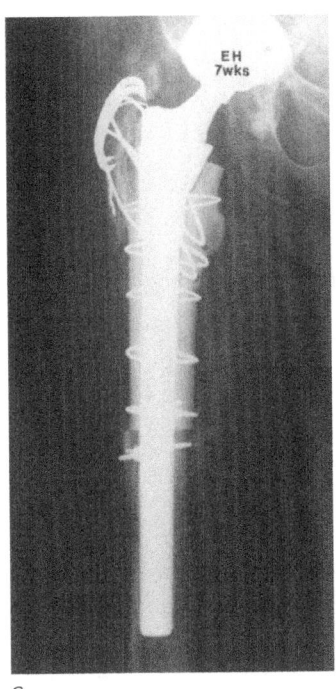

C

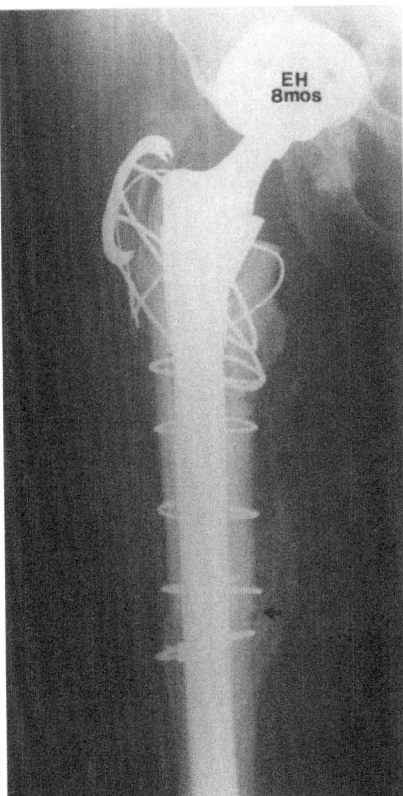

D

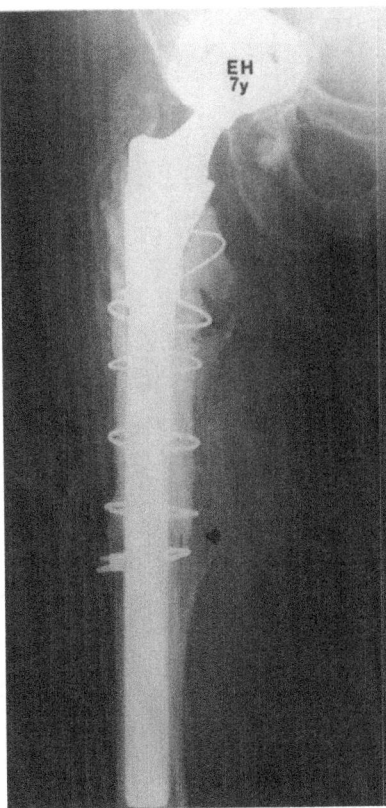

E

Figure 26.15. This 75-year-old woman had undergone seven previous total hip replacements before her index proximal femoral allograft reconstruction. A. Three weeks postoperatively she developed a *Staph aureus* infection. B. The allograft, femoral component, and acetabular liner were removed. An antibiotic-impregnated spacer was used. (We would now have used an articulating spacer.) The patient was treated with antibiotics for 6 weeks. Ten days after the antibiotics were discontinued, an aspiration showed no evidence of infection. C. A new proximal femoral allograft reconstruction was performed 10 weeks after the original debridement. The allograft–host junction is obvious at 7 weeks. The patient was encouraged to use a cane. D. At 8 months, the graft had united to the host femur. E. Seven years after the second allograft, the patient remains comfortable without evidence of pain. She uses a cane for outside walking (she is 82 years old at this point), but has a normal gait without support.

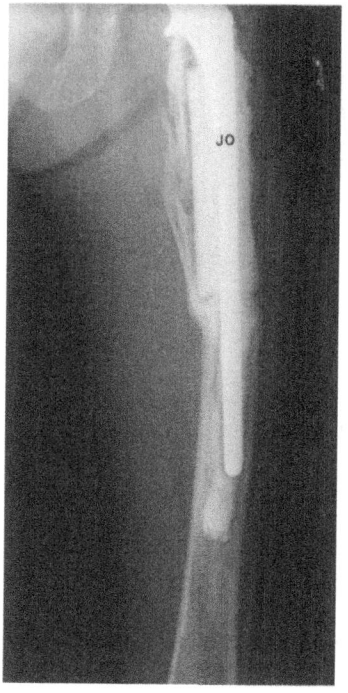
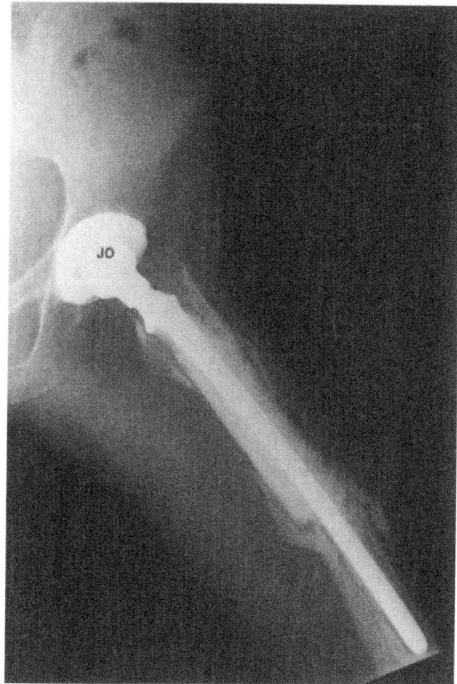
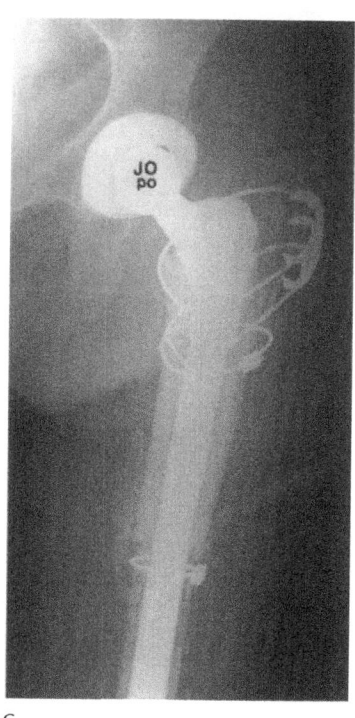
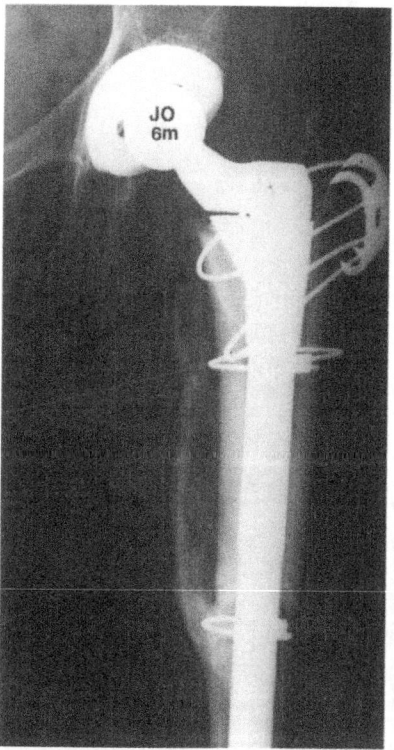
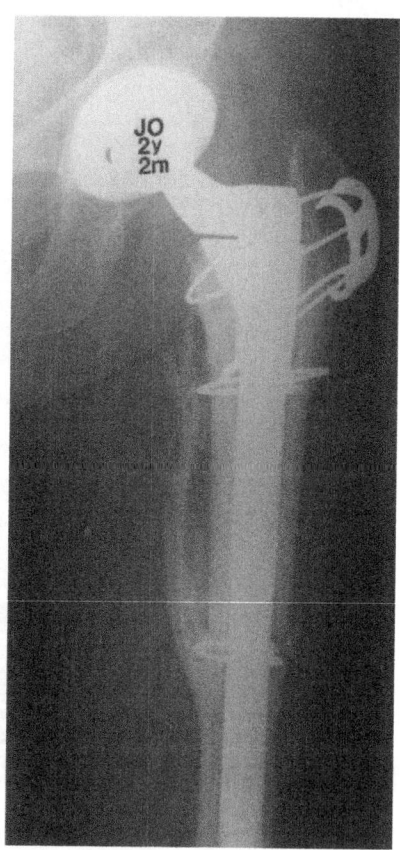

Figure 26.16. This 59-year-old woman had undergone three previous total hip replacements. An allograft was used at her last revision (at another institution). A. Cement was used in both allograft and host femur. Cement extruded at the graft–host interface, and she had a nonunion after 19 months of crutch protection. Loosening of the stem within the host femur is obvious on the AP view. B. There is also evidence of loosening of the stem seen on the lateral view. C. A new reconstruction was performed by using the current technique. An extended trochanteric osteotomy was used along with a trochanteric slide. At 6 weeks she discarded all support and walked without a limp. D. At 6 months, she was able to walk 2 miles without support and without a limp. E. At 2 years, 10 months, her Harris hip score is 100. The graft has united to the host femur, and the extended trochanteric osteotomy has also united to the allograft.

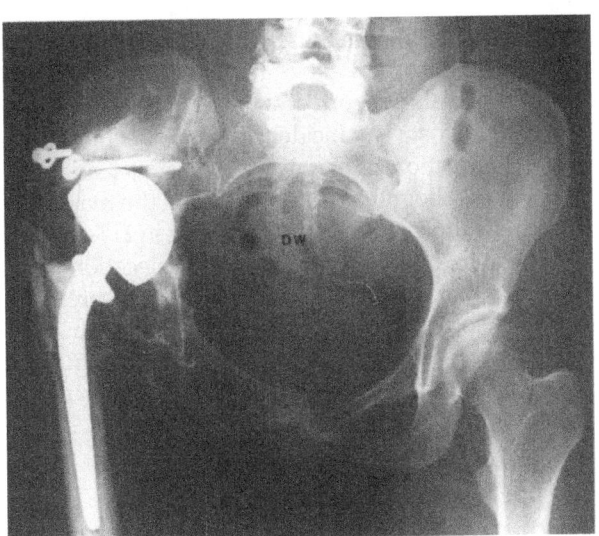

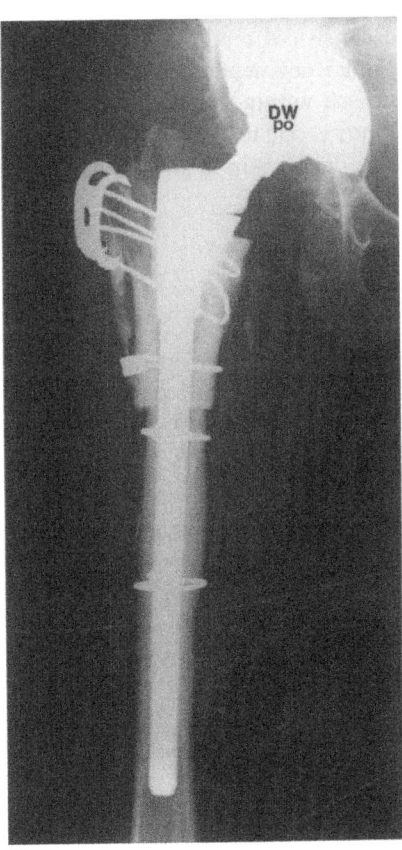

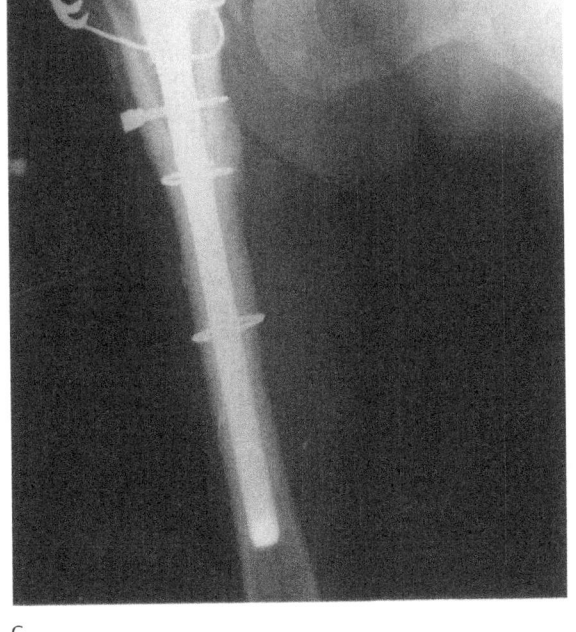

Figure 26.17. A. This 41-year-old woman had undergone two previous total hip replacements. B. At 7 weeks, she discarded support. C. At 2 years, she rates 100 on the Harris hip score. The graft has united to the host femur, and the extended trochanteric osteotomy has united to the graft.

femoral allografts. It seems logical to cement the femoral component to the graft routinely.

The third question involves the method of attachment of the allograft to the host bone. The options are (1) metal plates with screws in the graft and in the host bone, (2) long stems cemented to the graft and to the host, and (3) long stems cemented to the graft but press-fit to the host.

Plates that are held to the graft and to the host with screws have several disadvantages.[16,17,18] Screws above and below the junction of the graft to the host can prevent impaction of the graft to the host bone and inhibit union. Screws are difficult to place around the stem and can potentially compromise the cement mantle around the prostheses. Screw holes in either the graft or the host bone can potentially increase stress and cause fractures.

Long stems cemented to the graft and to the host also have several disadvantages.[13,19] Cement above and below the junction site can prevent the graft from impacting to the host. In addition, cement can extrude at the junction site and, because the diaphyseal bone has been altered by the previous stem, cement intrusion into the host bone is not optimal (Fig. 26.16A, B).

The best solution is to cement the proximal stem to the graft and to press-fit the distal stem to the host bone.[15,20,21,22] This construct is strong enough to permit early weight-bearing and it encourages impaction of the graft to the host bone (Fig. 26.16C, D, E and 26.17A, B, C).

The final technique question is how to obtain rotational stability at the graft–host junction. A step-cut provides good rotational control and heals rapidly because of the broad surface areas that are opposed.[23,24] However, a step-cut is technically more difficult than a transverse butt joint and it also determines the anteversion of the proximal femur. An oblique cut at the junction of the graft and the host also provides some rotational control.[14] However, the distal flutes of the S-ROM within the host canal and the proximal sleeve within the allograft provide enough rotational stability so that a simple transverse butt joint can be used with this particular stem. A butt joint is technically very easy to accomplish and a perfect fit is easily attained by using a thin oscillating saw to remove any high points just before final impaction. A butt joint also permits rotational adjustment before the flutes engage the host bone. If during final range-of-motion test the hip dislocates because of an error in anteversion, the stem and the allograft can be removed from the host bone, rotated at 10° increments into either more or less anteversion, and reinserted into the grooves that were previously cut by the flutes.

The incidence of complications in revision total hip replacement is greater than that in primary hip replacement. The infection rate encountered with proximal femoral allografts ranges from 5% to 20%.[16,18] In our series, it was 2%, despite the fact that 8 patients had experienced sepsis previously. Perhaps the low incidence of infection was related to the fact that all surgeries were performed in laminar flow operating rooms with the use of body exhaust systems. Nonunion of proximal femoral allografts has ranged from 6% to 13.6%.[15,16,18] In our series, the nonunion rate was 3%, perhaps because the patients were encouraged to walk early and so impacted their graft against the transverse butt joint. Fractures have occurred in 5% to 14% in other series using proximal femoral allografts held to the host bone with screws in the graft and in the host bone.[15,16,18] There were no fractures in our series, probably because the allograft was protected by the stem and there were no holes in the allograft itself. However, dislocations with proximal femoral allografts remain a major problem. Head et al.[15] reported an incidence of 23%, and Zmolek and Dorr,[14] an incidence of 58% of either instability or dislocation in their respective series using proximal femoral allografts. Dislocation was the major serious complication in our series, occurring in 21% of cases. We believe that the high incidence of dislocation is due to the fact that all patients were very short preoperatively and soft tissue tension at the index grafting procedure prevented complete restoration of length and myofascial tension. As soft tissues stretched out over time, the hips became more unstable.

Conclusion

Cementing the sleeve of the S-ROM prosthesis into a proximal femoral allograft and using the distal fluted stem press-fit within the host bone has proven to be a simple and consistent method of reconstructing major proximal femoral segmental bone loss. A cylindrical tibial allograft used within the medullary canal of a patulous host femur is one technique that permits the use of smaller stems. Follow-up is short but early results are encouraging.

References

1. Ballard WI, Lowery PA, Brand RA. Resection arthroplasty of the hip. *J Arthroplasty*. 1995;10:772–779.
2. Carangelo RJ, Schutzer S. Resection arthroplasty. In: Rubash H, Callaghan J, Rosenberg A, eds. *The Adult Hip*. Philadelphia, Pa: Lippincott-Raven Publishers; 1998:737–747.
3. Callaghan JJ, Salvati EA, Pelluci PM, Wilson PD Jr, Ranawat CS. Results of revision for mechanical failure after cemented total hip replacement, 1979–1982: a two to five year follow-up. *J Bone Joint Surg Am*. 1985;67:1074–1085.
4. Estok DM II, Harris WA. Long-term results of cemented femoral revision surgery using second generation techniques: an average 11.7 year follow-up evaluation. *Clin Orthop*. 1994;799:190–202.
5. Pelluci PM, Wilson PD Jr, Sledge CB, Salvati EA, Ranawat CS, Poss R. Long-term results of revision total hip replacement: a follow-up report. *J Bone Joint Surg Am*. 1985; 67:513–516.
6. Kerhaw CJ, Adkins RM, Dodd CA, Bulstrode CJ. Revision total hip arthroplasty for aseptic failure: a review of 276 cases. *J Bone Joint Surg Br*. 1991;73:564–568.
7. Engh CA, Bobyn JD. The influence of stem size and extent of porous coating on femoral bone loss resorption after preliminary cementless hip arthroplasty. *Clin Orthop*. 1988; 231:7–28.
8. Engh CA, Bobyn JD, Glassman AH. Porous coated hip replacements: the factors governing bone ingrowth, stress

shielding, and clinical results. *J Bone Joint Surg Br.* 1987;69: 45–55.
9. Bobyn JD, Glassman AH, Goto H, Krygier JJ, Miller JE, Brooks CE. The effect of stem stiffness on femoral bone resorption after canine porous coated total hip arthroplasty. *Clin Orthop.* 1990;261:196–213.
10. Bobyn JD, Mortimer ES, Glassman AH, Engh CA, Miller JE, Brooks CE. Producing and avoiding stress shielding: laboratory and clinical observations of noncemented total hip arthroplasty. *Clin Orthop.* 1992;274:79–96.
11. Paprosky WG, Jablensky W, Magnus RE. Cementless femoral revision in the presence of severe proximal bone loss using diaphyseal fixation. *Orthop Trans.* 1993;17:965–966.
12. Chandler H. Intramedullary grafting of the expanded canal in total hip replacement. *Tech Orthop.* 1993;7:33.
13. Head WC, Malinin T, Berklacich F. Freeze-dried proximal femoral allograft in revision total hip arthroplasty. *Clin Orthop.* 1987;215:109–121.
14. Zmolek JC, Dorr LD. Revision total hip arthroplasty: the use of solid allograft. *J Arthroplasty.* 1993;8:361–370.
15. Head WC, Berklacich FM, Malinin TI, Emerson RH Jr. Proximal femoral allografts in revision total hip arthroplasty. *Clin Orthop.* 1987;225:22–36.
16. Jofe MH, Gebhardt MC, Tomford WW, Mankin HJ. Reconstruction for defects of the proximal part of the femur using allograft arthroplasty. *J Bone Joint Surg Am.* 1988;70:507–516.
17. Johnson MF, Mankin HJ. Reconstruction after resection of tumors involving the proximal femur. *Orthop Clin North Am.* 1991;22:87–103.
18. Mankin HJ, Doppelt S, Tomford WW. Clinical experience with allograft implantation. *Clin Orthop.* 1983;174:69–86.
19. McGann W, Mankin HJ, Harris WH. Massive allografting for failed total hip arthroplasty. *J Bone Joint Surg Am.* 1986; 68:4–12.
20. Chandler H, Clark J, Murphy S, McCarthy J, Penenber B, Danylchuk K, et al. Reconstruction of major segmental loss of the proximal femur in revision total hip arthroplasty. *Clin Orthop.* 1994;298:67–74.
21. Allan DG, Lavoie GJ, McDonald S, Oakeshott R, Gross AE. Proximal femoral allografts in revision hip arthroplasty. *J Bone Joint Surg. Br* 1991;73:235–240.
22. Gross AE, Lavoie ME, McDermott P, Marks P. The use of allograft bone in revision of total hip arthroplasty. *Clin Orthop.* 1985;197:115–122.
23. Gross AE. Reconstruction of the femur in revision arthroplasty of the hip. In: Galante JO, Rosenberg AG, Callaghan JJ, eds. *Total Hip Revision Surgery.* New York, NY: Raven Press; 1995.
24. Gross AE, Allen G, Lavoie GJ. Revision arthroplasty using allograft bone. *Instr Course Lect.* 1993;42:363–380.

27
Revision of the Femoral Component Using Cement Fixation

John J. Callaghan

Early Results of Cemented Revisions

During the first fifteen years that total hip arthroplasty was performed extensively in the United States (1970–1985), revision surgery was limited because most primary procedures were done in older inactive patients and the time in service of most devices had been limited. Even at the Hospital for Special Surgery, by 1983 just over 250 revision procedures had been performed.[1] The studies of cemented revision total hip arthroplasty performed during the early evolution of revision hip surgery were not encouraging.[1-29] Pellicci et al.[18] demonstrated a 19% incidence of rerevision (18% femoral side), and a 29% incidence of loosening in revision cases followed for an average of 8.1 years. Results were more discouraging in patients who had required multiple revisions, with Kavanagh and Fitzgerald[30] reporting 50% clinical or radiographic failure at 3-year follow-up. In addition to a high incidence of aseptic rerevision, the early reports of revision surgery demonstrated a high incidence of complications when compared to primary cemented arthroplasty. Femoral canal perforation rates ranged from 4% to 13%. Femoral fracture rates ranged from 2.1% to 8%. Dislocation rates ranged from 8% to 10.6%. Infection rates ranged from 1.2% to 3.4%. Nerve injury rates ranged from .5% to 7%. Trochanteric problems ranged from 6.2% to 12.7% (Table 27.1).

Contemporary Femoral Canal Preparation and Cementing Techniques in Revision Hip Surgery

The initial frustrations with the revision total hip arthroplasty procedure became the ultimate challenge for the arthroplasty surgeon. As experience was gained, principles for canal preparation and cement technique, as well as femoral component design, evolved.[31-44] In the initial revision cases, the fibrous membrane between bone and cement was not adequately excised. The neocortex between the fibrous membrane and any residual cancellous bone was not removed. In the late 1970s and early 1980s surgeons began to recognize the need, in femoral canal preparation, to remove all femoral neocortex in areas where virgin cancellous bone could be obtained (Fig 27.1A & B). This is important when revising both the cemented and uncemented cases of loose femoral components as neocortex develops in both cases (Fig. 27.3 and 27.4). In addition, in areas where only cortical bone remains (especially in the proximal area where visualization is excellent) careful burring (proximally) or reaming (distally) of the bone to roughen the canal, in order to provide interdigitation of cement into bone, is imperative (Fig. 27.1C). Dohmae et al.[45] demonstrated (in a cadaveric human model) a 79% reduction in bone–cement interface sheer strength in revision surgery when compared with primary replacement if such preparation is not performed.[46]

After canal preparation, the femur is carefully examined for any perforations by placing a cannulated guide wire (used for cannulated reaming) down the femoral canal and palpating distally to ensure that the wire abuts the distal femur at the knee and not the soft tissues. It is especially important to palpate anterolaterally in the femoral canal, as 90% of perforations occur at that location.[1] In addition, this anterolateral aspect is the weakest area of the femur, as it is usually loaded in tension. If a perforation is noted, the femoral shaft is exposed by reflecting the posterior part of the vastus lateralis anteriorly. A rubber dam (a surgical glove is often convenient for this purpose) is placed over the perforation at the time of cementing (Fig. 27.8C & D) and, if the bone in that area is thinned, a cortical strut graft is applied over the defect after removing all excess cement. As a trial, femoral component is placed down the femoral canal; viewing it through the perforation can aid in determining the desired prosthesis length, which should bypass the defect by 1.5 to 3 times the outer shaft diameter[1,47] (Fig. 27.5).

	HSS and Brigham[17]	UCLA[67]	MAYO[68]	HSS[1]
Number of hips	110	66	166	139
Follow-up period (average)	3.4 yrs.	2.1 yrs.	4.5 yrs.	3.6 yrs.
Results (excellent/good)	60%	—	52%	66%
Loosening	13.6%	29%	20% a 40% f	12%
Rerevision	5.4%	9.0%	6.0%	4.3%
Femoral fracture	—	6.0%	7.8%	2.1%
Femoral perforation	—	—	4%	13%
Dislocation	—	10.6%	9.0%	8.2%
Infection	1.8%	1.5%	1.2%	3.4%
Nerve palsy	—	7.0%	.5%	.7%
Trochanteric problems	12.7%	7.6%	6.6%	6.2%

Table 27.1. Early results of revision cemented total hip arthroplasty.

a = acetabulum; f = femur

However, if no distal defect is present, standard-length stems (120 to 140 mm) are utilized. Better cement pressurization can be achieved when a shorter, rather than a longer, column of cement needs to be filled.

Removing cortical femoral windows, especially when cement extends distal to the femoral isthmus, is preferable to multiple uncontrolled perforations.[48,49] When making a window, it should be placed anteriorly to avoid the lateral tension surface, and the edges should be beveled to allow replacement of the window (before cementing) without much extrusion of the pressurized cement, and to avoid displacement of the fragment (Fig. 27.8). We perform more extended trochanteric osteotomies and make more cortical windows in the femur today than in the past to remove cement more easily and less traumatically, as maintenance of the femoral cortical tube and minimizing perforations allow for optimal cement pressurization. When cementing into a femur where an extended osteotomy has been performed, it is advisable to bevel the osteotomy bone edges, as is done for the cortical windows, to avoid cement extrusion. The femur is placed in the internally rotated position to take tension off the extended osteotomy, which has been reapproximated with cable prior to cement injection. Cement is pressurized into the canal with direct visualization of the osteotomy site to remove any cement that interdigitates between the osteotomized piece of the greater trochanter and the femur. Supplemental cancellous bone graft may be applied over the osteotomy site to aid in union.

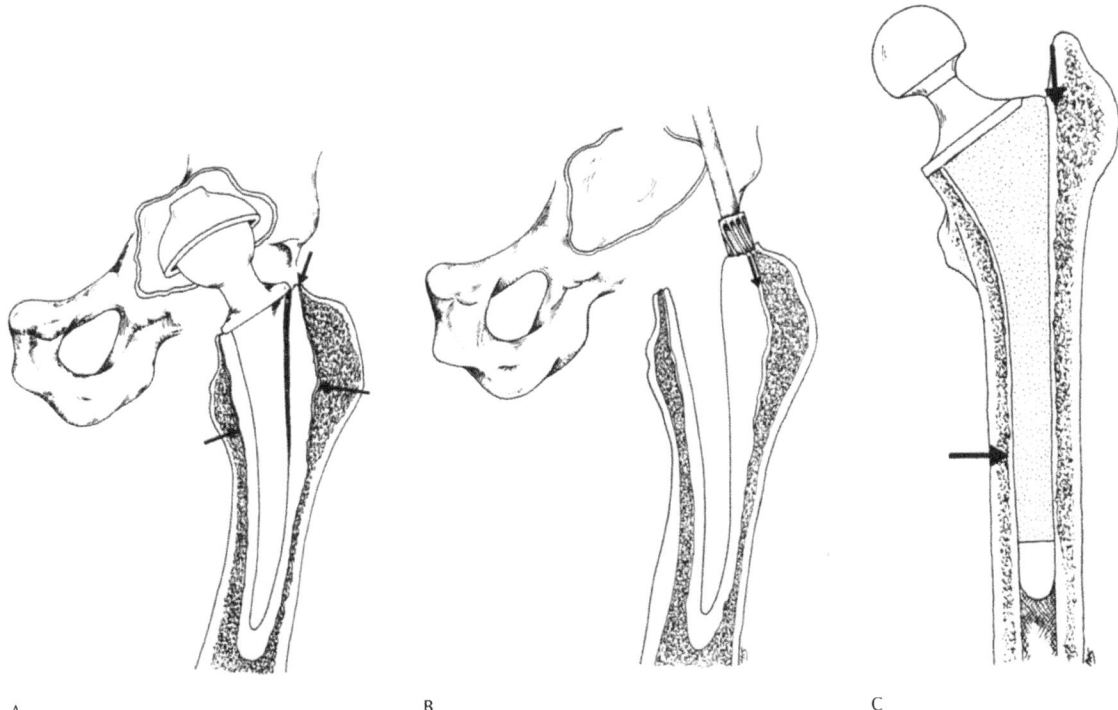

Figure 27.1. Removal of neocortex. A. Typical neocortex in cemented case (arrow). B. Burr removal of neocortex in previously cemented case. C. Typical neocortex in loose cementless case (arrow).

Figure 27.2. Contemporary cement technique. A. Distal cement plug inserted. B. Distal femoral shaft elevated (arrows) to allow blood to evacuate from proximal femoral canal opening. C. Three to five packs of antibiotic-impregnated cement pressurized into femoral canal using a reliable and powerful cement delivery system.

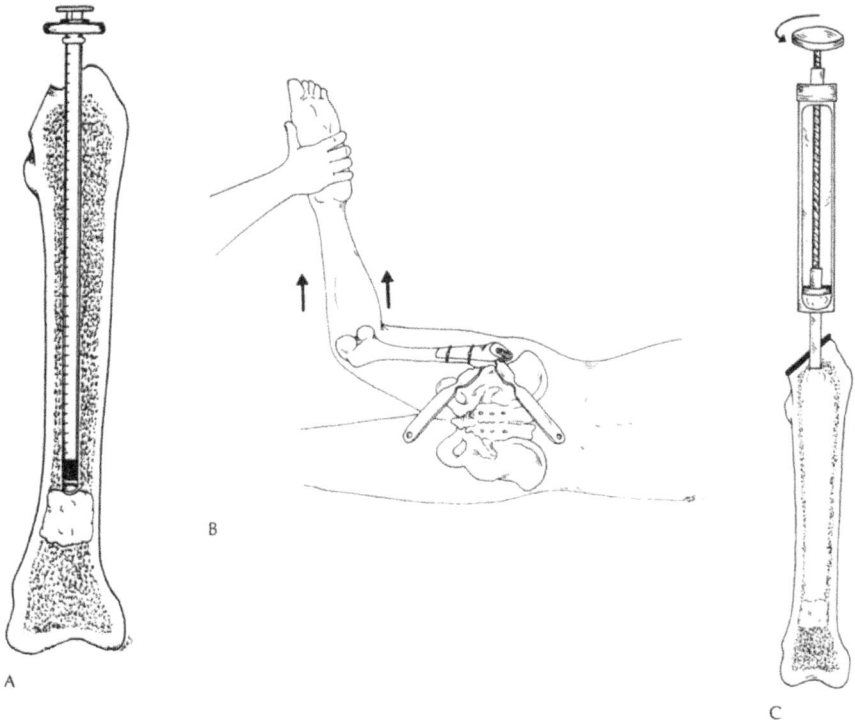

Figure 27.3. Cementing into femoral canal where cemented femoral component has loosened. Cement fixation achievable (B) when neocortex removed and contemporary cement technique used in a case where a cemented device had loosened (A).

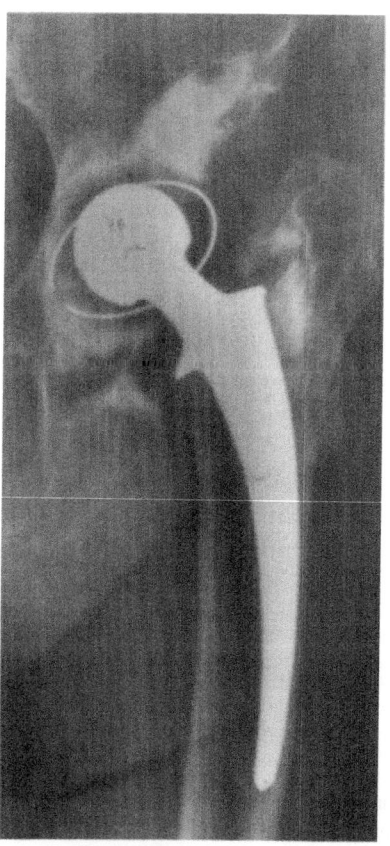
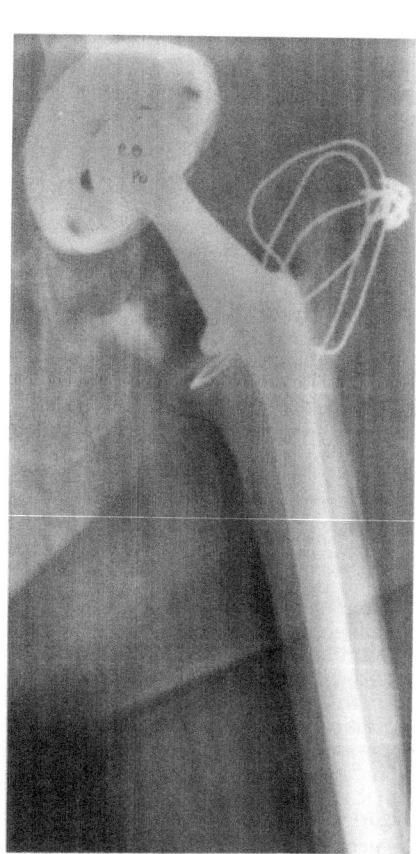

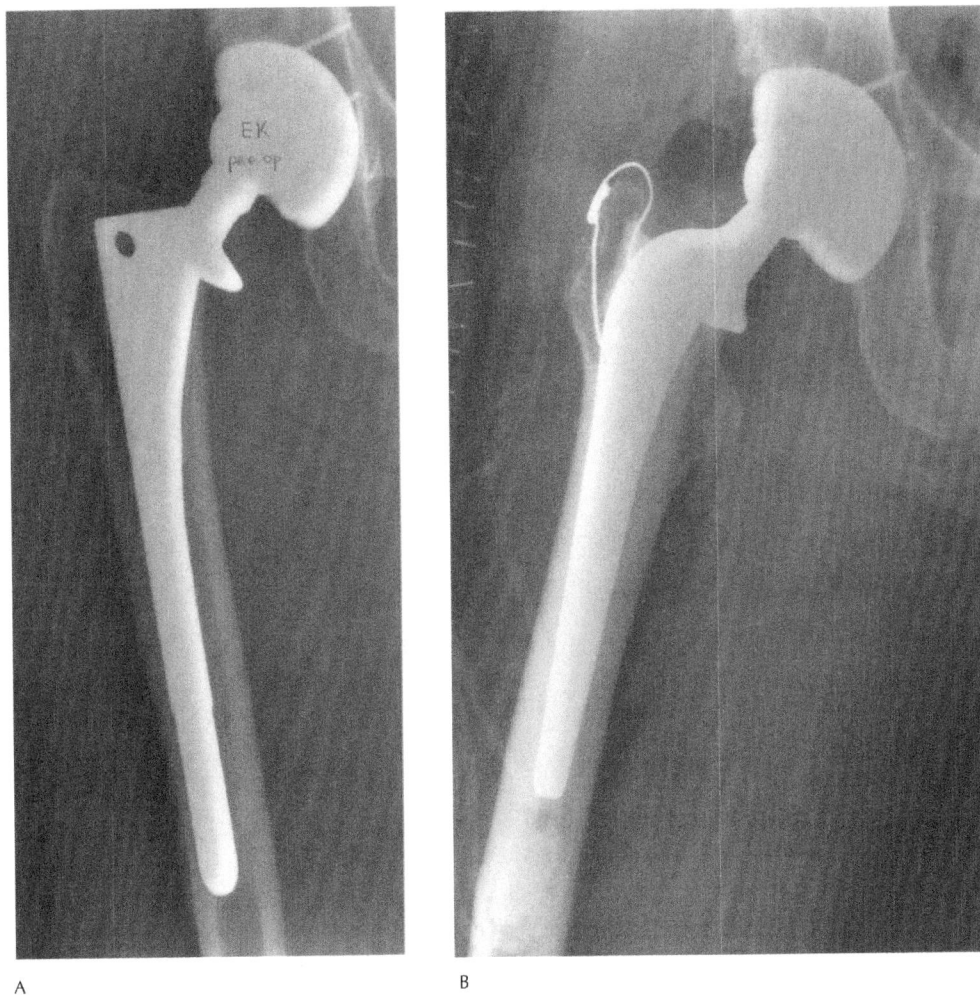

Figure 27.4. Cementing into femoral canal where uncemented femoral component has loosened: Cement fixation achievable (B) when neocortex removed and contemporary cement technique used in a case where bony ingrowth was not obtained in a porous coated femoral construct (A).

A disciplined operating room staff is essential for cementing the femoral component, especially in the revision situation. Initially, a half pack of cement is mixed and placed in the Oh-Harris™ syringe[38] (Fig. 27.2A). If the plug is to be placed distal to the isthmus, 6 to 8 cm of doughy cement is released from the syringe. After this cement has cured, three to six packs of cement are mixed, depending on the size of the femoral canal. In the revision situation especially, the surgeon should be sure that adequate cement is available for pressurization. Prior to mixing, 3.6 g tobramycin is introduced into each two packs of cement (1.8 g per pack). Studies have demonstrated minimal adverse effects on the mechanical properties of cement when less than 2.0 g of antibiotic powder (per pack) is introduced.[50] Lynch et al.[51] demonstrated a reduction in infection from 3.5% to 0.81% when antibiotics were added to cement in the revision situation. Porosity reduction of the cement by centrifugation or vacuum mixing is performed to optimize strength.[52–57] The author prefers centrifugation because it is more predictable in removing bubbles. One to two minutes is the optimal centrifugation time. If there is a long, capacious canal to fill, chilling the monomer (with sterile ice) will permit longer setup time. Custom-designed twisting guns rather than caulking guns are useful to introduce the cement, and the distal end of the femur can be elevated so that the gravitational force will cause any blood to exit the femur proximally rather than to interdigitate with cement (Fig. 27.2B & C). The canal is also dried with a sponge soaked in a 1:500,000 epinephrine solution prior to injecting cement into the femur. Pressurization can be applied with a proximal cement seal. The component is then placed down the femoral canal when the cement has cured to the doughy state. If a perforation has previously been noticed, it should be watched as the stem is introduced to avoid having the stem protrude through the defect in bone. Mechanical studies have demonstrated the

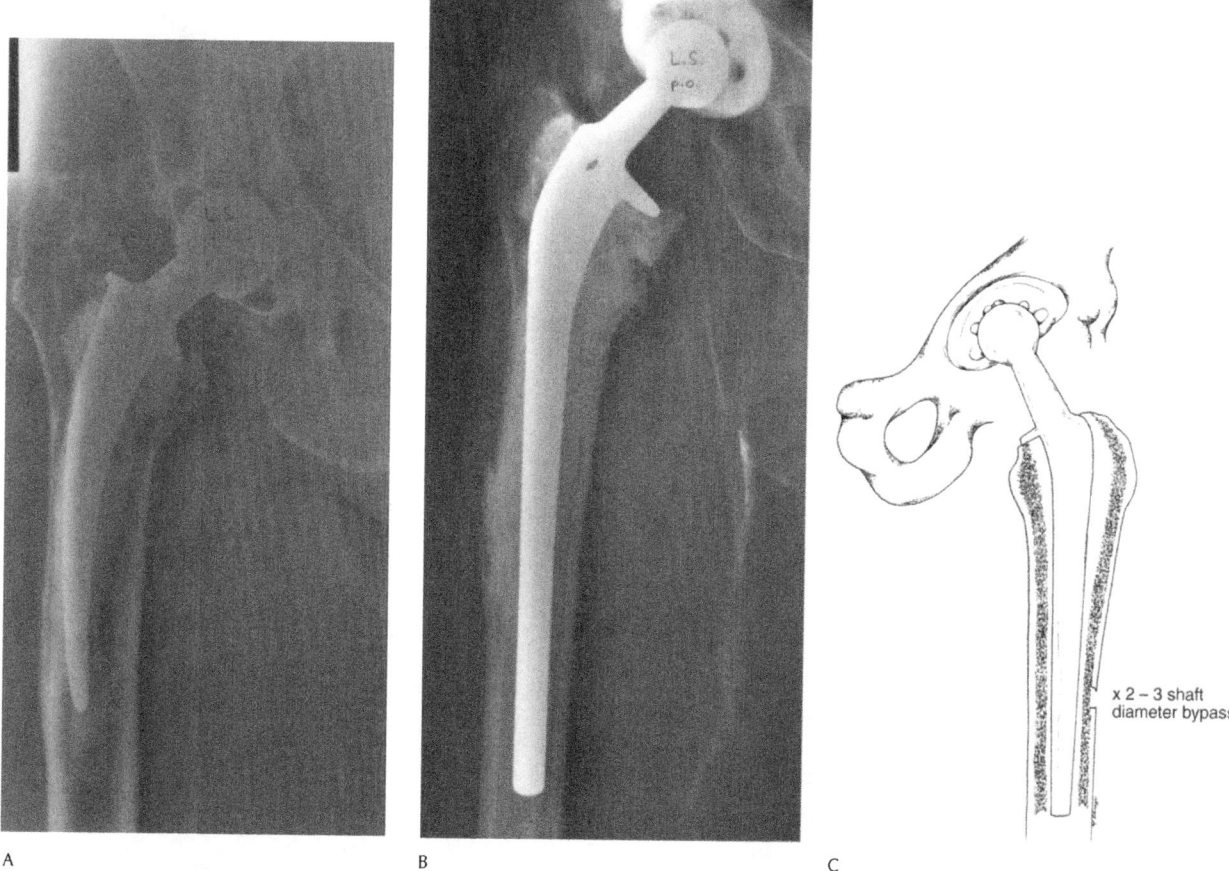

Figure 27.5. Bypass of femoral canal defect. A. A case of paper-thin lateral cortex at the tip of a loose cemented femoral component. B. The revision stem bypasses the defect by 2 or 3 shaft diameters. C. Illustration of revision construct.

need to bypass perforations with the femoral stem by two to three shaft diameters.[47] This amount of bypass negates any stress-riser effect from the perforation. If an adequate amount of cement is utilized and inadequate pressurization is obtained in the canal, the surgeon should check by means of an intraoperative radiograph or by direct femoral shaft exposure to ensure that a perforation with cement extrusion or femoral component canal penetration has not inadvertently occurred.

All cemented femoral components used today are made of chrome-cobalt and have wide, rounded medial surfaces to protect the cement mantle.[58,59] In addition, higher offset stems are available to help recreate the patient's natural femoral offset. This has become more important as surgeons attempt to perform revision surgery without removing the greater trochanter. In the past, offset adjustments were accomplished by distal and lateral advancement of the greater trochanter. In addition, calcar replacement prostheses should be available in cases with proximal femoral bone loss to allow adequate soft tissue tensioning.[60,61] In the revision setting, even

when offset and length have been adequately obtained, dislocation occurs in up to 10% of cases.[1] We apply some form of bracing postoperatively after many revisions to protect the reconstruction during the first 6 to 8 weeks while the patient is gaining leg control and while the soft tissues and bony trochanteric attachment sites are healing. Adherence to these technical details has reduced the rerevision rate of cemented revision femoral components to 10% at 10 to 15 years, even in cases with extensive femoral osteolysis (Table 27.2).[32,35,36,39–44]

Select Situations

Several situations warrant special technical consideration. If some or all of the cement mantle remains intact from the primary situation and if there are no signs of sepsis, the surgeon should consider hollowing out the cement column to slightly beyond the extent needed to introduce a new stem (Fig. 27.6). After drying the hollowed canal (with previous cement intact) and intro-

Table 27.2. Results of cemented femoral revision total hip arthroplasty using contemporary cementing techniques.

Author	# Hips	Average age	Average f/u	Rerevision incidence	Radiographic loosening
Raut et al.[41]	351	64 y	6 y	5.7%	9.4%
Weber et al.[44]	61	68 y	6.2 y	3%	8%
Katz et al.[35]	79	63.7 y	11.9 y	5.4%	16.6%
Mulroy et al.[36]	43	52.8 y	15.1 y	16%	23%
Calcar Replacements: in revisions surgery					
McLaughlin, J.R. et al.[61]	38	55 y	10.8 y	21%	32%

ducing cement in a slightly liquid phase, a prosthesis can be inserted. Greenwald et al.[50] have demonstrated excellent bonding strength of cement in these situations, and McCallum and Hozack[62] and Lieberman et al.[63] have demonstrated excellent clinical results with recementing into an intact cement column. As suggested by the former group, ultrasonic cement-removing tools work well in tunneling out the secure cement shell. This technique is applicable in cases of cement–prosthesis failure (the case with many Charnley prosthesis failures), femoral component fracture where the distal cement is intact, revision for instability or leg-length inequality, or in cases where the head size of an intact monolithic component needs to be changed (eg, a 32-mm head in a young patient). An even more intriguing method has been employed by the New England Baptist group in Boston. If a femoral cement mantle is completely intact and the stem is not bonded to cement (not precoated or grit blasted), the stem is tapped out during exposure and tapped back in after acetabular revision.

When the femoral canal is very narrow, as in congenital hip dysplasia, a narrow nozzle is needed to introduce cement to a more distal aspect of the femur past the final distal position of the prosthesis stem tip. When placing the acetabular component in the high hip cen-

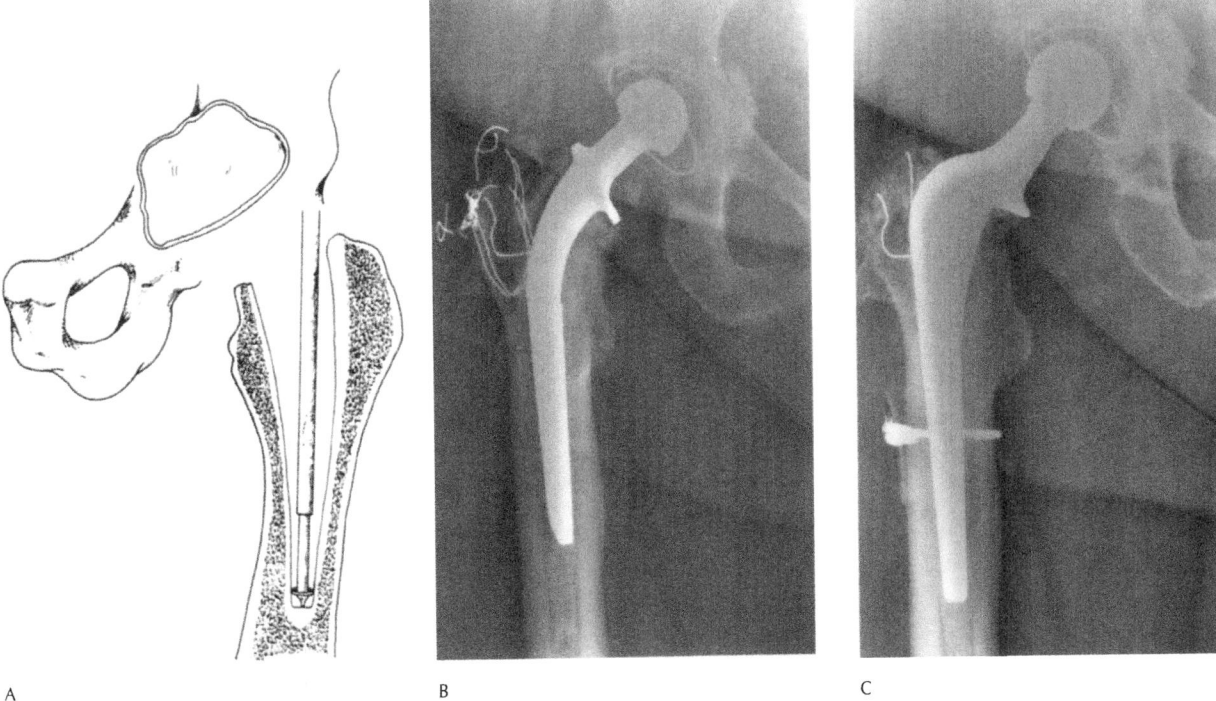

Figure 27.6. Recementing into old cement mantle. Cement mantle widened to accept new prosthesis. A. Ultrasound ski pole tool can be helpful to widen the cement mantle to accept a new prosthesis in these cases. Preoperative (B) and postoperative (C) case of a fractured stem revision in which the distal cement was intact. The distal cement mantle was widened to accept a new prosthesis. A cortical struct was placed over a proximal cortical window used to extract the distal stem with a carbide punch.

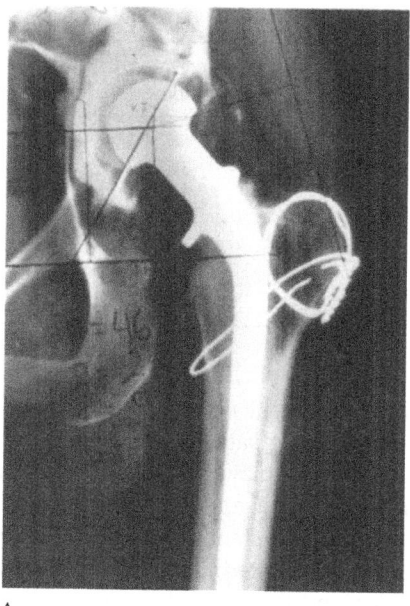
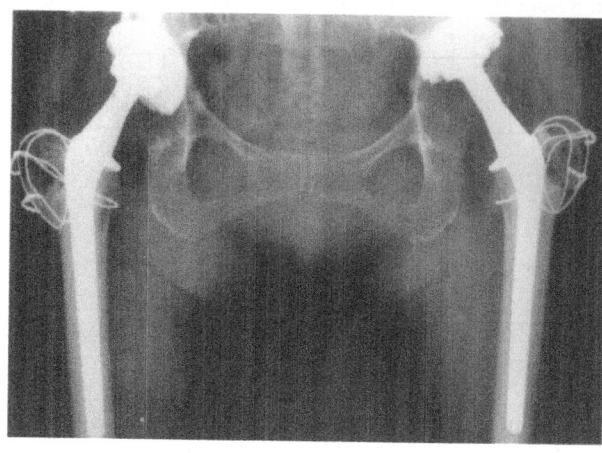

Figure 27.7. Use of calcar type replacement when high hip center utilized. Cemented calcar type femoral replacement used in a high hip center acetabular reconstruction on the left hip (B) in a patient with failed reconstruction (A) for a prior congenital hip dislocation.

ter position to avoid bone grafting, especially when using uncemented acetabular components, calcar and proximal femoral replacements are necessary to preserve leg length and to avoid the use of long-skirted head sizes that can hinder hip stability by early impingement[64] (Fig. 27.7). In these high hip center cases, partial ischial resection may be necessary to prevent anterior instability in hip extension. This instability can be caused by posterior ischial impingement on the femur when the hip is in the high hip center position.

Some fine technical considerations concern the rare use of segmental allografts in the cemented femoral revision construct.[65,66] If the surgeon is to cement the stem into the host bone, whether an oblique transverse or step-cut is created at the host–allograft junction makes little difference. However, to obtain adequate cement mantles in the allograft bone, the allograft should be sized to the endosteal surface of the proximal host femur (ie, oversized to the other shaft of the host femur) because the allograft usually has thick cortices (due to the young age of the donors). Reaming out the allograft should be avoided to maintain the strength of the allograft bone. The stem is first cemented into the allograft, and the distal stem is protected from cement ad-

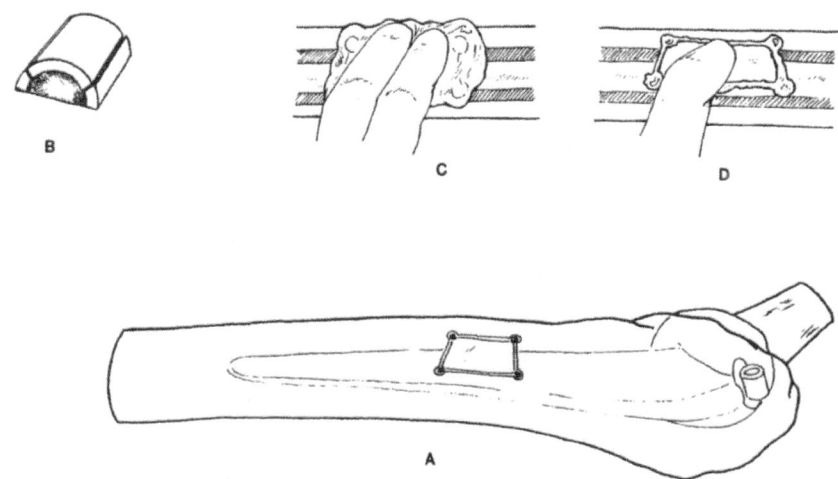

Figure 27.8. Schematic of cortical window to remove distal cement. A. Window positioned on anterior cortex. (B) Window beveled to prevent cement extrusion. C. Rubber dam placed over window when new cement pressurized. D. Excess cement needs to be removed. Cortical strut is applied if window is within 1.5 shaft diameters proximal to the new component tip.

herence by covering it with the manufacturer's wrapping before it is skewered through the allograft, which has been previously pressurized with very viscous cement. After cementing the allograft prosthesis composite into the host bone, cortical struts are placed at the host–allograft junction to add stability and to aid in the host–allograft junction healing. Some surgeons prefer press-fit fixation into the host bone rather than cement fixation to allow compression at the host–allograft bone junction.

Conclusion

When a better understanding of the complexities of the revision hip operation were recognized, the results of cemented femoral revision improved markedly. Nontraumatic cement removal and proper preparation of the femoral canal (removal of all neocortex that does not violate the femoral shaft cortical continuity) are essential. A chrome-cobalt femoral component with broad medial surfaces and no sharp corners, which bypasses any cortical defects, should be selected. A distal cement plug and adequate amount of cement to pressurize the cement in the canal is paramount. Although in cases with extensive osteolysis and in high-demand patients the author prefers the use of impaction grafting with cement[66] or the use of extensively coated porous stems, cemented femoral fixation can still provide durable long-term results in the less active patient with mild to moderate bone stock loss. These are the cases this author indicates for the use of cemented femoral fixation in revision surgery today.

References

1. Callaghan JJ, Salvati EA, Pellicci PM, Wilson PDJ, Ranawat CS. Results of revision for mechanical failure after cemented total hip replacement, 1979 to 1982. A two to five-year follow-up. *J Bone Joint Surg Am.* 1985;67:1074–1085.
2. Ballard W, Callaghan J, Johnston R. Revision of total hip arthroplasty in octogenarians. *J Bone Joint Surg Am.* 1995; 77:585–589.
3. Callaghan JJ. Total hip arthroplasty. Clinical perspective. *Clin Orthop.* 1992;276:33–40.
4. Eftekhar NS, Smith DM, Henery JH, Stinchfield FE. Revision arthroplasty using Charnley low friction arthroplasty technique. With reference to specifics of technique and comparison of results with primary low friction arthroplasty. *Clin Orthop.* 1973;95:48–59.
5. Ejsted R, Olsen NJ. Revision of failed total hip arthroplasty. *J Bone Joint Surg Br.* 1987;69:75.
6. Engelbrecht DJ, Weber FA, Sweet MB, Jakim I. Long-term results of revision total hip arthroplasty. *J Bone Joint Surg Br.* 1990;72:41–45.
7. Garcia-Cimbrelo E, Munuera L, Diez-Vazquez V. Long term results of aseptic cemented Charnley revisions. *J Arthroplasty.* 1995(April);10:121–131.
8. Hunter GA, Welsh RP, Cameron HU, Bailey WH. The results of revision of total hip arthroplasty. *J Bone Joint Surg Br.* 1994;76:419–422.
9. Iorio R, Eftekhar NS, Kobayashi S, Grelsamer RP. Cemented revision of failed total hip arthroplasty. Survivorship analysis. *Clin Orthop.* 1995;316:121–130.
10. Izquierdo RJ, Northmore-Ball MD. Long-term results of revision hip arthroplasty-survival analysis with special reference to the femoral component. *J Bone Joint Surg Br.* 1994;76:34–39.
11. Kershaw CI, Atkins RM, Dodd CAF, Bulstrods CJK. Revision total hip arthroplasty for aseptic failure: a review of 276 cases. *J Bone Joint Surg Br.* 1991;73:564–568.
12. Marti RK, Schuller HM, Besselaar PP, Vanfrank Haasnoot EL. Results of revision of hip arthroplasty with cement. A five to fourteen-year follow-up study. *J Bone Joint Surg Am.* 1990;72:346–354.
13. Michelson JD, Riley LH, Jr. Considerations in the comparison of cemented and cementless total hip prosthesis. *J Arthroplasty.* 1989;4:327–334.
14. Morrey BF, Kavanagh BF. Complications with revision of the femoral component of total hip arthroplasty. Comparison between cemented and uncemented techniques. *J Arthroplasty.* 1992;7:71–79.
15. Pellicci PM, Salvati EA, Robinson HJ. Mechanical failures in total hip replacement requiring reoperation. *J Bone Joint Surg Am.* 1979;61:28–36.
16. Pellicci PM, Wilson PD, Sledge CB, et al. Revision total hip arthroplasty. *Clin Orthop.* 1982;170:34–41.
17. Pellicci PM, Wilson PDJ, Sledge CB, Salvati EA, Ranawat CS, Poss R, et al. Long-term results of revision total hip replacement. A follow-up report. *J Bone Joint Surg Am.* 1985;67:513–516.
18. Kavanagh BF, Fitzgerald RH, Jr. Multiple revisions for failed total hip arthroplasty not associated with infection. *J Bone Joint Surg Am.* 1987;69:1144–1149.
19. Retpen JB, Varmarken JE, Jensen JS. Survivorship analysis of failure pattern after revision total hip arthroplasty. *J Arthroplasty.* 1989;4:311–317.
20. Retpen JB, Varmarken JE, Sturup J, Olsen C, Solund K, Jensen JS. Clinical results after revision and primary total hip arthroplasty. *J Arthroplasty.* 1989;4:297–302.
21. Retpen JB, Jensen JS. Risk factors for recurrent aseptic loosening of the femoral component after cemented revision. *J Arthroplasty.* 1993;8:471.
22. Snorrason F, Karrholm J. Early loosening of revision hip arthroplasty: a roentgen stereophotogrammetric analysis. *J Arthroplasty.* 1990;5:217.
23. Stromberg CN, Herberts P, Ahnfelt L. Revision total hip arthroplasty in patients younger than 55 years old. Clinical and radiographic results after 4 years. *J Arthroplasty.* 1988; 3:47–59.
24. Stromberg CN, Herberts P. A multicenter 10-year study of cemented revision total hip arthroplasty in patients younger than 55 years old. A follow-up report. *J Arthroplasty.* 1994; 9:595–601.
25. Stromberg CN, Herberts P, Palmertz B. Cemented revision hip arthroplasty. A multi-center 5–9 year study for 204 first revisions for loosening. *Acta Orthop Scand.* 1992;63:111–119.
26. Turner RH, Mattingly DA, Scheller A. Femoral revision total hip arthroplasty using a long-stem femoral compo-

nent. Clinical and radiographic analysis. *J Arthroplasty.* 1987;2:247–258.
28. Wilson PD. Revision total hip arthroplasty: current role of polymethylmethacrylate. *Clin Orthop.* 1987;225:218–228.
29. Wirta J, Eskola A, Hoikka V, Honkanen V, Lindholm S, Santavirta S. Revision of cemented hip arthroplasties. 101 hips followed for 5 (4–9) years. *Acta Orthop Scand.* 1993; 64:263–267.
30. Wirta J, Eskola A, Santavirta S, Tallroth K, Konttinen YT, Lindholm S. Revision of aggressive granulomatous lesions in hip arthroplasty. *J Arthroplasty.* 1990;5:S47–52.
31. Barrack R, Mulroy R, Harris W. Improved cementing techniques and femoral component loosening in young patients with hip arthroplasty. A 12-year radiographic review. *J Bone Joint Surg Br.* 1992;74:385–389.
32. Estok D, Harris W. Long-term results of cemented femoral revision surgery using second-generation techniques: an average 11.7-year follow-up evaluation. *Clin Orthop.* 1994;299:190–202.
33. Harris WH, McCarthy JC, O'Neill DA. Femoral component loosening using contemporary techniques of femoral cement fixation. *J Bone Joint Surg Am.* 1982;64:1063–1067.
34. Harris WH, McGann WA. Loosening of the femoral component after use of the medullary-plug cementing technique. Follow-up note with a minimum five-year follow-up. *J Bone Joint Surg Am.* 1986;68:1064–1066.
35. Katz R, Callaghan J, Sullivan P, Johnston R. Results of cemented femoral revision total hip arthroplasty using improved cementing techniques. *Clin Orthop.* 1995;319:178–183.
36. Mulroy WF, Harris WH. Revision total hip arthroplasty with use of so-called second generation cementing techniques for aseptic loosening of the femoral component. A fifteen-year-average follow-up study. *J Bone Joint Surg Am.* 1996;78:325–330.
37. Mulroy RD, Jr., Harris WH. The effect of improved cementing techniques on component loosening in total hip replacement. An 11-year radiographic review. *J Bone Joint Surg Br.* 1990;72:757–760.
38. Oh I, Bourne RB, Harris WH. The femoral cement compactor. An improvement in cementing technique in total hip replacement. *J Bone Joint Surg Am.* 1983;65:1335–1338.
39. Pierson JL, Harris WH. The effect of second generation techniques on the longevity of fixation in revision cemented femoral arthroplasties. Average 8.8 year follow-up. *J Arthroplasty.* 1995;10:581–591.
40. Raut VV, Siney PD, Wroblewski BM. Cemented revision Charnley low-friction arthroplasty in patients with rheumatoid arthritis. *J Bone Joint Surg Br.* 1994;76:909–911.
41. Raut VV, Siney PD, Wroblewski BM. Revision for aseptic stem loosening using the cemented Charnley prosthesis. *J Bone Joint Surg Br.* 1995;77:23–27.
42. Raut VV, Wroblewski BM, Siney PD. Revision hip arthroplasty. Can the octogenarian take it? *J Arthroplasty.* 1993;8:401–403.
43. Rubash HE, Harris WH. Revision of non-septic, loose, cemented femoral components using modern cementing techniques. *J Arthroplasty.* 1988;3:241–248.
44. Weber K, Callaghan J, Goetz D, Johnston R. Revision of a failed cemented total hip prosthesis with insertion of an acetabular component without cement and a femoral component with cement—A five to eight-year follow-up study. *J Bone Joint Surg Am.* 1996;78:982–994.
45. Dohmae Y, Bechtold JE, Sherman RE, Puno RM, Gustilo RB. Reduction in cement-bone interface shear strength between primary and revision arthroplasty. *Clin Orthop.* 1988;236:214–220.
46. Fornasier VL, Cameron HU. The femoral stem/cement interface in total hip replacement. *Clin Orthop.* 1976;116:248–252.
47. Panjabi M, Trumble J, Hult E, Southwick W. Effect of femoral stem length on stress raisers associated with revision hip arthroplasty. *J Orthop Res* 1985;3:447–455.
48. Klein AH, Rubash HE. Femoral windows in revision total hip arthroplasty. *Clin Orthop.* 1993;291:164–170.
49. Shepherd BD, Turnbull A. The fate of femoral windows in revision joint arthroplasty. *J Bone Joint Surg Am.* 1989;71: 716–718.
50. Greenwald AS, Narten NC, Wilde AH. Points in the technique of recementing in the revision of an implant arthroplasty. *J Bone Joint Surg Br.* 1978;60:107–110.
51. Lynch M, Esser MP, Shelley P, et al. Deep infection in Charnley low-friction arthroplasty: comparison of plain and gentamycin-loaded cement. *J Bone Joint Surg Br.* 1987; 69:355–360.
52. Burke DW, Gates EI, Harris WH. Centrifugation as a method of improving tensile and fatigue properties of acrylic bone cement. *J Bone Joint Surg Am.* 1984;66:1265–1273.
53. Davies JP, Harris WH. Optimization and comparison of three vacuum mixing systems for porosity reduction of Simplex P cement. *Clin Orthop.* 1990;254:261–269.
54. Davies JP, Burke DW, O'Connor DO, Harris WH. Comparison of the fatigue characteristics of centrifuged and uncentrifuged Simplex P bone cement. *J Orthop Res* 1987;5:366.
55. Davies JP, O'Connor DO, Burke DW, Jasty M, Harris WH. The effect of centrifugation on the fatigue life of bone cement in the presence of surface irregularities. *Clin Orthop.* 1988;229:156–161.
56. Davies JP, Jasty M, O'Connor DO, Burke DW, Harrigan TP, Harris WH. The effect of centrifuging bone cement. *J Bone Joint Surg Br.* 1989;71:39–42.
57. Wixson RL, Lautenschlager EP, Novak M. Vacuum mixing of methylmethacrylate bone cement. *Trans Orthop Res Soc.* 1985;10:327.
58. Crowninshield RD, Brand RA, Johnston RC, Milroy JC. An analysis of femoral component stem design in total hip arthroplasty. *J Bone Joint Surg Am.* 1980;62:68–78.
59. Crowninshield RD, Brand RA, Johnston RC, Milroy JC. The effect of femoral stem cross-sectional geometry on cement stresses in total hip reconstruction. *Clin Orthop.* 1980;146:71–77.
60. Harris WH, Allen JR. The calcar replacement femoral component for total hip arthroplasty: design uses and surgical technique. *Clin Orthop.* 1981;157:215–224.
61. McLaughlin JR, Harris WH. Revision of the femoral component of a total hip arthroplasty with the calcar-replacement femoral component. Results after a mean of 10.8 years postoperatively. *J Bone Joint Surg Am.* 1996;78:331–339.

62. McCallum J, Hozack W. Recementing a femoral component into a stable cement mantle using ultrasonic tools. *Clin Orthop.* 1995;319:232–237.
63. Lieberman JR, Moeckel BH, Evans B, et al. Cement-within-cement revision hip arthroplasty. *J Bone Joint Surg Br.* 1993;75:869–871.
64. Kelley SS. High hip center in revision arthroplasty. *J Arthroplasty.* 1994;9:503–510.
65. Allan DG, Lavoie G, McDonald S, et al. Proximal femoral allograft in revision hip arthroplasty. *J Bone Joint Surg Br.* 1991;73:235–240.
66. Zmollek JC, Dorr LD. Revision total hip arthroplasty: the use of solid allograft. *J Arthroplasty.* 1993;8:361–370.
67. Gie G, Linder L, Ling R, et al. Impaction cancellous allografts and cement for revision total hip arthroplasty. *J Bone Joint Surg Br.* 1993;75:14–21.
68. Retpen JB, Varmarken JE, Rock ND, Jensen JS. Unsatisfactory results after repeated revision of hip arthroplasty: 61 cases followed for 5 (1–10) years. *Acta Orthop Scand.* 1992;63:120–127.
69. Kavanagh BF, Ilstrup DM, Fitzgerald RH, Jr. Revision total hip arthroplasty. *J Bone Joint Surg Am.* 1985;67:517–526.

28
Cement within Cement Femoral Revision

Frank V. Aluisio and David A. Mattingly

Revision of failed cemented total hip arthroplasties represents a significant challenge to the hip surgeon, especially if the femoral component remains within a well-fixed cement column. Options for the femoral side include (1) cemented revision with a variety of prosthetic choices including standard, calcar replacement, and long stems; (2) cementless revisions; (3) impaction cancellous grafting; and (4) cementation of allograft–prosthetic composites. All of these options require removal of the preexisting cement mantle, which is associated with increased operative time, increased blood loss, increased cost, and increased intraoperative complications including femoral perforation and fracture.[1–3]

Another option, which bypasses the need for cement removal, is cement-within-cement revision. Prerequisites for the procedure include an intact cement mantle without evidence of fracture or loosening, a smooth stem (precoated or textured stems preclude use of this procedure), no preexisting thigh pain, and intraoperative confirmation that no cracks exist beyond the proximal 2 cm of the cement mantle.[2] This procedure may also eliminate the need for greater trochanteric osteotomy, which is associated with higher rates of nonunion in a revision setting[3] and which also potentially damages the bone–cement interface.

Indications

Indications for cement-within-cement femoral revision include removal of a broken stem in an intact distal cement mantle, component debonding in an intact mantle, recurrent dislocation secondary to component malposition, monoblock femoral components where femoral head diameter change is required (Fig. 28.1), and isolated acetabular revision with need for extensive exposure or increased offset.[1] The latter indication is probably the most frequent reason for utilizing this procedure (Fig. 28.2).

Contraindications include use of a textured or precoated stem, evidence of cement loosening, and pre- or intraoperative demonstration of a broken or cracked distal cement mantle.[1,2] In cases that involve damage to the proximal 2 cm of cement, the cement can be removed with a high-speed burr and new cement can be added at the time of reinsertion.[2]

Concerns exist over the strength and stability of the cement–cement interface and the ability of this technique to provide acceptable long-term results.

Technique[1,2]

The technique, referred to as the tap-out; tap-in procedure, begins with inspection of the prosthesis–femur composite for any evidence of gross loosening. All soft tissue is then cleared from the proximal portion of the prosthesis and prosthesis–cement interface. The prosthesis is subsequently removed without excess force. No torque is applied to the femur as this can cause cement column failure, and the head is well protected while disimpacting the prosthesis.

Once the prosthesis is removed, the cement mantle is inspected for cracks and irregularities. If any exist within the proximal 2 cm, this area of cement is removed and new cement is placed with reinsertion of the prosthesis. If irregularities occur in the distal mantle, all cement is removed and formal revision is performed.

The superficial layer of cement is roughened with a rasp and thoroughly cleaned and dried prior to recementing the prosthesis. It is essential that all blood and debris be removed from this surface as it has been shown to weaken the torsional strength of the cement–cement interface significantly.[4]

A new stem can be inserted if the offset of the component needs to be altered, or if it is needed to improve

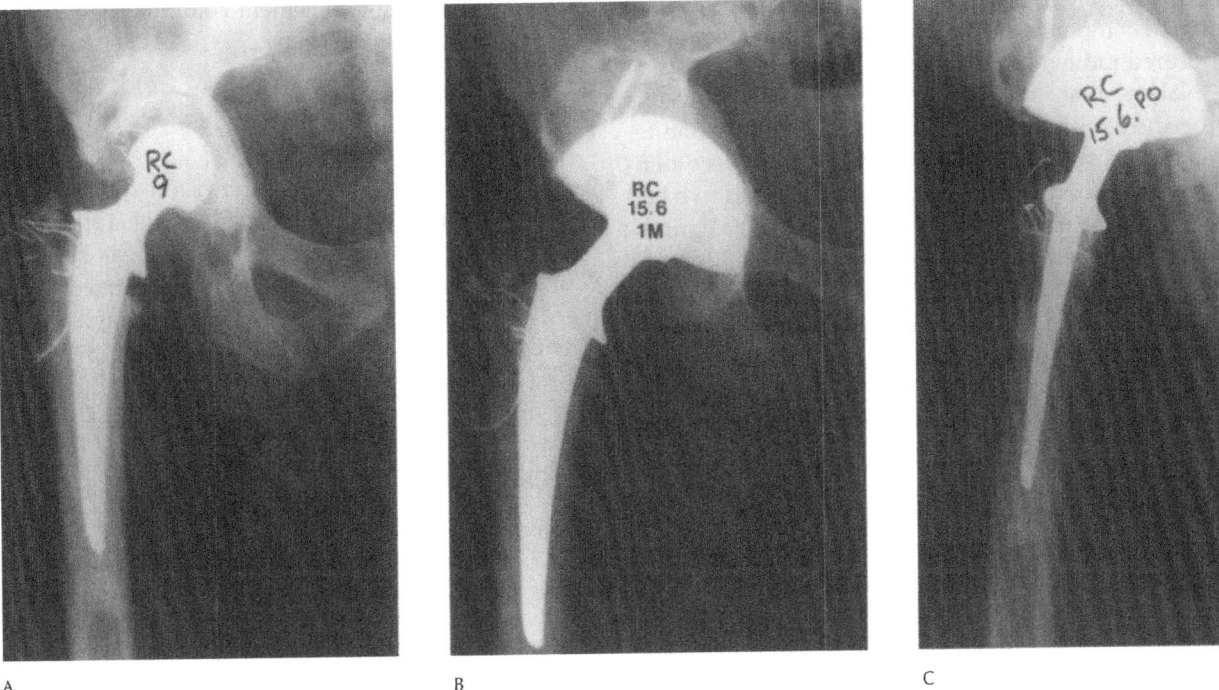

Figure 28.1. A. Anteroposterior radiograph 9 years after index arthroplasty with failed acetabular component. B. Anteroposterior radiograph 15 years after index arthroplasty and 6 years after acetabular revision with femoral component tap-out; tap-in procedure for improved exposure. C. Lateral radiograph 6 years after femoral component tap-out; tap-in procedure with acetabular revision.

stability. Utilization of a stem smaller than the original allows for a greater cement mantle and the option to change femoral component version, but the original stem may also be reinserted with no apparent difference in results.[2]

Results

Revision femoral surgery utilizing the cement-within-cement technique has not been widely reported in the literature. Lieberman et al.[1] reviewed 19 hips undergo-

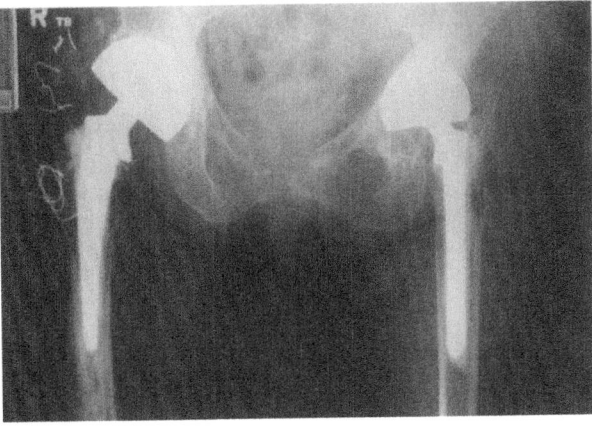
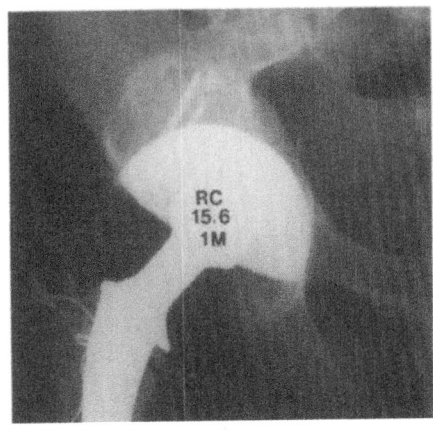

Figure 28.2. A. Prerevision AP radiograph of failed bipolar scheduled for acetabular revision; femoral component not loose but head size (29 mm I.D.) not anticipated. B. Postrevision AP radiograph with acetabular revision and cement-within-cement femoral revision with 28 mm head, prophylactic wires, and longer stem.

ing this procedure. With a mean 59-month follow-up, there were 7 excellent, 11 good, and 1 fair result. No femoral components were revised for loosening and all appeared radiographically stable.

Nabors et al.[2] reported on 42 hips undergoing this procedure with a mean 67-month follow-up. One femur was revised for joint instability, two were definitely loose (both patients asymptomatic), and two had distal cement fractures (one thigh pain, one asymptomatic). The average Harris hip score increased from 61 prerevision to 90 at the most recent follow-up examination. Both series have thus demonstrated good intermediate-term results utilizing this technique. The concerns of torsional weakness at the cement–cement interface have also been addressed in biomechanical studies.

Nabors et al.[2] performed in vitro testing of cementing into a cement column in eight cadaveric hips and found no significant increase in rotational micromotion with torque testing before and after removal and reinsertion of the prosthesis. Greenwald et al.[5] found that cementing into a clean rasped cement column led to a decrease in torsional (shear) strength of 6% compared with a uniform cement cylinder, whereas an unrasped surface had a 16% decrease and an unrasped surface with a bloody interface had a 37% decrease.

The importance of a clean interface was reinforced by Li et al.[4] who demonstrated an 80% to 85% decrease in torsional strength at the cement–cement interface when a thin layer of blood and marrow debris were present. When the interface was clean at the time of cementation, histologic sectioning revealed no evidence of an interface between the two cement columns suggesting a chemical bond between them.

Conclusion

Cement-within-cement femoral revision represents an effective surgical option if utilized for the appropriate indications. Intermediate-term results have been encouraging and mechanical testing has confirmed the integrity of the cement–cement interface as long as strict attention is paid to rasping the intact column and ensuring a bloodless field without debris.

References

1. Lieberman JR, Moeckel BH, Evans BG, Salvati EA, Ranawat CS. Cement-within-cement revision hip arthroplasty. *J Bone Joint Surg Br.* 1993;75:869–871.
2. Nabors ED, Liebelt R, Mattingly DA, Bierbaum BE. Removal and reinsertion of cemented femoral components during acetabular revision. *J Arthroplasty.* 1996;11:146–152.
3. Turner RH, Mattingly DA, Scheller A. Femoral revision total hip arthroplasty using a long-stem femoral component: clinical and radiographic analysis. *J Arthroplasty.* 1987;2:247–258.
4. Li PLS, Ingle PJ, Dowell JK. Cement-within-cement revision hip arthroplasty; Should it be done?. *J Bone Joint Surg Br.* 1996;78:809–811.
5. Greenwald AS, Narten NC, Wilde AH. Points in the technique of recementing in the revision of an implant arthroplasty. *J Bone Joint Surg Br.* 1978;60:107–110.

29
Distal Fixation

Charles A. Engh and Charles A. Engh, Jr.

The senior author has used extensively porous-coated femoral stems for revision of failed cemented stems for more than 20 years. This chapter describes the concept of distal fixation, presents the rationale for using this technique, and discusses the principles he believes are most important for a successful outcome.

Rationale

In 1984, the senior author participated in an NIH Consensus Panel on the Status of Total Hip Replacement.[1] Aseptic component loosening was identified as the most frequent cause of failure. It was also agreed that the use of cement in cases of rerevision of a loose cemented femoral component make loosening even more likely to occur.

This information stimulated clinical research into achieving better femoral implant fixation. Implants with sintered metal porous surfaces were a promising alternative. If implants could become fixed by bone growth into a sintered metal surface, a more durable fixation than that achieved with cement would be possible. Figure 29.1 illustrates this type of fixation. Although the clinical effectiveness of this method was documented as early as 1983,[2] advocates of the use of cement for revision cases expressed doubt that bone ingrowth would occur. If it did occur, they feared that these implants would stress-shield the adjacent bone, leading to an unacceptable level of bone atrophy. They also warned that if these implants became securely fixed to bone, it would be impossible to remove them. For these reasons the porous surface of most first-generation porous-coated implants was confined to the proximal part of the stem. These proximally porous-coated implants proved successful in primary surgery, but the limited amount of porous coating made them less successful in revision cases. The proximally damaged bone in the revision cases often had an abnormal shape that did not match the shape of the new implant. This damaged bone was also sometimes unable to generate the fracture-healing response necessary for bone ingrowth.

For these reasons, the author advocated using only extensively porous-coated prostheses for revision surgery. These implants achieve primary fixation in the femoral diaphysis where the bone is stronger, has a more consistent shape, and has better bone-ingrowth capabilities than those of proximally damaged bone. This technique became known as distal fixation, as opposed to the proximal fixation, which occurs with a proximally coated implant. The authors believe that the term *distal fixation* is misleading. Their goal is not distal fixation. It is fixation to the first 5 cm of the proximal femur, which appeared strong enough to support the implant and viable enough to provide a bone-ingrowth response. The idea is simply to bypass the proximally damaged bone that does not have this capability.

Patient Selection

Many revision surgeons use multiple techniques for revision surgery, basing their selection of the most suitable one on the condition of the femur. The authors believe that the technique of distal fixation can be used predictably in virtually all situations. This versatility is particularly important because bone damage can sometimes be difficult to evaluate on preoperative radiographs. It is even more difficult to judge how much bone stock will remain after removal of the failed implants and the cement. The author acknowledges that other techniques, which allow more proximal stress transfer, may potentially spare bone stock from stress-shielding, and may even increase bone stock in the case of proximal bone allografting. Because the authors' technique works for simple femoral revision cases as well as for complex cases, and because it can address complications that may occur during revision, every revision surgeon should be familiar with this technique. Although the technique is potentially applicable to all revisions, there are some patient selection considerations.

The surgeon should be particularly cautious about revising what appears to be a well-fixed cemented or ce-

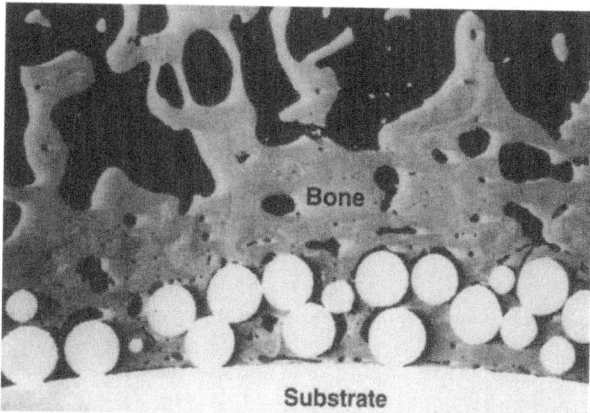

Figure 29.1. Twenty-five-times magnification backscatter electromicrograph of bone within the sintered metal beaded surface of a chrome cobalt femoral prosthesis.

mentless femoral stem because of unexplained stem pain. The surgeon should also be sure that the patient understands and will abide by postoperative physical restrictions. This means, particularly, that the patient must be willing to restrict postoperative activities to prevent dislocation of the hip. Even more specific to the technique is the recognition that the patient must follow weight-bearing restrictions required to provide an adequate mechanical environment for bone ingrowth. These weight-bearing precautions can range from as minor as immediate full weight-bearing to as major as non-weight-bearing for as long as 3 months, depending on the quality of the bone into which the prosthesis is to be implanted, the tightness of fit determined when the prosthesis is implanted, and the appearance of the immediate postoperative radiographs. Patients who are not compliant should not undergo this type of revision surgery.

Preoperative Planning

Before femoral revision hip surgery is begun, the surgeon must have a detailed knowledge of the damaged parts that need to be removed. The surgeon must know whether the part is modular; if it is modular, he or she needs to determine whether the bearing surface can be replaced with another part that meets current standards. The surgeon needs to plan a method for removing the existing parts, including the cement. This plan includes selection of a proper surgical approach and the decision as to whether a trochanteric osteotomy is needed. After the existing parts, including the cement, have been removed, the goal is to replace the failed prosthesis with one that can become more permanently fixed to the cortical bone of the proximal femur. When this new implant is seated in the femur, the shape of the prosthesis should correct for any reduction in leg length resulting from failure of the previous hip replacement.

For planning purposes, the implant templates are divided into two parts. The stem part of the template functions to fill the femoral diaphysis and become permanently fixed at this level. The upper part of the prosthesis functions to restore normal hip anatomy. The size and shape of the prosthesis are planned by applying these templates on anteroposterior radiographs of the pelvis. The lower half of the template (the stem) is placed over the femoral diaphysis at the level where the surgeon hopes to achieve primary stability, that is, the first 5-cm segment of the femoral diaphysis that appears radiographically normal. The template should be of a size that contacts both the medial and lateral endosteal cortices of the femoral diaphysis at this level. Figure 29.2 illustrates this fit.

Selection of the upper part of the prosthesis is the second step. To perform this step, the surgeon must first know exactly how much to change the patient's leg length and femoral offset. This measurement can be calculated by studying the preoperative radiographs (Fig 29.3 A–C). The leg length difference should also be calculated by physical examination. Blocks are placed beneath the patient's shorter leg until leg lengths are equal. By "femoral offset," we mean the amount that the femur is displaced laterally away from the acetabulum. As shown in Figure 29.3 A–D, the normal distance can

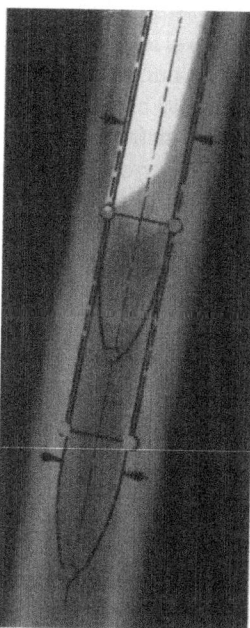

Figure 29.2. Radiograph showing the distal part of a prosthetic template overlaid on the femoral diaphysis. The medial and lateral borders of the template contact the medial and lateral borders of the intramedullary canal for more than 5 cm, beginning at a level just below the former prosthesis.

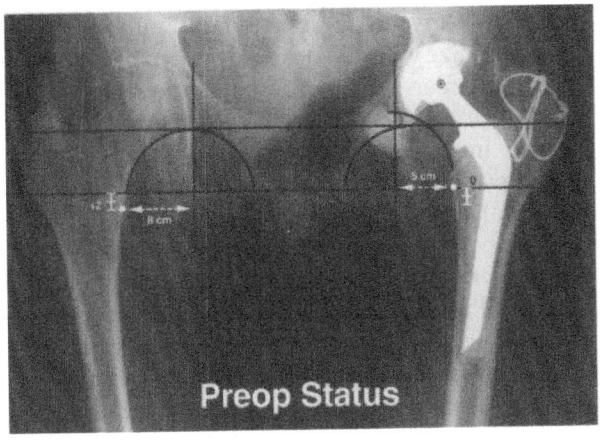
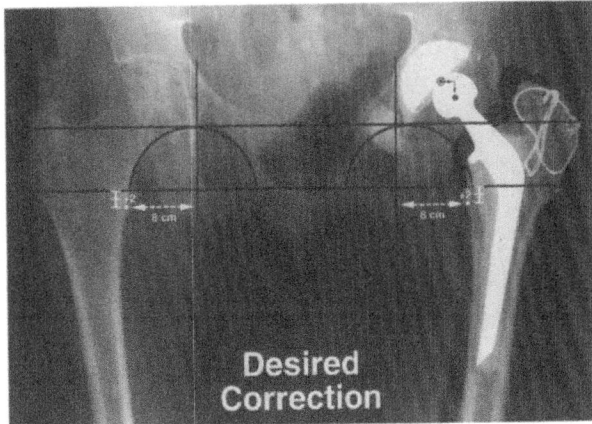
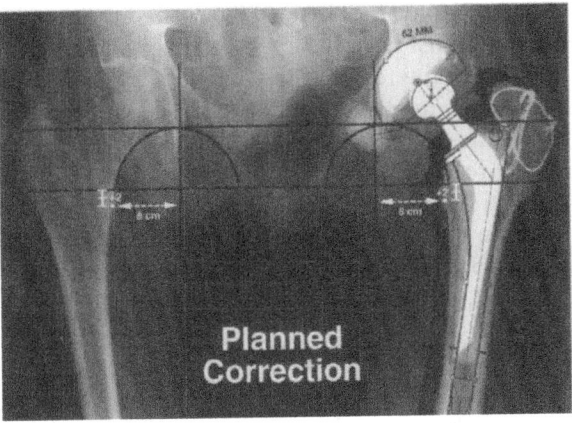
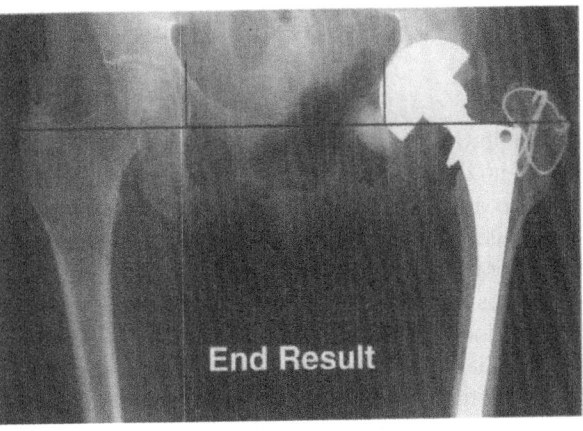

Figure 29.3. A. An AP pelvic radiograph of a failed total hip replacement. The cephalad and medial migration of the acetabular cup has shifted the femur upward and medially, placing the femur closer to the pelvis than to the contralateral normal hip. The differences in offset and length between the two sides can be calculated as shown. B. A computer-generated image in which the position of the femur shown in A has been changed to correct for the shortening and medial displacement of the femur also shown in A. The revision surgical procedure should ideally return the femur to this position. C. The same computer-generated image as shown in B with templates overlaid to show how the femoral width and offset corrections will be made. In this case, the connection has been made by using an acetabular cup that has moved the socket center the required distance laterally and distally. D. If the porous-coated components are placed in the stemmed position, the postoperative radiographs should appear similar to the plan.

be determined from the contralateral side of the anteroposterior (AP) radiograph if the contralateral hip is normal. In cases in which this is not possible, we assume that the offset on the failed side is decreased and plan to increase this distance by approximately 1 cm.

Templating for these changes in offset and leg length makes it necessary to know the position of the acetabular component and the seating level of the new femoral component. Once known, it is possible to select a femoral template with a femoral head that will reach enough cephalad and enough medial to the proposed socket so that when the hip is reduced, the desired increase in offset and leg length will have been obtained. This templating technique is shown in Figure 29.3 C. Figure 29.3 D illustrates the end result.

Surgical Technique

The surgical technique should closely follow the preoperative planning. Successful stem fixation involves precise cylindrical reaming and impacting of the appropriate stem into the femur. Revision surgery is routinely performed through a posterior approach. In cases in which cement removal appears difficult, an extended trochanteric sliding osteotomy is used. This osteotomy

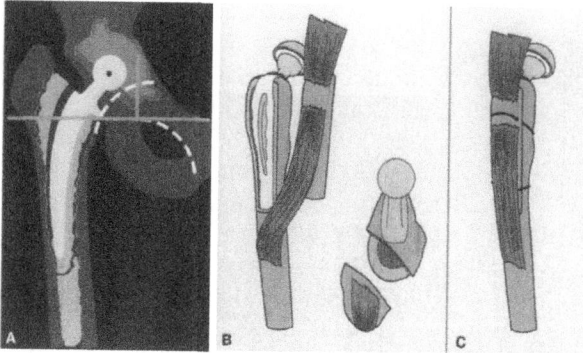

Figure 29.4. This schematic demonstrates the extended trochanteric slide used by the authors in cases in which on one radiograph the cement removal appears to be difficult. A. Removal of distal cement is facilitated with an extended trochanteric osteotomy. B. The osteotomy and exposure of the failed prosthesis and cement. C. The osteotomy is repaired with two cables.

is a longitudinal one involving the removal of the anterior lateral third of the femur from the greater trochanter above to approximately 10 cm below the trochanteric flare. This approach is illustrated in Figure 29.4. Because the femoral prosthesis is fixed in the femoral diaphysis below this level, the osteotomy does not compromise this fixation. Precise reaming over 5 to 10 cm in the femoral diaphysis below this osteotomy is the critical step in distal fixation. The only way to ensure precise reaming is to be certain that the diaphysis directs the reamer. In other words, the reamer cannot impinge on a distal bone plug or retained cement. In addition, the reamer must be free proximally and must not impinge on the greater trochanter or overlying proximal soft tissue. If there is any doubt about reamer direction, reamer impingement, retained cement, or bone plugs, AP and lateral radiographs should be obtained intraoperatively with a small-diameter reamer in place. The extended trochanteric osteotomy permits accurate machining of the diaphysis with straight reamers in cases that require a long stem or have excessive anterior femoral bow. Without the osteotomy, the presence of the femoral neck and greater trochanter could make distal reaming with a straight reamer impossible.

In the majority of cases, we advocate using only straight, rigid reamers. Occasionally we use the thin-shafted rigid reamers. We never use flexible reamers over a guide wire. The more rigid the reamer, the more precise the reaming. Such precise reaming is critical to prevent femoral fractures during prosthesis impaction and to ensure maximum contact between bone and porous coating on the prosthesis.

Reaming is accomplished in 0.5 mm increments. The appropriate reamer tightness requires both irrigation to prevent bone necrosis and frequent cleaning of cortical bone from the reamer tip. Excessive force should not be required to advance the reamer. Typically, reamers of increasing size will advance easily down the femur. The last two reamers to be used will require a gentle push. The last reamer may need to be removed and the tip cleaned multiple times to remove caked-on cortical bone. Reaming is stopped at a size 0.5 mm smaller than the actual size of the implant to be used.

After both the femur and the acetabulum have been prepared for the new implants, the orientation of the new prostheses should be checked by first using trial components. The trial acetabular component is positioned first. A damaged shape of the acetabulum often limits the ability to orient the trial acetabular cup perfectly. After the trial cup is seated, the trial femoral component is inserted. This component must be long enough to extend through the 5 to 10 cm segment of femoral diaphysis to achieve the desired fixation. In addition, it must have the appropriate proximal shape so that, when the femoral head is placed within the trial acetabular cup, the desired offset and length correction are attained.

The rotation of the femoral stem in the canal may need to be adjusted to improve hip joint stability. If, for example, it is necessary to place the trial acetabular component in less than the usual amount of anteversion, it may be necessary to increase the forward rotation or anteversion of the femoral component to improve the hip stability. Finally, if a trochanteric osteotomy had been performed, the surgeon must be certain that the size of the proximal part of the trial prosthesis does not interfere with the replacement of the trochanter. The slightly larger porous-coated components should be inserted only after all these requirements have been met.

In most cases, we use a porous-coated femoral stem that has a diameter in the femoral diaphysis 0.5 mm larger than the diameter of the channel that has been prepared. Use of this slightly oversized stem usually requires 30 to 40 blows with a 2-lb hammer to fully impact the prosthesis. With each impaction, the stem should drop approximately 2 to 3 mm. For the last 2 cm, it should drop only 1 mm with each forceful impaction. If greater than this amount of force is required, the stem should be removed and the intramedullary canal should be prepared with a drill the same size as the stem. In every case, the surgeon should have a stem removal instrument that creates a metal-to-metal, motion-free connection between the implant and the removal device to permit extraction of a stuck, partially seated stem. The potential of getting the stem stuck in a partially impacted position is another reason we advocate using a straight cylindrical prosthesis. We believe straight stem implants can be removed with less danger of fracturing the femur than can stems with a curved shape.

The final step in the surgical procedure is the trochanteric reattachment. This is usually accomplished using two cables. The upper cable is placed through drill holes in the greater and lesser trochanters. The lower cable is placed circumferentially around the femur and the trochanteric fragment. This method of reattachment is shown in Figure 29.4 C.

Complications

Modifications of the surgical technique described above can be made to reduce the possibility of postoperative complications. The most frequently encountered complications are (1) failure of bone ingrowth; (2) recurrent dislocations; (3) femoral perforation; and (4) distal femoral fractures, usually caused by using a stem that is either too long or too large in diameter.[3]

The failure of bone ingrowth is usually related to imperfect surgical technique, the condition of the bone stock, and the level of patient compliance. Insertion of stems that are undersized to the intramedullary canal or that do not fit tightly create a situation that is prone to ingrowth failure. These complications can be prevented by obtaining intraoperative radiographs with the tightest fitting drill in the canal to ensure that it fills the canal.

Postoperative dislocations as well as leg length inequality problems can be minimized by using trial components to check leg length and hip stability prior to inserting the trial components. When only the femoral component needs to be revised, the rasp that corresponds to the size of the porous-coated implant is seated. Different head and neck possibilities are tried until correct leg length and hip stability are obtained. If hip instability is a result of incompatability of the orientation of the well-fixed cup with the rotation of the stem, it may be necessary to remove the well-fixed cup and change its orientation to achieve stability. When the cup and the stem are well aligned but dislocation of the hip still occurs easily because of poor soft tissue tension, the surgeon must be prepared to advance the trochanter or use an acetabular cup that better captures the femoral head.

Femoral perforations can be prevented by obtaining intraoperative radiographs with a drill in place. Drilling too far down a curved femur with a straight drill usually is the cause of anterior perforations. Lateral perforations usually result from incomplete cement removal or incomplete removal of the bone pedestal beneath the previously failed stem. We routinely obtain intraoperative radiographs in cases requiring a stem longer than eight inches, in cases in which a bone pedestal or cement plug has been removed, and in cases in which a canal is larger than 16.5 mm in diameter. In these cases we have learned that it is difficult to assess how well the drill is filling the canal by the "feel" of the drill during the drilling process. In addition, the radiographs will indicate whether all retained cement or bone pedestals are removed and whether the reamer alignment and cortical contact are appropriate. Retained cement and poor stem alignment are usually associated with suboptimal stem fit and an increased possibility of bone ingrowth failure.

Femoral fractures occur after revision surgery when the stem is inserted too tightly. A precise surgical technique, the use of intraoperative radiographs, and experience can prevent such fractures. The most common type of fracture occurs during impaction. In this situation, the stem, which was advancing about 1 mm with every blow of the hammer, suddenly begins to advance 3 to 5 mm with each blow. This sudden decrease in resistance to stem impaction indicates that a femoral shaft fracture has probably occurred. The fracture should be confirmed with AP and lateral radiographs. If it is nondisplaced and the stem appears stable, no additional operative fixation is used. However, in this situation the patient is kept at less than 25% weight-bearing status for 6 weeks. When radiographs indicate that the fracture is displaced, it is treated with cables, strut allografts, and 3 months of protected weight-bearing. The frequency of all of these complications is directly related to the surgeon's attention to detail and his experience with this technique.

Results

Review of the published results of revision surgery confirms the success of our method. The first report from the author's institution by Lawrence[4] reviewed 81 patients revised between 1980 and 1986. All had a minimum 5-year follow-up with a mean follow-up of 9 years (range, 5–13 years). In this series, the femoral revision rate was 10% and the mechanical loosening rate was 11%. Function, physician-defined success, and patient satisfaction were measured to determine clinical success. In terms of pain and walking, 87% of patients improved and 93% of patients were satisfied with the outcome of their revision hip arthroplasty. Only 5% of these patients had an unstable implant at final follow-up (including all interim procedures). A more recent study by Moreland[5] reported on 175 patients who underwent femoral revision between 1984 and 1991. The mean follow-up was 5 years (range, 2–10 years).

The results in the Moreland report are considerably better, with a femoral rerevision rate of 4% and a mechanical loosening rate of 4%. In this series, the authors report improved pain and walking scores, and also address thigh pain and stress shielding. Although 8% of patients reported thigh pain, this pain was considered to be severe in only half of these patients. This pain was correlated with preoperative osteoporosis and failure of

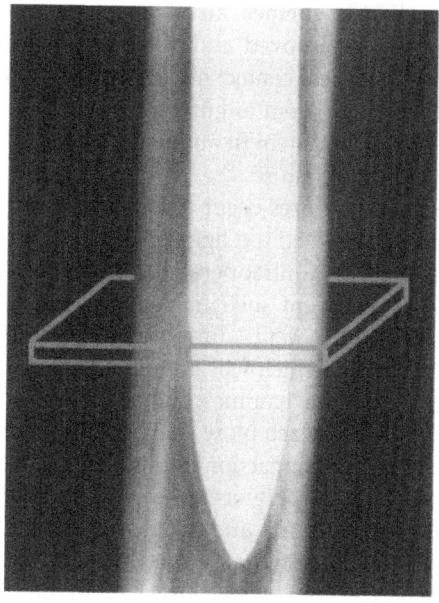
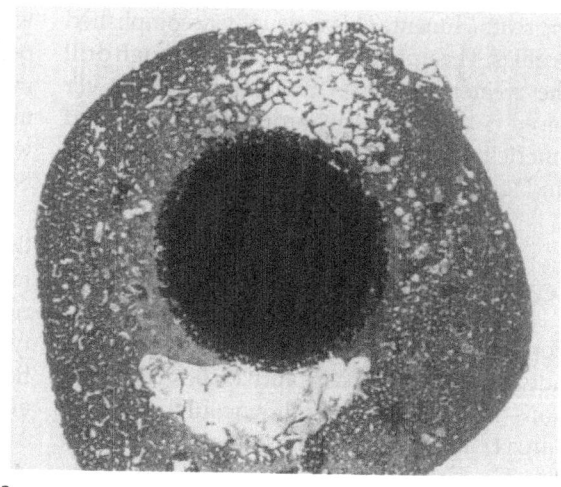

Figure 29.5. A. Radiographic signs of successful distal stem fixation by bone ingrowth. B. Five-times magnification of the hematoxylin- and eosin-stained plastic section of the femur as shown in A.

bone ingrowth. Severe stress-shielding was reported in 8% of the cases. However, no patient experienced a failure or complication attributed to stress-shielding. Rather, the stress-shielding was associated statistically with preoperative osteoporosis and large stem size.

It is important to note that the majority of published studies report on the revision of failed cemented femoral components. The authors recently reviewed the revision of failed porous-coated femoral stems with extensively porous-coated femoral revision components. In their series, 21 cases were followed for a mean 6.3 years (minimum 5 years). There were no femoral rerevisions or cases with mechanical loosening. The mean time to failure of the initial cementless femoral component was 2.6 years. In every case, the failure was diagnosed when pain was associated with migration or varus tilt of the stem. Since the failed cementless stem was easily disimpacted in each case, the revision procedure was uncomplicated. This straightforward situation differs from the procedure in which the failed cemented component loosens late and the revision is complicated by more extensive bone damage plus additional damage caused by cement removal.[4,6]

Conclusion

The authors believe that using extensively porous-coated femoral components in revision femoral surgery is applicable to many femoral revision situations. The reader should feel comfortable using this technique because the results have been well documented in the literature. The success of the procedure depends most on the surgeon's choosing the first 5 to 10 cm of normal-appearing diaphyseal bone and reaming to the precise shape of a cylindrical stem. With this method, surgical impaction is uncomplicated because the femoral diaphysis aligns the component and imparts a reproducible press-fit sensation during impaction. The complications of this technique are well documented and can be avoided with adequate exposure, intraoperative radiographs, and surgical experience. However, when extensive bone damage is present, when a stem longer than 8 inches is required, and when very large diameter stems are used, the procedure requires more particular attention.[3]

The authors acknowledge that to prove that fixation by this method is as good or better than cement fixation, they must show that bone ingrowth can be made to occur consistently. It is therefore necessary to be able to assess from postoperative radiographs whether bone ingrowth was actually present. Since it is impossible to show on a radiograph that bone is growing into an opaque metal surface, the process must be identified by the gradual changes in the appearance of the periprosthetic bone (bone remodeling). The bone remodeling signs indicating successful bone ingrowth include (1) narrowing of the intramedullary canal around the diaphyseal portion of the implant and (2) atrophy of bone around the proximal part of the stem. The signs of failed bone ingrowth include (1) a widening of this intramedullary space; (2) the formation of demarcation lines within the space; and (3) hypertrophy rather than atrophy in proximal bone, particularly the bone beneath the collar of the stem. Any signs of movement of the stem within the canal also indicate that biological fixation has not occurred and that the stem is loose.

Figure 29.5 shows the signs of bone ingrowth in a revision case. After documenting these signs, the authors in subsequent publications demonstrated repeatedly that bone ingrowth does occur consistently. In addition, they have documented that when osseointegration is diagnosed, femoral stability is exceptionally durable.[5,7] In fact, to the authors' knowledge, a case has never been demonstrated in which achieved bone ingrowth has loosened. This observation remains the strongest argument for using extensively porous-coated stems. The authors do acknowledge that there are occasional cases of fixation failure in which revision is indicated. In these cases, the procedure involving the removal and replacement of a loose uncemented stem is far less complicated than the one that requires removing cement.

References

1. Status of Total Hip Replacement. NIH Consensus Conference, National Institutes of Health, Washington, D.C., 1984.
2. Engh C. Hip arthroplasty with a Moore prosthesis with porous coating: a 5-year study. *Clin Orthop.* 1983;176:52–66.
3. Egan E, DiCesare P. Intraoperative complications of revision hip arthroplasty using a fully porous-coated straight cobalt-chrome femoral stem. *J Arthroplasty.* 1995;10 (Supp): S45–S51.
4. Lawrence J, Engh C, Macalino G, et al. Outcome of revision hip arthroplasty done without cement. *J Bone Joint Surg Am.* 1994;76(7):965–973.
5. Moreland J, Bernstein M. Femoral revision hip arthroplasty with uncemented, porous coated stems. *Clin Orthop.* 1995; 319:141–150.
6. Engh C, Culpepper WJ 2d, Kassapidis E. Revision of loose cementless femoral prostheses to larger porous coated components. *Clin Orthop.* 1998;347:168–178.
7. Engh Jr. C, Culpepper W, Engh C. Long-term results of the anatomic medullary locking prosthesis in total hip arthroplasty. *J Bone Joint Surg Am.* 1997;79:177–184.

30
Modularity in Total Hip Arthroplasty: The S-ROM® Prosthesis

Robert J. Carangelo and James V. Bono

Historical Perspective

The current S-ROM® system (stability, range of motion, (DePuy, a Johnson & Johnson Company, Warsaw, IN) represents the fourth generation in the evolution of the Sivash total hip system introduced in the early 1960s. Sivash introduced the concept of modularity in the earlier design with the use of titanium alloy for the femoral stem and chrome-cobalt for the head articulation, and titanium alloy proximal sleeves for enhanced collar calcar contact. The prosthesis was intended for cementless implantation. In 1972, however, the Food and Drug Administration approved the use of polymethylmethacrylate, which significantly diminished interest in cementless application.

The prosthesis underwent further modification by Noiles in 1975. The smooth femoral stem was changed by adding eight longitudinal flutes and an array of cross-notches or crenelations. This added feature was intended to reduce torsional failure by rotation of the implant. In addition, a distal coronal slot was placed in the stem. This reduced bending stiffness by 80%. The proximal circular sleeve was also made more eccentric. These changes created a new design called the SRN total hip system. In 1984 Meyers introduced a self-tapping threaded proximal sleeve that was used with the SRN system.

The final modifications occured under the direction of Cameron and Noiles, producing a stem that had distal flutes and a coronal slot without the cross-notches. There were also a large number of proximal taper-lock sleeves that enhanced proximal fixation. Furthermore, Noiles enhanced the design characteristics of the proximal sleeve. In addition to the threaded sleeve, there were now porous-coated conical sleeves (SPA), conical sleeves with an additional triangular spout with proximal ridges (ZT™, ZTT™). The ZTT™ sleeve has one layer of sintered titanium beads on its surface to enhance implant fixation and eventual osseointegration. The proximal ridges or steps were designed to convert the hoop stress into compressive rather then shear loads.

Thus was born the S-ROM® total hip system (Fig. 30.1). It defines modularity. It is a two-piece system that allows independent proximal and distal sizing of the femur. It has 6 different stem sizes with 10 proximal modular sleeves for each stem diameter (Fig. 30.2). It has 8364 possible combinations, making it one of the most versatile systems to handle a range of complexity in revision total hip reconstruction.

Why Modularity?

Revision surgery is often a complex procedure involving the use of bone grafts and modular or custom implants. The goals of revision and primary surgery are to achieve immediate implant stability, restore hip biomechanics by correcting offset and limb length discrepancy, restore femoral and acetabular integrity, and restore painless range of motion to the hip joint.

Immediate stability is an absolute necessity when using cementless components for revision. Because it has been shown that there is no proportional relationship between the metaphyseal and diaphyseal geometry in the proximal femur, the theory of "fit and fill" is often too difficult to achieve in practice.[1] This is even more true in a revision setting, where there is often altered anatomy and deficient proximal femoral bone stock. The conventional one-piece uncemented proximal porous-coated implants have compromised proximal bony contact because of the mismatch in stem geometry and bone loss in the proximal femur. Because most proximally sintered implants lack distal rotational stability, they may loosen if metaphyseal stability is not attained. Extensively porous-coated implants rely on distal fixation through an interference fit and then bone ingrowth. Proximal femoral geometry and bone deficiency is less of a concern. The tradeoff of distal fixation is further bone

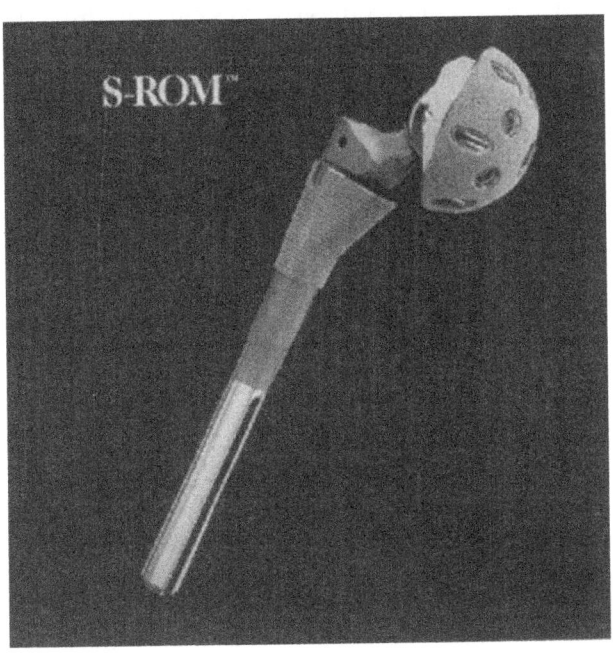

Figure 30.1. The two-piece stem design of the S-ROM prosthesis. (See color insert.)

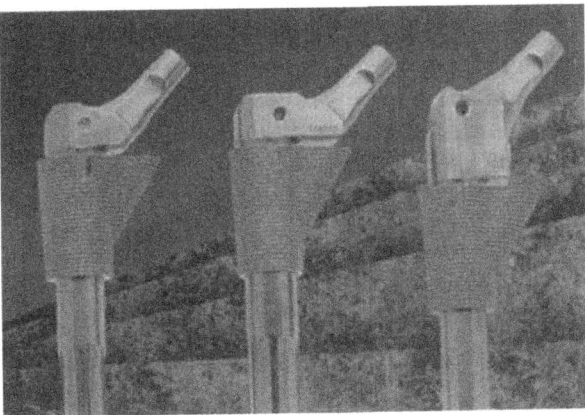

Figure 30.3. Variations in neck length and offset permit intraoperative customization to maximize stability. (See color insert.)

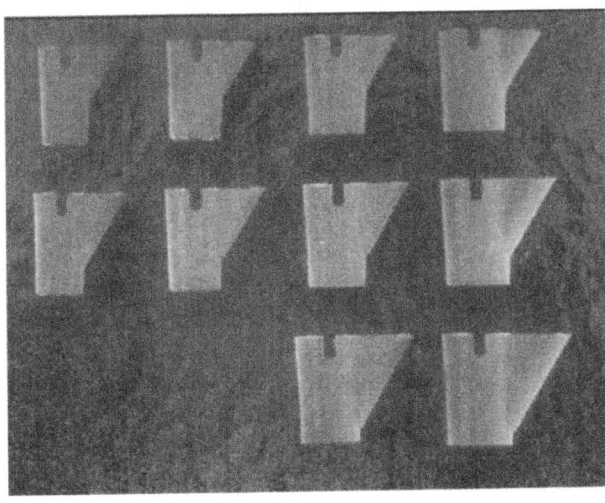

Figure 30.2. Ten proximal modular sleeve sizes are available for each stem. (See color insert.)

loss through stress-shielding and a more complicated revision.[2,3] Modularity allows increased surgical latitude, optimizing fixation, stability, version, and length.

Present options include modular head and necks that can modify head size, neck length, and offset (Fig. 30.3). Proximal sleeves and body allow for adjustments in the anterior/posterior and medial/lateral dimensions and calcar replacement. Proximal pads and distal sleeves satisfy differences in proximal fill and distal fit. Stems come in a plethora of lengths and diameters with variable proximal neck offset. Examples of modular systems include the Impact Mallory-Head (Biomet), Omniflex (Osteonics), APR-II (Intermedics), Richards Modular (Smith & Nephew, Richards), and the S-ROM® (DePuy, a Johnson & Johnson Company).

The evolution of the modular stem for revision surgery was stimulated by the acceptance of the modular head and neck Morse taper in primary surgery. In addition, an unsatisfactory rerevision rate of cemented total hip arthroplasty ranges between 8% and 30% at ten-year follow-up.[4–7] This was felt to be related to poor bone cement interface secondary to the smooth, sclerotic endosteal femoral surface. Results of revision with cementless prostheses are somewhat better, ranging from 3% to 7%, but only at 3 to 6-year follow-up.[8–10] Extensively porous-coated, long-stem prostheses that rely more on distal fixation for stability have a 6.7% revision rate at 5 years.[11] The complication of stress-shielding and the difficulty of implant retrieval compromising proximal femoral bone stock has made this a less attractive option for revision surgery.

The complexity of femoral revisions requires a versatile system that can adjust for proximal femoral bone loss, bone quality, altered anatomy, limb length discrepancy, and offset. A modular hip system like the S-ROM® allows the surgeon to assemble the implant at the time of surgery to provide maximal proximal femoral bone contact and optimal distal fit to satisfy the needs of the individual patient.

The S-ROM: Components, Technique, Indications

Femoral Stem

The titanium alloy stem has several characteristic features: 6 distal and proximal diameters ranging from

14 × 9mm to 24 × 19mm (also now available in other distal and proximal diameters through special order), variable stem lengths from 150 mm to 325 mm (the longer versions come right or left curved), and variable neck lengths and offsets (Fig. 30.4). All the stems have a 3° proximal taper, a fluted smooth distal portion with a coronal slot, and a taper lock neck for the modular femoral heads. Because the stem is not sintered, it is 100% stronger than sintered titanium and 50% stronger than chrome-cobalt.

The range of diameters and lengths should accommodate a small CDH-type femur, or a large patulous femur so frequently seen at revision. The low modulus titanium implant with the distal coronal slot increases stem flexibility and has been shown to be effective in reducing end-stem thigh pain.[12,13] Some authors believe that the larger diameter implants (24 × 19) have been implicated in thigh pain because of the increased bending stiffness.[14]

The longitudinal flutes provide distal stability and nonrigid fixation. Because the femur is reamed line-to-line and the flutes have a depth of approx. 0.5 mm, the implant firmly engages the endosteal cortex. If the femur is not very compliant, it may need to be reamed an additional 0.5 mm. For longer stems flexible reamers are used first for the distal portion of the femur, followed by straight reamers proximally. Because of the anterior bow and the curved implant, the femur is often over-reamed by 1 mm to 1.5 mm distally. Ohl et al.[15] demonstrated that the flutes provide more initial stability in torsion than a fully porous-coated stem. This distal stability allows for the use of extended trochanteric osteotomies (Fig. 30.5 and 30.6), subtrochanteric osteotomies, and cortical onlay and proximal femoral allografts.

The smooth surface of the distal portion of the stem also prevents bony ingrowth, thus preventing rigid distal fixation and proximal stress-shielding. In addition, it makes retrievability of the stem easier.

The Proximal Sleeve

The femoral intramedullary reaming determines the distal diameter of the implant and also the initial proximal size. Because there are 10 sleeves for every standard stem diameter, a wide variation in proximal femoral anatomy can be accommodated. The proximal femur is machined to a simple geometry that maximizes bony contact with the sleeve. Rather than broaching, a conical reamer is used to mill the proximal femur. This is more friendly to the osteoporotic or sclerotic bone often encountered during revision. It reduces the incidence of calcar fracture and preserves bone more effectively. Conical milling provides axial stability. Following this, the calcar is milled to accommodate the triangular spout of the sleeve. The unique aspect of this technique is that triangular milling is done where the best bone is located. This could be in the calcar in a primary hip or in the greater trochanter if the calcar is deficient in a revision situation. Triangular milling provides rotational stability to the construct. In addition, the steps or ridges alongside the sleeve reduce subsidence by acting as an internal collar and converting hoop stresses to compressive loads. Long-term stability is enhanced by bony ingrowth into the sintered titanium beads.

Neck Lengths and Offset

Prior to insertion of the implant, a trial prosthesis is used to determine the appropriate neck length and offset. If necessary, an intraoperative radiograph may be obtained to determine whether the size and position of the implant are satisfactory.

There are a array of neck choices, from a standard length with no additional offset to a calcar replacement with additional offset. With the addition of 0, +6-mm, or +12-mm heads, limb length can be adjusted depending upon the type of revision. This is especially useful, for example, during conversion of a girdlestone or a cup arthroplasty to a total hip arthroplasty (Fig. 30.7). The neck length and offset improve hip biomechanics by restoring abductor tension and reducing joint reactive force.

Implantation

When the machining of the proximal femur is complete the sleeve is inserted first, followed by the stem, until

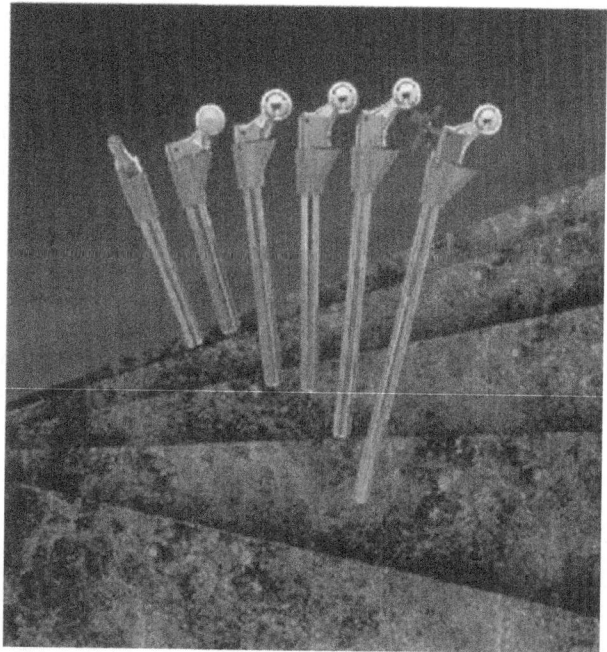

Figure 30.4. A wide assortment of stem options is essential in revision surgery. (See color insert.)

30. Modularity in Total Hip Arthroplasty: The S-ROM Prosthesis

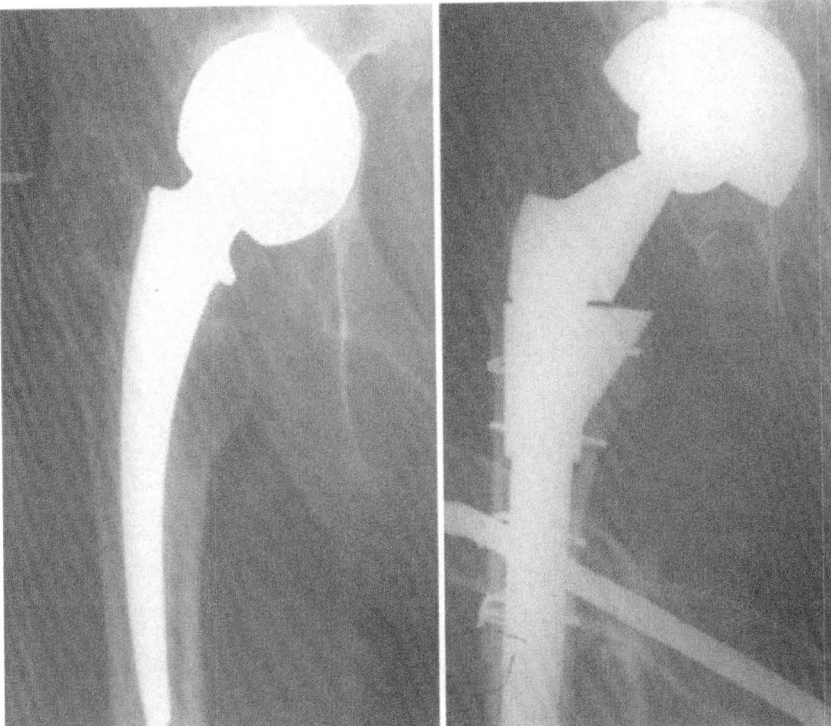

Figure 30.5. An extended trochanteric osteotomy is used to facilitate cement removal.

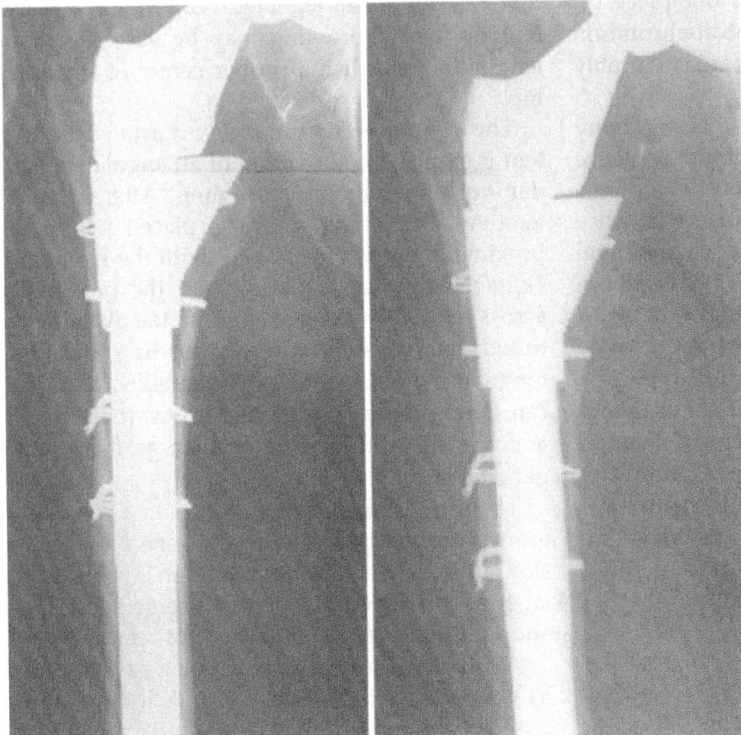

Figure 30.6. The osteotomy is seen at 6 weeks and again at 3 months, completely healed.

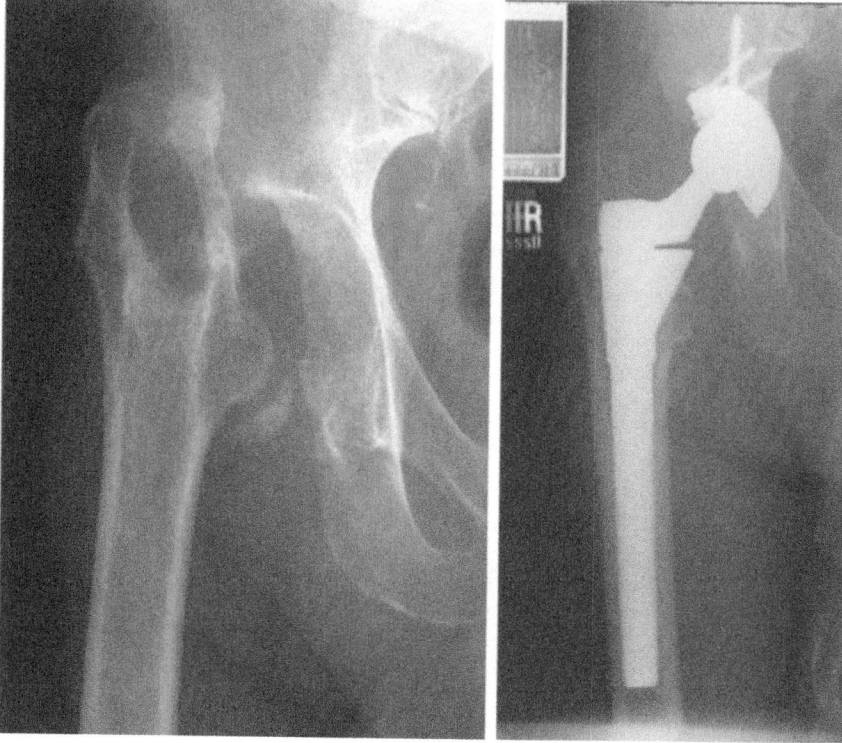

Figure 30.7. Adjustment of neck length is especially useful during Girdlestone conversion.

there is engagement of the taper lock. The stability of this construct was investigated by Ohl et al.[15] They found that when a tight metaphyseal and diaphyseal fit were obtained, load to failure was three times higher than that achieved with a conventional one-piece cementless prosthesis or a distally fixed, cobalt-chromium stem.[15–17] In fact, the load-to-failure compared favorably with a cemented stem.[17]

The sleeve can be oriented to the existing bony anatomy while the stem is positioned within the sleeve independent of bony anatomy or the position of the sleeve. This permits adjustment of version to enhance stability. This is especially helpful in developmental dysplasia or following osteotomy (Fig. 30.8). The sleeve is placed in a position to achieve maximal contact with the host bone and the stem is placed in the appropriate anteversion for stability. In a revision, the calcar may be deficient and the sleeve may need to be placed in a more retroverted position or into the greater trochanter. Again, the stem is placed with the proper amount of version to maintain stability. However, this applies primarily to straight stems because the curved stem is limited by the anterior femoral bow.

Special Indications

There are many indications for using the S-ROM® system. There are, however, unique instances that highlight its versatility. In complicated primary cases secondary to congenital problems, there may be proximal femoral deformity. In DDH there is often increased anteversion and leg length discrepancy. Treatment of the anteversion has been described previously. In a dislocated hip that has significant leg length difference, a femoral osteotomy and shortening may be necessary to restore length and establish a proper center of rotation of the hip.

The technique and rationale for using a modular system is similar for correction of an angular or rotational deformity or femoral shortening. After a femoral osteotomy, the ZTT™ sleeve is placed within the best proximal femoral bone. Then, with the femur properly aligned, the stem is placed into the proximal femur across the osteotomy site and into the distal femur. The fluted, curved stem controls bending and rotational forces and provides immediate stability. The osteotomy can therefore be transverse. Augmentation of the osteotomy site with a plate or strut graft is usually not necessary.

The same situation pertains when a structural bone graft is required for significant bone loss during revision surgery. In a patulous femur an intramedullary tibial graft can be combined with a cemented ZT™ sleeve and the stem press-fit into the host femoral diaphysis.

A proximal femoral allograft that can be brittle is easily prepared with milling tools. A hybrid stem, composed of a cemented ZT™ sleeve and a cementless stem, is placed into the allograft, and then the stem is im-

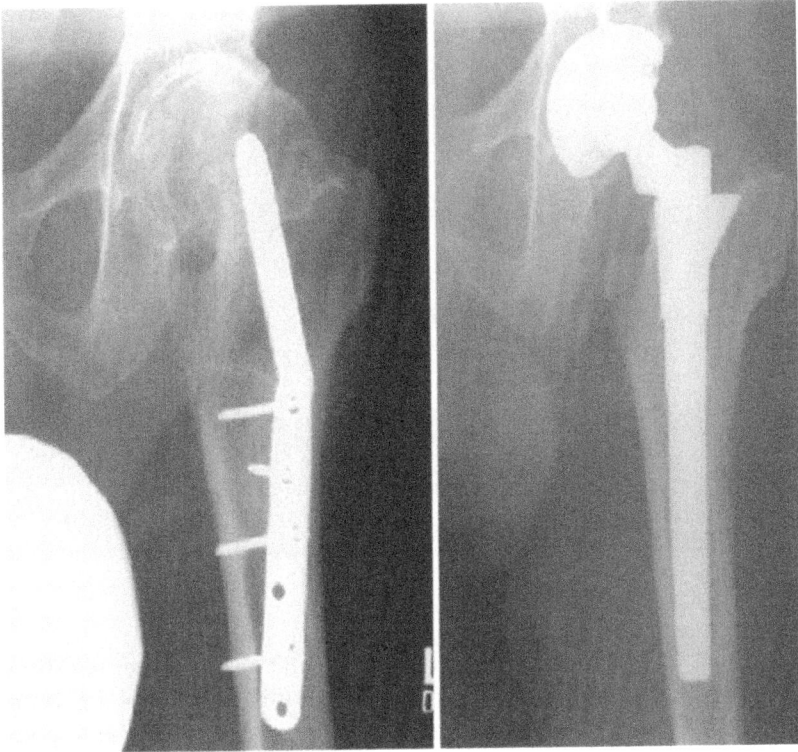

Figure 30.8. A previous osteotomy has distorted the proximal femoral anatomy. The sleeve is placed to maximize stability and ingrowth.

pacted into the distal host canal until the osteotomy site impacts (Fig. 30.9). Again, because the S-ROM® allograft composite has rotational and axial stability, a simple transverse osteotomy can be performed.

One of the main difficulties in hip revision surgery is retrievability of the implants. This can be quite difficult if the stem is osteointegrated. Because the distal portion of the stem is highly polished, there is minimal chance for bone apposition. With a series of wedges the taper lock can be dissociated and the stem removed. This is optimal if anteversion, neck length, or offset needs to be readjusted because of instability or because conversion

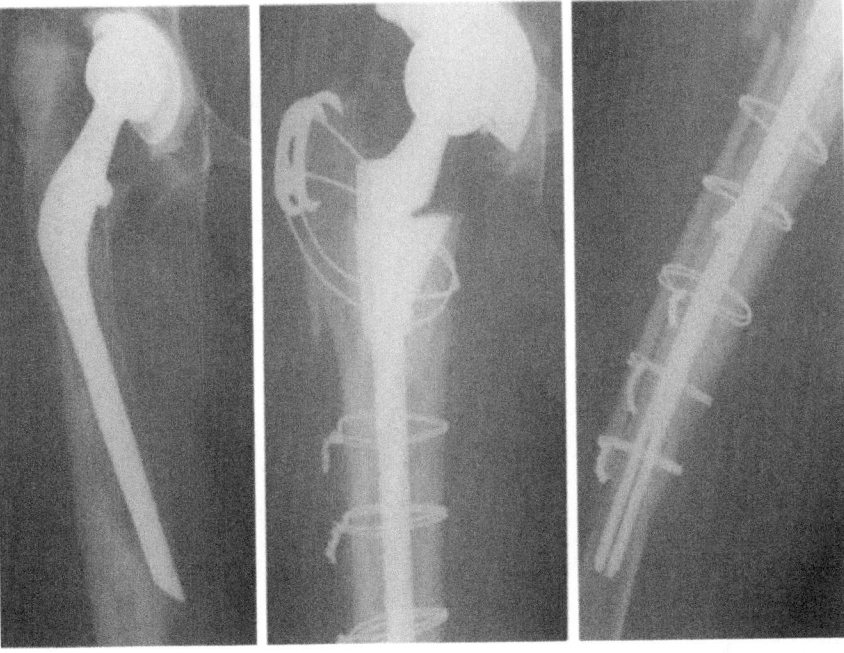

Figure 30.9. The proximal sleeve is cemented into a proximal femoral allograft; the remainder of the stem is inserted without cement.

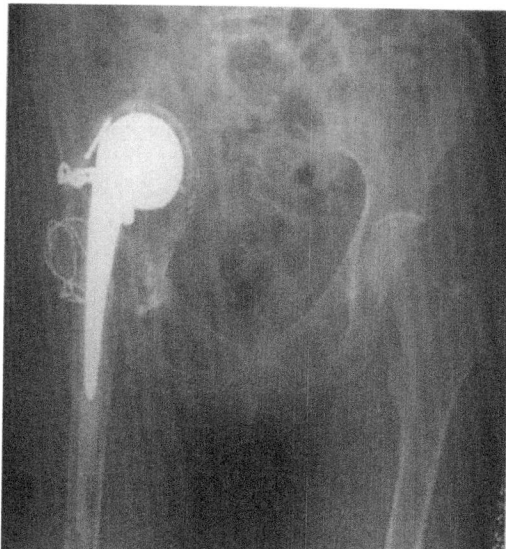
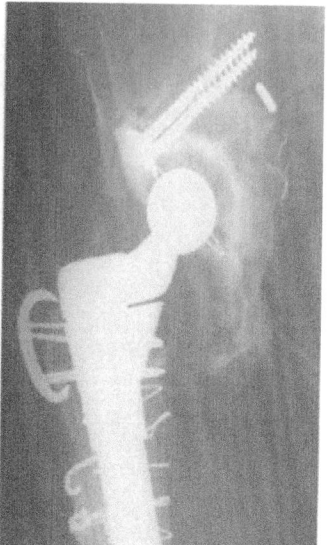

Figure 30.10. Complex revisions create the potential generation of particulate debris.

to a longer stem is required after a periprosthetic femur fracture. However, if there is a septic process, the sleeve can be removed with either flexible osteotomes or sectioned from within with a high-speed burr.

Disadvantages of Modularity

Theoretical questions concerning modularity include: Is micromotion occurring at the stem–sleeve interface sufficient to cause fretting and generation of metallic particulate debris, and will this particulate debris act as third body wear or cause osteolysis similar to polyethylene? (Fig. 30.10).

Bobyn et al.[18] investigated this with dry and wet laboratory testing and examination of *in vivo* prosthesis and reported that given sufficient load and loading cycles, fretting is an inevitable process. However, the generation of particle (1–3 μm) debris is minimal compared

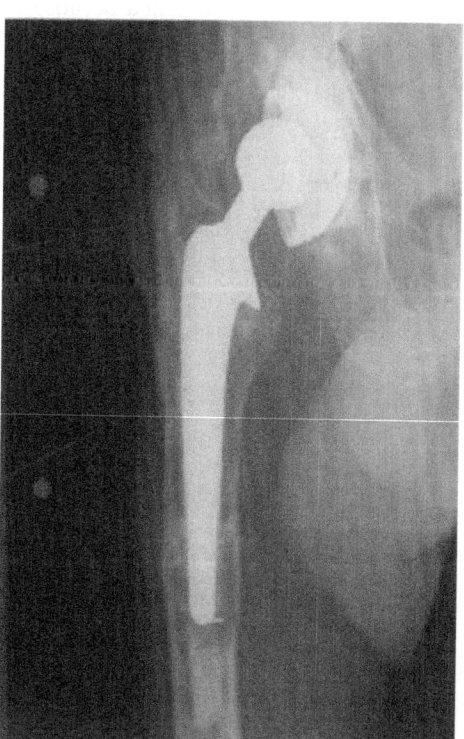
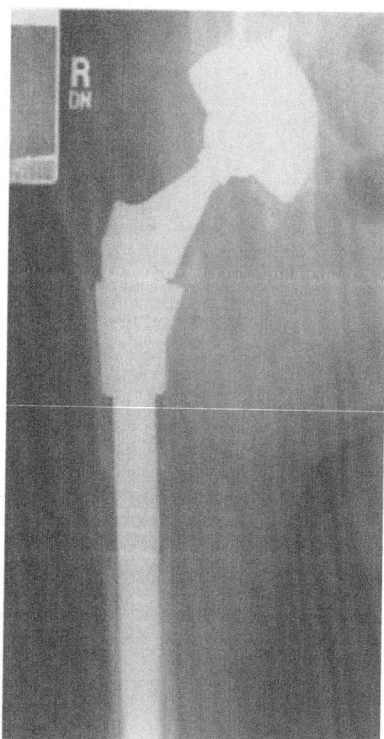

Figure 30.11. Bone reconstitution. An S-ROM femoral component is used (B) in a patient with femoral osteolysis (A) and loosening. At 3 months (C) and 6 months (D) endosteal hypertrophy is noted in response to proximal loading of the femur.

with that seen with polyethylene articulation.[18,19] It is not known, however, how many particles need to be released before there is macrophage-mediated osteolysis or increased third-body wear of the articular surface.

Another potential concern is over dissociation of the modular connections. This has never been reported in *in vivo* or *in vitro* testing. Furthermore, Bobyn reported that there was no gross movement of the stem–sleeve interface when loaded at 3 to 8 times body weight or at torque up to 50 Nm.[18]

Finally, there are situations during revision surgery in which the proximal and distal diameter of the femur are larger than the largest stem. Stability cannot be achieved with the implant alone and, therefore, alternative modalities must be used such as impaction grafting or an intramedullary structural allograft. If the diameter of the femur is the proper size for an implant and the cavitary expansion is moderate, there can be osteolytic defects distal to the sleeve. Interestingly, they tend to reconstitute with new bone over time (Fig. 30.11).[20] This is probably related, in part, to the initial debridement of the inflammatory tissue and later to the physiologic loading of the bone.

Results of Clinical Studies

Clinical trials began in 1984 by Hugh Cameron. Since that time several authors have reported on its use in primary and revision total hip surgery. Cameron reported on the 3- to 6-year results of the S-ROM® in primary arthroplasties. There were 48 cases with no revisions for mechanical failure. An excellent result was achieved in 94% of the cases, with only 4.4% complaining of thigh pain.[13]

Cameron also reviewed the 2- to 6-year results of the S-ROM® used in hip revisions. The results of 91 revisions with 29 primary stems and 62 long curved calcar replacement stems were presented. The mean follow-up was 3.5 years, with 80% of the primary cases reporting an excellent result. No patients had end-stem thigh pain, subsidence, or osteolysis. One case was rerevised for a loose acetabular component, for a rerevision rate of 6.8%. When there was sufficient proximal bone loss to require a long curved stem, the rerevision rate increased to 16.1% at 3.9 years. Of the 10 revisions, four were rerevised for anterior femoral perforation, three for sepsis, one for acetabular migration, and one for recurrent dislocation. There was no stem–sleeve failure, loss of rotational stability, subsidence, metallosis, or osteolysis. There was only 3% incidence of radiographic loosening with long stems.[20]

Chandler et al.[21] also reported on revision total hip arthroplasty using the S-ROM® component. Complex hip revisions were performed in 52 cases. Twenty-two patients required structural allograft because of severe bone deficiency. The mean follow-up was 3 years. Eighty-four percent of the patients were satisfied with

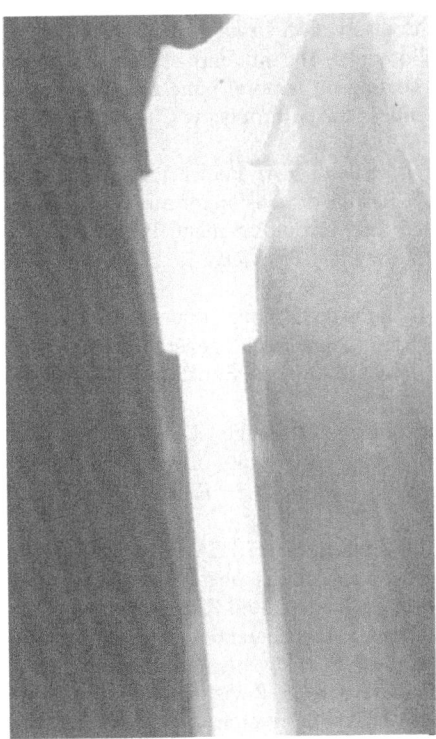
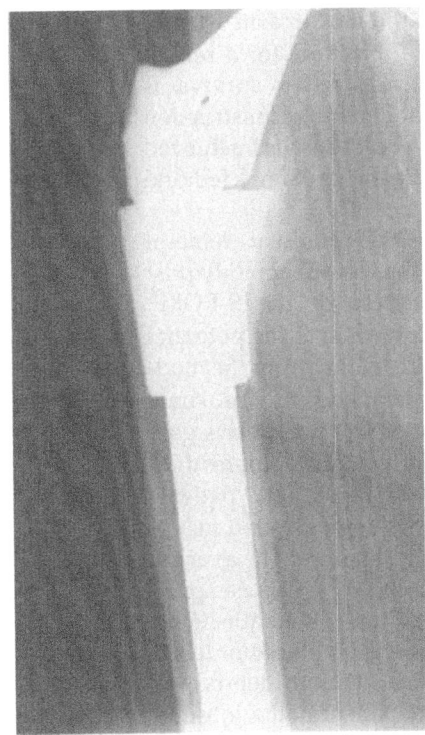

C

their outcome. Only two patients (4%) complained of thigh pain, and this was associated with a stem diameter greater than 17mm. There was no evidence of fretting at the modular stem–sleeve junction or osteolysis below the sleeve. While rerevision occurred in 25% of the patients, only two patients were rerevised for an undersized loose component. The overall mechanical loosening rate was 10%. The authors concluded that the S-ROM® is a unique system with the versatility to accommodate complex hip reconstruction.[14]

Chandler et al.[22] reviewed the results of reconstruction of major segmental bone loss of the proximal femur with an S-ROM® allograft composite. Thirty proximal femoral allografts were performed in 29 patients. The sleeve was cemented into the proximal femoral allograft, then a long-stem curved femoral implant was press-fit into the host femur. The host–allograft junction is created with a butt joint from a transverse osteotomy. At a mean follow-up of 22 months, all but two of the 30 allografts united to the host bone at the host-allograft junction.[21] This has since improved with 41 of 42 allografts achieving union.[22]

A recent clinical review was performed at the New England Baptist Bone and Joint Institute. Seventy-five patients underwent a revision total hip arthroplasty using the S-ROM® system. There was a minimum 5 year follow-up. A previously cemented stem was used in 75% of the patients. Femoral allograft was used in 30 cases. Calcar replacement stems were used in 66%; long curved stems, in 84%. Ninety-seven percent of the stems were found to be bony ingrown by Engh criteria.[23] No osteolysis was seen distal to the sleeve. Only two patients (2.6%) complained of thigh pain. Average prerevision HHS was 52 and the most recent was 82. One stem was revised for late infection, for a rerevision rate of 1.3%. The overall rate of stem survival is 98%. The authors conclude that femoral reconstruction using a proximally modular prosthesis has achieved excellent results despite significant proximal femoral deficiencies.

Since 1987, over 900 S-ROM® modular femoral stems have been implanted at the New England Baptist Hospital. Despite clinical success of the S-ROM® femoral component, concern lingers over the potential generation of metallic debris emanating from the modular junction between the stem and the proximal sleeve. To detect the presence of titanium debris generated by the S-ROM® modular femoral component, 19 synovial fluid specimens were examined in 19 patients in whom the S-ROM® prosthesis demonstrated no evidence of loosening or mechanical failure. The average length of implantation of the S-ROM® prosthesis prior to sampling of the synovial fluid was 38 months (6–89 months). In 17 of the 19 specimens no titanium debris was detected. In two specimens titanium debris was detected (250–400 mcg/L): one patient had a loose titanium cup with broken screws; the other had multiple broken wires from previous trochanteric reattachment. The authors conclude that the use of the S-ROM® modular femoral stem has not resulted in any significant accumulation of titanium debris.[24]

Conclusion

We believe and agree with other authors that the S-ROM® hip system is extremely versatile. The modularity provides intraoperative customization to address many problems encountered in primary and revision hip surgery. The concept of "fit and fill" is optimized by the S-ROM® component. The prosthesis provides maximum proximal bony contact with ingrowth potential while providing isthmic stability.

The theoretical risk of modularity must be balanced with the potential advantages. Longer follow-up studies are necessary to reveal whether the S-ROM® system and modularity are beneficial. Thus far it represents a unique solution to many complex problems in hip arthroplasty revision.

References

1. Noble PC, Alexander JW, Lindahl LJ, Yew DT, Granberry WM, Tullos HS. The anatomic basis for femoral component designs. *Clin Orthop.* 1988;235:148–165.
2. Bobyn JD, Mortimer ED, Glassman AH, Engh CA, Miller JE, Brooks CE. Producing and avoiding stress shielding. Laboratory and clinical observations of noncemented total hip arthroplasty. *Clin Orthop.* 1992;274:79–96.
3. Engh CA, Bobyn JD. The influence of stem size and extent of porous coating on femoral bone resorption after primary cementless hip arthroplasty. *Clin Orthop.* 1988;231:17–28.
4. Callaghan JJ, Salvati EA, Pellici PM, Wilson PD Jr, Ranawat CS. Results of revision for mechanical failure after cemented total hip replacement, 1979–1982: a two to five year follow-up. *J Bone Joint Surg Am.* 1985;67:1074–1085.
5. Estock DM, Harris WH. Long term results of cemented femoral revisions using second generation techniques. An average 11.7 year follow-up evaluation. *Clin Orthop.* 1994;299:190–202.
6. Pellicci PM, Wilson PD, Sledge CD, Salvati EA, Ranawat CS, Poss R. Long term results of revision total hip replacement: a follow-up report. *J Bone Joint Surg Am.* 1985;67:513–516.
7. Kershaw CJ, Adkins RM, Dodd CA, Bulstrode CJ. Revision total hip arthroplasty for aseptic failure: a review of 276 cases. *J Bone Joint Surg Br.* 1991;73:564–568.
8. Engh CA, Glasman AH. Cementless revisions of failed total hip arthroplasty. *Orthop Rev.* 1990;12(suppl):23.
9. Gustillo RB, Pasternak HS. Revision total hip arthroplasty with titanium ingrowth prosthesis and bone grafting for

failed cemented component loosening. *Clin Orthop.* 1988; 235:111.
10. Hungerford DS, Jones LC. The rationale of cementless revision of cemented arthroplasy failures. *Clin Orthop.* 1988; 235:12–24.
11. Lawrence JM, Engh CA, Macaline GE. Revision total hip arthroplasty. Long term results without cement. *Orthop Clin North Am.* 1993;24:635–644.
12. Cameron HU, Trick L, Shepard B, et al. An international multicenter study on thigh pain in total hip replacements. Scientific Exhibit AAOS. New Orleans, La. 1990.
13. Cameron HU. The 3–6 year results of a modular noncemented low-bending stiffness hip implant: a prelimiary study. *J Arthroplasty.* 1993;8:239–243.
14. Chandler HP, Ayer DK, Tan RC, Anderson LC, Varma AK. Revision total hip replacement using the S-ROM femoral component. *Clin Orthop.* 1995;319:130–140.
15. Ohl MD, Whiteside LA, McCarthy DS, White SE. Torsional fixation of a modular femoral hip component. *Clin Orthop.* 1993;287:135–141.
16. Sugiyama H, Whiteside LA, Engh CA. Torsional fixation of the femoral component in total hip replacement: the effect of surgical press-fit technique. *Trans Orthop Res Soc.* 1990;36:258.
17. Sugiyama H, Whiteside LA, Kaiser AD. Examination of rotational fixation of the femoral component in total hip arthroplasty: a mechanical study of micromovement and acoustic emission. *Clin Orthop.* 1989;249:122–128.
18. Bobyn DJ, Tanzer M, Krygier JJ, Dujovne AR, Brooks CE. Concerns with modularity in total hip arthroplasty. *Clin Orthop.* 1994;298:27–36.
19. Bobyn JD, Dujovne AR, Krygier JJ, et al. Surface analysis of the taper junctions of retrieved and *in vitro* tested modular hip prostheses. In: Morrey BF, ed. *Biological, Material, and Mechanical Considerations of Joint Replacement.* New York: Raven Press; 1993:287–301.
20. Cameron HU. The two-six year results with a proximally modular noncemented total hip replacement used in hip revisions. *Clin Orthop.* 1994;298:47–53.
21. Chandler HP, Clark J, Murphy S, McCarthy J, Penenberg B, Danylchuk K. Reconstruction of major segmental loss of the proximal femur in revision total hip arthroplasty. *Clin Orthop.* 1994;288:67–74.
22. Chandler HU, Carangelo RJ. The use of femoral allografts to reconstruct major segmental defects in revision total hip arthroplasty. In: Bono JV, McCarthy JM, Turner R, eds. *Revision Total Hip Arthroplasty.* New York: Springer-Verlag; 1998.
23. McCarthy JC, Bono JV, Turner RH, Tigges R, Krebbs V, Lee J. Bony response to a modular femoral revision component at mean 5.6 year follow-up. Presented at the 11th Annual Symposium of the International Society for Technology in Arthroplasty. Marseille, France; October 1998.
24. Bono JV, McCarthy JC, Turner RH. S-ROM femoral component: Does modularity create metallic debris? Presented at The Hip Society Summer Meeting London, Ontario, Canada; September 25, 1998.

31
Femoral Component Using the Impact Modular Total Hip Implant

Leo A. Whiteside

Revision of the femoral component in total hip replacement is a time-consuming and complicated procedure that requires an array of instrumentation and techniques. In some cases the cancellous bone and a cylindrical cortical structure remain intact and require no special grafting, fixation, or exposure techniques, whereas other cases require all three. Radiographic appearance is unreliable for preoperative planning in any case, and an elaborate array of instruments and an extensive implant selection should be available at the outset. Even cases that appear relatively simple often have angular deformity, complete loss of cancellous bone, peripheral defects, deficient cortical bone, patulous proximal femur, and fragile diaphyseal cortical bone. To deal with these challenges, proximal and distal fixation of the femoral component generally is considered necessary,[1-4] but proximal stress relief and subsequent osteoporosis are long-term issues that must be addressed when using these techniques.[5-9]

Osteotomy for extraction of the implant or for correction of deformity often is necessary before the revision femoral component can be inserted. Defects left in the proximal femur after extraction of the implant often require reconstruction with allograft. Special grafting techniques used to fill such defects are unique to the femoral side of total hip revision, and they often entail the use of special, rigid fixation devices to create a reliable construct of allograft, patient host bone, and an intramedullary implant. Complications with these devices, as well as the question of their structural integrity, are common challenges in revision arthroplasty.

Leg length inequality is not the least of the technically challenging issues to be dealt with in revision arthroplasty. This issue is the most common source of malpractice litigation involving total hip arthroplasty in this country. No arthroplasty system or technique is complete unless this aspect of clinical outcome is considered.

Surgical Technique

Exposure

Both the anterolateral and posterior approaches adequately expose the femur through virtually the same route. The linea aspera should be exposed posteriorly, and the perforating vessels should be suture ligated about 1 cm distal to the linea aspera. The vastus lateralis then can be elevated with its fascial covering almost intact, and the femoral shaft can be fully exposed without denervating or devascularizing the muscle groups that attach to the proximal femur.

Intraosseous exposure of the implant often requires an extended trochanteric osteotomy or bivalving of the femur. When the implant cannot be extracted proximally, bivalving the femur offers a direct and versatile means of extracting an implant that otherwise would be impossible to remove without destroying the proximal femoral bone stock. Bivalving the femur can be done without disrupting muscle attachments and vascular supply to the lateral cortex of the bone and greater trochanter. A straight osteotomy is made with an oscillating saw along the posterior aspect of the femur in line with the linea aspera. The muscle is elevated from a narrow band of the lateral cortex over the lateral side to the anterior aspect of the femur, and then the osteotomy is carried laterally across this denuded surface. A curved half-inch osteotome is used to penetrate the vastus muscle belly and to cut through the anterior cortex to free the lateral bone flap with its muscular attachments. This segment is elevated and the inner aspect of the femur is exposed.

Bone Preparation

Bone in the proximal femur nearly always is deficient in several areas. A general rule that improves the safety of working with this weakened proximal bone is to place two cables circumferentially around the femur. One cable is passed just below the lesser trochanter and one at the distal metaphyseal–upper diaphyseal junction. Since the bone is incapable of maintaining the hoop stresses that are essential for fixation of the implant, cables provide structure to maintain these stresses. But cable placement around the midshaft and upper femur is fraught with significant risk of major complications. The superficial and deep femoral arteries are within reach of the cable passer, but the deep femoral artery and its perforators are the most commonly damaged. The perforating vessels should be identified and suture ligated with approximately 1 cm of stump lateral to the intermuscular septum when the exposure is in the vicinity of the distal metaphysis–upper diaphysis of the femur. Elevating the thigh by lifting the knee helps the surgeon avoid damage to the deep femoral artery by allowing it to fall away from the femur.

The proximal femur is slow to heal after reconstruction and much of the structural material is dependent on the allograft healing, so meticulous cable fixation techniques must be used and composite structures that are robust enough to support early weight-bearing must be constructed. The cables should sit directly on bone around the entire circumference without fibrous or muscle tissue intervening between the cables and bone. This can be achieved by sawing the cable through soft tissue entrapped beneath the cable. A knife is used to cut through the fibrous tissue accessible in the operative field.

Placement of allograft struts along the proximal femoral cortical bone stock is an important adjunct to reconstruction. In areas of discontinuity between the remaining metaphyseal bone and the diaphyseal bone just distal to the defective area, allograft struts should be positioned carefully to abut the upper leading edge of the intact diaphyseal bone. These allograft struts are incorporated in the proximal femoral construct with the circumferential cable technique. They bear shear stresses and transmit axial load, so substantial, reliable approximation between the allograft struts and the distal bone is essential for creating a stable construct of the proximal femur and allograft material.

Reliable fixation can be achieved if a 3-cm cone is constructed in the metaphyseal area. This construct will accept the cone-shaped femoral component and will bear the axial load necessary for early weight-bearing. The hoop-stress bearing capacity of the cables and the axial-load bearing capacity of the butt-joint between the allograft and the diaphyseal cortical bone are more than adequate to bear the load in the proximal femur if the toggle in this load-bearing system can be attenuated through the distal stem.

Distal stem fixation is especially important.[1–4,6–9] Revision hip arthroplasty using proximally porous-coated stems without reliable distal fixation has not achieved great clinical success.[6,10,11] However, combined proximal and distal fixation, even in the presence of substantial bone structure compromise in both areas, has resulted in a high rate of success.[4,8,12] The longest and most extensive cementless clinical follow-up studies have been reported with fully porous-coated femoral stems.[6–9] However, the need for distal porous coating and long-term bone ingrowth into the distal portion of the stem has not been established with certainty.[2] In fact, the proximal stress relief may be disastrous for bone stock integrity if revision surgery later is necessary.[6–8] Of course, rigid early fixation of the implant distally is crucial to long-term success,[2] and torsional fixation of the femoral component traditionally has been the weak link in achieving clinical success in total hip arthroplasty of any type.[2,13–16] The biomechanical problems of achieving rigid torsional fixation in revision are even more challenging than in primary total hip arthroplasty. The quality of fixation achieved if rigid, scratch-fit fixation of the distal component is combined with tight press-fit in the metaphyseal region is greatly superior to that achieved by fixation in either of these regions alone.[1] The techniques for obtaining this type of fixation have been established for primary total hip arthroplasty, and are directly transferable to the revision situation. Although distal fixation is commonly associated with fully porous-coated femoral components, torsional fixation of the distal component is not dependent on porous-coating, but can be achieved equally well, or even better, with distal flutes.[4,12,17] The immediate advantage of flute fixation in the distal portion of the component is safety; it does not risk diaphyseal fracture nearly as often as a fully porous-coated stem. The late advantage of distally fluted stems is that they facilitate proximal, axial load bearing.[1,4] Stems that are smooth distally are incapable of bearing substantial axial load,[4] and thus do not shield the proximal bone from axial forces of weight-bearing. The ideal stem has proximal porous-coating, tight wedge-fit in the metaphyseal region, and distal flutes with parallel sides. This combination of features permits the stem to resist torsional load both proximally and distally, but applies most of the axial load of weight-bearing proximally in the metaphyseal bone, especially after bone ingrowth has occurred into the proximal porous coating.

The technique for achieving tight distal fixation requires underreaming of the diaphyseal cortical bone, cable fixation of the compromised diaphysis, and press-fit of the cylindrical stem into this prepared diaphysis.

Occasionally excision of bone cement or removal of an implant requires a transverse osteotomy of the femoral diaphysis. In other cases, transverse diaphyseal fracture occurs before surgery, or during extraction of the implant. This mechanical challenge is easily met by using a fluted diaphyseal stem and a proximal porous-coated wedge. When rotational correction is desired to this osteotomy, a simple transverse saw cut is used. If rotational correction is not planned through the diaphyseal osteotomy, then rotational fixation of this osteotomy can be enhanced by using an oblique transverse osteotomy. After the bone has been transected, a single cable above and below the osteotomy helps protect it from splintering as the bone is prepared with reamers. After final preparation of the bone, the two ends are held in correct rotational position while the fluted distal stem and conical proximal metaphyseal portion are inserted. Since tight fixation is achieved against torsional loads distally and proximally, additional fixation of this osteotomy usually is not necessary.

Allograft

Without strut allograft reinforcement the construct created with an intramedullary femoral component and the remaining proximal femoral bone stock usually would be weak and insufficient to allow early load bearing. Since early load bearing cannot be avoided after total hip replacement, the surgeon should reinforce the metaphysis with circumferential cables, and often should apply cortical strut allografts. Six- and twelve-inch cortical allograft struts and a cable system that allows multiple cables to be applied and tightened sequentially are necessary parts of the surgeon's armamentarium.

Often the operation cannot be designed so that the stem bypasses all the defects in the femur, so strut allograft fixation and augmentation of these areas are essential for revision of the femoral component.

When preparing for the allograft, circumferential stripping of the diaphyseal cortex should be avoided so that adequate blood supply remains to the intact bone stock. Cable passers should be minimally disruptive to the muscular and periosteal attachments. Although stronger fixation can be achieved with circumferential strut allografts, this procedure is destructive to bone circulation and leaves little access to the patient's remaining bone stock for attachment to soft tissues and reconstitution of blood supply.

In areas of severely deficient bone stock, two struts are necessary. When struts are applied over an irregular femur, cable wastage is inevitable unless the cables are sequentially tightened prior to the final crimping. This technique requires multiple tensioning devices to be placed and tightened repeatedly until all cables are tight. At least three cables should be applied to the allograft–femoral bone construct initially. Then each cable again is tightened sequentially until all three are fixed securely. Other cables then can be added as needed.

Trial Implantation and Leg Lengths

Trial reduction and leg length adjustment are done after the proximal femur has been reconstructed and a solid bone allograft construct has been established. The trial implant is assembled and inserted and is positioned relative to the tip of the greater trochanter or other preoperatively established femoral landmark. Neck length is adjusted accordingly. If the trial implant seats further distally than expected, then a longer neck length is needed. The opposite is done if the trial implants seat proximally to the preoperatively estimated position. Once the final position is achieved and the implant is positioned rotationally, trial reduction is done.

In cases in which the proximal femur is severely deficient and is composed of two or more disconnected segments of bone, reconstruction is impossible without the stabilizing effect of the femoral stem. In these cases, trial reduction is done before the proximal cables are applied. The trial is removed, the final component is inserted partially, then the remaining bone segments and allograft struts are applied around the cone-shaped portion of the femoral component. The cables are placed and the tensioners left attached to the cables as the implant is inserted. If further tensioning of the cables is necessary, or if inadequate positioning is achieved with the final component, the component is partially withdrawn from the femur and the cables are tightened as necessary until the final desired position is achieved. Once all of the cables are tight and the allograft and host bone construct is firmly fixed around the tapered portion of implant, the cables are crimped and cut. If the allograft struts are abutted against firm diaphyseal cortical bone, if the cables are tightly applied to the proximal tapered portion of the implant, and if the diaphyseal portion of the stem is rigidly engaged into a firm construct of bone and allograft distally, then adequate reconstruction is achieved and the patient can safely bear partial weight in the early postoperative period. (Fig. 31.1)

Clinical Results

In a recent study comparing the results of a fully porous-coated monolithic stem with a proximally porous-coated modular stem, similar fixation results were achieved, but the fracture rate was significantly lower when the proximally porous-coated implant was used. Also, proximal bone reconstitution was more readily achieved with the proximally porous-coated implant.

Twenty-eight hips with deformity and severe proximal bone loss had revision total hip arthroplasty between January 1985 and January 1994. Eighteen had fully porous-coated anatomic medullary locking (AML) (DePuy, Warsaw, IN) femoral components fixed with "scratch fit" of the porous surface into distal cortical bone. Ten had proximally porous-coated Impact Modular (Biomet, Warsaw, IN) femoral components with distal scratch fit of a fluted surface and proximal wedge fit of a porous surface.

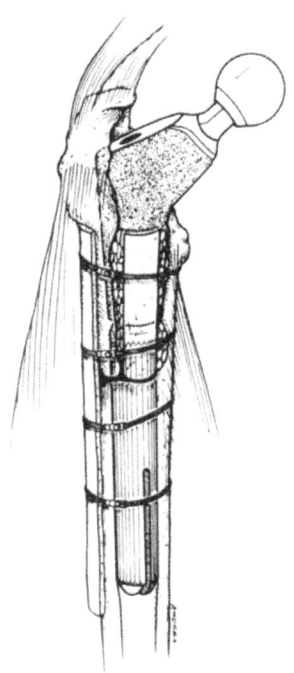

Figure 31.1. Graphic drawing of the reconstructed proximal femur and implant. Rigid distal fixation against torsional loads is achieved by the fluted stem. The porous metaphyseal segment of the stem is wedged into the reconstructed proximal femur. Axial load is borne primarily proximally through the construct composed of metaphyseal bone, strut allografts, and cables. The allograft struts abut the upper edge of the diaphyseal cylinder, and a long allograft strut bridges the junction between metaphyseal and diaphyseal bone. Morselized cancellous bone is packed into crevices and defects between the patient's bone and the allograft.

All 28 cases had more than 1.5 cm leg length shortening, the greatest being 4.5 cm. Six required osteotomy to decrease the diameter of the femoral medullary canal, four required osteotomy to expand the femoral canal enough to accept the femoral component, and eight required oblique osteotomy to correct angular deformity to accept a long femoral component. Strut allografts were used in all cases to cover deficient areas and to strengthen the transition zone at the stem tip. Cables were used to hold tensile stress as the implants were inserted. This construct provided surprisingly good stability, and early weight-bearing was started during the first week after surgery. Morselized cancellous allograft and demineralized bone powder were used to fill cracks and defects. Patients were evaluated at 1 month, 3 months, 6 months, and then yearly for pain, limb length, limp, and walking ability. Radiographs also were evaluated at these intervals for hypertrophy, atrophy, trabecular attachment, and radiographic healing of the bone and strut allograft.

Solid radiographic healing of the proximal construct occurred during the first year in all cases, and a solid tubular structure was achieved. Radiographic signs of bone attachment to the porous surface occurred in 26 of the 28 cases, and the other two had stable, fibrous support of the implant. Trabecular attachment was always distal in the fully porous-coated stems and was associated with hypertrophy of diaphyseal bone and atrophy of proximal metaphyseal bone. The two hips with stable fibrous attachment did not develop distal hypertrophy or proximal atrophy of bone. Trabecular attachment always occurred at the distal portion of the porous surface of the proximally coated implants (Fig. 31.2). Proximal atrophy and distal hypertrophy were less pronounced than in the fully coated components. Postoperative diaphyseal fracture occurred in 4 of the 18 hips with fully porous-coated implants, and in none of the 10 hips with proximally porous-coated implants. Leg length was restored to within 1.5 cm of the length of the opposite leg in all but one case, which remained 4 cm short. None of the patients could walk without limping. Two were moderately painful, and the rest had mild or no pain. The two groups differed significantly in their rates of severe proximal bone atrophy ($p < 0.01$) and in their rates of diaphyseal fracture ($p < 0.02$).

Conclusions

Secure fixation of revision femoral components can be achieved reliably with porous-coated, cementless im-

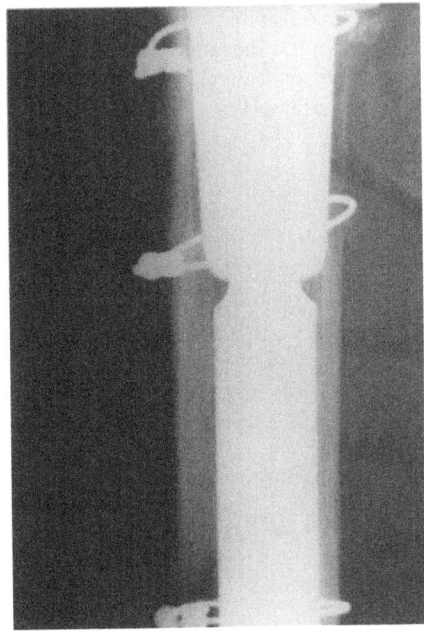

Figure 31.2. Radiograph of the metaphyseal–diaphyseal junction at two years after surgery. Trabecular attachment is apparent at the distal end of the porous-coated metaphyseal segment of the femoral component. Stress-relief atrophy of the metaphyseal bone is apparent above this point of attachment.

plants even in the face of severe deformity requiring osteotomy, strut allograft, and cable fixation. When only diaphyseal fixation is achieved through a fully porous-coated component, fracture rate is high.

Proximal femoral deformity accompanied by severe bone loss can be reconstructed with proximally porous-coated implants if diaphyseal fixation is achieved. When load is shared by the proximal femoral construct, fracture rate is low.

References

1. Ohl MD, Whiteside LA, McCarthy DS, White SE. Torsional fixation of a modular femoral hip component. *Clin Orthop.* 1993;287:135–141.
2. Sugiyama H, Whiteside LA, Engh CA. Torsional fixation of the femoral component in total hip arthroplasty. Effect of surgical press-fit technique. *Clin Orthop.* 1992;275:187–193.
3. Whiteside LA, Easley JC. The effect of collar and distal stem fixation on micromotion of the femoral stem in uncemented total hip arthroplasty. *Clin Orthop.* 1989;239: 145–153.
4. Whiteside LA, Arima J, White SE, Branam L, McCarthy DS. Fixation of the modular total hip femoral component in cementless total hip arthroplasty. *Clin Orthop.* 1994;298: 184–190.
5. Cook SD, Kalwitter JJ, Weinstein AM. The influence of design parameters on calcar stresses following femoral head arthroplasty. *J Biomed Mater Res.* 1980;14:133–144.
6. Engh CA, Bobyn JD, Glassman AH. Porous-coated hip replacement. The factors governing bone ingrowth, stress shielding, and clinical results. *J Bone Joint Surg Br.* 1987; 69:45–55.
7. Engh CA, Bobyn JD. The influence of stem size and extent of porous coating on femoral bone resorption after primary cementless hip arthroplasty. *Clin Orthop.* 1988;231:7–28.
8. Engh CA, Glassman AH, Griffin WL, Mayer JG. Results of cementless revision for failed cemented total hip arthroplasty. *Clin Orthop.* 1988;235:91–110.
9. Engh CA, Massin P. Cementless total hip arthroplasty using the anatomic medullary locking stem. *Clin Orthop.* 1989;249:141–158.
10. Khalily C, Whiteside LA. Early radiographic comparison of the femoral component in three cementless total hip replacement designs. Presented at the Congress of the European Federation of National Associations of Orthopaedics and Traumatology (EFORT), Barcelona, Spain. April 27, 1997.
11. Khalily C, Whiteside LA. Predictive value of early radiographic findings in cementless total hip arthroplasty femoral components: an eight-to-twelve year followup. *J Arthroplasty,* in process, 1998.
12. Whiteside LA. Comparison of two cementless fixation techniques in complex revision total hip arthroplasty. Abstract submitted for 1998 Annual Meeting of the American Academy of Orthopaedic Surgeons.
13. Crowninshield RD, Johnston RC, Andrews JG, Brand RA. A biomechanical investigation of the human hip. *J Biomech.* 1978;11:75–85.
14. Davy DT, Kotzar GM, Brown RH, Heiple KG, Goldberg VM, Heiple KG Jr., et al. Telemetric force measurements across the hip after total arthroplasty. *J Bone Joint Surg Am.* 1988;70:45–50.
15. Mjoberg B, Hansson LI, Selvik G. Instability of total hip prostheses at rotational stress. *Acta Orthop Scand.* 1984;55: 504–506.
16. Wroblewski BM. The mechanism of fracture of the femoral prosthesis in total hip replacement. *Int Orthop.* 1979;3: 137–139.
17. Cameron HU, Jung Y, Noiles DG, McTighe T. Design features and early clinical results with a modular proximally fixed low bending stiffness uncemented total hip replacement. Scientific exhibit at the annual meeting of the American Academy of Orthopaedic Surgeons, Atlanta, Georgia, Feb. 4–9, 1988.

32
Cemented Long-Stem Femoral Components in Revision Total Hip Arthroplasty

David A. Mattingly

Indications and Rationale

Although cementless reconstruction is indicated for most femoral revisions, there are exceptions where cemented, long-stem femoral revisions may be preferred.[1,2,3] These relative indications include: allograft–prosthetic composites (Fig. 32.1); failed cementless reconstruction (Fig. 32.2A, B); reimplantation for sepsis with antibiotic-impregnated bone cement (Fig. 32.3); elderly patients with poor proximal femoral bone; and medical conditions limiting life expectancy and activity level with pathologic remaining bone (rheumatoid arthritis, dialysis and transplantation patients, systemic lupus erythematosus, and metastatic disease). Relative exclusions include young, active patients with life expectancy greater than 10 years; and femora with fractures, perforations, and/or bone deficiencies requiring internal fixation or biologic bone graft reconstruction.

Cemented long-stem femoral components were initially found to be useful in the treatment of certain cases of femoral shaft fractures associated with total hip arthroplasty (THA).[4,5] With increasing knowledge of the anatomy, physiology, and biomechanics of cemented femoral revision arthroplasty (Fig. 32.4), combined with the poor long-term results reported for revisions utilizing a standard length cemented femoral stem,[6,7,8] the potential advantages of using a long-stem femoral prosthesis becomes evident.[3,5] The longer stem provides a longer cement fixation surface area, reducing the unit load on the prosthesis and cement.[3] It also bypasses bone deficiencies and stress concentrations in the pathologic proximal femur, permitting more rigid bone-cement fixation with distal bony trabeculae and reducing the incidence of cement and femoral shaft fracture. The constraint on the implant imposed by the femoral isthmus allows less potential for motion, which may lead to bone resorption and mechanical loosening. Disadvantages of the long-stem femoral component include the sacrifice of normal distal bone stock, increased technical difficulty with insertion and revision of a long-stem prosthesis, and the potential for stress shielding of an already compromised proximal femur.

Surgical Technique

Most standard revision surgical approaches can be utilized for insertion of a long-stem cemented femoral component. However, extended lateral trochanteric osteotomy windows, or distal osteotomies should be avoided to prevent nonunion from cement interposition and to improve cement pressurization. Trochanteric osteotomy is required in most cases where the previous cement mantle extends distally greater than 180 to 200 mm. All cases should be performed with the patient positioned over a fluoroscopy extension table to permit biplane fluoroscopic visualization when needed.

To minimize the risk of fracture or perforation, it is essential to obtain full length anteroposterior (AP) and lateral radiographs of the femur before surgery to determine the exact position of the femoral stem and distal cement column, the amount of femoral bow, and any areas of cortical thinning. Prophylactic cerclage wires are placed in areas of bony compromise prior to component removal. Trochanteric osteotomy, fiberoptic illumination of the femoral canal, and reflection of the vastus lateralis improve visualization and accurate instrumentation of the medullary canal. Standard techniques are used for cement removal. We attribute our low incidence of fractures and perforations to several techniques that aid in central placement of the distal stem in both the coronal and sagittal planes.[3] We re-

Figure 32.1. A. Prerevision AP radiograph demonstrating aseptic loosening and bone deficiency. B. Postrevision AP radiograph of allograft–prosthetic composite with femoral stem cemented into the allograft and host bone.

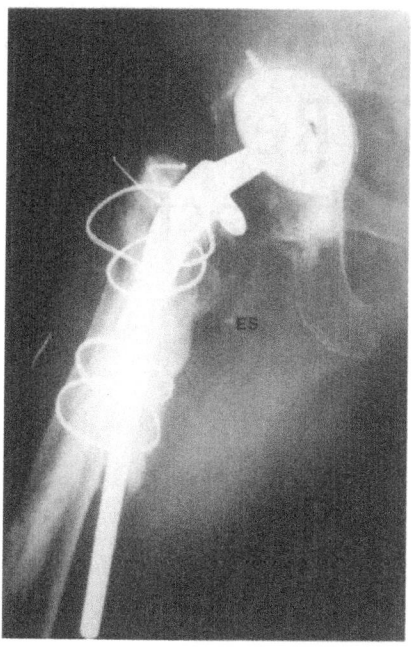
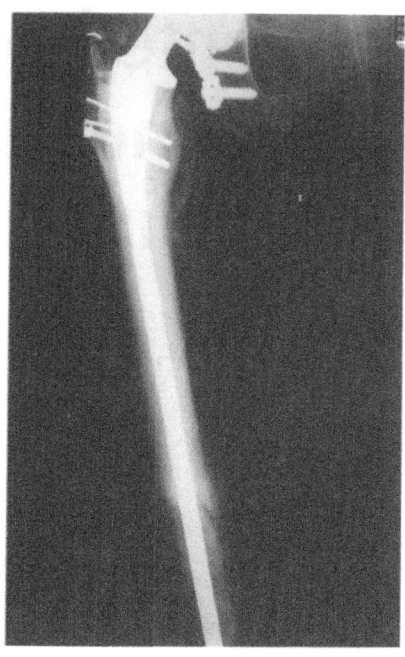

move as much proximal cement as possible and any obstructive endosteal bony projections to prevent impingement and misdirection of the implant. Flexible reamers are used to widen the intramedullary canal to at least 3 mm greater than the femoral stem, to permit easy passage of the stem past the isthmus into the canal, and provide an adequate cement mantle. A stem length is chosen that bypasses the distal most area of cortical weakening by 2 to 2.5 cortical diameters. The trial stem is placed into the distal canal with gentle hand pressure until either the prosthesis is fully seated or resistance is met; the position of the distal stem is then checked with the use of AP and lateral biplane fluoroscopy. Central stem placement in the coronal plane is usually not dif-

Figure 32.2. A. Failed, painful cementless femoral revision. B. Reconstruction of femur with long-stem cemented implant (6 years).

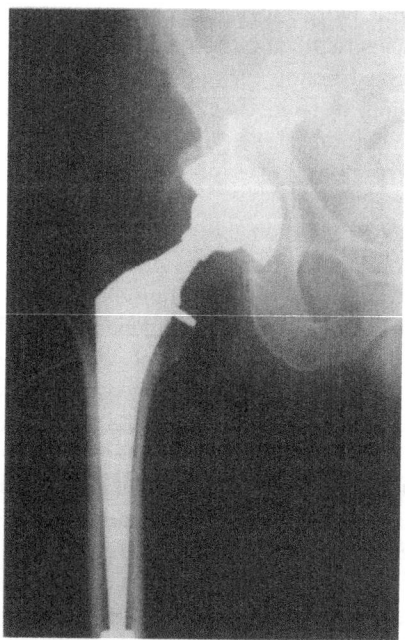
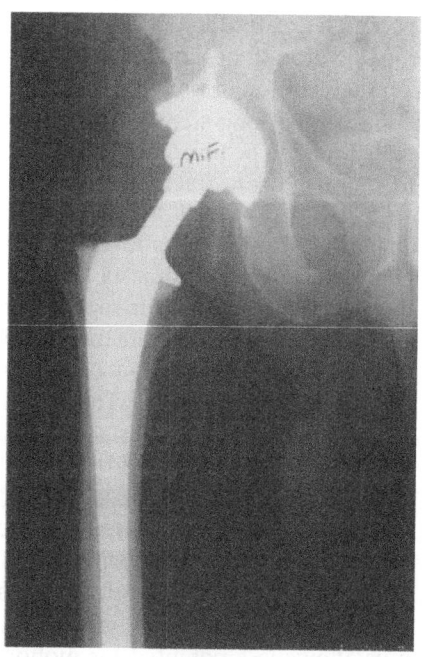

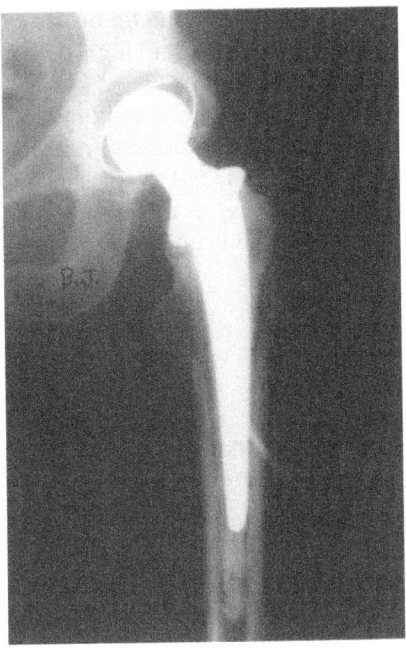
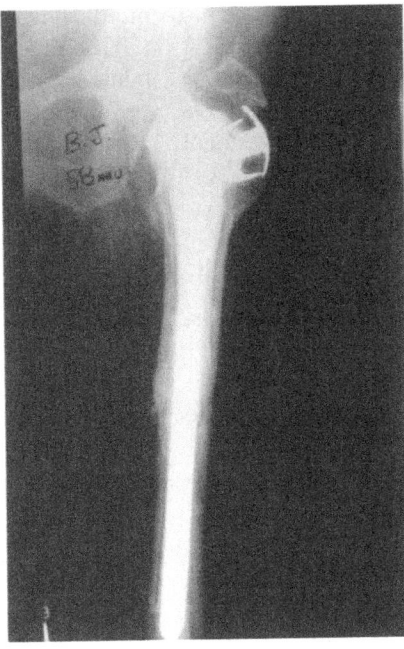

Figure 32.3. A. Elderly patient with septic total hip replacement and minimal bone loss. B. Staged reimplantation of long stemmed femoral component with antibiotic impregnated cement (58 months).

ficult; however, anterior femoral bowing may cause the prosthetic tip to abut the anterior cortex distally, increasing the risk of fracture and/or perforation. If this occurs, shortening of the stem or use of an anteriorly bowed prosthesis will usually solve this problem.

After reaming and broaching, the femoral canal is debrided by pulsatile lavage and thoroughly dried. A distal cement restrictor is prepared by injecting low viscous cement into a chest tube with a 10 mm silastic cement plug proximal to the cement. A long, thin rod is then used to push the plug and cement into the canal, at least 2 cm distal to the end of where the implant will seat. As this plug hardens, two bags each of room-temperature cement (four bags total) are mixed 2 minutes apart. The second batch is inserted first into the distal canal via a long-nozzled cement gun in a low viscous state. The first batch is then placed into the proximal femur when it reaches a doughy state. As the long-stem prosthesis is inserted, the proximal doughy cement contains the more distal low-viscous cement into the more

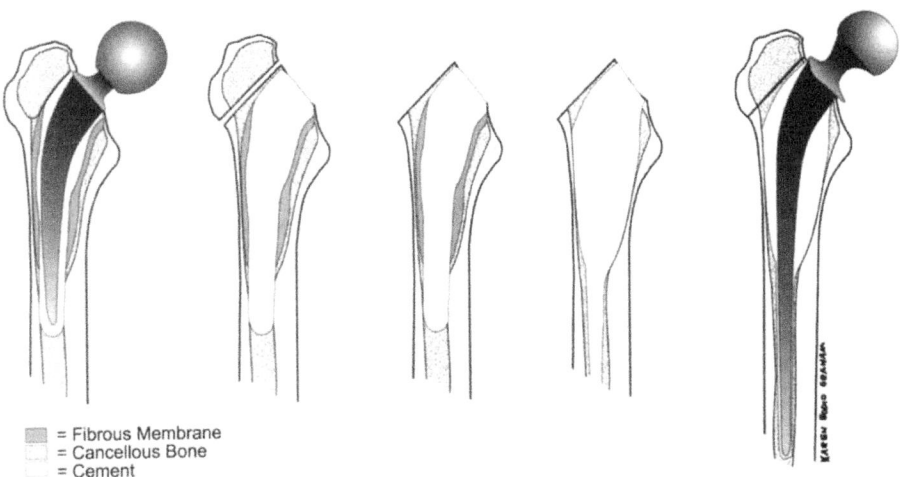

= Fibrous Membrane
= Cancellous Bone
= Cement

Figure 32.4. In femoral revisions, removal of the loose femoral component leaves the old cement and a thickened membrane at the bone–cement interface. The adjacent bone is thinning from endosteal resorption, with minimal remaining cancellous bone for cement binding. The revision prosthesis should come well below (2–2.5 cortical diameters) this area of pathologic bone to enhance the revision cementing and protect the weakened proximal bone.

distal femur. When allograft–prosthetic composites are performed, the long-stem implant is first cemented into the allograft prior to cementing into the distal canal. A transverse anastomosis between allograft and host bone allows for easy clearance of cement at the anastomosis site; rotational stability is provided for by the cement and onlay allograft bridging the anastomosis.

Results and Discussion

Results utilizing a long-stem femoral component during revision THA have been previously published.[1,2,3] In Turner's series,[3] clinical results for 110 patients (follow-up average 81 months) demonstrated on average Harris hip score of 84 points, with 70% good or excellent scores, 17% fair, and 13% poor. Only 10% of patients in this series felt that they had not benefited significantly from the revision arthroplasty. Radiographic bone cement lucencies are common in the compromised proximal one-third of the femur, but extent and progression of radiolucent lines was noticeably reduced when compared to other series. Callaghan et al.[1] also noted a significant difference in the incidence of progressive radiolucencies after revision with a long stem (25%) versus a conventional length (40%) femoral component. Turner et al.[3] reported that seventeen of 139 hips (12%) with follow-up were considered failures due to aseptic loosening (11 hips), sepsis (3 hips), component fracture (2 hips), and shaft fracture (1 hip). Intraoperative complication occurred in 38 hips (23%), the most common being femoral perforation of fracture (34 hips) during cement removal. It was also noted that the larger quantities of polymethylmethacrylate required for long-stem implants can produce severe hypotensive episodes, especially in patients with previous cardiovascular disease. Extreme care must be taken during revision to maintain an adequate blood volume, systemic pressure, and central perfusion. Swan–Ganz or central venous monitoring, arterial lines, and Foley catheter urine output monitoring are essential in elderly and high-risk patients.

When indicated, long-stem, cemented femoral components provide a useful solution to difficult revisions with satisfactory long-term results.[1,2,3] Patient selection, careful preoperative planning, and exact surgical technique are essential to successful outcomes that this type of implant can provide.

References

1. Callaghern JJ, Salvati EA, Pellici PM, et al. Results of revision for mechanical failure after cemented total hip replacement. *J Bone Joint Surg Am.* 1985;67:1074–1085.
2. McLaughlin JR, Harris WH. Revision of the femoral component of a total hip arthroplasty with the calcar replacement femoral component. *J Bone Joint Surg Am.* 1976;78:331–339.
3. Turner RH, Mattingly DA, Scheller AD. Femoral revision total hip arthroplasty using a long-stem femoral component. Clinical and radiographic analysis. *J Arthroplasty.* 1989;2(3):247–258.
4. Scott RD, Turner RH, Leitzes SN. Femoral fractures in conjunction with total hip replacement. *J Bone Joint Surg Am.* 1975;57:494.
5. Turner RH, Emerson RH, Jr. Femoral revision total hip arthroplasty. In: Turner RH, Scheller AD Jr., eds *Revision total hip arthroplasty.* New York: Grune and Stratton; 1982:75–106.
6. Amstutz HC, Ma SM, Jinwatt RH, Mai L. Revision of aseptic loose total hip arthroplasties. *Clin Orthop.* 1982;170:21.
7. Kavanagh BF, Ilstrup DM, Fitzgerald RH. Revision total hip arthroplasty. *J Bone Joint Surg Am.* 1985;67:517.
8. Pellicci PM, Wilson PD, Sledge CB, et al. Long term results of revision total hip replacement: a follow-up report. *J Bone Joint Surg Am.* 1985;67:513.

Section 1
Conclusions

Femoral reconstruction *remains* a formidable challenge and requires expertise in surgical planning, extensile exposure, implant removal, bone grafting, and rigid fixation methods for the new prosthesis. Since the actual soft tissue and bony abnormality is often more onerous than can be seen radiographically, the surgeon must be resourceful and plan accordingly. While both cemented and cementless component fixation can be successful, the principles of femoral reconstruction need to be observed. These include restoration of leg length and muscle balance, restoration of femoral bony integrity, prosthetic containment and rigid fixation, and secure bone graft coaptation. When combined with comprehensive preoperative planning, adherence to these principles gives the greatest prospect for a successful reconstructive procedure.

Section 2
Surgical Approaches

Unlike primary total hip replacement, revision surgery presents an additional challenge to the surgeon because of extensive tissue scarring. The previous skin incision may be located in a suboptimal position and may not be usable. The previous scar may have keloid formation or may have stretched considerably. If possible, the previous incision should be excised, including the skin and a wedge-shaped area of subcutaneous tissue to fresh margins. Scarring superficial to the fascia distorts tissue *planes* and can result in anterior or posterior translation of the iliotibial band fascial incision. Similarly, dense adhesions frequently occur between the fascia and the subjacent vastus lateralis fascia, further distorting the surgical approach. More ominously, the sciatic nerve posteriorly or the femoral nerve anteriorly can become intimately scarred to the hip joint margins and can potentially result in significant nerve injury, *neurotonesis* or axonotomesis if not recognized. If possible, the previous operative note should be obtained and reviewed.

This section examines the principal surgical approaches utilized for revision total hip surgery. It highlights methods used to address surgical scarring as well as techniques to make the approach extensile. The rationale and specific indications for each approach are provided. In addition, details of each surgical technique and surgical "pearls" are included.

33
Posterolateral Approach

David A. Mattingly

Extensile exposure of the pelvis, acetabulum, and femur is often required in revision total hip arthroplasty to manage fractures, discontinuities, bone deficiencies and deformities, and soft tissue contractures. The surgical approach selected should allow flexibility for extension of the exposure as needed. The posterolateral approach (Fig. 32.1) provides excellent exposure for most acetabular and/or femoral revisions, whereas providing easy conversion to more extensile approaches (eg, osteotomies, windows) where indicated. Decreased time of surgery, excellent exposure with minimal muscle damage, and fast rehabilitation make this approach attractive for most revisions in the active, cooperative patient.

Indications, Limitations

The posterolateral approach can be utilized for all revisions where conventional or extended trochanteric osteotomy are not required or indicated. Situations that may require trochanteric osteotomy include the following revisions: limb lengthening greater than 1 cm, or the need to shorten the operative extremity; marked soft tissue contracture or shortening; global acetabular deficiency requiring anterior column plating or whole acetabular grafting; removal of well-fixed porous or cemented femoral stems; and removal of long cement columns greater than 200 mm from the femoral neck. In this last situation, the posterolateral approach may be combined with a femoral window or distal femoral osteotomy. Also, the posterolateral approach can be combined with the ilioinguinal approach to treat global acetabular deficiencies where anterior and posterior column plating may be required.[1] The posterolateral approach is also preferred over trochanteric osteotomy where postoperative irradiation for heterotopic ossification is anticipated, eliminating the potential complication of trochanteric nonunion (Fig. 33.2).

Surgical Technique

Surgical anatomy for the posterolateral approach has been well defined.[2,3,4] This section highlights general principles and surgical tips to maximize exposure, avoid complications, and improve outcomes with the posterolateral approach. The patient is positioned in the direct lateral decubitus position. The pelvis is rigidly immobilized with the operative leg freely mobile and positioned over a fluoroscopy extension table to allow for x-ray visualization if needed. Old incisions are incorporated or excised where possible, usually extending the incisions proximally and distally to more easily define tissue planes for release of scar and to facilitate extensile exposure when needed. The iliotibial band (ITB) and gluteus maximus fascia are split in line with the skin incision, mobilizing the ITB from the scarred vastus lateralis and tensor fascia lata. The sciatic nerve is identified and palpated since it may be scarred or displaced from prior surgery; dissection away from the nerve is recommended to avoid devascularization and injury unless preoperative symptoms necessitate a neurolysis. With the leg maximally extended and internally rotated, the scarred extensor rotators are released and reflected posteriorly, protecting the sciatic nerve. The interval between the scarred abductors and pseudocapsule is developed superiorly and Cobra retractors are placed here and at the inferior neck. A posterior and superior capsulectomy is completed prior to posterior dislocation. In scarred or contracted hips, especially those with flexion contracture, anterior capsulectomy prior to posterior capsulectomy and dislocation may be necessary. The anterior capsule can be easily approached and excised by flexing and externally rotating the limb and developing the interval between the anterior gluteus medius and the origin of the vastus lateralis and vastus intermedius. Anterior capsulectomy at this point also provides a pocket to rest the prosthetic femoral head when isolated acetabular revision surgery is performed.

The prosthetic femoral component is dislocated posteriorly by applying traction, internal rotation, and slight flexion to the limb. After femoral component extraction, the anterior-inferior capsule is dissected from the iliopsoas tendon sheath and removed. This usually permits easy mobilization and retraction of the femur to complete acetabular revision arthroplasty. If further mobilization of the femur is required, partial or com-

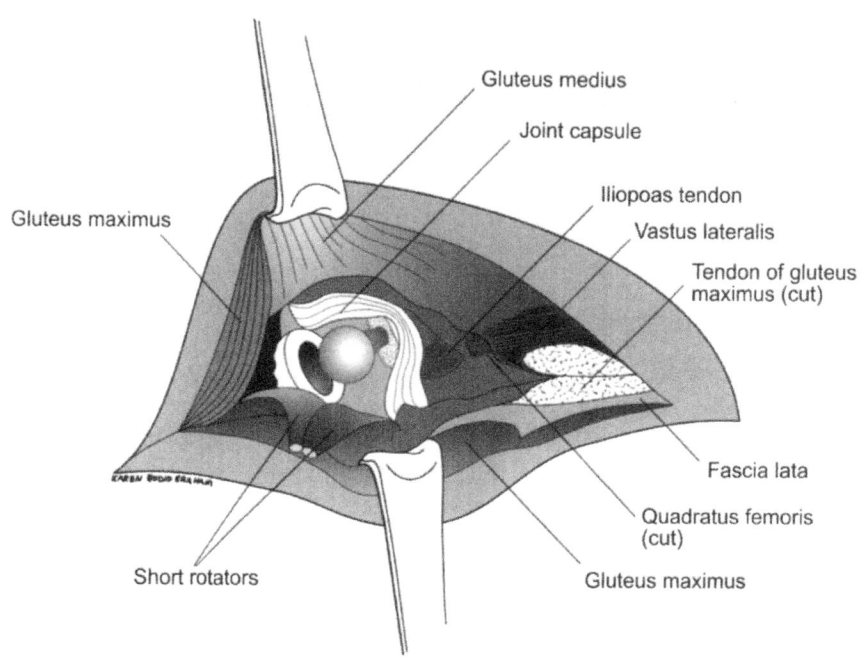

Figure 33.1. The posterolateral approach provides excellent exposure with minimal muscle damage. Release of the capsule, short rotators, iliopsoas and gluteus maximus tendon permits excellent exposure in contracted, shortened limbs requiring lengthening.

plete release of the iliopsoas and gluteus maximus tendon or skeletalization of the proximal 5 cm of the femur may be required (Fig. 33.1 and 33.2).

The posterolateral approach provides excellent exposure for complex acetabular reconstructions, including structural allografts (Fig. 33.3A), posterior column platings (Fig. 33.3A), and antiprotrusio cages (Fig. 33.3B). The anterior column is poorly visualized through this approach, but can be combined with the ilioinguinal approach for anterior column plating to fix whole acetabular allografts and/or discontinuities.

Most complex femoral reconstructions can be effectively managed through the posterolateral approach (Fig. 33.4A and B). This approach allows excellent visualization of the proximal 150 to 180 mm of the femoral canal. If the femoral canal needs to be exposed in the diaphyseal region, distal femoral windows and/or osteotomies can be combined with the posterolateral approach to adequately expose deformities, bone deficiencies or distal cement by elevation of the vastus lateralis from the lateral intermuscular system. When more extensile exposure is required, the posterolateral

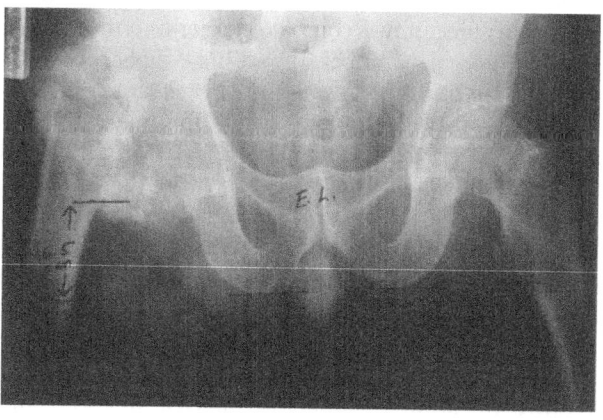
A

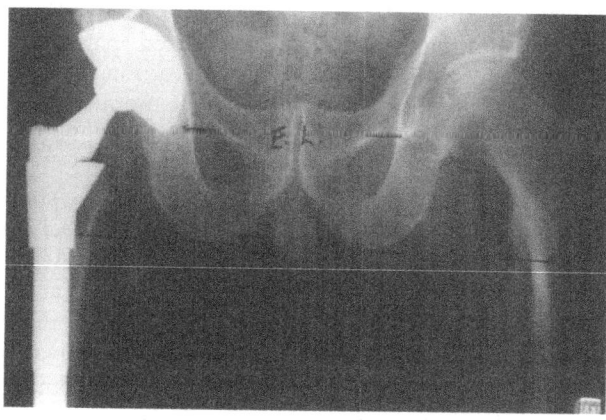
B

Figure 33.2. A. Preoperative resection arthroplasty with significant shortening and heterotopic ossification. B. Postoperative reconstruction with restoration of length after skeletalization of the proximal femur and release of the iliopsoas and gluteus maximum tendons through the posterolateral approach. Postoperative irradiation limited heterotopic bone formation and the posterolateral approach eliminates the potential morbidity of trochanteric nonunion associated with osteotomy and postoperative irradiation.

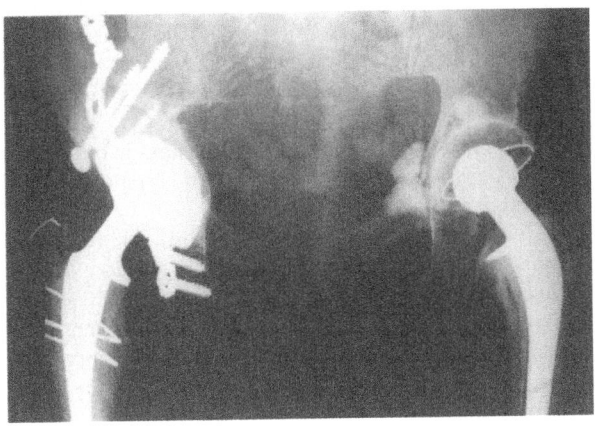
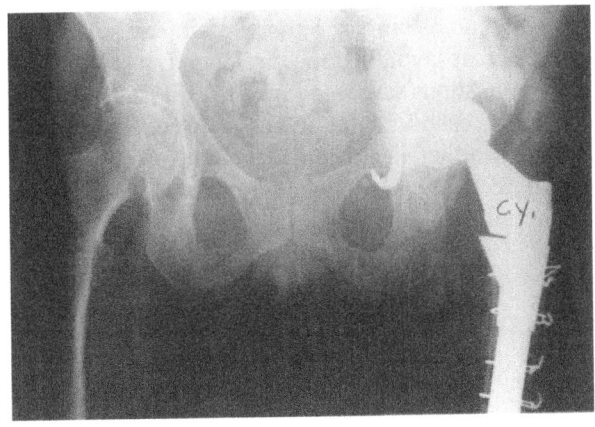

Figure 33.3. Complex acetabular reconstructions performed through posterolateral approach: A. Structural allograft and posterior column plating. B. Antiprotrusio cage with particulate bone graft.

approach permits easy conversion to the conventional trochanteric osteotomy, anterior trochanteric slide or extended lateral trochanteric osteotomy.

Conclusion

Data from several studies indicate an increased incidence of postoperative posterior dislocation when the posterolateral approach is compared to the anterolateral, lateral, and trochanteric osteotomy approaches using total hip arthroplasty.[5,6,7] This complication can be significantly reduced by careful positioning of the prosthetic components (usually 40° to 50° of combined acetabular and femoral anteversion); restoration of leg lengths, offset and myofascial tension; and strict adherence to hip precautions during the early postoperative rehabilitation phase. For most revision patients, we recommend partial weight bearing with two crutches and strict adherence to hip precautions for a minimum of two months; longer protection may be required for more complex revisions with bone or soft tissue deficiencies.

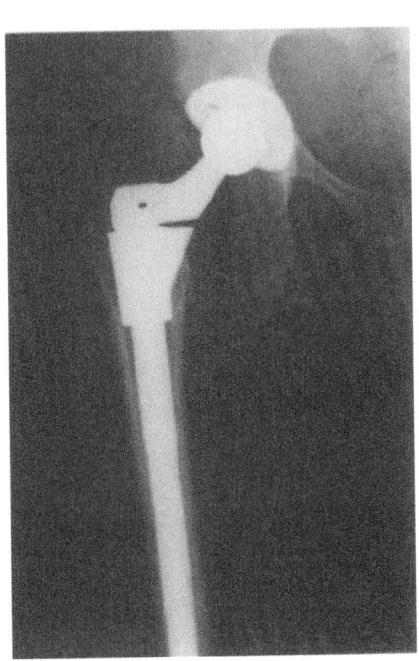
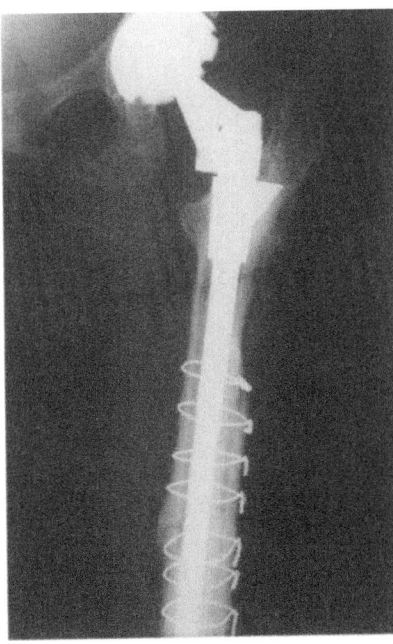

Figure 33.4. Complex femoral reconstructions performed through posterolateral approach: A. Postoperative cementless long stem for loose, cemented stem. B. Postoperative cementless long stem with cortical onlay graft to treat loose stem with periprosthetic fracture.

The posterolateral approach can be effectively used to manage most complex femoral and acetabular revisions whereas avoiding the prolonged rehabilitation and complications associated with the direct lateral and trochanteric osteotomy approaches. A cooperative patient, strict adherence to postoperative protocols, and surgical technique are essential to successful reconstruction utilizing this approach.

References

1. Mattingly DA. Surgical approaches to the hip. In: Callaghan JJ, Dennis DA, Paprosky WG, Rosenberg AG, eds. *Orthopaedic knowledge update: hip and knee reconstruction.* Rosemont Ill.: American Academy of Orthropaedic Surgeons. 1995:171–177.
2. Crenshaw AH. Surgical approaches. In: Crenshaw AH, ed. *Campbell's operative orthopaedics*, 8th ed. St. Louis, Mo: Mosby Year Book; 1992:23–116.
3. Cuckler JM. Surgical approaches. In: Steinberg ME, ed. *The hip and its disorders.* Philadelphia, Pa: WB Saunders; 1991:88–105.
4. Hoppenfled S, deBoer P. Surgical exposures in orthopaedics. *The anatomic approach.* Philadelphia: J B Lippincott Co, 1984.
5. Callaghan JJ, Dysnet SH, Savory CG. The uncemented porous-coated anatomic total hip prosthesis: two-year results of a prospective consecutive series. *J Bone Joint Surg Am.* 1988;70:337–346.
6. Carlson DC, Robinson HJ Jr. Surgical approaches for primary total hip arthroplasty: a prospective comparison of the Marcy modification of the Gibson and Watson-Jones approaches. *Clin Orthop.* 1987;222:161–166.
7. Mostardi RA, Askew MJ, Gradisar IA Jr, Hoyt WA Jr., Snyder R, Bailey B. Comparison of functional outcome of total hip arthroplasties involving four surgical approaches. *J Arthroplasty.* 1988:279–284.

34
The Direct Lateral and Vastus Slide Approach

Hugh P. Chandler and Robert J. Carangelo

Adequate exposure of the hip joint is of paramount importance in primary and revision hip surgery. It is the first and often the limiting step in the successful outcome of total hip replacement.

There are several anterolateral approaches to the hip joint. In 1935, Watson-Jones described an approach that develops the interval between the tensor fascia femoris and the gluteus medius.[1] Although this approach provides excellent exposure to the anterior aspect of the acetabulum, the posterior and superior acetabulum are not as well visualized with the Watson-Jones approach. The anterior muscle fibers of the gluteus medius, as well as the superior gluteal nerve to the tensor fascia femoris can be also be damaged.

In 1954, McFarland and Osborne described a new lateral approach to the hip, based on the fact that the gluteus medius and the vastus lateralis are in continuity with each other through a tendinous periosteal sleeve over the greater trochanter.[2] The patient is placed in the lateral position and the gluteus medius and vastus lateralis are detached from their posterior borders and are reflected anteriorly, remaining in continuity with the periosteal sleeve. The McFarland and Osborne approach has been more recently modified by the use of a trochanteric osteotomy, still keeping the abductors and the quadriceps in continuity with the greater trochanteric fragment. It is now known as the trochanteric slide.[3,4]

Bauer described a transgluteal lateral approach in 1979, and Hardinge modified Bauer's approach in 1982 and should be credited with the direct lateral approach as we know it today.[5,6] In Hardinge's approach, an anterior cuff of tissue, comprised of the medius, minimus, anterior capsule, and the anterior portion of the vastus lateralis is reflected anteriorly, exposing the femoral neck.

In 1986, Dall modified Hardinge's direct lateral approach. He advocated taking a thin wafer of bone from the anterior portion of the greater trochanter.[7] The entire gluteus minimus muscle and the anterior portion of the gluteus medius and capsule are reflected anteriorly with the wafer of bone. Dall felt that the proximal split in the abductor muscles should extend only 2 cm above the tip of the greater trochanter to make sure that the superior gluteal nerve was not damaged.

This chapter describes the surgical anatomy, surgical technique, and postoperative rehabilitation of the direct lateral approach which is the senior author's choice for most primary hip arthroplasties and for simple revisions. A modification of the direct lateral approach is the vastus slide that offers the proximal advantages of the direct lateral approach and provides an extensive and extensile exposure to the entire shaft of the femur.[3]

Surgical Anatomy

Although the gluteus medius is a much larger muscle then the gluteus minimus muscle, a significant portion of the medius is a flexor and internal rotator. The tendon of the gluteus medius attaches to the lateral and posterior aspect of the greater trochanter. The posterior muscle fibers of the gluteus medius are oriented almost vertically and the anterior fibers are transverse (Fig. 34.1).

The gluteus minimus is a smaller muscle but is a pure abductor and is probably similar in abductor strength to the gluteus medius. The tendon of the gluteus minimus inserts on the front of the greater trochanter, anterior to the vastus tubercle. Its fibers are oriented obliquely toward the anterior portion of the greater trochanter (Fig. 34.2). Proximal to the greater trochanter, the muscle belly of the gluteus minimus lies on the lateral capsule which is the inferior fascia of this muscle. The capsule and the muscle fibers of the minimus attach to the inferior and medial aspect of the greater trochanter just superior to the femoral neck. There is a consistent layer of fat between the gluteus medius and minimus (Fig. 34.3). It is not possible to close these two muscles back to the trochanter with a single suture because they arise from

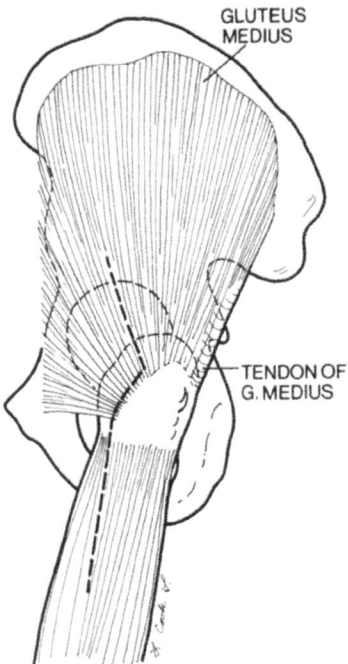

Figure 34.1. The posterior muscle fibers of the gluteus medius are oriented almost vertically and the anterior fibers are transverse.

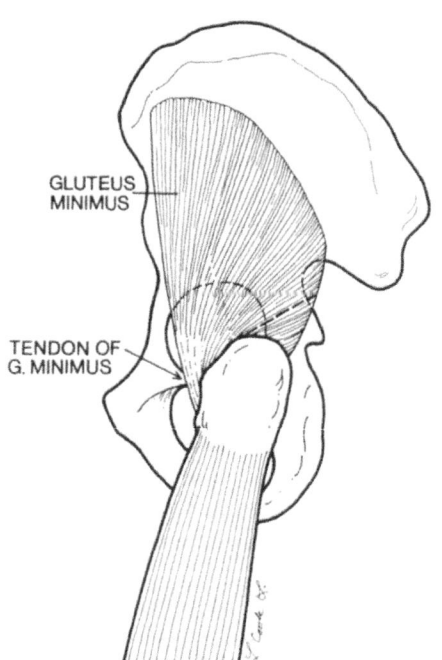

Figure 34.2. The fibers of the gluteus minimus are oriented obliquely towards the anterior portion of the greater trochanter. The gluteus minimus tendon inserts on to the front of the greater trochanter just anterior to the vastus tubercle.

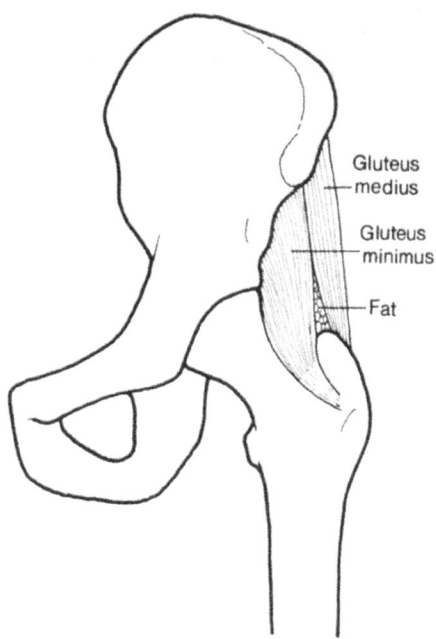

Figure 34.3. In between the gluteus medius and gluteus minimus there is a consistent layer of fat.

separate anatomic areas. If the minimus is not anatomically reattached to the anterior aspect of the greater trochanter, there will be a significant limp.

The superior gluteal nerve emerges from the pelvis through the greater sciatic foramen, superior to the piriformis muscle, and runs horizontally between the abductors. It is the motor nerve for the gluteus medius, minimus, and tensor fascia femoris. Jacobs and Buxton have described the pattern of branching and distribution of the superior gluteal nerve in reference to the greater trochanter.[8] They feel there is a 5 cm "safe-zone" between the top of the greater trochanter and the superior gluteal nerve (Fig. 34.4). Bos and others have shown that there is variability in the nerves innervation of the muscles, and that there may be an inferior branch as close as 3 cm from the greater trochanter.[8,9,10] The superior gluteal nerve is, therefore, at risk when the gluteus medius and minimus are split too far proximally. Injury to this nerve denervates that portion of the gluteus medius and minimus that are anterior to the injury as well as the entire tensor fascia femoris.

In some situations, where the center of rotation of the hip is high (developmental dysplasia or in some revision circumstances) the safe zone between the trochanter and the nerve is diminished (Fig. 34.5). The direct lateral approach is, therefore, contraindicated in the patient with a high center of rotation.

Surgical Technique

The direct lateral approach can be done in either the supine position as advocated by Hardinge or in the lateral position. We feel that it is preferable to use the lateral position as gravity pulls the subcutaneous fat away

34. Direct Lateral and Vastus Slide Approach

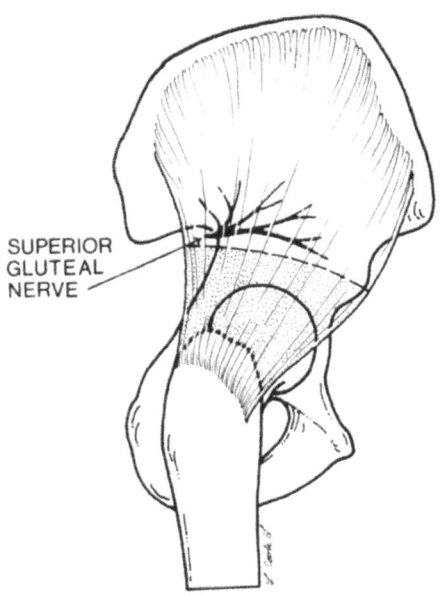

Figure 34.4. There is a safe area that is roughly 5 cm above the greater trochanter where a split in the gluteus minimus will not injure the superior gluteal nerve.

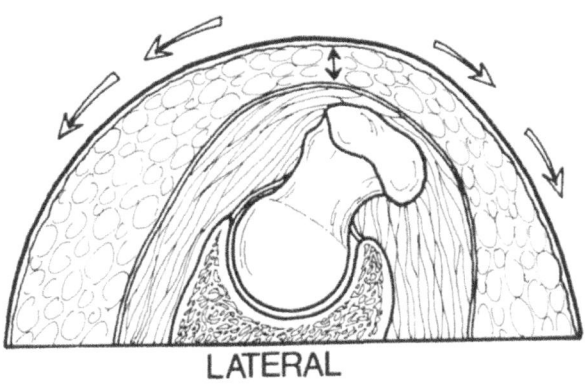

Figure 34.6. The thickness of the subcutaneous fat is diminished by the force of gravity with the patient in the lateral position.

from the area of the incision (Figs. 34.6 and 34.7). This is especially important when operating on the obese patient. In obese patients, undermining the fat anteriorly and posteriorly at the level of the deep fascia, dramatically increases exposure as the fat retracts itself by gravity (Fig. 34.8).

The skin incision begins 4 to 6 cm proximal to the greater trochanter and is centered over the interval between the gluteus maximus and tensor fascia femoris. It extends 10 to 12 cm distally over the midshaft of the femur (Fig. 34.9). The incision is made longer in the obese patient.

At the level of the deep fascia, the distal split in the fascia is begun over the shaft of the femur. It is extended proximally between the tensor fascia femoris and the gluteus maximus. This split can also be through the most anterior portion of the gluteus maximus. The trochanteric bursa should be divided slightly posterior to the midline to avoid the vascular plexus that lies within the anterior fatty portion of the bursa. Posteriorly, the tendon of the gluteus medius should be palpated. The muscle fibers of the gluteus medius should be split at the anterior border of the greater trochanter using two wing tipped or Cobb elevators. This split is roughly 4 to 5 cm anterior to the posterior border of the gluteus medius. Therefore, the majority of the abductor portion of the medius remains attached to the greater trochanter (Fig. 34.10). Care should be made to avoid splitting the gluteus medius more than 4 to 5 cm proximal to the greater trochanter to avoid injury to the superior gluteal nerve. If the split in the medius is made at the anterior border of the greater trochanter, only the anterior fibers (that are flexors and internal rotators) would be denervated if the nerve was inadvertently damaged and the portion of the medius that is a pure abductor would still be preserved. After splitting the medius, a fat pad is consistently encountered overlying the minimus (Fig. 34.11). The posterior border of the minimus and the pir-

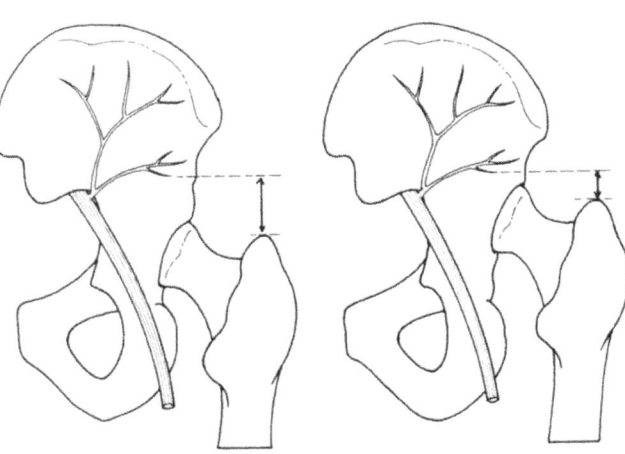

Figure 34.5. If the center of rotation of the hip is higher than normal, the safe zone between the trochanter and the superior gluteal nerve is diminished.

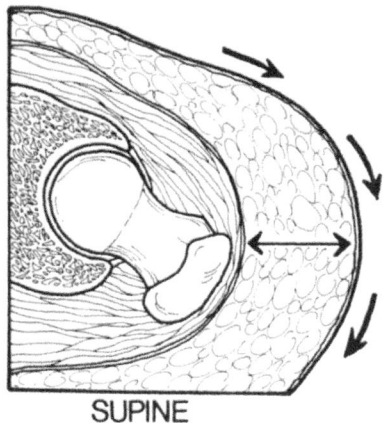

Figure 34.7. In the supine position, the thickness of fat is increased.

iformis tendon can be palpated. The split in the gluteus minimus fascia is made sharply, paralleling its fibers, and should be about 1 cm anterior to its posterior border (Fig. 34.2). After the fascia has been incised, the muscle fibers of the minimus can be separated with two wing-tipped elevators to expose the capsule. The incision in the capsule is made parallel to the split in the gluteus medius, and extends proximally to the acetabular labrum.

At the distal portion of the split in the gluteus medius, electrocautery is used to divide the anterior tendinous cuff of the gluteus medius from the front of the trochanter. Distally this incision should extend just anterior to the vastus tubercle, ensuring that a strong tendinous cuff of tissue will be left on the greater trochanter for later repair (Fig. 34.11). If this incision in the anterior portion of the medius is made too posteriorly on the greater trochanter, there will not be a cuff left on the trochanter for later repair. If the incision is made too anteriorly, the soft muscle fibers of the gluteus medius will not hold sutures.

Distally, the incision extends below the greater trochanter into the anterior fascia of the quadriceps for 5 to 6 cm. The quadriceps is split with two wing-tipped

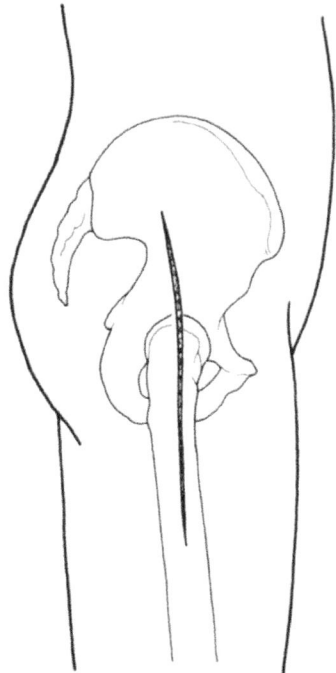

Figure 34.9. The skin incision is centered over the interval between the gluteus maximus and tensor fascia femoris. It begins 4 to 6 cm proximal to the greater trochanter and extends distally 10 to 12 cm over the midshaft of the femur.

elevators to expose the shaft (Fig. 34.11). Just distal to the vastus ridge, a consistent transverse branch of the lateral circumflex vessel should be identified and ligated (Fig. 34.11 and 34.12). A one-half inch curved osteotome is then used to subperiosteally dissect the anterior aspect of the vastus lateralis off the femur just anterior to the greater trochanter.

At this point, the soft tissues can be sharply dissected from the front of the trochanter, keeping the anterior cuff of the medius, minimus, capsule, and quadriceps in continuity. (Fig. 34.13) Alternatively a thin wafer of bone can be divided from the anterior trochanter as described by Dall.[7] (Fig. 34.14 to 34.16) For several years we used Dall's technique, but have had occasional prob-

Figure 34.8. To increase exposure in the obese patient, it is helpful to undermine the fat both anteriorly and posteriorly at the level of the deep fascia. The fat retracts itself by gravity.

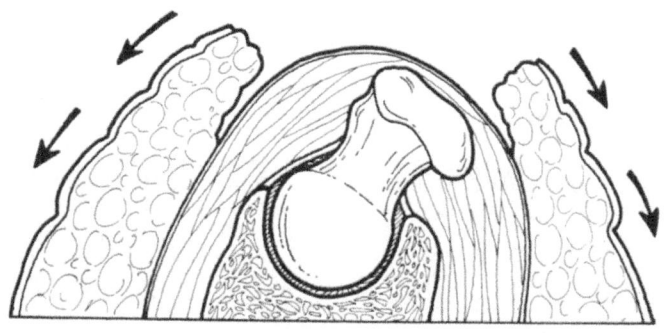

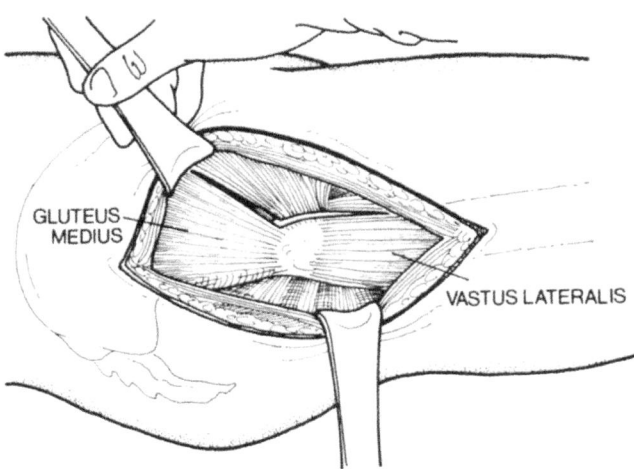

Figure 34.10. The muscle fibers of the gluteus medius should be split at the anterior border of the greater trochanter. This split is roughly 4 or 5 cm anterior to the posterior border of the gluteus medius. It should not be made more than 4 to 5 cm proximal to the greater trochanter to avoid injury into the superior gluteal nerve.

lems of nonunion of the anterior trochanteric fragment (even though this has not resulted in weakness) and have had a significant incidence of trochanteric bursitis from fixation wires or cables. On one occasion, a traumatic transverse fracture of the proximal tip of the greater trochanteric occurred postoperatively, resulting in abductor weakness and requiring reattachment. It is now the senior author's preference to remove the soft tissue cuff from the front of the trochanter rather than to remove a wafer of bone.

The hip is dislocated anteriorly with flexion, adduction and external rotation. A Bennett retractor is placed behind the inferior portion of the greater trochanter and just above the lesser trochanter, translating the femur forward so the neck can be resected. Care should be made to avoid placing this retractor under the proximal portion of the greater trochanter, as the trochanter could fracture if it is osteopenic.

After the head has been removed, the best exposure of the acetabulum is afforded by placing the femur in 25° of flexion, 20° of adduction and neutral rotation (to relax the iliopsoas). A bone hook, placed above the lesser trochanter, is helpful to translate the femur posteriorly. The labrum is excised circumferentially. A com-

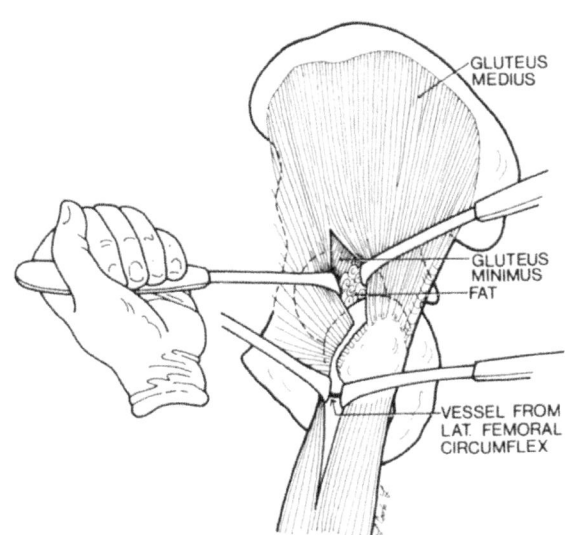

Figure 34.11. After splitting the gluteus medius with wing-tipped elevators, a fat pad is consistently found overlying the gluteus minimus. Wing-tipped elevators are also used to split the anterior portion of the vastus lateralis. A consistent transverse branch of the lateral circumflex vessels is routinely encountered at the anterior and inferior border of the greater trochanter.

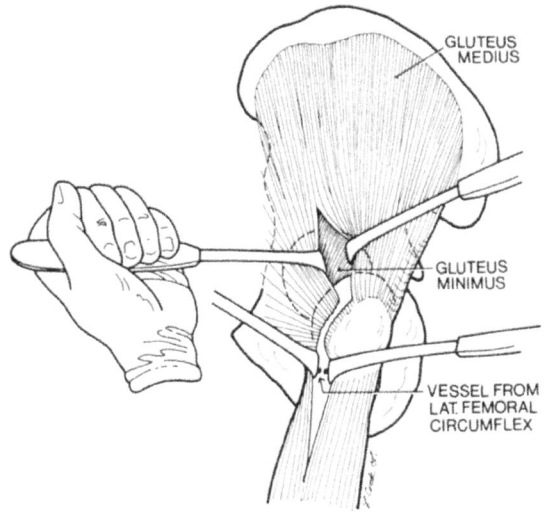

Figure 34.12. The split in the gluteus minimus fascia is made sharply paralleling its fibers and should be approximately 1 cm from its posterior border. Splitting the muscle fibers of minimus with two wing-tipped retractors, this will expose the capsule of the hip joint. The incision in the capsule is made parallel to the split in the gluteus medius. Note that the transverse vessel from the lateral femoral circumflex has been ligated.

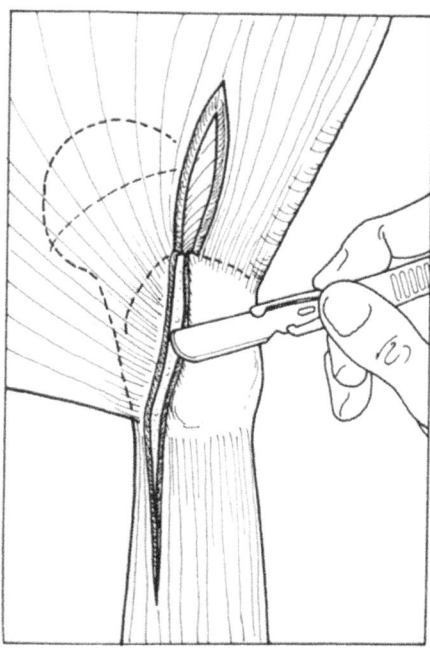

Figure 34.13. A scalpel is used to sharply dissect the soft tissues from the front of the greater trochanter. This anterior cuff includes the medius, minimus, anterior capsule and anterior portion of the vastus lateralis.

plete capsulotomy is performed. Anteriorly, the capsulotomy should extend at least one centimeter and one half. This anterior capsulotomy helps to release flexion contractures and greatly improves exposure. A capsulectomy is never necessary in primary total hip arthroplasty. Hip retractors, placed anteriorly and posteriorly are used to retract the capsule. A Cobra retractor placed

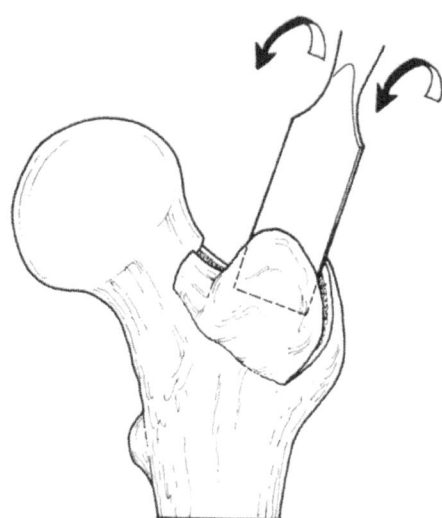

Figure 34.15. An osteotome is used to elevate the anterior portion of the trochanter. Attached to this anterior wafer of bone are the gluteus medius, minimus, anterior capsule and the anterior portion of the vastus lateralis.

anteriorly and inferiorly, just posterior to the iliopsoas tendon, helps to provide optimal exposure of the acetabulum.

Preparation of the femur is facilitated by positioning the limb within a sterile pouch in about 50° to 60° of flexion, 30° of adduction and neutral rotation. A Bennett retractor, placed at the inferior portion of the greater trochanter, translates the femur anteriorly. It may be necessary to release the inferior capsule from the femoral neck to facilitate anterior translation of the femur. Placement of a thin flat retractor over the gluteus medius protects this muscle during reaming of the femoral canal.

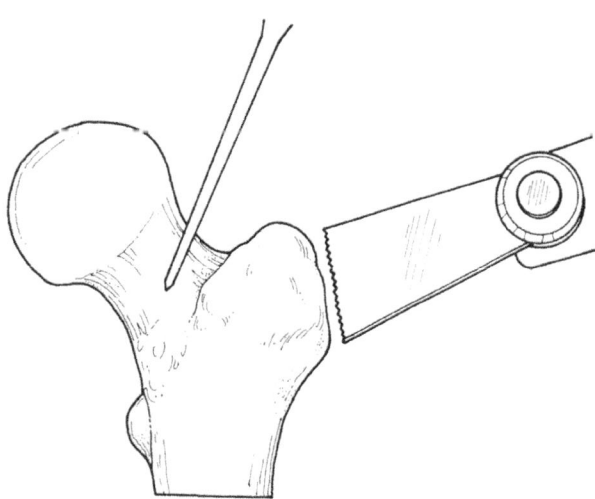

Figure 34.14. An alternative method is to take a thin wafer of bone from the anterior trochanter with an oscillating saw. A counter cut in the anterior portion of the neck is helpful.

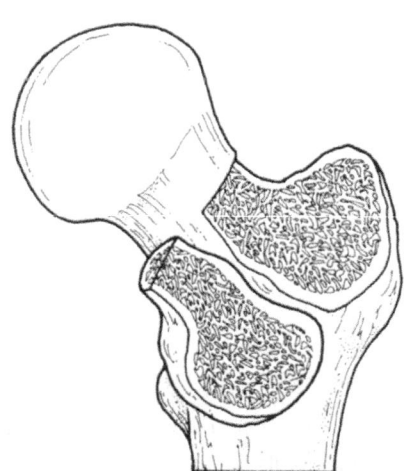

Figure 34.16. The wafer of bone is reflected anteriorly to expose the femoral neck.

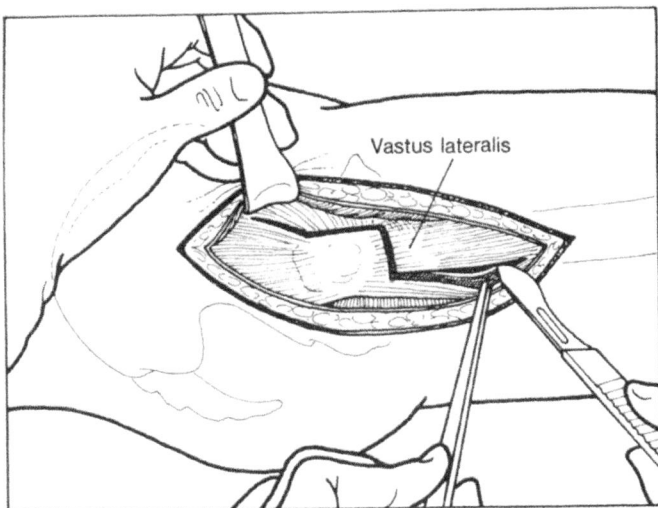

Figure 34.17. The vastus slide is a modification of the direct lateral approach. Proximally the dissection is the same but at the distal aspect of the greater trochanter, the incision in the quadriceps fascia is directed posteriorly leaving a one-quarter inch of cuff for reattachment. The incision then extends distally at the posterior border of the vastus fascia.

Vastus Slide

If more extensive exposure of the femoral shaft is required, the direct lateral approach can be modified. The proximal development of the anterior cuff of tissue remains the same, but at the distal aspect of the greater trochanter, a transverse posterior incision is made in the quadriceps fascia, leaving a 5 mm to 1 cm cuff of the vastus fascia attached to the greater trochanter for later closure. (Fig. 34.17) At the posterior border of the greater trochanter, the incision in the quadriceps fascia is directed distally about 1 cm from its posterior insertion. The quadriceps muscle fibers are initially dissected free from the investing fascia posteriorly, then from the intermuscular septum and finally from the femoral shaft (Fig. 34.18). Perforating vessels are isolated and ligated as the dissection is continued distally. The quadriceps musculature is then mobilized anteriorly in continuity with the proximal cuff of tissue (Fig. 34.19).

This approach provides the same acetabular exposure as the direct lateral approach, but has the advantage of wide and extensile exposure of the femur. The vastus slide is ideal when modest exposure of the acetabulum is required, but extensive exposure of the femur is necessary. In the revision situation, when the femoral component does not need to be removed, the vastus slide offers better exposure of the acetabulum, because the femur can more easily be translated posteriorly. The vastus slide is also helpful for hardware removal from the proximal lateral femur.

Intraoperative Testing for Stability

With either the direct lateral or the vastus slide, it is important to determine the stability of the hip with trial components prior to closure. The hip is first tested in extension, adduction, and external rotation. It is then

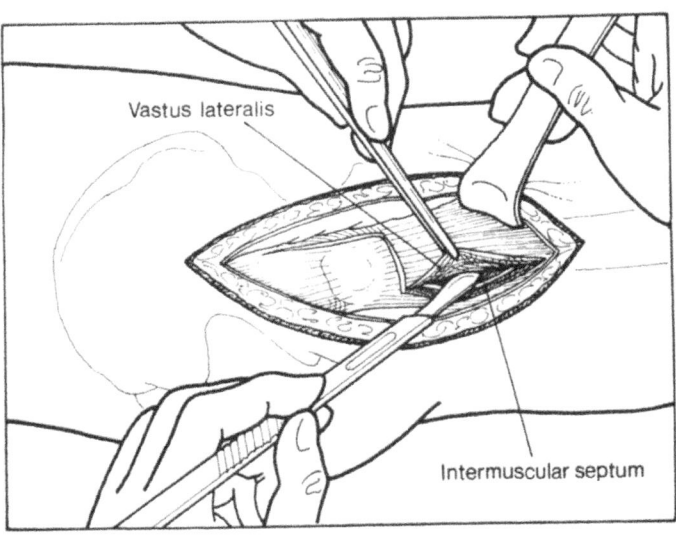

Figure 34.18. All quadriceps fibers are dissected first from the fascia, then from the intermuscular septum and then from the shaft of the femur. Perforating vessels are isolated and ligated as the incision is continued distally.

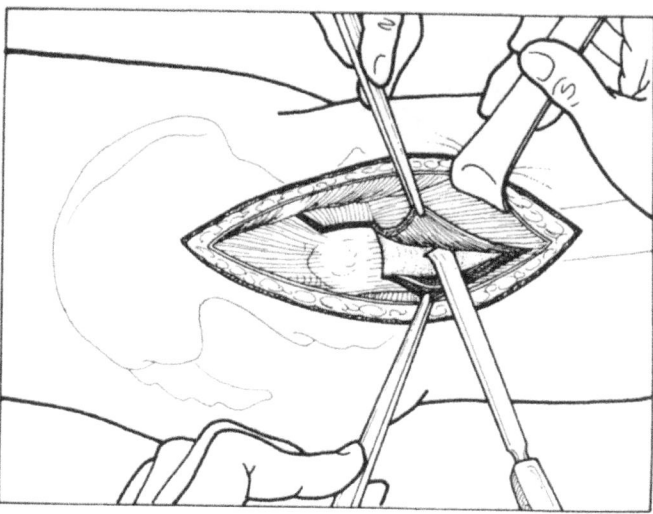

Figure 34.19. The entire quadriceps is mobilized anteriorly with the anterior cuff of the gluteus medius, gluteus minimus and capsule, exposing the anterior and lateral aspects of the femur as well as the anterior and superior acetabulum.

tested in flexion, adduction and internal rotation, looking specifically at the mid-range from 60° to 90° of flexion and the extreme range from 90° to maximum flexion, both combined with maximum adduction and internal rotation. If instability is noted, every attempt should be made to increase stability by improving the mechanics of the hip. The first step is to look for impinging osteophytes and to remove these. With modular components, a longer trial head can be used. If modular femoral components such as the S-ROM (Johnson and Johnson, Raynham, Massachusetts) have been used, more anteversion or retroversion can be tested with trial components. A lipped trial component can be used in the metal acetabular shell but if the shell is malpositioned, it should be changed to the optimal orientation.

Closure

It is important to anatomically close the soft tissues. The capsule is closed from proximal to distal with a running #1 resorbable suture, starting at the superior rim of the acetabulum. The fascia of the gluteus minimus is also closed from proximal to distal with a #1 resorbable suture (Fig. 34.20).

At this point if an anterior wafer of the greater trochanter has been removed, it can be reattached using three twisted #16 chrome-cobalt monofilament wires or three #5 nonresorbable sutures, placed through drill holes in the greater trochanter and passed around the anterior fragment. A circumferential Dall Miles cable, combined with Merciline tape (Ethicon, Johnson and Johnson, Somerville, NJ) can also be used.

When a soft tissue cuff has been utilized, it is helpful to first decorticate the anterior portion of the greater trochanter to ensure that the gluteus minimus can be reattached to bleeding cancellous bone (Fig. 34.21).

Superiorly, the cuff of the minimus and capsule should be anatomically reattached to the base of the trochanter using a #2 nonabsorbable mattress suture through bone. Three to five additional #2 nonabsorbable mattress sutures can be passed through the bone of the greater trochanter to anatomically reattach the anterior cuff of minimus (Fig. 34.22). With osteopenic bone these su-

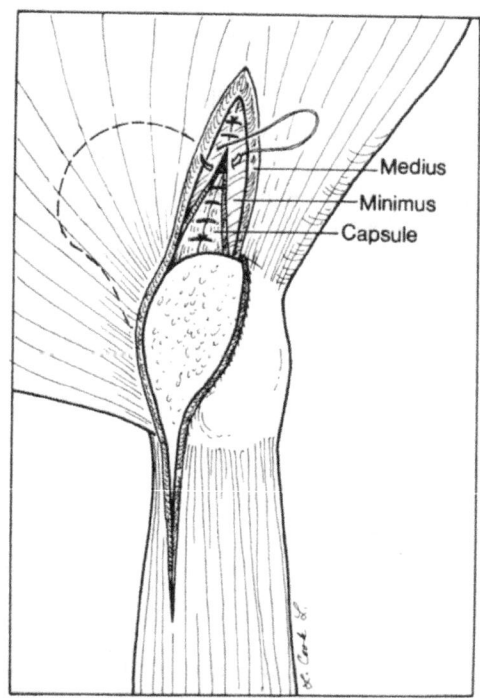

Figure 34.20. The closure begins with the capsule which is closed from proximal to distal with a running #1 resorbable suture. Following this, the fascia of the minimus is closed in a similar fashion.

34. Direct Lateral and Vastus Slide Approach

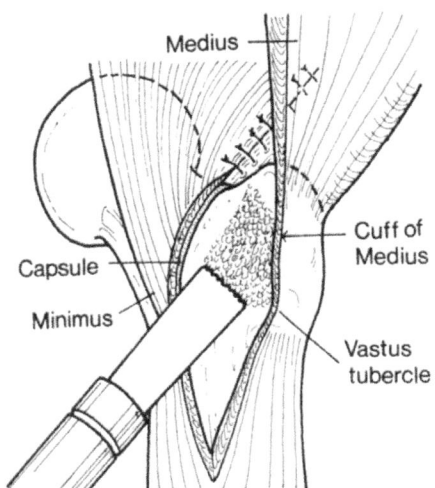

Figure 34.21. The anterior portion of the greater trochanter is decorticated with an oscillating saw to ensure reattachment of the gluteus minimus to bleeding cancellous bone.

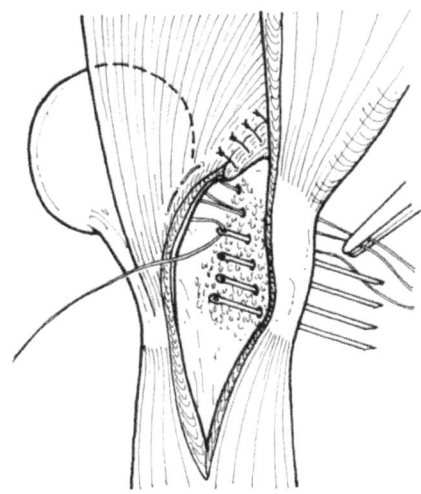

Figure 34.23. Keith needles passed through drill holes are an alternative method of reattaching the gluteus minimus and capsule to the anterior trochanter.

tures can be passed through the trochanter with a sharp trochar needle. With harder bone, it may be necessary to first make drillholes in order to pass these sutures. An alternative technique is to pass Keith needles through drillholes. If Keith needles are to be used, the drillholes are best made with smooth K-wires that are 5/64 inch in diameter (Fig. 34.23). These thin K-wires can be bowed as they are drilled, making it easier to place the holes anatomically. Suture anchors can also be used and work well, but are very expensive. The most distal of these sutures picks up the minimus, medius, and anterior cuff of the quadriceps, attaching all of these structures together to the area of the vastus tubercle (Fig. 34.24). The hip is abducted and internally rotated while these sutures are tied from proximal to distal.

The anterior cuff of the gluteus medius is closed with a separate #1 running resorbable suture, starting 1 cm proximal to the greater trochanter and running distally (Fig. 34.25). The fascia of the vastus lateralis is closed with the same running suture. If the vastus slide ap-

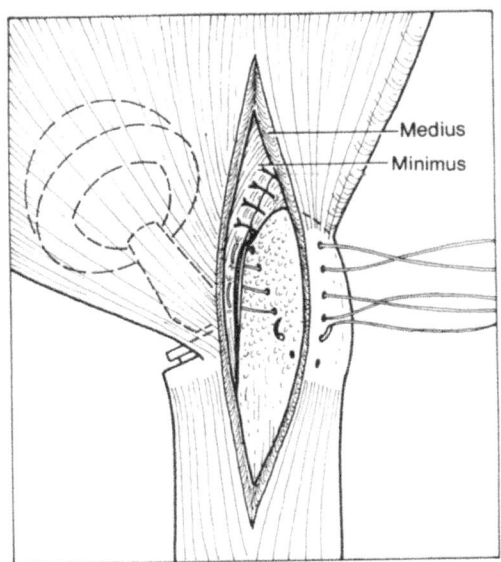

Figure 34.22. Superiorly the cuff of the minimus and capsule should be anatomically reattached to the base of the trochanter using #2 nonabsorbable mattress sutures through bone. Additional mattress sutures can be passed through the bone of the greater trochanter to anatomically reattach the minimus and capsule to the anterior trochanter.

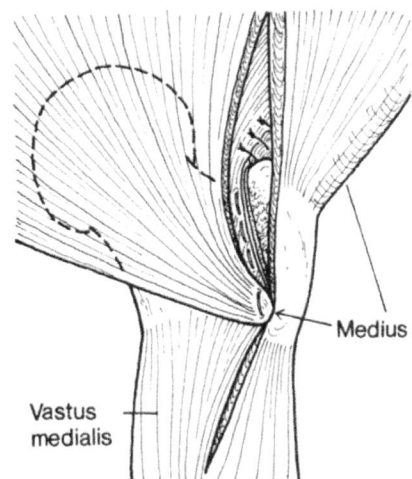

Figure 34.24. The most distal aspect of these nonabsorbable sutures picks up the minimus, medius, and anterior cuff of the quadriceps and attaches all of these structures to the area of the vastus tubercle.

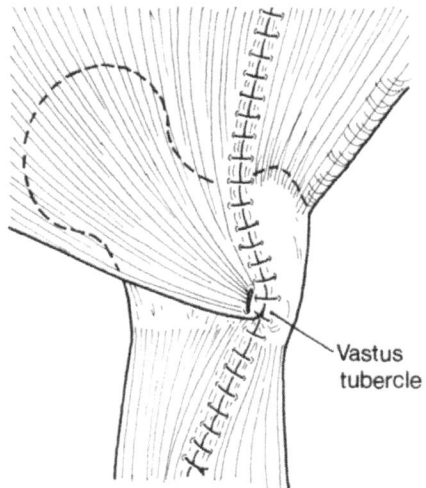

Figure 34.25. The anterior cuff of the gluteus medius is now reattached with a running number 1 resorbable suture. The fascia of vastus lateralis is included in this closure.

proach is used, the running suture stops at the vastus tubercle. The transverse incision in the quadriceps fascia is closed with interrupted pulley sutures and the distal posterior split is closed with a running number 1 suture.

The deep fascia is strongest in its mid-portion and becomes thinner proximally and distally. For this reason the closure of the deep fascia starts in the middle, just distal to the muscle fibers of the gluteus maximus. The fascia is run proximally with one number 1 resorbable suture. A second running suture also starts in the middle and is run distally.

Although drains are controversial, it is our preference to use a deep drain below the deep fascia and a second drain in the subcutaneous layer to prevent subcutaneous hematoma formation. The fat is closed with a deep layer of number 2.0 resorbable suture and then multiple interrupted number 2.0 sutures. We prefer to close the skin with a 3.0 subcuticular running suture and steri-stripes.

The postoperative dressing consists of sterile bandages about the hip and an ace bandage wrap that extends from the base of the toes to around the waist. This dressing is kept on for 48 hours and helps to compress any dead spaces which are also drained by the suction drains. The suction drains are not sutured in place and are removed 12 to 24 hours after the initial procedure without disturbing the compression dressing.

Postoperatively patients are placed in pillow suspension for the first night after surgery. This suspension is removed the following day, and ambulation begins with protective weight-bearing of 60 to 80 pounds. A walker is used initially, but the majority of patients move onto axillary crutches. Protective weight-bearing is continued for six weeks to allow the anterior cuff of tissue to become firmly attached to the greater trochanter. All patients are encouraged to flex maximally and many can flex as high as 120° while in the hospital. However, we do not encourage patients to flex their hip in combination with significant adduction and internal rotation. Patients are encouraged to dress their feet while in the hospital, flexing down in an abducted and externally rotated position as an exercise. The majority are shown how to cross the ankle of the operated leg on the opposite knee in order to dress the feet (abduction and external rotation). Most patients turn prone by the third day, and do active hip extension with their knee straight (hamstrings) and with the knee flexed 90° (gluteus maximus). They are not allowed to do side lying abduction for 6 weeks. The majority of patients are taught to get up on their hands and knees and to try to place their buttock on their heels and to flex the elbows so they can put their chin between their knees (Figs. 34.26 and 34.27).

At six weeks, patients are seen, and are weaned from support observing two rules: they are not allowed to limp or to have increased pain as they diminish support. The majority of patients walk without a limp at 6 weeks, and most are off of all support by 10 weeks. At six weeks, patients are encouraged to do active side lying abduction. It is important with side lying abduction that patients roll slightly toward their abdomen (about 20°) to ensure that the gluteus medius and minimus are being used and not the tensor fascia femoris. Patients continue with abductor and extensor strengthening until they can walk indefinite distances without support. Straight leg raising is discouraged because this exercise can so commonly cause groin pain and because it stresses the anterior repair.

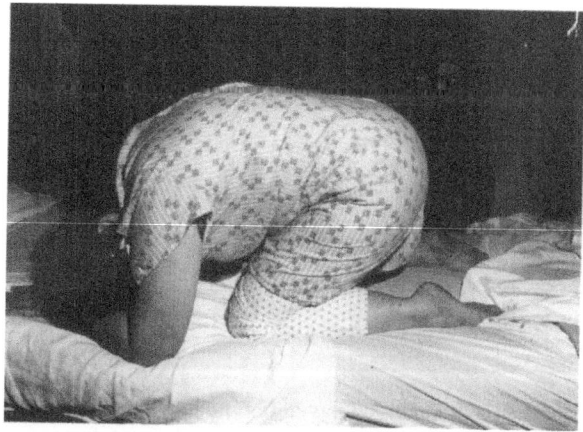

Figure 34.26. By the 3rd or 4th postoperative day, most patients are taught to get up on their hands and knees and to try to place their buttocks on their heels and to flex their elbows so they can put their chin between their knees.

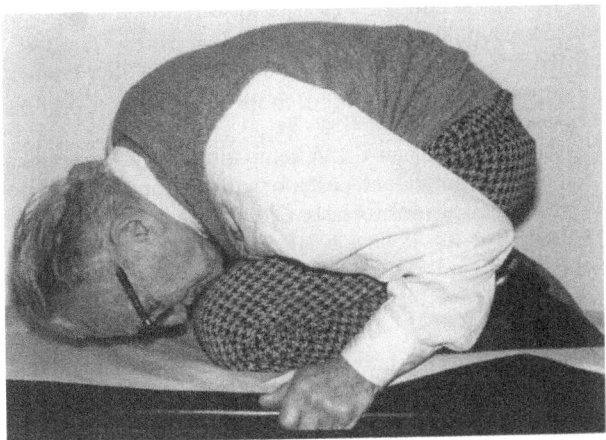

Figure 34.27. Some patients eventually achieve maximum flexion.

Discussion

The great advantage of the direct lateral approach is the low incidence of dislocation after total hip replacement. Vicar and Coleman reported a dislocation rate of 9.5% with the posterior approach and 2.2% with the Hardinge approach.[11] A higher rate of dislocation after the posterior approach is well recognized in the literature.[12,13,14] In our series of over 900 primary total hip replacements that have been done using the direct lateral approach, there have been only two dislocations. One heavy patient fell in a small bathroom two weeks postoperatively. The hip was forced into flexion adduction and internal rotation and she sustained a posterior dislocation. A closed reduction was performed, but she eventually required revision because of recurrent dislocation. One other 6'10" male had a single posterior dislocation because there were no standard components that matched his unusual offset. In retrospect we should have used a custom component. This patient remained stable after closed reduction and treatment with four weeks of a brace.

There is concern by many surgeons that patients have a limp after the direct lateral approach. This will surely be the case if the abductors are not meticulously repaired, and the proximal split in the abductors must be conservative in order to avoid super gluteal nerve damage. Baker and Bitounis found evidence of denervation of the abductor muscles in 15% of their patients after the direct lateral approach.[10] Using electromyography (EMG) studies, Ramesh et al. found superior gluteal nerve damage in 11% of their patients after the direct lateral approach. Patients with damage to the superior gluteal nerve in their series had a persistent Trendelenburg gait.[15]

However, Pai et al. found no difference in adbuctor weakness or limp when the Hardinge, the transtrochanteric, and the Liverpool approaches were compared.[16] This finding is similar to Minns' study of muscle strength after total hip arthroplasty, comparing trochanteric osteotomy and the direct lateral approach.[17] Mostradi also demonstrated superior abductor strength with the direct lateral approach compared to the transtrochanteric approach.[18] In our series, no patient has a limp that we feel is related to the approach. However, we have not done EMG studies, and perhaps there has been nerve damage that we have not recognized. If the split in the medius is made posteriorly and the nerve is damaged, all fibers of the abductors that are anterior to the damaged nerve will be denervated and the patient will clearly limp. If the split in the medius is made at the anterior portion of the greater trochanter, just at the junction of the abductor and flexor portion of the gluteus medius, only the anterior fibers of the medius will be denervated and a limp probably will not be present because the pure abductor portion of the medius still has a nerve supply. Flexion and internal rotation of the hip might still be possible using other muscles. Therefore, it is possible that the superior gluteal nerve has been damaged in some of our patients who had a negative Trendelenburg gait.

Heterotopic bone after direct lateral approach is common. Horwitz reported an incidence of 45% in patients after the Hardinge approach, but only 8% of their patients had Brooker class that was greater than two.[19] Vicar and Coleman found that heterotopic bone was three times more common in their patients who had a posterior lateral or transtrochanteric approach than with the direct lateral approach.[11] In our series, heterotopic bone in the area of reattachment of the abductors has been very common and approaches 30% to 40%. However, this bone is distal and over the trochanter. Only one patient in our series has had bone formation that limits motion.

Conclusion

The direct lateral approach provides excellent exposure of both the acetabulum and femur for primary hip arthroplasty and simple revisions. The vastus slide modifies the distal portion of the direct lateral approach and gives wide distal exposure of the shaft for complex femoral reconstruction during revision surgery. If extensive superior exposure of the acetabulum is required, the direct lateral approach is not recommended because any proximal extension of the split in the abductors will injure the superior gluteal nerve. The transtrochanteric, posterolateral, or trochanteric slide will afford greater exposure of the acetabulum for complex revisions and primaries, such as developmental dysplasia.

Closure of the anterior cuff of tissue, gluteus medius, minimus, capsule and vastus lateralis, must be meticulous and anatomic. If care is made to avoid damage to the superior gluteal nerve and careful closure is performed, the direct lateral approach provides excellent postoperative stability and early functional recovery.

References

1. Watson-Jones R. Fractures of the neck of the femur. *Br J Surg.* 1936;23:787.
2. McFarland B, Osborne G. Approach to the hip: a suggested improvement on kochers method. *J Bone Joint Surg Br.* 1954;36:364.
3. Chandler HP, Penenberg BL. Surgical approaches. In: Chandler HP, Penenberg BL, eds. *Bone Stock Deficiency in Total Hip Arthroplasty.* Thorofare, NJ: Slack; 1989:Chapter 4.
4. Glassman AH, Engh CA, Bobyn JD. A technique of extensile exposure for total hip arthroplasty. *J Arthroplasty.* 1987;2:11–21.
5. Bauer R, Kerschbaumer F, Poisel S, Oberthaler W. Transgluteal approach to the hip. *Arch Orthop Trauma Surg.* 1979;95:47–49.
6. Hardinge K. The direct lateral approach to the hip. *J Bone J Surg Br.* 1982;17–19.
7. Dall D. Exposure of the hip by anterior osteotomy of the greater trochanter: a modified anterolateral approach. *J Bone J Surg Br.* 1986;68:382–386.
8. Jacobs LGH, Buxton RA. The course of the superior gluteal nerve in the lateral approach to the hip. *J Bone J Surg Am.* 1989;71:1239–1243.
9. Bos JC, Stoeckart R, Klooswijk AI, van Linge B, Bahadoer R. The surgical anatomy of the superior gluteal nerve and anatomical radiologic basis of the direct lateral approach to the hip. *Surg Radiol Anat.* 1994;16:253–258.
10. Baker AS, Bitounis VC. Abductor function after total hip replacement: an electromyographic and clinical review. *J Bone J Surg Br.* 1985;71:47–50.
11. Vicar AJ, Coleman CR. A comparison of the anterlateral transtrochanteric and posterior surgical approaches in primary total hip arthroplasty. *Clin Orthop.* 1984;199:152–159.
12. Robinson RP, Robinson HJ, Salvati EA. Comparison of transtrochanteric and posterior approaches for total hip arthroplasty. *Clin Orthop.* 1980;149:143–147.
13. Lewinneck GE, Lewis JL, Tarr R., Compere CL, Zimmerman JR. Dislocation after total hip replacement arthroplasty. *J Bone J Surg Am.* 1978;60:217–220.
14. Woo RYG, Morrey BF. Dislocation after total hip arthroplasty, *J Bone J Surg Am.* 1982;64:1295–1306.
15. Ramesh M, O'Byrne JM, McCarthy N. Damage to the superior gluteal nerve after the Hardinge approach to the hip. *J Bone J Surg Br.* 1996;78:903–906.
16. Pai VS. Significance of the Trendelenberg test in total hip arthroplasty: influence of the lateral approach. *J Arthroplasty.* 1996;11:174–179.
17. Minns RJ, Crawford RJ, Porter MD, Hardinge K. Muscle strength following total hip arthroplasty: a comparison of trochanteric osteotomy and direct lateral approach. *J Arthroplasty.* 1993;8:625–627.
18. Mostardi RA, Askew MJ, Gradisar IA Jr., Hoyt WA Jr., Snyder R, Bailey B. Comparison of functional outcome of total hip arthroplasty involving four surgical approaches. *J Arthroplasty.* 1988;3:279–284.
19. Horwitz BR, Rockowitz NL, Goll SR. A prospective randomized comparison of two surgical approaches to total hip arthroplasty. *Clin Orthop.* 1993;281:154–163.

35
Modified Dall Approach

Desmond M. Dall

Approaches: Modified Dall

The anterior partial trochanteric osteotomy (APTO) approach was described in 1986.[1] In this approach, the anterior part of the greater trochanter is osteotomized (Fig. 35.1) and maintains the continuity of the tendinous junction between the anterior half of gluteus medius and the vastus lateralis and preserves intact the insertion of gluteus minimus into the anterior surface of the osteotomized trochanter (Fig. 35.2). The approach allows good exposure of the hip without sharp dissection of muscular insertions (gluteus medius and minimus) into the anterior trochanter, as is required in the direct lateral approach. Bony union restores full power in the abductors without the risk of tendons pulling away from bone.[2,3] Reattachment of the osteotomized fragment is simple and proximal detachment after operation, as sometimes seen after complete osteotomy of the greater trochanter, rarely occurs. In this approach, as in the direct lateral approach, splitting the gluteus medius carries the risk of superior gluteal nerve damage. For this reason, the approach has been modified by not splitting gluteus medius and keeping the muscle intact.[4] The osteotomy now extends posteriorly in the sagittal plane, to emerge deep to the posterior fibers of the insertion of gluteus medius, incorporating the whole lateral aspect of the greater trochanter. In this way, insertions of the whole gluteus medius and minimus and the origin of vastus lateralis from the vastus ridge remain attached to the fragment, and muscle integrity and strength is maintained.

The osteotomy is made with a Gigli saw, commencing anteriorly, deep to gluteus minimus tendon, thereby ensuring that the tendon is protected. This is in contrast to the usual trochanter slide approach technique that utilizes an oscillating saw from posterior to anterior, increasing the risk of damage to the gluteus minimus tendon.[5] The preservation of the attachment of vastus lateralis distally ensures that proximal detachment of the greater trochanter is unlikely to occur. Fixation of the fragment can be achieved with two cerclage, wires or cables and crimp sleeves, or if the limb is lengthened, with the Dall–Miles cable-grip system. The risk of superior gluteal nerve damage is almost abolished, and abductor function remains preserved. At the same time, the posterior capsule is not violated, and the incidence of postoperative dislocation is extremely low.

The approach can be used for revision total hip arthroplasty (THA) and provides excellent mobilization of the proximal femur for visualization and orientation. The approach also provides excellent visualization of the posterior and superior acetabulum but is slightly limited for anterior acetabular exposure as might be required in cases of pelvic discontinuity. In the latter, a classic trochanteric osteotomy with proximal mobilization of the fragment and the abductor muscles would be a preferable approach.

Technique

The patient is positioned in the lateral position. Make a straight lateral skin incision extending along the center of the shaft of the femur and greater trochanter to at least 7 cm proximal to the tip of the greater trochanter. The fascia lata is incised in line with the incision along the posterior margin of tensor fascia lata. The gluteus maximus muscle is split in the proximal part of the incision and the anterior margin of the gluteus medius is defined by blunt section. A Charnley initial incision retractor is inserted to provide wide exposure with the greater trochanter in the center of the wound. Using electrocautery, the posterior attachment of the vastus lateralis to the femur (close to the linea aspera) is incised longitudinally commencing from a point approximately 8 cm distal to the vastus ridge (Fig. 35.3). This incision is extended proximally along the posterior margin of the trochanter through the thick periosteum. The incision terminates at the posterior tip of the trochanter just behind the edge of the posterior tendinous insertion of gluteus medius. An angled Hohmann retractor is placed deep to the proximal rectus femoris, with its tip over the anterior margin of the acetabulum providing exposure of the anterior capsule. The plane between the su-

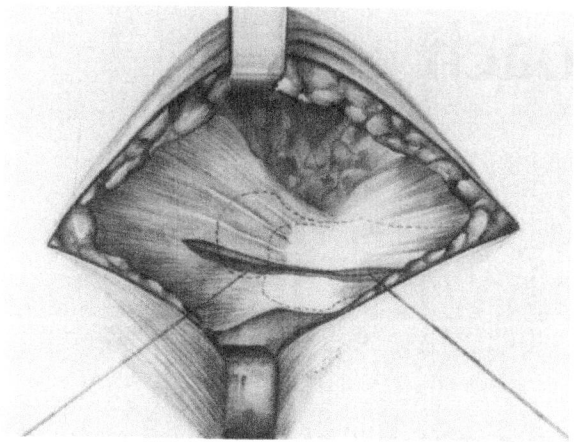

Figure 35.1. Original APTO approach. The anterior half of the greater trochanter is osteotomized using a Gigli saw passed deep to the tendons of gluteus minimus and the anterior half of gluteus medius. The saw is also passed deep to the vastus lateralis. (From Dall DM[1]- by permission of *J Bone Joint Surg*)

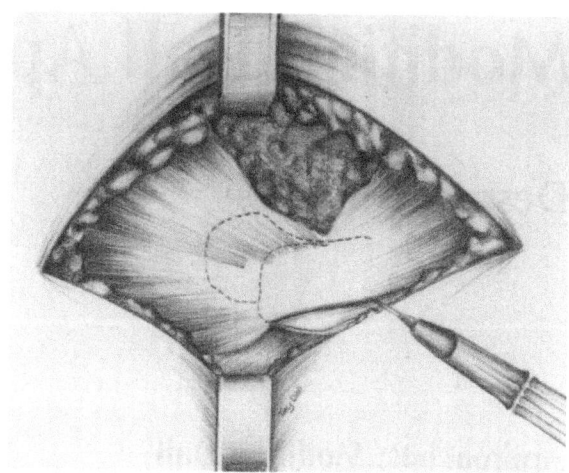

Figure 35.3. Modified approach. Incision through posterior fibers of vastus lateralis and periosteum along the posterior margin of the trochanter.

pero lateral capsule and the deep fibers and tendon of gluteus minimus is identified. A strong curved cholecystectomy forceps is passed deep to gluteus minimus in this plane from below, over the neck of the femur, outside the capsule deep to the whole of gluteus minimus. Remove the Hohmann retractor to facilitate this step. The tip of the forceps is then directed posteriorly to emerge behind the tip of the greater trochanter to grasp a Gigli saw. The saw, preferably of the long thin Stille type, is drawn back through to emerge at the anterior edge of gluteus medius. The cholecystectomy for-

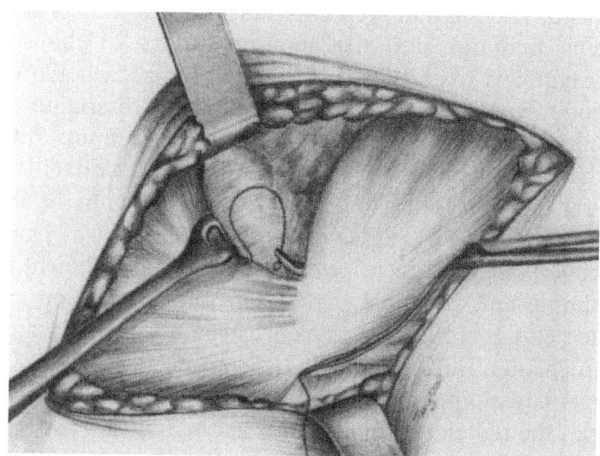

Figure 35.4. Modified approach. Gigli saw passed deep to vastus lateralis using a cholecystectomy forceps.

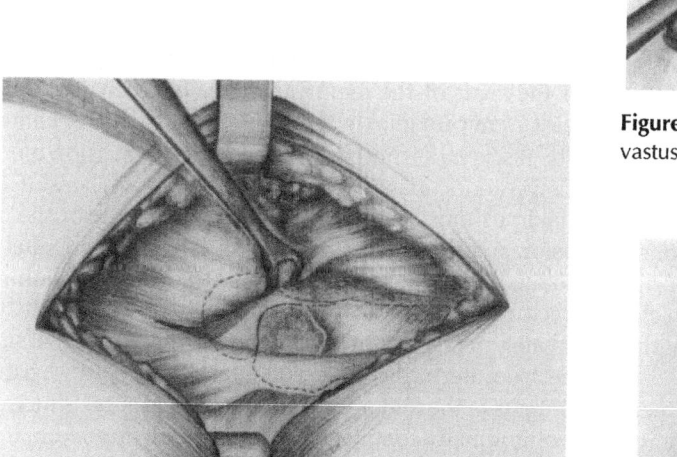

Figure 35.2. Original APTO approach. The osteotomized portion of the greater trochanter is mobilized anteriorly maintaining the continuity of the tendinous junction between the anterior half of gluteus medius and the vastus lateralis and preserves intact the insertion of gluteus minimus into the anterior surface of the osteotomized trochanter. This approach requires splitting the gluteus medius. (From Dall DM[1]- by permission of *J Bone Joint Surg*)

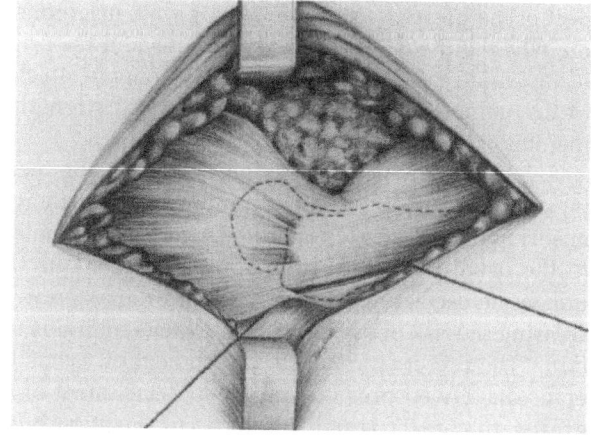

Figure 35.5. Modified approach. Osteotomy performed with a Gigli saw passed deep to gluteus minimus and medius as well as vastus lateralis. Gluteus medius is not split.

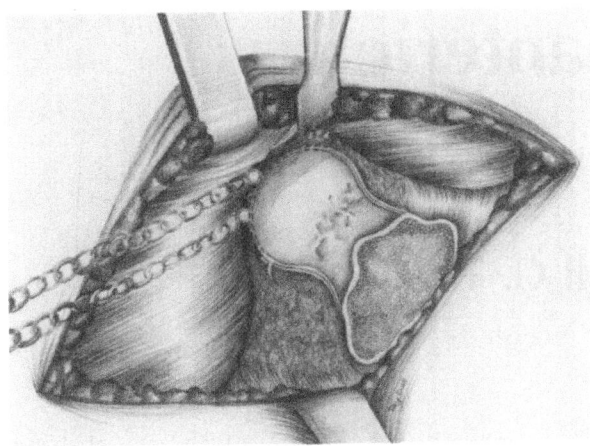

Figure 35.6. Modified approach. Mobilization of the trochanter anteriorly and medially retracted by the Hohmann retractor and Charnley pin retractors. The whole of gluteus medius and minimus as well as vastus lateralis remain intact and attached to the trochanter.

ceps are then passed, keeping close to the bone, from the incision along the posterior margin of the vastus lateralis to penetrate the vastus intermedius at a point just distal to the anterior distal insertion of gluteus medius (Fig. 35.4). The end of the Gigli saw is pulled back through and drawn against the bone. The trochanteric osteotomy is now performed with the Gigli saw (Fig. 35.5). The femur is fully internally rotated so that the osteotomy can be made almost in the sagittal plane. The ideal trochanteric fragment should not be more than 10 to 12 mm thick. In order to achieve this, the cut should commence as lateral as possible just medial to the insertion of the tendon of gluteus minimus. Sawing is begun with the hands as far apart as possible pulling in a posterior direction with the saw emerging at the posterior margin of the greater trochanter through the original electrocautery incision of the periosteum. At the completion of the osteotomy, the trochanteric fragment will have the whole of gluteus medius, gluteus minimus and vastus lateralis attached to it.

The femur is then externally rotated. In so doing, the trochanter naturally tends to shift forward. The trochanter and its muscle attachments are then mobilized anteriorly and medially (Fig. 35.6). The angled Hohmann retractor, passed deep to the trochanteric fragment is replaced deep to rectus femoris with its tip over the anterior rim of the acetabulum and used to retract forward the gluteus medius and minimus. The plane between the capsule and the deep fibers of gluteus minimus (which often gain origin from the capsule) is developed using sharp dissection with scissors. In this way, the deep fibers of gluteus minimus can be mobilized superiorly to expose the lateral margin of the acetabulum. The gluteus minimus and medius are retracted superiorly and anteriorly with Charnley pin retractors placed in the lateral wall of the ilium proximal to the acetabulum. The anterior and lateral portions of the capsule are now fully exposed and can be excised. The capsulectomy incision begins medially at the inferior margin of the anterior rim of the acetabulum, extending along the inferior margin of the femoral neck in a lateral direction. It then extends along the lateral femoral attachment of the capsule to the base of the trochanter and proximally through the lateral capsule to the lateral acetabular margin. Finally, it is excised off the lateral and anterior acetabular margins. If there is shortening and contracture, the femoral attachment of the inferior capsule is incised from anterior to posterior to mobilize the proximal femur. The hip is now ready for anterior dislocation by adduction and lateral rotation of the femur. The major posterior capsular attachments are kept intact. More extensive capsulectomy might be required in revisions with particulate synovial reactions and thickened capsules. Acetabular exposure is obtained by levering the proximal femur posteriorly with a strong Charnley horizontal self retaining retractor. Alternatively, an angled Hohmann or similar retractor, with its tip under the posteroinferior lip of the acetabulum, can be used.

Reattachment of the trochanteric fragment is best obtained using the Dall-Miles cable-grip system. Anchorage of the horizontal cables is obtained through or below the lesser trochanter. The correctly positioned grip will prevent proximal migration of the fragment especially if the limb is being lengthened. The incision in the posterior margin of vastus lateralis may require one or two interrupted sutures. The fascia lata is sutured and finally the skin closed.

References

1. Dall DM. Exposure of the hip by anterior osteotomy of the greater trochanter. *J Bone Joint Surg Br*. 1986;68:382–326.
2. Mostardi RA, Hoyt Jr WA, Askew MJ, et al. Comparison of trochanteric osteotomy techniques in total hip arthroplasty. 33rd Annual Meeting, Transactions Orthopaedic Research Society, Jan 19–22, 1987, San Francisco, CA.
3. Baker AS, Bitounis VC. Abductor function after total hip replacement. *J Bone Joint Surg Br*. 1989;71:47–50.
4. Dall DM. Modification of the anterior partial trochanteric osteotomy approach for total hip replacement. Scientific exhibit, SICOT World Congress, September 9–14, 1990, Montreal, Canada.
5. Glassman AH, Engh CA, Bobyn JD. A technique of extensive exposure for total hip arthroplasty. *J Arthroplasty* 1987;2:11–21.

36
Conventional Trochanteric Osteotomy

Benjamin E. Bierbaum and Russell G. Tigges

Conventional trochanteric osteotomy was first described by Charnley[1] as the standard approach for low-friction arthroplasty. Currently other approaches are used in the majority of primary joint replacements due to the complications[2] that occur with the transtrochanteric approach. We will describe our indications for trochanteric osteotomy, techniques for reattachment, and the complications associated with it.

Indications

The authors agree on the following recommendations about trochanteric osteotomy and transplantation:

1. Most primary hip operations can be adequately performed by a careful surgical approach without trochanteric osteotomy. We prefer the posterolateral approach; those well schooled in the anterolateral approach may prefer it.
2. Complex hip problems with distorted anatomy, contractual deformity, or a severe loss of motion are best approached with trochanteric osteotomy, even for primary surgery. (Examples: developmental dysplasia of the hip (DDH), ankylosed hips, severe protrusio acetabulae.)
3. Trochanteric osteotomy facilitates exposure in the morbidly obese patient.
4. Trochanteric osteotomy is helpful in many revision total hip arthroplasties.
5. Distal transplantation of the trochanter for treatment of the recurrent dislocation when the components are aligned correctly.
6. Whenever the trochanter is transplanted, the surgeon should have a careful preoperative plan for reattachment and be certain fixation is secure prior to wound closure.
7. Trochanteric osteotomy allows exposure for plating with or without grafting of both anterior and posterior columns of the acetabulum.

Techniques

After skin and subcutaneous exposure, the vastus lateralis fascia is incised 0.5 cm distal to the vastus tubercle. A small elevator is inserted in the interval between the tendon of the gluteus minimus and the superior part of the hip capsule at the junction of the greater trochanter with the superior part of the femoral neck. The osteotomy cut traverses the sulcus between the lateral portion of the origin of the vastus intermedius muscle and the insertions of the gluteus medius and minimus. As the osteotomy progresses posteriorly, the direction is more transverse so that the short rotators can be left attached to the trochanter. In very tight, deformed hips, the short rotators need to be released to facilitate proximal retraction of the greater trochanter. The osteotomy can be performed with an osteotome or oscillating saw aimed at the small elevator. The trochanter can then be retracted proximally. Sharp, blunt dissection is used to free the muscular origin of the minimus from the capsule and the psoas. The capsule is thus exposed from the lesser trochanter to the posterior-inferior aspect and is incised.

Many techniques have been devised for securing the trochanter to the host femur,[3-12] which leads to the realization that no single method is perfect. Among the securing devices used are bolts, screws, tension wires, cerclage wires, and synthetics sutures and tapes. The most popular methods use 16-gauge stainless steel or cobalt-chrome wire or multifilament cables. Some techniques imbed the wire in cement; in others, the wires are wrapped around the proximal femur and/or femoral component (Fig. 36.1). Clark et al.[4] showed that the usual cause of wire breakage is fatigue fracture rather than tension failure. This breakage is seen primarily when a wire is kinked or subjected to a stress-riser when it exits the cement.

Careful preparation of the trochanter and adjacent femoral bed for reattachment is critical to successful

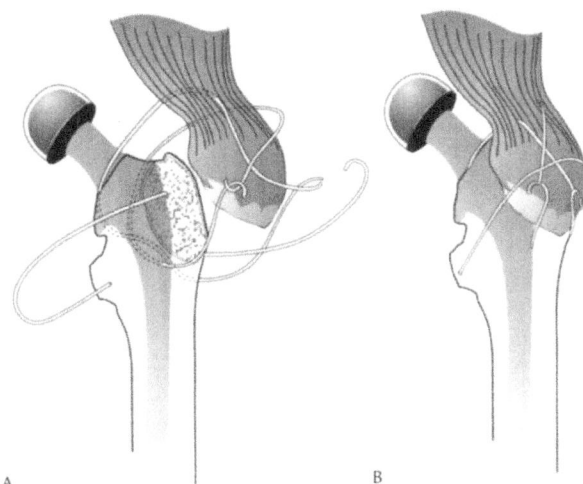

Figure 36.1. Diagram showing the three-wire technique used at the NEBH. A. Two vertical wires are crossed and passed prior to stem insertion. The third wire is transverse and is passed after stem insertion. The wires are tightened sequentially, starting with the vertical wire against the trochanter and ending with the transverse wire. B. A radiograph demonstrating the three-wire technique.

trochanteric repairs. Meticulous soft tissue debridement of both the trochanter and femoral bed is important. Obtaining a flat bone-to-bone contact surface is ideal but not often possible. The use of cancellous bone graft may be necessary to fill gaps in the bony surfaces.

Certain patients represent substantially increased risk for trochanteric problems. Included are patients with marked osteopenia, revision patients, bilateral arthroplasty patients, and obese and noncompliant patients.

Currently, when conventional trochanteric osteotomy is needed, our preferred reattachment technique involves using Dall-Miles (Howmedica, Rutherford, NJ) cables and grip system. A grip is placed over the trochanteric fragment and secured to the host femur using two cables passing under the lesser trochanter and through a drill hole placed in the lesser trochanter (Fig. 36.2). Care is taken to ensure no wire is in contact with the femoral component to prevent generation of metal debris. Krakow has described a method of fixation with the cable-grip system to allow better distal translation and fixation without drilling holes in the host femur (Fig. 36.3). Several techniques utilizing a range of one to four wires have been described extensively in the literature.[3,4,6,9–11,13–17]

When the trochanter is to be advanced in DDH or instability surgery or when a chronically migrated trochanter is to be reattached, it may be difficult to approximate the trochanter to the host femur. The first step is to remove all the superior capsule and scar tissue down to the muscle and tendon of the gluteus minimus. The origins of the minimus and medius can be stripped from the lateral face of the ilium with an elevator, beginning at the lateral lip of the acetabulum. In rare instances, a secondary incision is utilized along the crest of the ilium and the gluteus medius, and minimus and tensor fascia are stripped off the ilium and then left to slide distal.

Postoperatively the patient should be partial weight-bearing for 6 weeks with no active abduction of the leg to protect the abductor fixation.

Results and Complications

Trochanteric osteotomy can result in excellent exposure for the hip surgery performed and will often heal without incident. In two of the few randomized simultaneous clinical studies, Mallory[18] and Murray[19] reported equal or better abductor strength in patients who had trochanteric osteotomy when compared to those whose surgery was done without trochanteric osteotomy. Thompson et al.[20] reported fewer postoperative complications in patients whose surgery was done without trochanteric osteotomy when compared to patients with an osteotomy. It must be noted that Thompson's most difficult cases often required trochanteric osteotomy, and is not a truly comparable series.

In several published series with various fixation techniques, the complication rate due to the trochanteric fixation ranged from 0 to 37.5%.[3–5,11–15,17,21,22] Some

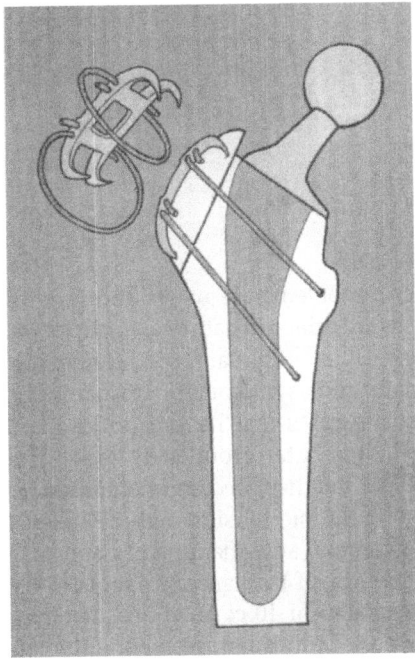

Figure 36.2. The trochanter can be fixed with a grip and multifilament cables with drill holes through the lesser trochanter and/or the medial cortex to prevent proximal migration.

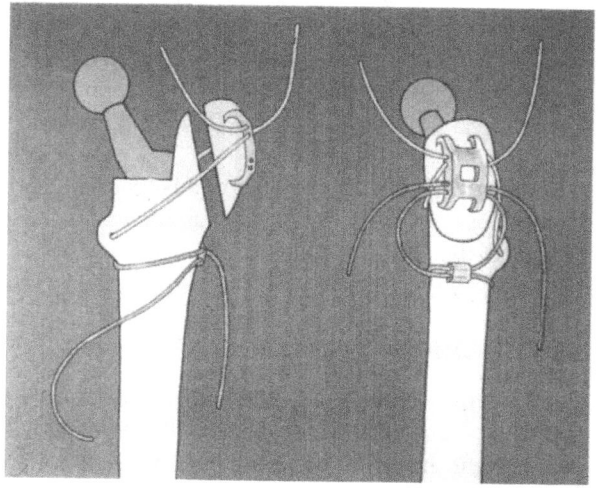
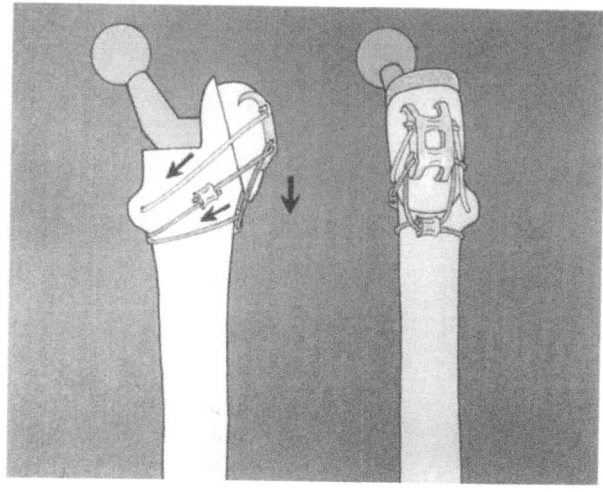

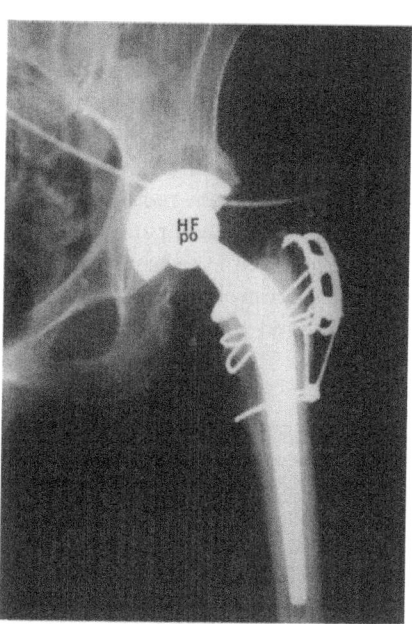

Figure 36.3. The trochanter can also be fixed with a grip and cables to maximize distal translation as described by Krackow.[13] A. A grip is applied to the trochanter fragment and a proximal cable is passed through the lesser trochanter. A second distal wire is secured around the femur below the lesser trochanter and tightened and crimped. This second wire is then passed through the distal grip and tightened, pulling the grip and trochanter distal. B, C. This second wire is then passed around the femur again to result in (1) distal force and (2) compressive forces holding the trochanter in place (C).

trochanteric problems are major and require reoperation; others are minor in nature and can be treated nonoperatively. It is important to differentiate between symptomatic and asymptomatic trochanteric problems, and to isolate cases that have significant trochanteric pathology. This latter group may range from simple bursitis to painful displaced and nonunited trochanters. Patients with simple bursitis may be relieved by systemic nonsteroidal antiinflammatory agents.

If the etiology of trochanteric pain is in doubt, a diagnostic injection of 10 cc local anesthetic may clarify the issue. If the pain is not relieved within 20 minutes, the surgeon must be suspicious that the etiology of the pain is not trochanteric bursitis. If the local anesthetic relieves the pain, then an injection into the bursal sac with steroids may give prolonged or even permanent relief.

If trochanteric fixation devices such as wires or bolts protrude prominently, they may cause a chronic bursitis that responds to injections only temporarily. Repeated trochanteric injections are not advised because of the remote but serious risk of infection.

Surgical removal of any offending devices is indicated if symptoms are not relieved after a few injections. At surgery, only the prominent offending portion of the device should be removed. Wires that are solidly embedded should be cut flush where they exit the bone. Heavier devices, such as bolts, can be cut with metal cutting instruments, such as the diamond wheel attachment available with the Midas Rex drill. Attempts to forcefully extract metal embedded in cement risks unnecessary immediate cement fracture or creates cement defects that can lead to future fatigue fracture of the cement.

The most common complication found with conventional trochanteric osteotomy is nonunion. The nonunion rate has been reported in the range of 0 to 32%.[3-5,11-15,17,21,22] Delayed union of the greater trochanter is present when there is x-ray evidence of separation 3 months following surgery. Patients with proven delayed union should be kept on crutches and should have a 1/2-inch lift added to their contralateral heel. If union is not achieved by 6 months, then nonunion of the trochanter is present and further crutch protection is based solely on the presence or absence of symptoms.

Nonunion of the greater trochanter can lead to abductor weakness, pain, instability of the hip joint, and decreased walking ability. The amount of trochanteric migration has been shown to have a significant influence on the functional outcome of the patients with nonunion,[16,23] with a displacement of >3 cm leading to a poorer result. The most likely cause for nonunion is a poor initial reduction and fixation at the time of surgery.[7]

Management of the trochanteric nonunion is complicated by shortening of the abductor sleeve, poor bone bed, and metallosis or granulation from prior fixation. Treatment carries a low success rate and will be addressed elsewhere.

Other less common complications reported with trochanteric osteotomy and fixation include heterotopic ossification[6] around the hip and sciatic nerve injury.[24]

Conclusion

Conventional trochanteric osteotomy is an excellent way to increase exposure in difficult primary or revision total hip arthroplasty. Careful replacement and fixation of the fragment is mandatory to avoid the many possible complications associated with it.

References

1. Charnley J. Total hip replacement by low-friction arthroplasty. *Clin Orthop.* 1970;72:7–21.
2. Glassman AH. Complications of trochanteric osteotomy. *Orthop Clin N Am.* 1992;23(2):321–333.
3. Browne AO, Sheehan JM. Trochanteric osteotomy in Charnley low-friction arthroplasty of the hip. *Clin Orthop.* 1986;211:128–133.
4. Clarke RP Jr, Shea WD, Bierbaum BE. Trochanteric osteotomy: analysis of pattern of wire fixation failure and complications. *Clin Orthop.* 1979;141:102–110.
5. Dall DM, Miles AW. Re-attachment of the greater trochanter. The use of the trochanter cable-grip system. *J Bone Joint Surg Br.* 1983;65:55–59.
6. Errico TJ, Fetto JF, Waugh TR. Heterotopic ossification. Incidence and relation to trochanteric osteotomy in 100 total hip arthroplasties. *Clin Orthop.* 1984;190:138–141.
7. Gottschalk FA, Morein G, Weber F. Effect of the position of the greater trochanter on the rate of union after trochanteric osteotomy for total hip arthroplasty. *J Arthroplasty.* 1988;3:235–240.
8. Hersh CK, Williams RP, Trick LW, Athanasiou K. Comparison of the mechanical performance of trochanteric fixation devices. *Clin Orthop.* 1996;329:317–325.
9. Markolf KL, Hirschowitz DL, Amstutz HC. Mechanical stability of the greater trochanter following osteotomy and reattachment by wiring. *Clin Orthop.* 1979;141:111–121.
10. McGrory BJ, Bal BS, Harris WH. Trochanteric osteotomy for total hip arthroplasty: six variations and indications for their use. *J Am Acad Orthop Surg.* 1996;4:258–267.
11. Nercessian OA, Newton PM, Joshi RP, Sheikh B, Eftekhar NS. Trochanteric osteotomy and wire fixation. a comparison of 2 techniques. *Clin Orthop.* 1996;333:208–216.
12. Rozing PM. Trochanter fixation with the Dutchman's hook. *Acta Orthop Scand.* 1983;54:174.
13. Krackow K. A technique for improved Dall Miles trochanteric re-attachment. *J Ortho Techniques.* 1994;2(1):37–40.
14. Hodgkinson JP, Shelley P, Wroblewski BM. Re-attachment of the un-united trochanter in Charnley low friction arthroplasty. *J Bone Joint Surg Br.* 1989;71:523–525.
15. Jensen NF, Harris WH. A system for trochanteric osteotomy and reattachment for total hip arthroplasty with a ninety-nine percent union rate. *Clin Orthop.* 1986;208:174–181.
16. Nutton RW, Checketts RG. The effects of trochanteric osteotomy on abductor power. *J Bone Joint Surg Br.* 1984;66:180–183.
17. Schutzer SF, Harris WH. Trochanteric osteotomy for revision total hip arthroplasty. 97% union rate using a comprehensive approach. *Clin Orthop.* 1988;227:172–183.
18. Mallory TH. Total hip replacement with and without trochanteric osteotomy. *Clin Orthop.* 1974;103:133–135.
19. Murray MP, Gore DR, Brewer BJ, Gardner GM, Sepic SB. Comparison of Muller total hip replacement with and without trochanteric osteotomy. Kinesiology measurements of 82 cases 2 years after surgery. *Acta Orthop Scand.* 1981;52:345–352.
20. Thompson RC, Culver JE. Role of trochanteric osteotomy in total hip replacement. *Clin Orthop.* 1975;106:102–106.
21. Frankel A, Booth RE, Balderston RA, Cohn J, Rothman RH. Complications of trochanteric osteotomy. Long-term implications. *Clin Orthop.* 1993;288:209–213.
22. Ritter MA, Eizember LE, Keating EM, Faris PM. Trochanteric fixation by cable grip in hip replacement. *J Bone Joint Surg Br.* 1991;73:580–581.
23. Ritter MA, Gioe TJ, Stringer EA. Functional significance of nonunion of the greater trochanter. *Clin Orthop.* 1981;159:177–182.
24. Mallory TH. Sciatic nerve entrapment secondary to trochanteric wiring following total hip arthroplasty. A case report. *Clin Orthop.* 1983;180:198–200.

37
The Anterolateral Surgical Approach

Thomas H. Mallory

The incidence of revision total hip replacement in the United States is significantly increasing relative to the number of primary total hip replacements performed, the age of the patient receiving the primary total hip replacement, and the longevity/life expectancy of the overall population. As in primary total hip replacement, the goals of revision total hip replacement include the relief of pain, the development of a stable prosthetic composite, the restoration of function, and the return of as normal an activity of daily living for the patient as possible. However, the joint replacement surgeon must be aware of an additional set of problems specific to the revision procedure.

The hip musculature has been previously invaded and there exists the issues of altered anatomy. The previously altered soft tissue envelope may be bound in scar, heterotopic bone, or encased in a granulomatous mass of reactive tissue from foreign body debris from component wear. There may have been a previously performed trochanteric osteotomy that may have created muscle disruption, nonunion of the greater trochanter, and residual broken wire debris.[1] The prosthetic composite may be compromised, and removal of the components demands certain requirements of the surgical approach. There may be marked bone lysis that has created large cavitary defects requiring extensile exposure for reconstruction. Also, once the revision procedure is completed, the surgical approach must allow restoration of function as well as facilitate prosthetic stability. Therefore, any surgical approach clearly prejudices the subsequent revision procedure.

Given the above issues, the anterolateral approach, which has been described as a primary total hip replacement exposure, is versatile in revision hip replacement.[2,3] The anterolateral approach is expansile and can easily be developed, proximally and distally, exposing the hip joint as well as the periarticular region in an all-inclusive manner.[4] It is a muscle splitting incision rather than a muscle resection. Historically, the work of McFarland et al. identified that the hip abductor muscle mass was connected distally through a myofascial sleeve to the quadriceps complex.[5] By splitting the abductor muscle and continuing distally into the substance of the vastus lateralis, two prominent muscle cuffs develop. The anterolateral approach, therefore, maintains muscle continuity, allowing for early restoration of muscle function. Moreover, the closure of the muscle split creates a side to side anastomosis with maintenance of muscle continuity. With appropriate tension of the involved muscle envelope, prosthetic stability is assured and function quickly restored.

Since it is not a frequently used surgical approach for the index procedure, the anterolateral approach offers a new entry pathway into the previously invaded hip joint. Failed trochanteric osteotomy can be managed appropriately even though it may have been avulsed, fractured, or complicated by broken trochanteric wires. The option for extensile exposure offered by the anterolateral approach allows the surgeon to appropriately manage the excision of scar tissue, granulation tissue, and heterotopic bone while avoiding major areas of anatomical risk and danger. Prosthetic extraction is enhanced by an extensile exposure. Major bone deficits can be adequately visualized and reconstructive procedures enhanced.

There are limitations to the anterolateral approach. The continuity of the myofascial sleeve, as it passes over and about the greater trochanter, is important and requires an understanding of the involved anatomy. Also, if the location of the muscle split is inappropriate through the abductor muscle mass, exposure is compromised and neurovascular damage can occur.[6] In certain clinical series, increased heterotopic bone has been reported with the anterolateral approach.[7] For the most part, this approach creates a stable environment for prosthetic integrity. The incidence of prosthetic dislocation is characteristically low. However, failure to develop a proper muscle tension within the residual envelope can create an unstable prosthetic composite.

37. The Anterolateral Approach

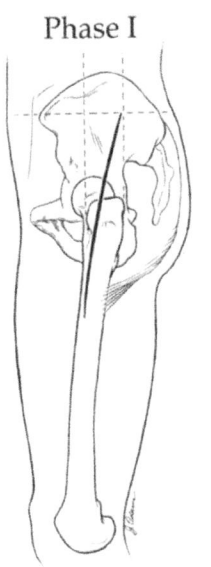
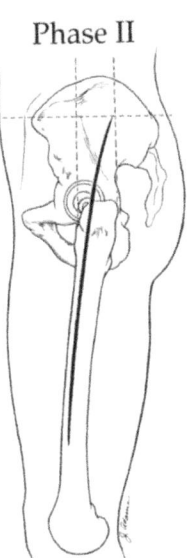
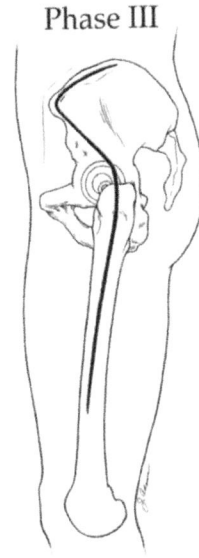

Phase I   Phase II   Phase III

Figure 37.1. The skin incisions of the three phases of the anterolateral approach in revision surgery. (Reprinted with permission, Lippincott-Raven Publishers, Philadelphia, 1993; and W.B. Saunders Company, Philadelphia, 1992.)

Three Phases of the Anterolateral Approach

The anterolateral approach in revision surgery encompasses three phases (Fig. 37.1);

Phase I: The preliminary use of the anterolateral approach in situations which require only exposure of the specific region of the hip most frequently associated in reconstructive procedures which are simple and straight forward.

Phase II: Revision surgical procedures that require extensive exposure of the proximal femur.

Phase III: An exposure which requires a circumferential view of the acetabular region.

All three phases of the anterolateral approach are interconnected, but allow the development of each portion of the exposure as needed.

Phase I: Basic Surgical Approach

The patient is positioned in a full lateral attitude with a slight inclination posteriorly. The hip area is prepped and draped in the usual manner, allowing exposure of the surgical area extending from the crest of the iliac to the midportion of the thigh. Identifying proximal landmarks include the superior anterior and posterior iliac spine. The anterior border of the greater trochanter as well as the anterior border of the femoral shaft are important landmarks. The incision should be drawn out with a marking pencil to be sure that these landmarks are clearly identified and utilized. The incision should extend proximally from the tip of the greater trochanter cephalad to the level of the superior anterior and posterior iliac spines. As the incision moves distally it extends along the anterior border of the greater trochanter paralleling the anterior shaft of the femur to the midshaft. The incision of subcutaneous tissue and the fascia should duplicate the skin incision. The incision through the fascia must lie between the posterior border of the tensor fascia lata muscle and anterior to the insertion of the tendon of the gluteus maximus. Generally, this portion of the fascia is thin and is easily incised. As the fascial incision is extended proximally, a simple muscle

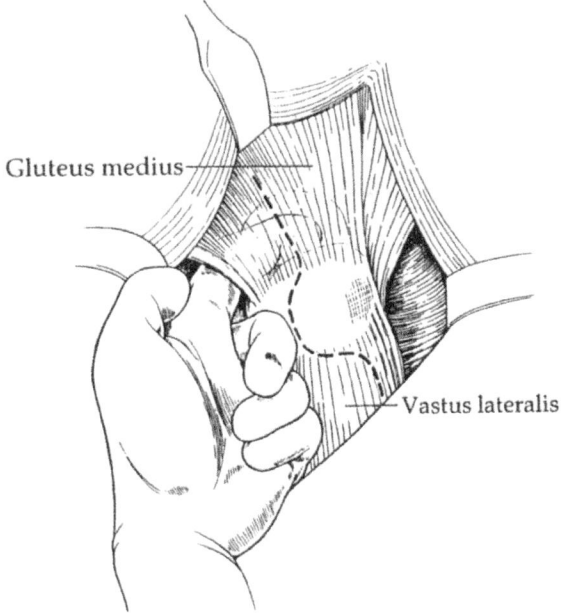

Figure 37.2. The surgeon palpates beneath the inferior medial border of the abductor muscle to determine the point of entry for the abductor muscle split. (Reprinted with permission, Lippincott-Raven Publishers, Philadelphia, 1993.)

splitting phenomena occurs within the fibers of the gluteus maximus muscle. With the fascia incised and the gluteus maximus muscle split performed, ample vision of the abductor muscle mass is accomplished. If the abductor muscle mass is not fully visualized, then simply splitting the tensor fascia lata vertically will expand the exposure anteriorly.

At this point, one of the most important developments of anterolateral approach must occur involving a specific identification of the location of the muscle split within the abductor muscle mass. Placing the exploring finger beneath the inferior medial border of the abductor medius muscle, the location of the prosthetic composite can be identified (Fig. 37.2). This is the point of entry for the abductor muscle split. Meanwhile, the abductor muscle fiber pattern is observed so that the muscle split parallels natural cleavage planes. The abductor muscle fibers are simply split as they course over the prosthetic complex as predetermined. The proximal extension of the muscle split must not extend beyond 2.5 cm superior to the acetabulum.[6] This avoids injury to the neurovascular bundle of the gluteal artery and nerve. Proximal development of the muscle split should be slow and careful to avoid injuring this particular neurovascular structure.

The muscle split creates a substantial amount of muscle mass in both an anterior and lateral cuff. Developing the muscle split along the anterior border of the greater trochanter allows the development of the exposure distally. With sharp dissection the anterior cuff proceeds distally along the anterior lateral border of the greater trochanter to the level of vastus tubercle ridge. This surgical maneuver involves elevating the insertion of the gluteus minimus tendon. At the level of the vastus tubercle, distal to the greater trochanter, the muscle dissection proceeds posterior and then distally along the linea aspira, thus elevating the vastus lateralis muscle. The importance of moving the incision posteriorly is advantageous because it minimizes blood loss and tends to maintain definitive muscle cuffs.

Phase II: Distal Expansion

When the revision total hip replacement procedure requires extensile exposure of the proximal femur, the anterolateral approach is quite appropriate. The distal exposure is accomplished by elevating the vastus lateralis muscle from the linea aspera incorporating this muscle group into the extended anterior cuff. If complete femoral exposure is necessary, elevation of the lateral cuff is accomplished by releasing the short rotators, the conjoined tendon of the gluteus maximus and the remaining musculature along the border of the linea aspera. By extending the medial and lateral muscle sleeves, a complete circumferential view of the femur is accomplished. This exposure must deal with the status of the greater trochanter. If the trochanter has been previously elevated and has been sufficiently reattached, the substance of the trochanter is left *in situ*. However, if the trochanter is avulsed, simply excising the trochanter fragment from the muscle cuff does not compromise the muscle envelope.

If the abductor muscle involved in the lateral muscle cuff remains well attached to the greater trochanter, then two options exist. It is possible to perform an extended trochanteric osteotomy. However, an alternative method involves elevating the lateral muscle cuff along the posterior border of the greater trochanter maintaining the lateral muscle sleeve. Subsequent reattachment of the muscle group to the greater trochanter is easily accomplished with the use of heavy, nonabsorbable suture.

The distal extension of the this exposure is all inclusive. It allows for a complete extirpation of the femur, should it be necessary (such as in total femoral replacement). At the completion of the surgical procedure, closure is easily accomplished by reattaching the split muscle envelope to the shaft of the femur in a conventional manner.

Phase III: Proximal Expansion

Phase III exposure can be combined with Phase II and may well be necessary where cases merit an extensile exposure of both the acetabulum as well as the femur. The specific nature of the Phase III exposure concentrates on acetabular visualization. It is well recognized that the course of the gluteal neurovascular bundle transects the region approximately 2.5 centimeters proximal to the acetabulum. To continue the muscle split proximally in an indefinite direction could inadvertently sever this particular neurovascular group, which could seriously affect the long term function of the abductor complex. In order to avoid such a catastrophe, the muscle split is redirected in an anterior superior direction towards the anterior superior iliac spine. This particular course assures that encountering the neurovascular bundle is subsequently avoided. Through this cleavage plane the interval between the tensor fascia lata and the medial border of the gluteus medius is developed. With exposure developed to the level of the anterior superior iliac spine, the direction of the incision proceeds superiorly along the crest of the ileum in a posterior direction. The abductor muscle is lifted subperiosteally from the wing of the ilium, the extent of which depends on the exposure needed. It is possible to extend the muscle mass elevation in a posterior direction to the level of the sciatic notch thus exposing the posterior column of the acetabulum. If entry into the intrapelvic cavity is necessary, it is accomplished with blunt dissection, entering the cavity anteriorly beneath the iliacus muscle. This particular maneuver allows the surgeon to manage protruded intrapelvic cement masses.

Finally at the completion of the surgical procedure, the abductor muscle mass is reattached to the crest of the ilium by incorporating the abdominal fascia. The patient is placed in a postoperative program of muscle rehabilitation. Within 3 to 6 months independent abductor function is consistently observed.

Conclusion

The anterolateral approach is indeed versatile. This is quite obvious when the surgical exposure is divided into the appropriate three phases of development. By following anatomic cleavage planes, muscle continuity is maintained and the muscular envelope rapidly reattaches to the osseous substrate. In complex revision total hip arthroplasty (THA), the anterolateral exposure can be developed rapidly, which shortens operative time, decreases the associated risks, and avoids prolonged anesthesia. It facilitates a direct exposure to the anatomical site, avoids major neurovascular structures, and minimizes blood loss. The anterolateral approach consistently leaves a stable construct allowing maximum functional activity in the early postoperative period.

References

1. Amstutz HC, Maki S. Complications of trochanteric osteotomy in total hip replacement. *J Bone Joint Surg Am.* 1978; 60:214–316.
2. Frndak PA, Mallory TH, Lombardi AV Jr. Translateral surgical approach to the hip. The abductor muscle "split." *Clin Orthop.* 1993;295:135–141.
3. Hardinge K. The anterolateral approach to the hip. *J Bone Joint Surg Br.* 1982;64:17–19.
4. Head WC, Mallory TH, Berklacich FM. Extensile exposure of the hip for revision arthroplasty. *J Arthroplasty.* 1987;2: 265–273.
5. McFarland B, Osborne G. Approach to the hip: a suggested improvement on Kocher's method. *J Bone Joint Surg Br.* 1954; 36:364.
6. Abitbol JJ, Gendron D, Laurin CA, Beaulieu MA. Gluteal nerve damage following total hip arthroplasty. A prospective analysis. *J Arthroplasty.* 1990;5:319–322.
7. Morrey BF, Adams RA, Cabanela ME. Comparison of heterotopic bone after anterolateral, transtrochanteric, and posterior approaches for total hip arthroplasty. *Clin Orthop.* 1984;188:160–167.

38
Trochanter Slide Surgical Approach

Joseph C. McCarthy

Extensile exposure of the hip greatly improves the likelihood of a consistently successful outcome in revision surgery. Although some repeat procedures can be accomplished without trochanteric removal, many surgical situations are encountered that make osteotomy desirable.[1-5] Potential indications for a trochanteric slide approach to the hip include:

- Fracture of the femur about a femoral prosthesis.
- Identification of the extent and location of femoral bony deficiency. Preoperative radiographs frequently fail to visualize the presence or underestimate the number of cortical violations.
- Removal of extraosseous bone cement.
- Removal of preexisting hardware (screws, plates, wires).
- Osteotomy of the femur to correct varus/valgus or deformity.
- Correction of rotational malalignment from prior malunion.
- Osteotomy for leg lengthening or shortening.
- Osteotomy to correct excessive anterior femoral bowing.
- Access to facilitate cortical onlay or proximal femoral allografting.
- Trochanteric repositioning in patients with excessive anteversion.
- Trochanteric lengthening.
- Trochanteric lateralization for biomechanical advantage.
- Cement removal.
- Extensile acetabular exposure.
- Structural acetabular bone grafting.
- Insertion of modular bilobed cup.
- Vertical relocation of acetabular hip center congenital dysplasia of the hip (CDH), girdlestone conversion).
- Removal of heterotopic bone.
- Excessive scarring that prevents adequate exposure of the acetabulum or femur.

Despite the myriad advantages of the trochanteric slide approach there are some limitations. Removal of the trochanter initiates the potential for bony nonunion, especially if there has been a previous trochanteric procedure.[6-9]

The inferior branch of the superior gluteal nerve and artery exit the pelvis through the greater sciatic notch and then course from posterior to anterior between the gluteus minimus and medius. This neurovascular bundle may be tethered by excessive anterior translation of the trochanteric myosseous composite. For this reason procedures requiring extensive superior pelvic access are better served by conventional trochanteric osteotomy.[1,7,3,10-13]

In revision hip surgery this could include the exposure necessary for insertion of an acetabular cage device (G.A.P., Burch-Schneider, Link), whole acetabular allograft, pelvic plating to correct dissociation, or distal translation of a very high hip center.[4,13-15]

Thorough preoperative planning helps to identify these situations. Should the revision procedure become more complex than originally planned, the surgeon can readily convert a trochanteric slide to a conventional osteotomy by merely detaching the vastus lateralis fibers from the inferior edge of the greater trochanter bone

Approach

The patient is placed in the lateral decubitus position and held securely on a peg board or similar padded device. These devices help to prevent pelvic tilt during the revision procedure. The previous skin incision is excised. The fascia is incised directly above the center of the greater trochanter. Scar tissue between the iliotibial band and the underlying vastus lateralis fascia is carefully resected, using a combination of blunt and sharp dissection. The vastus lateralis fascia is then incised one finger breadth anterior to the linea aspera. While carefully protecting the fascia, the lateralis muscle is re-

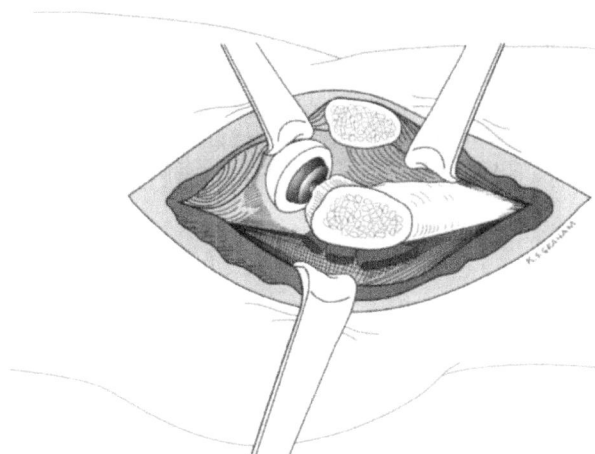

Figure 38.1. The osteotomized greater trochanter is displaced anteriorly with the vastus lateralis attached inferiorly and the gluteus minimus/medius intact superiorly.

flected anteriorly, off the linea. Perforator vessels are carefully identified and ligated. Bennet retractors displace the muscle anteriorly, allowing visualization of the femoral shaft below the vastus lateralis tubercle.

Attention is directed proximally. The posterior tendinous edge of the gluteus medius and minimus is identified and retracted anteriorly with a hip retractor. At the surgeon's discretion, a Cushing elevator is passed between the abductors and the underlying joint capsule from posterior to anterior. This instrument helps to provide visual reference as to the depth of the desired bone cut.

With the patient's leg slightly internally rotated and the retractors in place, the osteotomy is initiated just deep to the abductor tendons. The oscillating saw is advanced from posterior to anterior aiming at the Cushing elevator. The leg may be externally rotated during the most anterior extent of the osteotomy cut. With the lower leg now positioned perpendicular to the floor within a sterile pocket drape, the surgeon then displaces the osteotomized trochanter anteriorly (Fig. 38.1). Scar tissue is resected and a cobra retractor is positioned just over the anterior edge of the pelvic brim. A complete capsulectomy is easily accomplished, and joint cultures and tissue samples are sent for analysis.

Acetabular reaming can be completed with the femur displaced either anteriorly or posteriorly. Preparation of the femur for the new implant is greatly facilitated by anatomic orientation, the ability to elevate the femur up out of the surgical wound and by ready access to the lateral trochanteric bed. In addition, direct visualization of the femur facilitates cement removal, especially from extraosseous locations, improves the likelihood of neutral axial implant alignment, and is requisite for fixation and grafting of fractures and bone deficiencies.

Following femoral implant insertion, reattachment of the trochanter is made easier by having the myosseous sleeve (abduction–bone–vastus lateralis) intact. Drill holes in the lesser trochanter will allow passage for wire or cable bony fixation (see section on trochanteric reattachment). The integrity of the muscle–bone–muscle composite greatly lessens the risk of vertical migration in the event of trochanteric nonunion.

Results

In a series of 251 revision hip surgeries the trochanteric slide approach was employed. When reviewed at a minimum of 4 years postoperative, trochanteric healing was accomplished in 96% of cases.[3] This healing rate is more impressive since, preoperatively, 109 hips had a previous trochanteric osteotomy and the nonunion rate was 45%. In addition, this series included 13 cases of proximal femoral allografts where trochanteric nonunion and translation are common. Preservation of the abductor–bone–vastus lateralis insert greatly facilitated trochanteric coaptation and healing.

References

1. Chandler HP, Penenberg BL. *Bone stock deficiency in total hip replacement, classification and management.* Thorofare, N.J.: Slack, 1989.
2. Engh CA, Bobyn JD, *Biological fixation in total hip arthroplasty.* Thorofare, NJ: Slack, 1985.
3. McCarthy JC, Turner RH, Bono JV, Krecheck T, O'Donnell PJ. Trochanteric reattachment after revision total hip replacement using the Dall-Miles cable grip system: minimum six year follow-up. publication pending. *J Arthroplasty.*
4. Scher MA, Jakim I. Trochanter re-attachment in revision hip arthroplasty. *J Bone Joint Surg Br.* 1990;72:435–438.
5. Younger TI, Bradford MS, Magnus RE, Paprosky WG. Extended proximal femoral osteotomy. A new technique for femoral revision arthroplasty. *J Arthroplasty.* 1995;10:329–338.
6. Clarke RP, Shea WD, Bierbaum BE. Trochanteric osteotomy. Analysis of pattern of wire fixation failure and complications. *Clin Orthop.* 1979;141:102–110.
7. Ekelund A. Trochanteric osteotomy for recurrent dislocation of total hip arthroplasty. *J Arthroplasty.* 1993;8:629–632.
8. Gottschalk FA, Morein G, Weber F. Effect of the position of the greater trochanter on the rate of union after trochanteric osteotomy for total hip arthroplasty. *J Arthroplasty.* 1988;3:235–240.
9. Markolf KL, Hirschowitz DL, Amstutz HC. Mechanical stability of the greater trochanter following osteotomy and reattachment by wiring. *Clin Orthop.* 1979;141:111–121.
10. Dall DM, Miles AW. Re-attachment of the greater trochanter. The use of the trochanter cable-grip system. *J Bone Joint Surg Br.* 1983;65:55–59.
11. Jensen NF, Harris WH. A system for trochanteric os-

teotomy and reattachment for total hip arthroplasty with ninety-nine percent union rate. *Clin Orthop.* 1986;208:174–181.
12. Kaplan SJ, Thomas WH, Poss R. Trochanteric advancement for recurrent dislocation after total hip arthroplasty. *J Arthroplasty.* 1987;2:119–124.
13. Peters PC Jr, Head WC, Emerson RH Jr. An extended trochanteric osteotomy for revision total hip replacement. *J Bone Joint Surg Br.* 1993;75:158–159.
14. English TA. The trochanteric approach to the hip for prosthetic replacement. *J Bone Joint Surg.* 1975;57A:1128–1128.
15. McGrory BJ, Bal BS, Harris WH. Trochanteric osteotomy for total hip arthroplasty: six variations and indications for their use. *J Am Acad Orthop Surg.* 1996;4:258–267.

39
Extended Trochanteric Osteotomy

Roger H. Emerson, Jr. and William C. Head

From the inception of total hip replacement surgery the role of osteotomy of the greater trochanter has been debated. Charnley felt that it was essential to move the trochanter laterally as an integral part of the low friction principle of his procedure.[1] Comparison of surgeries with and without osteotomy clearly show that trochanteric osteotomy prolongs the surgery, is associated with more blood loss, and causes a slower postoperative rehabilitation course.[2] Most hip surgeons have found that many hips can be approached without osteotomizing the trochanter, but it is an invaluable technique in the more difficult and previously operated hip.[3] Glassman concluded in a review of trochanteric osteotomy that it is an important adjunct in selected cases, but is not necessary in every instance. The major benefit in his opinion was improved exposure.[4]

The two main problems with osteotomy, as reported by Clarke et al.,[5] have been nonunion, with a prevalence of 9% and migration of the trochanteric remnant, with a prevalence of 15.5%, defunctionalizing the abductors. Although Ritter et al.[6] found very little overall morbidity from nonunion of the greater trochanter, there was a significant finding of less subjective walking ability and a trend for more pain (in the previously operated group) in the nonunion group compared with the united group. The extent of the gap between fragments was not associated with any diminished function. Others do not agree with the latter finding. Both Clarke et al.[5] and Glassman et al.[7] found that over 2 cm of fibrous gap was associated with a significant alteration in function. Frankel et al. noted a Trendelenburg gait in 17% of the nonunions compared to 6% of the united patients.[8] Later successful reattachment of a nonunited trochanter is unreliable[5] making primary union all the more important.

Methods to Improve Trochanter Osteotomy

Several traditional wiring methods have been used for reattachment of the trochanter. Mechanical testing of these various methods by Markolf et al.[9] showed that no technique provided for completely rigid fixation. Avoiding damaging kinks and bends in the wire will prevent premature wire breakage from fatigue injury to the wire, and radiographic evidence of delayed union requires continued protection of the hip with a walking aid.[5] Schutzer and Harris have described a new four-wire technique with a reported 3% rate of nonunion.[10] Cable fixation of the trochanter has been another approach to enhance the strength of trochanteric fixation. Concerns about cables have arisen, especially fraying of the cable with resulting debris production, which can migrate into the bearing surface of the joint causing acetabular failure.[11]

A trochanteric slide approach has been described that leaves both the abductors and quadriceps attached to the bony trochanter, thus keeping the abductor mechanism in continuity. Glassman reports that this technique diminishes the amount of fragment separation (4 mm) when loss of trochanter fixation develops, and makes any degree of separation less clinically significant because the lateral soft tissue sleeve remains intact.[7]

Extended Trochanter Osteotomy

Many of the complications of trochanter osteotomy, especially in the revision setting, are due to the compromised nature of the underlying bone stock with osteopenia due to both stress-shielding and osteolysis from the prior implant. In this setting, a more extended osteotomy has a number of advantages. The underlying concept is to create a larger trochanter fragment to permit more reliable fixation. Better exposure of the femoral component for ease of removal is an added benefit. This technique differs from the traditional in that a tongue of lateral cortex is left attached to the trochanter (Fig. 39.1 and 39.2). The method of fixation of this fragment can vary, but due to the larger size of the trochanteric piece, additional wires can be used for more stable and rigid fixation. The longer tongue of cortex makes rotational stability more secure compared to a wafer fragment. Additional fixation can be obtained by means of

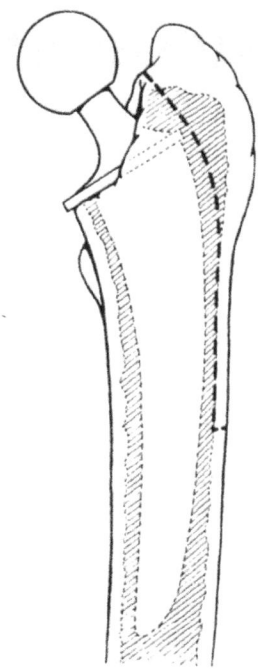

Figure 39.1. Depiction of the extended osteotomy prior to completing the cuts in a revision of a short-stemmed femoral component. Note the access to the cement mantle of the femoral component.

ing or, if the leg has been lengthened, left slightly short of its anatomic position. As depicted in the figures, this osteotomy lends itself to a calcar deficient implant with a trochanteric surface and reattachment device (Fig. 39.2). The traditional wiring should be augmented with several cerclage wires over the extended tongue of bone. Postoperative management is no different than for any osteotomy. Protection with a walking aid is important until union has been demonstrated radiographically.

Clinical Results

Out of a series of 169 revision total hip arthroplasties done between 1988 and 1991, 21 extended osteotomies were done in this fashion, with 9 requiring struts to augment the repair.[13] All 21 of these trochanters united.

a cortical onlay graft as depicted in Figure 39.2. The extended osteotomy can be combined with a trochanteric slide method or done with the traditional transection of the vastus lateralis at the vastus tubercle. This differs from the longer lateral shaft osteotomy as described by Younger et al.,[12] which entails a much larger trochanteric and diaphyseal piece of bone with attached quadriceps muscle.

The key to this technique is to maintain a very thick piece of trochanter, encompassing the entire lateral femur. The rim of the trochanter and femur are maintained for bony apposition and union. The osteotomy should be started posteriorly with an oscillating saw, coming down the lateral cortex for several centimeters, usually 3 to 5 centimeters is sufficient. The anterior cut is more difficult. It can be started with the saw, but must be completed with an osteotome. Often the anterior cut is incomplete, but will allow the trochanter to be gently levered, hinging on the anterior bone, cracking the osteotomy to completion. If a trochanteric slide is used, the lateral and anterior soft tissues will need to be retracted out of the way. No attempt is made to keep the vastus lateralis attached to the tongue of lateral cortex.

At closure, the trochanter can be positioned at the desired level, advanced for better soft tissue tension-

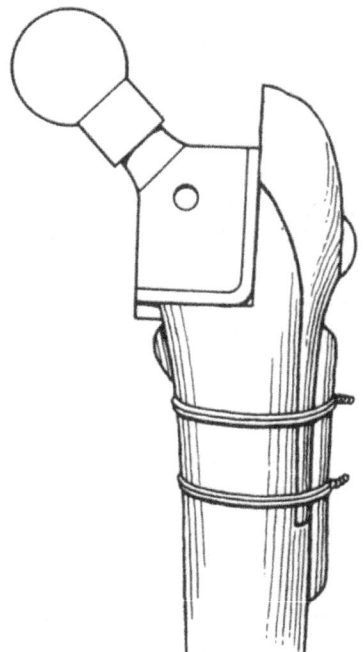

Figure 39.2. Completion of the revision with reattachment of the extended osteotomy using a reattachment "bolt" with the calcar deficient femoral revision component. The bolt traverses the calcar portion of the implant and lags the bone to the surface of the implant and the lateral shaft of the femur. Two additional wires and a short onlay allograft are shown augmenting the fixation postoperatively. The onlay graft is optional depending on the strength of the bone stock.

References

1. Charnley J. Total hip replacement by low-friction arthroplasty. *Clin Orthop.* 1970;72:7–21.
2. Parker HG, Wiesman HG, Ewald FC, et al. Comparison of preoperative, intraoperative and early postoperative total hip replacements with and without trochanteric osteotomy. *Clin Orthop.* 1976;121:44–49.
3. Thompson RC Jr, Culver JE. The role of trochanteric osteotomy in total hip replacement. *Clin Orthop.* 1975;106:102–106.
4. Glassman AH. Complications of trochanteric osteotomy. *Orthop Clin North Am.* 1992;23:321–333.
5. Clarke RP, Shea WD, Bierbaum BE. Trochanteric osteotomy. Analysis of pattern of wire fixation failure and complications. *Clin Orthop.* 1979;141:102–110.
6. Ritter MA, Gioe TJ, Stringer EA. Functional significance of nonunion of the greater trochanter. *Clin Orthop.* 1981;159:177–182.
7. Glassman AH, Engh CA, Bobyn JD. A technique of extensile exposure for total hip arthroplasty. *J Arthroplasty.* 1987;2:11–21.
8. Frankel A, Booth RE Jr, Balderston RA, et al. Complications of trochanteric osteotomy. Long-term implications. *Clin Orthop.* 1993;288:209–213.
9. Markolf KL, Hirschowitz DL, Amstutz AC. Mechanical stability of the greater trochanter following osteotomy and reattachment by wiring. *Clin Orthop.* 1979;141:111–121.
10. Schutzer SF, Harris WH. Trochanteric osteotomy for revision total hip arthroplasty. *Clin Orthop.* 1988;227:172–183.
11. Kelley SS, Johnston RC. Debris from cobalt-chrome cable may cause acetabular loosening. *Clin Orthop.* 1992;285:140–146.
12. Younger TI, Bradford MS, Magnus RE, et al. Extended proximal femoral osteotomy. A new technique for femoral revision arthroplasty. *J Arthroplasty.* 1995;10:329–338.
13. Peters PC, Head WC, Emerson RH Jr. An extended trochanteric osteotomy for revision total hip replacement. *J Bone Joint Surg Br.* 1993;75:158–159.

40
Extended Lateral Femoral Osteotomy

Wayne G. Paprosky, Todd D. Sekundiak, and Terry I. Younger

Revision total hip arthroplasty presents a myriad of difficulties to the surgeon attempting to obtain a functional, predictable, long-term result. Difficulties initially arise from attempts at exposing a multiply operated hip. The next challenge arises in attempting removal of components without destroying significant bone stock.[1-3] One is further challenged by attempting to place preformed components in bone that has now remodelled secondary to loosening, osteolysis, and the redistribution of stresses.[4-6] Once components are placed, balancing of soft tissues is essential to prevent instability at the joint. This must all be performed with a minimum of complications to the patient and without hindering the postoperative course and future possible rerevisions. The extended lateral trochanteric osteotomy addresses all of the above hurdles.

Rationale

In the revision total hip arthroplasty, scarring can lead to significant limitations in exposing the hip. A routine trochanteric osteotomy allows for significant ease in exposure of the hip joint but does not aid in distal exposure.[7] Exposure can be also limited when the femur has shortened or where the greater trochanter has expanded secondarily to remodelling from osteolysis. In these cases, an osteotomy is essential to dislocate the hip and to prevent fracturing of the bone. A routine trochanteric osteotomy allows for this exposure but is limited by the fact that healing is poor with nonunion rates being very high.[8-14] The nonunion rate for the extended trochanteric osteotomy is essentially zero as the fragment is long enough to allow for stable cable or wire fixation.[15] Healing rates are also improved because of the extended bony contact surface between the fragment and remaining intact femur. The vascularity of the component is maintained, as minimal soft tissue dissection is required.

Attempting to remove a loose femoral component or cement mantle is not routinely a technically demanding feat. In cases where trochanteric remodelling or overgrowth obscures the femoral intramedullary canal, retrieval of components or cement can be challenging with the additional concern of fracturing the bone. An osteotomy can eliminate this problem by clearing the intramedullary canal and allowing complete visualization distally. In cases where the component or cement mantle is well fixed, the extended trochanteric osteotomy allows for safe rapid removal of materials as opposed to other methods where distal visualization can be difficult.[16-18] Similar concerns are raised for removal of a loose porous coated stem with justification of the osteotomy to prevent bone–prosthesis impingement on removal. For components that are ingrown, the osteotomy is required to debond the prosthesis from the host bone and allow for controlled, safe extraction.

With components removed, the ectatic distorted femur must accept new components. Commonly, we see components fail in varus with the femur assuming a secondary varus deformity secondary to remodelling. An extended trochanteric osteotomy allows visualization of the remaining structural diaphyseal bone and prevents component malpositioning or bone fracturing[1] by allowing a straight trajectory for insertion. In addition, this prevents under or oversizing the component and the possibility for this mode of failure.

Soft tissue balancing is essential in the revision arthroplasty to ensure that properly positioned components have a stable range of motion. The extended trochanteric osteotomy allows for distal advancement of the abductor musculature to increase the resting tension and improve contractile force. Correcting the femoral varus deformity also lateralizes the abductor insertion point, to increase the lever arm, and improve the abductor force that can be generated. Anterior or more commonly posterior advancement can also improve stability by a mechanism undetermined, but likely from tightening noncontractile capsular tissues. In fact, for recurrent dislocations of a well-positioned, well-fixed total hip arthroplasty, an extended trochanteric osteotomy with advancement and temporizing fixation is the first step to assessing and managing the problem in our institution.

Preoperative Planning

The surgical technique begins with preoperative templating to determine the length of the osteotomy, how the bone will be osteotomized, and when the bone will be osteotomized. Multiple factors must be considered in determining the length of the osteotomy. First, the osteotomy must be long enough to ensure that two cables can be passed around the fragment to control the traction and rotational forces which occur during healing. Cable fixation occurs around the diaphyseal bone where adequate compressive forces can be applied without the risk of fracturing bone or causing proximal migration of the cable. The most proximal cable needs to be placed at the metaphyseal–diaphyseal junction with the second cable approximately 3 cm distal to it. Therefore a minimum of 5 cm of diaphyseal bone is needed to be attached to the fragment for safe fixation. The maximum length of the osteotomy is only limited by the ability of the revision stem to obtain fixation in the remaining distal diaphyseal bone. Length of the osteotomy is measured on the preoperative radiograph and correlated to the loose femoral stem or radiographic bony landmarks to help confirm length intraoperatively.

For components that are loose and that can be removed without risk of damaging bone on dislocation of the joint or with removal, removal should precede the osteotomy. If the press-fit component is fixed, then one must determine the extent of the porous coating.[19] Proximal coated devices must have the osteotomy extend past the coating to allow for effective removal. Extensively coated devices must have the osteotomy extend past the metaphyseal flare portion of the stem with only the cylindrical diaphyseal portion remaining distal to the osteotomy. For cemented components, it is commonly the cement mantle that determines the length of the osteotomy. A well bonded cement plug must be approached cautiously. The osteotomy must be carried down to a point that allows easy access to the proximal and distal cement yet retains a portion of intact diaphyseal femur for revision implant fixation.

The width of the osteotomy can be better controlled with the component initially removed as there is no concern of the cutting tool impinging on the lateral shoulder of the prosthesis. Removal of the component prior to the osteotomy, however, is not indicated if it risks fracturing the femur with removal. On average, one-third of the femoral circumference should be included in the osteotomy fragment. Where bone has been significantly weakened from osteolysis, infection or disuse, the width can be more generous.

Use of an oscillating saw to perform the osteotomy can proceed if the component has been removed prior or if the distance between the lateral aspect of the component and the exosteal surface of the lateral femoral cortex is ample enough to accept the blade. The swath of bone removed by an oscillating saw can be excessive with the multiplanar motion of a vibrating blade, leaving the osteotomy fragment fragile or fragmented. A pencil tipped burr on a high speed pneumatic rotating tool allows for better control and allows the operator to feel over the lateral shoulder of the prosthesis.

Timing of the osteotomy is determined by the reason for its use. For exposure, there is no choice but to perform the osteotomy initially. If exposure is possible but the osteotomy is being performed for femoral component removal or femoral deformity correction, then the osteotomy can be performed at a later time. Later timing of the osteotomy is indicated to prevent exposing the raw bony surfaces for extended periods that can lead to some increased blood loss.

Operative Technique

Revision procedures are commonly performed through an extensile posterolateral approach. The femur is held in an internally rotated position to bring the posterior aspect of the femur into view. The gluteus maximus insertion is identified and can be partially released to allow for better exposure. The vastus lateralis is then released off the lateral intermuscular septum to expose the posterolateral aspect of the femur for a distance predetermined by the length of the osteotomy. As exposure proceeds distally, the perforating arteries must first be identified and then cauterized to prevent excess bleeding from retraction behind the intermuscular septum. A small cuff of vastus lateralis can be left on the intermuscular septum that will prevent the cut arteries from retracting. Stripping of the muscle off the femur is avoided and its origin on the vastus ridge is maintained. The distal extent of the osteotomy is then measured either with preoperative length determinants or by correlating to intraoperative markers such as bony defects or the removed prosthesis.

A blunt retractor is placed around the anterior aspect of the femur to determine overall width of the femur and to assess extent of the distal transverse cut. The transverse cut is performed first to prevent inadvertent extension of a fracture of the femur from indiscriminate rotation of the extremity. It is wise to mark the direction of the posterior cut to ensure that the osteotomy is ample enough to maintain structural integrity. The cutting tool is then used as advised above. First pass of the cutting tool will breach the posterior cortex and posterior cement mantle, if present. Cues are then taken by feeling the anterior proximal femoral cortex, feeling the lateral aspect of the femoral component with the cutting tool, and by visualizing the shoulder of the prosthesis and proximal bone to determine the direction in the sagittal plane to complete the anterior femoral cortex bone cut (Fig. 40.1). These cues help to ensure that the

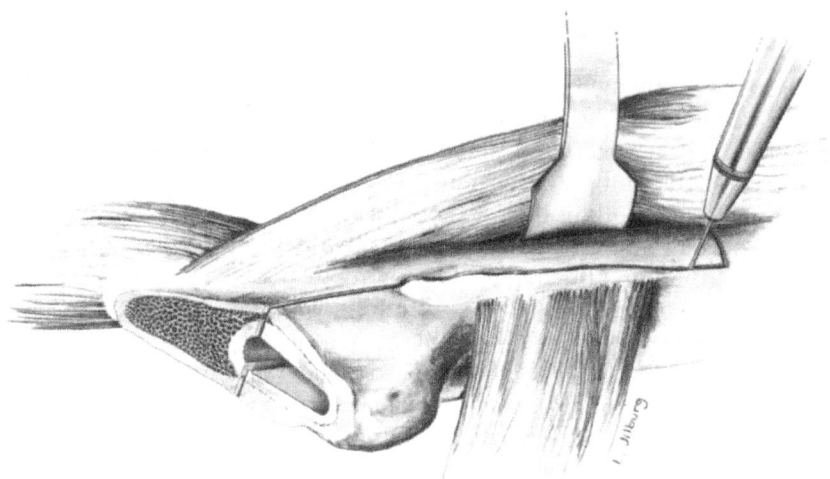

Figure 40.1. The posterior and transverse extent of the osteotomy.

fragment is structurally sound enough to accept cable. The anterior bony cut can be completed with the oscillating saw or burr with a second pass.

Completion of the osteotomy occurs with wide osteotomes opening the fragment from posterior to anterior. The osteotomy is hinged open on its anterolateral hinge of periosteum and muscle (Fig. 40.2). At this stage, anterior capsular and scar need to be assessed. If taut and if the fragment is immobile, then soft tissue release is required to prevent fracturing of the osteotomy fragment. Blunt retractors are then placed around the anterior aspect of the remaining intact proximal femur to keep the trochanter and attached musculature out of the field.

Removal of components then proceeds in a specific manner. Proximal coated ingrown stems can be removed by channelling on the anterior and posterior aspects of the component-bone interface with a high speed burr. A Gigli saw is then passed around the proximal calcar and passed through the remaining medial ingrowth areas. Extensively-coated ingrown stem removal proceeds in a similar manner. Once the metaphyseal flare portion of the component is released, the component is transected with a metal cutting burr.[20] The cylindrical diaphyseal portion is then trephined and extracted. Cemented components, if not yet removed, can be tapped out after patiently extracting some impinging proximal cement mantle. Distal cement plugs must be prudently drilled and tapped for removal.

Preparation of the femoral canal then proceeds for reimplantation. Cementing a femoral revision component dictates that the osteotomy fragment must be returned to its anatomic bed to prevent cement extrusion. Soft tissue tension must be accepted. By ensuring 4 to 6 cm of diaphyseal endosteal bone remains, the canal can then be reamed and prepared for a fully coated or a fluted stem. Fixation of a proximal coated device will

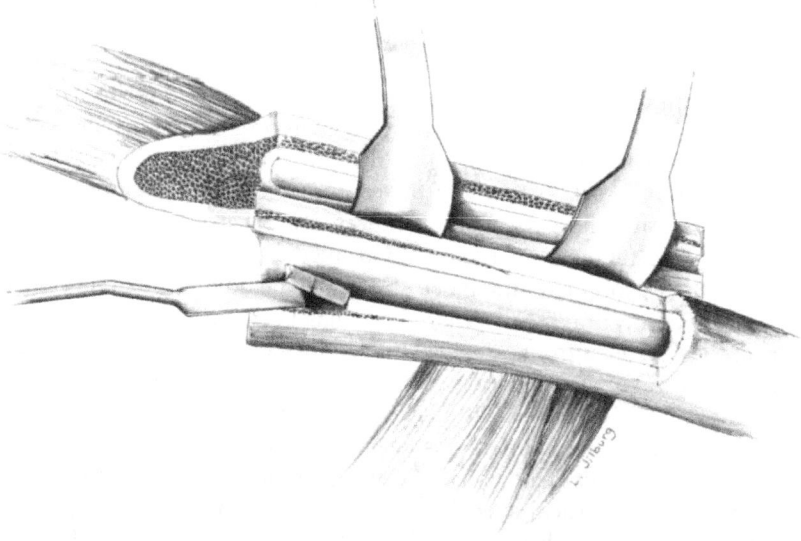

Figure 40.2. Osteotomes are used to open the osteotomy on its anterior hinge.

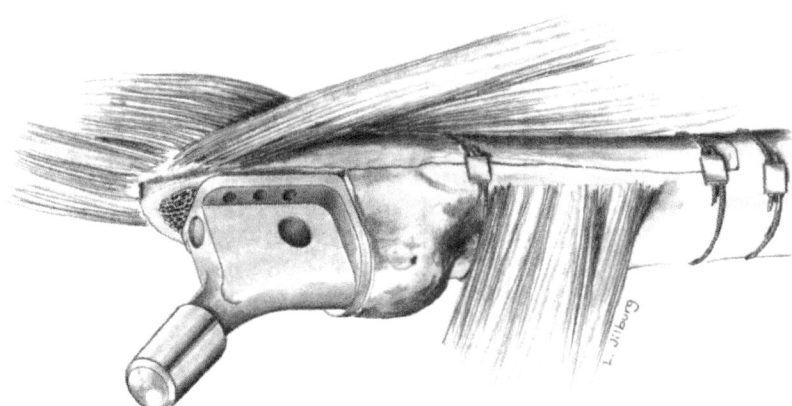

Figure 40.3. Osteotomy is closed over lateral aspect of prosthesis and cabled.

rely on the integrity of the remaining intact proximal femur. Stability of the joint is assessed initially with trial components in place and then with the actual components and the osteotomy fragment temporarily reduced. The endosteal surface of the osteotomy fragment can be debrided and shaped to fit the lateral aspect of the component. The osteotomy fragment is reduced and held in position by two cerclage cables passed prior. Adjustment of the osteotomy is done and retrialed by simply loosening and retightening the cable tighteners. Particulate graft can be placed at defect sites to promote healing. Cortical strut graft can also be used to supplement a weakened osteotomy.[21,22] Cables are crimped and cut (Fig. 40.3). Closure goes routinely.

Results

In reviewing the extended trochanteric osteotomy, union was achieved in 100% of the cases.[15] No fractures occurred from removal of old implant or materials. Fracture of the osteotomy did occur in a few cases but can commonly be prevented by releasing adherent anterior scar and capsule. Forces from the cable can be dissipated throughout the osteotomy fragment by placing a cortical onlay graft between the bone fragment and the cable when needed. Postoperative rehabilitation proceeds as if no osteotomy had been performed. Importantly, bone distal to the osteotomy site has been preserved which can support the new femoral revision stem, and because deformity is corrected, the optimal implant can be selected. Stability of the joint is further improved by fine tuning the soft tissue tension upon replacing the osteotomy fragment to its bed.

References

1. Harris WE. Revision surgery for failed, nonseptic total hip arthroplasty: the femoral side. *Clin Orthop.* 1982;170:8–20.
2. Shepherd BD, Turnbull A. The fate of femoral windows in revision joint arthroplasty. *J Bone Joint Surg Am.* 1989;71:716–718.
3. Turner RH, Emerson RH. Femoral revision total hip arthroplasty. *Revision total hip arthroplasty.* New York: Grune and Stratton; 1982:75–104.
4. Cameron HU. Femoral windows for easy cement removal in hip revision surgery. *Orthop Rev.* 1990;19:909–912.
5. Dennis DA, Dingman CA, Meglan DA, et al. Femoral cement removal in revision total hip arthroplasty: a biomechanical analysis. *Clin Orthop.* 1987;220:142–147.
6. Sydney SV, Mallory TH. Controlled perforation: a safe method of cement removal from the femoral canal. *Clin Orthop.* 1990;253:168–172.
7. Glassman AH, Engh CA, Bobyn JD. A technique of extensile exposure for total hip arthroplasty. *J Arthroplasty.* 1987;2:11–21.
8. Amstutz HC, Ma SM, Jinnah RH, et el. Revision of aseptic loose total hip arthroplasties. *Clin Orthop.* 1982;170:21–28.
9. Callaghan JJ, Salvati EA, Pellicci PM, et el. Results of revision for mechanical failure after cemented total hip replacement, 1979 to 1982: a two to five year follow-up. *J Bone Joint Surg Am.* 1985;67:1074–1085.
10. Kavanaugh BF, Ilstrup DM, Fitzgerald RH Jr. Revision total hip arthroplasty. *J Bone Joint Surg Am.* 1985;67:517–526.
11. Kavanagh BF, Fitzgerald RH. Multiple revisions for failed total hip arthroplasty not associated with infection. *J Bone Joint Surg Am.* 1987;69:1144–1149.
12. Pellici PM, Wilson PD Jr, Sledge CB, et el. Revision total hip arthroplasty. *Clin Orthop.* 1982;170:34–46.
13. Pellicci PM, Wilson PD Jr, Sledge CB, et el. Long-term results of revision total hip replacement: a follow-up report. *J Bone Joint Surg Am.* 1985;67:513–516.
14. Wroblewski BM, Shelley P. Reattachment of the greater trochanter after hip replacement. *J Bone Joint Surg Br.* 1985;67:736–740.
15. Younger TI, Bradford MS, Magnus RE, Paprosky WG. Extended proximal femoral osteotomy: a new technique for femoral revision arthroplasty. *J Arthroplasty.* 1995;10:329–338.
16. Chin AK, Moll FH, McColl MB, et al. An improved technique for cement extraction in revision total hip arthro-

plasty. *Contemp Orthop.* 1991;22:255-264.
17. Klapper RC, Caillouette JT, Callaghan JJ, Hozack WJ. Ultrasonic technology in revision joint arthroplasty. *Clin Orthop.* 1992;285:147-154.
18. Schurman DJ, Maloney WJ. Segmental cement extraction at revision total hip arthroplasty. *Clin Orthop.* 1992;285:158-163.
19. Engh CA, Massin P, Suthers KE. Roentgenographic assessment of the biologic fixation of porous-surfaced femoral components. *Clin Orthop.* 1990;257:107-127.
20. Glassman AH, Engh CA. The removal of porous-coated femoral stems. *Clin Orthop.* 1992;285:164-180.
21. Emerson RH, Malinin TI, Cuellar AD, et al. Cortical strut allografts in the reconstruction of the femur in revision total hip arthroplasty: a basic science and clinical study. *Clin Orthop.* 1992;285:35-44.
22. Pak JH, Lawrence JM, Jablonsky WS, Paprosky WG. Use of femoral strut allografts in cementless revision hip arthroplasty. *Clin Orthop.* 1993;295:172-179.

41
The Cameron Anterior Osteotomy

Hugh U. Cameron

Removal of a fully porous-coated, fully ingrown stem can be exceedingly difficult. This can frequently be avoided by using custom neck extensions[1] or constrained sockets.[2] However, occasionally the challenge has to be faced because of infection, implant malposition, or severe, unrelieved end of stem pain.

A straight stem can be removed by means of an extended trochanteric osteotomy,[3] implant section, and a crown drill or hollow mill. Unfortunately, if the stem is bowed, a crown drill cannot be used as the current models are not flexible and will therefore not follow the curve of the implant.

The problem can be handled either by transverse osteotomies[4] or by an anterior femoral osteotomy.[5] The transverse osteotomy technique first involves a very long extended trochanteric osteotomy, which is then freed from the implant by means of sharp curved osteotomes. The metal is transected and the proximal end removed. Tiny high-speed burrs are used to free the remaining implant as far distally as possible. A transverse femoral osteotomy is then made at the stem tip and the burrs are passed proximally in retrograde fashion. This

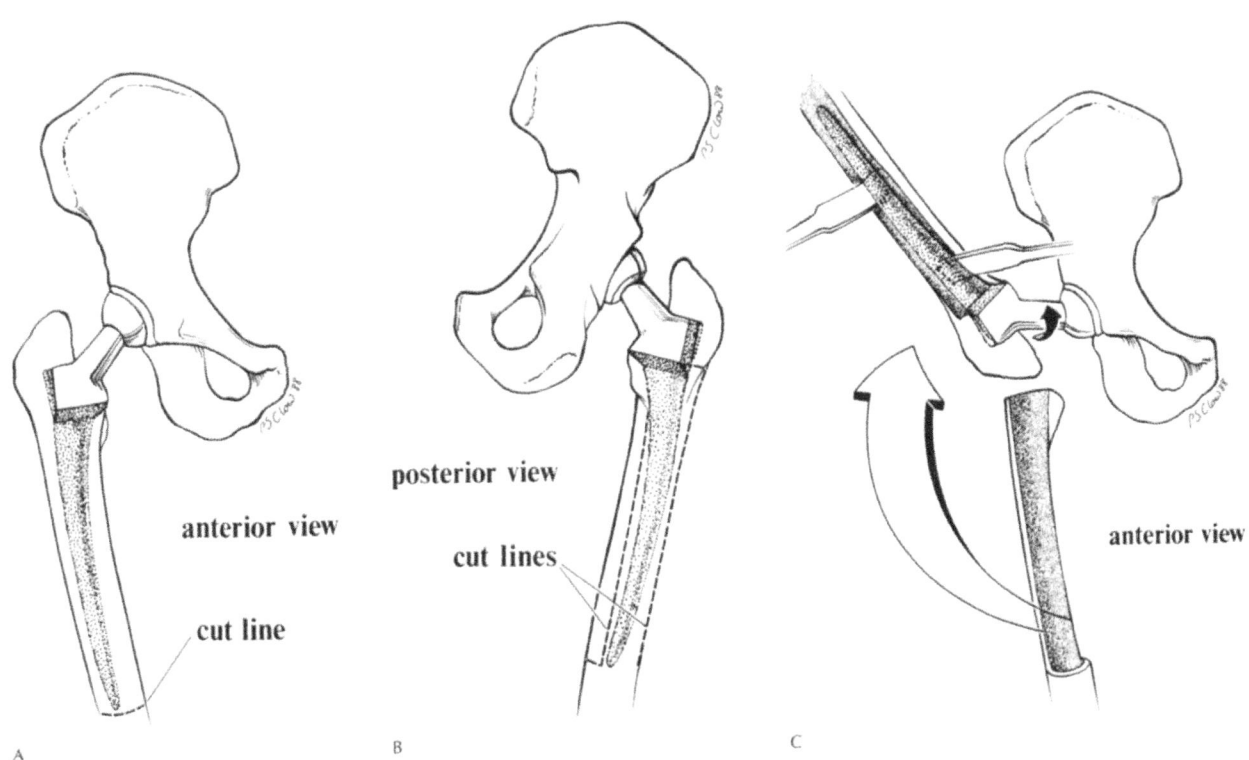

Figure 41.1. A. A femoral osteotomy is performed at the tip of the implant leaving the posterior one-third of the femur intact. B. The greater trochanter remains attached to the proximal fragment. C. The proximal fragment is loosened from the posterior fragment and turned up, giving access to all ingrowth surfaces. (Figures courtesy of Contemporary Orthopaedics 1989; 28:565–572)

is exceedingly time-consuming, but it does leave some blood supply attached to the proximal femur.

The alternative procedure is an anterior femoral osteotomy, which starts by skeletonizing the femur down to the tip of the implant. A transverse saw cut is made at the tip going around two-thirds of the anterior femur (Fig. 41.1). Vertical cuts are then made by going up either side of the rough line posteriorly leaving the posterior third of the proximal portion of the femur attached to the distal part. Thin curved osteotomes are then used to free the attachment of the implant to the posterior third of the femur, and the whole osteotomy bearing the implant is turned up. This gives access to all faces of the implant; that is the tip, collar, and sides. With gentleness and patience, the implant can be removed with tiny, high speed burrs and flexible osteotomes.

The proximal fragment of the femur is wired back to the distal fragment with a few cerclage wires and is surprisingly stable. Because of the large area of contact, in spite of the damage to the blood supply, bone union is rapid. This osteotomy should only be used in desperate situations where there is no other alternative. The main complication is infection. Should this occur, because the whole proximal femur is initially devascularized, loss of the whole anterior bone flap can occur. This occurred in one case, and salvage proved exceedingly difficult, requiring massive allografting after the infection had been relieved.

Implant choice following an anterior osteotomy is limited. Cement obviously should not be used as it will fill the osteotomy site preventing union. Similarly, a short ingrowth implant will gain no attachment, at least initially, to the devascularized femur, and bending forces will be resisted only by the cerclage wires until union occurs. A straight long-stem should not be used as it will prevent approximation of the proximal part of the osteotomy. A long-bowed stem is therefore required, bypassing the distal cut by at least two canal diameters. Optimally, at least 5 cm of full cortical contact should be obtained distally to unload the osteotomy site, and a proximal collar or sleeve overhang is required to allow vertical load transmission to the upper end of the femur.

References

1. Cameron HU. Use of a neck extension sleeve in total hip replacement. *Contemp Orthop.* 1990;21:67–69.
2. Cameron HU. Use of a constrained acetabular component in revision hip surgery. *Contemp Orthop.* 1991;23:41–49.
3. Cameron HU. Use of a distal trochanteric osteotomy in hip revision. *Contemp Orthop.* 1991;23:235–241.
4. Cameron HU. Further notes on removal of an extensively ingrown hip prosthesis. *Contemp Orthop.* 1993;27:329–333.
5. Cameron HU. Proximal femoral osteotomy in difficult revision hip surgery: how to revise the unrevisable. *Contemp Orthop.* 1989;28:565–572.

42
Retroperitoneal Approach

Steven J. Camer and Joseph C. McCarthy

Intrapelvic extension of polymethylmethacrylate (PMMA) poses a dilemma for the surgeon during revision arthroplasty. Its presence indicates that the medial wall has been compromised, either during the previous joint procedure or from trauma or osteolysis. When the medial acetabular wall has been violated the intraabdominal contents of the pelvis become at risk. These structures include the ureter, vagina, rectum, and most importantly, the iliac vessels.[1] (See Part 5, Chapter 59.)

Indications

During the era when cemented acetabular components were inserted with the Charnley medialization technique or with 3.5 inch recess holes in the ilium, ischium, and pubis there were many occasions when PMMA extruded intrapelvically. When the cement bolus was isolated, small in size and not symptomatic, it could usually be left *in situ*. At other times however, the cement should be removed during revision surgery. These situations include:

- Encroachment or fistula formation with intrapelvic organs, including the bladder, vagina and rectum.
- Voluminous cement mass > 2 cm within pelvis especially if symptomatic.
- Dislodgement or displacement of PMMA from trauma or protrusio.
- Mushroom configuration of PMMA where component removal may result in tethering vessels.
- Cement or medial screw positioning resulting in vessel distortion.
- In massive protrusio to affix a medial wall bone graft.

Imaging

When intrapelvic protrusion of cement, component or screw risks injury to the pelvic contents radiographic imaging is essential to identify its proximity to neurovascular and organ structures. Plain radiographs with pelvic inlet and outlet views will define the bony architecture. Soft tissue definition however will require CT scanning, vascular ultrasound studies, venography or, more recently, MR arthrography (see Chapter 7). The ultimate determination of whether a retroperitoneal approach is necessary will in large part be determined by the 3-D locatization of the intrapelvic material as defined by these studies.

Surgical Approach

This approach can be performed as an isolated or two-stage procedure for cement or hardware removal. When done as part of a one-stage revision arthroplasty, the pa-

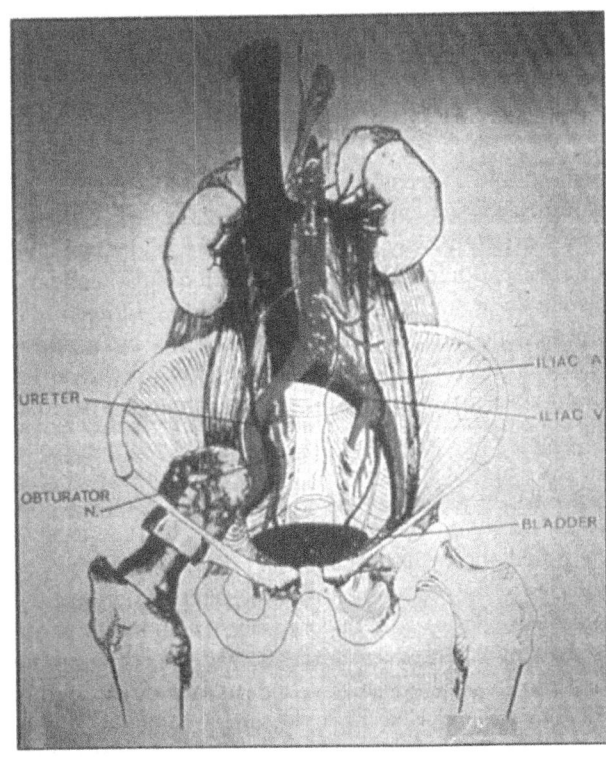

Figure 42.1. Retroperitoneal cement adjacent to neurovascular bundle. (See color insert.)

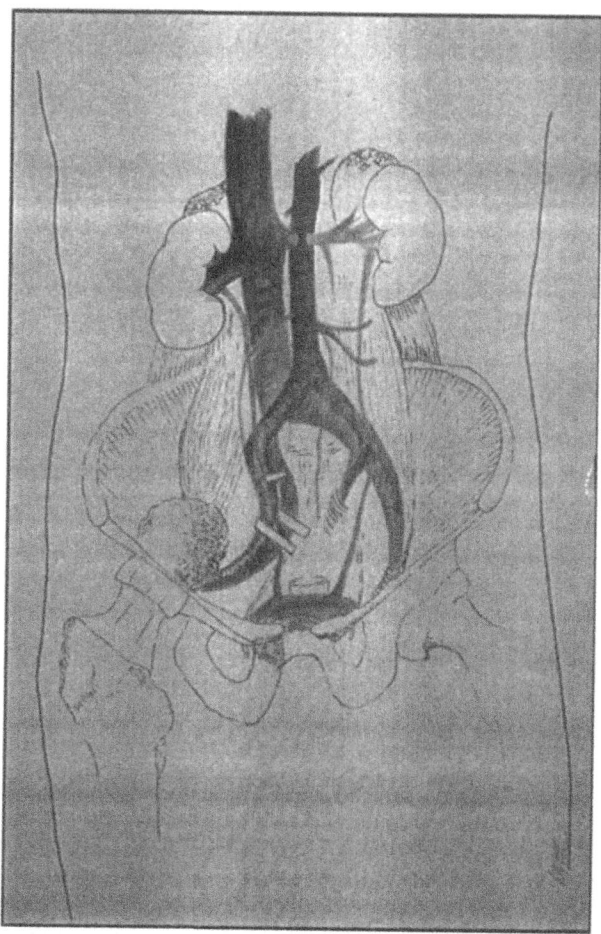

Figure 42.2. Retroperitoneal approach exposing and protecting iliac vessels. (See color insert.)

and genitourinary contents. For a left hip approach, the aorta will be the nearest great vessel; for a right hip, the vena cava. Both of these great vessels are anchored in place by an arcade of lumbar arteries and veins. When approaching the right pelvic cavity, retraction should be gentle to avoid injury to the vena cava. The genitofemoral nerve is located on the anteromedial side of the iliopsoas and the ureter between the peritoneum and psoas. Neither should be encountered if the psoas is protected.

The external iliac artery branches from the common iliac artery anterior to the sacroiliac joint and extends obliquely downward along the medial border of the psoas muscle. Beneath the inguinal ligament it continues as the femoral artery. Control of this vessel and its tributaries is accomplished by placement of a spaghetti ligature both proximally near the SI joint and distally near the inguinal ligament. Once this is completed, the protruding cement can be morselized and removed. Alternatively, should a screw be abutting the vessel adventitia, it can now be slowly and safely be backed out. Finally, should a medial segmental bone graft be necessary for a massive defect, it an be safely secured under direct vision.

tient should be positioned on the side and then rolled back to a 45° semilateral position.[2] This allows the pelvic contents to fall away from the operative field. The pelvis and chest should be securely supported on a pegboard, bean bag, or similar padded device. The perineal nerve on the dependent leg should be protected and all bony prominences should be padded. The operative leg should be draped free and the perineum sealed off from the operative field.

The incision is initiated over the iliac crest, stopping anteriorly at the lateral border of the rectus tendon. The fascia overlying the medial border of the iliac crest is identified and incised in line with the skin incision. The muscles of the abdominal wall, the external oblique, the internal oblique, and the transversus abdominus are split sequentially. Every effort is made to continue the dissection subperiosteally along the medial iliac wing. The iliopsoas muscle and peritoneal contents are reflected medially. Further blunt dissection will allow visualization over the pelvic brim into the quadrilateral space. A deep Dever retractor will protect the abdominal

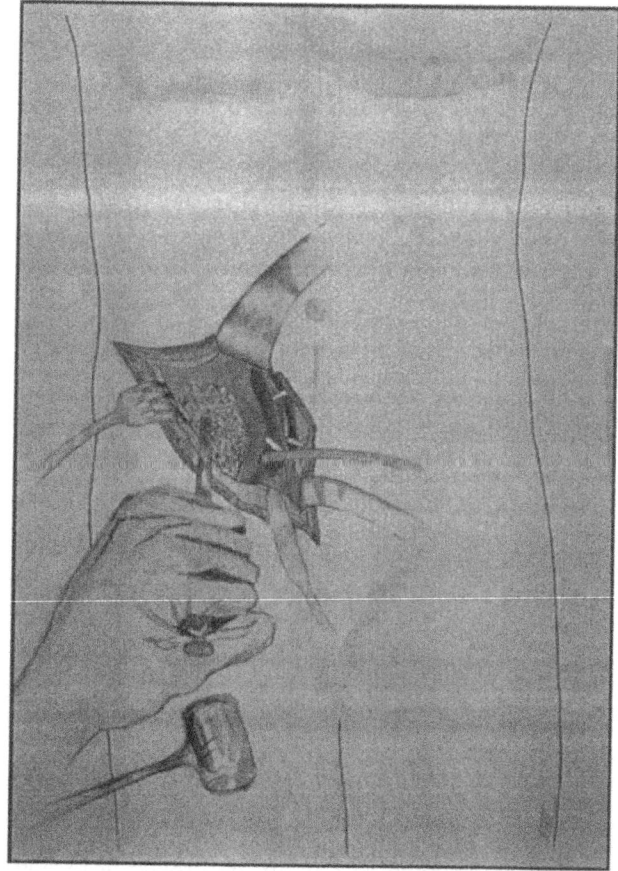

Figure 42.3. With vessels protected, intrapelvic cement is removed with an osteotome. (See color insert.)

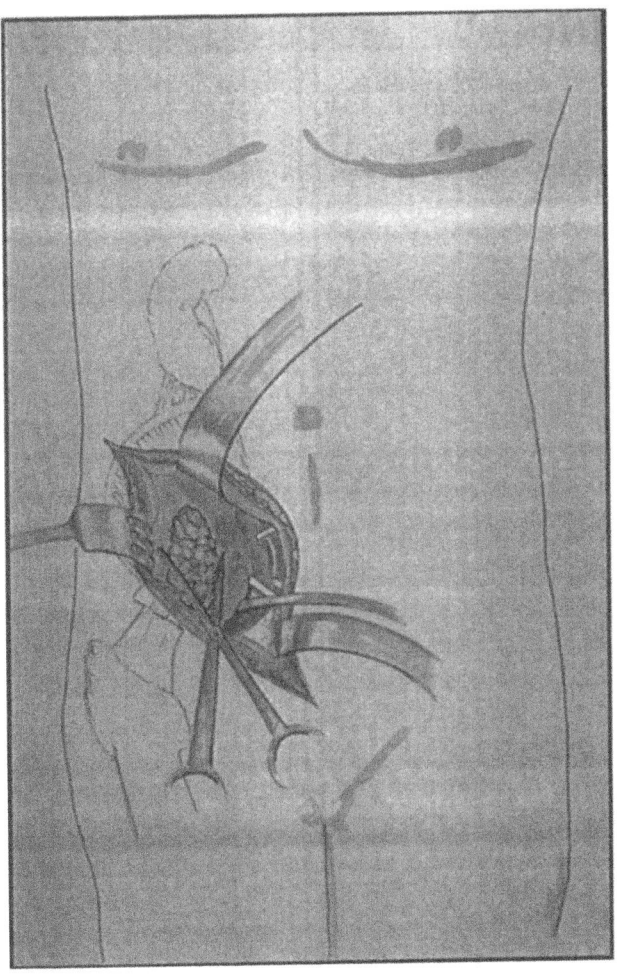

Figure 42.4. Kocher clamp around intrapelvic cement prior to removal from wound. (See color insert.)

The wound is then drained and the fascia closed in layers to avoid hernia formation. Postoperatively the patient should remain on intravenous fluids until bowel sounds return. On occasion a nasogastric tube will be necessary to treat paralytic ileus. If the patient is having a simultaneous hip exposure for revision surgery, keep the skin bridge as far apart as possible. All posterior and trochanteric approaches can be accommodated with this technique.

Conclusion

The retroperitoneal approach is an expeditious and safe approach to the inner pelvis. When faced with a revision procedure that may compromise the pelvis structures, the operating surgeon should consider this approach in concert with a vascular surgery colleague. A thorough understanding of the anatomy, combined with appropriate preoperative studies and good surgical technique will result in safe extraction of intrapelvic hardware. The new acetabular reconstruction can then be completed with considerably less potential morbidity.

References

1. Agur AM, Lee MJ. *Grants Atlas of Anatomy*. 9th ed, Baltimore: Williams & Wilkins, 1991.
2. McCarthy JC, Camer S. Retroperitoneal Approach to the Hip for Removal of Protruded Cement. American Academy of Orthopaedic Surgeons 60th Annual Meeting, San Francisco, CA, February 1993.

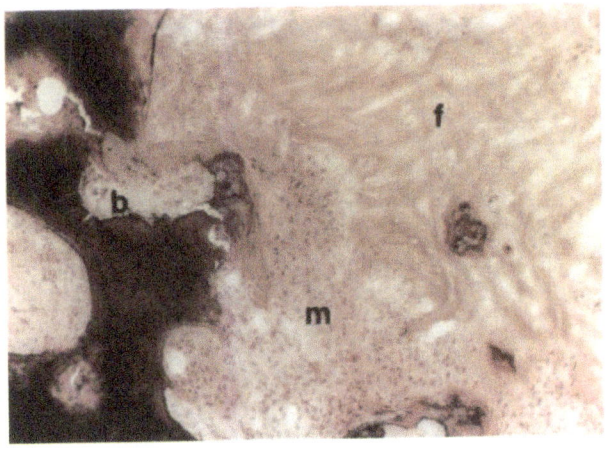
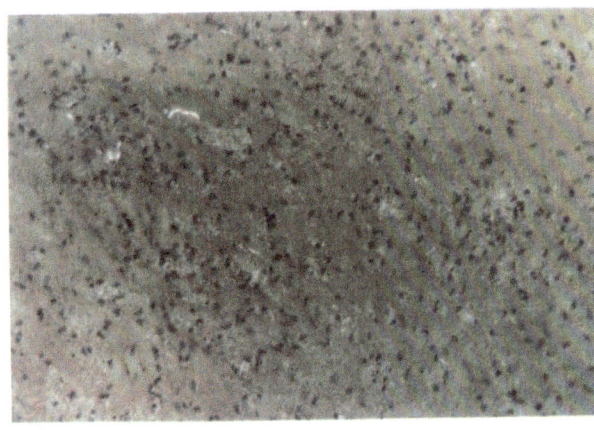
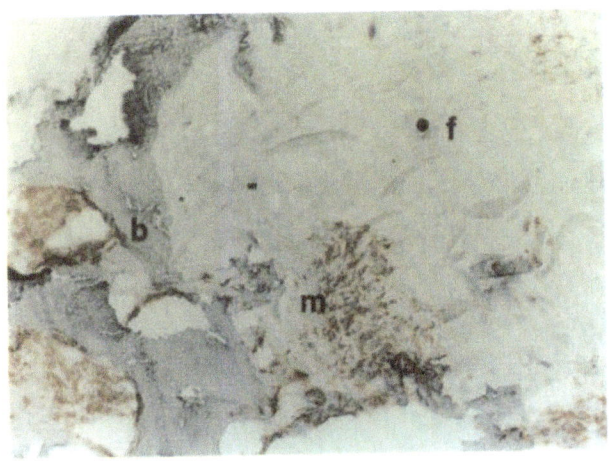
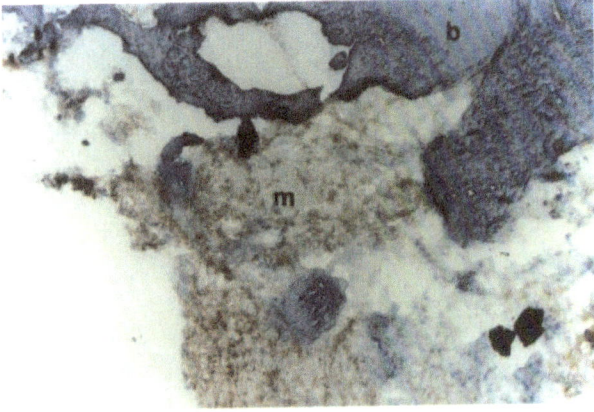
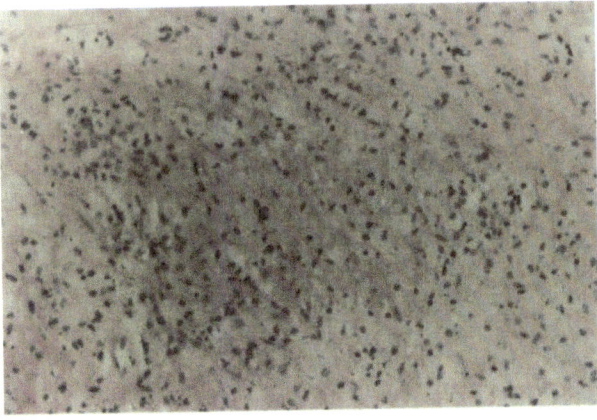

Figure 3.2. 2A. Linear osteolysis demonstrating the three layers: trabecular bone to the left (*b*), a macrophage infiltrate in the center (*m*), and the reparative fibrous layer to the right (*f*). X200, H&E. 2B. Linear osteolysis: a serial section to A treated with MAC 3 antibody (*red staining*) showing pockets of macrophages adjacent to bone but no staining in the fibrous tissue. X100, Hematoxylin. 2C. Transitional osteolysis, from a case of moderate erosive osteolysis around a cementless titanium component. The cells are primarily macrophages, there is less fibrous tissue (*pink*) and it is disorganized, and there is a large amount of titanium debris. 2D. Transitional osteolysis: a serial section from C taken under polarized light showing a large number of birefringent polyethylene particles. 2E. Aggressive osteolysis. This section is treated with MAC 3 antibody (specific for activated macrophages) showing virtually all cells are macrophages, with little reparative fibrous tissue response. There is a large amount of cell necrosis. X1200, Hematoxylin.

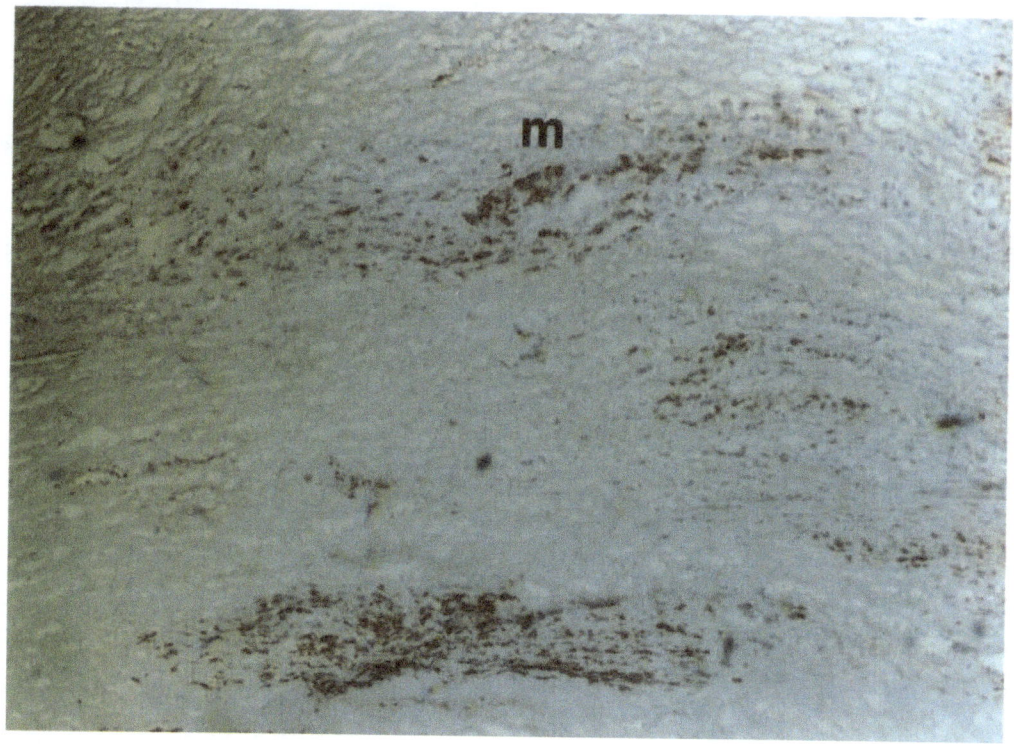

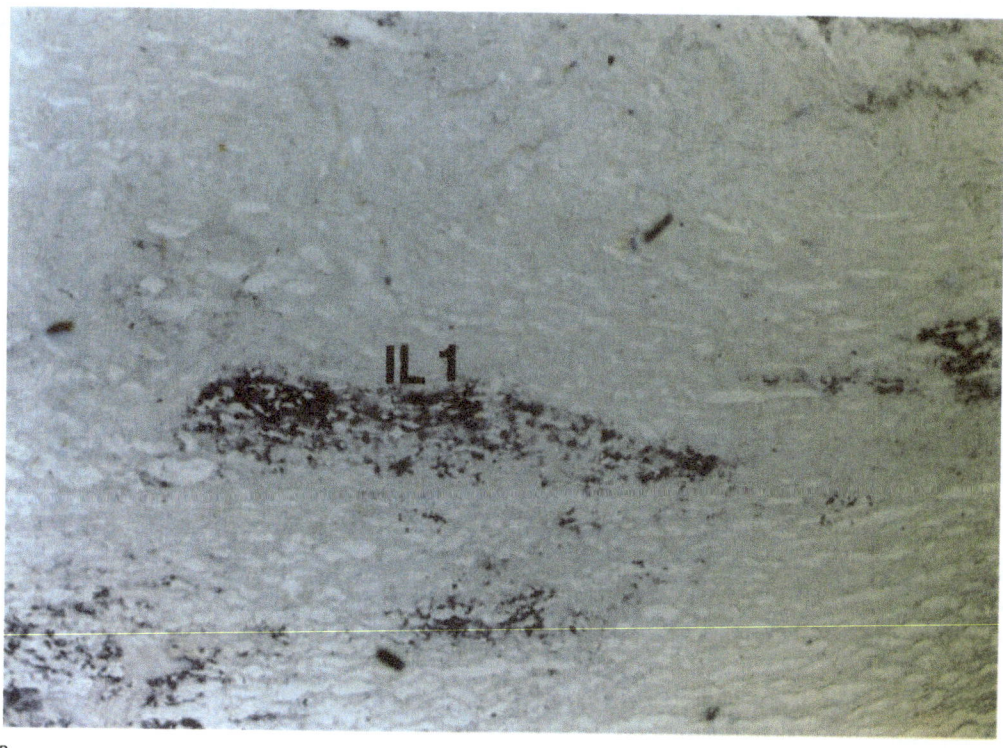

Figure 3.3. A. From a case of linear osteolysis, treated with MAC 3 antibody showing collections of macrophages (*red staining*) contained within well organized fibrous tissue. X40, H&E. B. A serial section, treated with a probe specific for interleukin 1B messenger RNA (*purple color*), showing that IL1 is being produced by the macrophage populations.

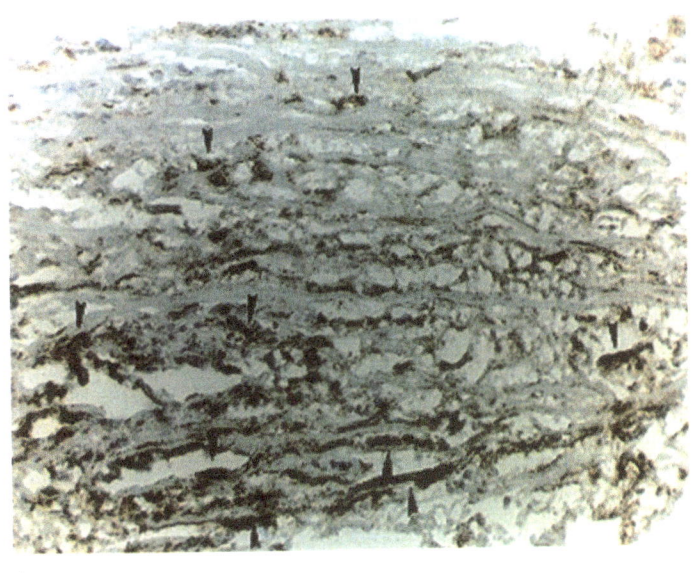

Figure 3.4. A. Specimen from linear osteolysis treated with antifibroblasts antibody, demonstrating a preponderance of positive cells. (AEC chromagen, X100). B. Serial section from Figure 4A, hybridized with Interleukin 1B probe, showing limited localization to fibroblasts. (X100).
C. Serial section from Figure 4A, hybridized with Interleukin 6 probe, showing large amount of localization to fibroblasts. (X100).

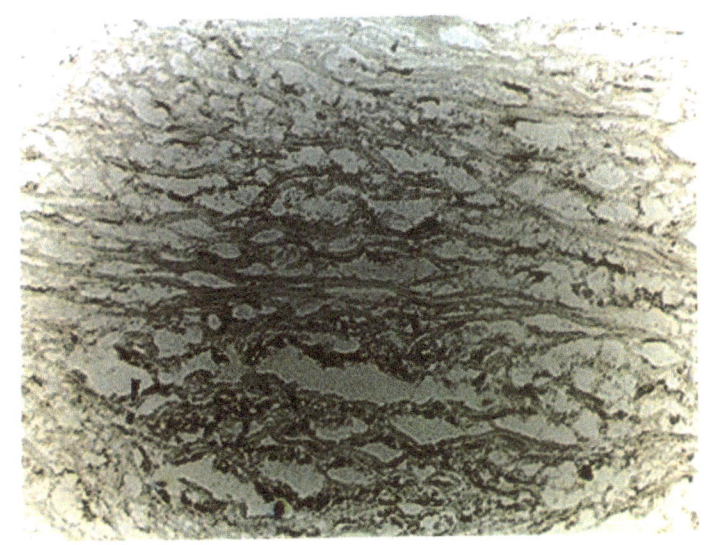

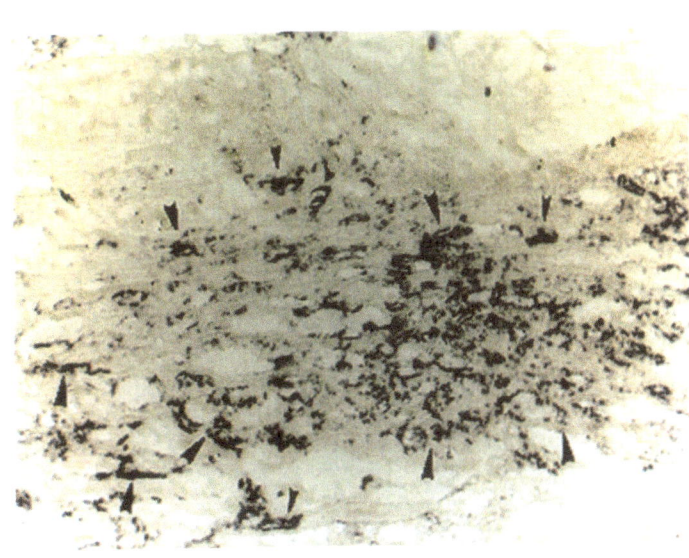

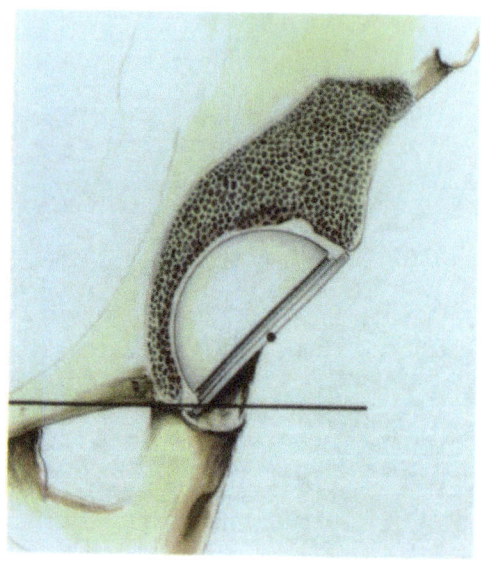

Figure 9.1. Type I acetabular defect.
Teardrop Lysis: None
Ischial Lysis: None
Kohler's Line: Grade I
Migration: None

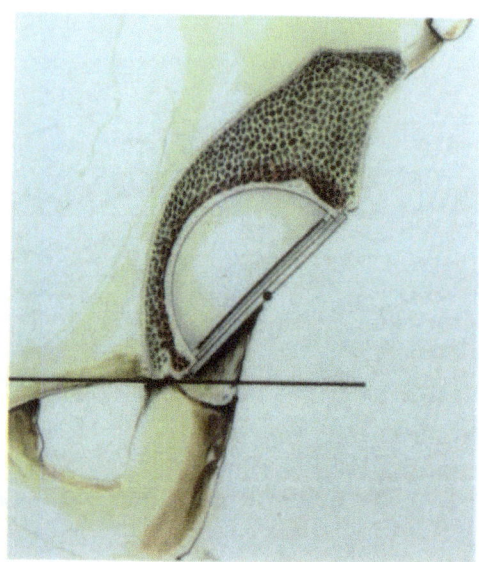

Figure 9.2. Type IIA acetabular defect.
Teardrop Lysis: Mild
Ischial Lysis: Mild
Kohler's Line: Grade I
Migration: <3.0 cm

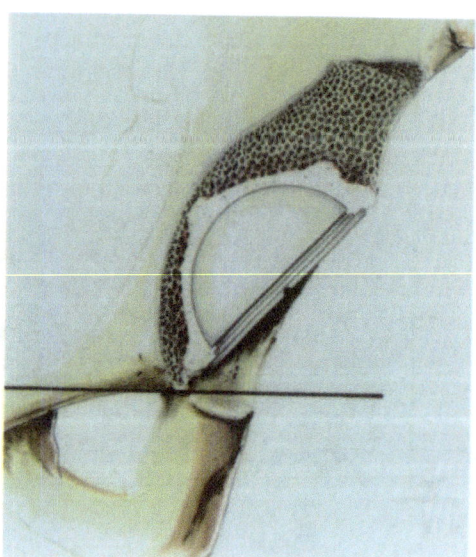

Figure 9.3. Type IIB acetabular defect.
Teardrop Lysis: Mild
Ischial Lysis: Mild
Kohler's Line: Grade I-II
Migration: <3.0 cm

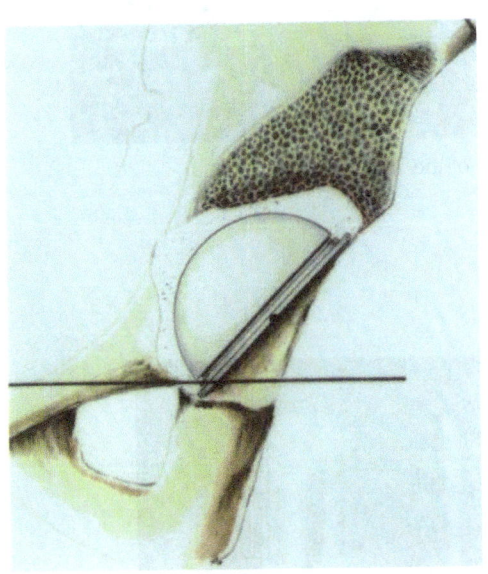

Figure 9.4. Type IIC acetabular defect.
Teardrop Lysis: Moderate/Severe
Ischial Lysis: Mild
Kohler's Line: Grade III
Migration: <3.0 cm

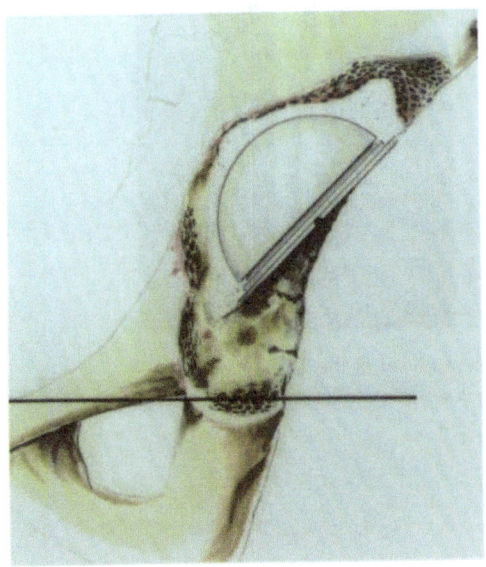

Figure 9.5. Type IIIA acetabular defect.
Teardrop Lysis: Moderate
Ischial Lysis: Mild/Moderate
Kohler's Line: Grade II, II+
Migration: >3.0 cm

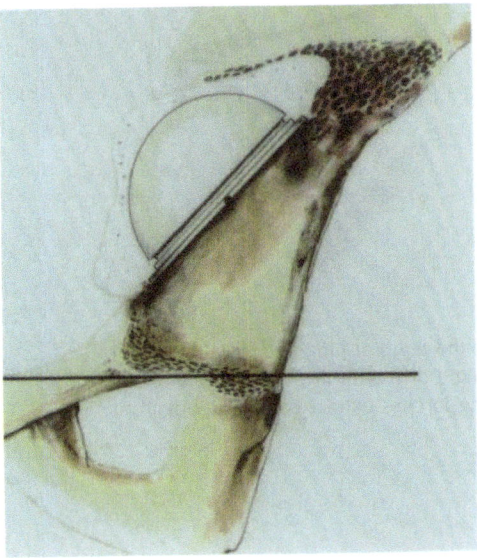

Figure 9.6. Type IIIB acetabular defect.
Teardrop Lysis: Severe
Ischial Lysis: Severe
Kohler's Line: Grade III+
Migration: >3.0 cm

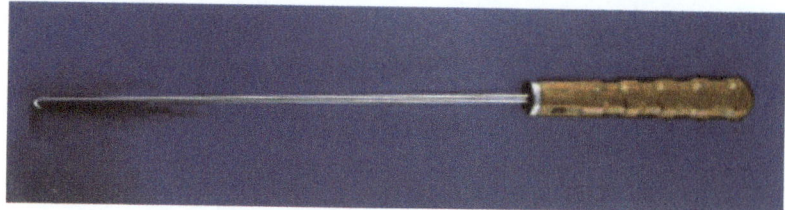

Figure 18.3. Cement removal tool of the Trebay system.

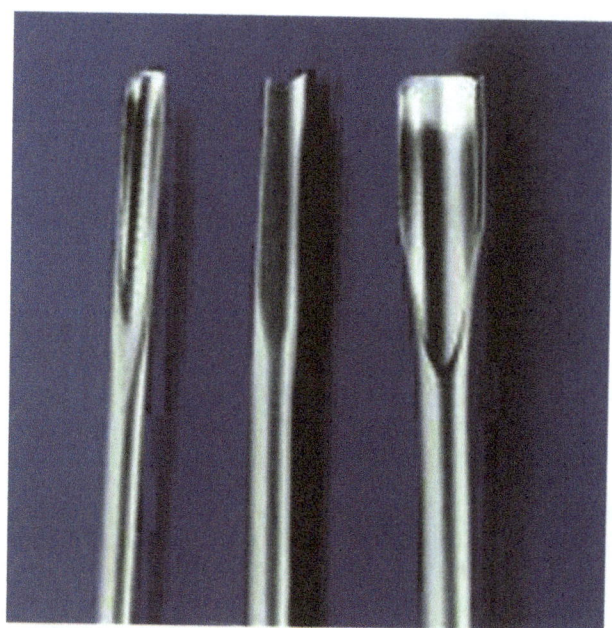

Figure 18.4. Circular cement chisel of the Trebay system.

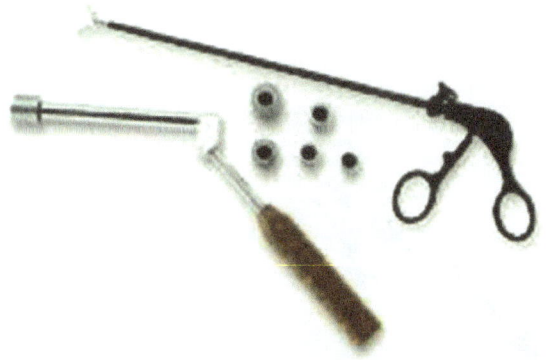

Figure 18.5. Extraction of the femoral plug and distal cement can be accomplished using a drill with the Trebay system centering handle. Grasping forceps extract cement debris from the distal canal.

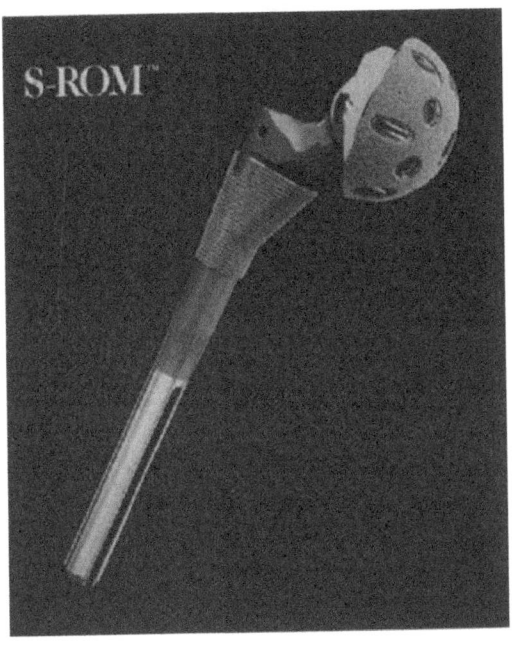

Figure 30.1. The two-piece stem design of the S-ROM prosthesis.

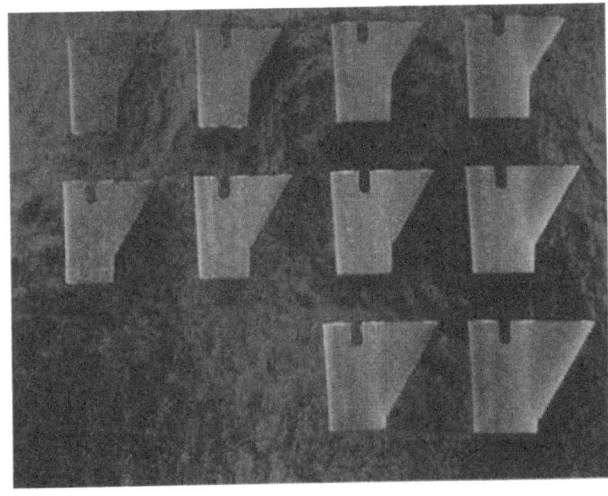

Figure 30.2. Ten proximal modular sleeve sizes are available for each stem.

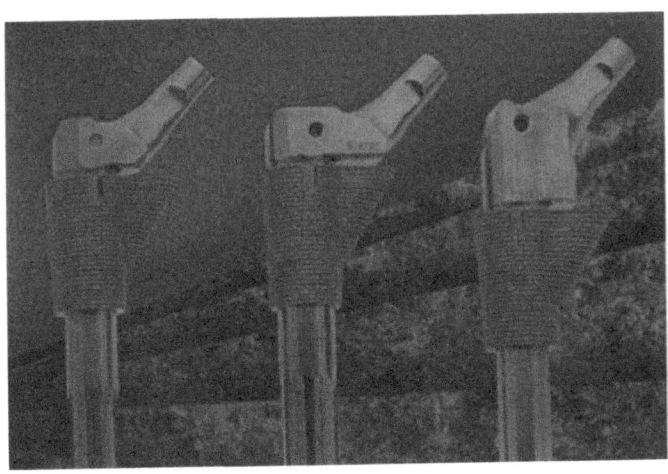

Figure 30.3. Variations in neck length and offset permit intraoperative customization to maximize stability.

Figure 30.4. A wide assortment of stem options is essential in revision surgery.

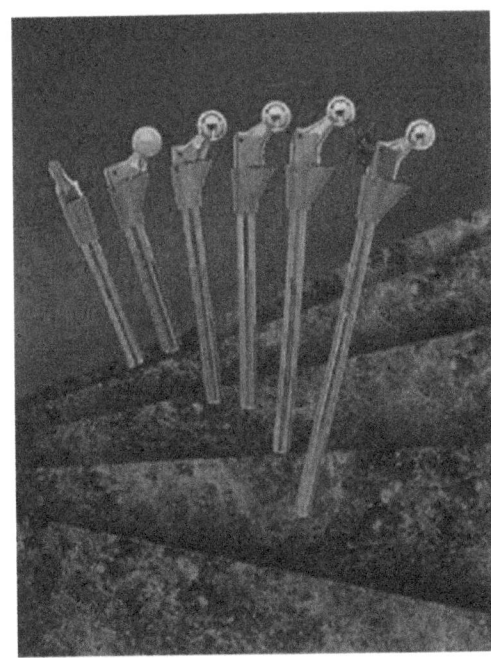

Figure 42.1. Retroperitoneal cement adjacent to neurovascular bundle.

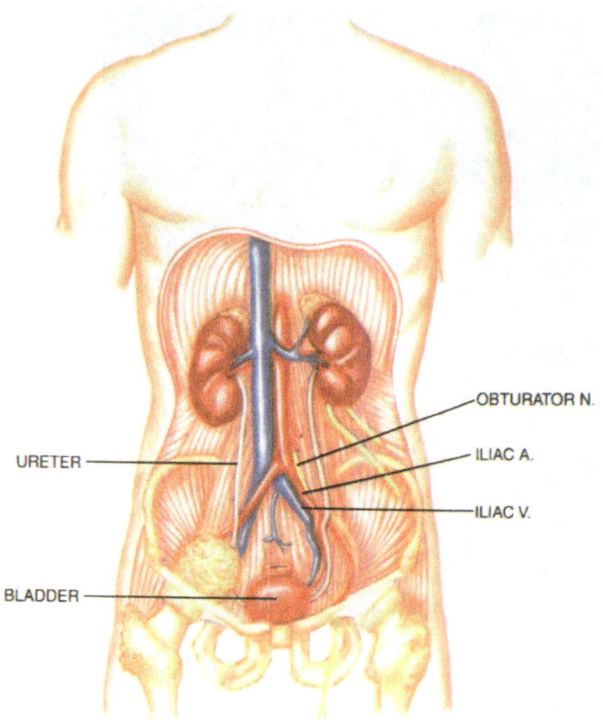

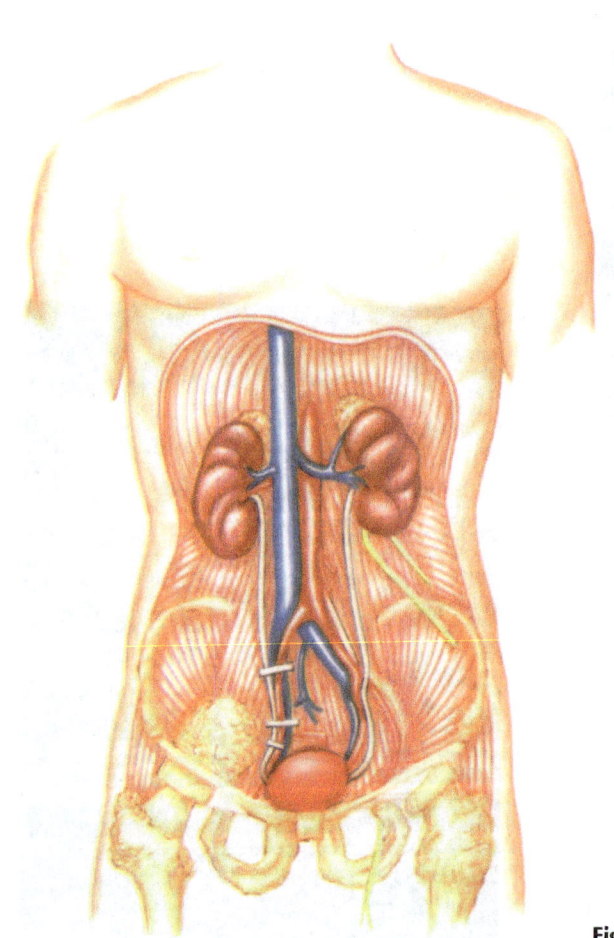

Figure 42.2. Retroperitoneal approach exposing and protecting iliac vessels.

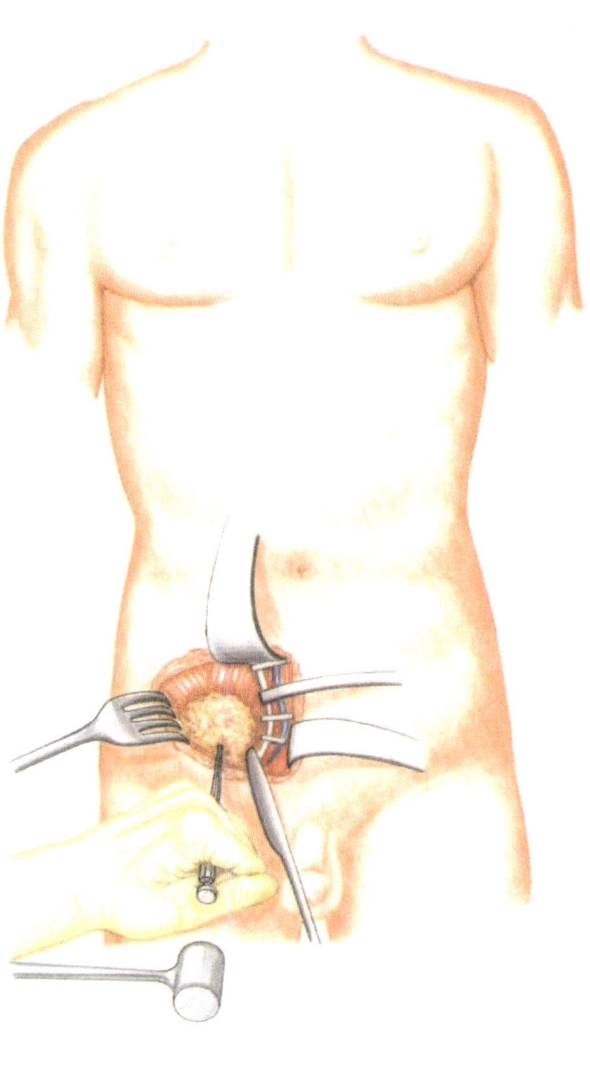

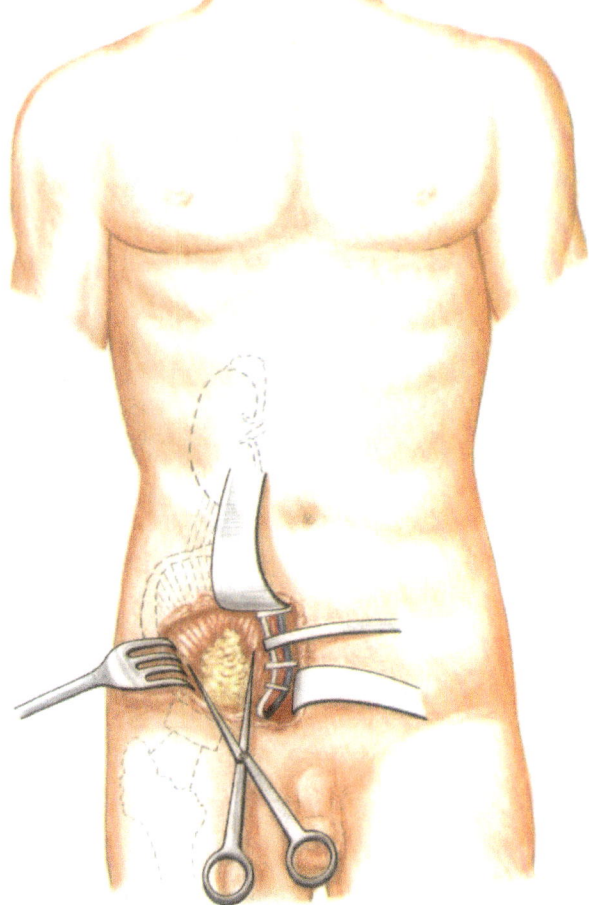

Figure 42.3. With vessels protected, intrapelvic cement is removed with an osteotome.

Figure 42.4. Kocher clamp around intrapelvic cement prior to removal from wound.

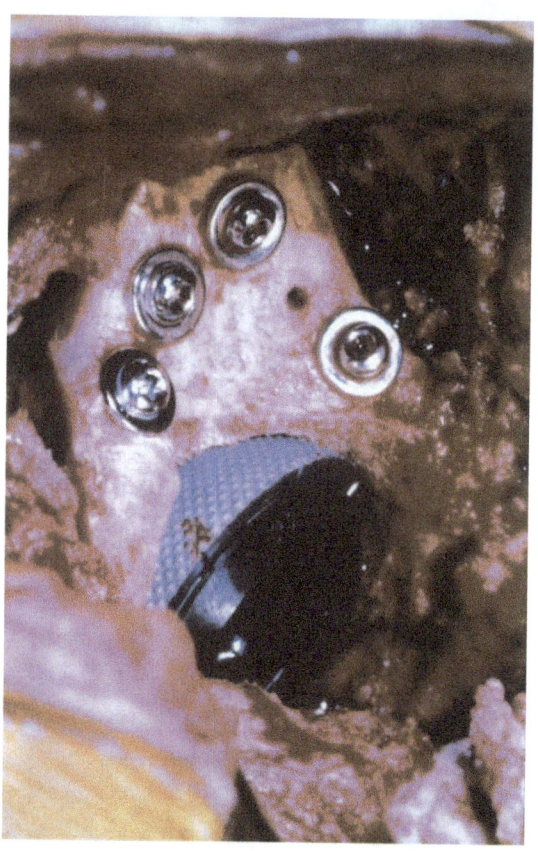

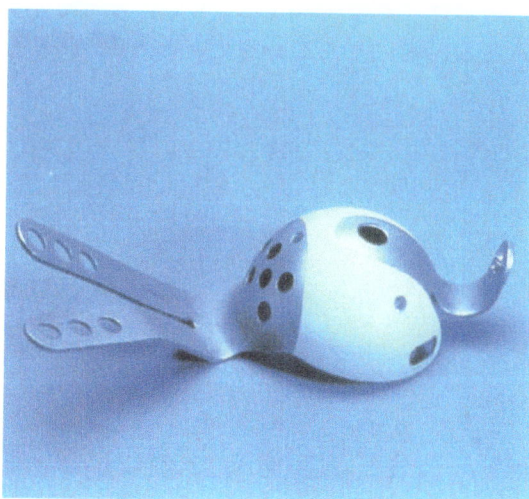

Figure 51.5. Graft augmentation prosthesis (GAP) with hydroxyapatite coating.

Figure 51.4. B. Intraoperative photograph showing bulk allograft in place.

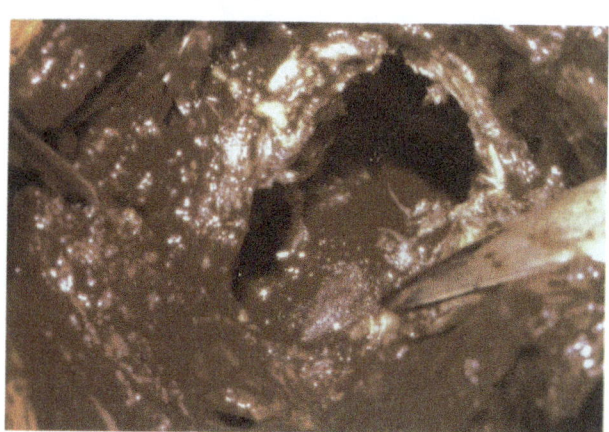

Figure 51.6. B. Intraoperative photograph showing acetabular defect.

Figure 51.6. C. Amount of morselized bone graft needed to fill defect.

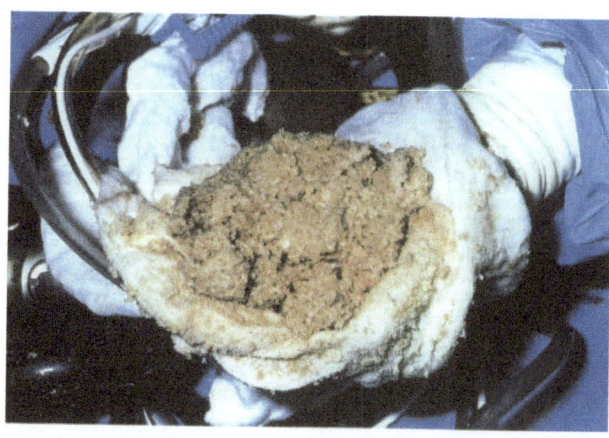

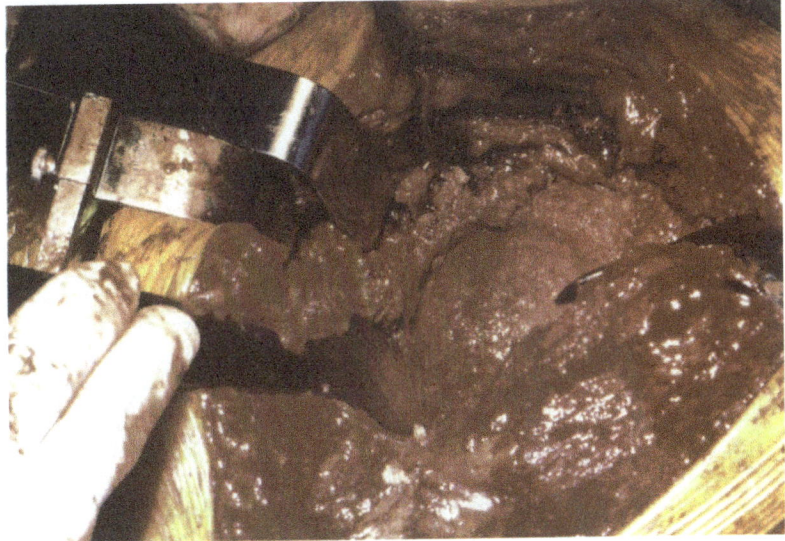

Figure 51.6. D. Intraoperative photograph showing defect filled with packed morselized bone graft.

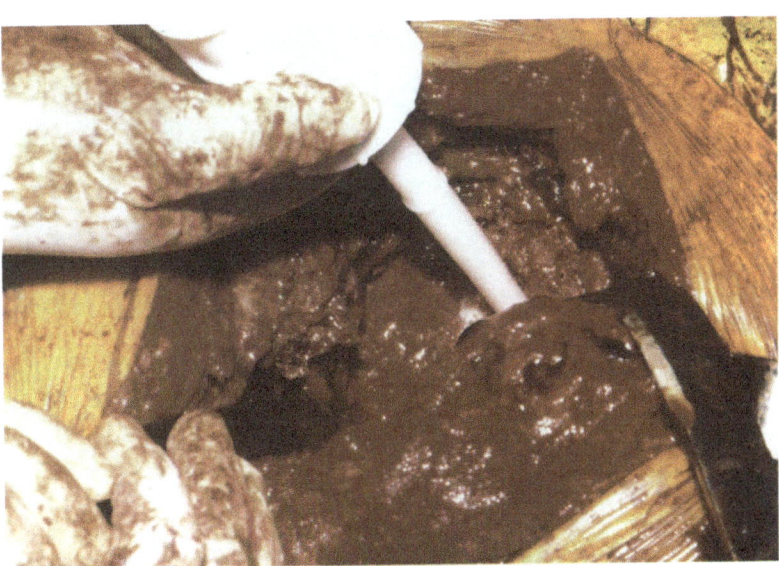

Figure 51.6. E. Intraoperative photograph showing cement pressure injected into packed bone graft.

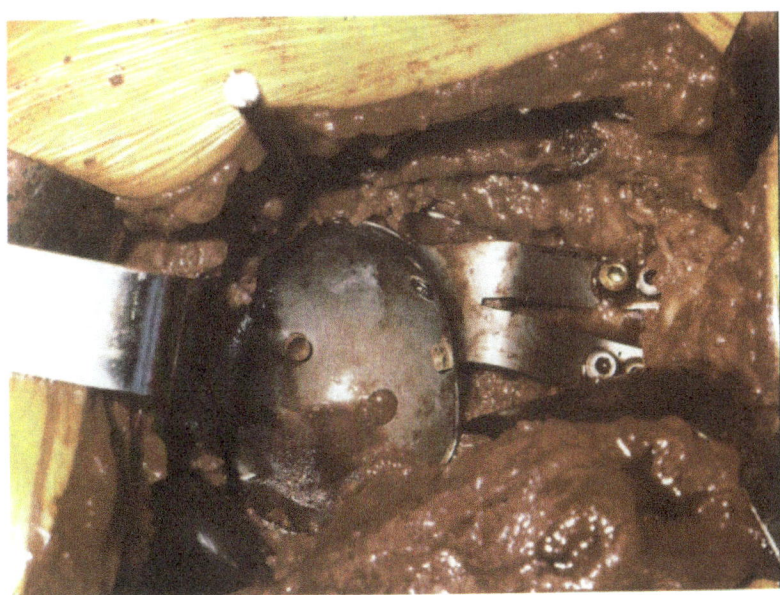

Figure 51.6. F. Intraoperative photograph of GAP cup in place.

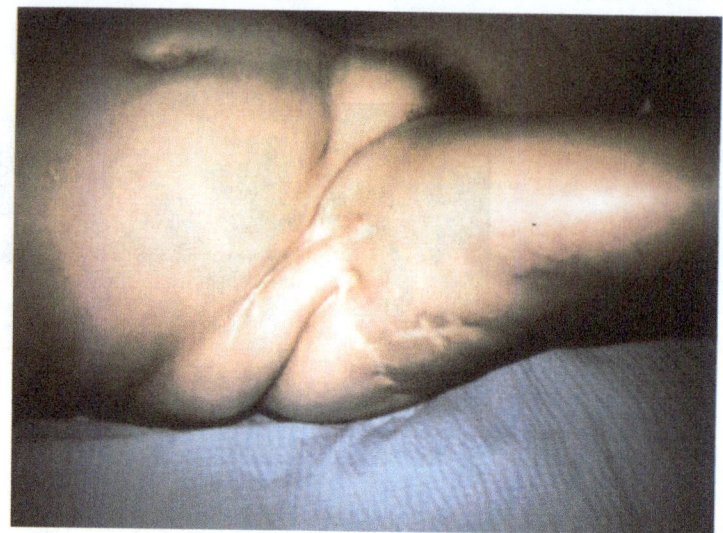

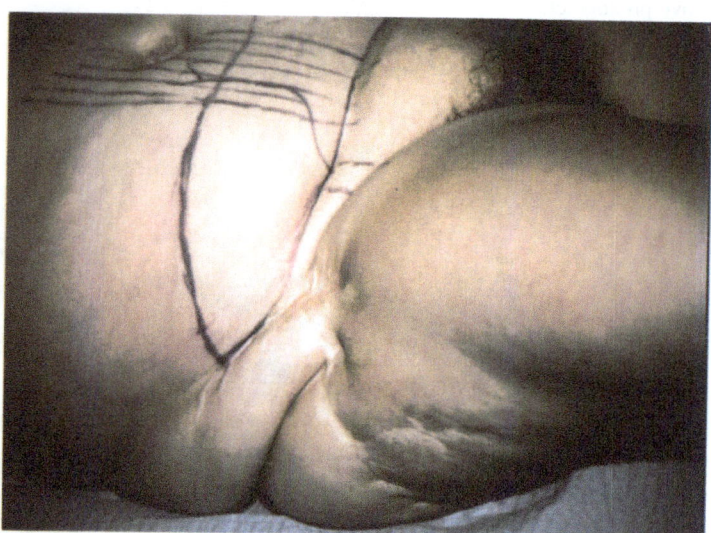

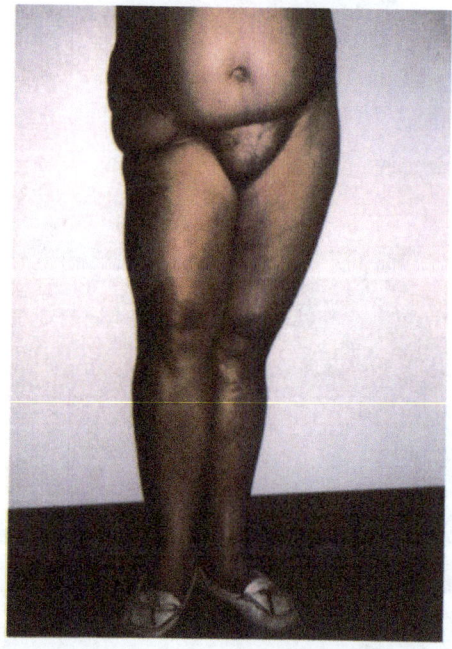

Figure 61.1. A. Scar contracture right hip status post multiple hip procedures. B. Design of inferiorly based rectus abdominis myocutaneous flap. C. Healed flap.

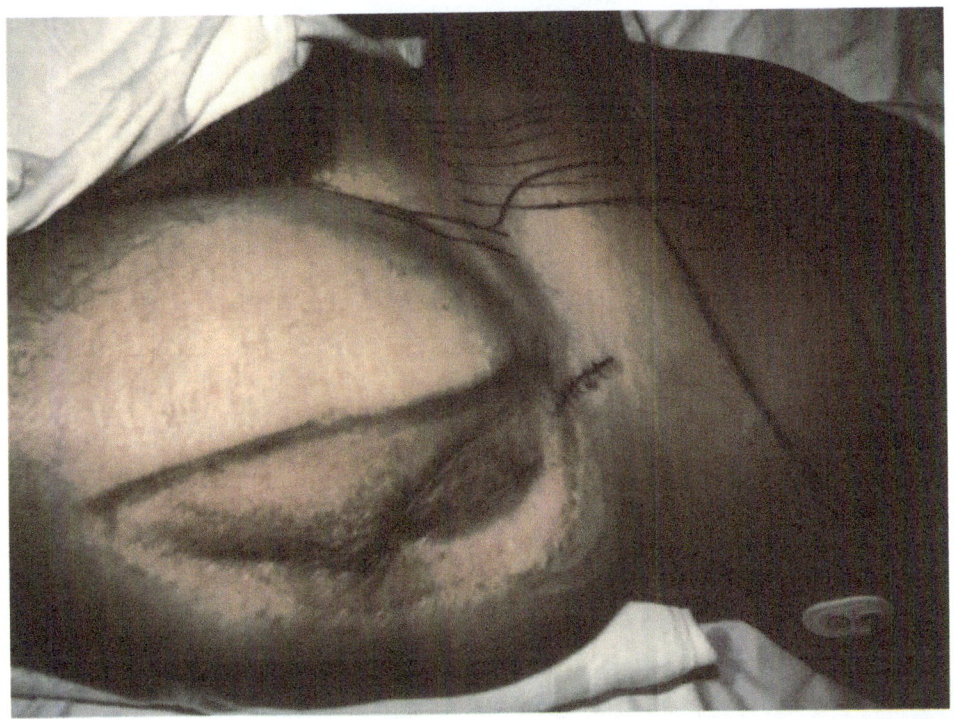

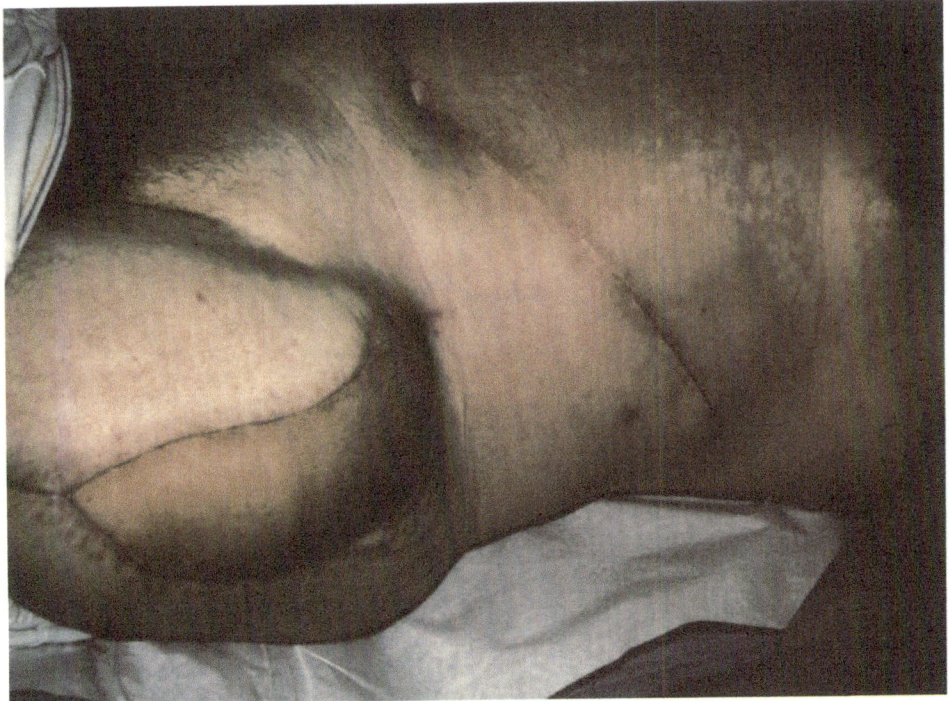

Figure 61.2. A. Traumatic wound left hip adjacent osteomyelitis of femur. C. Inferiorly based rectus abdominis myocutaneous flap following debridement.

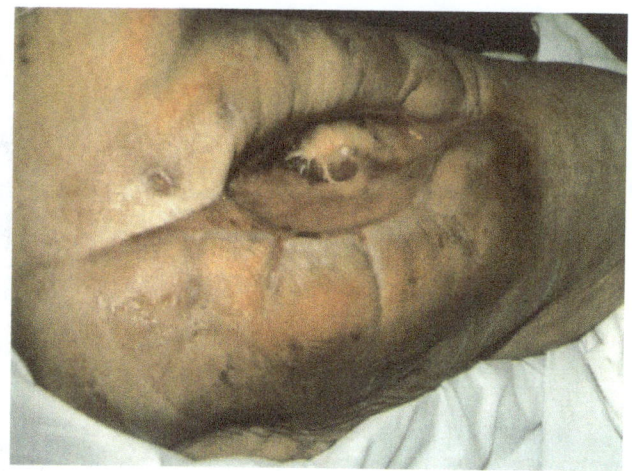

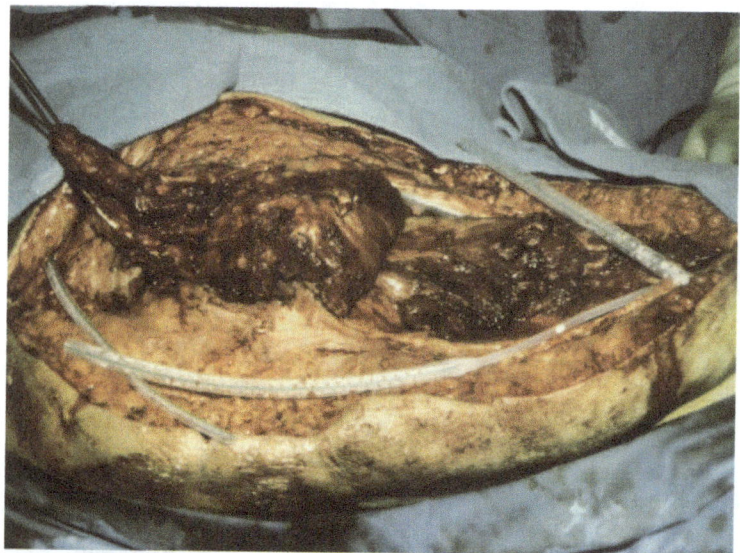

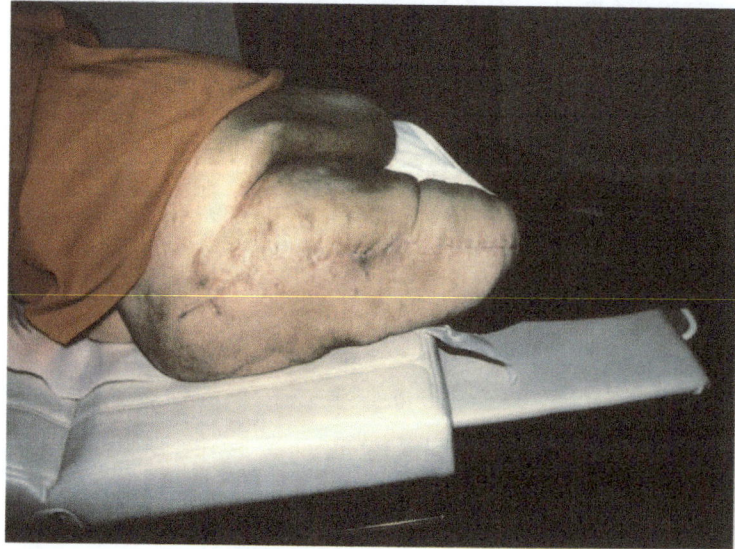

Figure 61.3. A. Infected girdlestone hip wound. C. Vastus lateralis muscle flap. D. Healed wound 6 months later.

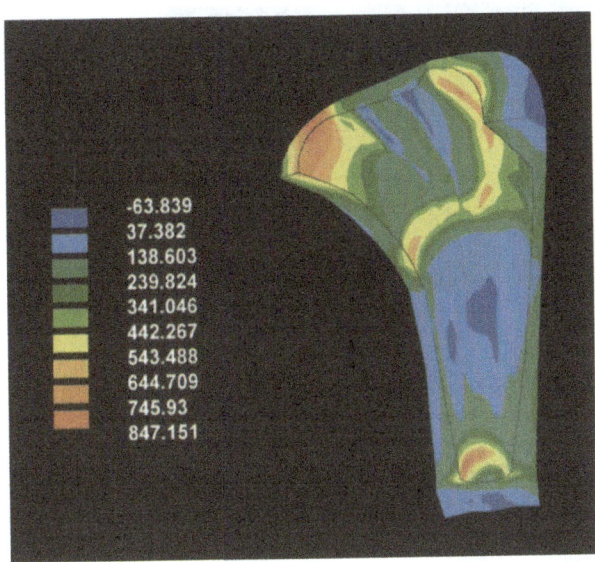

Figure 74.3. Finite element model and result showing location of maximum principal stress in the region of the distal tip of a femoral component. The bone and prosthesis have been removed and the cement mantle has been cross-sectioned along the M/L plane.

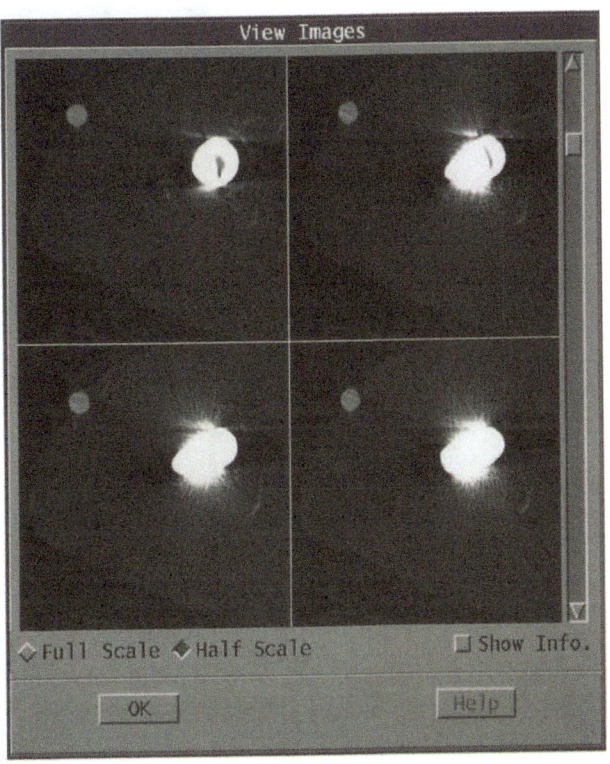

Figure 75.1. Cross-sectional ORTHODOC views of a CT study of a failing implant.

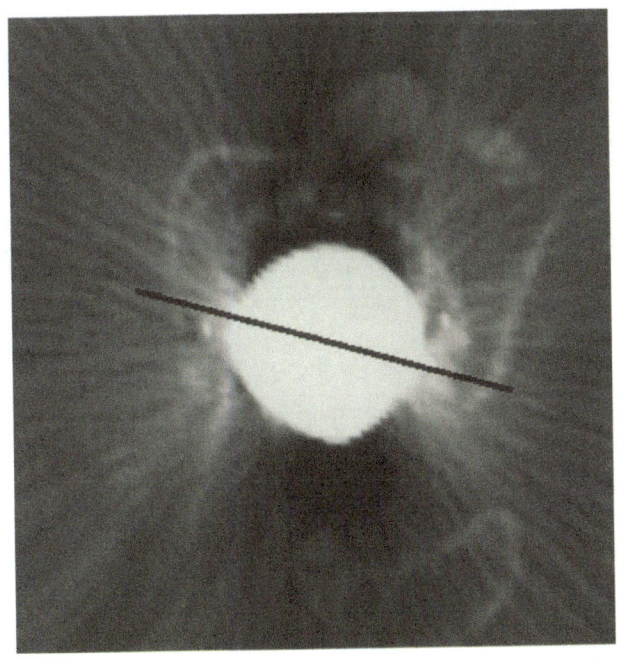

A

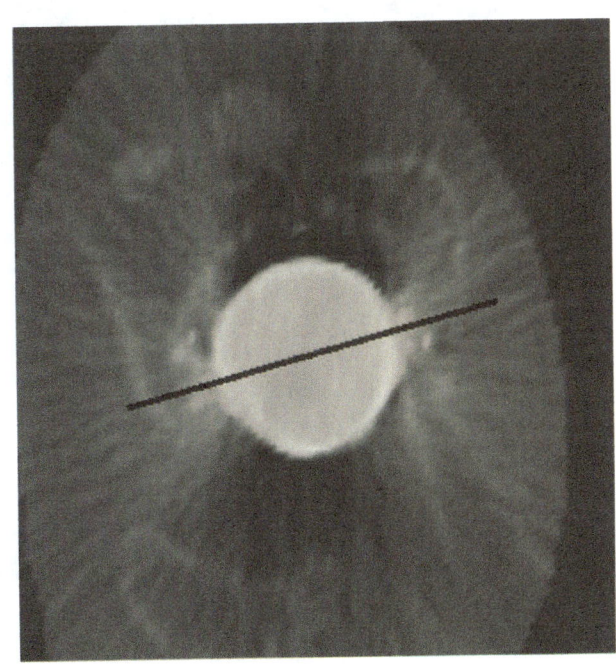

B

Figure 75.2. A. Original CT axial image of bone with implant. B. Artifact reduced image of bone with implant.

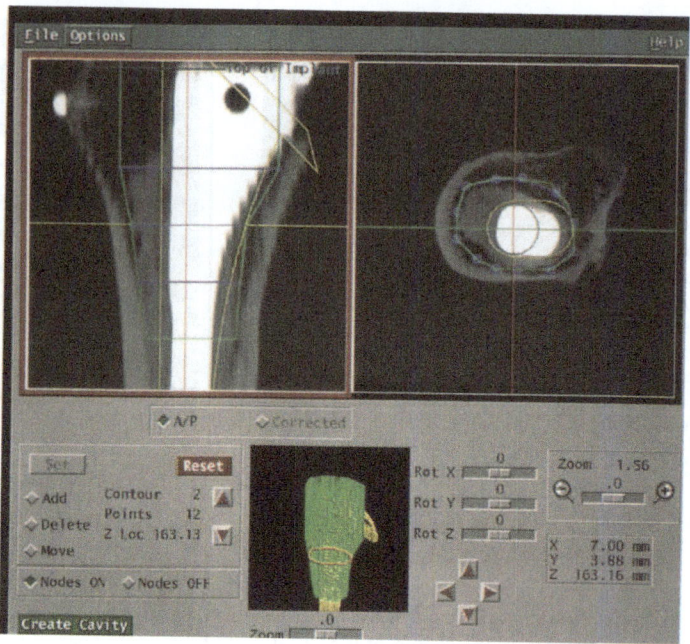

Figure 75.3. Example of user interface surgeon uses to interactively define cut cavity for robot.

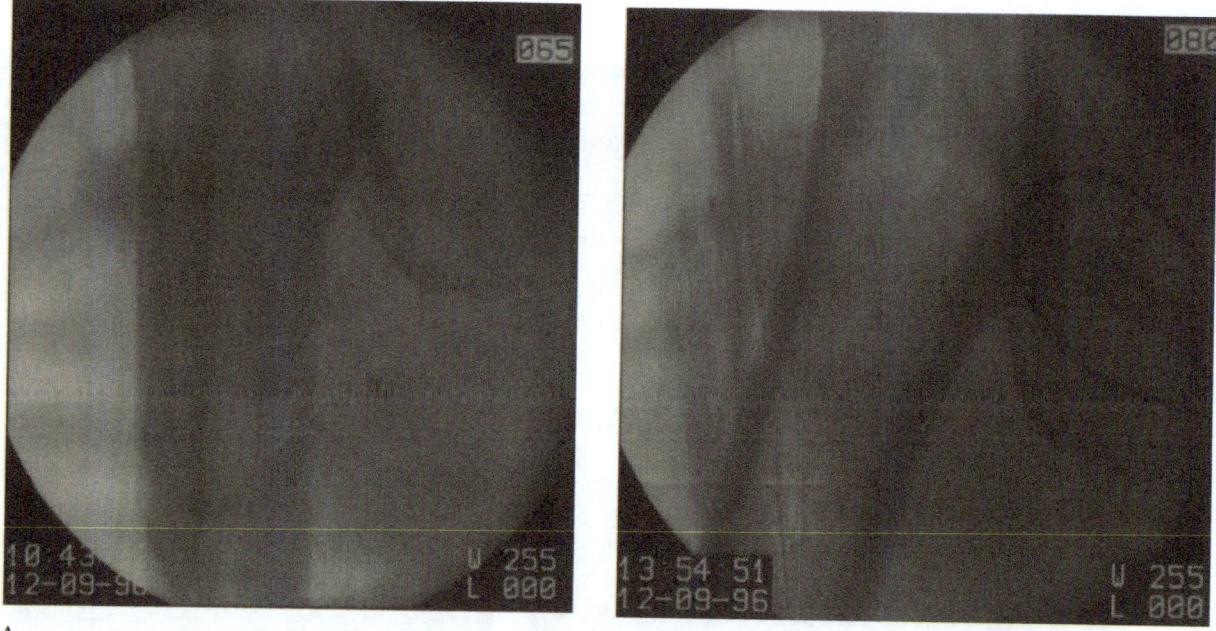

Figure 75.4. A. Inter-Op fluoroscope after implant removed, cement mantel is still intact. B. Inter-Op fluoroscope after robot removed bone cement.

Section 3
Acetabulum

Joseph C. McCarthy

Failure of the acetabular component is a frequent reason precipitating revision surgery. Early experience with cemented cup fixation demonstrated a marked increase in loosening rates, both radiographic and clinical, beyond 10 years (Charnley, Sutherland). Failure of these implants resulted from wear, fixation failure, migration, malposition, infection, trauma, or bone stock loss. When revision surgery was necessary, the surgeon needs to address three areas: component removal, cement extraction, and replenishment of bone stock. Cement removal on occasion could be quite difficult. This was particularly true if there were multiple acetabular recess holes containing mushroom shaped methylcrylate pieces, if there was sepsis, or if the cement was intrapelvic.

More recently cementless acetabular fixation methods have been developed. The first generation modular components, whether porous or threaded, however, have experienced a high failure rate (Harris, Collier, Jasty, Bono). Metal backing, although advantageous for bony ingrowth fixation, often resulted in thin or unsupported polyethylene, thus significantly increasing the likelihood of wear, third body particle debris, component dissociation or dislodgement and osteolysis. During the revision procedure, the surgeon may be faced with the prospect of removing broken screws, extracting a malpositioned threaded implant or retrieving a protruded prosthesis such as a bipolar.

The complexities involved with acetabular component revision thus require considerable preoperative planning (see Section 3). Proper understanding of the type of failed implant present, the specific equipment that will facilitate its removal, and an assessment of the available bone stock both before and after component removal will result in a more successful revision surgical outcome. This section investigates each of these issues. It focuses on specific surgical techniques for management of bone stock deficiency as classified by the American Academy of Orthopedic Surgeons Committee on the Hip. Each of the authors highlight surgical tips and pearls that facilitate bone stock restoration and rigid component fixation.

43
Management of Cavitary Deficiencies

Richard D. Scott and Christopher W. Olcott

The management of a failed acetabular component presents many challenges to the hip surgeon. The goals of revision surgery include: (1) restoration of the anatomic hip center, (2) preservation or restoration of bone stock, (3) acetabular containment and stability and (4) durability or long-term fixation.[1] In the case of a Type II cavitary or a Type III combined acetabular defect (AAOS Classification),[2] the surgeon encounters an enlarged, smooth, sclerotic acetabulum with some degree of bone deficiency. Alternatives for acetabular revision include: cemented cup, threaded cup, bipolar cup, and porous ingrowth cup. Although some investigators report low rerevision rates with cemented cups,[3] most results with cemented sockets in the setting of revision surgery have been poor even with more modern cement techniques.[4,5] Likewise, threaded cups have shown high failure rates in both primary and revision surgery.[6,7] The results of bipolar cups combined with morselized autograft and allograft have been less consistent.[8-10] Wilson and Scott[10] reported good results with bipolar cups whereas Brien et al.[8] showed over a 60% failure rate and discouraged use of bipolar cups in revision surgery. More recently Padgett et al.[11] and Tanzer et al.[12] reported excellent results with uncemented acetabular components in revision surgery. In these reviews, the majority of acetabular defects were packed with morselized autograft or allograft. This morselized bone graft acts as a nonstructural filler for contained or cavitary defects and provides a scaffolding for osteoconduction or bone ingrowth. In addition, the morselized graft enhances bone stock for possible future surgery.[13]

Acetabular revision surgery requires thorough preoperative evaluation. Since morselized bone graft will not offer structural support for uncontained defects, it is imperative to identify segmental acetabular defects that may require bulk structural allograft. Preoperative radiographs such as an anteroposterior pelvis, an anteroposterior and lateral of the hip, and oblique or Judet views are helpful in assessing acetabular coverage.[1] A computerized tomography (CT) scan of the pelvis with 3-D reconstructions may be necessary in complex cases. Evaluation of acetabular integrity in revision surgery is similar to assessment of acetabular fractures in trauma situations. Paprosky et al.[14,15] identified radiographic findings useful in determining acetabular coverage. For example, ischial lysis represents posterior column insufficiency and disruption of Kohler's line demonstrates anterior column insufficiency.[14] Absence of the teardrop represents an inferomedial defect and superior migration of the acetabular component more than 2 cm suggests significant loss of superior wall coverage.[14] Overall, at least 40% to 50% host–bone contact is required for use of an uncemented, porous ingrowth cup.[14,16] Therefore, acetabular defects with adequate rim support and column coverage can be managed with morselized bone graft and large, uncemented acetabular components. The appropriate amount of allograft bone and inventory of acetabular components must be ordered preoperatively.

Technique

Intraoperatively, a wide, extensile exposure is required for adequate visualization and assessment of acetabular coverage. A trochanteric osteotomy or slide may be helpful in cases where exposure and dislocation are difficult. Upon entering the hip capsule, fluid is sent for immediate gram stain, tissue may be collected for frozen section, and both fluid and tissue are sent for at least aerobic and anaerobic cultures. If the femoral component requires revision, its removal will facilitate acetabular exposure. If the femoral component is being retained, a complete capsulectomy improves exposure and allows translocation of the proximal femur. Some older nonmodular femoral stems can be safely tapped out of their cement mantle and reinserted at the end of the procedure.[17] The femoral head of a modular component should be removed to aid exposure. Either the retained nonmodular femoral head or the trunion of a modular component should be protected from being scratched by an instrument throughout the procedure. It should also be noted that patients undergoing isolated socket revision are at a high risk for postoperative dis-

Figure 43.1. Schematic of cavitary acetabular deficiency packed with morselized graft prior to cup insertion. A. Cavitary deficiency with large voids. B. Placement of morselized graft to fill voids. C. Insertion of acetabular shell.

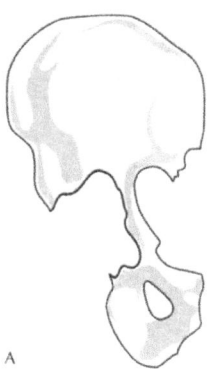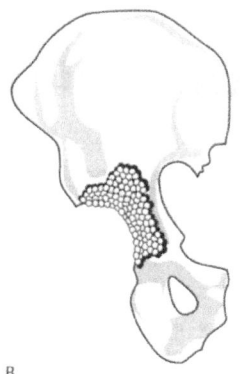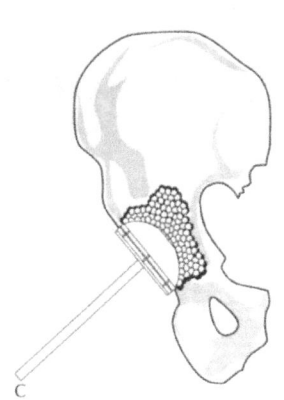

location and should be counseled and braced if necessary.

A complete, careful removal of the failed acetabular component, cement, and fibrous membrane is followed by thorough irrigation with the pulsatile lavage. Complete excision of the fibrous membrane is especially important since this membrane contains the degradative enzymes responsible for aseptic loosening. During removal of the failed component and preparation of the acetabulum, care must be taken to preserve existing bone stock. Visual and manual inspection of anterior and posterior column coverage as well as viability of the superior, medial, and inferior walls allows final determination of the type of acetabular reconstruction required. Adequate posterior and superior coverage are mandatory for success of an uncemented acetabular component.[1]

Next, acetabular reamers are used to prepare the bony bed and to obtain a peripheral fit. An attempt is made to restore the anatomic hip center, rather than use a high hip center, in order to recreate normal joint forces and decrease abnormal stresses across the acetabulum. An undersized reamer is used first to lightly ream the medial bone. Sequentially larger reamers are applied until at least 50% of the outer rim is engaged. The integrity of the acetabular walls are periodically evaluated to guard against over reaming and compromising coverage. Depending upon bone stock, the surgeon may elect to utilize a shell 1 to 2 mm larger than the final reamer for better peripheral contact. Of note, since the acetabular bed is often sclerotic, it may be helpful to make small drill holes or use a burr to promote bleeding before packing the morselized bone graft. The morselized bone graft may be prepared on a back table

Figure 43.2. Radiographs of a sixty-six-year-old man with a failed cup arthroplasty. A. Preoperative radiograph demonstrating large cavitary defect of acetabulum. B. Postoperative radiograph showing well-incorporated packed morselized autograft and a large acetabular shell.

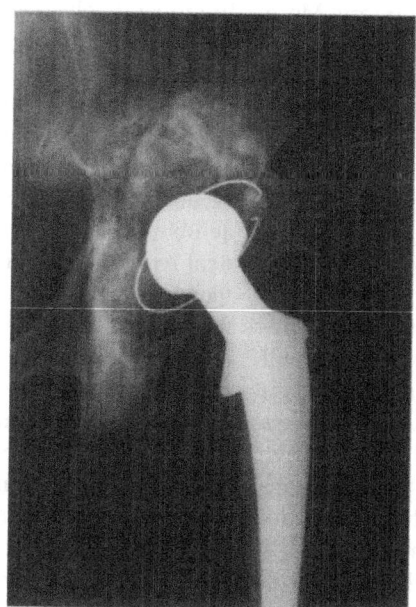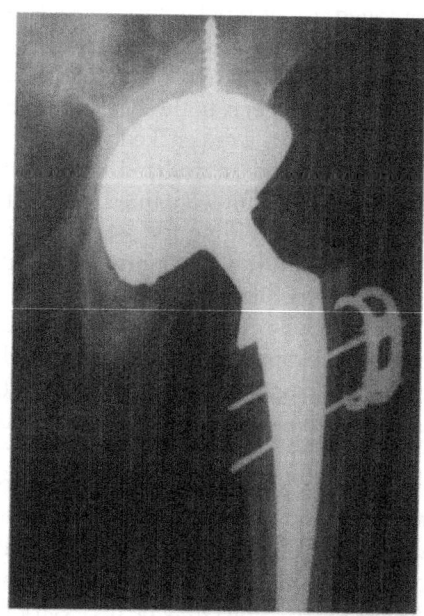

by another member of the surgical team. If autograft from acetabular reamings is adequate to fill defects, no allograft may be necessary. However, most often a small amount of autograft is combined with allograft from femoral or humeral heads. If possible, female femoral or humeral heads should be used for morselized bone graft so as to save stronger, male allograft bone for use as bulk, structural allografts.[16] The bone may be morselized with a bone mill, acetabular reamers or manually with a rongeur. Gross et al.[16] feel that bone mills and reamers make the allograft too mushy to fill defects and prefer using rongeurs to create chunks of allograft bone which retain some structural integrity. Next, the morselized bone graft is packed tightly into defects using a bone tamp and mallet. A wafer of allograft bone may be necessary to cover a defect in the medial wall and allow containment of morselized bone graft.[1] The last acetabular reamer used or a smaller one is then reversed to pressurize and contour the morselized graft. The above steps may need to be repeated to ensure tight packing of the morselized bone graft (Fig. 43.1).

Intraoperative radiographs with trial components in place may be helpful to assess component fit, position, and filling of defects with morselized bone graft. The real acetabular component is then impacted into anatomic position. If there is rigid rim contact and secure primary fixation, no ancillary screws are necessary. If indicated, 6.5 mm cancellous dome or peripheral screws provide increased support (Fig. 43.2 and 43.3). Immediate acetabular stability with screw fixation prevents component migration and micromotion so as to allow for bone ingrowth.[18] Emerson et al.[19] confirmed that nonstructural morselized allograft fares significantly better under stable acetabular components. A bipolar cup remains a controversial alternative to an uncemented acetabular component with screw fixation. A bipolar cup may be helpful in a salvage situation with poor soft tissue tensioning and a high risk for dislocation.

Postoperatively the patient is kept on antibiotics for 48 hours and in balanced suspension until regaining protective muscle control. Mobilization occurs on either postoperative day one or two and the patient is maintained on partial weight-bearing for 3 to 6 months with trochanteric precautions if indicated. Gross et al.[16] continue intravenous cephalosporin for 2 to 5 days postoperatively followed by 5 additional days of cephalosporin by mouth. Gentamicin is given and continued for 24 hours if the patient is catheterized during the procedure.[16] Bactrim is used afterwards until the catheter is removed.[16] The patient is kept partial weight-bearing until union of the allograft, usually 3 to 6 months.[16]

Results

The use of morselized autograft or allograft depends upon the availability of each and the size of the contained acetabular defect. Autograft represents the gold standard in bone graft materials because it offers osteoconductive and osteoinductive properties as well as viable cells with osteogenic potential.[20] Therefore, the autograft not only provides the collagen framework or scaffolding for bone ingrowth but also contains living osteoprogenitor cells and growth factors responsible for promoting differentiation to osteoblasts.[20] It is always used in primary cases such as protrusio where the pa-

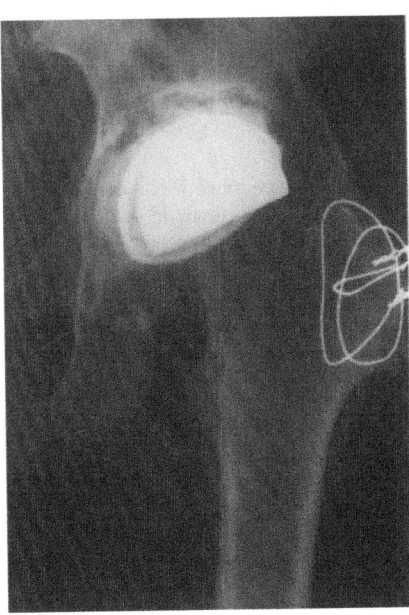
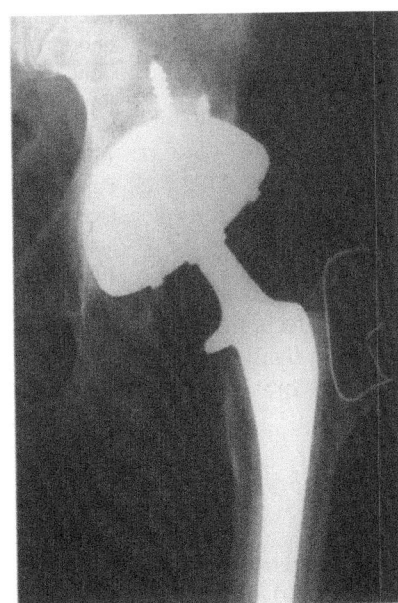

Figure 43.3. Radiographs of a sixty-one-year-old man with a failed cemented, all-polyethylene cup. A. Preoperative radiograph of a loose cemented, all-polyethylene component with an extensive superior cavitary defect. B. Postoperative radiograph demonstrating well-incorporated morselized allograft and an oversized acetabular shell.

A   B

tient's own femoral head is available. Freeze-dried allograft retains its osteoconductive quality but lacks osteoprogenitor cells and contains only minimal amounts of growth factors.[20] However, whereas the incorporation of allograft by creeping substitution occurs slower than that of autograft, both graft types are completely incorporated over time.[21] A postmortem retrieval analysis demonstrated that morselized allograft had almost completely incorporated by 83 months.[22] The investigators added that the extent of graft incorporation histologically correlates poorly with postoperative radiographs.[22] Although morselized autograft possesses qualities superior to those of allograft, an adequate amount of autograft is often lacking in the revision situation. Therefore, morselized allograft provides an effective alternative bone graft material to fill acetabular defects. It can be used independently or mixed with existing autograft.

Good to excellent intermediate results with uncemented acetabular components and morselized autograft and/or allograft in revision surgery have been reported in the literature. Tanzer et al.[12] reviewed 140 acetabular revisions and found a 1% rerevision rate at a mean follow-up of 3.4 years. Morselized autograft was combined with an uncemented acetabular component in 97 hips whereas allograft was utilized in six others. Padgett et al.[11] reported a 5% rerevision rate among 138 acetabular revisions at a mean follow-up of 3.6 years. A combination of morselized autograft and allograft was used in approximately 80% of cases.[11] Both investigators identified a high incidence of incomplete radiolucent lines especially in regions of allograft.[11,12] However, both studies showed incorporation of all autografts and allografts.[11,12] Woolson and Adamson[23] reported a 9% rerevision rate in 32 hips with a bone-ingrowth acetabular cup and morselized autograft and/or allograft at a mean follow-up of almost 5 years. Silverton et al.[18] updated the findings of Padgett et al.[11] and found that of 111 acetabular revisions no further rerevisions had been performed for aseptic loosening or migration at a follow-up of 7 to 11 years.

Conclusion

Overall, morselized autograft and/or allograft provides an effective filler of contained acetabular defects in revision surgery and contributes to long-term fixation of uncemented acetabular components and restoration of acetabular bone stock.

References

1. D'Antonio JA. Periprosthetic bone loss of the acetabulum. Classification and management. *Orthop Clin N Am.* 1992; 23:279–290.
2. D'Antonio JA, Capello WN, Borden LS, et al. Classification and management of acetabular abnormalities in total hip arthroplasty. *Clin Orthop.* 1989;243:126–137.
3. Azuma T, Yasuda H, Okagaki K, Sakai K. Compressed allograft chips for acetabular reconstruction in revision hip arthroplasty. *J Bone Joint Surg Br.* 1994;76:740–744.
4. Callaghan JJ, Salvati EA, Pellicci PM, Wilson PD, Ranawat CS. Results of revision for mechanical failure after cemented total hip replacement, 1979 to 1982. *J Bone Joint Surg Am.* 1985;67:1074–1085.
5. Marti RK, Schuller HM, Besselaar PP, VanfrankHaasnoot EL. Results of revision of hip arthroplasty with cement. *J Bone Joint Surg Am.* 1990;72:346–354.
6. Ayerza M, Pierson R, Sheinkop M, et al. A clinical review of a conical screw-in acetabular design. *Orthop Trans.* 1988;12:662.
7. Engh CA, Glassman AH, Griffin WL, Mayer JG. Results of cementless revision for failed cemented total hip arthroplasty. *Clin Orthop.* 1988;235:91–110.
8. Brien WW, Bruce WJ, Salvati EA, Wilson PD, Pellicci PM. Acetabular reconstruction with a bipolar prosthesis and morseled bone grafts. *J Bone Joint Surg Am.* 1990;72:1230–1235.
9. Ochsner JL, Penenberg BL, Dorr LD, Conaty JP. The bipolar endoprosthesis and bone graft in the management of aseptic acetabular component loosening. *Orthopedics* 1990;13:45–49.
10. Wilson MG, Scott RD. Reconstruction of the deficient acetabulum using the bipolar socket. *Clin Orthop.* 1990;251: 126–133.
11. Padgett DE, Kull L, Rosenberg A, Sumner DR, Galante JO. Revision of the acetabular component without cement after total hip arthroplasty. Three to six year follow-up. *J Bone Joint Surg Am.* 1993;75:663–673.
12. Tanzer M, Drucker D, Jasty M, McDonald M, Harris WH. Revision of the acetabular component with an uncemented Harris-Galante porous-coated prosthesis. *J Bone Joint Surg Am.* 1992;74:987–994.
13. Papagelopoulos PJ, Lewallen DG, Cabanela ME, McFarland EG, Wallrichs SL. Acetabular reconstruction using bipolar endoprosthesis and bone grafting in patients with severe bone deficiency. *Clin Orthop.* 1995;314:170–184.
14. Paprosky WG, Magnus RE. Principles of bone grafting in revision total hip arthroplasty. *Clin Orthop.* 1994;298:147–155.
15. Paprosky WG, Perona PG, Lawrence JM. Acetabular defect classification and surgical reconstruction in revision arthroplasty. A 6 year follow-up evaluation. *J Arthroplasty.* 1994;9:33–44.
16. Gross AE, Allan DG, Catre M, Garbuz DS, Stockley I. Bone grafts in hip replacement surgery. *Orthop Clin N Am.* 1993; 24:679–695.
17. Nabors ED, Liebelt R, Mattingly DA, Bierbaum BE. Removal and reinsertion of cemented femoral components during acetabular revision. *J Arthroplasty.* 1996;11:146–152.
18. Silverton CD, Rosenberg AG, Sheinkop MB, Kull LR, Galante JO. Revision of the acetabular component without cement after total hip arthroplasty. *J Bone Joint Surg Am.* 1996;78:1366–1370.
19. Emerson RH, Head WC, Berklacich FM, Malinin TI.

Noncemented acetabular revision arthroplasty using allograft bone. *Clin Orthop.* 1989;249:30–43.
20. Gazdag AR, Lane JM, Glaser D, Forster RA. Alternatives to autogenous bone graft: efficacy and indications. *J Am Acad Orthop Surg.* 1995;3:1–8.
21. Burchardt H. The biology of bone repair. *Clin Orthop.* 1983;174:28–42.
22. Heekin RD, Engh CA, Vinh T. Morselized allograft in acetabular reconstruction. A postmortem retrieval analysis. *Clin Orthop.* 1995;319:184–190.
23. Woolson ST, Adamson GJ. Acetabular revision using a bone-ingrowth total hip component in patients who have acetabular bone stock deficiency. *J Arthroplasty.* 1996;11:661–667.

44
Management of Acetabular Deficiency with a Bipolar Prosthesis at Revision THA

Steven Robert Wardell

Acetabular deficiency in hip arthroplasty can exist in different clinical situations including developmental dysplasia of the hip, protrusio acetabulae, posttraumatic acetabular fracture, and most commonly anteversion total hip arthroplasty. Causes of bone loss at revision hip arthroplasty include wear debris induced osteolysis, prosthetic loosening with bony erosion, infection, multiple revision procedures, and iatrogenic causes such as overreaming.

The principles of acetabular reconstruction at revision total hip arthroplasty include restoring hip biomechanics, restoring acetabular integrity and continuity, and both prosthetic and bone graft containment and fixation. The options for treatment of acetabular deficiency include utilization of large oversized porous coated hemispherical components, oblong or custom porous coated components, bipolar component, acetabular reinforcement rings or cages, or cemented hemispherical components all with or without the use or particulate or structural bone graft.

The guidelines for management of specific acetabular defects at revision hip arthroplasty has been described elsewhere. This section reviews the benefits and techniques of the bipolar prosthesis at revision hip arthroplasty with clinical correlation.

Why a Bipolar Prosthesis?

The bipolar prosthesis was first described by Bateman[1] in 1974 as a single-assembly total hip prosthesis that would address the acetabular wear seen with the unipolar Austin-Moore hemiarthroplasty and as an alternative to Charnley's low friction total hip arthroplasty. The creation of a "mobile head element and the addition of another head surface for motion in the acetabulum" was thought to provide for a greater distribution of bearing forces, thus minimizing implant and acetabular wear.[1] In addition, the bipolar prosthesis was described as a self-aligning system that provided improved stability and range of motion.

The bipolar prosthesis has several advantages over traditional fixed cup total hip arthroplasty in revision hip arthroplasty. The bipolar prosthesis is inherently more stable than a fixed acetabular component given adequate acetabular coverage, and several authors[2,3] have advocated the use of the bipolar prosthesis with recurrent dislocation. Trochanteric nonunion, abductor insufficiency, and superior gluteal nerve palsy would lead to a high risk for postoperative instability after revision total hip arthroplasty. The bipolar prosthesis is a viable alternative to provide postoperative stability as compared to a fixed acetabular component in the patient who is at high risk for postoperative instability. These same patients might also be candidates for use of a constrained liner if a fixed acetabular component is preferred.

Another advantage of the bipolar prosthesis at revision hip arthroplasty includes the ability to mold or shape particulate bone graft utilized for cavitary or segmental bone deficiencies of the acetabulum. Several authors[4-6] have noted difficulties with migration of the bipolar prosthesis when particulate and/or structural allograft is utilized. A staged acetabular reconstruction is effectively performed with shaping and incorporation of the bone graft over time. If subsequent revision hip arthroplasty is required secondary to pain, conversion to a fixed acetabular component is easier with previous bone graft incorporation which effectively converts a segmental AAOS (American Academy of Orthopedic Surgeons) Type I or III defect or large cavitary AAOS Type II defect to a much smaller residual defect which is easily managed with hemispherical components. Other advantages of the bipolar prosthesis at revision hip arthroplasty include shortened operative time and ease of use as compared to a fixed acetabular component.

The disadvantages of the bipolar prosthesis in both primary and revision hip arthroplasty have been cited by many authors.[7-10] Schaffer[7] noted inconsistent clinical results with primary bipolar hemiarthroplasty with persistent groin pain postoperatively. The authors noted hip capsular impingement about the bipolar component and recommended complete capsulectomy at surgery to prevent the situation postoperatively. Several authors[8-11] have noted significant polyethylene wear with early bipolar prostheses in primary bipolar hemiarthroplasty secondary to thin polyethylene with the use of smaller diameter components. Notching and impingement of the femoral neck on the polyethylene and metal bipolar outer shell has also been implicated as a cause of polyethylene wear. Furthermore, several authors[12-14] have noted that over time the bipolar prosthesis can act effectively as a unipolar prosthesis as the inner bearing becomes locked with scar or capsule that leads to persistent groin pain from accelerated acetabular cartilage degeneration and wear.

Surgical Technique

Circumferential visualization of the bony acetabulum is achieved with a complete capsulectomy and careful retractor placement. The failed acetabular component is removed along with any other debris including cement and fibrous membrane between the bone–cement or bone–metal interface. Acetabular bony deficiencies are reconstructed utilizing structural or particulate bone graft, depending on the type of bony deficiency present. Concentric hemispherical acetabular reaming is performed in a sequential fashion with careful attention to both the anterior and posterior columns of the acetabulum throughout reaming so that an iatrogenic segmental defect is not created. The anterior and posterior columns of the pelvis provide essential stability to the acetabular component be it bipolar or a fixed cup. Hemispherical bipolar prosthetic coverage is essential and reaming should stop once purchase has been obtained in both the anterior and posterior columns of the acetabulum after bony reconstruction. Cavitary defects within the acetabulum should be packed with particulate bone graft and reversed reamed as popularized by Scott.[15]

Selection of a bipolar prosthesis 1 to 2 mm larger than the last reamer allows maximum rim contact and load transfer to the anterior and posterior columns of the acetabulum to prevent significant migration, depending upon the patient's bone quality and type of bone graft utilized. Finite element analysis[16] noted underreaming of press-fitting a fixed acetabular component is better tolerated with larger diameters than with smaller diameter hemispherical components. Undersizing of the bipolar prosthesis leads to early migration and possible protrusio defect of the acetabulum.

Trial bipolar components should be utilized to assess stability, range of motion, and limb length prior to final implant selection. Implants and trial components should be available in 1 mm-incremental diameters to allow optimal sizing and stability without compromising further bone stock. In addition, polyethylene thickness within the bipolar component should be maximized with utilization of a 22- or 26-mm femoral head, especially in smaller diameter bipolar prostheses. Well-supported polyethylene of maximal thickness within the bipolar prosthesis decreases the rate of polyethylene wear and early aseptic failure.

Postoperatively weight-bearing is dictated by the extent of acetabular and/or femoral reconstruction required. Structural bone grafts, and possibly particulate bone grafts, should be protected postoperatively with a period of limited weight-bearing or traction to allow graft incorporation prior to weight-bearing.

Results

Even though the bipolar prosthesis was originally theorized as a two-stage acetabular reconstructive procedure in revision hip arthroplasty, several authors[5,6,17] have demonstrated satisfactory results both clinically and radiographically without the need for a subsequent surgery in short-term follow-up. Most reports required the use of allogeneic bone graft either for cavitary or segmental defects.

Most cavitary acetabular deficiencies (AAOS type II) require the use of particulate bone graft to restore bone stock and hip biomechanics. Several authors[4,18,19] have noted favorable results with the bipolar prosthesis in contained acetabular defects. Wilson[4] reported on a group of 47 cases in which a cavitary acetabular defect was revised with a bipolar prosthesis and particulate allograft. They noted some early migration with stabilization and incorporation of the allograft at one year postoperatively. Namba[18] reported on 32 hips revised with a bipolar prosthesis for both segmental and cavitary acetabular defects at a minimum five-year follow-up. They noted arrested migration with all cavitary defects. However, they noted progressive migration with all segmental defects. Postoperative functional scores did not deteriorate with bipolar migration. Segmental acetabular defects were not reconstructed with structural allograft and were treated with particulate bone graft and an oversized bipolar prosthesis. They noted progressive migration with segmental defects of the peripheral rim or medial wall even with apparent particulate graft incorporation. No structural bulk allograft was utilized in these patients with segmental deficiency, therefore, particulate allograft alone may be contraindicated in segmental deficiencies of the acetabulum.

Most segmental acetabular deficiencies (AAOS Type I or III) require the use of structural bulk allograft to restore bone stock and hip biomechanics. Restoration of the true hip center of rotation[20] has been shown by several authors to decrease the risk of aseptic failure. Restoration of bone stock will augment the host acetabulum and ease revision hip arthroplasty in the future. Several authors[5,21,22] have noted favorable results with the bipolar prosthesis in segmental or combined cavitary and segmental acetabular defects. Cameron[5] reported 37 cases of which 15 required minimal grafting and 22 cases that required massive structural allografting, and they noted only 55% good to excellent results at 1 to 3 years follow-up. There was no major migration noted even in the structural allograft group at this short-term follow-up. Cameron advocated the use of a bipolar prosthesis at revision hip arthroplasty even with the use of bulk allografts since reconstruction of the acetabulum at subsequent revision would be much easier in these complex patients. Roberson[17] reported on 27 patients revised with massive allografting and bipolar prosthesis. They noted satisfactory results in all patients with incorporation of the bone graft at 2 to 6 year follow-up. McFarland[21] reported on 81 hips revised with a bipolar prosthesis and allograft bone for failed total hip arthroplasty. They noted graft resorption universally over time, with 83% satisfactory results and 17% incidence of postoperative complication at a mean 16 months follow-up.[6] Murray reported on 101 hips revised with a bipolar prosthesis for failed hip arthroplasty. They utilized a bipolar prosthesis when contact between host bone and acetabular component was less than 50%. Structural bulk allograft was utilized in these patients to restore bone stock and biomechanical hip center. All grafts were incorporated radiographically with average cephalad migration of 2.4 mm at average 35 month follow-up. Significant migration or subluxation requiring revision was noted in only 19% (19/101) hips and there was a 10% (10/101) postoperative infection rate.

Although the above reports have only short-term follow-up, our experience with the bipolar prosthesis at revision hip arthroplasty with cavitary and/or segmental acetabular bony deficiencies has been favorable at a minimum six-year follow-up.[23] Our retrospective review examined 37 hips revised for aseptic loosening (35 hips) or recurrent instability (2 hips) after total hip arthroplasty. A bipolar prosthesis was utilized in all patients to reconstruct the acetabulum with particulate or structural allograft depending on the type of acetabular deficiency present. Particulate bone graft alone was utilized to reconstruct AAOS Type II cavitary defects in 25 hips (Group A) and structural bulk allograft with particulate allograft was utilized to reconstruct AAOS Type I or III segmental defects in 12 hips (Group B). Group A had a mean age of 56 years and demonstrated a mean cephalad migration of 3.5 mm and medial migration of 2.0 mm. Intermittent groin pain was noted in 25% (5/20 hips) and no patients required rerevision. Group B had a mean age of 58 years and demonstrated a mean cephalad migration of 5.3 mm and medial migration of 1.4 mm. There was a 33% (4/12 hips) rerevision rate secondary to groin pain and migration. All patients were independent ambulators with or without a cane. There was no evidence of dislocation or instability noted postoperatively and all bone grafts demonstrated consolidation over time. The greatest rates of migration were noted over the first 12 months postoperatively in all patients with decreased migration rate thereafter with graft incorporation.

Conclusion

The bipolar prosthesis is a useful adjunct in the management of severe acetabular bony deficiency at revision hip arthroplasty because of the advantages of operative flexibility, allograft molding, and postoperative stability in these complex patients. When host bone coverage is less than 50% at revision hip arthroplasty, structural bulk allograft with a bipolar prosthesis or cemented acetabular component is recommended. Bipolar migration is not synonymous with a poor clinical result and previous poor reports of acetabular reconstruction with a bipolar prosthesis may be related to limited prosthetic size selection and surgical technique. The bipolar prosthesis was originally recommended to be utilized as part of a two-stage acetabular reconstruction in revision hip arthroplasty. If subsequent rerevision is required, allograft incorporation converts a previously large segmental or cavitary bony deficiency to a smaller more easily manageable defect over time.

References

1. Bateman JF. Single assembly total hip prosthesis: a preliminary report. *Orthop Digest.* 1974;2:15.
2. Giliberty RP. A new concept of bipolar endoprosthesis. *Orthop Review.* 1974;3:40.
3. Ries MD, Wiedel JD. Bipolar hip arthroplasty for recurrent dislocation after total hip arthroplasty: a report of three cases. *Clin Orthop.* 1992;78:121–127.
4. Wilson MG, Scott RD. Reconstruction of the deficient acetabulum using the bipolar socket. *Clin Orthop.* 1990;251:126–133.
5. Cameron HU, Jung YB. Acetabular revision with a bipolar prosthesis. *Clin Orthop.* 1990;251:100–103.
6. Murray WR. Acetabular salvage in revision total hip arthroplasty using the bipolar prosthesis. *Clin Orthop.* 1990;251:92–99.

7. Schaffer JL, Wilson MG, Scott RD. Capsular impingement as a source of pain following bipolar hip arthroplasty. *J Arthroplasty*. 1991;6:163–168.
8. Scarcella JB, Cohn BT. Mechanical failure of a Bateman bipolar prosthesis. *Orthopaedics*. 1992;15:1343–1345.
9. Herzenberg JE, Harrelson JM, Campbell DC, Lachiewicz PF. Fractures of the polyethylene insert in Bateman bipolar hip prostheses. *Clin Orthop*. 1988;228:88–93.
10. Incavo SJ, Ninomiya J, Howe JG, Mayor MB. Failure of the polyethylene liner leading to notching of the femoral component in bipolar prostheses. *Orthop Rev*. 1993;22:728–732.
11. Cameron HU, Cha EJ, Jung YB. An examination of factors contributing to failure of bipolar prostheses. *Clin Orthop*. 1989;240:206–209.
12. Mess D, Barmada R. Clinical and motion studies of the Bateman bipolar prosthesis in osteonecrosis of the hip. *Clin Orthop*. 1990;251:44–47.
13. Vazquez-Vela E, Vazquez-Vela G. Acetabular reaction to the Bateman bipolar prosthesis. *Clin Orthop*. 1990;251:87–91.
14. Bateman JE, Berenji AR, Bayne O, Greyson ND. Long-term results of bipolar arthroplasty in osteoarthritis of the hip. *Clin Orthop*. 1990;251:54–66.
15. Scott RD. Use of a bipolar prosthesis with bone grafting in revision surgery. *Tech Orthop*. 1987;2:84.
16. Ries MD, Harbaugh M, Shea J, Lambert R. Acetabular bone stains produced by oversized press fit cup. Presented at the 64th Annual Meeting of the American Academy of Orthopaedic Surgeons, San Francisco, California, February 1997.
17. Roberson JR, Cohen D. Bipolar components for severe periacetabular bone loss around the failed total hip arthroplasty. *Clin Orthop*. 1990;251:113–118.
18. Namba RS, Clarke A, Scott RD. Bipolar revisions with bone-grafting for cavitary and segmental acetabular defects: A minimum 5-year follow-up study. *J Arthroplasty*. 1994;9:263–268.
19. Brien WW, Bruce WJ, Salvati EA, Wilson PD Jr., Pellicci PM. Acetabular reconstruction with a bipolar prosthesis and morselized bone grafts. *J Bone Joint Surg Am*. 1990;72:1230.
20. Callaghan JI, Salvati EA, Pellici PM, Wilson PD, Ranawat CS. Results of revision for mechanical failure after cemented total hip replacement: Analysis of recent cases with two to five year follow-up. *J Bone Joint Surg Am*. 1985;67:1074.
21. McFarland EG, Lewallen DG, Cabanela ME. Use of bipolar endoprosthesis and bone grafting for acetabular reconstruction. *Clin Orthop*. 1991;268:128–139.
22. Chang JK, Wu JC, Yei SM, Lin SY. Reconstruction of the severely deficient acetabulum with the bipolar prosthesis and allo-autograft. *Kaohsiung J Med Sci*. 1992;8:82–88.
23. Wardell SR, VanFlandern G, Stamos VP, Mason JB, Bono JV, McCarthy JP, Turner RH. Acetabular revision utilizing a self-centering bipolar prosthesis. Presented at the New England Orthopaedic Society Fall Meeting, Boston, Massachusetts, November, 1996. Submitted for Publication, 1997.

45
Management of Segmental Deficiencies

Wayne G. Paprosky, Michael S. Bradford, and Todd D. Sekundiak

Extensive acetabular bone loss in the revision setting is becoming an increasing problem. Bone loss can occur from the patient's premorbid condition, previous operative procedures, infection, and osteolysis. This degree of loss can be massive, secondary to the asymptomatic nature of the osteolytic process. Once the acetabular defect has been assessed, one must then collect the armamentarium of instruments, prostheses, and bone graft required to remove the old components, reconstruct the bony acetabulum, and reinsert the new prosthesis. This entails a technically demanding process that becomes more complex as the acetabular bone defect increases.

Many techniques are described for acetabular revision, however the majority of the studies do not correlate the reconstruction to the type of defect. Those defects that only have cavitary or minor segmental defects have excellent results with the utilization of porous-coated implants.[1-13] Components that have 50% to 70% of host bone contact will ingrow into the host but require augmentation to obtain stable initial fixation.[1,3,9,11,14-19] Augmentation may include a modification of the acetabular cup or a structural bone allograft. When there is less than 50% host-bone contact, biologic fixation of the implant to the host is not possible as initial stable fixation cannot be obtained.[11,15,17,18] Many options have been assessed for acetabulae with massive bony deficiencies, unfortunately follow-up at a long-term period is still pending. For any size of defect, cemented components have generally met with poor results and are not being recommended in the revision setting.[20-34] Similarly, threaded acetabular components have had poor results.[35-38] For larger size defects, attempts at salvaging the hip joint with a bipolar prosthesis has met with component migration and graft failure.[39-43] Attempts at ingrowth with a structural allograft and either a cemented or porous ingrowth cup has also met with failure.[44-51] Results can be disputed, with some authors admitting to good results if strict adherence to technique and patient selection is followed.[1,2,11,14,15,16,52-56] Acetabular impaction grafting is having promising results but success is likely secondary to the less severe acetabular defects.[57] Use of a high hip center for placement of the component is again a viable alternative but also has variable results.[47,58-61] Ultimately, success of the implant is determined by the amount of host-bone contact, and where significant contact cannot be had, alternatives are required.

Although very controversial, two options remain for the severe acetabular defect. The use of an acetabular reconstruction ring, with morselized or bulk graft, has been employed with the initial series by Berry et el.[62] and Schatzker[63] demonstrating acceptable results but with concomitant high loosening and infection rates. Recent studies have had more favorable results.[64-66] The final alternative that has not previously been mentioned is the use of a whole pelvic transplant, into which an acetabular cup is cemented.

Preoperative Planning

Technique begins with preoperative templating to ensure one recognizes the defect to be reconstructed. We use a previously described classification that can be easily implemented as it uses only four radiographic criteria found on the anteroposterior radiograph of the pelvis.[11] These criteria are the level of superior migration of the hip center, the amount of ischial lysis below the superior obturator line, the degree of acetabular tear drop destruction, and the degree of disruption of Kohler's line. In cases where an allograft hemipelvis transplant is to be considered, all these parameters should be most severely affected. The hip center has migrated 2 cm superior to its normal location. Ischial lysis extends 15 mm below the superior transverse obturator line. The acetabular tear drop and Kohler's line have been completed disrupted. This degree of radiographic alteration in the acetabulum has been clinically correlated to a minimum of 50% loss of the host acetabulum. Thus, the use of a press-fit component in this situation is not a viable option.[68]

Having templated and determined the severity of the acetabular defect, one then obtains an ipsilateral hemipelvis allograft from their tissue bank. If possible, an allograft from a young male donor is requested. This ensures that the graft is of adequate structural integrity, which may prevent early collapse of the graft and allow acceptance of screw fixation. The graft will also be large enough to bridge the bony defects. This type of hemipelvis also ensures that the acetabulum will be large enough to accept an acetabular component. In smaller individuals, it is important not to have an oversized component. In general, a hemipelvis with an acetabulum of 50 to 56 mm diameter is adequate.

Operative Technique

A posterolateral approach is standard for this procedure. This exposure allows for complete visualization of the acetabular rim without the need for a more extensile and complex dissection. Debridement of the acetabular pseudocapsule is continued until the acetabular rim is encountered. Dissection proceeds judiciously in the posterior direction to prevent sciatic nerve transection. Use of the electrocautery provides warning to the surgeon when the nerve is in close proximity to the dissection. The entire acetabular rim, along with the component–bone or cement–bone interface is exposed by subperiosteal dissection. Removal of the component and biomaterials proceeds in a routine manner and may include sectioning of the component. Once all debris and reactive membrane have been removed, the acetabulum is assessed and correlated to the preoperative radiograph. It is essential to systematically assess the acetabulum to determine the viability of fixing a component to the host bone versus transplanting an allograft acetabulum.

One must thoroughly examine the columns and ensure that a pelvic dissociation does not exist. Because the dissociation occurs from degenerative and not traumatic causes, the dissociation can be insidious. All type IIIB acetabular defects have complete violation of Kohler's line with significant superior migration of the head center. This makes pelvic dissociation a possibility. Subperiosteal dissection continues to expose the columns and ensure bony integrity exists. If it does not, stabilization of the discontinuity must precede the transplantation. This can be performed by use of a pelvic reconstruction plate. It is transfixed onto the posterior column with extension to the ischium and ilium.

At this stage minimal acetabular reaming proceeds to determine the degree of host bone contact with the prosthesis. Acetabular trialing is essential to assess coverage and degree of support from the anterior and posterior columns. At this stage, a decision of acetabular allograft transplanting is made. Sizing of the acetabular defect with the acetabular reamers not only sizes the defect, but also creates a hemispherical shape to the remaining bone for acceptance of the transplant. This is performed by reaming in a superomedial direction. It is essential to remember that reaming is minimal with minimal host bone being removed. The diameter of the remaining host rim is now determined and used for sizing the transplant. Exposure of the posterior column and lateral aspect of the iliac crest is required for fixation of the graft and is performed by subperiosteal stripping above the acetabulum in a posterior and superior direction. Stripping in a superoposterior direction will expose branches of the superior gluteal vessels and can cause significant bleeding if not cauterized. The superior gluteal nerve is uninvolved if one remains subperiosteal and does not enter the greater sciatic notch.

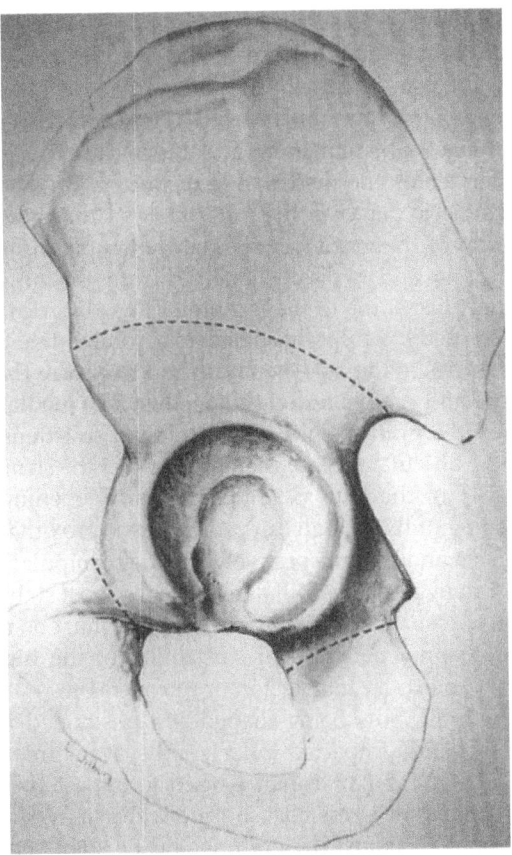

Figure 45.1. This diagram of the hemipelvis graft shows the initial cuts on the graft.

The aim in preparing the graft is to create a tongue and groove mortise that ensures intimate contact of the graft bone to the host. This allows for transfer of load from the graft and to the host, which may aid in biologic incorporation. The acetabular allograft is shaped to buttress against the host bone (Fig. 45.1). The superior pubic and ischial rami are cut at a point distal to the structural acetabulum with a length remaining to fill the defects present in the host pelvis. This will allow host–graft bone contact inferiorly, which will distribute stresses through the construct and provide for better stability. The graft iliac crest is cut in a curvilinear manner from the greater sciatic notch to the anterior inferior iliac spine. This gives ample room for the graft to accept fixation without the bulk of excess bone. The iliac crest flange that is created can vary in its superior–inferior height depending on where host–bone fixation can be obtained. For example, the anterior height of the flange can be increased to obtain purchase in the anterior iliac crest host bone or increased posteriorly if there is better structural bone in this vicinity for fixation. Initial trialing of the graft for fit is now performed.

The tongue and groove mortise is created on the medial aspect of the graft by creating a groove in the graft's inner table at a point where contact is being made with the host's superior acetabular rim (Fig. 45.2). A high-speed cylindrical burr and female reamer, sized 2 mm larger than the last male reamer previously used to shape the acetabulum, create the trough in the graft bone. By using a reamer 2 mm larger than the estimated diameter of the acetabular defect, one is able to estimate the diameter of remaining acetabular rim. The female reamer scores the medial side of the graft to create a hemispheric defect in the inner table of the graft. The position of the groove is marked by templating to the host bone and typically extends from the anterior-inferior iliac spine to the ischium. The cylindrical burr is then used to sculpt this defect to accommodate the irregularities in the host–bone rim and to ensure that the tongue and groove fit tightly together. The medial portion of the graft should not be thinned so extensively that the articular surface is entered or that the structural integrity of the graft is compromised. Deepening and widening of the trough can proceed to approximately 1 to 1.5 cm and 1 cm respectively. Gentle manipulation of the graft in all planes will determine the most stable position. Gross malpositioning of the graft must be monitored to prevent iatrogenic instability of the hip secondary to excess anteversion or retroversion.

The graft, now being shaped and positioned in the host, is gently impacted to lock and seat its final position. An acetabular reamer is used to impact the graft and to prevent stress concentrations that may fracture host or graft bone. The graft should be stable enough that no significant macromotion occurs with gentle manipulation. Fixation now proceeds with 6.5-mm cancellous screws to lag the graft to the host bone (Fig. 45.3). Washers are placed on the screws to distribute forces on the graft and to obtain better compression at the host-graft interface. Placement of screws into the remaining host bone has been determined by the initial dissection of the superior acetabular dome and iliac crest. The graft's iliac crest has also been shaped into a flange to cover this remaining structural bone. Screws are introduced in a superomedial direction. By inserting screws parallel to the normal reactive forces of the hip and by lag technique, the graft can settle to its most stable position against the host. This promotes the greatest surface area of contact between the graft and host and aids in promoting incorporation of the graft. A minimum of four cancellous screws is required for fixation. At this stage, if fixation is questionable, one should not hesitate to use a pelvic reconstruction ring or plate to augment fixation of the graft. In the case of an associated pelvic discontinuity, one may be required to extend a pelvic reconstruction plate along the posterior column—from the host ischium, over the defect, and onto the graft's posterior column and flange. These latter screws enter the graft bone and exit through the host ilium. This will allow for augmentation of graft fixation while bridging the pelvic dissociation.

Only once secure fixation of the graft has been achieved can preparation of the graft acetabulum proceed. The graft acetabulum is prepared for component insertion by sequential reaming to remove cartilage but to leave subchondral bone. Trial reductions ensure stability of the hip and determine orientation of the cup to

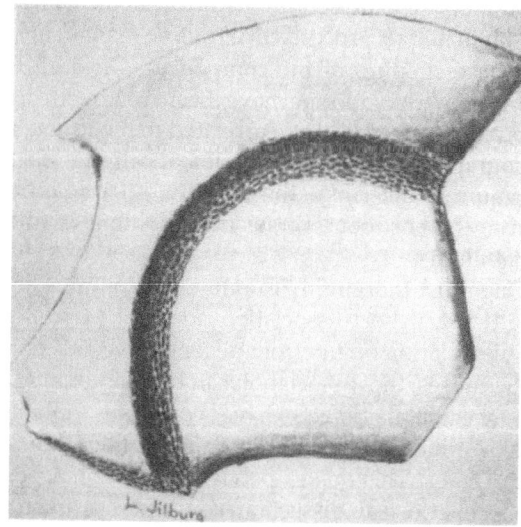

Figure 45.2. The medial surface of the graft is shaped with a trough to lock into the defect.

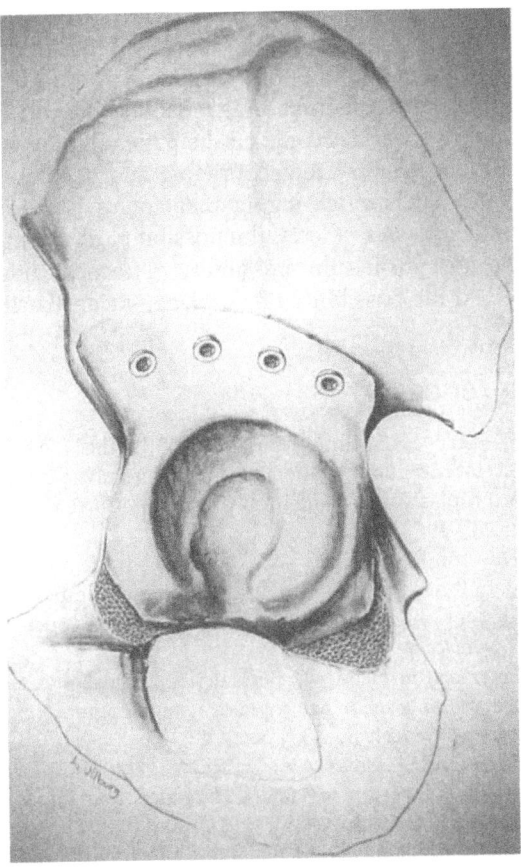

Figure 45.3. The graft is secured to the host pelvis with cancellous screws.

the graft acetabulum. The acetabular component is selected to allow for 2 to 3 mm of cement mantle. Anchor holes are drilled but placed so as not to violate the medial wall or the sculpted medial trough. Doing so would cause cement intrusion at the host-graft interface and prevent bony union from occurring. The bone is pulse lavaged, dried, and then cemented with pressurization.

The type of component will be dependent on the trial reduction and the stability required. Rarely does one find improved stability with a hooded component. Instability is usually secondary to soft tissue imbalance or localized areas of impingement. It is essential to remove any scar that may be acting, in its contracted state, as a force to lever the head out of position. Scar may also act by mass effect in conjunction with bony blocks to lever components out of their reduced state. Continued instability is likely secondary to the soft tissue imbalance from muscular insufficiency. A constrained acetabular liner has been used in this situation, although the long term sequelae have not yet been determined.

Postoperative Regimen

Postoperative rehabilitation initially consisted of protected weight-bearing for a period of 6 months with a hip–knee–ankle–foot orthosis for the initial 4 months. Depending on the fixation and the patient's overall soft tissue status, the rehabilitation can be slightly altered. If bony fixation is adequate with good interdigitation at the host–graft interface then touch weight-bearing will continue for 3 months versus a normal 4-month protocol. One-third weight-bearing then continues for an additional 1 to 2 months. All patients are braced because of the inherently poor soft tissue tension and increased soft tissue exposure. If the abductor musculature has some type of tension and contractility, then a hip abduction brace will be used during the period of touch weight-bearing. If there has been severe damage and scarring of the abductor musculature then a knee-ankle-foot extension will be added to the brace. The transplant patients are then followed clinically and radiographically at 1, 2, 3, 6, 12, 18 and 24 months, and then annually. Radiographs are assessed with anteroposterior pelvis and lateral hip films. Radiographs are assessed for component and graft migration, graft–host union, and graft resorption. A hip is considered a radiographic failure if migration exceeds 4 mm or if greater than 10° of angular change in the component occurs.

Results

Acetabular transplant allograft is reserved for the worst acetabular defects where other modes of fixation are not possible. Patients have had multiple surgical procedures with resultant poor soft tissue mass and severe bone deficiency. Gross has previously reported on a series of eleven cases of acetabular transplants with a two year success rate of 71%.[15] Paprosky et al. have reported on 19 cases with a minimum 2 year follow-up. All had a Paprosky Type IIIB defect which meant less than 50% of host bone is available for contact with a proposed press-fit acetabular shell. At an average follow-up of 33 months, 3 patients failed with the remaining 14 available for follow-up having good results.[68] The failure rate with bulk structural allografts and porous acetabular components is 6% versus 64% for type IIIA and type IIIB acetabular defects respectively at an average follow-up of 6.1 years.[67] All good results had union of the graft with the failures remaining ununited secondary to sepsis. All grafts showed some degree of resorption with one occurring to a more significant degree at 8 months follow-up. This graft was placed in a more lateral position which meant graft-host interdigitation and loading contact was poor. No acetabular components loosened or migrated. According to the modified D'Aubigne and Postel pain and walking score patients improved from 3.7/12 to 8.9/12 at last follow-up.[69]

Complications

The most common complication noted is dislocation. In the Paprosky group,[68] six patients dislocated postoperatively. Two occurred anteriorly from excessive anteversion of the graft and resultant cup position. One occurred secondary to patient noncompliance and the other three occurred in patients with poor musculature, multiple previous operative procedures, and a history of recurrent dislocation. Consideration is now given to constrained acetabular liners if abductor musculature is absent or if stability is not within an acceptable safe range with trial reduction.

Infections occurred in four patients with one patient being successfully treated with antibiotic suppression. The other three patients had a resection arthroplasty as a curative procedure. One of these patients also had irradiation induced osteonecrosis, which likely contributed to nonunion and failure. For this reason, transplant reconstruction can not be recommended with severe pelvic osteonecrosis.

Conclusion

Revision of the severely deficient acetabulum is a demanding procedure, which is becoming more prevalent secondary to the increased prevalence of joint arthroplasties in general. Certainties for reconstruction do not exist, but whole hemipelvis acetabular allografts provide a systematic approach with acceptable results. Previous revision results have not determined the degree of acetabular defect and correlated it to the type of reconstruction. This makes comparison difficult. Certainly cemented acetabular components have met with poor results. Bipolar acetabular components with and without structural allografts have performed as poorly as threaded components. Bulk structural allografts in conjunction with a porous coated component have been reported to have had variable results as have porous cups with high hip centers. This has been proposed to be secondary to differences in technique but also may be secondary to different defects being treated. In our hands these grafts work for less severe defects but continue to have a high failure rate in more significant defects.

Acetabular reconstruction rings have been suggested and have been reported with favorable results. Their technique and complications, however, are significant. Presently, we reserve this technique for the older individual who tends to have a lesser defect, that is a type IIIA.[17] Obtaining a stable construct with a ring is a difficult if not unobtainable feat in the severe defects. A 27% failure rate at five years must also be recognized.[62]

The hemipelvis allograft has provided acceptable results for reconstruction of the severely deficient acetabulum where no other option may exist. It must be realized that the reconstruction is a demanding procedure that places great demands on the patient, surgeon, and institution. Results are encouraging and despite a failure rate that is much higher than for revisions of acetabulae of lesser defects, the possibility of graft union to the host means the possibility of reconstitution of bone and the possibility of simpler re-reconstructions.

References

1. Convery FR, Minter-Convery M, Devine LSD, et al. Acetabular augmentation in primary and revision total hip arthroplasty with cementless prostheses. *Clin Orthop.* 1990; 252:37–49.
2. Emerson RH Jr, Head WC. Dealing with the deficient acetabulum in revision hip arthroplasty: the importance of implant migration and use of the jumbo cup. *Semin Arthroplasty.* 1993;4:2–8.
3. Emerson RH, Head WC, Berklaich FM, et al. Noncemented acetabular revision arthroplasty using allograft bone. *Clin Orthop.* 1989;249:30–43.
4. Engh CA, Glassman AH, Griffin WL, et al. Results of cementless revision for failed cemented total hip arthroplasty. *Clin Orthop.* 1988;235:91–110.
5. Harris WH, Krushell RJ, Galante JO. Results of cementless revisions of total hip arthroplasties using the Harris–Galante prosthesis. *Clin Orthop.* 1988;235:120.
6. Harris WH, Schmalzried TP. The Harris–Galante porous-coated acetabular component with screw fixation. *J Bone Joint Surg Am.* 1992;74:1130–1139.
7. Lachiewicz PF, Hussamy OD. Revision of the acetabulum without cement with use of the Harris–Galante porous coated implant. *J Bone Joint Surg Am.* 1994;76:1834–1839.
8. McGann WA, Welch RB, Picetti GD III. Acetabular preparation in cementless revision total hip arthroplasty. *Clin Orthop.* 1988;235:35.
9. Oakeshott RD, Morgan DAF, Zukor DJ, et al. Revision total hip arthroplasty with osseous allograft reconstruction: a clinical and roentgenographic analysis. *Clin Orthop.* 1987;225:37–49.
10. Padgett DE, Kull L, Rosenberg A, et al. Revision of the acetabular component without cement after total hip arthroplasty. *J Bone Joint Surg Am.* 1993;75:663–674.
11. Paprosky WG, Magnus RE. Principles of bone grafting in revision total hip arthroplasty. *Clin Orthop.* 1994;147–155.
12. Silverton CD, Rosenberg AG, Sheinkop MB, Kull LR, Galante JO. Revision total hip arthroplasty using cementless acetabular component: technique and results. *Clin Orthop.* 1995;319:201–208.
13. Tanzer M, Drucker D, Jasty M, et al. Revision of acetabular components with an uncemented Harris–Galante porous-coated prosthesis. *J Bone Joint Surg Am.* 1992;74:987–994.
14. Chandler HP, Penenberg BL. *Bone stock deficiency in total hip replacement. Classification and management.* Thorofare, NJ: Slack; 1989.

15. Gross AE, Allan DG, Catre M, et al. Bone grafts in hip replacement surgery: The pelvic side. *Orthop Clin North Am.* 1993;24:679–687.
16. McAllister CM, Borden LS. Allograft reconstruction of the acetabulum in revision hip surgery. *Semin Arthroplasty.* 1993;4:80–86.
17. Paprosky WG, Perona PG, Lawrence JM. Acetabular defect classification and surgical reconstruction in revision arthroplasty. A 6 year follow-up evaluation. *J Arthroplasty.* 1994;9:33–44.
18. Patch DA, Lewallen DG. Reconstruction of deficient acetabula using bone graft and a fixed porous ingrowth cup: a 5 year roentgenographic study. *Orthop Trans.* 1993;17:151.
19. Trancik TM, Stulberg BN, Wilde AH, et al. Allograft reconstruction of the acetabulum during revision total hip arthroplasty. *J Bone Joint Surg Am.* 1986;68:527.
20. Amstutz HC, Ma SM, Jinnah RH, et al. Revision of aseptic loose total hip arthroplasties. *Clin Orthop.* 1982;170:21–28.
21. Broughton NS, Rushton N. Revision hip arthroplasty. *Acta Orthop Scand.* 1982;53:923–928.
22. Callaghan JC. Total hip arthroplasty: clinical perspective. *Clin Orthop.* 1992;298:47–54.
23. Callaghan JJ, Salvati EA, Pellicci PM, et al. Results of revision for mechanical failure after cemented total hip replacement, 1979 to 1982: a two to five year follow-up. *J Bone Joint Surg Am.* 1985;67:1074–1085.
24. Hoogland T, Razzano CD, Marks KE, et al. Revision of Mueller total hip arthroplasties. *Clin Orthop.* 1981;161:180–185.
25. Hunter GA, Welsh RP, Cameron HU, et al. The results of revision of total hip arthroplasty. *J Bone Joint Surg Br.* 1979;61:419–427.
26. Kavanagh BF, Ilstrup DM, Fitzgerald RH Jr. Revision total hip arthroplasty. *J Bone Joint Surg Am.* 1985;67:517–526.
27. Kavanagh BF, Fitzgerald RH. Multiple revisions for failed total hip arthroplasty not associated with infection. *J Bone Joint Surg Am.* 1987;69:1144–1149.
28. Marti RK, Schuller HM, Besselaar PP, Vanfrank Haasnoot EL. Results of revision hip arthroplasty with cement. *J Bone Joint Surg Am.* 1990;72:346–354.
29. Mulroy RD, Harris WH. The effect of improved cementing techniques on component loosening in total hip replacement. An 11-year radiographic study. *J Bone Joint Surg Br.* 1990;72:757–760.
30. Pellicci PM, Wilson PD Jr, Sledge CB, et al. Revision total hip arthroplasty. *Clin Orthop.* 1982;170:34–46.
31. Pellicci PM, Wilson PD Jr, Sledge CB, et al. Long-term results of revision total hip replacement: a follow-up report. *J Bone Joint Surg Am.* 1985;67:513–516.
32. Repten JB, Varmarken J-E, Rock ND, Jensen JS. Unsatisfactory results after repeated revision of hip arthroplasty. 61 cases followed for 5 (1–10) years. *Acta Orthop Scand.* 1992;63:120–127.
33. Stromberg C, Herberts P, Palmertz B. Cemented revision hip arthroplaty. A multicenter 5–9 year study of 204 first revisions for loosening. *Acta Orthop Scand.* 1992;63:111–119.
34. Stromberg C, Herberts P. A multicenter 10-year study of cemented revision total hip arthroplasty in patients younger than 55 years old. A follow-up report. *J Arthroplasty.* 1994;9:595–601.
35. Ayerza M, Pierson R, Sheinkop M, et al. A clinical review of a conical screw-in acetabular design. *Orthop Trans.* 1988;12:662.
36. Cameron HU, Bhimji S. Design rationale in early clinical trials with a hemispherical threaded acetabular component. *J Arthroplasty.* 1988;3:399–310.
37. Mallory TH, Vaughn BK, Lombardi V, et al. Threaded acetabular components: design rationale and preliminary clinical experience. *Orthop Rev.* 1988;17:305–316.
38. More RC, Amstutz HC, Kabo JM, et al. Acetabular reconstruction with a threaded prosthesis for failed total hip arthroplasty. *Clin Orthop.* 1992;282:114–122.
39. Cameron HU, Jung YB. Acetabular revision with a bipolar prosthesis. *Clin Orthop.* 1990;251:100–103.
40. Murray WR. Acetabular salvage in revision total hip arthroplasty using a bipolar prosthesis. *Clin Orthop.* 1990;251:92–99.
41. Namba RS, Clarke A, Scott RD. Bipolar revisions with bone-grafting for cavitary and segmental acetabular defects. *J Arthroplasty.* 1994;9:263–272.
42. Scott RD. The use of a bipolar prosthesis with bone grafting in revision surgery. *Tech Orthop.* 1987;2:84–93.
43. Wilson MG, Nikpoor N, Aliabadi P, et al. Failure of support allografts: unacceptable migration of bipolar components. *J Bone and Joint Surg Am.* 1989;71:1469–1479.
44. Harris WH, Crothers O, Oh I. Total hip replacement and femoral head bone-grafting for severe acetabular deficiency in adults. *J Bone Joint Surg Am.* 1977;59:752–759.
45. Hooten JP, Engh CA Jr, Engh CA. Failure of structural acetabular allografts in cementless revision hip arthroplasty. *J Bone Joint Surg Br.* 1994;76:419–422.
46. Jasty M, Harris WH. Salvage total hip reconstruction in patients with major acetabular bone deficiency using structural femoral head allografts. *J Bone Joint Surg Br.* 1990;72:63–67.
47. Kwong LM, Jasty M, Harris WH. High failure rate of bulk femoral head allografts in total hip acetabular reconstruction at 10 years. *J Arthroplasty.* 1993;8:341–350.
48. Mulroy RD, Harris WH. Failure of acetabular autogenous grafts in total hip arthroplasty: increasing incidence, A follow-up note. *J Bone Joint Surg Am.* 1990;72:1536–1540.
49. Pollock FH, Whiteside LA. The fate of massive allografts in total hip acetabular revision surgery. *J Arthroplasty.* 1992;7:271–276.
50. Whiteside LA, Pollack FH. Failure of support allografts. *J Arthroplasty.* 1992;7:3–12.
51. Young SK, Dorr LD, Kaufman RL, et al. Factors related to failure of structural bone grafts in acetabular reconstruction of total hip arthroplasty. *Arthroplasty.* 1991;6 Suppl: 573–582.
52. Huo MH, Friedlaender GE, Salvati EA. Bone graft and total hip arthroplasty. *J Arthroplasty.* 1992;7:109–117.
53. Knight JL, Fujii K, Atwater R, et al. Bone-grafting for acetabular deficiency during primary and revision total hip arthroplasty—A radiographic and clinical analysis. *J Arthroplasty.* 1993;8:371–382.
54. Paprosky WG. Allograft reconstruction in massive acetabular defects. *Tech Orthop.* 1993;4:44–53.
55. Paprosky WG, Lawrence J, Cameron HU. Acetabular defect classification: clinical application. *Orthop Review (supp).* 1990;19:3–12.

56. Zmolek JC, Dorr LD. Revision total hip arthroplasty—the use of solid allograft. *J Arthroplasty*. 1993;8:361–370.
57. Azuma T, Yasuda H, Okagaki K, Sakai K. Compressed allograft chips for acetabular reconstruction in revision hip arthroplasty. *J Bone Joint Surg Br*. 1994;76:740–744.
58. Harris WH. Management of the deficient acetabulum using cementless fixation without bone grafting. *Orthop Clin North Am*. 1993;24:663–671.
59. Kelley SS. High hip center in revision arthroplasty. *J Arthroplasty*. 1994;9:503–511.
60. Russotti GM, Harris WH. Proximal placement of the acetabular component in total hip arthroplasty. A long-term follow-up study. *J Bone Joint Surg Am*. 1991;73:587–592.
61. Schutzer SF, Harris WH. High placement of porous-coated acetabular components in complex total hip arthroplasty. *J Arthroplasty*. 1994;9:359–367.
62. Berry DJ, Muller ME. Revision arthroplasty using an antiprotrusio cage for massive acetabular bone deficiency. *J Bone Joint Surg Br*. 1992;74:711–720.
63. Schatzker J, Glynn MK, Ritter D. A preliminary review of the Muller acetabular and Burch-Schneider anti-protrusio support rings. *Arch Orthop Trauma Surg*. 1984;103:5.
64. Peters CL, Curtain M, Samuelson KM. Acetabular revision with the Burch-Schneider anti-protrusio cage and cancellous allograft bone. *J Arthroplasty*. 1995;10:307–312.
65. Rosson J, Schatzker J. The use of reinforcement rings to reconstruct deficient acetabulae. *J Bone Joint Surg Br*. 1992; 74:716–720.
66. Zehntner MK, Ganz R. Midterm results (5.5–10 years) of acetabular allograft reconstruction with the acetabular reinforcement ring during total hip revision. *J Arthroplasty*. 1994;9:469–479.
67. Paprosky WG, Bradford MS, Jablonsky WS. Acetabular reconstruction with massive acetabular allografts. *Inst Course Lect*. 1996;45:149–159.
68. Bradford MS, Paprosky WG. Total acetabular transplant allograft reconstruction of the severely deficient acetabulum. *Semin Arthroplasty*. 1995;2:86–95.

46
Use of Structural Allografts in Hip Reconstruction

Hugh P. Chandler and Robert J. Carangelo

In years past, only three sizes of cemented acetabular components were available, and structural acetabular grafts were commonly necessary to reconstruct deficient bone stock in hip surgery. There are now many sizes of uncemented acetabular components, ranging from as small as 44 mm outer diameter to 80 mm. If the rim will successfully support an uncemented component, contained defects can often be grafted using allograft or autograft morselized bone.[1,2] Small uncemented components can be used in a high hip center of rotation.[3–5] Oblong porous-coated acetabular components can also be used in situations where the columns are intact and there is an isolated superior defect. For major central defects, there is a place for protrusio shells, combined with morselized bone and cemented, all-polyethylene components.[6]

Therefore, there is now little need for the use of structural acetabular grafts. However, there are still two major indications for the use of structural acetabular grafts. The first is the deficient rim that will not support an uncemented component. The second indication is global acetabular deficiency where there is no bone stock. Factors that affect the results of structural grafts include: exposure, choice of graft material, trabecular orientation, fixation of the graft, fixation of the acetabular component, and postoperative management.

Techniques for Acetabular Grafting

Surgical Exposure

Wide exposure is necessary for major hip reconstruction. The standard transtrochanteric approach is adequate for most structural grafting procedures. The trochanteric slide is not as helpful because the superior gluteal nerve tethers the abductors from translating anteriorly and limits exposure of the anterior and superior acetabular rim. The extended iliofemoral approach provides extensive exposure of the entire rim and of the iliac wing. The ilioinguinal approach, combined with the extended iliofemoral approach, permits exposure of the entire hemipelvis and is helpful in those rare situations in which the anterior and posterior columns both need to be plated (Fig. 46.3D). If the extended iliofemoral and the ilioinguinal approach are combined, care should be taken to make sure that the skin incision of the ilioinguinal approach intersects the iliofemoral incision at right angles to diminish the potential for skin loss.

Choice of Graft Material

In developmental dysplasia (DDH), autogenous femoral heads are ideal for subluxed hips in a false acetabulum.[1,7–9] If allograft femoral heads are used in revision, they should be of good quality. Osteopenic bone is adequate only to use as morselized bone. We used an autogenous femoral head that had been used beneath a surface replacement on one occasion and beneath a mold arthroplasty in another as a structural graft. Both heads were osteopenic and may have been avascular, and both failed very quickly.

Allograft distal femoral condyles and proximal tibias can be used for larger defects, but perhaps the most helpful source for global acetabular deficiency is an acetabular allograft, harvested from an allograft pelvis (Figs. 46.1, 46.2, and 46.3).[10–13]

Trabecular Orientation

In life, the trabeculae of all lower-extremity bones are aligned with weight-bearing forces in response to stress (Fig. 46.4). If a structural graft is used, the trabeculae must be similarly aligned with weight-bearing forces or the trabeculae will routinely fracture and the graft will fail (Fig. 46.5, 46.6).[14,15]

Fixation of the Graft

The graft must fit the host defect accurately, or union cannot occur. In DDH, with a subluxed hip in a false ac-

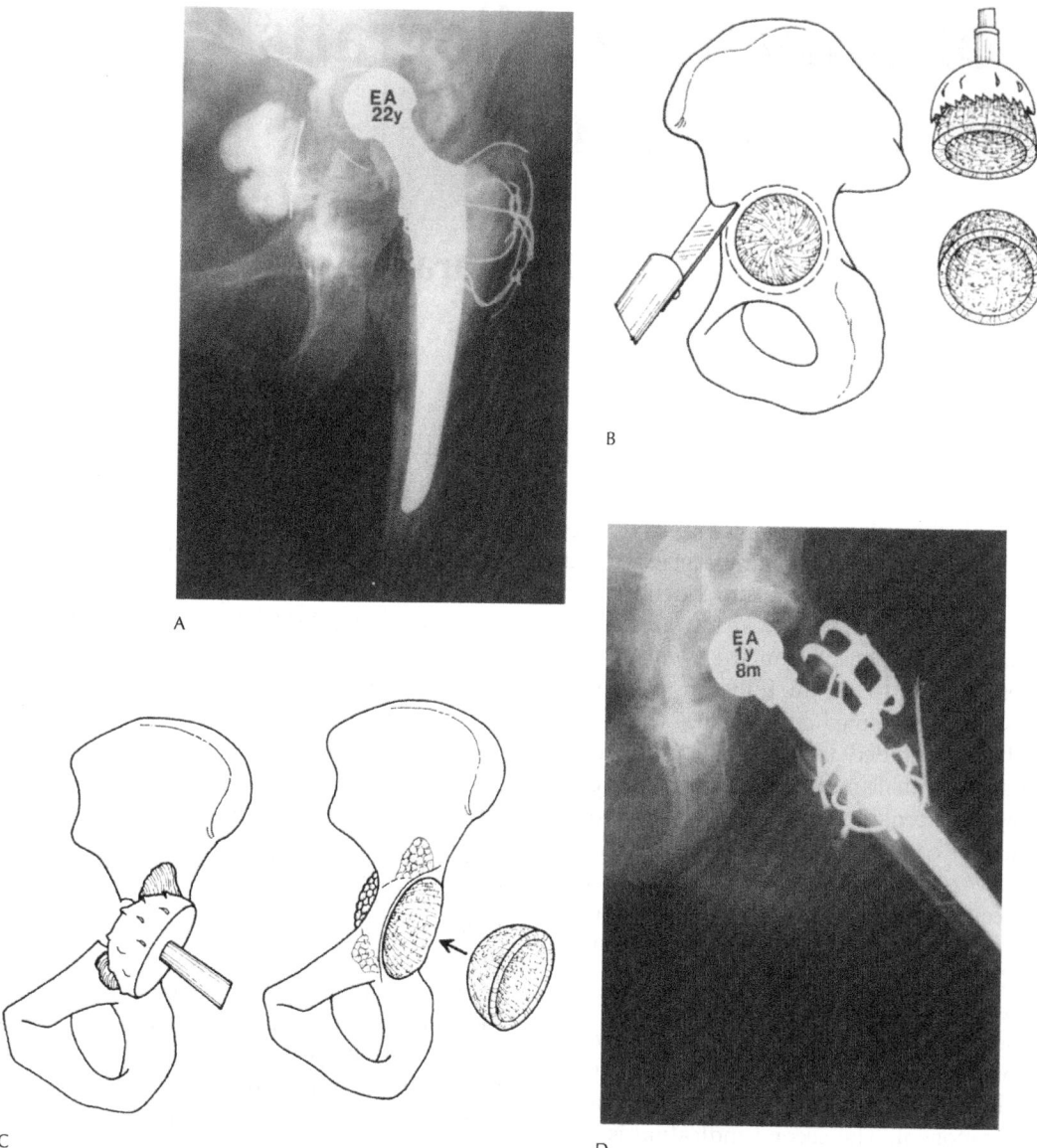

Figure 46.1. A. This 50-year-old woman presented with a loose acetabulum component 22 years after her index total hip replacement for developmental dysplasia. B. The acetabulum from an allograft hemipelvis was first reamed with hemispherical male reamers. The acetabulum was then cut out using a saw. The back portion of the graft was first shaped with a saw and then with female hemispherical reamers. C. The rim of the patient's acetabulum was reamed with a male reamer that was 1 mm smaller than the female reamer that had been used for the back of the acetabular graft. Host intraacetabular defects were filled with morselized allograft bone. The allograft acetabulum was impacted within the patients's acetabulum, achieving a press fit. Supplementary fixation was provided by countersunk lag screws. A polyethylene acetabular component with methacrylate studs was cemented into the allograft acetabulum. D. At 1 year, 8 months, radiographs show probable union of the graft. The patient is doing well, but follow-up is short.

etabulum, the fit is already established (Fig. 46.7A). In this circumstance, the head fits the acetabulum best in the position that it assumes with the hip in extension (Fig. 46.7D). The trabeculae are also optimally oriented in this position (Fig. 46.7F and G). With allografts, it is easier to change complex host or graft geometries to simple hemispherical shapes using male–female reamers or to flat surfaces using a saw or an osteotome (Fig. 46.3C and Fig. 46.9B). The graft must be supported by a host bone buttress. Initial fixation of the graft against the buttress can be achieved by three crossed K-wires. Final fixation is best maintained by cancellous lag screws that do not have threads in the graft and are oriented in line with weight-bearing forces. It is important

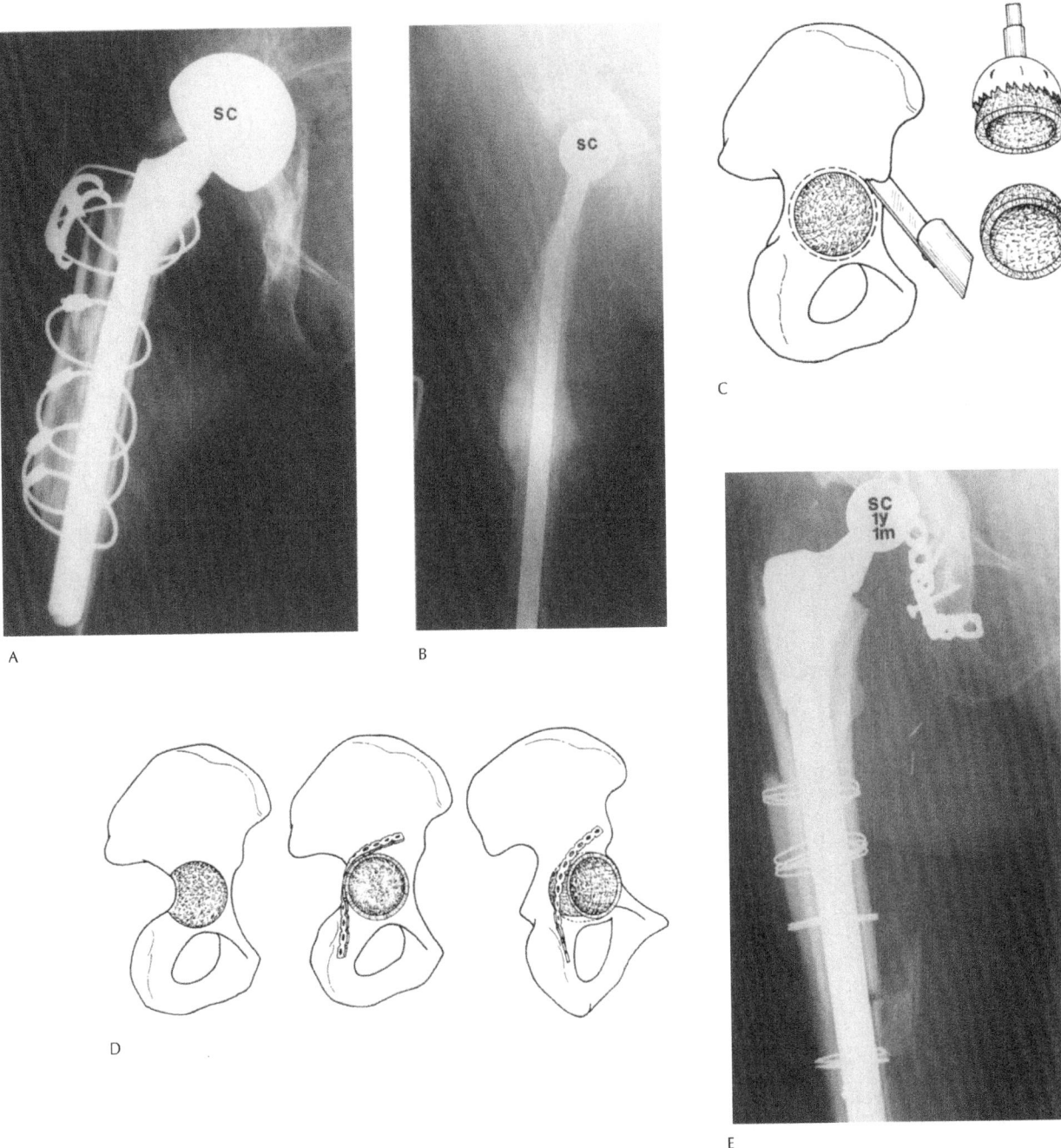

Figure 46.2. A. This 70-year-old woman had four previous operations for developmental dysplasia. She presented with a dislocated bipolar prosthesis that had eroded through the superior and posterior rim of her acetabulum. B. She presented with *S aureus* infection and required removal of all components and of her proximal femur, which was involved with osteomyelitis. An antibiotic-impregnated articulating spacer component was utilized. C. She was treated with appropriate intravenous antibiotics for 6 weeks. An aspiration 10 days later was negative and the hip was reconstructed. An allograft acetabulum was shaped with a saw and a female reamer. D. The rim of her acetabulum was reamed with a male reamer that was 1 mm smaller than the female reamer that had been used to shape the acetabular graft. The acetabular graft was impacted into the patient's acetabulum. Additional fixation was achieved by means of a posterior acetabulum reconstruction plate and three countersunk lag screws. E. A cemented polyethylene acetabular component with methacrylate studs was used within the acetabular graft. She required a proximal femoral segmental allograft as well. Radiographically, both the acetabular and femoral reconstruction appear to be doing well at short follow-up of a year and a month. She requires a single crutch because of abductor weakness, probably secondary to superior gluteal nerve injury related to the dislocated bipolar prosthesis.

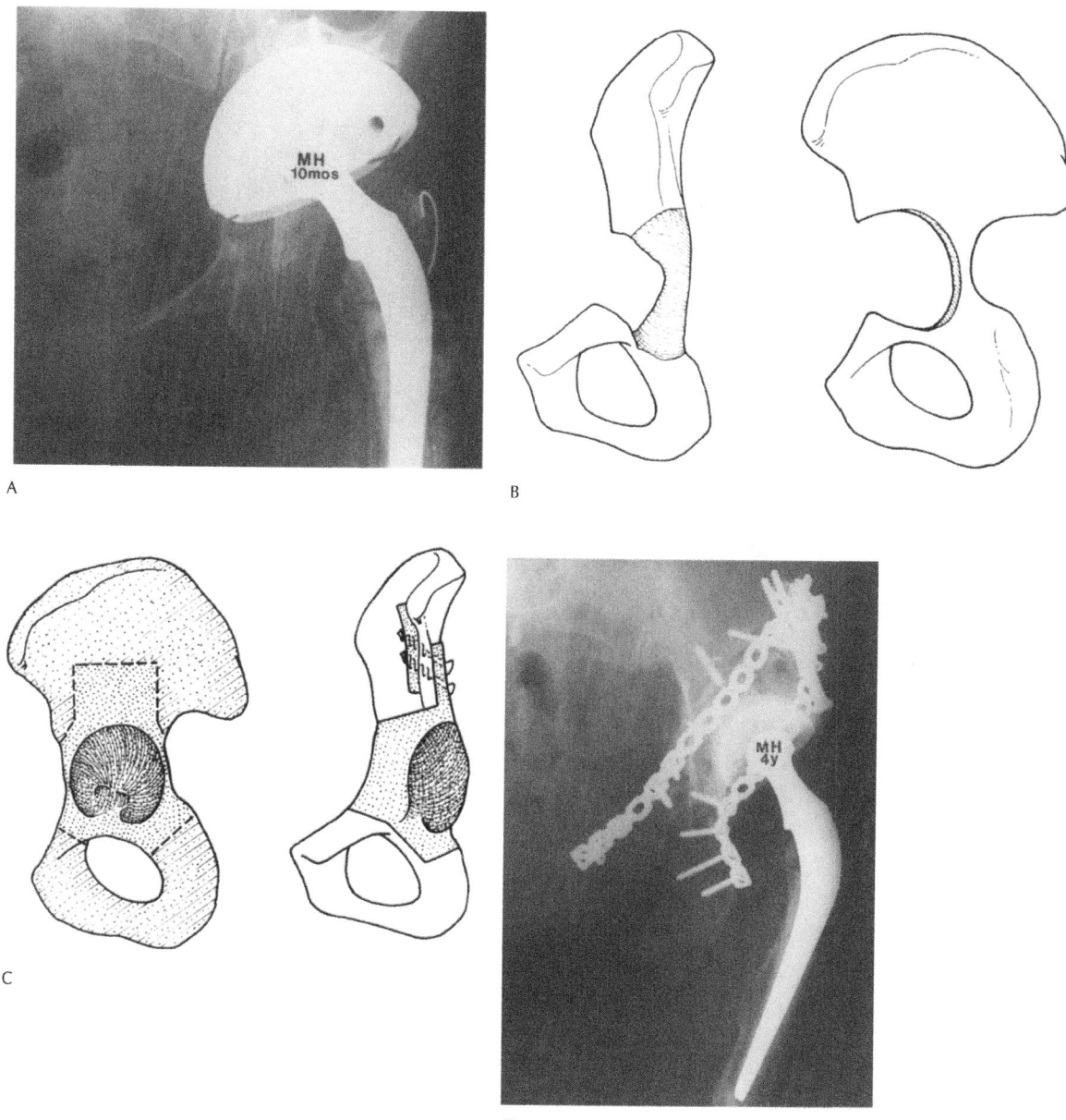

Figure 46.3. A. This 79-year-old woman had three previous total hip replacements. An 80 mm uncemented component was used at the last revision. She had residual pain because of acetabular loosening. B. The anterior column was deficient. The posterior column was very thin. C. A hemi-allograft acetabulum was used. A transverse shelf above the allograft acetabulum contacted a buttress of host bone. The outer table of the allograft ilium was placed outside the weak iliac wing of the host. Oblique screws were placed through the osteopenic ilium of the host pelvis and engaged strong allograft bone on the inside of the pelvis. An anterior and posterior column plate provided additional stability. D. X-rays at 4 years showed union. The patient has no pain, but unfortunately has a femoral nerve palsy and requires support because of knee instability.

that fixation screws be used only to hold the graft against the buttress and in themselves bear no weight. Such screws allow the graft to impact against the buttress, stimulating healing and later remodeling (Fig. 46.7 and 46.8). Reconstruction plates are occasionally necessary as additional fixation, but it is best to use lag screws first to impact the graft to the host buttress before acetabular plates are added.

Choice of Acetabular Components

Our initial experience was with cemented components used with structural grafts, because these were the only type available. When uncemented components proved to be helpful in primary and uncomplicated revision, these were also tried in conjunction with structural grafts. Since uncemented components can never achieve ingrowth

46. Structural Allografts in Hip Reconstruction

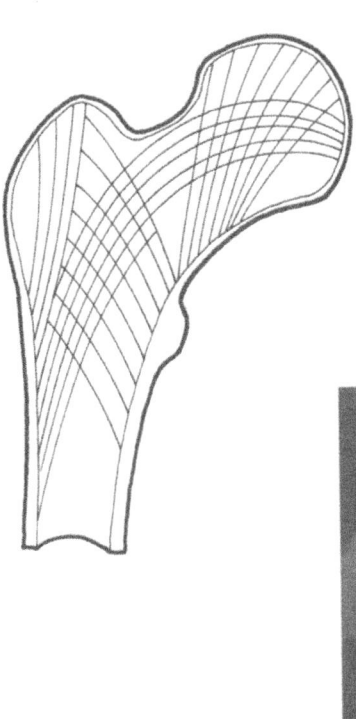

Figure 46.4. In life, the trabeculae of all lower-extremity bones are aligned with weight-bearing forces in response to stress.

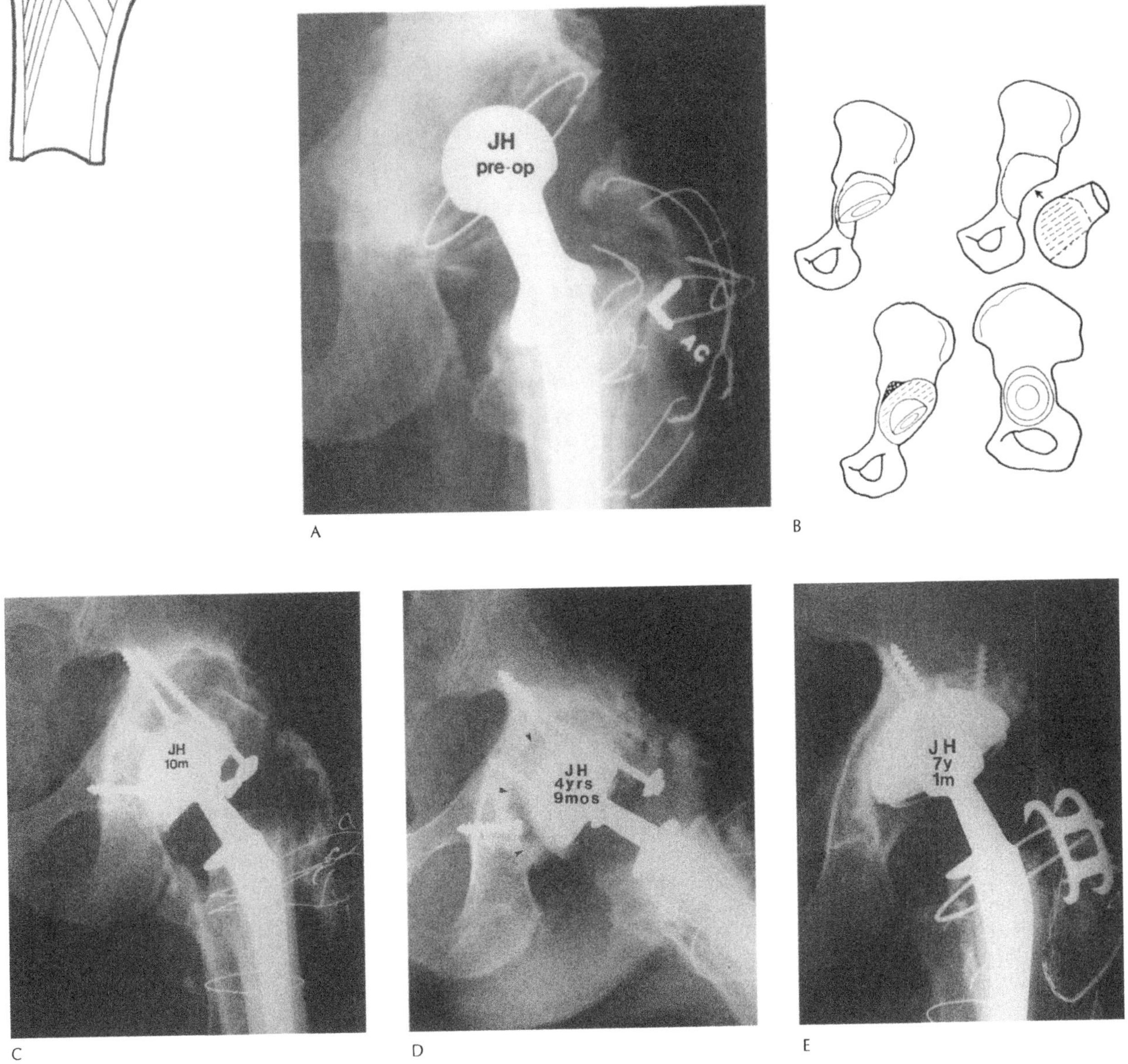

Figure 46.5. A. This 43-year-old man had undergone five previous left hip operations, including a mold arthroplasty that was revised once and a total hip that was also revised once. He presented with a loose polyethylene acetabular component with an outer diameter of 74 mm. B. A distal femur, including both condyles, was used to reconstruct the defect. The trabeculae of the graft were inadvertently placed transverse to the weight-bearing axis. We would now have used a jumbo uncemented acetabular component rather than a graft, but these components were not available then. C. At 10 months, the graft appears to have united to the host bone. The inferior screw is transverse to the weight-bearing axis. D. At 4 years and 9 months, there is evidence of resorption of the graft. E. At 5 years, revision was required. The majority of the graft had resorbed. An uncemented component was used and remains stable at 7 years.

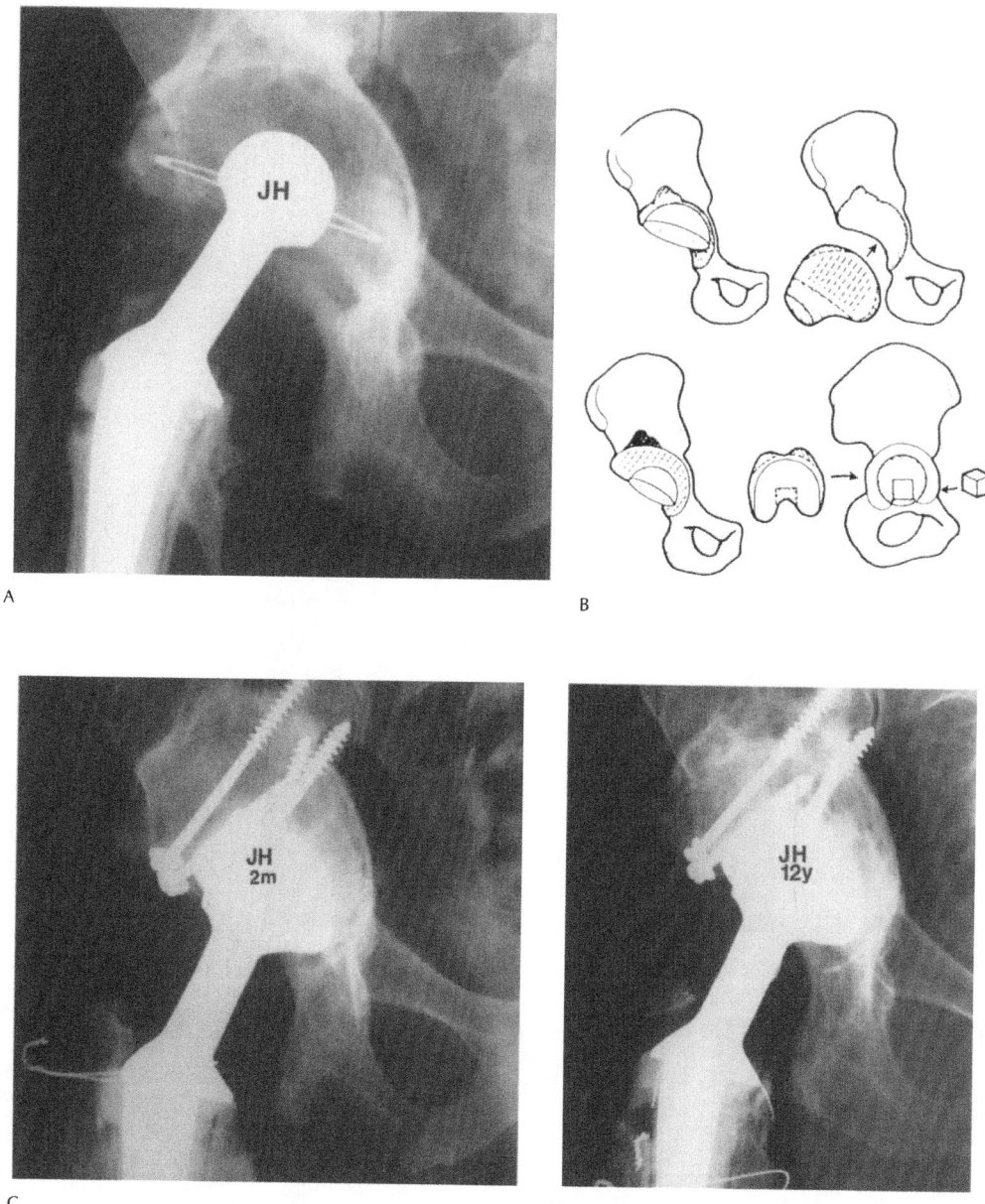

Figure 46.6. A. Three years after the left hip was done, the patient required revision of his right hip for an identical acetabular problem. He had undergone nine previous operations on this hip, including a Moore prosthesis, an arthrodesis, four cup arthroplasties, and three total hip replacements. B. The reconstruction was the same as that performed on the left hip except for the fact that the trabeculae of the femoral allograft on the right side were properly aligned with weight-bearing stresses. C. At 2 months, he was doing well and began to use a cane. The screws were in proper alignment. The cemented acetabular component is 100% covered by the graft. D. At 12 years, the acetabular component remains well fixed. Note the difference in the behavior of this graft compared to the graft in the left hip. The only difference in technique is the fact that the trabeculae of the graft was transverse in the left hip and properly aligned in the right.

against dead structural grafts, failure of these components used with structural grafts has been high in our experience (Figs. 46.10).[1] Similar results have been experienced by other reconstructive surgeons.[11,16–18] We now feel that if the acetabular component would be unstable without the support of the graft, cement should always be used. The unusual exception would be the rare circumstance in which an uncemented component would be stable without the use of a graft, and the graft would be used only for additional security. For practical purposes, the great majority of acetabular components should be cemented if used in conjunction with structural

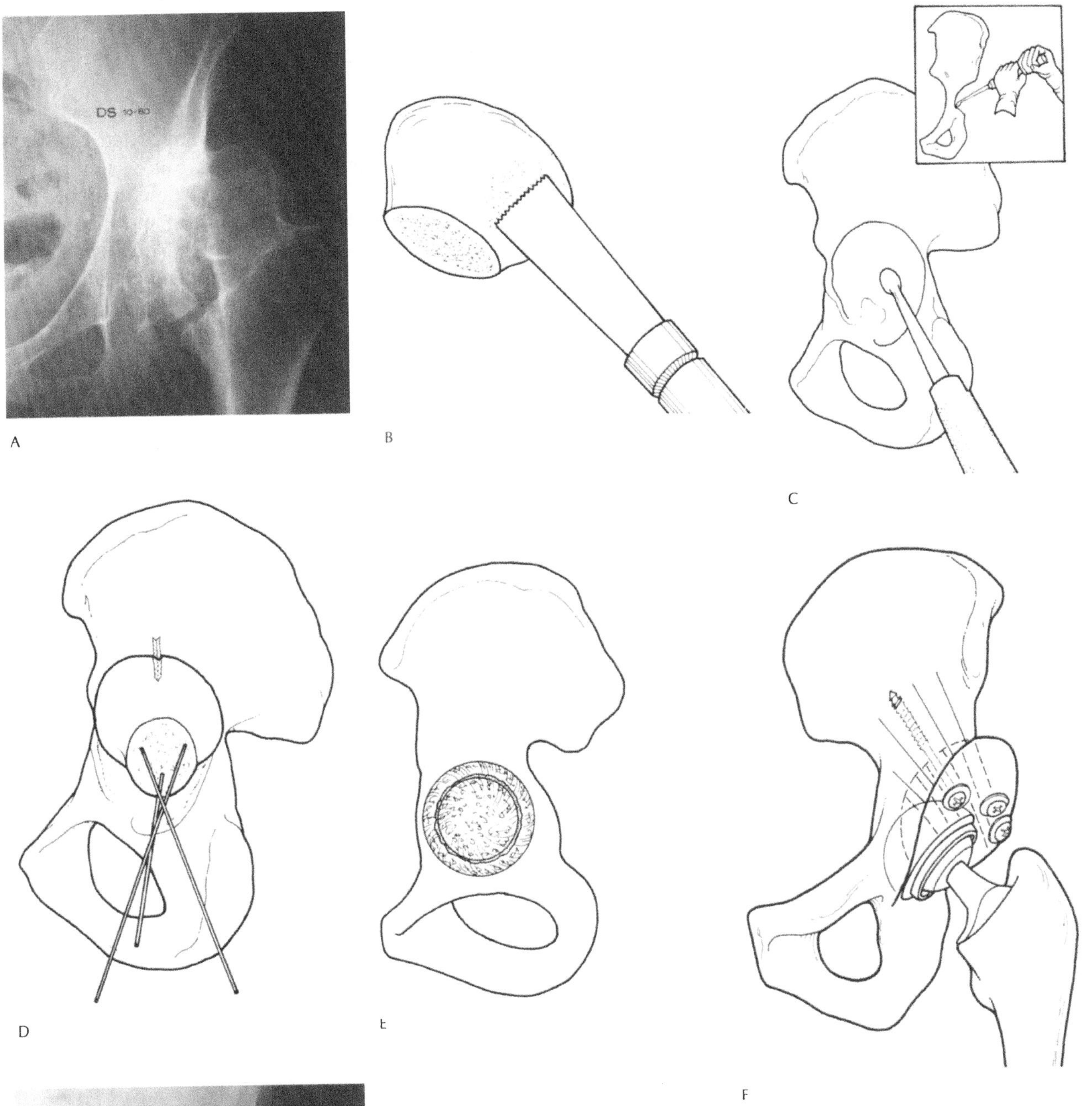

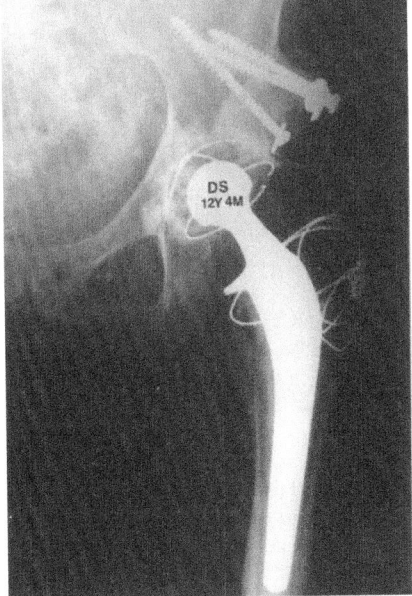

Figure 46.7. A. This 76-year-old woman had degenerative arthritis secondary to DDH. The femoral head is in a false acetabulum. B. The head was scuffed with an oscillating saw to remove soft tissues. It is not necessary to remove the cortex. C. The acetabulum was curetted to remove soft tissues. D. The relationship of the head to the acetabulum was previously marked with the hip in extension, prior to dividing the neck. The head was placed back in the acetabulum, matching these marks, to ensure that the trabeculae were anatomically aligned. The head was temporarily fixed with three smooth wires in the area where the new acetabulum was eventually placed. E. After the acetabulum had been reamed, a preliminary thin bead of cement was placed at the graft–host junction and allowed to harden to prevent the final cement from intruding between the graft and the host. F. The false acetabulum acts as a buttress. The trabeculae of the head are anatomically aligned with weight-bearing forces. Three cancellous screws have been placed in the periphery of the head. The screws are parallel and aligned with weight-bearing forces. There should be no threads in the graft so the head can impact against the buttress. The acetabular component should be cemented. G. Radiographs at 12 years, 4 months show that the graft and the acetabular component are stable. She is now 16 years, 9 months postoperative and reports by phone that she is doing well. She is 92, lives in a nursing home, and is too frail to get a new x-ray or return for follow-up.

grafts. Our preference now is to use all-polyethylene, cemented components with methacrylate studs to ensure a uniform cement mantle. A preliminary bead of cement should be used at the junction of the graft and the host to ensure that the second batch of cement does not intrude between the graft and the host bone (Fig. 46.7E). Some authors feel that bipolar components should not be used in conjunction with a structural graft, as they may erode through the graft.[19,20]

Postoperative Management

A cancellous structural acetabular graft that has the trabeculae oriented properly and is supported by a host buttress can support immediate full weight-bearing without risk of collapse. As the graft incorporates, new bone is added to the dead trabeculae and the graft becomes even stronger.[14] Weight-bearing forces impact the graft against the host buttress, stimulating healing of the

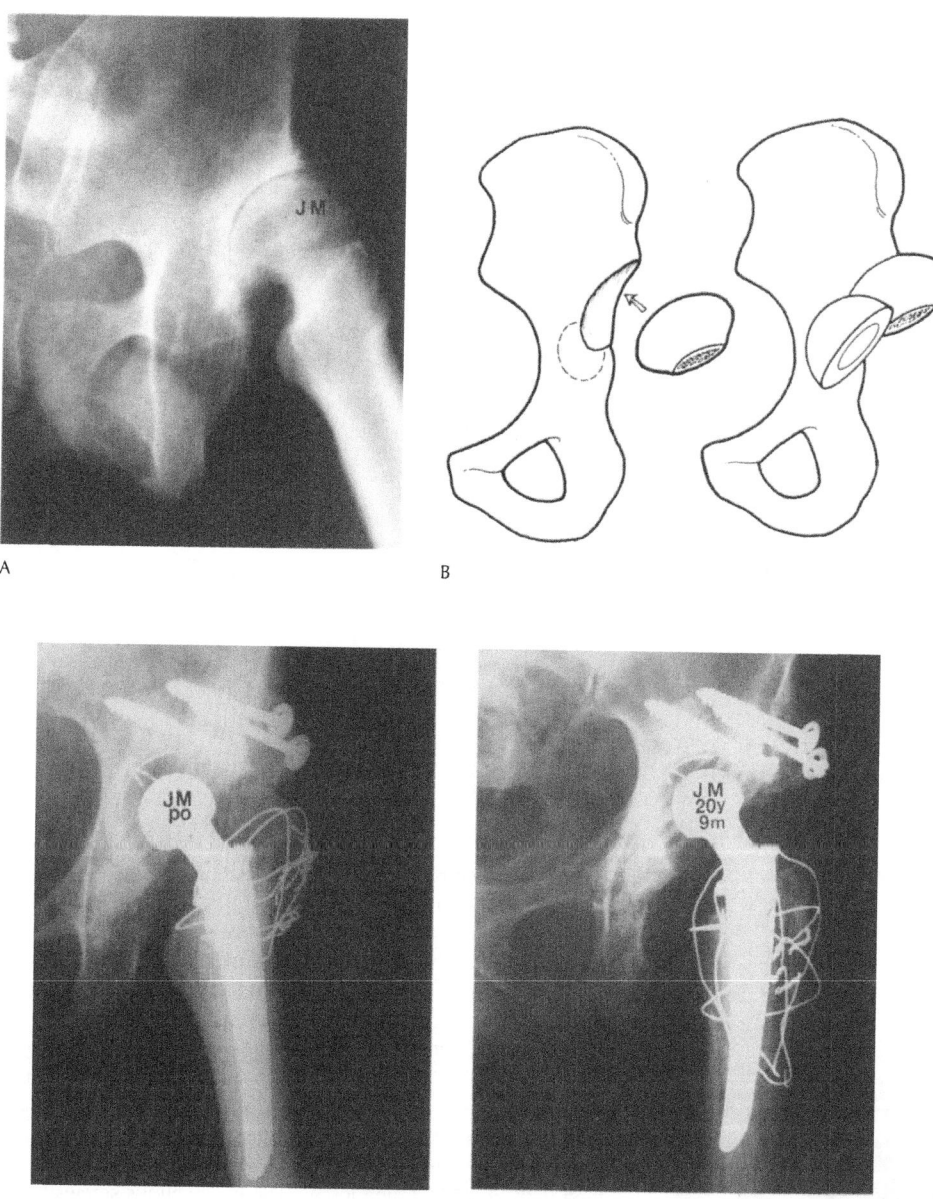

Figure 46.8. A. This 60-year-old man had developmental dysplasia with degenerative arthritis. B. His femoral head was used to reconstruct the superior rim. C. The junction between the graft and the host is hard to determine in the postoperative x-rays. The screws are more transverse than ideal. D. At 20 years and 9 months, the graft and the patient continue to do well.

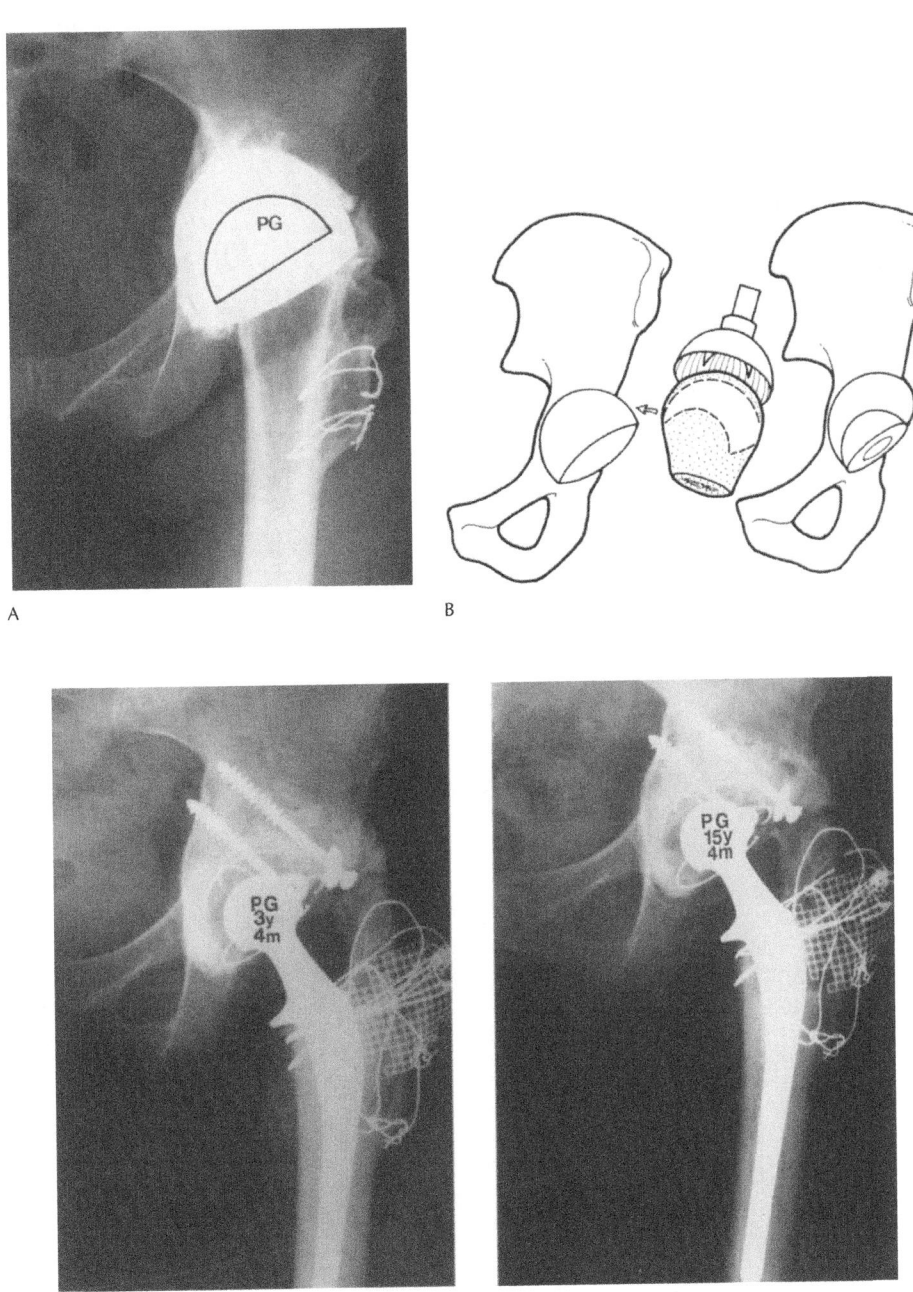

Figure 46.9. A. This 40-year-old woman had a painful left hip after two failed mold arthroplasties. B. The acetabulum was reamed with a male reamer. A very large allograft femoral head was reamed with a female reamer of the same size. The trabeculae are properly oriented. The acetabular component was cemented. C. At 3 years and 4 months, there was mild peripheral resorption of the graft in the area that is not stressed, and the washers had migrated medially a bit. D. At 15 years and 4 months, the graft and the patient continue to do well. The acetabular component is entirely supported by the graft. There is no further migration of the washers.

graft to the host and later remodeling of the graft. Sixty to 80 pounds of protected weight-bearing is encouraged if a trochanteric osteotomy has been performed to allow healing of the greater trochanter. Thereafter, weight-bearing as tolerated is encouraged, regardless of whether the graft has united or not. Prolonged protection from weight-bearing is detrimental.

Conclusion

It is clear that structural acetabular grafts are rarely necessary because other methods of managing bone deficiency are now available and are technically easier. There is some controversy as to whether structural acetabular grafts should ever be used.[16–18] However,

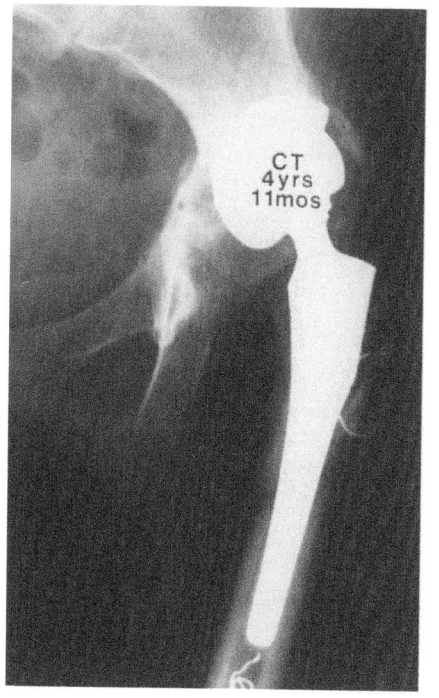
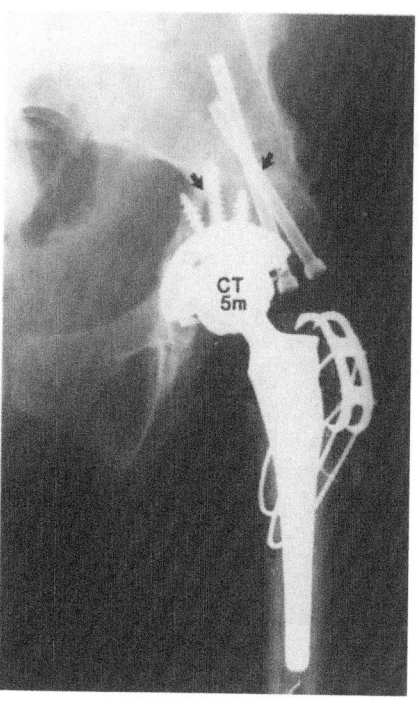
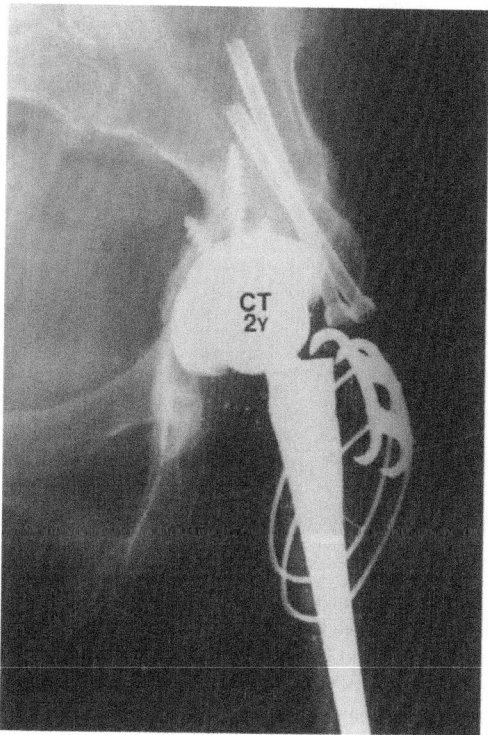
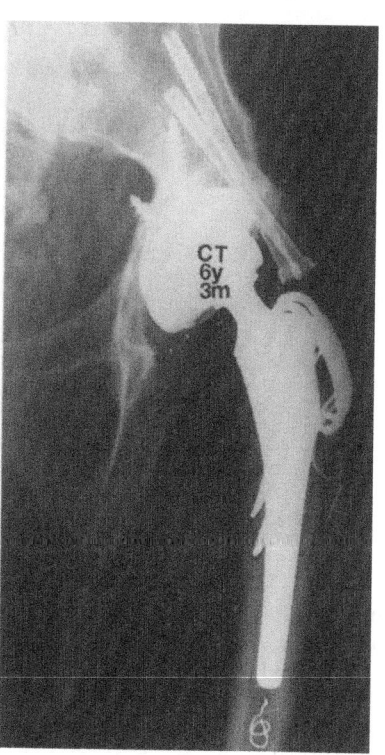

Figure 46.10. A. This 46 year-old-woman had a left total hip replacement 4 years, 11 months previously. She had pain because of acetabular loosening. B. The femoral head allograft was shaped with female reamers that matched the male reamers that had been used to prepare the patient's acetabulum (see Fig. 46.9B). The graft was of good quality, the fit was excellent, and the trabeculae were properly aligned. However the acetabular component was used without cement. At 5 months, the graft and the patient were doing well. Arrows outline the graft. C. X-rays at 2 years, show the graft has united but the acetabular component has migrated proximally. D. X-rays at 6 years, 3 months show further migration of the acetabular component. There is significant lysis of the proximal femur, probably related to metal debris from contact between the acetabular shell and the screws. The patient is scheduled for revision.

based on our long-term experience with structural grafts, it is obvious that their success or failure is distinctly related to technique.

It is always necessary to have good exposure, the graft must be of good quality, the trabeculae must be oriented in line with weight-bearing forces, the graft–host fit must be accurate, the graft must be supported by a host buttress, and the acetabular component must be cemented.

Of 29 surgical acetabular grafts followed for a minimum of 10 years and an average of 12 1/2 years, six grafts (20%) failed. Two failed because of sepsis, and four nonseptic failures resulted from technical errors. These included a poor choice of bone on two occasions, failure to use cement in two grafts, and transverse trabeculae in all. There was no correlation between the percentage of coverage of the acetabular component and failure of the graft.[21]

References

1. Chandler HP, Lopez C, Murphy S, Van Eenenamm DP. Acetabular reconstruction using structural grafts in total hip replacement: a 12 1/2 year follow-up. *Semin Arthroplasty.* 1995;6:118–130.
2. Padgett DE, Kuff L, Rosenberg A et al. Revision of the acetabular component without cement after total hip arthroplasty: 3–6 year followup. *J Bone Joint Surg Am.* 1995;75:663–673.
3. Pagnano MW, Hanssen AD, Lewallen DG, Shaughnessy WJ. The effect of superior placement of the acetabular component on the rate of loosening after total hip arthroplasty. Long term results in patients who have Crowe type II congenital dysplasia of the hip. *J Bone Joint Surg Am.* 1996;78:1004–1014.
4. Russotti GM, Harris WH. Proximal placement of the acetabular component in total hip arthroplasty—A long term follow-up study. *J Bone Joint Surg Am.* 1991;73:587–592.
5. Schutzer SF, Harris WH. High placement of porous coated acetabular components in complex total hip arthroplasty. *J Arthroplasty.* 1994;9:359–368.
6. Berry DH, Mullen ME. Revision arthroplasty using an protrusio cage for massive acetabular bone deficiency. *J Bone Joint Surg Br.* 1992;74:711–715.
7. Gross AE, Catre MG. The use of femoral head autograft shelf reconstruction and cemented acetabular component in the dysplastic hip. *Clin Orthop.* 1994;298:60–66.
8. Hasegawa Y, Iwata H, Iwase T, Kawamoto K, Iwasada S. Cementless total arthroplasty with autologous bone grafting for hip dysplasia. *Clin Orthop.* 1996;324:179–186.
9. Rodriquez JA, Huk OL, Pellicci PM, Wilson PD. Autogenous bone grafts from the femoral head for the treatment of acetabular deficiency in primary total hip arthroplasty with cement, long-term results. *J Bone Joint Surg Am.* 1995;77:1227–1233.
10. Bradford MS, Paprosky WG. Total acetabular transplant allograft reconstruction of the severely deficient acetabulum. *Sem Arthroplasty.* 1995;6:86–95.
11. Paprosky WG, Magnus RE. Principles of bone grafting in revision total hip arthroplasty; acetabular technique. *Clin Orthop.* 1994;298:147–155.
12. Paprosky WG, Perona PG, Lawrence JM. Acetabular defect classification and surgical reconstruction in revision arthroplasty; a six year follow-up evaluation. *J Arthroplasty.* 1994;9:33–44.
13. Chandler HP, Penenberg BL. *Surgical approaches: bone stock deficiency in total hip replacement.* Chandler HP, Penenberg BL, eds. Thorofare, NJ: Slack, 1989.
14. Evans FC. *Mechanical properties of bone.* Springfield, Ill.: Charles C. Thomas, 1973.
15. Springfield DS. Massive autogenous bone grafts. *Ortho Clin North Am.* 1987;18:249–256.
16. Hooten JP, Engh CA Jr, Engh CA. Failure of structural acetabular allografts in cementless revision hip arthroplasty. *J Bone Joint Surg Br.* 1994;76:419–422.
17. Kwong LM, Jasty M, Harris WH. High failure rate of bulk femoral head allografts in total hip acetabular reconstructions at ten years. *J Arthroplasty.* 1993;8:341–346.
18. Shinar AA, Harris WH. Bulk structural autogenous grafts and allografts for reconstruction of the acetabulum in total hip arthroplasty. Sixteen year average followup. *J Bone Joint Surg Am.* 1997;79:159–169.
19. Papagelopoulos PJ, Lewellen DG, Cabanela ME, McFarland EG, Wallrichs SL. Acetabular reconstruction using bipolar endoprosthesis and bone grafting in patients with severe bone deficiency. *Clin Orthop.* 1995;312:170.
20. Wilson MG, Nipoor N, Alibadi P, Poss R, Weisman B. The fate of acetabular allografts after bipolar revision arthroplasty of the hip. A radiographic review. *J Bone Joint Surg Am.* 1989;71:1469–1479.
21. Chandler HP, Tigges RG. Structural grafting in acetabular reconstruction. In: *The adult hip.* Callaghan JJ, Rosenberg AG, Rubash HE, eds. Philadelphia: Lippincott-Raven, 1988:1425–1438.

47
Determination of the Hip Center

Edward C. Brown III and Scott S. Kelley

The management of superior acetabular deficiency is controversial. Superior defects can be treated with anatomic centers,[1-5] as previously discussed, or high hip centers.[6-8] High hip centers can be created by two methods, either a small cup placed in the region of superior deficiency (Fig. 47.1), or an oversize cup filling the entire acetabular defect (Fig. 47.2). Oversize cups can only be used when there is enough bone available in the anteroposterior columns to contain the increased diameter.

Although hip centers can inadvertently be placed high in cemented arthroplasties, the use of high hip centers in revision arthroplasty infers the use of an uncemented acetabular component. High hip centers allow direct contact of the acetabular component to native host bone without the need for augmentation with a superior filler[1,3,4] (Figure 47.3).

This chapter will discuss the definition of a high hip center and review the literature and technical considerations at the time of surgery for high hip centers.

Definitions

The normal hip center has been measured in several studies.[6,7,9] The center of rotation of the anatomic hip is reported to be 12 to 14mm above the interteardrop line and 33 to 43mm lateral to the acetabular teardrop.

A high hip center is determined radiographically, and its definition is an arbitrary one. Although definitions vary, most authors accept and use 30 mm of hip center elevation above the interteardrop line as a minimal criteria. Ideally, this measurement should be corrected for magnification by using a measurement of femoral head size. In addition, pelvic rotation should be noted as 10° of hip flexion results in 2 mm of apparent hip center elevation.[7]

A criticism of the use of an arbitrary distance is the lack of accounting for normal variance in pelvic size. Ranawat proposed a technique to determine the true acetabular region based on pelvic size with a proportional assessment of the anatomic hip position.[10] However, in review of the literature of hip center height for normal hips,[6-9] the maximum elevation reported was below 20 mm, suggesting that the arbitrary use of 30 mm is a reasonable definition for a high hip center.

Review of the Literature

The effect of relocation of the hip center on hip forces and component longevity is controversial. Theoretical and clinical studies show that superolateral relocation increased hip loads[11] and were associated with increased acetabular component failure rates.[10,12-14] Other studies suggest that joint reaction forces and acetabular loosening rates remain low for superior relocation without concomitant lateralization.[6-8,15,16]

Johnston et al.[11] reported that location of the hip center was the most important factor affecting load on the hip joint, based on a mathematical analysis. Loads were minimized by placing the center as far medially, inferiorly, and anteriorly as possible. Movement of the hip center to a position 20 mm superior, 20 mm lateral, and 10 mm posterior from the anatomic position was calculated to increase the joint contact force 20%. An experimental study by Doehring et al.[16] reported that hip joint total force significantly increased only when the hip center was relocated superolaterally from the normal hip position for both single-leg stance and stair climbing positions. A mathematical analysis by Brand and Pedersen[15] also attempted to isolate these effects. Superior placement was determined to increase hip joint forces 5% per centimeter and superior placement alone did not increase the hip joint forces as much as lateral placement alone.

Several clinical studies reported the adverse effects of nonanatomic placement on cemented acetabular components in both primary and revision hip arthroplasties.[10,12-14] In studies of patients with rheumatoid arthritis, both Ranawat and Lachiewicz reported a high incidence of loosening for cemented cups at a nonanatomic position. Ranawat et al.[10] found a 93% (16 of 17 hips) radiographic loosening rate for components po-

47. Determination of Hip Center

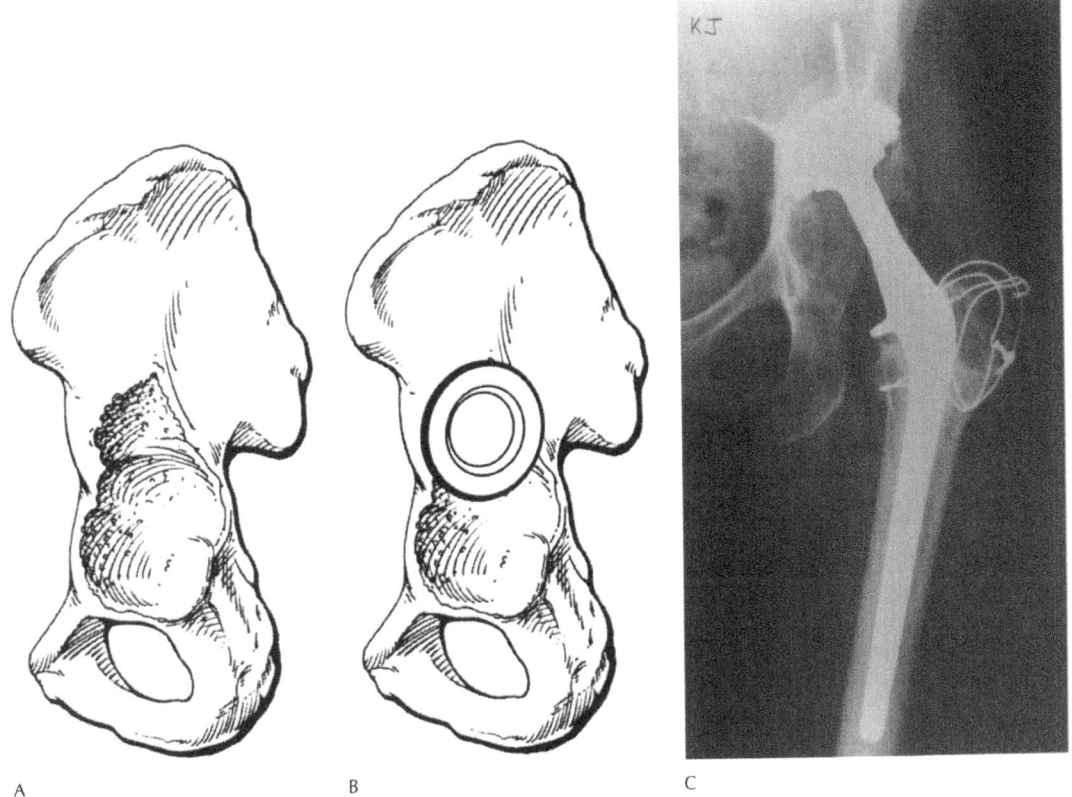

Figure 47.1. A. Superior acetabular defect. B. Superior placement of small acetabular component. C. Radiograph of small acetabular component placed in superior defect.

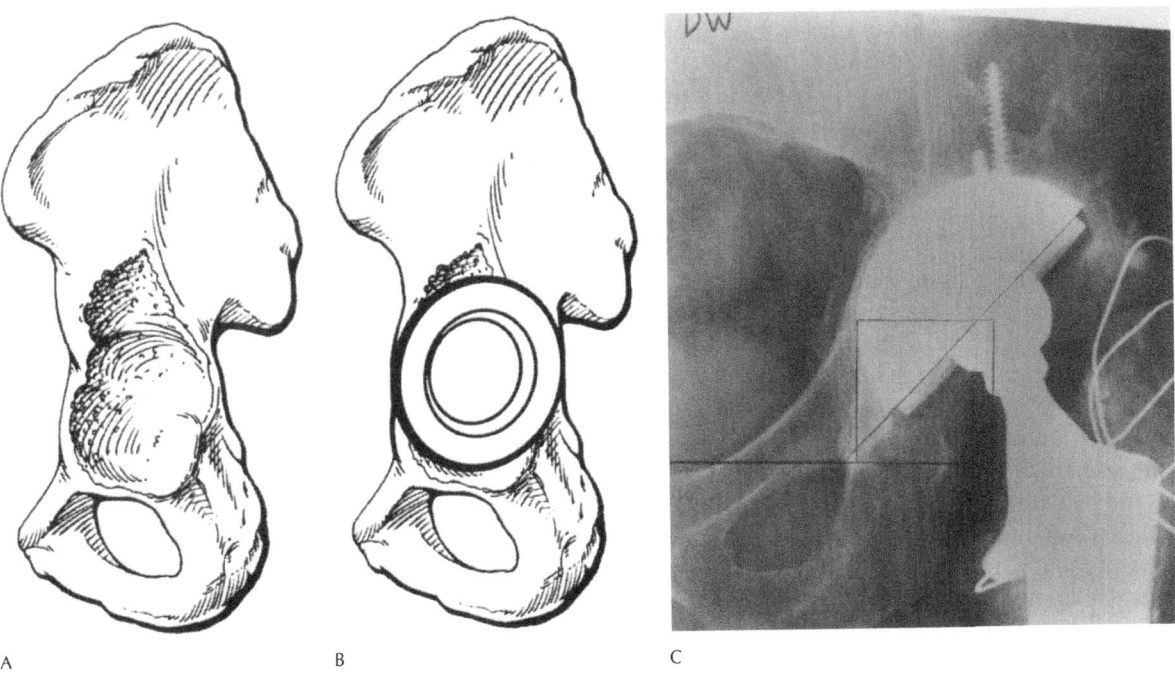

Figure 47.2. A. Superior acetabular defect. B. Central placement of oversize acetabular cup. C. Radiograph of oversize acetabular component filling acetabulum and superior defect.

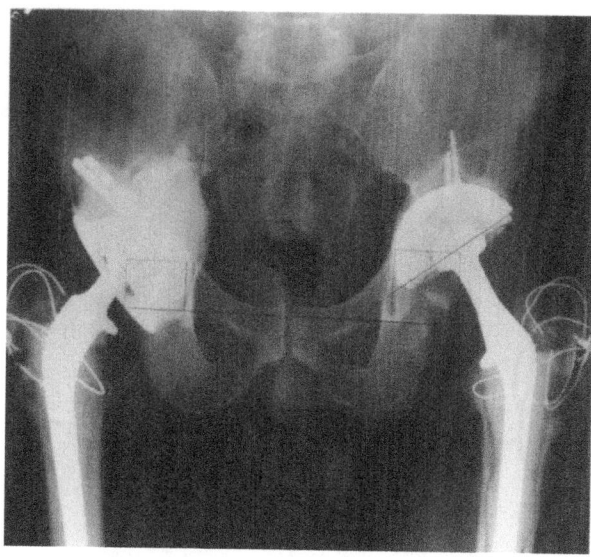

Figure 47.3. Radiograph of patient with bilateral total hip arthroplasties illustrating two separate methods to address acetabular deficiency. Large right acetabular deficiency treated with anatomic hip center and bulk cement filler. Large left acetabular deficiency treated with high hip center and oversize cup.

sitioned 1 cm superomedially beyond the anatomic position compared to a 0% (0 of 13 hips) for anatomically placed hips. In a study of 62 hips, Lachiewicz et al.[13] found a 42% (11 of 26 hips) loosening rate for components positioned 5 cm superior–medially beyond the anatomic position compared to a 14% (5 of 35 hips) for anatomically placed hips. In a study of patients with Crowe type-II congenital hip dysplasia, Pagnano et al.[14] reported on 145 cemented arthroplasties. Significantly increased acetabular loosening rates were found for cups in a superior position (hip center height greater than 35 mm), even without lateral displacement. However, specific rates of loosening at an anatomic versus superior hip position were not identified. Callaghan et al.[12] also proposed superior placement as a risk factor for early acetabular loosening. They reported 30 of 73 (41%) failed cemented acetabular components at 3.6 years had a cup center height more than 53 mm.

Several clinical studies reporting on isolated superior displacement without horizontal displacement have reported low radiographic loosening and revision rates for the acetabular components in an elevated position. In a study of cemented primary and revision components, Russotti and Harris[7] reported a 16% (6 hips) acetabular loosening rate and 2.7% (1 hip) revision rate for 37 hips with high hip centers at 11 years. McQueary and Johnston,[17] in a study of 61 hips with congenital dysplasia followed 8.5 years, showed that isolated superior displacement did not contribute to loosening, whereas isolated horizontal displacement significantly increased the loosening rate. Two studies report short-term results on ingrowth acetabular components in revision total hip arthroplasties.[6,8] Kelley[6] reported a 5% (one hip) acetabular loosening rate and a 0% revision rate for 20 hips at 3 years. Schutzer and Harris[8] reported a 0% loosening and revision rate for 56 uncemented acetabular components at 3.5 years.

The literature is less clear on the results of femoral longevity with elevated hip centers. There appears to be a high rate of femoral loosening, with failure rates reported in the 20% to 50% range.[6,7,9,14] Failure rates for modern primary cemented femoral components are typically less than 3% at more than 5 years[18–20] and for cemented femoral revisions with second-generation techniques are approximately 10% at 10 years.[21,22] Russotti and Harris[7] noted a 21% femoral loosening rate and 11% femoral rerevision rate (4 hips) at 11 years. Yoder et al.[9] found a 50% radiographic loosening rate (22 of 44 hips) for femoral components with hip centers greater than 3 cm compared to a 26% loosening rate (19 of 76 hips) for femoral components with hip centers less than 3 cm at 9 years. Both superior placement alone and superolateral displacement were significantly associated with an increased femoral loosening rate, up to 4.1 times increased risk of loosening. Pagnano et al.[14] similarly found significantly increased loosening and revision rates for the femoral component in cemented arthroplasties with hip center heights more than 35 mm, but did not comment on specific rates. Kelley[6] reported a 25% femoral loosening rate and 5% (one hip) revision rate for at 3 years for 20 arthroplasties with high hip centers.

All femoral failures in one study occurred in patients younger than 65 years of age.[6] Although age is a recognized risk factor for femoral loosening, particularly in cemented arthroplasties, studies of older patients with hip arthroplasties revealed hip joint forces consistently lower than those predicted for healthy adults.[23,24] Increased hip forces in younger patients could be a risk factor contributing to loosening in this population.

With a wide range of femoral components used in regards to both fixation and design, it is difficult to assess whether the reported high femoral component loosening rates are due to elevation of the hip center or some factor related to previous surgery, femoral component design, or proximal bone stock. When evaluating the effect of hip center location in revision, it will be important to continue to study the effects on the femoral component.

Technical Considerations

Numerous technical problems related to the acetabular component, the femoral component, and soft tissue management need to be considered with hip reconstruction using a high hip center. Acetabular issues include horizontal placement, proper component orientation, and cup size. Femoral component issues include the status of femoral fixation, femoral modularity, and femoral neck length. Soft tissue issues include abductor muscle length and hip stability.

When relocation of the hip center is necessary, care must be taken to minimize lateral displacement of the acetabular component. As reviewed previously, theoretical and clinical studies indicate superolateral relocation is detrimental to the longevity of the reconstruction whereas several studies report good results with superior only position. Criticism of superior hip placement has assumed that a proximally placed hip center must also mean concomitant lateral displacement. The literature reports that the cup can be placed in a high location without being lateralized. Several studies demonstrate the majority of cups can be placed in a superior position without lateral displacement.[6,7,9] Russotti and Harris[7] reported 33 of 37 hips (89%) in a superior only position and Schutzer and Harris[8] reported 47 of 56 hips (84%) in a superior or superomedial position. Pagnano et al.[14] reported that 35 cups in a superior position were not positioned significantly more laterally than cups placed at other positions.

There are no formal recommendations regarding cup angles with high hip centers as there is a fair amount of controversy regarding cup position in the anatomic position. Schutzer and Harris[8] aimed for 30° of abduction in high hip centers whereas Charnley originally suggested 45° of abduction for increased range of motion without impingement and 20° of forward flexion for anatomic centers. Petrera and Rubash[25] suggest a similar positioning for acetabular revisions. In general, we have found that positioning both the small and oversize cups at 45° to the interteardrop line with 10 to 30° of anteversion has resulted in adequate hip stability.

Geometry of the acetabular defect and the surrounding bone affects the choice of cup size. A smaller acetabular component is well suited to a narrow or elliptical acetabulum, as seen with congenital hip dysplasia, or to an acetabulum with anterior or posterior column deficiency[26] (Fig. 47.1). Acetabular defects that are broadened or widened with intact anterior and posterior columns, are ideal situations for a large or oversized ingrowth cup (Fig. 47.2).

High placement of a smaller cup potentially increases the risk of impingement and instability. In addition, the risk for dislocation may be increased with the smaller 22-mm femoral heads, frequently necessary with small acetabular cups or when polyethylene thickness is 8 mm or less. In a prospective, randomized study, Kelley and Lachiewicz[27] report a significantly increased dislocation rate with 22-mm heads compared to 28-mm heads, however, this was only seen with outside cup diameters 56 mm or greater. When 22-mm heads were used with smaller acetabular components, the dislocation rate was not increased. Impingement may also contribute to dislocation. At revision, prominent bone of the anterior or posterior column adjacent to the cup should be excised.

No formal definition of oversized or jumbo cups exists. Previous studies in primary total hip arthroplasty have shown a range of 46 mm to 66 mm for acetabular components.[28,29] We choose 70 mm as the outer diameter at which the component should be viewed as an oversize cup. Acetabular components 70 mm or more in size are available from several suppliers. The two largest available off-the-shelf acetabular components, the Trilogy cup (Zimmer) and the Duralock cup (DePuy), are available in outer diameters to 80 mm. Other cups available include the Vitalock cup (Howmedica) to 76 mm, the Arthrophor-II cup (Joint Medical Products) to 75 mm, and the PFC cup (Johnson & Johnson), to 70 mm.

An oversize cup can easily result in the creation of a high hip center as little margin for vertical displacement exists for these components. The hip center height (Hhc) is equal to the distance of the inferior edge of the acetabular component from the interteardrop line (Ditd) added to the product of the sine of the abduction angle [sin(Abd angle)] and the outer diameter of the acetabular component (OD): Hhc = Ditd + sin(Abd angle) × OD. A cup placed at the level of the inter-teardrop line and at 45° abduction will have a hip center above 30 mm if the diameter is 80 mm or greater. Although few cups approach this size, one can see that the margin of error is greatly diminished with oversize cups. Increased abduction or small amounts of elevation above the interteardrop line will result in high hip centers with smaller cups. For instance, a 70 mm cup placed with its inferior edge placed at the interteardrop line and at 45° of abduction already has a hip center at 25 mm, leaving a margin of error for further vertical displacement of only 5 mm. Larger cups potentially also lateralize the hip center.

The status of femoral component fixation is a crucial component in the evaluation for revision surgery when considering creation of a high hip center. A loose femoral component obviously requires revision. The status of the proximal femur, particularly in regards to available bone stock, must be considered prior to choices for a femoral component design and mode of fixation. Calcar-replacing femoral components, or even proximal femoral-replacing components, may be necessary for satisfactory reconstruction.

Long femoral neck lengths are often necessary with a high hip center to restore leg length, abductor length, and hip stability. In a computer simulation study, femoral neck length was identified as the most important variable to restore force-generating capacity of muscles after total hip arthroplasty with a high hip center.[30] A 2 cm superior displacement of the hip center was calculated to reduce abductor force-generating capacity 43%.[30] An equal increase in neck length to coincide with the superior displacement fully restored the moment-generating capacity of the muscle by increasing muscle length and force-generating capacity.[30] Kelley[6] used an average femoral neck length of 52 mm (36 to 56 mm) in a series of 20 high hip center reconstructions. The average standard femoral component may not have sufficient neck length to restore these properties. Calcar-replacing prostheses are typically used for proximal femoral bone loss. However these prostheses are often needed with high hip centers, even in instances of minimal bone loss, for overall soft-tissue balancing and maintenance of leg length.

Distal transfer of the greater trochanter also has a significant biomechanical benefit when the hip center has been placed superiorly. Using a 3-D computer model, Free and Delp[31] calculated that although distal transfer of the greater trochanter did not restore the moment arm for a superiorly displaced hip center, distal transfer did restore the muscle lengths and force-generating capacities of the gluteus medius and minimus. This is consistent with the findings of Gore et al.,[32] who reported that distal positions of the greater trochanter could increase abductor strength by elongating the muscles along their lines of action. The role of trochanteric advancement, therefore, is particularly important for restoration of abductor strength in high hip centers when femoral neck length can not be restored.

A well-fixed component requires assessment of modularity and the possibility of femoral neck lengthening. A well-fixed nonmodular component left unrevised in the setting of a newly created high hip center will create a leg-length discrepancy. In this situation, a trochanteric advancement will improve the biomechanics. A modular component that allows for longer neck placement may still require trochanteric advancement for proper abductor tension and function.

Conclusion

Superior acetabular defects create a situation that places revision hip components at risk for loosening. High hip center reconstructions without concomitant lateralization have been reported to have good results, particularly with uncemented acetabular components. Femoral component longevity is an unknown factor and needs to be closely evaluated when assessing the results of hip center location.

An extended femoral neck length is often required to restore leg-length, abductor strength, and hip stability in revision arthroplasty at a high hip center. Calcar-replacing femoral components, or even proximal femoral-replacing components, may be necessary for satisfactory reconstruction.

An older population with lower activity levels may be more likely to achieve good results with this technique.

References

1. Kwong LM, Jasty M, Harris WH. High failure rate of bulk femoral head allografts in total hip acetabular reconstructions at 10 years. *J Arthroplasty*. 1993;8:341–346.
2. Miyanaga Y, Tagawa H, Ninimiya S, et al. A new socket design for the dysplastic acetabulum in total hip replacement. *Clin Orthop*. 1980;149:194–200.
3. Mulroy RD Jr., Harris WH. Failure of acetabular autogenous grafts in total hip arthroplasty. Increasing incidence: a follow-up note. *J Bone Joint Surg Am*. 1990;71:1536–1540.
4. Pollock FH, Whiteside LA. The fate of massive allografts in total hip acetabular revision surgery. *J Arthroplasty*. 1992;7:271–276.
5. Sutherland CJ. Early experience with eccentric acetabular components in revision total hip arthroplasty. *Am J Orthop*. 1996;25:284–289.
6. Kelley SS: High hip center in revision arthroplasty. *J Arthroplasty*. 1994;9:503–510.
7. Russotti GM, Harris WH. Proximal placement of the acetabular component in total hip arthroplasty. *J Bone Joint Surg Am*. 1991;73:587–592.
8. Schutzer SF, Harris WH. High placement of porous-coated acetabular components in complex total hip arthroplasty. *J Arthroplasty*. 1994;9:359–367.
9. Yoder SA, Brand RA, Pedersen DR, et al. Total hip acetabular component position affects component loosening rates. *Clin Orthop*. 1988;228:79–87.
10. Ranawat CS, Dorr LD, Inglis AE. Total hip arthroplasty in protrusio acetabuli of rheumatoid arthritis. *J Bone Joint Surg Am*. 1980;62:1059–1065.
11. Johnston RC, Brand RA, Crowninshield RD. Reconstruction of the hip. A mathematical approach to determine optimum geometric relationships. *J Bone Joint Surg Am*. 1979;61:639–652.
12. Callaghan JJ, Salvati EA, Pellicci PM, et al. Results of revision for mechanical failure after cemented total hip replacement, 1979 to 1982, A two to five-year follow-up. *J Bone Joint Surg Am*. 1985;67:1075–1085.
13. Lachiewicz PF, McCaskill B, Inglis A, et al. Total hip arthroplasty in juvenile rheumatoid arthritis. Two to eleven-year results. *J Bone Joint Surg Am*. 1986;68:502–508.
14. Pagnano MW, Hanssen AD, Lewallen DG, et al. The effect of superior placement of the acetabular component on the rate of loosening after total hip arthroplasty. *J Bone Joint Surg Am*. 1996;78:1004–1014.
15. Brand RA, Pedersen D. Hip forces resulting from altered hip joint center location—Revisited. Presented at the Annual Meeting of the Hip Society, Scottsdale, AZ, Sept. 1990.
16. Doehring TC, Rubash HE, Shelley FJ, et al. High hip center: experimental measurements of joint force magnitude and direction in normal, superior, and superolateral hip-center positions (submitted manuscript).
17. McQueary FG, Johnston RC. Coxarthrosis after congenital dysplasia. Treatment by total hip arthroplasty without acetabular bone-grafting. *J Bone Joint Surg Am*. 1988;70:1140–1144.
18. Barrack RL, Mulroy RD Jr, Harris WH. Improved cementing techniques and femoral component loosening in

young patients with hip arthroplasty: a 12-year radiographic review. *J Bone Joint Surg Br.* 1992;77:385–389.
19. Oishi CS, Walker RH, Colwell CW. The femoral component in total hip arthroplasty. Six to eight-year follow-up of one hundred consecutive patients after use of a third-generation cementing technique. *J Bone Joint Surg Am.* 1994;76:1130–1136.
20. Mohler CG, Kull LR, Martell JM, et al. Total hip replacement with insertion of an acetabular component without cement and a femoral component with cement. Four to seven-year results. *J Bone Joint Surg Am.* 1995;77:86–96.
21. Estok DM II, Harris WH. Long-term results of femoral revision surgery using second-generation techniques: an average 11.7 year follow-up evaluation. *Clin Orthop.* 1994; 299:190–202.
22. Katz RP, Callaghan JJ, Sullivan PM, Johnston RC. Cemented revision total hip arthroplasty using contemporary techniques: a minimum ten year follow-up study. *J Arthroplasty.* 1994;9:103.
23. Davy DT, Kotzar GM, Brown RH, et al. Telemetric force measurement across the hip after total arthroplasty. *J Bone Joint Surg Am.* 1988;70:45–50.
24. Kotzar GM, Davy DT, Goldberg KG, et al. Telemeterized in vivo hip joint force data; a report on two patients after total hip surgery. *J Orthop Res.* 1991;9:621–633.
25. Petrera P, Rubash HE. Revision total hip arthroplasty: the acetabular component. *J Am Acad Orthrop Surg.* 1995;3: 15–21.
26. Crowe JF, Mani VJ, Ranawat CS. Total hip replacement in congenital dislocation and dysplasia of the hip. *J Bone Joint Surg Am.* 1979;61:15–23.
27. Hickman JM, Lachiewicz PF, Kelley SS. Increased risk of dislocation with small femoral head size. (unpublished manuscript)
28. Brown EC III, Lachiewicz PF: Primary total hip arthroplasty with a precoated femoral component: four-to-seven year results. (unpublished manuscript).
29. Latimer HA, Lachiewicz PF: Porous-coated acetabular components with screw fixation: five to ten-year results. *J. Bone Joint Surg Am.* 1996;78:975–981.
30. Delp SL, Komattu AV, Wixson RL. Superior displacement of the hip in total joint replacement: effects of prosthetic neck length, neck-stem angle, and anteversion angle on the moment-generating capacity of the muscles. *J Orthop Res.* 1994;12:860–870.
31. Free SA, Delp SL. Trochanteric transfer in total hip replacement: effects on the moment arms and force-generating capacities of the hip abductors. *J Orthop Res.* 1996;14:245–250.
32. Gore DR, Murray MP, Gardner GM, et al. Roentgeno-graphic measurements after Muller total hip replacement. Correlations among roentgenographic measurements and hip strength and mobility. *J Bone Joint Surg Am.* 1977;59:948–953.

48
Use of Oblong or Modular Cups

Philip A. G. Karpos

The challenges of acetabular revision in total hip arthroscopy can be met, in the majority of cases, with the use of hemispheric, porous-coated components. An anterior, medial, and inferior socket position is ideal to restore hip biomechanics and utilize the biomechanically optimal bone of the anterior and posterior columns.[1] This usually can be accomplished by using standard hemispheric components, occasionally oversized (jumbo), in combination with nonstructural allografting to cavitary defects and supplemental screw fixation if required.[2,3] Mid and now long-term results using these techniques are good to excellent in multiple series, and are certainly superior to the results of cemented acetabular revisions.[4-9] Therefore, when feasible, noncemented, porous-coated, hemispherical acetabular components should be utilized.

Not all acetabular defects, however, can be easily managed with a hemispheric component. When there has been significant cephalad migration of the hip center on the anteroposterior (AP) radiograph, large superior or superior-posterior defects are often encountered (AAOS Type III),[10,11] (Fig. 48.1). Historically, these defects have been treated with structural allografts to support the acetabular component or jumbo hemispherical components to maximize bony contact. These techniques, however, are labor intensive and often quite technically demanding. Concerns have also arisen about the long-term success of acetabular allografts.[12-14] Shinar et al. noted failure in 9 of 15 components supported by allografts at 16 years, whereas Hooten et al. reported a 44% failure rate with cementless sockets at only 29 months.[15,16] This has led some authors to advocate placement of the revision acetabular component in a superior but not lateral position rather than trying to reconstruct bone stock.[17] Good results at intermediate term have been reported with this technique.[18-20] However, abnormal hip biomechanics, leg length inequality and instability are concerns. In addition, this technique cannot be utilized when a monolithic femoral stem is retained.

Despite the overall success of hemispherical components, on occasion there is insufficient superior support for the component. Although the degree of acceptable unsupported acetabular component is debatable, studies by Shinar et al. and Gross et al. indicate that 30% superolateral uncoverage is acceptable.[15,21] However, when reaming to place a hemispherical component, if the length of the defect is significantly greater than the anterior to posterior diameter of the native acetabulum, adequate coverage cannot be obtained without violating the crucial anterior and posterior columns of the native acetabulum (Fig. 48.2).

Because of concerns regarding the use of structural allograft, high hip centers, and hemispheric components with inadequate structural support, the use of oblonged shaped components has become a viable option (Fig. 48.3).

History of Eccentric Acetabular Components

The use of eccentric acetabular components originated with the fabrication of CT-based custom components. This has evolved into off-the-shelf implant systems that allow intraoperative customization of a patient's defect to the implant. Presently, two systems are available for this purpose. The Johnson and Johnson S-ROM Oblong Cup system and the Biomet Modular Acetabular Reconstruction System. In theory, these components can normalize the hip center, provide optimum implant-bone contact for ingrowth, and eliminate the concerns of allograft by serving as a "metallograft".

Technique

S-ROM Oblong Cup (Johnson and Johnson Orthopedics, Raynham, MA) and Modular Acetabular Reconstruction System (Biomet, Inc. Warsaw, IN).

1. Preoperative assessment of anticipated acetabular defect via plain radiographs. Routine use of CT scanning is not indicated but may be useful in certain situations.

48. Oblong or Modular Cups

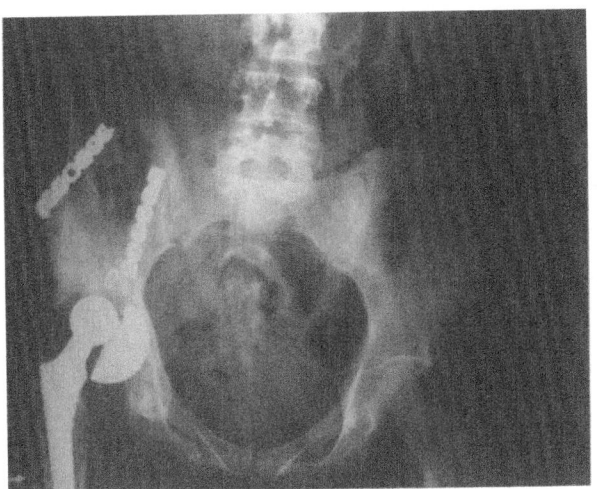

Figure 48.1. Loss of acetabular fixation due to infection. Following resection, replantation accomplished with an eccentric component to avoid use of allograft.

2. Availability of appropriate implants at time of revision.
3. Intraoperative assessment of defect after removal of failed component. Specifically, status of anterior and posterior columns and length of defect vs. anterior to posterior diameter.
4. Preliminary reaming of native acetabulum. Select a hemispheric component if greater than 70% contact with host bone can be obtained without violating the anterior and posterior columns, at or near the anatomic hip center.
5. If unable to use a hemispheric component, prepare the native acetabulum using hemispheric reamers to the appropriate size to establish the anatomic center of rotation. Select the appropriate base shell diameter. (J&J S-ROM range = 51 mm to 66 mm, Biomet M.A.R.S. = 56 mm to 72 mm).
6. Preliminarily size the defect with undersized trial components. Options include +15 mm and +25 mm oblong cups with the S-ROM system. The +25 mm buildup is oriented at 20° of adduction. The Biomet system offers half or full metallografts.
7. Prepare the defect, using contained, particulate allograft if required, with the system dependent defect reaming instrumentation. Attention must be paid to proper component anteversion. Note, the defect is enlarged slightly to allow for precise implant fit.
8. Trial reduction if felt to be necessary.
9. Select and assemble (if required) the appropriate implant and impact until seated. Note, even with excellent contact, the press-fit will be inferior to a hemispherical component. Supplemental screw fixation is required.
10. Following screw insertion, select and insert the appropriate liner. With the S-ROM oblong cup, the liner is fixed with a minimum of two screws or pins.

Results

The long-term results of hemispherical, porous-coated, acetabular components are well established. Silverton et al. reported, at a mean of 8.9 years, the results of 115

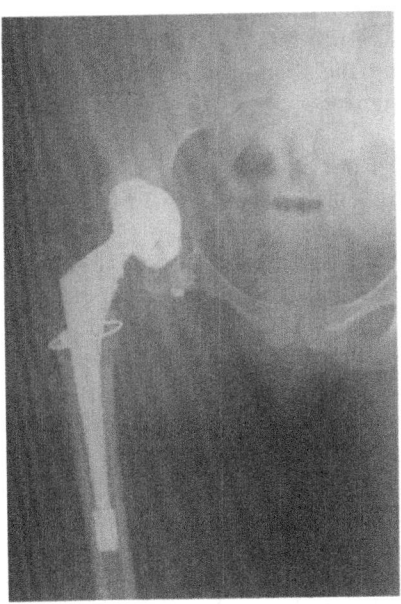
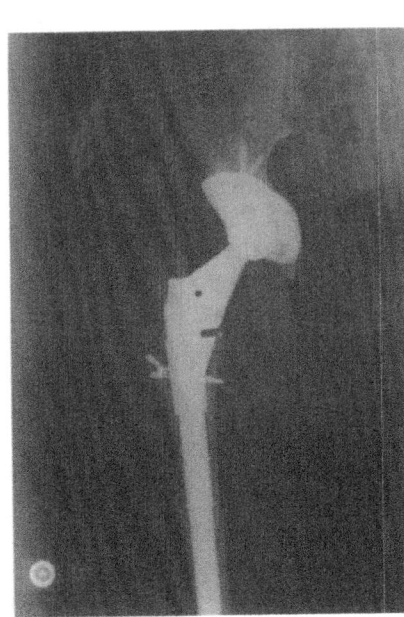

Figure 48.2. A. Fracture through pelvis osteolytic defect. Defect measured 50 mm wide × 65 mm long. B. One year followup, reconstructed with S-ROM Oblong Cup and particulate allograft.

A   B

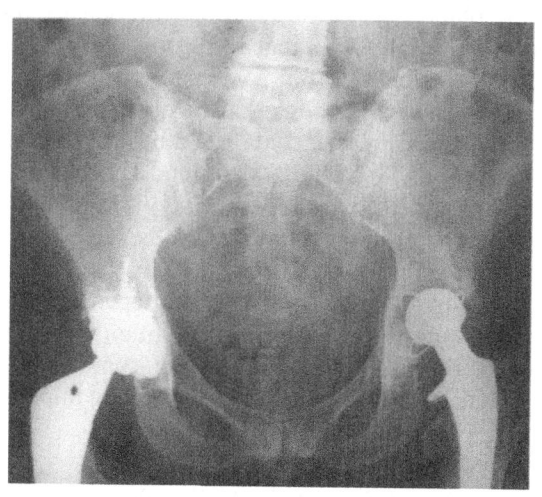 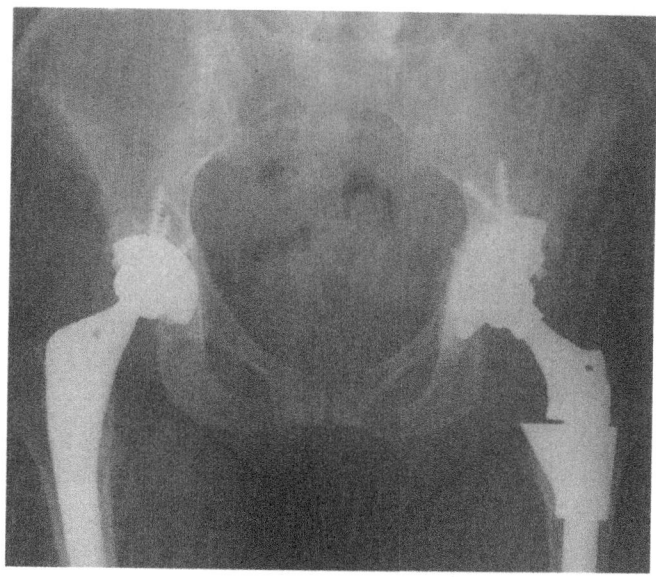

Figure 48.3. A. Significant cephalad migration of a loose, cemented acetabular component. B. Two year follow-up with restoration of leg length and no migration.

revision acetabular surgeries performed without bulk allografting. There were no repeat revisions for aseptic loosening, except in one patient who had radiation necrosis of the pelvis.[5] Multiple other studies have demonstrated good to excellent intermediate results using hemispherical components as well, as has been discussed in previous chapters.

The data supporting the use of eccentric acetabular components, although preliminary and limited, is encouraging. Early experience with eccentric acetabular components involved custom implant technology. Ure et al. reported good results in 10 patients at a mean of 6.6 years with a 70% survivorship rate.[22] Sutherland, however, reported failure in three of four patients at 4 years in whom custom eccentric components were used to reconstruct type III defects.[23] The shortcomings of custom components include the increased expense of a preoperative CT scan, the lack of specific instrumentation, the lack of intraoperative adaptation, and the increased expense of the component itself.[24] This led to the development of "off-the-shelf" eccentric components, either solid or modular. In the same series, Sutherland reported good results at 4 years in two patients treated with off-the-shelf eccentric components.

As experience with the use of eccentric components has increased, early and intermediate term results are becoming available. In 1997, Newman et al. reported a multi-center series of 64 patients using the S-ROM off-the-shelf oblong acetabular component.[25] Many cases required particulate allograft, however none required bulk allografting for implant stability. No progressive migration was seen and at the forty-four month follow-up, survivorship was 97%. In a single surgeon subset of the same study population, Deboer and Christie noted excellent mechanical stability and significant improvement in the average vertical displacement of the hip center at average follow-up of 4.5 years.[26] In a consecutive series of thirty-four patients from the Mayo Clinic using the S-ROM oblong cup, Berry also reports significant improvement in the vertical displacement of the hip center, however, three patients developed partial peroneal nerve palsies. At mean 2.6-year follow-up after revision, survivorship of implant was 100%. Two implants migrated greater than 2 mm, both with mild or no pain. (Berry, personal communication).

To date, no follow-up data has been presented or published regarding the Biomet Modular Acetabular Reconstruction System.

Conclusion

Intermediate and long-term data support the use of hemispherical, porous-coated acetabular components in revision total hip arthroplasty. However, certain acetabular defects may preclude their use. In these situations, the use of an eccentric acetabular component (either oblong or bi-lobed) may be useful. Indications include a desire to avoid a high hip center, structural allografting or compromise of the anterior or posterior columns with a hemispherical component. Short-term results with off-the shelf, eccentric acetabular components are very encouraging. Long-term results, however, are still needed to fully validate the use of these components for the management of segmental acetabular deficiencies.

References

1. Youder SA, Brand RA, Peterson DR, O-Gorman TW. Total hip acetabular component position affects component loosening rates. *Clin Orthop.* 1988;228:79–87.
2. Emerson RE, Mallory TH, Head WC. Principles of cementless acetabular reconstruction in primary revision cases. *Orthop Rev.* (Oct) 1990;32–37.
3. Emerson RE, Head WC. Dealing with the deficient acetabulum in revision hip arthroplasty: the importance of implant migration and the use of the jumbo cup. *Semin Arthroplasty.* 1993;4:2–8.
4. Woolson ST, Adamson GJ: Acetabular revision using a bone-ingrowth total hip component in patients who have acetabular bone stock deficiency. *J. Arthroplasty.* 1996;11:661–667.
5. Silverton CD, Rosenberg AG, Sheinkop MB, et al. Revision total hip arthroplasty using a cementless acetabular component. Technique and results. *Clin Orthop.* 1995;319:201–208.
6. Tanzer M, Drucker D, Jasti M, et al. Revision of the acetabular component with an uncemented Harris-Galante porous-coated prosthesis. *J Bone Joint Surg Am.* 1992;74:987–994.
7. Tanzer M, Drucker D, Jasti M, et al. Revision of the acetabular component with an uncemented Harris-Galante porous-coated prosthesis. *J Bone Joint Surg Am.* 1992;74:987.
8. Padgett DE, Kuff L, Rosenberg A, et al. Revision of the acetabular component without cement after total hip arthroplasty. 3–6 year followup. *J Bone Joint Surg Am.* 1993;75:663–673.
9. Callaghan JJ, Calvati EA, Pellici PM, et al. Results of revision for mechanical failure after cemented total hip replacement 1979–1982. *J Bone Joint Surg Am.* 1985;67:1074–1085.
10. Proprosky WG, Perona PG, Lawrence JM. Acetabular defect classification in surgical reconstruction in revision arthroplasty. *J Arthroplasty.* 1994;9:33–44.
11. Proprosky WG, Magnus RE. Principles of bone grafting in revision total hip arthroplasty; acetabular technique. *Clin Orthop.* 1994;298:147–155.
12. Mulroy RD, Harris WH. Failure of acetabular autogenous grafts in total hip arthroplasty. *J Bone Joint Surg Am.* 1990;72:1536–1540.
13. Mulroy RD Jr., Harris WH. Failure of acetabular autogenous grafts in total hip arthroplasty. Increasing incidence; a followup note. *J Bone Joint Surg Am.* 1990;72:1536–1540.
14. Kwong LM, Jasti M, Harris WH. High failure rate of bulk femoral head allografts in total hip acetabular reconstructions at ten years. *J Arthroplasty.* 1993;8:341–346.
15. Shinar AA, Harris WH. Bulk structural autogenous grafts and allografts for reconstruction of the acetabulum and total hip arthroplasty. Sixteen year followup. *J Bone Joint Surg Am.* 1997;79:159–168.
16. Hooten JP, Engh CA, Jr., Engh CA. Failure of structural acetabular allografts in cementless revision hip arthroplasty. *J Bone Joint Surg Br.* 1994;76:419–422.
17. Harris WH. Management of the deficient acetabulum using cementless fixation without bone grafting. *Orthop Clin North Am.* 1993;24:663–665.
18. Kelly SS. High hip center in revision arthroplasty. *J Arthroplasty.* 1994;9:503–510.
19. Russoti GM, Harris WH. Proximal placement of the acetabular component in total hip arthroplasty. *J Bone Joint Surg Am.* 1991;73:587–592.
20. Schutzer SF, Harris WH. High placement of porous-coated acetabular components in complex total hip arthroplasty. *J Arthroplasty.* 1994;9:359–367.
21. Gross AE, Allan DG, Catre M, et al. Bone hips in hip replacement surgery; the pelvic side. *Orthop Clin North Am.* 1993;24:663–665.
22. Ure KJ, Amstuts HC, Doshi TR, et al. Custom eccentric shells for complex acetabular defects in revision hip surgery. Presented 1996. American Academy of Orthopedic Surgeons, Atlanta, GA.
23. Sutherland CJ. Early experience with eccentric acetabular components in revision total hip arthroplasty. *Am J Orthop.* 1996;25:284–289.
24. Sutherland CJ. Treatment of Type III acetabular deficiencies in revision total hip arthroplasty without structure bone graft. *J Arthroplasty.* 1996;11:91–98.
25. Newman MA, Bargar WL, Christie MJ, et al. Multicenter study of acetabular reconstruction using an oblong cup; 2–7 year results. Presented 1997. American Academy of Orthopaedic Surgeons, San Francisco, CA.
26. DeBoer DK, Christie MJ. Reconstruction of the deficient acetabulum with an oblong-shaped prosthesis; 3–7 year results. *J Arthroplasty.* 1998;13:674–680.

ic # 49
Management of Medial Deficiencies

Christopher W. Olcott

Cavitary Deficiencies

Although several classification systems exist for acetabular deficiencies in revision total hip arthroplasty, the American Academy of Orthopedic Surgeons (AAOS) defines cavitary or type II defects as those with an intact, viable rim.[1] Although varying degrees of volumetric loss may exist, the peripheral rim and central wall remain intact[1] (Fig. 49.1). Paprosky and Magnus classify cavitary or contained acetabular defects with a complete, supportive rim as type I.[2] These investigators describe several key radiographic features of a type I or cavitary defect that should be assessed preoperatively.[2] On an anteroposterior view of the pelvis, a cavitary deficiency demonstrates no significant osteolysis of the teardrop and ischium, an intact Kohler's line, and superior component migration of less than 2 cm.[2]

Despite the method of classification, hemispheric, porous-coated acetabular components have demonstrated excellent short-[3-8] and intermediate-term[9-13] results in the management of cavitary acetabular deficiencies. Unlike reports of loosening of cemented acetabular components,[14] these studies show no correlation between loosening of the acetabular shell and the presence of radiolucent lines. Silverton et al.[12,13] note a partial, nonprogressive radiolucency in 54% of acetabular revisions, but add that no cups have been revised for aseptic loosening at a mean follow-up of over 8 years.

The principles of acetabular revision surgery include a thorough preoperative evaluation, extensile surgical exposure, preservation of bone stock, restoration of the anatomic hip center, and component stability. Preoperative preparation involves defining the acetabular deficiency with adequate radiographic and imaging studies, templating for prosthetic type, size and hip center, and ordering special equipment.[1] Radiographs should include an anteroposterior view of the pelvis and an anteroposterior and lateral view of the hip.[1] A Lowenstein lateral further delineates the extent of an acetabular defect and aids in templating for femoral revision. Oblique of Judet views determine the integrity of anterior and posterior columns and walls. Additional radiographs, such as pelvic inlet and outlet views, and imaging studies, such as a pelvic CT scan, may be helpful in complex cases, but are usually not warranted. The final and most accurate assessment of acetabular deficiency occurs intraoperatively.[1] Preoperative templates permit an estimation of acetabular component position and size, and a determination of the anatomic hip center. The hip center can be located by using the opposite normal hip as comparison[1] or the method of Ranawat et al.[15] in cases of bilateral deformed acetabulae. Special equipment needs, such as oversized or jumbo cups and allograft bone for morselized graft, can be planned for and ordered in advance.

Intraoperative management of a cavitary acetabular deficiency requires wide surgical exposure, careful component extraction, and proper preparation and reaming of the acetabular bed. Regardless of the surgical approach, exposure must include an adequate capsulectomy in order to position retractors and translocate the femur away from the acetabulum. The acetabular rim is then outlined by meticulous subperiosteal dissection.[16] This helps to define the extent of the deficiency and to visualize the implant–cement and/or implant–bone interface.[17] In many cases, the acetabular component will be grossly loose and easy to remove. However, an organized approach is mandatory in order to extract more well-fixed cemented and cementless sockets. To remove cemented acetabular components, gouges of differing sizes may be used at the implant-cement interface.[17,18] An alternative method for all-polyethylene, cemented sockets involves sectioning the polyethylene into pieces with an osteotome or high-speed burr.[17,18] In both cases an attempt is made to remove the component first and then to disrupt the cement–bone interface so as to maintain bone stock.[17] To remove cementless acetabular components with a modular polyethylene insert, the polyethylene and screws are removed first. The liner is either extracted with a special device, lifted out with a 4.5 mm or 6.5 mm screw or tap, or sectioned into pieces.[17] The metal shell is removed by disrupting the implant–bone interface with gouges, osteotomes, drills, or burrs.[17] It is imperative not to attempt extraction of the acetabu-

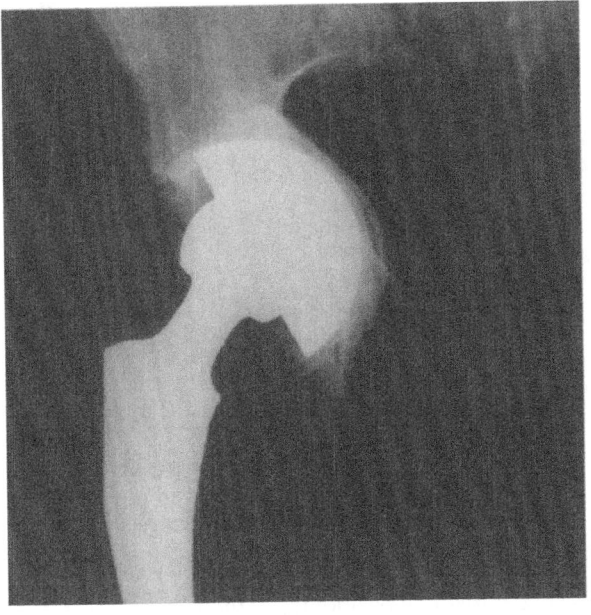 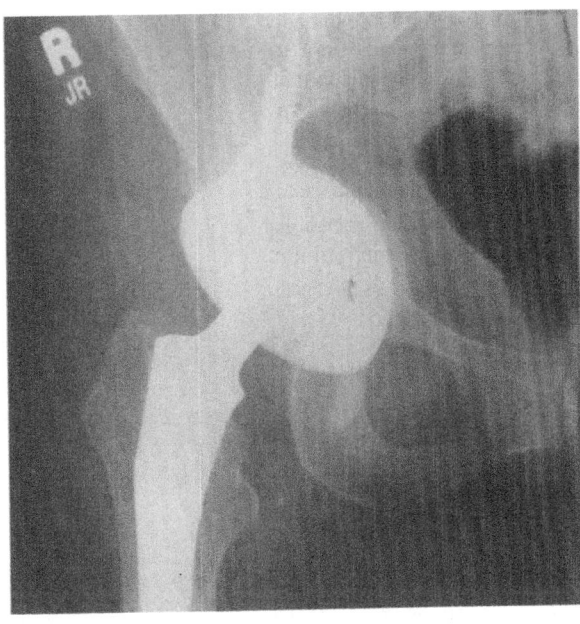

Figure 49.1. Radiographs of a 64-year-old man with a loose cemented metal-backed cup. A. Preoperative radiograph showing a complete radiolucent line and a cavitary acetabular defect. B. Postoperative radiograph with a jumbo acetabular shell secured with dome screws; morselized allograft was packed medially.

lar shell until motion is evident between the cup and bone.[17] Premature extraction may result in removing large segments of bone that have grown into the shell.[17]

Good exposure and organized, careful removal of the acetabular component should ensure preservation of existing bone stock. Once the acetabular component has been withdrawn, all fibrous tissue, cement, and polyethylene debris are scraped free with a curette. The sclerotic acetabular bed is then copiously irrigated. At this point, an assessment of acetabular bone stock is made by palpating the rim and columns. Defects created by cement, anchor holes, osteolytic lesions, and component migration are evaluated, and the need for morselized bone graft is determined. The thickness of the medial wall can be determined with a small drill and depth gauge.[16] An understanding of the bony integrity aids in correct reamer placement and prevents overreaming of one of the columns or walls.

Preparation of the acetabulum is begun with sequential reamers to obtain maximum apposition between implant and host-bone.[6,8] Proper preoperative templating and an understanding of hip joint biomechanics help guide the surgeon to correct component positioning. In order to restore the anatomical hip center and decrease joint reactive forces, the acetabular component should be placed as anterior, medial, and inferior as possible.[19,20] In a deep cavitary deficiency the acetabular introitus or opening is often narrower in the anterior–posterior or superior–inferior plane than the defect itself. Therefore, a decision must be made whether to simply engage the acetabular component with the peripheral rim and fill the remaining defect with morselized autograft and/or allograft (Fig. 49.2), or to deepen the socket to the medial wall and thereby inset the component deep into the anterior and posterior columns. In the latter case, a deep profile socket or lateralized polyethylene liner allows deepening of the acetabular shell without overmedialization of the hip center (Fig. 49.3). In a cavitary defect with a shallow socket, a low-profile acetabular component provides peripheral contact without overhang of the metal shell outside of the bony rim. Dorr and Wan[3] describe a technique of controlled medialization in cases with a shallow socket. The authors point out that, since the medial wall is not critical for acetabular support, reamers can be used to violate the medial wall and deepen the socket so as to attain adequate peripheral contact.[3] In other cases of cavitary deficiencies without a narrow acetabular introitus, reamers are used until good rim contact is established. This often involves use of a jumbo-sized acetabular component (Fig. 49.1). The acetabular component chosen is usually 1 to 2 mm larger than the last reamer in order to ensure solid peripheral contact.

Once reaming is completed, the acetabular bed is irrigated and morselized autograft and/or allograft is packed into cavitary voids. At the present time, there is no literature to support the use of synthetic bone graft substitutes to fill cavitary defects in revision surgery.

Figure 49.2. Radiographs of a 53-year-old man with a loose threaded cup. A. Preoperative radiograph demonstrating a threaded cup that has migrated superiorly creating a large cavitary defect. B. Postoperative radiograph in which cavitary defect is filled with morselized allograft and acetabular shell engages intact peripheral rim.

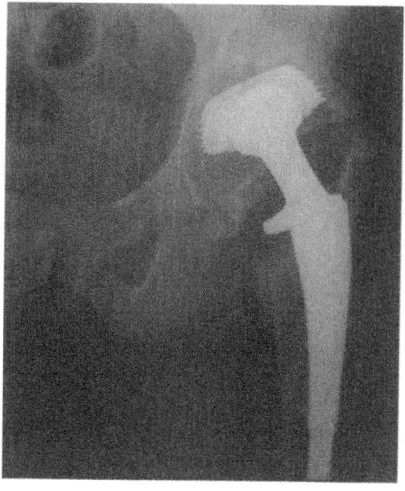
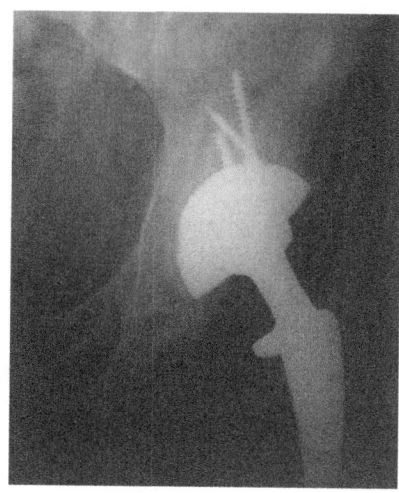

The last reamer is reversed to contour the morselized graft. Dorr and Wan[3] warn against placing too much morselized graft into the prepared acetabulum, which can prevent complete seating of the component. In their series, Dorr and Wan[3] noted better fixation when slurry bone graft was not used.

The oversized, hemispheric, acetabular component is impacted into the prepared acetabular bed. Investigators such as Knight et al.[21] recommend a cup abduction angle of less than 40° in order to reduce forces directed laterally on the cup that can lead to loosening. Anteversion or flexion of the cup should be between 20° and 30°. Engh et al.[5] support the hemispheric design of the acetabular component since it facilitates preparation of the implant site, minimizes the amount of resected bone, and allows slight adjustment in final positioning of the implant. Emerson et al.[4] add that the hemispheric design permits more consistent horizontal positioning of the acetabular component compared to other designs.

Another advantage of a hemispheric, porous-coated, acetabular component is the option for supplemental screw fixation.[8] Most authors recommend screw fixation in the revision setting.[8,11,12,22] However, placement of screws may jeopardize neurovascular structures and the surgeon must be familiar with the "safe-zones" for screw positioning.[23] Dorr and Wan[3] and Hedley et al.[24] did not use screw fixation to secure revision acetabular components and noted no increase in loosening rates. Since rigid peripheral contact is not always possible, screws provide initial component stability, which prevents micromotion and allows for more effective bony ingrowth and long-lasting durability. Acetabular components with both dome and peripheral screw holes can be helpful in cases with compromised bone stock. When

Figure 49.3. Radiographs of a 66-year-old male with a loose acetabular shell. A. Preoperative radiograph showing medial migration of cup. B. Postoperative radiograph after revision with a deep-profile acetabular component.

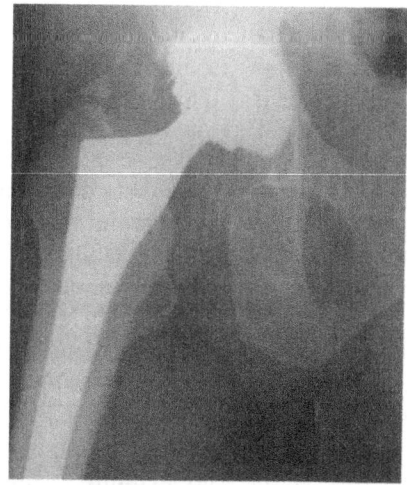
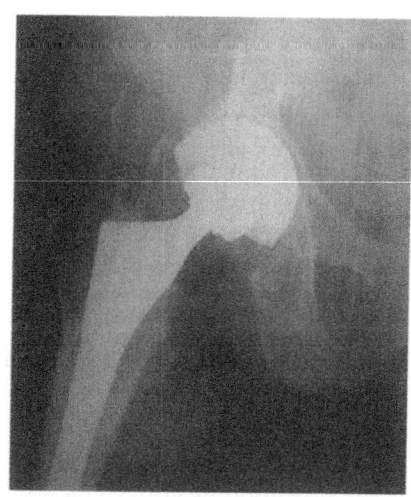

a large superior cavitary defect exists, dome screws may not provide adequate fixation. Instead, peripheral screws can be used to attain excellent purchase in the intact rim. Final positioning of the cup and screws can be checked with an intraoperative radiograph.

Management of cavitary acetabular deficiencies with a fixed, hemispherical cup has shown superior intermediate-term results.[9–13,25] Success requires thorough preoperative evaluation to define the acetabular defect and to plan for component size and any special equipment needs, wide exposure, component extraction with minimal bone damage, proper component orientation so as to restore the anatomic center of rotation and to provide stability, and rigid component fixation.

Segmental Deficiencies

Of the segmental acetabular deficiencies encountered in revision surgery, isolated bone loss of the medial wall is uncommon. Instead, loosening and migration of an acetabular component often leads to medial bone loss in conjunction with other segmental and/or cavitary defects. When a medial defect exists with a completely intact peripheral rim and no volumetric bone loss, the cause is often iatrogenic. The medial portion of a failed acetabular component can be difficult to reach with osteotomes and gouges. Failure to circumferentially disrupt the cement and/or bone interface may result in a portion of the medial wall being extracted along with the component. In addition, excessive reaming of the medial wall during acetabular preparation may also result in an isolated defect of the medial wall.

The American Academy of Orthopedic Surgeons (AAOS) subclassifies medial or central wall defects under type I, or segmental deficiencies.[1] In a type I central segmental deficiency the medial wall is absent, whereas in a type II cavitary central deficiency the medial wall is intact.[1] Paprosky et al.[25] classify medial wall defects as type 2C, in which preoperative radiographs demonstrate loss of the teardrop.

Preoperative planning involves obtaining adequate radiographs (AP Pelvis; AP/lateral of hip; Judet views) and computed tomographic imaging studies (CT scan) in order to define the acetabular defect. Templating allows for an estimation of prosthetic size, anatomic hip center, and need for supplemental bone graft. Paprosky et al.[2] note that medial wall integrity can be assessed by the presence of Kohler's line and the teardrop on preoperative radiographs. Kohler's line coincides with the integrity of the anteromedial acetabulum, whereas the teardrop corresponds with the status of the inferomedial acetabulum.[2] In a cadaveric study, Goodman et al.[26] claim that the teardrop is the most consistent marker for the status of the medial wall. The teardrop is located in the inferomedial acetabulum above the obturator foramen. On radiographic examination, the lateral side of the teardrop refers to the exterior acetabular wall and the medial side the interior acetabular wall. Absence of the medial lip of the teardrop corresponds with an inferomedial wall defect. Goodman et al. found that Kohler's or the ilioischial line shifted position relative to pelvic rotation or radiographic projection and remained radiographically intact despite creating a perforation of the medial wall. Therefore, since it is difficult to standardize radiographic examinations, the teardrop provides a consistent and accurate marker of the integrity of the medial wall of the acetabulum (Fig. 49.4).

The goals of acetabular revision surgery include: (1) component support and stability, (2) reapproximate normal anatomy, (3) restore hip center of rotation and leg lengths, and (4) restore bone stock.[5] A wide, extensile exposure with or without trochanteric osteotomy or slide is mandatory. Before addressing the acetabular component, the hip is dislocated and the stability and position of the femoral component is determined. If unstable, it is removed to aid in acetabular exposure. If stable, the anteversion is noted and taken into consideration when implanting the acetabular component. With good visualization, the acetabular component can be extracted safely with preservation of existing bone stock. All fibrous, cement and metal debris is removed and the acetabular bed is copiously irrigated. An assessment is then made regarding the integrity of the peripheral rim and acetabular walls and columns. Once the extent of the medial wall defect has been determined, the proper amount of allograft bone can be obtained for either morselized or structural graft. The segmental medial wall defect is dealt with first and then acetabular bed is prepared for component implantation.

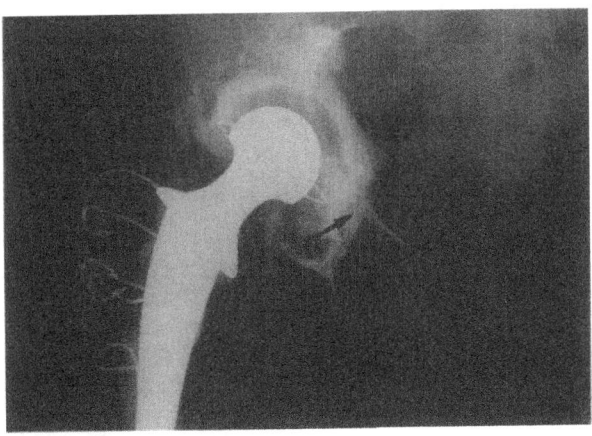

Figure 49.4. Anteroposterior radiograph of a loose cemented, all-polyethylene cup. Loss of teardrop (*arrow*) denotes defect of medial wall.

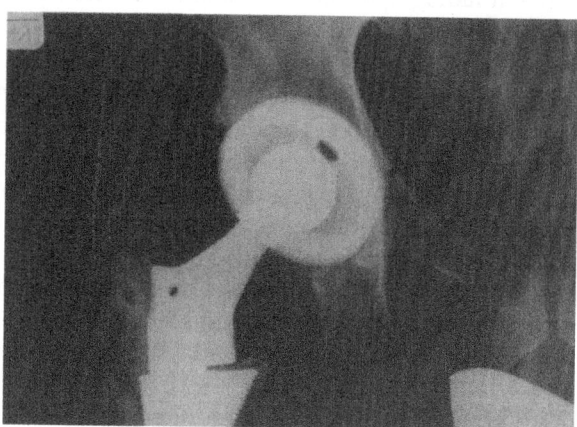

Figure 49.5. Anteroposterior radiograph of a small defect in medial wall (*arrow*) ignored and managed with a fixed, hemispherical cup. Note the loss of the teardrop and the violation of Kohler's line.

In acetabular revision surgery several options exist to address medial segmental bone loss. The deficiency can be either ignored or reconstructed using cement, morselized autograft/allograft or structural allograft. Dorr and Wan[3] stress that the medial wall is not vital to acetabular component support. In fact, they describe a technique of controlled medialization in revision surgery in which the medial wall is purposefully penetrated so as to obtain solid peripheral support for a fixed acetabular shell.[3] If the medial defect is small and an adequate peripheral rim is present, the defect can be either ignored or packed with morselized autograft/allograft[27] and a fixed, hemispherical, porous-coated component implanted (Fig. 49.5). Jasty and Harris[28] defined small medial wall defects as less than 1 cm and large defects as greater than 1 cm. The short and mid-term results of fixed, hemispheric, porous-coated acetabular shells in revision arthroplasty have been excellent when the component attains at least 50% of host–bone contact.[6,8,11,12,22] A large (>1 cm) medial wall defect requires either morselized graft or a structural graft. Since the periosteum and iliacus muscle provide both support and abundant blood supply, morselized graft packed tightly into the defect will remain in place and reconstitute a medial wall (Fig. 49.6). Likewise, no supplemental fixation is necessary for structural grafts such as a wafer[25,29] or "hat" graft, which is fashioned for the medial defect. A wafer of allograft taken from the dome of a femoral or humeral head contours well with the medial wall and attains support from the iliacus muscle medially and the acetabular component laterally. A hat graft is created by transecting a femoral or humeral head several centimeters above and 1 to 2 cm below the narrow portion of the neck. The graft is then wedged into the defect with the proximal or neck portion directed medially. The hourglass shape allows an interference fit within the defect so that supplemental fixation is unnecessary. The head portion is subsequently reamed to conform with the shape of the acetabular bed (Fig. 49.7).

The use of cement to augment medial defects has been unsuccessful. Jasty and Harris[28] found the use of acetabular mesh and cemented acetabular components ineffective in managing small or large medial wall defects. The sclerotic acetabular bed provides poor sup-

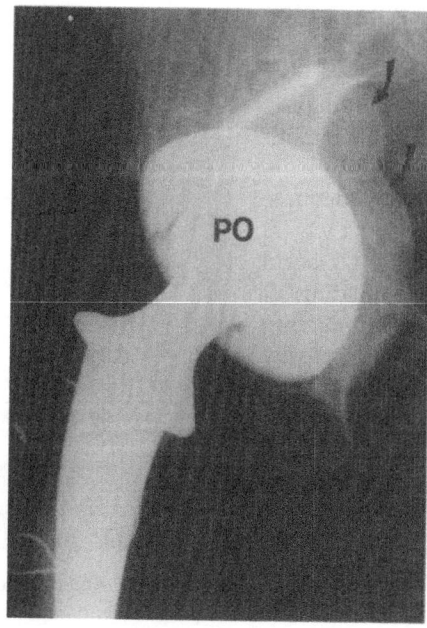
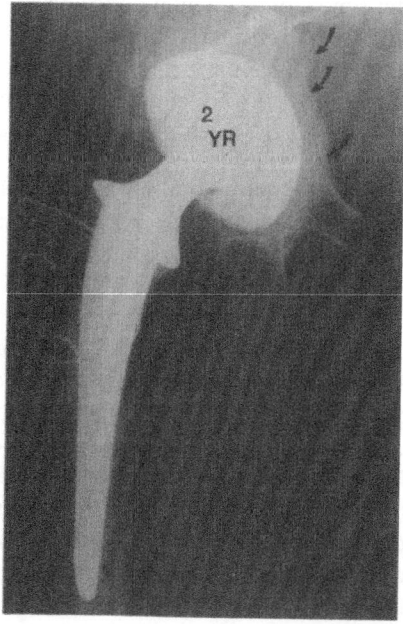

Figure 49.6. Anteroposterior radiographs of a large medial wall defect managed with morselized allograft and a porous-coated acetabular component. A. Postoperative radiograph demonstrating a massive amount of morselized allograft packed into medial defect (*arrows*). B. At 2 years postoperatively radiograph shows consolidation of allograft and reconstitution of medial wall (*arrows*).

49. Management of Medial Deficiencies

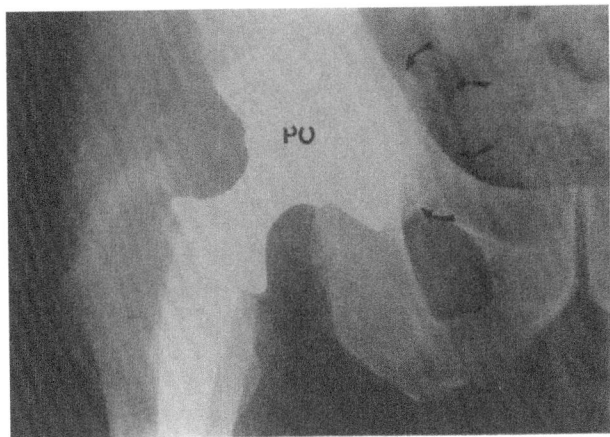

Figure 49.7. Radiograph showing "hat" graft (*arrows*) wedged into medial defect.

port for cement, and loosening can result from cement shrinkage and thermal bone injury.[30] Furthermore, use of cement precludes reconstitution of acetabular bone stock.

Once the medial segmental defect is augmented with either morselized graft (auto/allo) or structural allograft, the acetabular component is implanted. Cemented acetabular components have shown fair durability in revision situations.[31] Bipolar sockets perform well in the short-term in some instances,[32] but most show high rates of loosening and migration and are not recommended in most revision scenarios.[33–35] Wilson et al.[35] emphasize that bipolar components must obtain rim contact and that high loosening rates are seen when used in the presence of noncontained defects. Fixed, hemispheric, porous-coated acetabular shells with or without supplemental screw fixation represent the best option for isolated medial wall defects augmented with bone graft. The fixed acetabular component allows for restoration of the anatomic hip center and stabilization of the bone graft. The bone graft, protected from high stresses by a stable acetabular component, incorporates readily along the vascular medial wall and reconstitutes medial wall bone stock (Fig. 49.8).

In cases with massive medial wall defects, antiprotrusio cages or reinforcement rings offer an alternative to fixed, hemispheric sockets (Fig. 49.9). In a small series, Dartee et al.[36] showed good short-term results with an antiprotrusio cage, morselized allograft and a cemented polyethylene cup in revision cases with acetabular protrusion and medial wall defects greater than 2 cm. Garbuz et al.[9] reported a successful outcome for seven of eight hips that had reinforcement rings and cemented cups at an average 7 year follow-up. The reinforcement rings were used in cases where less than 50% host-bone support was available. Reinforcement rings have demonstrated better or comparable results to bulk structural allograft with severe acetabular bone loss.[37–41] Examples of reinforcement rings include: the Burch–Schneider antiprotrusio cage, the Muller reinforcement ring, and the Ganz ring. Peters et al.[38] and Berry and Muller[37] report good short- and mid-term results, respectively, with the Burch–Schneider antiprotrusio cage. A reinforcement ring is advantageous because it contacts only host bone and serves as a bridge across acetabular defects.[37,38] In

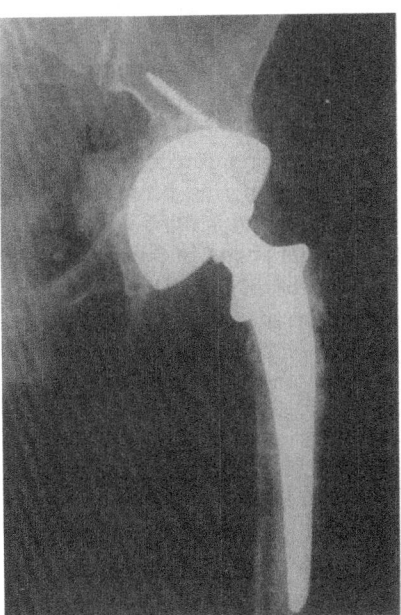
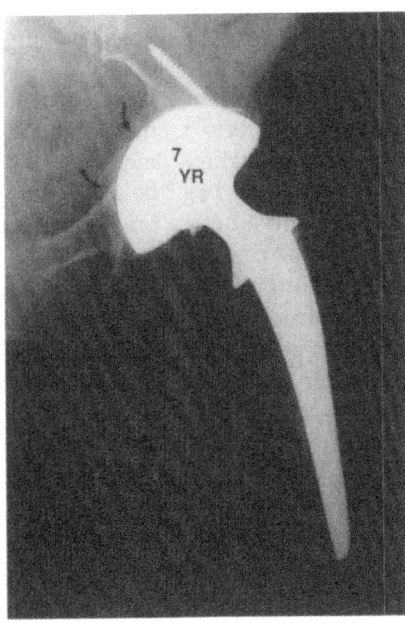

A   B

Figure 49.8. Anteroposterior radiographs of medial wall defect managed with bulk and morselized allograft. A. Postoperative radiograph with bulk, wafer allograft and morselized allograft packed into medial wall defect. B. At seven years postoperatively the graft has remodeled and reconstituted a medial wall (*arrows*).

Figure 49.9. Pre- and postoperative radiographs of a large medial wall defect managed with a reinforcement ring. A. Preoperative radiograph demonstrating large medial wall defect after resection arthroplasty. B. Postoperatively the reinforcement ring bridges the gap in the medial wall (*open arrows*) and is supported by only cement superiorly (*solid arrow*).

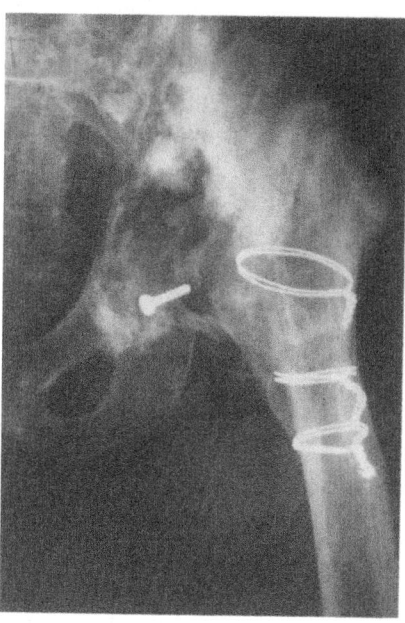
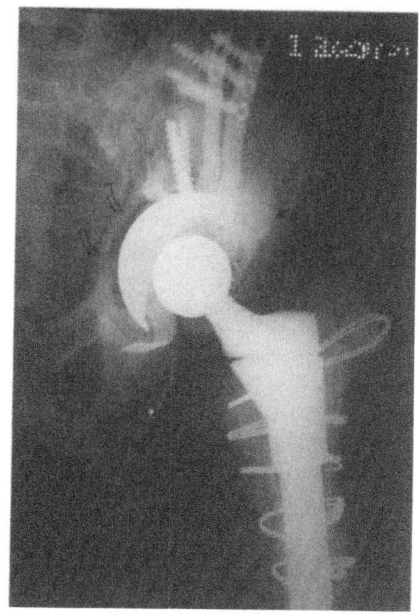

addition, morselized or structural graft used to fill a medial wall defect is stabilized behind the reinforcement ring and protected from excessive forces. Rosson and Schatzker[39] found the Burch–Schneider antiprotrusio cage more effective than the Muller ring at mid-term follow-up. They felt that the Burch–Schneider antiprotrusio cage was indicated with medial segmental defects as the Muller ring failed in two cases with medial bone loss.

Possai et al.[42] reviewed various types of reinforcement rings and felt they were indicated in low demand, physiologically elderly patients, or in salvage situations where a fixed, hemispheric, porous-coated shell cannot obtain adequate rim fit. The Burch–Schneider antiprotrusio cage seemed most effective in situations where the posterior column was intact but the medial and/or anterior wall was absent. The Muller ring relies on an intact superior rim, but can be used for cavitary defects[39] or when the anterior wall is absent.[42] The Ganz ring, which obtains inferior fixation via a hook placed beneath the cotyloid notch, is useful in cases with a deficient superior rim.[42] Neither the Muller or Ganz ring require excessive stripping of the abductors off of the ilium, unlike the Burch–Schneider antiprotrusio cage.

The use of a reinforcement ring requires adherence to several key technical aspects. First, like a fixed, hemispheric socket, the ring must obtain a press-fit within the acetabulum. Second, morselized allograft should be packed tightly behind the ring. Third, supplemental fixation is attained with screws into the ilium and/or ischium. Fourth, the reinforcement ring is usually vertically oriented so that the cemented polyethylene cup must be positioned independently. In order to keep the cup abduction angle less than 45°, up to one-third of the superior portion of the cup is covered only by cement. Fifth, unlike the superior portion of the polyethylene cup, the posterior part must be completely supported by metal. This may entail tilting the reinforcement ring posteriorly or using a smaller polyethylene component.[42]

Although isolated medial segmental deficiencies are not common in revision surgery, they are often encountered in conjunction with other defects. In general, any size medial wall defect can be packed with morselized graft since the iliacus muscle offers medial support. A small (<1 cm) medial wall deficiency can be either ignored and filled with the metal of the acetabular shell[43] or packed with morselized autograft/allograft and supported by a fixed acetabular shell. A larger defect (1 to 2 cm) may require more structural support in the form of a bone wafer or hat graft to prevent overmedialization of the acetabular component. For massive medial wall defects (>2 cm) a reinforcement ring may be necessary. The reinforcement ring provides a rigid bridge across a medial defect that is filled with graft. It is ideal in low demand patients and in those situations where a combined type acetabular defect (AAOS Type III)[1] prevents rim fixation of a fixed, hemispheric, porous-coated acetabular shell.

References

1. D'Antonio JA, Capello WN, Borden LS, et al. Classification and management of acetabular abnormalities in total hip arthroplasty. *Clin Orthop.* 1989;243:126–137.
2. Paprosky WG, Magnus RE. Principles of bone grafting in revision total hip arthroplasty. *Clin Orthop.* 1994;298:147–155.

3. Dorr LD, Wan Z. Ten years experience with porous acetabular components for revision surgery. *Clin Orthop.* 1995;319:191–200.
4. Emerson RH, Head WC, Berklacich FM, Malinin TI. Noncemented acetabular revision arthroplasty using allograft bone. *Clin Orthop.* 1989;249:30–43.
5. Engh CA, Bobyn JD, Glassman AH. Theory and practice of cementless revision total hip arthroplasty. *Hip.* 1987: 271–317.
6. Padgett DE, Kull L, Rosenberg A, Sumner DR, Galante JO. Revision of the acetabular component without cement after total hip arthroplasty: Three to six year follow-up. *J Bone Joint Surg Am.* 1993;75:663–673.
7. Samuelson KM, Freeman MA, Levack B, Rassmussen GL, Revell PA. Homograft bone in revision acetabular arthroplasty: A clinical and radiographic study. *J Bone Joint Surg Br.* 1988;70:367–372.
8. Tanzer M, Drucker D, Jasty M, McDonald M, Harris WH. Revision of the acetabular component with an uncemented Harris-Galante porous-coated prosthesis. *J Bone Joint Surg Am.* 1992;74:987–994.
9. Garbuz D, Morsi E, Mohamed N, Gross AE. Classification and reconstruction in revision acetabular arthroplasty with bone stock deficiency. *Clin Orthop.* 1996;324:98–107.
10. Incavo SJ, Ames SE, Difazio FA, Howe JG. Cementless hemispheric acetabular components: A 4-to 8-year follow-up. *J Arthroplasty.* 1996;11:298–303.
11. Lachiewicz PF, Hussamy OD. Revision of the acetabulum without cement with use of the Harris-Galante porous-coated implant: Two- to eight-year results *J Bone Joint Surg Am.* 1994;76:1834–1839.
12. Silverton CD, Rosenberg AG, Sheinkop MB, Kull LR, Galante JO. Revision total hip arthroplasty using a cementless acetabular component: Technique and results. *Clin Orthop.* 1995;319:201–208.
13. Silverton CD, Rosenberg AG, Sheinkop MB, Kull LR, Galante JO. Revision total hip arthroplasty using a cementless acetabular component: Technique and results. *Semin Arthroplasty.* 1995;6:109–117.
14. Hodgkinson JP, Shelley P, Wroblewski BM. The correlation between the roentgenographic appearance and operative findings at the bone-cement junction of the socket in Charnley low friction arthroplasties. *Clin Orthop.* 1988;228: 105–109.
15. Ranawat CS, Dorr LD, Inglis AE. Total hip arthroplasty in protrusio acetabulae of rheumatoid arthritis. *J Bone Joint Surg Am.* 1980;62:1059–1065.
16. Volz RG, Karpman RR. Revision of the cemented acetabular cup: preparation of the acetabular bed. *Hip.* 1984:271–285.
17. Pierson JL, Jasty M, Harris WH. Techniques of extraction of well-fixed cemented and cementless implants in revision total hip arthroplasty. *Orthop Rev.* 1993;22:904–916.
18. Gray FB. Total hip revision arthroplasty: Prosthesis and cement removal techniques. *Orthop Clin North Am.* 1992; 23:313–319.
19. Greenwald AS. Biomechanical considerations in revision arthroplasty. *Hip.* 1984:254–270.
20. Johnston RC, Brand RA, Crowninshield RD. Reconstruction of the hip: a mathematical approach to determine optimum geometric relationship. *J Bone Joint Surg Am.* 1979;61:639–652.
21. Knight JL, Fujii K, Atwater R, Grothaus L. Bone-grafting for acetabular deficiency during primary and revision total hip arthroplasty: A radiographic and clinical analysis. *J Arthroplasty.* 1993;8:371–382.
22. Woolson ST, Adamson GJ. Acetabular revision using a bone-ingrowth total hip component in patients who have acetabular bone stock deficiency. *J Arthroplasty.* 1996;11: 661–667.
23. Wasielewski RC, Cooperstein LA, Kruger MP, Rubash HE. Acetabular anatomy and the transacetabular fixation of screws in total hip arthroplasty. *J Bone Joint Surg Am.* 1990; 72:501–508.
24. Hedley AK, Gruen TA, Ruoff DP. Revision of failed total hip arthroplasties with uncemented porous-coated anatomic components. *Clin Orthop.* 1988;235:75–90.
25. Paprosky WG, Perona PG, Lawrence JM. Acetabular defect classification and surgical reconstruction in revision arthroplasty: A 6 year follow-up evaluation. *J Arthroplasty.* 1994;9:33–44.
26. Goodman SB, Adler SJ, Fyhrie DP, Schurman DJ. The acetabular teardrop and its relevance to acetabular migration. *Clin Orthop.* 1988;236:199–204.
27. Johnsson R, Pettersson H, Lidgren L. Revision of total hip replacement with solid cortico-spongious bone graft for medial acetabular disruption. *Scand J Rheumatol.* 1986;15: 119–123.
28. Jasty M, Harris WH. Results of total hip reconstruction using acetabular mesh in patients with central acetabular deficiency. *Clin Orthop.* 1988;237:142–149.
29. McCollum DE, Nunley JA, Harrelson JM. Bone grafting in total hip replacement for acetabular protrusion. *J Bone Joint Surg Am.* 1980;62:1065–1073.
30. Sotelo GA, Charnley J. The results of Charnley arthroplasty of the hip performed for protrusio acetabuli. *Clin Orthop.* 1978;132:12–18.
31. Callaghan JJ, Salvati EA, Pellicci PM, Wilson PD, Ranawat CS. Results of revision for mechanical failure after cemented total hip replacement, 1979 to 1982. *J Bone Joint Surg Am.* 1985;67:1074–1085.
32. Scott RD. Use of a bipolar prosthesis with bone grafting in acetabular reconstruction. *Contemp Orthop.* 1984;9:35–41.
33. Brien WW, Bruce WJ, Salvati EA, Wilson PD, Pellicci PM. Acetabular reconstruction with a bipolar prosthesis and morseled bone grafts. *J Bone Joint Surg Am.* 1990;72:1230–1235.
34. Papagelopoulos PJ, Lewallen DG, Cabanela ME, McFarland EG, Wallrichs SL. Acetabular reconstruction using bipolar endoprosthesis and bone grafting in patients with severe bone deficiency. *Clin Orthop.* 1995;314:170–184.
35. Wilson MG, Nikpoor N, Aliabadi P, Poss R, Weissman B. The fate of acetabular allografts after bipolar revision arthroplasty of the hip: A radiographic review. *J Bone Joint Surg Am.* 1989;71:1469–1479.
36. Dartee DA, Huij J, Tonino AJ. Bank bone grafts in revision hip arthroplasty for acetabular protrusion. *Acta Orthop Scand.* 1988;59:513–515.
37. Berry DJ, Muller ME. Revision arthroplasty using an antiprotrusio cage for massive acetabular bone deficiency. *J Bone Joint Surg Br.* 1992;74:711–715.
38. Peters CL, Curtain M, Samuelson KM. Acetabular revision with the Burch-Schneider antiprotrusio cage and cancellous allograft bone. *J Arthroplasty.* 1995;10:307–312.

39. Rosson J, Schatzker J. The use of reinforcement rings to reconstruct deficient acetabula. *J Bone Joint Surg Br.* 1992;74:716–720.
40. Stockl B, Beerkotte J, Krismer M, Fischer M, Bauer R. Results of the Muller acetabular reinforcement ring in revision arthroplasty. *Arch Orthop Trauma Surg.* 1997;116:55–59.
41. Zehntner MK, Ganz R. Midterm results (5.5–10 years) of acetabular allograft reconstruction with the acetabular reinforcement ring during total hip revision. *J Arthroplasty.* 1994;9:469–479.
42. Possai KW, Dorr LD, McPherson EJ. Metal ring supports for deficient acetabular bone in total hip replacement. *Instr Course Lect* 1996;45:161–169.
43. Sutherland CJ. Treatment of type III acetabular deficiencies in revision total hip arthroplasty without structural bone-graft. *J Arthroplasty.* 1996;11:91–98.

50
Management of Posterior Acetabular Deficiencies

Viktor E. Krebbs, Joseph C. McCarthy, and Lester S. Borden

Isolated posterior acetabular deficiencies encountered during revision and complex primary total hip arthroplasty have been reported only uncommonly. More frequently, posterior wall and column defects occur as part of a global deficiency. These salvage situations have historically been treated with implant resection, but over the last 20 years the evolution of acetabular allografting techniques and cages has made possible reconstructive arthroplasty. Evaluation and management of isolated posterior deficiencies has not been specifically addressed in the literature, although cases have been noted in series of acetabular revisions and in the treatment of end-stage developmental dislocation.[1–5,7–12,14–16,22–25,27,28,32,40] Because of relative infrequency and variability, there is no consensus as to the best and most durable method of treating these defects. This chapter will present our evaluation and treatment rationale, surgical techniques, and experience with these challenging reconstructions.

Posterior wall or column deficiencies may occur in isolation, or in combination with other areas of acetabular bone loss (Table 50.1). In revision total hip arthroplasty, the most likely cause is erosion of acetabular bone stock after aseptic component loosening and/or progressive osteolysis (Fig. 50.1). Identification and appreciation of the magnitude of the posterior defect is of paramount importance in planning acetabular revision. Deficiencies in this portion of the acetabulum should be treated differently than those encountered in anterior, superior, or medial locations. Great mechanical force transmission through the posterior and posteriosuperior acetabulum has been demonstrated by Hodge et al. using a telemetric endoprosthesis.[13] In the first postoperative year, posterior forces can reach up to 9 times body weight when patients climb stairs and rise from a seated to a standing position. In cases of defects in this high-stress area not being fully supported during reconstruction, premature or accelerated failure has been observed.[3,13]

Lack of posterior support has been identified in numerous studies as a cause of failure in revision and complex primary acetabular reconstruction. Harris modified his surgical technique to account for these deficiencies by extending bulk femoral head allografts onto the ischium. He noted posterior cement fractures in this area and radiographic evidence of loosening when allograft support was not present.[9,13] Posterior plating techniques to address these forces have been presented,[1] and successful use of this method has been included in reports addressing acetabular deficiencies.[5,7,8,12,22,40] Emerson et al. identified and reconstructed 9 posterior segmental defects in a series of 106 acetabular revisions. Of these 9 allograft reconstructions, the 5 that were supported with a buttress plate did better and showed graft incorporation.[7,8] Capello, in a series of acetabular revisions using the GAP cup, noted four failures when massive posterior defects were filled with morselized graft only prior to fixation of the cage. The technique has been subsequently modified to include structural distal femoral allograft with posterior buttress plating, followed by placement of the GAP cup and cemented polyethylene acetabular prosthesis.[3]

Classification and Preoperative Planning

Classification of acetabular deficiency according to the system proposed by the American Academy of Orthopedic Surgeons assists in reconstructive planning and selection of the operative approach.[6] The AAOS classification system defines three types of posterior defects: Type I—posterior cavitary, Type II—segmental posterior, and Type III—combined. Noncontained Type II and III posterior defects can range from very mild, requiring no special treatment, to very complex geometrical challenges necessitating large structural allografts supported by rigid internal fixation. Systematic evaluation and classification permits anticipation of implant,

Table 50.1. Causes of posterior acetabular defects.

Osteolysis surrounding failed acetabular implants (cemented and uncemented)
Long-standing and high-riding developmental dislocations
Infection
Erosion after resection arthroplasty
Component removal with failure to disrupt fixation
Eccentric reaming
Chondrodysplasias
Malreduced or nonunited acetabular fractures

bone graft, and fixation needs, and also helps avoid unexpected intraoperative difficulties.

The global requirements of individual patients should be the first and major consideration when planning major acetabular reconstruction. Age, activity level, medical status, and patient expectations should all be taken into account. These factors may necessitate deviation from complex and extensive treatment options. A debilitated Charnley class C patient may be better served with a Burch–Schneider cage and particulate grafting, conversion to an oversized bipolar (if containment can be achieved), creation of a high hip center, or resection arthroplasty, whereas physiologically young and active patients may benefit from bulk structural allografting and reestablishment of bone stock.[4,5] All these factors, in addition to the surgeons experience and training, need to be considered in planning complex acetabular revision.

Initially, classification is based on a series of radiologic studies that can be used to progressively clarify details of the defect (Table 50.2). This series of studies permits sequential acquisition of higher levels of detail, and should be utilized until the operating surgeon is comfortable with the size, location, and complex geometry of the deficiency. Once these factors have been delineated preoperatively, the most appropriate surgical approach can be selected. Intraoperative assessment provides the final classification and implant/bone graft selection. Classification and careful planning help the surgeon avoid situations in which inadequate resources are available at the time of the procedure. The importance of identifying pelvic discontinuity preoperatively cannot be overemphasized. Failure to identify or preoperatively plan for the dissociated pelvis results in considerably longer operating time, blood loss, postoperative morbidity, and often a less than optimal reconstruction.

Goals and Principles of Posterior Acetabular Deficiency Reconstruction

The goals of acetabular reconstruction, regardless of type, include: (1) restoration of hip mechanics, center of rotation, and acetabular integrity; (2) reestablishment of acetabular component coverage; and (3) installation of secure, rigid prosthetic and graft fixation. The foundation for posterior or posterior-superior acetabular deficiency reconstruction is initial and long-term component stability in host bone. When noncontained segmental and combined deficiencies are encountered in this quadrant, allograft reconstruction is usually necessary. Despite reports of poor long-term results with the use of bulk acetabular allografting,[9,11,15,16,22,34] in cases of posterior deficiency no other anatomic reconstructive options have proven superior.

The high stresses realized by the posterior wall and column make reconstruction in this area particularly susceptible to loosening. Failure to recognize a lack of component or allograft support in this quadrant has resulted in premature acetabular cement mantle fracture and premature component failure.[13] Posterior stresses realized in the immediate recovery period peak during rehabilitation 6 to 12 months postoperatively.[13] These posterior forces are not only great; they are also repeti-

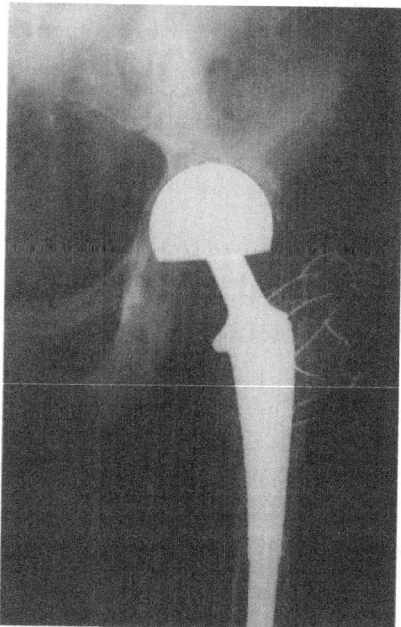

Figure 50.1. AP radiograph of a left bipolar hemiarthroplasty illustrating a significant posterior wall and column defect secondary to osteolysis.

Table 50.2. Radiographic studies used to sequentially define bony details of acetabular deficiencies.

1. AP pelvis, AP/lateral hip
2. Judet views
3. Inlet/outlet views
4. Arthrogram
5. CT scan
6. CT with 3D reconstruction

tive and impact-loading, and they occur with simple daily activities. During this critical rehabilitation period, allograft resorption, vascularization, incorporation, and remodeling are also occurring. In our opinion, failure to address these unavoidable forces and support the healing allograft have contributed to failures. Although proper graft selection, orientation, biological buttressing, and fixation have been successful in the hands of some,[4] these results have been unpredictable in the hands of others. Poor bone graft and host bone qualities are other variables that may be adversely affected by strong, concentrated posterior forces. Use of a posterior buttress plate, by providing more rigid fixation and graft support during healing, may decrease the contribution of these variables to graft failure and component loosening.

Treatment Options

The majority of posterior deficiencies encountered during acetabular revision can be successfully reconstructed with hemispherical uncemented porous-ingrowth components.[5–8,12,18,19,21,22,25,28,35–37] Contained posterior Type I cavitary lesions and some Type II segmental defects can be reconstructed with standard hemispheric press-fit acetabular components, particulate bone graft, and supplemental dome screw fixation. Segmental defects that do not compromise component stability, yet maintain the center of hip rotation within 2 cm of anatomic and contain the prosthesis fall into this category. The use of supplemental dome screw fixation is advised, and has been shown to be effective in revision situations.[18,19,21,25,28,35,37] If the posterior segmental defect is of the minor rim variety, medialization to the subchondral plate with careful preservation of the anterior and posterior columns permits stable fixation of a large press-fit cup and increases host bone-implant contact.[1,5]

In contrast to deficiencies that can be reconstructed with porous-ingrowth components, there are circumstances in which high failure rates have been reported.[22,28,31,33] Type III posterior combined deficiencies and large segmental defects require consideration of the use of bulk structural allograft and/or a Burch-Schneider cage. Type II defects that involve the supporting rim have poor quality remaining host bone and/or compromise the prosthetic stability, requiring additional support in our experience. Preoperative classification and planning provide the reconstructive framework from which the final reconstruction evolves. Ultimately, intraoperative assessment of defect geometry, volume, location, and initial component stability determine the type of reconstruction required to support the component.

When a massive posterior defect is encountered, the reconstructive options are limited (Table 50.3). We do not favor the creation of a nonanatomic high hip center. In these cases, the use of bulk structural allograft can be justified because no other treatment or implant has proven superior. The advantages of bulk structural allograft include: (1) restoration of bone stock, (2) restoration of hip mechanics and a more normal center of rotation, and (3) improved reconstructive options if rerevision is necessary. The disadvantages include: (1) increased operative time and postoperative morbidity, (2) the possibility of disease transmission, (3) a higher incidence of deep infection, and (4) the need for dissection in proximity of the sciatic notch for graft and hardware placement. The alternatives listed in Table 50.3 have all been mentioned in the revision literature for posterior deficiency reconstruction, but case numbers have been few and follow-up results have been similar to those for allograft, without the benefit of bone reconstitution. In certain situations these alternatives may be more feasible than embarking upon allograft reconstruction.

In older low-demand patients, implantation of a Burch-Schneider cage with a cemented polyethylene cup may be beneficial because of significantly reduced operating time, blood loss, and postoperative morbidity.[32] In addition to these advantages, the short- to medium-term results may be more predictable. Pain relief has been excellent and patients are able to bear weight sooner—both important factors when treating older patients. Disadvantages include a significant postoperative dislocation rate, the risk of gluteus medius denervating during exposure for the superior flange, and cage support dependent on screw fixation in bone stock that is usually poor.[30,32,33]

Surgical Techniques

Surgical Approach

The approach chosen should be based on the acetabular defect size and location as determined by the preoperative assessment and plan. Type I and minor Type II deficiencies can be exposed and reconstructed using standard anterolateral or posterior approaches. Severe Type II and Type III deficiencies require a more extensile exposure when allografting, cage placement, and/or posterior plating is anticipated. A carefully planned trochanteric slide provides excellent acetabular visual-

Table 50.3. Options for reconstruction of extensive unsupported posterior acetabular deficiencies.

Bulk acetabular allografting
Bulk acetabular allografting with posterior buttress plating
Burch-Schneider cage and particulate allografting
Creation of a high hip center to achieve bony support
Resection arthroplasty

ization in most posterior deficiency situations. There are situations where the trochanteric slide is not advantageous; the abductors, tethered by the superior gluteal nerve, limit anterior translation of the tissue and the extent of anterior exposure. Assessment of the proximal femur and femoral component are also critical before using the slide. Extensive proximal femoral osteolysis and the presence of or planned use of a proximal canal filling component increase the likelihood of an intraoperative or postoperative fracture after thinning the trochanteric–proximal femoral junction. In these situations a combined anterior transgluteal/posterior exposure or a formal trochanteric osteotomy should be undertaken. In cases of excessive shortening (greater than 2–3 cm), trochanteric osteotomy, soft tissue release, and advancement can be helpful.

Surgical Evaluation and Decision Making

The final reconstruction is based on thorough visualization and exploration of the defect at the time of surgery. After adequate exposure and removal of components, cement, and osteolytic membranes, the remaining host bone is extensively debrided. The true level of the acetabulum and center of rotation are then determined. This is facilitated by placing retractors inferior to the transverse acetabular ligament and just over the anterior rim of the socket below the anterior inferior iliac spine. It is also essential that the true medial wall be defined by removing the inferior portion of the subchondral plate between the inferior and anterior retractors, or carefully tapping a navicular gouge through the

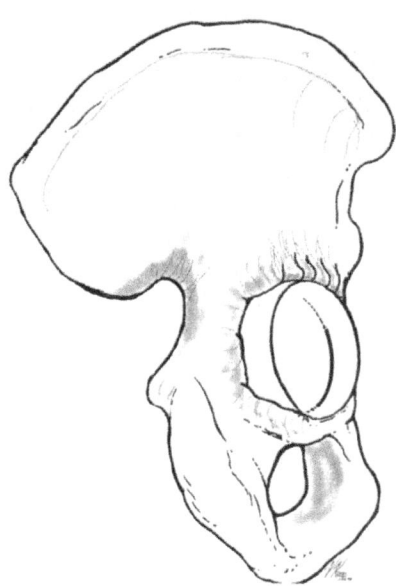

Figure 50.3. The need for posterior acetabular support can be visualized by placing an anatomically oriented trial acetabular component into the defect.

medial bone and then probing with a depth gauge. Correct placement of the component should be at these limits, regardless of the acetabular position preoperatively.

Correct implant sizing and the extent of the posterior defect is then determined by the distance between the anterior wall at its junction with the pubis and the posterior ischial wall (Fig. 50.2). Regardless of the size and location of the bone loss, the first step in reconstruction is to ream the floor of the true acetabulum to the depth of the medial wall. Johnston et al. have shown that medial, inferior, and anterior placement of the acetabular component minimizes prosthetic loading, whereas lateralizing the socket relative to the normal center greatly increases joint reactive forces.[17] The level at which reaming is started is determined by orienting the reamer between the anterior and inferior retractors. Preparation with progressively larger reamers at this level is carried out until the bone between the anterior and posterior limits of the socket is prepared. Care must be taken to avoid eccentric reaming and overreaming. The anterior and posterior columns or walls, when present, should be palpated intermittently to ensure that they are not being thinned precariously.

The largest reamer that was used to prepare the bone between the pubis and the ischium determines the size of the component to be implanted. A trial prosthesis is then inserted at the level of the true acetabulum and oriented in 20° flexion and 30° to 40° abduction. The bone graft requirements for adequate support of the acetabular component can then be readily visualized (Fig. 50.3). Determination of the need for bone grafting, with

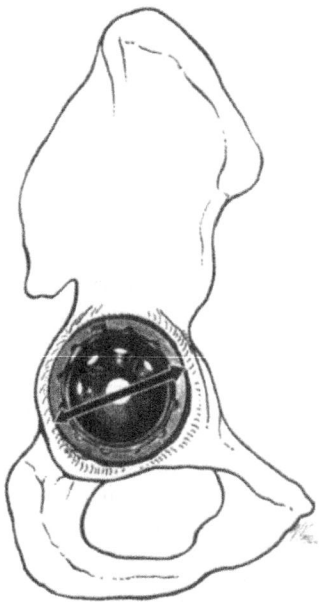

Figure 50.2. The distance between the anterior wall and the ischium may be of help in determining the appropriate acetabular component diameter.

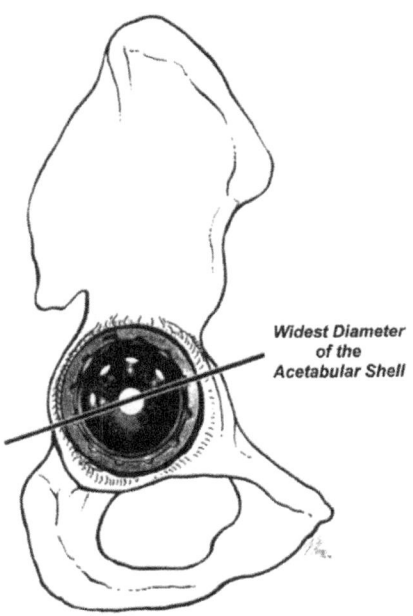

Figure 50.4. The position and containment of the widest diameter of the acetabular component or trial when placed anatomically provides a way to evaluate the need for bone grafting with or without additional posterior support.

or without posterior support, can be facilitated by visualizing the extent of the defect in relation to the widest diameter of the acetabular component or trial (Fig. 50.4). If posterior segmental bone loss does not extend below the widest portion or transverse diameter of the trial acetabular component, placed in the anatomic location and position, screw fixation of a bulk allograft is sufficient to provide containment and to restore bone stock (Fig. 50.5A). In this situation the host bone provides structural support. If the remaining posterior bone is of poor quality, or there is a question as to its ability to provide support for forces 9 times greater that the patient's body weight, a posterior buttress plate should be added. When posterior column bone loss is more extensive and does not extend superior to the transverse diameter of the trial, very little inherent stability of the component exists (Fig. 50.5B). In this situation a bulk structural allograft with a supporting posterior buttress plate should be used to fill the defect, contain the prosthesis, and reinforce the construct.

Surgical Technique: Posterior Allografting and Plating

Once the decision to use bulk structural allograft has been made, the reconstruction is carried out in the following sequence: (1) reconstituting and supporting the segmental defect, (2) determining the amount of host bone coverage of the implant, and then (3) filling the cavitary lesions with cancellous bone graft.

Fresh frozen allograft femoral head, proximal femur, or distal femur is selected based on the geometry and volume of the defect. The majority of posterior defects are best reconstructed using a femoral head. There is little space posteriorly for larger grafts, and the dense cortico-trabecular structure of the allograft femoral head theoretically provides more support than the metaphyseal distal femur. Regardless of the source of graft material, great care must be taken to provide congruity between the graft and host bone. After the graft has been prepared by denuding it of all remaining articular cartilage with a cup reamer, its diameter is measured and a similar-sized acetabular reamer is used to prepare the base of the defect (Fig. 50.6). This reamer may be larger

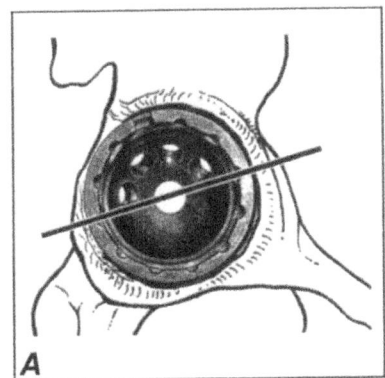 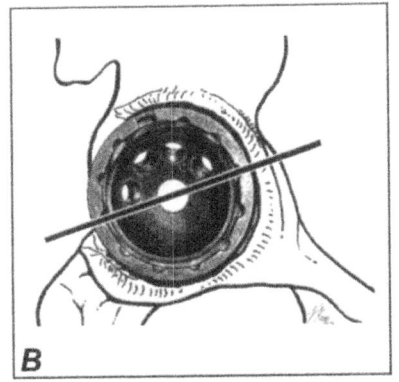

Figure 50.5. A. Posterior segmental bone loss that does not extend below the transverse diameter of the acetabular component. When an acetabular shell is placed in the anatomic location and position, the use of a bulk allograft fixed with screws alone is sufficient to provide containment and to restore bone stock. B. Extensive posterior column bone loss with a defect margin that does not extend superior to the transverse diameter of the cup. In this situation, very little inherent stability exists; a bulk structural allograft with a supporting posterior buttress plate should be used to fill the defect, contain the prosthesis, and reinforce the construct.

Figure 50.6. Preparation of a posterior acetabular defect to accept a bulk femoral head allograft. A. Details of an irregular posterior column defect. B. Eccentric reaming of the defect to create a hemispheric bed. C. Prepared hemispheric bed of bleeding host bone ready to accept a femoral head allograft prepared with a cup reamer.

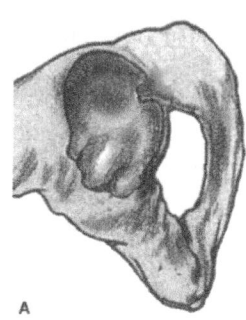 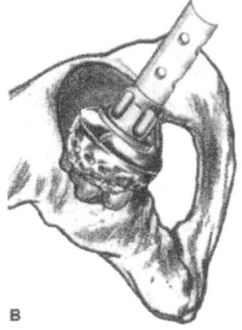 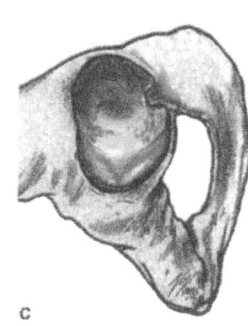

or smaller than the acetabular component to be used, depending on the size of the defect and femoral head. It is important to ream the defect so that the cortical portion of the allograft can be inset within the confines of the host acetabular rim.[4] Reaming the defect in this manner produces excellent graft–host bone conformity, enhances graft stability, and provides the optimal situation for graft incorporation and healing. For complex shapes, a high-speed burr is often useful to maximize congruity, and also allows conservation of the remaining host bone. Once the graft has been shaped, it is provisionally fixed in the defect with guidewires so that two cannulated, terminally threaded 6.5 mm or larger cancellous lag screws can be placed. Cannulated screws are recommended, and should be directed away from the sciatic notch.

At this point, posterior plating is carried out if required for additional support. A 4.5 mm pelvic reconstruction plate is selected to completely cover the graft and extend onto the ilium above and the ischium below. The plate should be contoured for maximum contact with the external surface of the graft, ilium, and ischium. It is often possible to pass one or two screws through the plate and graft into the underlying host bone to improve fixation, but extreme caution is necessary to avoid misdirecting the screw and injuring vital structures in the pelvis and sciatic notch. Problems with screw placement and fixation are usually a function of the adequacy of the exposure. Additional 6.5-mm cancellous screws can be countersunk through the superior portion of the graft into the ilium.

The final preparation of the graft is then accomplished once it is rigidly fixed by reaming to the predetermined size at the anatomic level and orientation (Fig. 50.7). Morselized graft is added to the host–graft interface and to fill any cavitary defects (Fig. 50.8). The trial component should now be contained completely within the reconstructed acetabulum. Use of a larger graft and a smaller acetabular component should be avoided, as maximum contact between the component and the host bone is a key factor in providing a long-lasting construct. It has been our experience that fewer failures occur when the component size is determined by the distance between the pubis and ischium of the patient's true acetabulum.

The type of acetabular component fixation is determined at this stage, after the bony reconstruction has been completed. It is currently our choice to cement the acetabular component when greater than 50% of the peripheral support is established by the allograft. In most revision cases with posterior column deficiencies, the amount of bone loss, and therefore the amount of allograft required, is less than 50% of the peripheral rim. In this most common scenario, we now use cementless porous-coated acetabular implants. Bipolar implants have also been used with positive short- to medium-term follow-up. However, in response to reports at longer follow-up that show increased component mi-

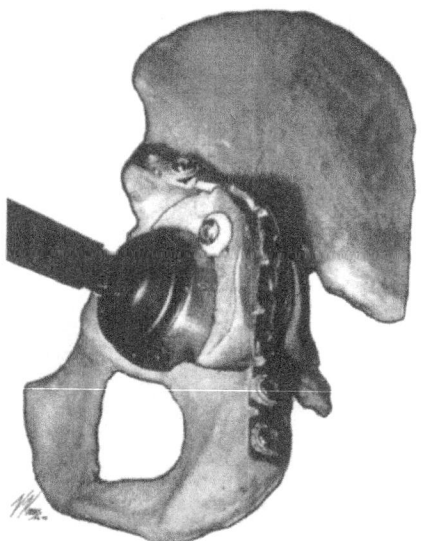

Figure 50.7. Reaming of the allograft buttress plate construct is performed after it is rigidly fixed to assure maintenance of graft–host bone conformity and a hemispheric socket. A contoured 4.5 mm pelvic reconstruction plate provides maximum contact with the external surface of the graft, ilium, and ischium.

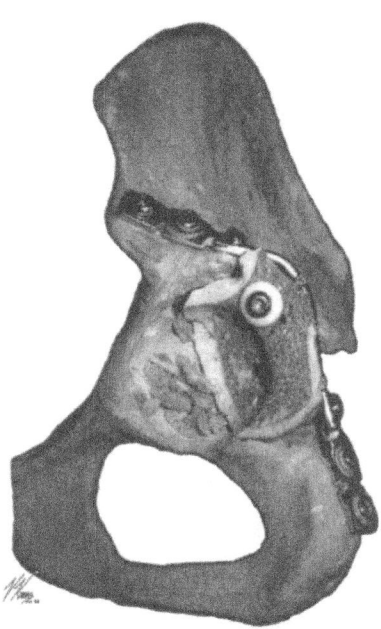

Figure 50.8. Appearance of the final posterior column reconstruction with morselized graft added to the graft–host interface and cavitary defects. Other key features of the reconstruction include inset of the femoral head allograft into the native acetabulum and restoration of the anatomic hip center.

gration and failure when bipolar articulates with allograft,[2,26] they have been reserved for low-demand patients in circumstances in which stability is tenuous due to poor muscular integrity.

Surgical Technique: Burch-Schneider Cage

The Burch-Schneider cage is well suited for reconstruction of posterior acetabular deficiencies due to its geometry and the fixation flanges, which attach to the ilium superiorly and the ischium inferiorly. Ischial fixation may be achieved with screws or by inserting the plate's inferior flange into the bone. When well fixed, with the cup portion in direct apposition with the remaining host bone in the acetabular dome, the posterior buttress function of this device is similar to a posterior reconstruction plate. Particulate allografting behind the device permits reconstitution of the acetabular bone stock.[30,32] In young patients, this method of reconstruction cannot be advocated because the long-term survival rate and results of rerevision are unknown.

The exposure, previous component extraction, membrane removal, and defect assessment are the same as discussed for the posterior plating technique. The presence of discontinuity needs to be ruled out. If present, posterior reconstruction with a plate prior to cage placement may be required. In some situations, the configuration of the cage itself may be enough to restore pelvic continuity. Light reaming of the acetabulum should then be performed to assess the bone quality and create a bleeding bed for incorporation of bone graft. Creation of a hemisphere is unnecessary if a cage is to be employed. The purpose of reaming is to obtain conformity in the superior dome for stable host bone-cage apposition. The defects present are then bone grafted completely to provide additional prosthetic support after healing and graft incorporation have occurred. We do not use bulk structural allograft beneath the cage. The cage should be impacted snugly into place to further compress the graft. It is critical to orient the cage so that complete posterior coverage of the polyethylene cup is achieved by the metal ring while maintaining anatomic cup position to prevent instability and dislocation.[30,32] Once in place, multiple screws are placed through the flanges in both the ilium and ischium.

The cup is then cemented into place. Use of a smaller cup with a 10° hood placed posteriorly is recommended; the hood does not need to be covered by the cage. When a posterior defect is present, there is a tendency to retrovert the cage to maintain bony apposition. This placement will result in significant instability if the cup is cemented correctly with complete posterior metal coverage. Superior cup coverage is not as critical, and up to one-third may be left uncovered by the metal support in order to obtain the correct abduction. Possai and Dorr have also used a protrusio plastic or a lateralized cup to avoid impingement on the ring.[32]

Postoperative Care and Rehabilitation

In cases of bulk structural allografting having been used to reconstruct a posterior defect and impart component stability, prolonged protective weight-bearing with crutches is necessary. The patient should be strict non-weight-bearing for the first six weeks postoperatively, and then partial/touch down weight-bearing to help minimize further abductor atrophy. Evidence of progressive graft union on serial radiographs determines the amount of activity and weight-bearing the patient is allowed. Clear evidence of graft union usually takes 3 to 6 months, and at that time progression to a cane is permitted. Stair climbing is discouraged, and using the leg to move from seated to standing is forbidden until the graft has healed. A cane should be used until the abductors have been rehabilitated to their maximum potential.

Results

Between 1987 and 1991, 16 patients underwent revision total hip replacement using a pelvic reconstruction buttress plate (Fig. 50.9). All patients had extensive segmental acetabular bone loss, involving primarily the posterior acetabular rim. There were 10 females and 6

Figure 50.9. Radiographs of a 69-year-old male with massive pelvic and femoral osteolysis 18 years after primary hip arthroplasty. A&B. AP and Lateral of the right hip illustrating a significant cavitary acetabular defect, with minimal posterior column bone stock. C. Postoperative AP of acetabular reconstruction with bone grafting and posterior column buttress plating. D. AP of acetabular reconstruction 5 years postoperatively.

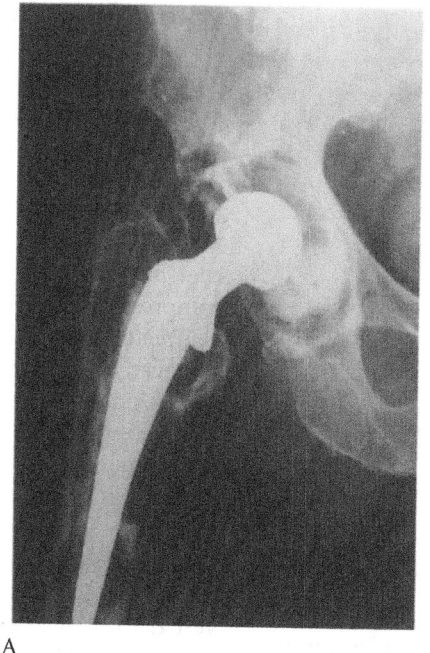
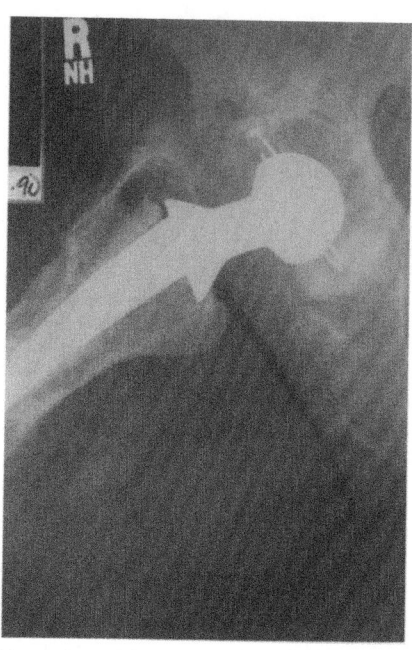
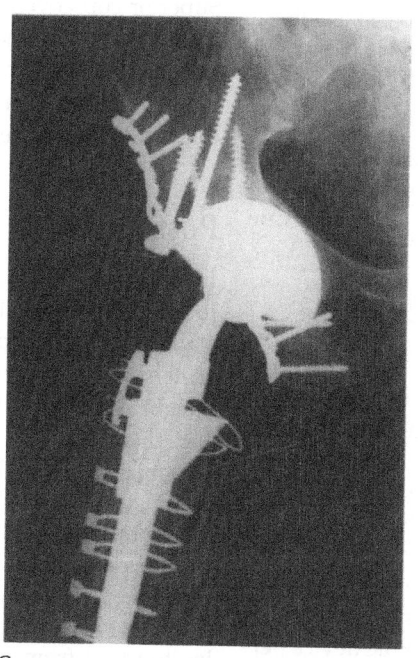
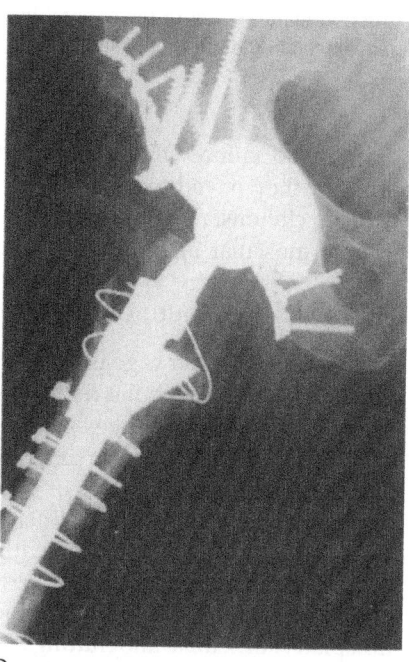

A B C D

males. The average age was 67 years (range 51–82). All 16 patients were severely disabled prior to surgery. Their average preoperative Harris hip score was 41 points (range 18–59). They all required the use of analgesics and an supportive device for ambulation. The patients had undergone an average of 2.7 hip operations (1–6) prior to this revision. Fifteen of the hips had previous cemented acetabular components, while 1 had an uncemented implant. At the index revision procedure, 14 patients had reconstruction using a femoral head allograft with pelvic plate, and 2 patients had fixation using a distal femoral allograft and plating. The implants used for reconstruction were uncemented: 14 bipolar and 2 press-fit porous ingrowth components.

Patients were followed a minimum of 4 years (4–7 years). All grafts had incorporated at an average of 13 months. All buttress plates remained well fixed, and no acetabular components have failed. At most recent follow-up, migration of the bipolar components averaged 1.9 mm medial (range 0–12 mm) and 7.5 mm superior (range 0–36 mm). These numbers include one patient who fell within 6 weeks of the reconstruction, resulting in bipolar translation of 12 mm medial and 36 mm superior. Aside from this patient, average medial migration was 1.5 mm and average superior migration was 5.9 mm. No further migration occurred after graft incorporation. Migration was not correlated with pain, HHS, or noticeable leg length discrepancy except for the one patient noted above. The Harris hip score improved 39 points, from 41 to 80 (range 71–87). There have been no revisions of the bone graft or acetabular components to date. Complications included one femoral nerve palsy in a patient who also had a femoral allograft. There were two peroneal palsies, one of which resolved fully and the other partially. One patient developed Grade IV heterotopic ossification, which was later resected and has not recurred. The bone graft was well incorporated.

Conclusion

Posterior bony deficiency does occur in association with failed total hip arthroplasty. This defect may occur alone or, more frequently, in combination with superior and/or medial acetabular bone loss. It is vital for the operating surgeon to anticipate this deficiency preoperatively. Since radiographs tend to underestimate the frequency and extent of bone loss, it is advisable to have the resources on hand to address pelvic discontinuity and segmental column loss. A full array of acetabular components, allograft bone, pelvic buttress plates, and reconstruction cages are invaluable if a significant deficiency is encountered. Radiographic studies such as Judet views and on occasion CT scan modeling may assist in the preoperative planning process. Once recognized, an extensile surgical exposure, use of a reconstruction cage or technically precise grafting with or without plating, and ultimately a rigidly fixed acetabular component give the patient the greatest potential for a long-lasting, successful outcome in the face of this complex and difficult reconstructive problem.

References

1. Borden LS, Greenky SS. The difficult primary total hip replacement: Acetabular problems. In Steinberg ME, ed. *The Hip and its disorders*. Philadelphia: WB Saunders; 1991: 1007–1019.
2. Brien WW, Bruce WJ, Salvati EA, Wilson PD, Pellici PM. Acetabular reconstruction with a bipolar prosthesis and morselized bone grafts. *J Bone Joint Surg Am.* 1990;72: 1230–1235.
3. Capello WM. Personal communication.
4. Chandler HP, Peneberg BL. *Bone stock deficiency in total hip replacement: Classification and management*. Thorofare, NJ: Slack; 1989.
5. D'Antonio JA. Periprosthetic bone loss of the acetabulum: Classification and management. *Orthop Clin North Am.* 1992;23:279–290.
6. D'Antonio JA, Capello WN, Borden LS, Bargar WL, Bierbaum BE, Goettcher WG, Steinberg ME, Stulberg SD, Wedge JH. Classification and management of acetabular abnormalities in total hip arthroplasty. *Clin Orthop.* 1989; 243:126–137.
7. Emerson RH, Head WC. Dealing with the deficient acetabulum in revision hip arthroplasty: The importance of implant migration and use of the jumbo cup. *Semin Arthroplasty.* 1993;4:2–8.
8. Emerson RH, Head WC, Berklacich FM, Malinin TI. Noncemented acetabular revision arthroplasty using allograft bone. *Clin Orthop.* 1989;249:30–43.
9. Gerber SD, Harris WH. Femoral head autografting to augment acetabular deficiency in patients requiring total hip replacement. *J Bone Joint Surg Br.* 1986;68:1241–48.
10. Gross AE, Lavoie MV, McDermott P, Marks P. The use of allograft bone in revision of total hip arthroplasty. *Clin Orthop.* 1985;197:115–122.
11. Harris WH. Bulk versus morselized bone graft in acetabular revision total hip replacement. *Semin Arthroplasty.* 1993;4:68–71.
12. Headley AK, Gruen TA, Ruoff DP. Revision of failed total hip arthroplasties with uncemented porous-coated anatomic components. *Clin Orthop.* 1988;235:75–90.
13. Hodge WA, Carlson KL, Fijan RS, Burgess RG, Riley PO, Harris WH, Mann RW. Contact pressures from an instrumented hip endoprosthesis. *J Bone Joint Surg Am.* 1989;71: 1378–1386.
14. Hozack WJ. Techniques of acetabular reconstruction. *Semin Arthroplasty.* 1993;4:72–79.
15. Jasty M, Harris WH. Salvage total hip reconstruction in patients with major acetabular bone deficiency using structural femoral head allografts. *J Bone Joint Surg Br.* 1990;72:63–67.
16. Jasty M, Harris WH. Total hip reconstruction using frozen femoral head allografts in patients with acetabular bone loss. *Orthop Clin North Am.* 1987;18:291–299.
17. Johnston RC, Brand RA, Crowninshield RD. Reconstruction of the hip, a mathematical approach to determine optimum geometric relationship. *J Bone Joint Surg Am.* 1979; 61:639–652.
18. Kavanagh BF, Fitzgerald RH. Multiple revisions for failed total hip arthroplasty not associated with infection. *J Bone Joint Surg Am.* 1987;69:1144–1149.
19. Kavanagh BF, Ilstrup D, Fitzgerald RH. Revision total hip arthroplasty. *J Bone Joint Surg Am.* 1985;67:517–526.
20. Kwong LM, Jasty M, Harris WH. High failure rate of bulk femoral head allografts in total hip acetabular reconstructions at 10 years. *J Arthroplasty.* 1993;8:341–346.
21. Lachiewicz PF, Hussamy OD. Revision of the acetabulum without cement with use of the Harris-Galante porous-coated implant. *J Bone Joint Surg Am.* 1994;76:1834–39.
22. McAllister CM, Borden LS. Allograft reconstruction of the acetabulum in revision hip surgery. *Semin Arthroplasty.* 1993;4:80–86.

23. Mulroy RD Jr, Harris WH. Failure of acetabular autogenous grafts in total hip arthroplasty, *J Bone Joint Surg Am.* 1990;72:1536–1540.
24. Oakeshott RD, Morgan DAF, Zukpr DJ, Rudan JF, Brooks PJ, Gross AE. Revision total hip arthroplasty with osseous allograft reconstruction. *Clin Orthop.* 1987;225:37–61.
25. Padgett DE, Kull L, Rosenberg A, Sumner DR, Galante JO. Revision of the acetabular component without cement after total hip arthroplasty. *J Bone Joint Surg Am.* 1993;75:663–673.
26. Papagelopoulos PJ, Lewallen DG, Cabanela ME, McFarland EG, Wallrichs SL. Acetabular reconstruction using bipolar endoprosthesis and bone grafting in patients with severe bone deficiency. *Clin Orthop.* 1995;314:170–84.
27. Paprosky WG, Magnus RE. Principles of bone grafting in revision total hip arthroplasty: Acetabular technique. *Clin Orthop.* 1994;298:147–55.
28. Paprosky WG, Perona PG, Lawrence JM. Acetabular defect classification and surgical reconstruction in revision arthroplasty. *J Arthroplasty.* 1994;9:33–44.
29. Patch DA, Lewallen W. Reconstruction of deficient acetabula using bone graft and a fixed porous ingrowth cup: a 5 year roentgenographic study. *Orthop Trans.* 1993;17:151.
30. Peters CL, Curtain M, Samuelson KM. Acetabular revision with the Burch-Schnieder antiprotrusio cage and cancellous allograft bone. *J Arthroplasty.* 1995;10:307–12.
31. Pollock FH, Whiteside LA. The fate of massive allografts in total hip acetabular revision surgery. *J Arthroplasty.* 1992;7:271–276.
32. Possai KW, Dorr LD, McPherson EJ. Metal ring supports for deficient acetabular bone in total hip replacement. *Instr Course Lect.* 1996;45:161–169.
33. Rosson J, Schatzker J. The use of reinforcement rings to reconstruct deficient acetabula. *J Bone Joint Surg Br.* 1992;74:716–20.
34. Shinar AA, Harris WH. Bulk structural autogenous grafts and allografts for reconstruction of the acetabulum in total hip arthroplasty: sixteen year average follow-up. *J Bone Joint Surg Am.* 1997;79:159–168.
35. Silverton CD, Rosenberg AG, Sheinkop MB, Kull LR, Galante JO. Revision of the acetabular component without cement after total hip arthroplasty. *J Bone Joint Surg Am.* 1996;78:1366–70.
36. Sutherland CJ. Treatment of type III acetabular deficiencies in revision total hip arthroplasty without structural bone graft. *J Arthroplasty.* 1996;11:91–98.
37. Tanzer M, Drucker D, Jasty M, McDonald M, Harris WH. Revision of the acetabular component with an uncemented Harris-Galante porous-coated prosthesis. *J Bone Joint Surg Am.* 1992;74:987–994.
38. Trancik TM, Stulberg BN, Wilde AH, Feiglin DH. Allograft reconstruction of the acetabulum during revision total hip arthroplasty. *J Bone Joint Surg Am.* 1986;68:527–533.
39. Wilson MG, Scott RD. Reconstruction of the deficient acetabulum using the bipolar socket. *Clin Orthop.* 1990;251:126–133.
40. Young SK, Dorr LD, Kaufman RL, Gruen TA. Factors related to failure of structural bone grafts in acetabular reconstruction of total hip arthroplasty. *J Arthroplasty.* 1991;6 supl:S73–82.

51
Use of Cages

William N. Capello, Edward J. Hellman, and Judy R. Feinberg

Revision of the acetabular component presents a challenge to the arthroplasty surgeon. Severe bone loss secondary to acetabular component migration and osteolysis often results in major segmental and/or cavitary defects. Complex reconstructions are necessary to manage these bony defects on the acetabular side.

The principles of acetabular reconstruction are similar to femoral reconstructions. The specific aims are: (1) to provide a stable, durable, and painless reconstruction; (2) to reconstitute bone stock; and (3) to restore mechanics. A variety of options are currently available, but because of the complexity of many reconstructions results are variable.

Options for Complex Acetabular Revisions

One current option is the hemispheric jumbo cup, that is, an acetabular component larger than 60 mm in diameter (Fig. 51.1). The jumbo cup is intended to span acetabular defects with rigid fixation to remaining viable bone stock. The potential advantages of the jumbo cup is that it is relatively easy to implant and is available off the shelf. The potential disadvantages of the jumbo cup are that: (1) it does not address segmental defects; (2) poor acetabular bone quality can make fixation tenuous; and (3) because of the size of these components, massive stress shielding is likely to occur. Jasty, in a report of 32 hips revised with jumbo cups and followed for an average of 4 years, reported only one rerevision in a type IV defect and no loose cups.[1]

Another option is the high hip center, that is, superior displacement of the acetabular component greater than 3 cm from a line drawn through the most inferior portion of the teardrop (Fig. 51.2). According to Harris, a high hip center that is also lateral is adverse, but a high hip center that is not lateral is not adverse.[2] The potential advantages of using a high hip center are: (1) less operative time; (2) an off-the-shelf component; and (3) host–bone prosthesis contact. The potential disadvantages of a high hip center are: (1) no potential for restoration of bone stock or mechanics; (2) leg length equalization is difficult; (3) a nonstandard femoral component may be required; and (4) greater potential for dislocation. At a minimum 2-year follow-up, Schutzer and Harris reported no migration and no acetabular revisions in a group of 49 high hip center acetabular revisions.[3] However they did report a 10% dislocation/subluxation rate, with no cases requiring subsequent surgery for recurrent instability. Kelley reported a 25% femoral loosening and a 5% acetabular loosening rate in a group of 20 hips with high hip centers at a 2-year minimum follow-up.[4]

The oblong cup is another option in reconstruction of the deficient acetabulum (Fig. 51.3). This implant is designed for use in situations where a large superior defect exists but the posterior columns are intact. The potential advantages are host–bone prosthesis contact and maintenance of an anatomic hip center. The potential disadvantages are the possibility of stress shielding and the limited application relative to the presence of segmental defects. At a recent American Association of Orthopedic Surgeons presentation, Newman reported on 64 cases followed for an average of 44 months with no failures.[5]

Anatomic positioning with block allograft with or without the use of a plate is another option (Figs. 51.4). The potential advantages are the restoration of bone stock and the restoration of mechanics. The potential disadvantages are increased operative time, morbidity, cost, and unpredictable results. Recent literature suggests that the greater the bone graft surface area, the higher the failure rates, regardless of the method of cup fixation. Patch, in his report of 73 porous-coated cups used in conjunction with allografting, found increasing failure rates based on percent of bone graft surface area, ranging from a 15% mechanical failure rate if the bone graft surface area was less than 25% to a 73% mechanical failure rate if the bone graft area exceeded 50%.[6] Similarly, Iida et al., in a study of 132 cemented cups at 10-year follow-up, reported a failure rate of 7% if the bone graft area was less than 25% and 67% if the bone graft area exceeded 70% of the implant surface area.[7]

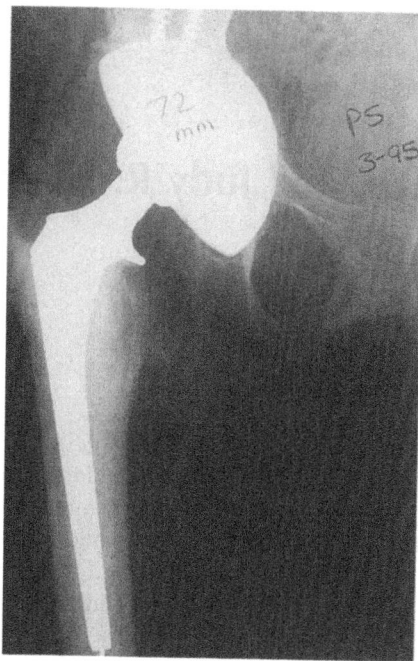

Figure 51.1. Example of jumbo cup.

Reinforcement rings may be the best option in the face of large cavitary and segmental defects. The reinforcing ring allows the defect to be spanned or bypassed by attaching to host bone. The ring provides support for particulate or morselized bone graft during the healing process and, even if bulk allografts are necessary, the ring may protect them from collapse and prevent early migration.[8] There are two general designs of reinforcing rings: rings that are fixed to the ilium with screws (eg, Muller) or with screws and a hook (eg, Ganz, Link, GAP), and cages that are fixed to both the ilium and ischium (eg, Burch–Schneider). The potential advantages of reinforcing rings are: (1) they can address significant cavitary and segmental defects; (2) they can restore mechanics; and (3) they can restore bone stock by providing support for morselized bone graft. The potential disadvantages are increased operative time and technical difficulty of the operative procedure. With follow-up periods of 5 years or less, reports of these devices have a collective rerevision rate of 3.3% in 418 hips.[9–14] Of note is the fact that only two (0.5%) of the 418 reconstructions had failed at the cement (ie, polyethylene-reinforcement ring) interface.

Several designs of reinforcing rings aimed at addressing varying bony deficits are currently available. We believe, as previously reported by Zehntner and Ganz,[15] that it is important to obtain maximal stability on host bone rather than bone graft. If the acetabulum has an intact rim or only a small segmental defect, such devices as the Muller ring will provide adequate fixation to host bone. A porous-coated hemispherical component may also be used with cavitary defects only. In cases of significant posterior or superior defects, a more extensive type of reinforcing ring is needed. A device such as the GAP cup, with an inferior hook around the teardrop and additional fixation superiorly on the ilium by means of plates, allows for maximum fixation to host bone. The GAP cup has a hydroxyapatite coating to enhance subsequent integration. The size of the ring should be chosen to maximize contact with host bone superiorly along the acetabular dome.

GAP Reinforcing Ring: Surgical Technique

The graft augmentation prosthesis (GAP) features hydroxyapatite coating or multiple holes for cement integration, dome screws, and an attached inferior hook and superior plates that can be fashioned to the pelvic anatomy for added stability (Fig. 51.5). In all cases the screw fixation of the reinforcing ring is through host bone, thus bypassing the bony defect. This provides sta-

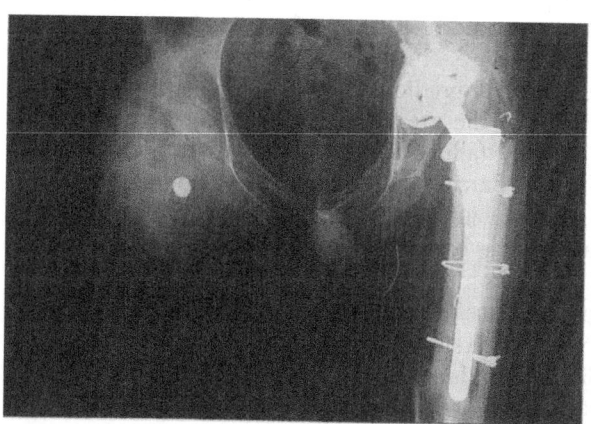

Figure 51.2. Example of high hip center.

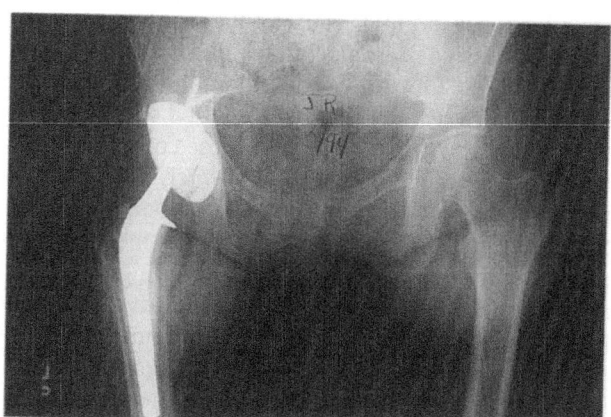

Figure 51.3. Example of oblong cup.

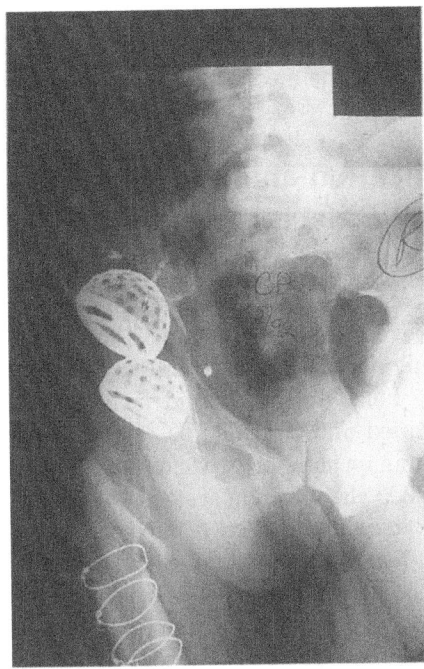
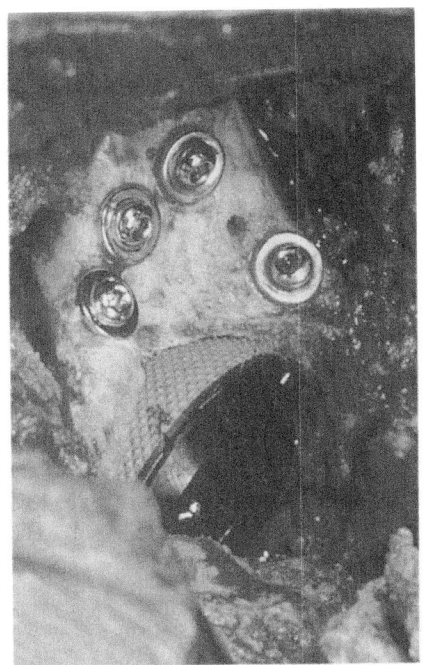

Figure 51.4. A. Intraoperative radiograph showing magnitude of acetabular defect (two reamer heads fit into defect). B. Intraoperative photograph showing bulk allograft in place. C. Postoperative radiograph showing anatomic positioning of cup with bone graft superior. (See color insert.)

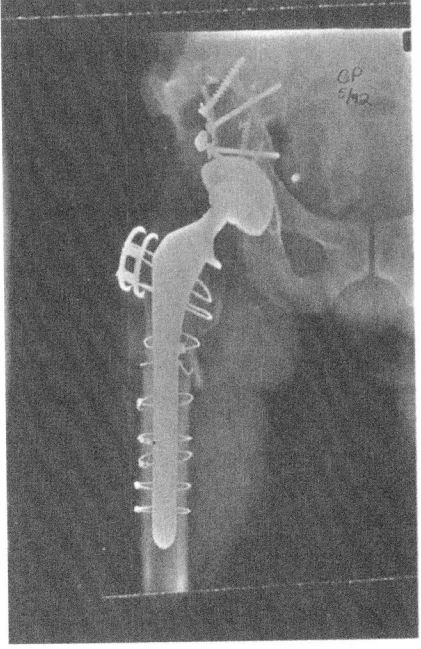

bility of the construct so bone graft incorporation is promoted. A polyethylene insert is cemented into the metal ring to complete the construct. Manufacturer's testing of six hybrid cups (polyethylene liner cemented into a GAP metal shell) under simulated in vitro ten million cycle fatigue loading with a grafted superior defect showed no shell, cement, or insert failures. Cyclic loading of 60 to 600 pounds at 10 Hz was applied through a 32 mm head at 45° from the cup centerline. (Osteonics Corporation, R & D Internal Tech Report #940620, Allendale, NJ).

Exposure

Any standard approach to the hip that provides excellent acetabular exposure can be used, but our preference

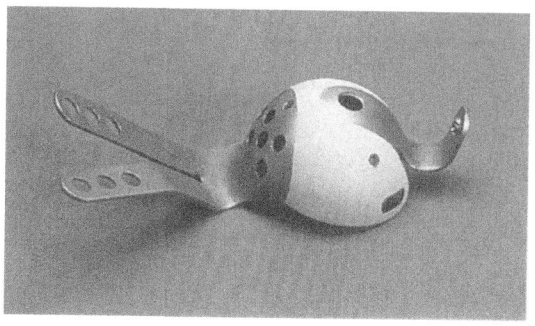

Figure 51.5. Graft augmentation prosthesis (GAP) with hydroxyapatite coating. (See color insert.)

is the posterolateral approach. When using this approach, it is necessary to displace the femur anteriorly to visualize the acetabulum. We find that this is facilitated by a complete release of the bony insertion of the gluteus maximus tendon. In addition, the entire anterior capsule must be cut to permit anterior translation.

It is necessary to expose the ilium anterior and superior to the acetabulum itself, since the GAP prosthesis obtains significant fixation from the ilium. Electrocautery can be used to provide exposure from the acetabular rim to the outer table of the ilium. The outer rim needs to be cleared sufficiently to allow for placement of the superior extension of the reinforcing ring. A periosteal elevator can then be used to elevate the abductor musculature superiorly and anteriorly from the acetabulum. In order to avoid damage to the gluteal vessels and nerves in the sciatic notch area, the dissection should not extend posteriorly.

It is necessary to obtain excellent exposure inferiorly as well when implanting a GAP prosthesis. The first landmark to identify during the course of this dissection is the superior pubic ramus. This is done by dissecting along the anterior wall in an inferior direction until a finger can be placed over the acetabular rim onto the pubic ramus. It is not necessary to visualize the ramus directly. Dissection continues along the posterior wall until the ischium is easily palpable. Dissecting the posterior hip capsule for a short distance from the posterior wall will allow for placement of a spike retractor into the ischium. The soft tissues can then be retracted while protecting the sciatic nerve from excessive tension. The next landmark to identify is the acetabular teardrop that marks the inferior-medial extent of the anatomic acetabulum and is located along the medial wall between the pubic ramus anteriorly and the ischium posteriorly. The medial wall is followed inferiorly until the bone starts to curve medially at the inferior margin of the acetabulum. The obturator foramen is entered by dissecting around this usually stout bone with a curved periosteal elevator. The acetabular branch of the obturator artery is present in this area and usually requires cautery. To adequately position the hook of the prosthesis, it is usually necessary to gain exposure sufficient to place a finger through the obturator foramen along the medial wall of the acetabulum.

Identification and Management of Bony Defects

Once the acetabulum has been adequately exposed, preexisting components, cement, and any osteolytic membranes are removed. The remaining bony acetabulum is thoroughly debrided with curettes removing incompetent bone. Following this debridement the bony defects are identified and classified as cavitary, segmental, a combination or both, or pelvic discontinuity according to the AAOS classification system.[16]

The acetabulum is then reamed lightly with hemispherical reamers to determine the necessary implant size. The bony defects are then addressed with the use of bone graft. If only modest cavitary defects exist, then morselized bone graft and a hemispheric porous-coated acetabular component may be all that is necessary. In cases with segmental defects, the membranous tissue and muscle medial to the acetabulum is usually sufficient to contain morselized bone graft. Prolene mesh may be necessary to contain the graft in cases of true rim defects. It can be cut to the size and shape of the existing rim defect and stapled to the existing bony rim. Fresh frozen allograft bone can then be morselized in a bone mill and tightly packed into the defect. Our preferred technique has been to use hemispheric tamps and a mallet to firmly pack the bone graft. Our current technique for managment of pelvic discontinuity has been to plate the posterior column with a pelvic reconstruction plate and to then use the GAP-reinforcing ring with its inferior and superior fixation. We do not believe it is necessary to plate the anterior column since the GAP does not depend on hoop stress for initial stability of the component.

Occasionally, posterior defects are massive. It has been our experience when trying to manage these massive posterior defects with prolene mesh, morselized graft, and cement alone that this is insufficient and the cup has failed. Our current approach to these large defects is to use structural bone graft, using the form of the distal femur, fix the graft to the host, and then reinforce that fixation with a plate. Once this is accomplished, the graft can be machined with a reamer and then the GAP cup is placed in the usual fashion. We believe that this method aids in reconstitution of bone stock posteriorly. At the same time, the GAP cup may minimize the loads on the structural graft and thereby facilitate incorporation and eventual revascularization.

In some of the larger cavitary defects where the GAP cup will be in contact with more than 50% of the grafted bed, our current approach is to use the morselized bone graft as described, but to then pressure inject cement into the grafted bed and then place the GAP cup into the cement, thereby integrating the GAP cup through the cement into the graft. In addition to securing the cup, the cement in this situation will reinforce the rather poor physical qualities of the cancellous bone, yet will still allow for graft–host bone contact for incorporation and reconstitution of defects. We frequently do this with superior cavitary defects. As the cement cures, we place our dome screws through the cup, through the setting cement, and into the host bone. We then secure the screws, adding further compression to the construct and further interdigitating the cement with the graft and compressing the graft against the host.

Placement of the GAP Cup

After packing the acetabular defects with bone graft, the construct should appear almost as a normal acetabulum. It is important that the reinforcing ring fits adequately into the acetabulum. Using the GAP cup, it is necessary to prebend the plates to fit against the ilium with the hemispherical portion of the ring supported by the dome. The reinforcing ring can then be positioned for final fixation by sliding the plates under the abductor muscles along the ilium and tapping the hemispherical portion into the grafted acetabulum. It is important that the hemispherical portion be tightly inserted against the rim of the acetabulum as well as against the packed or cement impregnated morselized bone graft. Screws (6.5 mm in diameter) are then placed through the ring into the existing superior bone to further compress the graft. Inferior fixation can then be obtained by crimping the hook around the teardrop. Once the hook is secure, the screw holes into the plates can be exposed and one or more screws used to secure the plates to the ilium. The screw heads within the ring are filled with bone wax to facilitate their removal, should that be necessary in the future. A polyethylene acetabular component is then cemented into the ring. At times it is necessary to place the acetabular reinforcing ring in an orientation that may not be optimal for joint mechanics in order to obtain maximal contact with the remaining existing acetabular bone stock. To compensate for this compromise in joint mechanics, the polyethylene cup can be oriented independent from the ring, should it be necessary to obtain proper abduction and anteversion for joint stability. In cases of muscle imbalance, a constrained liner may be used to prevent dislocation.

Clinical Experience With Reinforcing Rings

We have performed 72 acetabular reconstruction procedures in the past 40 months at Indiana University. These include 18 Ganz rings, 7 Link Pelvic Reconstruction rings, and 47 graft augmentation prostheses (GAP). Forty-four (61%) have follow-up between 12 and 40 months. The majority of these reconstructions were performed for aseptic loosening, and more than half had both cavitary and segmental defects (ie, Type III acetabular deficiencies). The most common areas of deficiency were superior and medial. Complications have been similar to those summarized in other reports for reconstruction of major acetabular bone loss. Component removal was necessary following deep joint infection in three hips, and a reoperation for placement of a constrained insert was required in three hips for repeated dislocations. There have been five rerevisions (6.9%) for aseptic loosening. In two of the five rerevision cases, bone graft technique had been noted to be inadequate on early postoperative radiographic analysis. There have also been four component failures requiring rerevision. Those four cases each had large posterior defects managed with morselized bone graft. As a result of these early failures, we have now modified our approach as previously described to include the use of a structural graft.

Patient Example

O.S. is a 70-year-old female with a history of a total hip replacement 22 years prior. She presented with a recent onset of hip pain. Radiographic assessment indicated an obviously loose and migrated acetabular component and signifcant osteolytic changes in the pelvis (Fig. 51.6A). Her femoral component appeared possibly loose with radiolucencies noted at the bone–cement interface medially. She underwent revision surgery in November, 1995. Acetabular defects identified at the time of surgery included superior segmental, superior cavitary, medial cavitary, and posterior cavitary defects (type III) (Fig. 51.6B). Two distal femurs and two femoral heads were morselized to fill these defects (Figs. 51.6C,D). Following pressure injection of cement into the packed allograft (Fig. 51.6E), a GAP cup was secured (Fig. 51.6F). The femoral component was secure but was revised because of concern for overlengthening from the acetabular reconstruction. At 1-year postreconstruction, she is painfree and walks with a mild limp. Her radiographs show good position of the prothesis and incorporation of the bone graft (Figs. 51.6G,H).

Discussion and Summary

Acetabular revision surgery, particularly in cases with large bony defects, can be quite complex, and positive results are often short-lived. Reinforcing rings are one option, however the use of reinforcing rings is not without challenges technically. Adequate exposure is needed both inferiorly and superiorly. The amount of morselized bone graft must be adequate to support the implant. A rigid support must be created from the dome of the cup to the host bone.

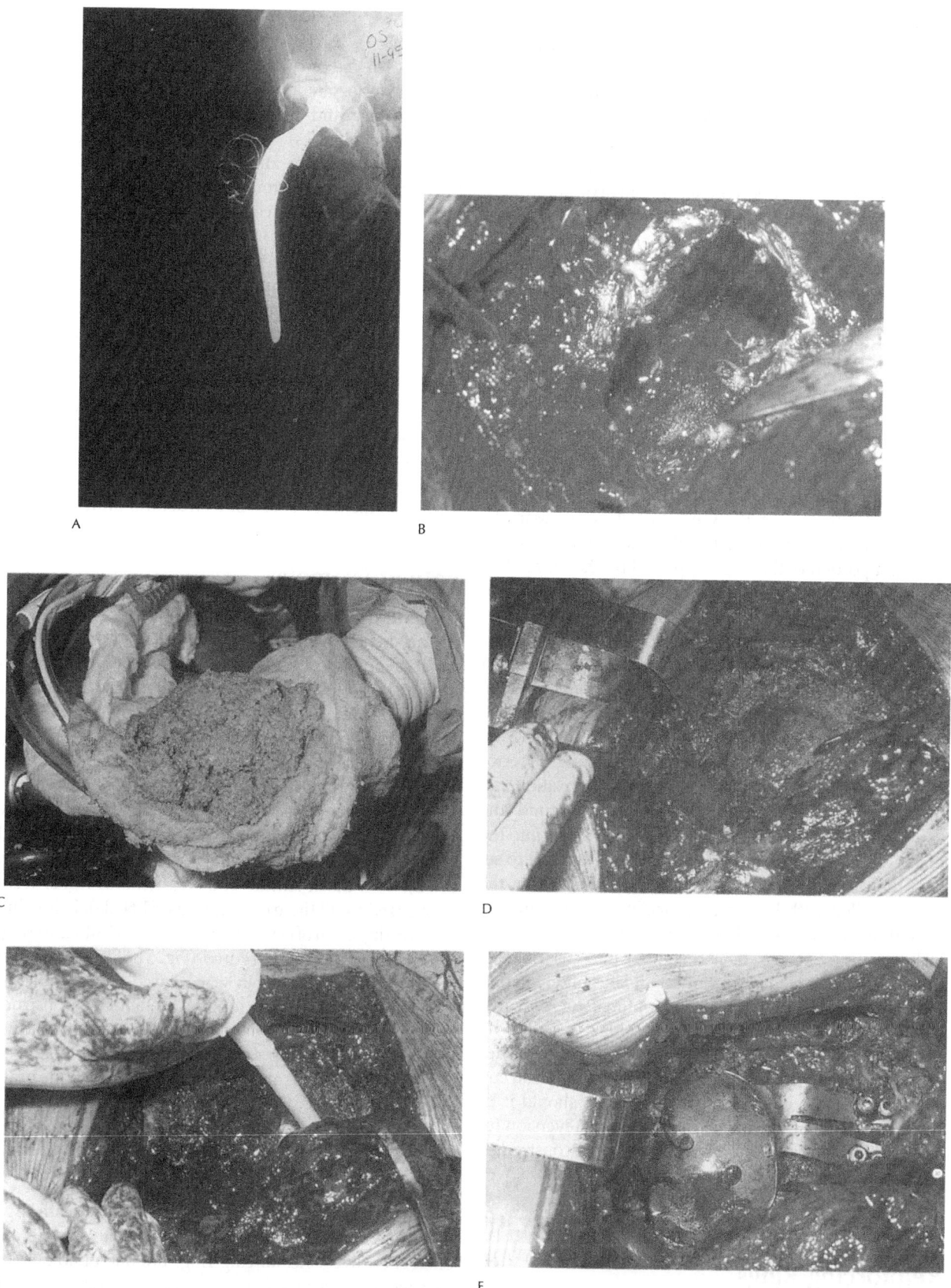

Figure 51.6. A. Preoperative radiograph (AP view). B. Intraoperative photograph showing acetabular defect. C. Amount of morselized bone graft needed to fill defect. D. Intraoperative photograph showing defect filled with packed morselized bone graft. E. Intraoperative photograph showing cement pressure injected into packed bone graft. F. Intraoperative photograph of GAP cup in place. (See color insert.)

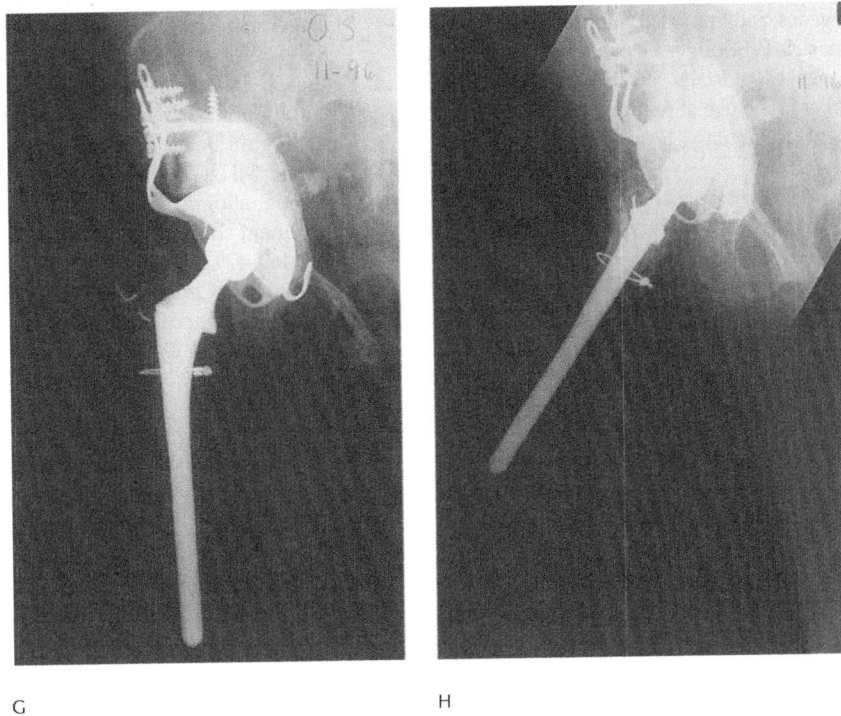

Figure 51.6. (continued) G. Radiograph at 1-year postoperative (AP view). H. Radiograph at 1-year postoperative (lateral view).

Frequently the morselized bone graft needs to be reinforced with PMMA to accomplish this. And attachment of the plates and hooks can be a frustrating exercise for the surgeon. However, if the entire procedure can be done well, the results—at least early results—are encouraging.

In summary, management of the pelvis with major bone loss poses a difficult problem for the arthroplasty surgeon. To date we have not found the perfect solution. No single technique or component is likely to provide the solution to the full spectrum of acetabular defects. If no or minimal defects exist, one may use a cemented or cementless cup. Larger defects may require the use of a jumbo cup or reinforcing ring with bone grafting. With each failure and subsequent revision, the patient is often left with greater bone loss and the surgeon is left with a more difficult and challenging reconstruction. Rerevision rates for reconstruction of severely deficient acetabula will no doubt be higher than those with intact or nearly intact bone.

Conceptually the use of a reinforcing ring in conjunction with bone grafting (morselized and/or structural) appears to be a sound solution for the patient with cavitary and segmental acetabular defects. Short-term failure rates are acceptable, but long-term data is needed. We do know that adequate bone graft technique is critical and that short-term failures at the cement interface have been rare. Long-term follow-up will determine if this use of reinforcing rings will provide an effective means of reconstruction of severely deficient acetabula.

References

1. Jasty M. Jumbo revisions. Presented at the 22nd Annual Hip Course, Boston, MA, September 16–19, 1992.
2. Harris WH. The high hip center concept. Presented at the 22nd Annual Hip Course, Boston, MA, September 16–19, 1992.
3. Schutzer SF, Harris WH. High placement of porous-coated acetabular components in complex total hip arthroplasty. *J Arthroplasty*. 1994;9:359–367.
4. Kelley SS. High hip center in revision arthroplasty. *J Arthroplasty*. 1994;9:503–510.
5. Newman MA, Bargar WL, Christie MJ, et al. Multicenter study of acetabular reconstruction using an oblong cup: 2 to 7-year results. Presented at the 64th Annual Meeting of the American Academy of Orthopaedic Surgeons, San Francisco, February 13–17, 1997.
6. Patch DA. Bone grafting about porous ingrowth aetabular components: A five-year roentgenographic review. Presented at the 61st Annual Meeting of the American Academy of Orthopaedic Surgeons, New Orleans, February 24–March 1, 1994.
7. Iida H, Matsusua Y, Kawanabe K, et al. A 5 to 20-year follow-up of cemented total hip arthroplasty with acetabular bone graft: Correlation between graft size and socket loosening. Presented at the 64th Annual Meeting of the American Academy of Orthopaedic Surgery, San Francisco, February 13–17, 1997.
8. Cabanela ME. Hemispherical large sockets and reinforcement cages. Presented at Instructional Course #242: Revision total hip arthroplasty: Management of acetabular bone loss,

64th Annual Meeting of the American Academy of Orthopaedic Surgeons, San Francisco, February 13–17, 1997.
9. Korovessis P, Spastris P, Sdougos G, et al. Acetabular roof reinforcement rings. *Clin Orthop*. 1992;283:149–155.
10. Rosson J, Schatzker J. The use of reinforcement rings to reconstruct deficient acetabula. *J Bone Joint Surg Br*. 1992;74:716–720.
11. Berry DJ, Muller ME. Revision arthroplasty using an antiprotrusio cage for massive acetabular bone deficiency. *J Bone Joint Surg Br*. 1992;74:711–715.
12. Haentjens P, DeBoeck H, Handelberg F, et al. Cemented acetabular reconstruction with the Mueller support ring. *Clin Orthop*. 1993;290:225–235.
13. Morscher EW. Management of the bone-deficient hip: Management of acetabular deficiency. *Orthopedics*. 1995;18:859–862.
14. Peters CL, Curtain M, Samuelson KM. Acetabular revision with the Burch–Schneider anti-protrusio cage and cancellous allograft bone. *J Arthroplasty*. 1995;10:307–312.
15. Zehntner MK, Ganz R. Midterm results (5.5–10 years) of acetabular allograft reconstruction with the acetabular reinforcement ring during total hip revision. *J Arthroplasty*. 1994;9:469–479.
16. D'Antonio JA, Capello WN, Borden LS, et al. Classification and management of acetabular abnormalities in total hip arthroplasty. *Clin Orthop*. 1989;243:126–137.

Part 4
Conclusions

Reconstruction of the acetabular component in revision surgery is a challenging undertaking. Extensive prior scarring, bone stock loss, leg length discrepancy, screw breakage or intrapelvic cement all make this procedure a formidable task. A comprehensive understanding of the bone stock deficiency classification system and preoperative planning are necessary to accomplish a successful outcome. The principles of reconstruction include restoration of bone stock, rigid component, and bone graft fixation, reestablishing the hip center of rotation and improving the biomechanical environment of the hip joint.

Twenty-five years of surgical experience as well as retrieval analysis have taught us that certain maxims should be adhered to. The newly chosen polyethylene component should be of high quality and have at least 6 to 8 mm of thickness on either side of the femoral head. To accommodate this, a smaller modular femoral head size may be necessary. Skirted femoral heads should be avoided to maximize range of motion and prevent impingement.

When an acetabular reconstruction can be performed with an enlarged hemispherical component rather than a solid allograft, that is preferable. However, when a solid allograft is required, it needs to be rigidly fixed and have a bony trabecular and screw orientation along the line of weight-bearing forces for optimal long term performance (Chandler & JMC). An allograft that occupies more than 50% of the surface area of the acetabulum should preferably be mated with a cemented prosthesis to avoid early failure of fixation.

Finally, on rare occasions, reconstruction may not be advisable. These unfortunate situations may include the patient with multiple socket failures, irradiated pelvis, pelvic discontinuity, metastatic tumor, multiple joint contractures, or a charcot joint. For these patients, supportive care or a girdlestone resection are the most compassionate treatment methods.

Part 5
Evaluation and Prevention of Postoperative Complications

Roderick H. Turner

The most devastating complication that can occur following major hip surgery is death. This rare postoperative event usually occurs in conjunction with one or more of the following conditions:

1. Anesthetic complications
2. Cardiac disease with crisis
3. Intra-abdominal crisis, especially cholecystitis
4. Thrombo-embolic disease with pulmonary embolus
5. Sepsis
6. CNS and (or) carotid artery disease

The sixth factor can be minimized by thorough preoperative work-up. Factors 1 through 5 will be discussed in the appropriate chapters in this section.

We will also deal with other complications which, although almost never fatal, can be very vexatious, both to the surgeon and to the patient, that is, broken stems, dislocations, heterotopic ossification, nerve damage, gastrourinary problems and problematic soft tissue contractures.

Each author was asked to review alternative treatment plans, but to focus on his or her preferred approach to both prevention and treatment.

52
Neurological Injury

Peter P. Anas and Brent Felix

The nervous system exemplifies the highest level of anatomic and physiologic development. It serves to simultaneously choreograph complex musculoskeletal movements, while receiving, deciphering, and transmitting efferent sensory stimuli. Neurologic complications associated with revision total hip arthroplasty are rare occurrences. Their periodic appearance provide dramatic evidence of the serious dysfunction that severely compromises the outcome of total hip arthroplasty. As orthopedic surgeons, we are trained to isolate, protect, and avoid nerves during all surgical procedures, demonstrating great reverence for their fragility and functional significance. Appropriate attention to anatomic detail, awareness of risk factors associated with revision arthroplasty, and avoidance of inappropriate mechanical and postural maneuvers all serve to limit the neurologic complications associated with revision hip arthroplasty. An understanding of neurophysiology and neurodiagnostic technique allow for prompt recognition of neurologic complications and may serve to limit the severity and impact.

Peripheral Nerve Morphology

The morphology of peripheral nerves is relevant to injury, repair, and regeneration. Each nerve is composed of an axon, myelin, connective tissue, and blood vessels. The individual central nerve cell is termed the neuron. Sensory neurons lie in the dorsal root ganglia, autonomic neurons lie in para vertebral ganglia and the motor neurons lie in the anterior horn of the spinal cord. The neurons maintain a precise intraneural environment and produce neurotransmitters that are released upon stimulation. Axons are peripheral extensions of neurons. An axon is commonly classified as either myelinated or unmyelinated with larger axons typically displaying myelination provided by the Schwann cell. Schwann cells are neuroglial cells that surround all peripheral axons and are arranged adjacent on them. An axon is myelinated when it reaches a diameter of over 1 to 2 μm. In this case, one Schwann cell is associated with one axon. Myelinated axons are heavily laden with myelin and have a fast conduction velocity. In contrast, several unmyelinated axons are associated with only one Schwann cell. Unmyelinated axons are lightly covered with myelin and subsequently have a slower conduction velocity. An axon's response to injury is proportional to the severity of injury to the axon and its connective tissue envelopes.[1]

Connective and supporting tissue layers surround the axon complex and include the epineurium, perineurium, and endoneurium. Epineurium is the outer layer of connective tissue that defines the gross structure of peripheral nerves. This collagenous tissue surrounds and cushions the fascicles of the nerves and absorbs stress. Perineurium surrounds individual fascicles and, through selective permeability, maintains the intraneural environment. It is an analogue of the blood-brain barrier and helps to limit the spread of infection and maintain a positive intrafascicular pressure. Perineurium provides the strongest resistance to longitudinal stretch. Endoneurium provides a loose packing of collagen around individual axons within the perineurium. It forms the Schwann cell tube and, following injury, provides a tunnel for regenerating axons.

The blood supply to the nerve enters through the mesoneurium, which is the connective tissue extending from the epineurium to the surrounding tissues. There is an intrinsic blood supply that extends longitudinally and an extrinsic blood supply that is segmental. The intrinsic blood supply is largely responsible for allowing mobilization of nerves without endangering their blood supply. Anastomoses between the intrinsic and extrinsic vascular systems are also important in maintaining collateral circulation. Pure infarction of a nerve is rare, if it ever occurs. Compression or traction of a nerve, however, may produce ischemic injury through vascular compromise or direct injury to neurons.

Each peripheral nerve, in general, is composed of neurons that originate from multiple levels of the spinal cord. Spinal nerves are the continuation of axons from the ventral and dorsal roots of a single spinal cord level. Once the spinal nerve leaves the dura, it combines with adjacent roots to form a regional nerve plexus, that is, brachial, lumbar, and sacral plexi. It is within these plexi that the actual peripheral nerves coalesce and proceed distally to innervate the extremity. In the lower extremity lumbar and sacral nerve roots exit the spine and recombine into lumbar and sacral plexi from which emerge the sciatic, femoral, and obturator peripheral nerves.

Nerve Degeneration and Regeneration

Once part of an axon is detached from its cell body, both axon and Schwann cells are destroyed by phagocytosis. This process is called secondary or Wallerian degeneration. The axon will often degenerate a short distance proximal to the injury. This has been termed retrograde degeneration. After 2 to 3 days, the distal neuronal segment becomes fragmented and involutes. Shrinkage and fragmentation of the myelin sheath parallels the degeneration of the axon. The time course for degeneration varies with the size and myelination of the fiber and therefore, differs with motor and sensory neurons. Macrophages continue to reach the injured area and by 15 to 30 days the axonal debris is virtually cleared. The endoneurial basement membrane cells can then differentiate to form new Schwann cells and prepare the way for regenerating sprouts from the axonal stump. If the endoneurial tube of connective tissue has remained intact, the axonal sprout passes along its previous course and innervates the original end organs. If the endoneurial tube has been disrupted, the result is much less predictable. Each axon may have as many as 100 sprouts which wander aimlessly around the site of injury and never reach an endoneurial tube. These sprouts may then form a neuroma. Axonal sprouts may regenerate through endoneurial tubes other than their own. However, axons appear to regenerate toward their own appropriate end organs as if they are influenced by certain neurotrophic substances contained within the distal nerve tissue. Brushart[2] has shown that this neurotrophic effect is present except when a gap of more than 2 mm exists between the injured ends of the axon.

The distance from the site of injury to the end organ is important as there is a time limit placed on reinnervation. Axon sprouts migrate at a rate of 1 to 4 mm per day with a faster rate occuring in younger patients. Several histologic changes occur over time in both the regenerating axonal pathway and the muscle awaiting reinnervation. In the nerve's pathway, the Schwann cell basement membrane within the endoneural tube undergoes degeneration. Consequently, the axonal sprout may lose its way and never reach its end-organ. With time, the motor endplates and muscle fascicles begin to atrophy. If the axon does not reach them before atrophy occurs, reinnervation may be ineffective. Furthermore, if the axon fails to reach the muscle endplate within approximately 2 years, the scarring and atrophy of the denervated muscle will render the muscle functionless. Sensation does not have such a strict time constraint. The quality of reinnervated sensation may diminish with time. Even after two years, however, the reinnervated region may provide some protective sensation. Factors which compromise regeneration include: distance from injury to end-organ, age of patient, coexistence of peripheral neuropathy, and overall poor medical health of the patient. Conversely, physical therapy and bracing help maintain residual muscle strength, tissue flexibility, joint motion, and skin integrity. This provides an environment that will maximize functional return following reinnervation.

Nerve Injury Pathology

The most commonly used classification for nerve injuries was that described by Seddon[3] during World War II. He classified these injuries into three groups: neurapraxia, axonotmesis, and neurotmesis. Neurapraxia is a mild injury of the nerve which produces a physiologic block rather than an anatomic disruption. The injury may be due to localized ischemic demyelinization and, therefore, motor fibers are usually more affected than sensory fibers. Spontaneous recovery usually occurs. Axonotmesis occurs after a greater injury to the nerve and involves physical disruption of the axon and myelin sheath. The endoneurial tube remains intact and the regenerating axons have the potential to retrace their peripheral connections. Thus, spontaneous recovery is possible and a good functional outcome can be anticipated. In neurotmesis, there is either complete anatomic disruption of the nerve; or the axon, myelin sheath, and endoneurium are so badly damaged that no spontaneous recovery can be expected.

Although the Seddon classification may be commonly used, a more precise classification is that of Sunderland.[4,5] In his classification, nerve injuries are classified from I to V in ascending order of severity and each degree corresponds with a greater anatomic disruption and altered prognosis. Anatomically, the degrees of severity corresponds to injury affecting (1) myelin, (2) axon, (3) endoneurial tube, (4) perineurium, and (5) the entire peripheral nerve.

A first degree injury corresponds with neurapraxia of Seddon's classification. There is a physiologic block of nerve conduction at the site of injury, but no anatomic lesion. No Wallerian degeneration occurs and the recovery is usually spontaneous within a few days or weeks. Motor function is usually more affected than sensory function. Sensory modalities are affected in order of increasing frequency as follows: pain, temperature, touch, and proprioception. Proprioception and motor are usually the last to return. A characteristic of this injury is simultaneous return of motor function in both the proximal and distal musculature and electrical excitability of the nerve distal to the lesion is preserved. There is no axonal damage, no regeneration, no Tinel's sign and complete restoration of function. This injury points to the necessity for painstaking examination of both motor and sensory modalities since any residual motor or sensory function indicates an improved prognosis.

Second degree injury corresponds with axonotmesis in Seddon's classification. There is disruption of the axon but the integrity of the endoneurial tube remains intact. Wallerian degeneration of the axon ensues and clinically there is complete neurologic deficit in motor, sensory and sympathetic function. Motor reinnervation occurs from proximal to distal in the order which the nerve branches leave the trunk. There is commonly a Tinel's sign advancing along the course of the nerve as it regenerates. Functional outcome is usually very good with modest or no residual impairment and the time course is dependent upon distance of end-organ from the site of injury.

In a third degree injury, there is damage to axons and endoneurial tubes, but the perineurium remains intact. Scar tissue may form within the endoneurial tube and divert the regenerating axons to paths other than there own. This results in disorganization of the axons and, in most instances, incomplete neurologic recovery. If the injury is not complete, there may be an advancing Tinel's sign, the duration of loss is longer than in second degree injury and there is incomplete recovery of function with significant residual impairment. The time course is again dependent upon the distance between the end-organ and the site of injury. The degree of recovery depends upon the number of axons that successfully cross the injury site and reach their appropriate end-organs.

A fourth degree injury is produced by disruption of the axon, endoneurium, and most if not all of the perineurium. The epineurium remains intact. Scar tissue prevents the axons from proceeding down the distal endoneurial tubes and the axonal sprouts may advance aimlessly around the site of injury. There is no advancing Tinel's sign and return of function is poor without operative intervention, which is aimed at reapproximating the nerve's respective fascicles.

A fifth degree injury corresponds to neurotmesis in Seddon's classification. In this injury, there is complete anatomic transection of the nerve as will only occur in an open wound or surgical site. Regenerating axons must traverse the transected section of nerve prior to proceeding down the endoneurial tubes. Thus, the prognosis for good functional recovery is poor without surgical intervention to reapproximate or graft nerve fasicles and connective tissues. The results of nerve repair cannot be accurately predicted. We do know that full return of function is unlikely especially when the factors that influence recovery are unfavorable, that is, older age of patient, longer distance from injury to end-organ, gap between nerve ends, condition of nerve ends, and delay between injury and repair. According to Sunderland, the results of sciatic nerve repair are poor.[4,5] This is due to the extended period of time required for nerve regeneration to the end muscle, extensive retrograde axonal degeneration, and intraneural mixing of regenerating fibers.

It is important to appreciate that the various classifications of nerve injury imply a homogeneous injury to all axons composing a given peripheral nerve. Clinical experience, however, indicates that heterogeneous patterns usually occur.

Nerves are injured through several means, that is endogenous or exogenous toxins, malignancies, metabolic or collagenous disorders. Only injuries caused by operative and perioperative trauma, however, are considered here. Causes of nerve injury in this situation are ischemia, compression, traction, and laceration. One of the first and most prominent experiment on the effects of ischemia on neuronal tissue was by Lundborg in the early 1970s.[6,7] Using an animal model, a tourniquet was used to produce complete ischemia of extremities. The intraneural circulation was then evaluated at variable intervals. Two hours of ischemia was well tolerated and resulted in almost immediate return of normal circulation. Nerves having sustained ischemia of 4 to 6 hours required 2 to 3 minutes before restoration of blood flow occurred. This restoration was followed by hyperemia and continued perfusion. After 8 to 10 hours of ischemia, however, the blood flow was restored only after 5 to 20 minutes and was never restored completely. After this prolonged ischemia, there was no recovery of nerve function and the injury was apparently irreversible.

Numerous experiments have been performed to study the conduction across a compressed area of nerve. It has been unclear, however, if the deterioration in nerve function is due to the direct mechanical damage of the nerve or the ischemia produced by the tourniquet. Lundborg[8] examined the effects of compression by tourniquet and reported that there is an increase in the permeability of endoneurial vasculature and irreversible nerve injury after only 2 to 4 hours of compression by the cuff. He concluded that local compression was of greater significance for the development of nerve injury than ischemia induced in the distal segments. These studies demonstrate the resilience of peripheral nerve structures to ischemic injury and parallel the orthopedic experience operating under tourniquet control.

Another source of operative nerve injury is traction during maneuvers such as lengthening and manipulations of the extremity. Several studies of nerve injury associated with lengthening have been published. Each has reported differing amounts of elongation associated with nerve damage. Nerve damage has been seen with as little as 4% to 11%[9,10] elongation and conduction failure was found in rabbit sciatic nerves after 25% elongation.[11] Neural vasculature, as well, can be damaged by stretch. Lundborg[12] showed that there was complete cessation of perfusion after 15% elongation. Nerves are more susceptible to stretch effects when lying in scar, tethered by bone or other prominence. During revision arthroplasty, scarring from previous surgery, anatomical distortion of bone and soft tissues, and the duration of the procedure add to the susceptibility of neurologic structures.

Clinical Diagnosis of Nerve Injuries

Clinical evaluation of peripheral nerve injury demands precise knowledge of the sensory and motor innervation patterns and anatomic course of the affected nerve. Transection or complete physiologic disruption of a peripheral nerve produces loss of all motor and sensory function distal to the injury. Less severe injury may preserve partial innervation to a muscle and residual function will persist. Any residual function following neurologic injury signifies an improved prognosis. If the strength of each muscle in the extremity is graded, a baseline clinical assessment can be made. Highet has recommended a 0 to 5 grading system and it has been widely accepted: 0—paralysis; 1—muscle flicker; 2—muscle contraction; 3—muscle contraction against gravity; 4—muscle contraction against gravity and resistance; and 5—normal muscle contraction. Sensory loss will follow a specific anatomic distribution, although there can be some overlap of dermatomes.

Clinical evaluation depends largely upon physical examination and may be aided by electrodiagnostic studies. There are significant limitations upon the extent of information imparted by electrodiagnostic study and they must be integrated into the overall clinical picture. Several features of electrodiagnostic study need to be appreciated for proper interpretation of data. Significant electromyographic changes are not evident for at least 8 to 14 days following injury. After this period of time, spontaneous fibrillations may become evident and coincide with the onset of atrophic changes in the muscle. Transient fibrillation potentials on needle insertion may be seen. Denervation fibrillations cannot determine if a second, third, fourth, or fifth degree injury occurred. No motor unit potentials are seen during attempted volitional contraction. Furthermore, reinnervation potentials may indicate that only a few muscle fibers are reinnervated and does not guarantee that a good outcome will be achieved. Immediate electromyography can be helpful in demonstrating residual innervation or retained motor unit potentials during volitional contraction, which suggests that complete nerve injury did not occur and prognosis is favorable.

Nerve conduction studies distal to the site of injury will demonstrate a normal response for 2 to 3 days after injury. Thereafter, the physiologic result of Wallerian degeneration impedes further conduction. This failure of nerve conduction is the earliest neurophysiologic evidence of the severity of injury and can exclude neuropractic type of injury. A slow nerve conduction across a specific point can confirm the diagnosis of compression neuropathy as opposed to other types of nerve damage. The sympathetic fibers of a nerve are among the most resistant to mechanical trauma. The presence of sweating within an autonomic zone suggest that these fibers are intact and functioning. Iodine starch can be placed on the limb and sweating can be induced by various means. The powder will change to a deep purple in areas with sweat and remain gray if no sweat is present.

In summary, an immediate EMG can be used to demonstrate residual innervation or retained motor unit potentials during volitional contracture. After 8 to 14 days, an EMG can help to localize the nerve injury and to follow recovery. Nerve conduction studies can be used 3 days after injury to localize the lesion and determine if the injury is neurapraxia or a more severe injury.

Nerve Injury in Revision Hip Arthroplasty

Although peripheral nerve injury during total hip arthroplasty is uncommon, this complication can be troublesome, and at times, devastating to the patient. Although most of these patients have return of function, many are left with severe impairment and disability. To avoid and better manage this complication, the surgeon should have knowledge about the patients at risk, the mechanisms of injury, how to diagnose and treat a peripheral nerve injury, and their prognosis.

Numerous reports in the literature indicate the incidence of nerve palsies following total hip arthroplasty ranges from 0 to 3% in primary total hip arthroplasty and 2.9 to 7.6% in revision total hip surgery. These figures include injury to all major nerves around the hip joint, which include the sciatic, femoral, and obturator nerves. Each of these studies demonstrate that injury to the peroneal division of the sciatic nerve is the most common palsy seen in both primary and revision surgery. Isolated injuries to the femoral and obturator nerves are rare and generally account for less than 10% of the total number of nerves injuries. Because nerve injury during total hip arthroplasty is uncommon, individual experience with operative neuropathy is limited. One of the largest and most comprehensive studies is that by Schmalzreid et al.[13] who reviewed 3126 consecutive total hip replacements and found an overall nerve palsy rate of 1.7%. The rate in primary replacement was

1.3% compared to 3.2% in revision hip surgery. Approximately 80% of injuries were isolated to the sciatic nerve alone (47% to peroneal division alone, 30% to peroneal and tibial divisions, and 3% to the tibial division alone). Concommittent injuries to the sciatic and femoral nerves accounted for 13% of injuries. The remaining 7% were to the femoral nerve alone. Obturator nerve injury was not documented in this series.

Patients undergoing revision hip surgery have been shown to have an increased risk of nerve injury. Amstutz et al.[14] previously reported a nerve injury incidence of 7.6% in patients undergoing hip revision surgery. More recently, Schmalzreid et al., in their report of 3126 patients, found an overall incidence of nerve injury in revision surgery of 3.2%.[13] This was compared to an overall incidence of 1.3% in those patients undergoing primary total hip replacement. Revision arthroplasty undertaken for different diagnoses had similar incidences of nerve palsy, that is, failed total hip arthroplasty had an incidence of 2.6%, failed hemiarthroplasty had an incidence of 3.6%, and failed surface replacement had an incidence of 2.9%. Thus, revision surgery is accepted as a risk factor for nerve injury during total hip replacement.

Several studies have reported additional risk factors for nerve injury in patients during total hip arthroplasty. These risk factors include: (1) patients with a primary diagnosis of developmental dislocation of the hip, (2) female patients, although this has recently been disputed, (3) lateral approach to the hip, (4) peripheral neuropathy, (5) leg lengthening, and (6) hip arthroplasty after a previous arthrodesis. Schmalzreid et al. found that patients with a primary diagnosis of DDH had a 5.8% incidence of nerve injury. This was compared to a 1.0% incidence in osteoarthritic patients, 1.2% incidence in rheumatoid arthritis patients and an incidence of 0.8% in patients with a primary diagnosis of osteonecrosis.

Several studies have reported increased rates of nerve injury among female patients. Solheim[15] reported six peripheral neuropathies after total hip replacement, five of which were women. He speculated that this was from peculiarities in the vasculature of the sciatic nerve in women. Furthermore, pelvic width and soft tissue mass have also been forwarded as potential explanations. Weber et al.[16] reported an increased incidence of nerve palsy in women patients after total hip surgery and that patient gender was the only factor that correlated with the development of neuropathy. Schmalzreid et al. also reported an increased incidence of nerve palsy in women. After correction for other risk factors, however, there was no difference in the incidence in men and women. Therefore, females appear to be at greater risk for operative nerve palsy, but this may be related to the association with developmental dysplasia of the hip rather than other gender specific anatomic issues.

There has been no conclusive evidence that a specific surgical approach creates more of a risk than another. Some studies, however, suggest that a lateral or transtrochanteric approach creates more of a risk than a posterior approach. Johanson et al.[17] found a 50% decrease in incidence of nerve palsies when the frequency of using trochanteric osteotomies for exposure was greatly reduced. Robinson et al.[18] compared 130 patients who had hip replacement through a trantrochanteric approach to 138 patients who underwent replacement through a posterior approach. Of these patients, two developed sciatic nerve palsy and both of these patients had had a transtrochanteric approach. More recently, Weale et al.[19] compare nerve injuries in the lateral and posterior approaches. Forty-two consecutive patients underwent total hip arthroplasties, one half of the patients via a posterior approach and the other half via a lateral approach. Pre- and postoperative EMGs and nerve conduction velocities were done. None of the patient had clinically symptomatic nerve palsies, but five of the patients who had a lateral approach performed had nerve injuries detected on electrophysiologic tests. Thus, the above studies suggest that the transtrochanteric or lateral approach carries more of a risk for nerve injury that a posterior approach.

The precise mechanism of nerve injury following total hip replacement is often difficult to ascertain. Johanson et al.[17] reported that only 16 of 34 nerve injuries could be attributed to a specific cause. Similarly, Schmalzreid et al.[13] found that in 55% of patients in their series the exact mechanism of injury was unknown. The proposed and known etiologies include: compressive trauma during exposure and retraction, dislocation or limb position during the procedure, leg lengthening, direct surgical trauma, compression over a bony prominence or prosthesis, methylmethacrylate extrusion, intraneural hemorrhage, compression by hematoma, constriction by trochanteric wire or suture, acetabular screw penetration, and a prominent protusio ring.

Neural ischemia can occur due to direct damage of the neurovascular supply.[5] This can occur during exposure of the nerve or by intraneural hemorrhage. Nonetheless, Stillwell[20] reported on using sciatic neurolysis in complex revisions in order to allow direct visualization and protection of the nerve. There were no cases of neuropathy in his report. The etiology of direct damage of the local neurovascular supply remains uncertain.

Traction and compression may produce direct injury to the nerve by the application of force in excess of the tissue capacity to absorb such force either crushing or tearing the tissues. Alternatively, traction and compression may cause vascular compromise to the affected nerve. It is likely that both mechanisms play a role and efforts should be made by surgeon and assistants to periodically relax the amount of force applied to retractors or the amount of force applied to hold a dislocated limb in a given position. Similarly, the positioning of any retractor must take into account its relationship to surrounding neurovascular structures. Retractors placed anteriorly over the brim of the pelvis are potential sources of femoral nerve trauma where as retractors placed posterior to the acetabulum are potential sources of injury to the sciatic nerve.

Traction injuries may occur intraoperatively during limb manipulation or after leg lengthening. Black et al.[21] monitored 100 consecutive patients with intraoperative somatosensory-evoke potentials and found that latency was significantly increased in 18 patients. Sixteen of the 18 patients had return to baseline latency after repositioning of the limb or replacement of the retractors. Furthermore, Nercessian et al.[22] noted deterioration of the evoked potentials during 12 of 25 revision total hip arthroplasties. There was return to baseline after repositioning of the limb in 5 of the 12 affected patients and after replacing the retractors in 7 of the 12 patients. Examination of lower extremity anatomy reveals that the intraoperative limb position that places the greatest tension on the sciatic nerve is a dislocated hip in flexion with the knee in extension.

Traction injuries can also be caused by limb lengthening. Edwards[23] reported on 23 nerve injuries after total hip arthroplasty. Fourteen of the 23 occurred after lengthening of the operated extremity. Schmalzreid[13] found that leg lengthening accounted for 13 of the 53 patients with nerve injuries in that series and may have been a contributing factor in 12 other patients. The reported amount of lengthening which caused a neuropathy has varied between 1.9 to 5.1 cm in these reports and it is generally accepted that a limb should not be lengthened over 2.0 to 2.5 cm.

Of special interest are those patients who awaken from anesthesia with normal nerve function, but develop a nerve deficit in the immediate postoperative period. Hematoma formation and anticoagulation must be implicated as a possible cause of the neuropathy in this group of patients.[24,25] Correction of the coagulopathy and evacuation of the hematoma may help restore nerve function. Pressure on the peroneal nerve by tight antithrombotic stockings or by external rotation of the leg during the convalescence period has been found to contribute to palsies of that nerve.[24] Removing pressure from the nerve will improve the prognosis in these patients. Contralateral nerve palsy is most likely secondary to intraoperative positioning and local pressure.

The specific cause for the increased incidence of nerve palsies in revision hip surgery appears to be multifactorial. In the multiply operated hip, the nerves may be bound in scar, which lessens their mobility. This immobility increases the risk of an inadvertant injury to the nerve. Johanson[17] found an increased blood loss and operative time in patients who develop a nerve palsy.

Schmalzreid et al.[13] similarly found an increased operative time and blood loss in primary cases complicated by a nerve injury. In revision cases, however, only increased blood loss seemed to correlate with nerve injury, and did not correlate with increased operative time. Both authors believed that it reflected technical difficulties encountered, possibly indicating increased time duration or force needed for exposure.

Diagnosis and Management

In order to eliminate potentially reversible causes, minimize the consequences and hasten recovery, an accurate diagnosis of nerve injury complicating hip surgery is essential. Accurate diagnosis of a neurologic lesion requires that a complete preoperative assessment of nerve function be accomplished and documented. This assessment is best done with a thorough knowledge of hip anatomy and lower extremity innervation.

The sciatic nerve is a continuation of the sacral plexus roots of L4, L5, S1, S2, and S3 and includes the tibial and common peroneal nerves, which are anatomically separate fascicles within the sciatic nerve. As the sciatic nerve exits the sciatic notch, the fibers of the nerve are spatially oriented with the fibers of the common peroneal being more lateral. The descent of the common peroneal nerve is more superficial and thus may predispose the nerve to a greater chance of injury. The tibial nerve innervates the semimembranosus, semitendonosis, long head of the biceps, anterior aspect of the adductor magnus and then proceeds distally to innervate the muscles in the posterior compartment of the lower leg. It then terminates as the medial and lateral plantar branches of the foot. The only muscle the common peroneal innervates in the thigh is the short head of the biceps. This nerve then proceeds distally to innervate the anterior and lateral compartments of the lower leg and terminates by supplying sensation to the dorsum of the foot.[26] The sympathetic fibers, in general, follow the fibers of sensation. Injury to the sciatic nerve is typically not complete or homogeous. This results in a nonuniform pattern of motor and sensory dysfunction among the muscle groups and sensory distributions supplied. Furthermore, each division may have a partial injury and this may further complicate the clinical picture. Thus, a careful motor and sensory exam is important to evaluate and determine the location and extent of injury. It is important to make this differentiation, as the location and extent of injury may have prognostic value.

The femoral nerve is a continuation of the spinal roots of L2, L3, and L4. It overlies the iliopsoas as it passes through the femoral triangle and proceeds down the thigh. The femoral triangle is a tight fascial compartment immediately anterior to the hip rendering the nerve vulnerable to direct trauma from retractors or compression from hematoma. The femoral nerve's motor fibers innervate the iliacus, pectineus, sartorius, and quadriceps muscles. The sensory fibers of the nerve innervate the anteromedial aspect of the thigh and the medial aspect of the lower leg. Decreased weakness of the quadriceps, decreased patellar tendon reflex and decreased sensation the femoral nerve distribution suggests a femoral nerve lesion. At times, this lesion is overlooked due to the small area of sensory innervation supplied by the femoral nerve. Furthermore, the neurological assessment in the recovery room or floor is often confined to "wiggling the toes". Physicians, nurses, and therapists must assess quadriceps strength independently.

The obturator nerve has two branches (anterior and posterior) that are a continuation of the L2, L3 and L4 nerve roots. It passes over the obturator internus, which lies on the quadralateral surface of the acetabulum. It innervates the obturator externus, gracilis and adductor muscles, but customarily has no sensory innervation. Decreased strength of adductors and persistent groin or thigh pain suggest injury to the obturator nerve. This is a rare injury and has usually been attributed to methylmethacrylate protrusion inferior to the acetabulum.

In addition to physical examination, electrodiagnostic studies can be helpful in localizing the nerve injury and quantifying the extent of damage. For example, when a patient has a palsy of the peroneal nerve, an EMG can determine if the lesion has occurred at the level of the hip or the knee. The key to this determination is innervation of the short head of the biceps femoris, which is the only muscle above the knee to be innervated by the peroneal nerve. An EMG can also determine if the tibial division, peroneal division or both are affected. Moreover, electrodiagnostic examination is helpful in determining if the patient had a preexisting subclinical peripheral neuropathy that may impact on the patient's prognosis. As discussed earlier, one disadvantage is that the EMG has limited usefulness during the first 2 to 3 weeks following injury. During this time, the test will only show decreased or absent motor unit potiential patterns during volitional contraction. One must be aware that decreased or absent motor unit potentials may be due to a lack of voluntary effort.

Nerve conduction velocity tests can also be helpful in determining the location of the nerve lesion. Nerve conduction studies distal to the site of injury will demonstrate normal conduction for 3 days after injury. After that period of time, if the nerve injury is severe, and Wallerian degeneration begins, the nerve conduction velocity test will be abnormal. Thus, nerve conduction velocity is the first test that can determine if the injury is neuropraxia or a more severe nerve injury.

Imaging studies are helpful to evaluate various etiologies of nerve injury. The plain film must be scrutinized for conditions such as dislocation, leg lengthening, extruded methylmethacrylate, prominent prosthetic devices, and penetrating hardware. More detailed evaluation by computed tomography (CT) scan or magnetic resonance imaging (MRI) may be obtained if plain films are suspicious or if hematoma is suspected.

Once a patient has been diagnosed with a nerve palsy, the first step in management is to determine if immediate reoperation is appropriate. Some reversible causes of nerve palsy include: hematoma formation, extruded cement, encircling wire or suture material, and external compression. Initially, external compression should be evaluated by addressing the bandages, traction apparatus, compressive stockings, and posture. The optimal position of the limb to alleviate traction is flexion of the hip and knee. If the surgeon suspects any of the other causes of reversible neuropathy, he or she should consider diagnostic scanning, re-exploration, and removal of the offending agent as soon as possible. Birch et al.[27] reported a series of 38 sciatic and 10 femoral nerve injuries. Urgent reexploration was performed in 7 of the patients permitting evacuation of hematoma, removal of extruded cement, and encircling suture material. All seven patients had early pain relief and useful neurological recovery. Furthermore, Mont et al.[28] reviewed 31 patients with peroneal nerve palsies who were treated with operative decompression. Ninety-seven percent reported subjective and functional improvement and were able to discontinue the use of the ankle–foot orthosis. Thus, reexploration and decompression has a role in perioperative nerve palsies.

Once a potentially reversible cause has been ruled out, the treatment for patients with postoperative nerve injury is supportive. Patient education is one of the most important aspects of treatment. Thus, a clear and thorough review of the injury, supportive treatment and prognosis should be discussed with the patient. The patient should be aware of the uncertainty in the prognosis and that the goal of treatment is to maximize remaining muscle strength and maintain range of motion of joints until nerve function returns. These patients should also be aware that this return of nerve function may require weeks, months or years. Patients should be fitted with orthotics within a few days postoperatively and physical therapy should proceed as normally as possible. The physical and occupational therapists should be aware of the injury and the patient's deficits as they can help strengthen weakened muscles, stretch affected muscles and assist in helping the patient to adapt. They can also reinforce to the patient the importance of examining the anesthetic areas of the limb. One may also consider neurologic consultation to assist and reinforce the patients understanding. The psychological impact of neurologic complications should be addressed with the patient and counseling should be offered and encouraged.

Prognosis

The recovery of patients sustaining a nerve injury has been reviewed in multiple studies. Many of these studies focus on the functional recovery of the lower extremity and demonstrate that a residual deficit is present in most cases. In our experience, the residual deficits will often have great impact on the patient's self image and perception. A failure by the surgeon to appreciate this impact may compound the patient's displeasure.

Because of the rarity of nerve palsies following hip surgery, the number of patients used in reporting outcomes is small. Nonetheless, most authors report a majority of patients will have a good or excellent functional outcome. Weber et al.[16] reported that the prognosis for recovery is good even though only 4 of 14 patients in their series had full recovery. Soheim and Hagen[15] had similar results and agreed with the above conclusion except when the nerve had been severely damaged. Johansen et al.[17] reported that 24 of 34 patients who had a sciatic nerve injury had good or excellent results at an average of 3.7 year follow-up. Seventy-nine percent of the patients, however, had incomplete recovery of nerve function. They believed that this persistent neurologic deficit, with the exception of causalgic pain, did not create a significant disability as evaluated by the Hospital for Special Surgery rating system.

Edwards et al.[23] reported the one year follow-up outcomes of 19 patients with nerve palsy following total hip arthroplasty. Only three patients in this series had complete functional recovery. Eleven patients had a mild and five had a major deficit. All patients who had a major functional deficit had injury to both tibial and peroneal divisions of the sciatic nerve. They concluded that those patients who sustain an injury to the peroneal nerve alone have a better outcome than when the entire sciatic nerve is involved. Simmons et al.[29] reported the results of 10 femoral nerve injuries in 440 patients after total hip arthroplasty. They reported that all affected patients had significant initial disability. However, full functional recovery occurred within the first postoperative year.

Schmalzreid et al.[13] at a minimum of 1 year and a maximum of 16½ years, used a modification of the Sunderland scale to grade 53 extremities affected by nerve injury. Recovery was complete in seven limbs and had attained that status by 21 months after the operation. Mild weakness, sensory loss, mild dysesthesias, or a combination of the above was found in 18 extremities. Fifteen limbs had a greater degree of deficit and required an orthosis. Thirteen extremities had a severe deficit and in 6 of these limbs, the deficit was so severe that it limited the patients ability to walk. Thus, 15% fully recovered, 61% had a mild deficit and 24% had a major deficit. The ability to walk was decreased in all of the subgroups who had a nerve injury. It was especially decreased in younger patients who had a primary total hip replacement. There was a statistically significant association with normal or near normal recovery of function if the patient had residual motor function or recovered some motor function while hospitalized. Moreover, of the seven patients who had full recovery, all but one of them had full recovery by seven months. These authors did not use a poor, fair, good and excellent scale in evaluation, but did report that the outcome for the patients in their study was not dramatically different than those outcomes previously reported.

There does appear to be some author's bias as to what amount of disability is considered an excellent, good and poor result. Each patient who sustains a nerve injury may have good objective findings consistent with a successful arthroplasty, such as hip range of motion and joint stability. These findings, however, do not consider the amount of dissatisfaction commonly seen in patients with a nerve palsy and this discontent may hamper the claim of a good result.

Prevention

In order to prevent nerve injuries during total hip arthroplasty, one must determine the patients at risk and take the measures necessary to avoid nerve palsies. Those who have a history of prior arthrodesis, developmental dysplasia of the hip, marked inequality of leg lengths, previous nerve injury, multiple procedures or underlying neuropathy have an increased risk of neurological injury. Situations which require complex revision arthroplasty, major allografting, or extensive pelvic dissection and reconstruction are also at greater risk. Once the patient is identified as being at increased risk, preoperative planning is mandatory. This plan will help to minimize operative time, reduce blood loss, prevent intraoperative problems and allow the surgeon to forewarn those patients at risk.

A familiarity of different approaches and a willingness to vary the exposure if difficulties arise during surgery will help to avoid neurological complications. A comprehensive knowledge of pelvic anatomy, meticulous dissection, identification and constant attention to the major nerves during surgery is essential. This will allow the necessary caution needed for placement of retractors and protection of the neural structures. In order to prevent cement migration, all acetabular and femoral bone defects should be grafted or restricted. Moreover, acetabular screws, reconstruction plates, trochanteric clamps and cerclage wires need to be applied with attention to all adjacent neural structures.

Limb-length equalization is an important concept in total hip arthroplasty. Unfortunately, there are no exact guidelines that will allow a surgeon to safely lengthen an extremity.[30] Johanson et al.[17] stated that it is impossible to retrospectively determine the amount of lengthening a patient could tolerate, especially as numerous factors are probably involved in the injury. Edwards et al.[23] correlated the amount of lengthening to the type of palsy. They found that limbs which had been lengthened more than 3.8 cm sustained an injury of both divisions of the sciatic nerve. Lengthening of less than 3.8 cm were associated with a peroneal nerve palsy only. Schmalzreid et al.[13] found that in six of nine patients with congenital dysplasia or dislocation of the hip, the limb had been lengthened at least 3.0 cm. They found, however, that the incidence of palsy in this patient population when the leg had not been lengthened, was still double the incidence of those patients with a preoperative diagnosis of osteoarthrosis. They found a similar situation in those patients with a nerve palsy after revision surgery, in that, leg lengthening only partially accounted for the increased incidence of nerve palsy. When they disregarded the four patients who had over 3.3 cm of lengthening, the incidence of nerve palsy was still 2.6%. The increased incidence in revision surgery is probably a result of distorted anatomy and scarring about the anatomic structures. Furthermore, revision cases tend to be more complex, often requiring bone grafting and reconstruction. This may predispose these patients to direct nerve injury.

In revision and complex primary cases, the surgeon should consider somatosensory-evoked potential monitoring, which is presently an investigational tool. Stone et al.[31] first reported the use of SSEP in 50 patients. In these 50 patients, there were 12 instances of temporary nerve compromise in 10 patients. Six instances were due to limb positioning, two were due to limb lengthening during trial reduction, three were due to retractor positioning and one was due to acetabular reamer slippage. In all cases, the potential returned to normal after the offending stimulus was removed. Similarly, Nercessian[22] reported using SSEP monitoring in 25 patients undergoing revision surgery and reported 32% incidence of nerve compromise. Corrective actions were taken to restore the evoked-potential and no patient had postoperative nerve palsy. Black et al.[21] reported monitoring 100 consecutive patients. Eighteen of the 100 patients had intraoperative changes in evoked potential. Corrective measures were taken to improve the potentials. Nonetheless, two of the one hundred patients had persistant nerve palsy postoperatively. They compared this 2% incidence with monitoring with their 2.6% incidence without monitoring and concluded that intraoperative monitoring was not indicated on a routine basis.

In summary, nerve palsies are distressing and potentially devastating injuries. The risk of nerve injury can be minimized by preoperative planning and by having a comprehensive knowledge and experience of surgical anatomy. This will allow accurate and safe placement of retractors and instruments. Bone grafting defects and good cementing techniques should be used to avoid extrusion. Screws in the anterior quadrants should be avoided. If an extremity is planned to be lengthened or if the case is suspected to be complex, consideration should be given to SSEP monitoring.

References

1. Anderson AF, Brushart TM, Harner CD, Pagnani MJ, Ticker JB. Soft-tissue physiology and repair. In: Kasser JR, ed. *Orthopaedic knowledge update 5*. Rosemont: American Academy of Orthopaedic Surgeons, 1996:3–20.
2. Brushart TM. Selective reinnervation of distal motor stumps by peripheral motor axons. *Exp Neurol*. 1987;97: 289.
3. Seddon HJ. Three types of nerve injury. *Brain*. 1943;66: 237–288.
4. Sunderland S. Factors influencing the course of regeneration and the quality of the recovery after nerve suture. *Brain*. 1952;75:19.
5. Sunderland S. *Nerves and nerve injuries*. 2nd ed. Edinburgh: Churchill-Livingstone, 1978.
6. Lundborg G. Ischemic nerve injury: experimental studies on intraneural microvascular pathophysiology and nerve function in a limb subjected to temporary circulation arrest. *Scand J Plast Reconstr Surg Suppl*. 1970;6:3–113.
7. Lundborg G. Limb ischemia and nerve injury. *Arch Surg*. 1972;104:631.
8. Lundborg G. Structure and function of the intraneural microvessels as related to trauma, edema formation, and nerve function. *J Bone Joint Surg Am*. 1975;57:938–948.
9. Highest WB, Sanders FK. The effects of stretching nerves after suture. *Br J Surg*. 1943;30:355.
10. Liu CT, Benda CE, Lewey FH. Tensile strength of human nerves: an experimental physical and histologic study. *Arch Neurol Psychiatry*. 1948;59:390.
11. Mitchell SW. *Injuries of nerves and their consequences*. JB Lippincott: Philadelphia, 1972.
12. Lundborg G, Rydevik B. Effects of stretching the tibial nerve of the rabbit: a preliminary study of the intraneural circulation and the barrier function of the perineurium. *J Bone Joint Surg Br*. 1973;55:390.
13. Schmalzreid TP, Amstutz HC, Dorey FJ. Nerve palsy associate with total hip replacement. *J Bone Joint Surg Am*. 1991;73:1074–1080.
14. Amstutz HC, Ma SM, Jinnah RH, Mai L. Revision of aseptic loose total hip arthroplasties. *Clin Orthop*. 1982;170:21.
15. Solheim LF, Hagen R. Femoral and sciatic neuropathies after total hip arthroplasty. *Acta Orthop Scand*. 1980;51:531.
16. Weber ER, Daube JR, Coventry MB. Peripheral neuropathies associated with total hip arthroplasty. *J Bone Joint Surg Am*. 1976;58:66.
17. Johanson NA, Pellicci PM, Tsairis P, Salvati EA. Nerve injury in total hip arthroplasty. *Clin Orthop*. 1983;179:214.
18. Robinson RP, Robinson HJ, Salvati EA. Comparison of the transtrochanteric and posterior approaches for total hip replacement. *Clin Orthop*. 1980;147:143–147.
19. Weale AE, Newman P, Bannister GC. Nerve injury following total hip replacement. Lateral and posterior approaches compared. *J Bone Joint Surg Br*. 1996;78:Supp I.

20. Stillwell WT. Sciatic neurolysis: an adjunct to complex total hip arthroplasty. In: Stillwell WT, ed. *The art of total hip arthroplasty.* Orlando: Grune & Stratton, 1987;437.
21. Black DL, Reckling FW, Porter SS. Somatosensory-evoked potential monitored during total hip arthroplasty. *Clin Orthop.* 1991;262:170–177.
22. Nercessian OA, Gonzalez EG, Stinchfield FE. The use of somatosensory evoked potentials during revision or reoperation for total hip arthroplasty. *Clin Orthop.* 1989;243:138–142.
23. Edwards BN, Tullos HS, Noble PC. Contributory factors and etiology of sciatic nerve palsy in total hip arthroplasty. *Clin Orthop.* 1987;218:136.
24. Leonard MA. Sciatic nerve paralysis following anticoagulant therapy. *J Bone Joint Surg Br.* 1972;54:152.
25. Fleming RE, Michelsen CB, Stinchefield FE. Sciatic paralysis: a complication of bleeding following hip surgery. *J Bone Joint Surg Am.* 1979;61:37.
26. Agur AMR, Lee MJ. *Grants atlas of anatomy.* 9th ed. Baltimore: Williams and Wilkins, 1991.
27. Birch R, Unwin A, Chen L. Iatropathic lesions of sciatic and femoral nerve from hip arthroplasty. *J Bone Joint Surg Br.* 1996;78:Supp I.
28. Mont MA, Dellon AL, Chen F, Hungerford MW, Krackow KA, Hungerford DS. The operative treatment of peroneal nerve palsy. *J Bone Joint Surg Am.* 1996;78:863–869.
29. Simmons C Jr, Izant TH, Rothman RH, Booth RE, Balderston RA. Femoral neuropathy following total hip arthroplasty. *J Arthroplasty.* 1991;6:S59–S66.
30. Harris WH. Revision for failed, non-septic total hip arthroplasty: the femoral side. *Clin Orthop.* 1982;170:8.
31. Stone RG, Weeks LE, Hajdu M, et al. Evaluation of sciatic nerve compromise during total hip arthroplasty. *Clin Orthop.* 1985;201:26.

53
Postoperative Infection

Geoffrey H. Westrich, Eduardo A. Salvati, and Barry Brause

Total hip arthroplasty is considered one of the most successful procedures for alleviation of pain and restoration of hip function, with good to excellent results reported in over 90% of cases. The experience of the past two decades has contributed to a significant improvement in prosthetic design, materials, cementation, and the surgical technique of total joint replacement.[1] Unfortunately, postoperative complications still exist in a minority of patients.[2] The most common complications are thromboembolic disease, dislocation, aseptic loosening, osteolysis, and postoperative sepsis. Historically, Wilson et al. noted an infection rate of 14% after total hip arthroplasty without perioperative antibiotic prophylaxis; however, more recent data reveals that the incidence of infection has been greatly reduced.[3,4] In 1992, The Health Care Financing Center reported the incidence of postoperative infection after total hip arthroplasty to be 1% to 2% in the Medicare patient population.[5] Fitzgerald et al. suggests that specialized centers have reduced rates of infection in patients with primary osteoarthritis and reports infection rates as low as 0.5%.[3]

The careful selection of patients, the preoperative elimination of remote infections, perioperative prophylactic antibiotics, and the improvement in operating room sterility and antisepsis contributed to the above success. Improvements in ultraclean laminar air flow, sterile draping, limiting operating room personnel and traffic, impervious exhaust suits for the surgical team, the use of ultraviolet light and more expeditious surgery, covering skin margins to prevent skin edge contamination with meticulous closure over closed section, and avoiding dead spaces are all factors that contribute to a lower infection rate.

When pain develops after total joint arthroplasty and no clear explanation for the persistent symptoms is found, the surgeon should be aware of the possibility of infection. Diagnosing acute severe infections that present with local and general symptoms is usually of no particular difficulty. However, most of the delayed, insidious, latent infections are manifested mainly by hip pain, with very little local and no general symptomatology. The usual radiologic findings and laboratory tests, including white blood cell count, differential, left shift, and erythrocyte sedimentation rate, may prove of no help.

Establishing the diagnosis of infection and isolating the causal organism is essential to the successful treatment of the infected total hip arthroplasty. Classification of the type of infection may also prove useful in assisting with the proper treatment algorithm. While treatment with antibiotics alone is rarely successful in the treatment of an infected total hip arthroplasty, this modality may be considered in a small group of patients that are not able to tolerate surgical intervention. Currently, the mainstay of a successful treatment includes surgical options such as irrigation and debridement alone, resection arthroplasty, primary exchange arthroplasty, two-stage reimplantation, and in rare instances three-stage reimplantation.[6-11] Unfortunately, the increasingly restrictive economics of our healthcare system are beginning to affect the choice of the two latter treatment options.

Sequence of Infection

The proliferation of a significant number of pathogenic microorganisms in viable tissue produces local edema, necrosis, and inflammation, which in turn impair local tissue circulation, with consequent reduction of the local levels of antibodies, leukocytes, oxygen, and tissue nutrients. Waste products and bacterial toxins accumulate, and the acidity increases. The phagocytes, unable to function in this environment, eventually die, releasing cytolytic enzymes that increase suppuration and tissue destruction. The bacteria persist at a phase of stationary growth on the surface of the prosthesis and/or cement. Incision, drainage, and debridement permit a fresh serous exucate to reach the lesion, starting a new cellular and humoral immunologic process.

Certain patients have been identified as predisposed toward periprosthetic infection, including those with prior hip surgery, rheumatoid arthritis, corticosteroid therapy, diabetes mellitus, poor nutritional state, obesity, and patients who are immunosuppressed, on dialysis, or with renal and liver transplants.[12-15] Elderly individuals experience a diminution in their immune response, further increasing their susceptibility to infection.[16]

Deep periprosthetic infections are dependent, as any other infections, on the interplay between the microorganism and the resistance of the host. Factors such as type, number, and virulence of infecting bacteria, and cellular and humoral immune mechanisms play an essential role.

The indwelling prosthesis and the polymethylmethacrylate cement represent foreign bodies and predispose to septic processes. Foreign materials contribute to local sepsis experimentally by decreasing the quantity of bacteria necessary to establish infection and by permitting pathogens to persist on the surface of the avascular material, sequestered from circulating immune factors (leukocytes, antibody, and complement) and systemic antibiotics.[17] Polymethylmethacrylate cement appears to predispose toward infection by effects beyond those of inert foreign materials. The cement in unpolymerized form has been shown to inhibit lymphocytic phagocytosis and complement function in vitro.[3] The in vivo polymerization process itself appears to enhance the risk of infection in an experimental dog model. In this study, in vivo polymerized polymethylmethacrylate significantly reduced the quantity of *Staphylococcus epidermidis*, *Staphylococcus aureus*, and *Escherichia coli* necessary to establish osteomyelitis, in comparison with prepolymerized methylmethacrylate, polyethylene, cobalt–chromium, and stainless steel. In an effort to avoid the use of polymethylmethacrylate, porous and press-fit cementless prostheses have been implanted, but the infection rate has remained unchanged.

Host responses to polymethylmethacrylate may also play a role in the pathogenesis of infection. Fibronectin, a connective tissue and plasma glycoprotein, appears to enhance *S. aureus* adherence to polymethylmethacrylate in vivo and thus may contribute to the occurrence of sepsis.[18] In the presence of prosthetic devices, many bacteria elaborate a recently defined fibrous exopolysaccharide material called glycocalyx.[3,19] Organisms growing within this matrix, form thick biofilms. The glycocalyx modifies the environment in favor of the microbe by concentrating nutrients and by protecting them from surfactants, opsonic antibodies, phagocytes, and antimicrobial agents (antiseptics and antibiotics). These conditions enhance the density of colonization on the surface of foreign materials (including metallic prostheses) in vivo and may play a role in predisposing toward tissue invasion. The presence of these protected biofilms may also result in persistence of infection, despite treatment with systemic antibiotic therapy (especially in the absence of extensive debridement of tissue at the bone-cement interface).

The particulate debris and toxicity of metals, which dissolve in the body fluids, can also favor infection by producing localized tissue necrosis and alterations in the immune response.[20-22] The potentially most harmful components of metal alloys appear to be cobalt in cobalt-chromium alloy, nickel in stainless steel, and vanadium in titanium alloy.[23] Early deep infections tend to be more virulent, with local signs of inflammation and systemic symptoms. Late, latent, or delayed infections usually follow a more silent course, persistent hip pain being the main indication of its presence. Metastatic or hematogenous infections can produce a more acute and severe symptomatology, resembling early deep infections in their manifestations in spite of their late onset.*

Routes of Infection

Two different pathogenic routes of infection are recognized: blood-borne and introduced. Approximately twenty percent of prosthetic joint infections arise by the hematogenous route with the remainder being introduced.[24,25] Any bacteremia can produce infection of a total joint replacement. Dental manipulations are known causes of infection by viridans, streptococcal, and anaerobic organisms (*Peptococcus*, *Peptostreptococcus*).[26,27] Pyogenic skin processes can cause staphylococcal (*S. aureus*, *S. epidermidis*) and streptococcal (group A and B streptococcus) infections. Genitourinary and gastrointestinal tract procedures or infections are associated with Gram-negative bacillary, enterococcal, and anaerobic infections. These bacteremic events usually cause joint sepsis with a single pathogen.

The introduced form of infection is the result of operative contamination or wound sepsis, contiguous to the prosthesis. Delayed wound healing, especially when associated with ischemic skin necrosis, infected wound hematomas, wound infection (with or without identifiable cellulitis), and suture abscesses are common preceding events for joint-replacement infection. During the early postimplantation period, when these superficial infections develop, fascial healing has not yet occurred and the deeply placed periprosthetic tissue is unprotected by the usual anatomic barriers. Most often, these infections are caused by a single pathogen, but polymicrobial sepsis with as many as five different organisms is occasionally observed, particularly when a

---

*Prophylactic antibiotics—American Heart Association Standards: Patients should take Amoxicillin 3 gm 1 hour before the procedure and 1.5 gm 6 hours after the procedure. If you are unable to take Amoxicillin, use Erythromycin 1 gm 1 hour before the procedure and 500 mg 6 hours after the procedure.

wound with delayed healing is contaminated by feces. Infrequently, latent foci of old osteomyelitis are reactivated by the local tissue disruption associated with implantation surgery. Despite sterile operative cultures, old, quiescent S. aureus and Mycobacterium tuberculosis osteomyelitis have reactivated in this setting.

Microbiology of the Infected Total Hip Arthroplasty

Adherence to Listerian principles has reduced virulent postoperative infections. Currently, coagulase negative Staphylococci and Staphylococcus aureus are the most commonly found pathogens.[28] A combined study from The Hospital for Special Surgery and the Mayo Clinic isolated 97 pathogens from 76 patients with periprosthetic hip infection.[3,29,30] In 80.3% (61 of 97) of the hips, a single organism was identified, while in 18% (14 of 97) hips a polymicrobial infection was noted and in 1.3% (one patient) the culture was sterile. Gram-positive bacteria accounted for 74%, gram-negative organisms 11%, and anaerobes 12%. (Table 53.1).

Staphylococcus epidermidis and Staphylococcus aureus accounted for more than one half of the pathogens. Other gram-positive organisms included Streptococcus viridans, group-D Streptococcus or Enterococcus, and β-hemolytic sero-groups. Eleven percent of the specimens were identified as gram-negative aerobic and facultative organisms including: Escherichia coli, Proteus mirabilis, Pseudomonas aeruginosa, Salmonella choleraesuis, and Campylobacter intestinalis. While Klebsiella, Serratia, Acinetobacter species, and other Pseudomonas species are commonly reported, they were not observed in this study. Anaerobic bacteria accounted for 12% and included: Propionibacterium acnes, Peptococcus asaccharides, Peptococcus magnus, Peptostreptococcus microsphore, and Clostridium bifermentans. Anaerobic bacterium of the Bacteriodes genus, Mycobacterium, atypical Mycobacterium, and fungi can also be responsible for periprosthetic infections.[31,32]

Strains of common staphylococcus pathogens have been reported as resistant to previously used antibiotics. Brown identified β-lactam antibiotic and oxacillin-resistant Staphylococcus aureus and Staphylococcus epidermidis.[33] Resistant pathogens such as these originate from the patient, the operating room environment, colonized hospital personnel, or prolonged admission to intensive care units. Usually all foreign biomaterial will need to be removed in order to resolve the infection. Gristina et al. suggests that biomaterials might act as a substrata encouraging bacterial adhesion and proliferation, resulting in resistant infection.[19,34-37] If bacteria can bind to the surface of the biomaterial, they can secrete a biofilm with an outer glycocalyx, protecting the pathogen from antibiotics and immune defense. As a result, an infected total hip arthroplasty with a microorganism that produces a biofilm may be resistant to antibiotic treatment alone. Fitzgerald uses the presence of a biofilm as a marker for resistance to treatment, and considers a biofilm producing organism a relative contraindication for primary exchange.[3]

Table 53.1. Microorganisms isolated from specimens taken at the time of resection arthroplasty.

Organisms	%	Number of isolates
Gram-positive bacteria	74%	
Staphylococcus epidermidis		36
Staphylococcus aureus		18
Streptococcus		14
Alpha-hemolytic-7		
Beta-hemolytic-3		
Enterococcus-4		
Diptheroids (corynebacterium, bacilli, and unknown species)		4
Unknown gram-positive cocci		1
Unknown bacillus species		1
Gram-negative bacteria	11%	
Escherichia coli		5
Proteus mirabilis		2
Pseudomonas aeriginosa		2
Salmonella choleraesuis		1
Campylobacter intestinalis		1
Anaerobes	12%	
Peptostreptococcus		6
Proprionibacterium acnes		5
Clostridium bifermentans		1
Unknown		1
Negative culture		1

Classification

Several classifications are available for periprosthetic hip infection. At The Hospital for Special Surgery, we use the following categories based upon the time of onset of infection: *early postoperative infection (diagnosed within 3 months of surgery)*, *late chronic infection*, and *acute hematogenous infection*.

An *early postoperative infection* is diagnosed within 3 months after the original total hip arthroplasty. Classically, patients have continuous pain after the operation that does not abate. A *late chronic infection* is apparent after 3 months from the index total hip arthroplasty. This type of infection is associated with a pain-free interval followed by the insidious onset of hip pain. One must exercise caution in evaluating a patient with signs and symptoms as described above, since postoperative heterotopic ossification may mimic a *late chronic infection*. An *acute hematogenous infection* is characterized by the acute onset of hip pain in a previously asymptomatic total hip arthroplasty. This infection is most notably caused through a hematogenous spread of the infecting organism. One should obtain a history of previous infections unrelated to the hip joint such as urinary tract, dental, respiratory, or skin lesions.

Other classification systems based on the time of onset of infection are proposed by Coventry and subsequently modified by Estrada.[38,39] The first three stages were originally described by Coventry in 1975, and include acute postoperative infections (stage I), delayed deep infections (stage II), and late hematogenous infections (stage III). Stage I infections include acute post operative infections (within 3 months from surgery), while stage II infections are more indolent and are diagnosed between 6 months and 2 years after surgery, usually in patients with a painful total hip since the index procedure. Stage III infections are diagnosed after 2 years in patients with a previously asymptomatic total hip arthroplasty, and are thought to occur via a hematogenous route.[38] The classification system was later modified and expanded by Estrada to include a fourth category, namely positive intraoperative culture. This category is established during revision hip arthroplasty when two or more intraoperative specimens are cultured positive for the same organism.[39]

At The Hospital for Special Surgery, we developed our own criteria for the establishment of deep hip infection.[40] In this system, points are assigned to several categories such as clinical diagnosis, wound condition, laboratory results, radiographic findings, bacteriology, intraoperative observations, and histopathology (Table 53.2). Out of a total of twenty nine points, fifteen or more points are consistent with a deep hip infection.[40]

Diagnosis

The most common presenting symptom in patients with an infected total hip arthroplasty is persistent pain. Pain that has not resolved since the operation or pain at rest are ominous symptoms of an inflammatory process that may be consistent with a deep infection. Unfortunately, early postoperative pain may also result from other conditions including wound healing, hematomas, soft tissue tension, or heterotopic ossification. However, the burden of proof that this type of pain is *not* from infection is the responsibility of the examining physician. Such aforementioned pain after total hip arthroplasty should be considered a deep infection until proven otherwise.

The second most common sign of an infected total hip arthroplasty is persistent drainage. In a patient with a wound that continues to drain postoperatively, one must suspect the possibility of infection. In the immediate postoperative period, wound drainage may be sanguinous, from a hematoma; serous, from fat necrosis; or purulent from frank infection. In a postoperative wound in which drainage persists, the sterile skin barrier is violated. As such, a portal of entry for skin bacteria is established that may subsequently result in colonization and infection of the wound. Therefore, it is essential to promptly evaluate a draining wound and determine if operative intervention or local wound care is necessary. Early diagnosis and treatment can prevent an acute deep infection of invading the bone–implant interface and diminishing the possibility of a successful debridement.[41]

In order to decrease the morbidity of infection, a prompt evaluation of the painful total hip arthroplasty patient is essential. A thorough history and physical examination may suggest the diagnosis of infection, while laboratory investigation and radiologic assessment are also useful.[65] In our experience, however, the most expeditious way of diagnosing an infection is by performing a hip aspiration under sterile conditions with a local anesthetic, preferably under fluoroscopy to assure accurate needle placement. If no fluid is aspirated, then a repeat aspiration is performed. If enough synovial fluid is obtained and processed, the cell count, differential, gram stain, and culture are likely to be diagnostic. If a culture is positive for a relatively avirulent organism or one frequently considered a contaminant, such as coagulase negative *staphylococcus* or diptheroids, then a second aspiration should be performed to confirm the pathogen. Aspiration of a potentially infected total hip arthroplasty should be performed in a patient who has been off antibiotics for several weeks. When the diagnosis remains elusive, arthroscopy of the painful hip for biopsy, tissue culture, and histopathology is also useful. While many modalities exist to aid in the diagnosis, ultimately, the prompt diagnostic acumen

Table 53.2 Criteria for deep hip infections.

Category	Point distribution	Subcategory
I. Clinical diagnosis	2 points	History of previous hip infection within 3 years
	1 point for any subcategory	Clinical signs & symptoms of infection
II. Condition of wound	3 points	Draining wound or sinus communicating with hip joint
III. Laboratory	2 points	Sedimentation rate greater than 30 mm
	1 point for each positive subcategory	Leukocytosis greater than 11000 with a shift to the left (greater than 5% bands)
IV. Roentgenographic findings	3 points	Plain films showing loosening, settling, wandering or bony resorption adjacent to the hardware or prosthesis
	1 point for each positive subcategory	Arthrogram or sinogram showing sinus tracts or soft tissue abscess communicating with the joint or the demonstration of contrast agent between acrylic and bone suggesting septic loosening
		Scan showing increased uptake compatible with infection or loosening
V. Bacteriology	10 points	A) Hip aspirations 1. Gram stain 2. Culture
	4 points for the initially positive gram stain or culture from aspiration or intraoperative specimen with 2 additional points for each subsequent specimen positive for the same organism	B) Intraoperative specimens 1. Gram stain 2. Culture
VI. Intraoperative observations	6 points	A) Gross periprosthetic infection 1. Purulent fluid in joint
	4 points for subcategory A and 2 points for subcategory G	B) Appearance of tissue suggestive of infection 1. Boggy edematous capsule 2. Inflamed synovium
VII. Histopathology	3 points	A) Acute inflammation on surgical specimen

of the evaluating physician is essential to the successful treatment of an infected total hip arthroplasty.

Laboratory Tests

While laboratory tests may be helpful in the diagnosis of an infected total hip arthroplasty, patients may have normal laboratory results in spite of a deep infection, particularly if the infection is indolent. Such tests are dependent on the systemic response to the local infection. Specific tests that may be useful include a complete blood count with differential, erythrocyte sedimentation rate, and C-reactive protein. While some authors have noted the peripheral neutrophil count to be elevated in periprosthetic infections,[30,42] others have observed this to be within the normal range in many instances.[3]

At The Hospital for Special Surgery, we rarely use the acute phase reactants to assist in the diagnosis of infection, since we found that the erythrocyte sedimentation rate and C-reactive protein, while sensitive, lack specificity for infection. Usually, both the erythrocyte sedimentation rate and C-reactive protein are elevated postoperatively and return to normal as the inflammatory process abates. However, the erythrocyte sedimentation rate may remain elevated for many months after surgery. In a study of forty postoperative total hip arthroplasty patients, Alto et al. noted that the erythrocyte sedimentation rate achieved a maximum level at 6 days, but remained elevated even after one year. In contrast, the C-reactive protein level peaked after only two days, and normalized after three weeks. Thus, the authors concluded that the C-reactive protein was more sensitive in evaluating an inflammatory process after total hip arthroplasty. Bauer and Saltarelli also reported that the C-reactive protein returns to normal more quickly after total hip arthroplasty, and that it was more accurate in identifying patients with a deep periprosthetic infection.[42] Unfortunately, these acute phase reactants lack specificity and are not useful in patients with systemic diseases that cause a baseline elevation of these markers, such as rheumatoid arthritis or malignancy. According to Garvin et. al., the C-reactive protein is the most sensitive test for diagnosing infection; repeated monitoring of C-reactive protein is recommended to evaluate the response to treatment.[63]

Some authors question the utility of the erythrocyte sedimentation rate. Fitzgerald et. al. has observed that up to one fourth of his painful total hip arthroplasty patients have a normal erythrocyte sedimentation rate, and recommend only the C-reactive protein.[3] Furthermore, in patients with a periprosthetic hip infection, Sanzén and Carlsson have observed that neither the erythrocyte sedimentation rate nor the C-reactive protein are universally elevated, although they recommend both studies in the evaluation of a painful total hip arthroplasty.[43] Due to the small prevalence of periprosthetic infections at each institution, a determination as to the appropriate diagnostic test may be possible only with a multicenter evaluation.

Radiography

Plain radiographs, when studied serially, can be an informative but nonspecific method of evaluation, particularly if obtained using standardized position and technique.[44] The original postoperative radiographs provide the baseline for future comparison with serial radiographs obtained later at yearly intervals. Therefore, radiographic evaluation of the painful total hip arthroplasty may be useful in the diagnosis of infection. In general, the longer the duration of the infection, the more striking the radiographic findings. In a patient with persistent pain despite normal radiographs, the possibility of infection should not be excluded, and further evaluation either with hip aspiration or scintigraphy is warranted. While an early infection may not reveal any radiographic abnormality, a chronically infected total hip arthroplasty may have obvious findings suggestive of infection. Although periosteal reaction is a hallmark finding for infection, radiolucency, osteolysis, and endosteal erosions are also observed. Unfortunately, many of the observed radiographic findings of periprosthetic infection are also noted with aseptic loosening; generation of particulate debris, and radiographic analysis is sensitive, but not specific for infection.[45]

While there is no single pathognomonic radiographic finding of deep infection, gross loosening of the prosthesis, periosteal reaction, and osteolysis, especially around screws and wires, are consistent with infection. Aseptic loosening of any prosthesis should be a diagnosis of exclusion, having eliminated infection as the source of the radiographic findings.

Radioactive Isotope Scanning (Scintigraphy)

While a bone scanning has been reported as an accurate and reliable method of demonstrating infection, it not specific for the diagnosis of an infected total hip arthroplasty.[46-48] Technetium 99m methylene diphosphonate (^{99m}Tc-MDP) is believed to be absorbed into the hydroxyapatite crystal of bone, and its uptake is proportional to the degree of vascularity and rate of bone remodeling. Three-phase bone scan in infection demonstrates increased uptake during the early vascular phase and diffuse uptake around the components in the static phase.[49] Unfortunately, the uptake of Technetium is usually increased in the presence of both mechanical loosening and infection. As such, the utility of a bone scan at our institution has been limited. Other institutions, however, advocate the use of bone scanning to aid in the diagnosis of the painful endoprosthesis more routinely.

In reviewing our experience with periprosthetic hip infections at The Hospital for Special Surgery, we noted that for acetabular loosening, the sensitivity and specificity of bone scanning were 87% and 95%, respectively, with an accuracy of 90%. For serial plain radiography, in contrast, the sensitivity was 95%, the specificity 100%, and the accuracy 97%. For femoral component loosening, bone scan sensitivity was 85%, the specificity 100%, and the accuracy 89%. The sensitivity of plain radiography was 100%, with a specificity of 92%, and accuracy of 98%.[50] Therefore, bone scan did not provide additional information with regard to loosening, and its routine use in the assessment of a painful total hip arthroplasty was questioned. At our institution we do not routinely order a bone scan on every patient with a painful total hip arthroplasty, and we reserve this test for patients that have persistent pain, despite radiographs that reveal good position and fixation of the components and equivocal laboratory and bacteriologic analysis. In addition, the expense of scintigraphy as an adjunctive diagnostic tool should be considered, since it cost approximately $440 at our institution. A negative bone scan, however, should rule out the possibility of infection.

The leukocyte scan, in which the patient's polymorphonuclear cells are labeled with Indium-111, appears to be sensitive and more specific for the diagnosis of infection.[51] In a canine model, Merkel et. al. noted that scintigraphy with Indium-111 labeled autologous neutrophil was able to distinguish between septic and aseptic loosening, and a well fixed prosthesis in 93% (14 of 15) of the study population.[52] Furthermore, in a prospective study of forty-two patients with suspected musculoskeletal infection, Merkel et. al. also noted that with Indium-111 labeled autologous neutrophil scintigraphy correctly identified the presence or absence of sepsis in 87% (37 of 42) of the patients. In the same study, Technicium-99m scintigraphy was only accurate in 62% (26 of 42) of patients.[52] As a result, the authors concluded that a negative Indium-111 neutrophil scan should rule out the possibility of infection. Unfortunately, this is an expensive test and should not be utilized in every patient. Fitzgerald states that this test should be limited to patients with either an elevated erythrocyte sedimentation rate or C-reactive protein level.[3]

Due to its affinity for polymorphonuclear leukocytes, Gallium GA 67 uptake is also increased in the presence of infection.[53] While this test has been used in the diagnosis of periprosthetic hip infections, it is expensive and lacks specificity. Certainly, in our present healthcare environment, the judicious use of any screening test should be encouraged, and more rigid criteria determined as to the applicability and usefulness of such diagnostic tools. With rapidly advancing technology, however, more accurate and cost effective diagnostic modalities may be available in the future to assist in the diagnosis of the periprosthetic infection. Two new tests, namely 111-labeled Ig G and Technetium 99m monoclonal antibody, are currently being evaluated both in the United States and Europe.

Hip Aspiration

The recommended and most expeditious procedure to establish the presence of infection is a joint aspiration performed with local anesthesia, under strict antiseptic precautions, preferably under fluoroscopic control to confirm intraarticular needle placement.[54-57] The patient should not have had antibiotic treatment within the past few weeks. The fluid aspirated is sent immediately to the bacteriology laboratory for direct smear (gram stain), aerobic, anaerobic, mycobacterial, and fungal cultures and sensitivities. Occasionally, the infecting organism can be a fastidious type of bacteria. In order to increase the chances of bacterial growth, the aspirate should be inoculated as soon as possible into the appropriate broth and culture medium. We favor the use of a transport system with a culture medium to support the bacteria during the time of transport. We believe that so-called sterile infections (a contradictory expression) are attributable to difficulty in culturing fastidious and anaerobic types of bacteria, which require careful culturing techniques and oxygen-free environment, respectively. Incubating cultures for 1 week can increase the isolation and identification of fastidious organisms of low virulence that may require longer time to grow.

If enough fluid is aspirated, a complete cell count and differential may also give valuable information. If the complete count shows more than 25,000 leukocytes/mL, and the differential count reveals that more than 25% are polymorphonuclear leukocytes, the greater the possibility of infection. Fluid should also be analyzed for glucose and protein levels. In normal synovial fluid, protein levels are about one-third serum levels. Glucose values in synovial fluid are similar to those of plasma. In the presence of infection, the synovial glucose levels are lowered due to an alteration in transport mechanisms. Thus, a low glucose and high protein level are suggestive of infection.

In patients with an infected total hip arthroplasty, the aerobic and anaerobic bacterial cultures are successful in identifying the causal organism in 88% to 93% of the cases in which fluid was successfully aspirated.[44,58,59] In the majority of cases and considering the most common pathogens, a negative culture following an aspiration in which fluid was obtained should exclude the possibility of infection, provided adequate bacteriologic techniques were used without delay. However, in approximately 20% of the cases of periprosthetic infection at our institution, the hip aspiration is unsuccessful in identifying the offending organism. One factor that may be responsible for a negative culture is a patient that received antibiotics prior to the hip aspiration. Ideally one should wait three to four weeks prior to hip aspiration to ensure that the culture is not inhibited by the antibiotic. Other causes of a negative culture from a hip aspiration include more indolent types of infection with mycobacterium, TB, fungi, and certain anaerobes.[60] In the very early stages of infection, the actual infection may involve the bone cement interface and not communicate with the joint space. In this scenario, a joint space aspirate would also be negative. Finally, with a single negative culture after hip aspiration, one may consider a few week interval with subsequent re-aspiration of the painful hip.

Some authors have stated that the routine use of hip aspiration with arthrography is not cost effective, and that careful selection of patients is necessary. Fitzgerald asserts that such a test should be reserved for patients with laboratory abnormalities that implicate an inflammatory process.[3] As a result, he reserves hip aspiration for patients with a painful total hip arthroplasty in whom either the erythrocyte sedimentation rate or the C-reactive protein are elevated.

Selective hip aspiration is also recommended by Barrack and Harris who studied routine aspiration in a cohort of 270 consecutive revision hip arthroplasty patients. They noted a 13% rate of false positive cultures in patients that had a noninfected prosthesis.[61] They concluded that selective aspiration was indicated in evaluating the painful total hip arthroplasty and that this test should be employed in patients with a history or radiographic findings suggestive of infection. Such findings, they stated, included global radiolucency, focal osteolysis, nonfocal osteolysis, and periosteal reaction.

Arthrography

Hip aspiration may be combined with hip arthrography, both to confirm that the needle is located within the intracapsular space of the hip joint, and to rule out pocketing of the radiopaque medium in a periprosthetic abscess. The communication of sinus tracts with the intra-articular space may be better demonstrated by arthrography than by sinogram. However, a false-negative arthrogram can be observed despite radiographic evidence of loosening, due to the presence of granulation tissue at the bone-cement interface, which prevents the seeping of contrast agent. Furthermore, if abscesses are present, the contrast agent tends to collect at these sites, failing to penetrate at the bone–cement interface. The injection of a larger quantity of contrast agent could outline the loosening, but in infection the increased pressure is contraindicated, as it can produce septicemia.

At our institution, we have recently utilized ultrasound where the aspiration was negative and the arthrogram nondiagnostic. In this setting, loculated effusions and abscesses have been observed, thus allowing redirection of the needle under ultrasonic guidance. Our experience to date is favorable, but limited. Further experience will help define the role of ultrasound in the diagnosis of the infected total hip arthroplasty.

Biopsy and Reoperation

In the rare case in which the diagnosis is still unclear once all this information has been gathered, and if the clinical suspicion of infection is strong, a biopsy might be indicated, either open or closed, with needle, trocar, or arthroscopic techniques.[62] The final diagnosis is established at the time of reoperation. Antibiotics should not be given prior to surgery, to maximize the chances of isolating and identifying the infecting organism. Antibiotics are given intravenously, as soon as several cultures have been obtained from joint fluid and suspicious inflamed tissue specimens. At surgery, the macroscopic observation of the wound by an experienced surgeon and frozen tissue sections will give a good idea of the acuteness of inflammation. The finding of more than five to ten polymorphonuclear leukocytes per high-power field in the tissues, excluding those found in fibrin, has been considered a reliable indication of infection.[63] Repeat gram stains, cultures of joint fluid and several tissue specimens, the macroscopic appearance of the wound, and the histopathology demonstrating inflammatory granulation tissue should provide diagnostic and definite bacteriologic information.

Occasionally, the surgeon is confronted with the dilemma of deciding whether an isolated positive culture is of pathologic significance. This problem emphasizes the importance of obtaining multiple cultures. One positive culture might represent a contaminant if several other cultures fail to grow the same organism. This is particularly true if the growth occurs only in a liquid medium (broth). Growth on plates is less likely to represent contamination. The organisms usually encountered as contaminants are those mostly found in the perioperative environment and include *S. epidermidis* and diptheroids.

In order to define whether we are dealing with a contaminant as opposed to infection, we established a classification for the establishment of deep hip infection.[40] In this system, points are assigned to several categories such as clinical diagnosis, wound condition, laboratory results, radiographic findings, bacteriology, intraoperative observations, and histopathology. Out of a total of twenty nine points, fifteen or more points are consistent with a deep hip infection (Table 54.2).

Frozen Section

Lonner et al. recently reviewed frozen sections for the intraoperative diagnosis of an infected total hip arthroplasty, and noted that five to ten polymorphonuclear leukocytes per high-power field in the tissues was suggestive of infection, but not definitive. However, when greater than ten polymorphonuclear leukocytes per high-power field were observed, the diagnosis of infection was conclusive. This study revealed a sensitivity of 84% and a specificity of 90%.[63] Other authors have found that five to ten polymorphonuclear leukocytes per high-power field is strongly correlated with pathologic evidence of acute inflammation and presumptive evidence of infection.[64]

While frozen section has a high specificity for infection (approximately 90%), the sensitivity of this test may be quite low (approximately 20%). Therefore, the routine use of isolated frozen section as a screening tool for infection is questionable. When evaluated independently, Frank et al. found that frozen section was the most specific test for the diagnosis of infection and that C-reactive protein was the most sensitive. In a paired test protocol, the combination of these two tests demonstrated a sensitivity of 100% and a specificity of 94%.[65]

Prevention of the Joint Prosthesis Infection

Since infection of a prosthetic joint replacement prosthesis is catastrophic, prevention is of paramount importance. Before scheduling elective total joint replacement the patient should be evaluated for a history of infection and treated for pyogenic dental processes, obstructive urinary tract conditions, and dermatitis, which might predispose to infection.[66-68]

In patients with indwelling joint prostheses, early recognition and prompt therapy of infection in any location are critical to reduce the ever-present risk of hematogenous seeding of the joint implant. Situations likely to cause bacteremia should be avoided, and prophylactic antibiotics should be considered in anticipation of a bacteremic event. In performing dental manipulations, genitourinary and gastrointestinal procedures, and surgery on infected or contaminated tissues, one should consider prophylactic antibiotic use in a manner similar to that for patients with abnormal cardiac valves. No studies are available to determine the adequacy of prophylactic antibiotic regimens for these situations, and they are not likely to be forthcoming.

Clean Air

The incidence of infection is reduced by prophylactic measures. Sir John Charnley reduced exogenous operative wound contamination by the use of an enclosure, unidirectional air flow, ultrafiltered air, rapid air changes, ultrafine fabrics for clothing and draping, and air-exhaust systems for the operative teams.[69]

We have studied the effect of clean air at The Hospital for Special Surgery. The air flowing over the wounds of patients operated on in the enclosure with horizontal unidirectional filtered airflow was noted to be more sterile than in conventional operating rooms. The organisms most frequently recovered in these studies from incisions, surgical field and air flowing over the wound were coagulase-negative staphylococci.[70]

In 1982, a definitive study was published on the efficacy of ultraclean air. In a multicenter, prospective, randomized study of sepsis over a 7-year period, after more than 8000 total hip and knee replacements, Lidwell et al. concluded that the infection rate was about one-half when operations were done in ultraclean air systems compared with those operated on in conventional operating rooms.[71] Furthermore, when whole-body exhaust-ventilated suits had been worn in a theater ventilated by an ultraclean air system, the incidence of sepsis was about one-fourth that found in conventional operating rooms. A significant reduction of infections was also observed in those patients who received prophylactic antibiotics.

However, a study performed by us in 1982 at The Hospital for Special Surgery outlined that horizontal laminar airflow may produce either beneficial or adverse effects, depending on whether the surgical procedure can be performed in accordance with the theory of operation of the airflow system.[72] We demonstrated a significant reduction of infection in total hip replacement, but in total knee replacement the infection rate was increased, probably because during the knee surgery members of the surgical team must stand in positions which create a turbulent air flow between the source of the horizontal laminar airflow and the open wound.

Prophylactic Antibiotics

Certainly from our own experience and that of others, the use of prophylactic antibiotics has been highly efficacious. At The Hospital for Special Surgery, a prophylactic antibiotic program was instituted in December 1969, after our early experience with total hip replacement had shown a 14% incidence of infection. As most of these infections were due to gram positive organisms, particularly coagulase-negative S. epidermidis, a semisynthetic penicillin (oxacillin) was selected so as to control penicillinase-producing organisms. Currently, we use cefazolin as the primary antibiotic for prophylaxis in patients without a penicillin allergy. In patients allergic to penicillin, intravenous Vancomycin is administered, and thus far we have not encountered any significant difficulty. Of all the first-generation cephalosporins, cefazolin reaches a higher serum peak and has the longest half-life (1.8 hours), as it is cleared more slowly by the kidney and is more tightly bound to serum proteins. This permits administration at a lower dose, every 8 hours. Effective prophylaxis has been shown with only two doses of ceforanide, an antibiotic with a longer half-life, providing sustained plasma and bone levels during the perioperative period. However, ceforanide is less effective against staphylococci than cefazolin.[73]

A prospective double-blind randomized placebo-controlled study performed on 2137 total hip arthroplasties demonstrated that cefazolin significantly reduced the infection rate (from 3.3% to 0.9%). However, the reduction of infection was not statistically significant when performed in ultraclean operating rooms.

There is much experimental and clinical evidence to show that the use of short duration, bactericidal prophylactic antibiotics in clean surgery is beneficial in lowering the infection rate.[74] Sandusky reported more than 30 studies in the surgical literature that demonstrated a reduction in the infection rate when prophylactic antibiotics were used. He recommended that their use be routine when implants were utilized.[75]

Burke was able to show the optimum time to administer prophylactic antibiotics with an experimental dermal model.[76] His work showed that for antibiotics to be effective they must be present in the tissues at adequate levels before the bacteria arrive. This prevents the rapid exponential growth of the bacteria and allows the host to eradicate the infection. The pharmacokinetics of these drugs enables them to be given no more then one hour preoperatively, and they should be discontinued after 24 to 48 hours. Drainage tubes, intravenous lines, and urinary catheters do not necessitate prolonged use of prophylactic antibiotics.

Bone Penetration by Antibiotics

Bactericidal antimicrobial agents that produce significant serum levels also penetrate bone by readily transversing the capillary membrane. The bone level of most antibiotics approximates 10% to 30% of the serum level. Antimicrobial regimens for bone infections are usually designed to produce serum bactericidal activity several multiples higher than the quantitative susceptibility of the pathogen to the therapeutic agent (minimum bactericidal concentration).[77,78] In our experience, a post peak serum bactericidal titer of at least 1:8, measured 25% into the time interval between dosages constitutes effective antimicrobial therapy for prosthetic joint infections.

Joint, Synovium, and Hematoma Penetration by Antibiotics

Most antimicrobial agents diffuse easily from the blood into infected joint spaces. Synovial fluid bactericidal activity bears a linear relationship to the serum bactericidal activity.[79,80] Synovial fluid antibiotic levels are substantially higher in infected joints than in noninfected joints. Intravenous administration of antimicrobial agents has been shown to penetrate hematomas up to 4 days after their formation.[81] This penetration may be dependent on the size of the collection, since larger hematomas may not have demonstrable antibiotic, unless the hematoma occurred while the patient was receiving prophylactic antibiotics.

Local Antibiotics

As antibacterial agents diffuse readily from the blood into infected joints, it is not necessary to employ intra-articular antibiotic therapy in the standard treatment of septic arthritis. Intra-articular antibiotics can be irritants to the synovium, inducing a severe chemical synovitis. In addition, intra-articular antibiotics are readily absorbed systemically, which can result in toxic serum levels. Moreover, intra-articular administration may predispose to contamination and superinfection of the involved joint. These principles also apply to the use of antibiotics in irrigation tubes in postoperative orthopedic patients.[82]

The rapid penetration of bacteria into the tissues appears to defeat the purpose of surface therapy. Recent studies have shown that antibiotic solutions failed to eradicate bacteria from wounds even when irrigation was commenced 1 minute after contamination. The mechanical cleansing of irrigation appears to be more beneficial than the activity of the antimicrobial agent.

Surgical Technique

The importance of meticulous, gentle surgical technique cannot be overemphasized. Good aseptic technique is absolutely essential and requires strict discipline by the surgical team. Operative time should be kept to a minimum, without jeopardizing the quality of surgery. Gentle tissue handling, coverage of skin margins, maintenance of moist tissue surfaces by repeated irrigation, avoidance of tissue-crushing clamps, and rough or excessive retraction, unnecessary use of electrocautery and frequent mechanical lavage to remove clots and tissue particles, careful hemostasis and suction drainage to avoid hematoma formation, and meticulous closure to obliterate dead space (but without excessive tension) are all crucial factors in reducing the risk of infection.[82,83]

Treatment

The treatment of the infected total hip arthroplasty has evolved considerably in the last three decades.[3,84–91] Several treatment options are reported with varying indications and success. Antibiotic suppression, debridement with component retention or removal, primary exchange arthroplasty, two stage reimplantation, and exceptionally a three stage protocol, are all considerations in treating an infected total hip arthroplasty. Each of the above options has specific indications and associated results.[92] In considering the above treatment plans, the decision is multifactorial and relies upon the patient, the surgeon, the type of organism, and unfortunately, lately the cost.

With any of the above treatment options, the goals of treatment should be the eradication of the infection with preservation of limb function. The functional results of reimplantation, either primarily or secondarily, are preferable to a resection arthroplasty or Girdlestone procedure.[93] In general, antibiotic therapy combined with surgical débridement of the infected tissues, prosthesis and cement removal, are the mainstays of treatment and have the greatest likelihood of success. If a patient has more than one prosthetic joint replacement, prompt diagnosis and treatment is imperative to prevent metachronous infection.[94]

Antibiotic Suppression

Antibiotic therapy might suppress the symptoms of an infected total hip replacement and may be indicated as a temporizing measure if surgery is contraindicated due to medical reasons or if the patient does not accept it. However, it is unlikely to cure the infectious process. Its use can also complicate the problem by selecting genetically resistant strains or by inducing spontaneous mutation to resistant strains, while still not resolving the underlying infection. Sinuses will not heal where they serve as tracts for the passage of purulent material that is being continually manufactured by a pyogenic membrane.

The effectiveness of antibiotic therapy is closely related to the intensity of the bacterial metabolism. Wood and Smith demonstrated in 1956 that bacteria were killed promptly when penicillin was added early, during the logarithmic phase of bacterial growth, but failed to occur if the addition of antibiotics was delayed until the stationary growth phase.[95] In thick purulent exudates, penicillin exerted only a slow bactericidal effect. The bacteria tended to persist at a stationary growth phase.

Bactericidal oral antibiotic (suppressive) therapy may permit prosthesis retention when surgery is contraindicated in the elderly patient who has neither systemic manifestations nor prosthetic loosening, and in cases where the bacteria is avirulent, sensitive to oral antibiotic therapy, and well tolerated by the patient. All these prerequisites are rarely present; thus, suppressive antibiotic therapy is infrequently indicated at our institution. However, Goulet et al. reviewed 19 patients treated at our institution in the early 80s by suppressive antibiotic therapy, following infected total hip arthroplasty. An average follow-up of 4.1 years, of 7 of the 19 prosthesis had failed. Therefore, a 63% (12/19) success rate was reported.[96] The authors stipulated that antibiotic suppression was indicated in patients with well fixed components and a highly sensitive and relatively avirulent organism. If an infection involving an implant is diagnosed, the ideal treatment is early, adequate, and prolonged bactericidal antibiotic therapy combined with incision, drainage, and thorough debridement of involved tissues.

Recently, two studies reported more successful results with combined antibiotic suppression, administered for 6 months.[97,98] By combining rifampin with a flouroquinolone (i.e. ciprofloxacin), Drancort et al. noted 81% (17 of 21) successful treatment.[97] Widmer et al. also observed similar success with multi-modal therapy, however, his average follow-up was only 6 months.[98] Clearly, longer follow-up is essential to determine the true efficacy of such antibiotic therapy.

In treating a periprosthetic infection with prolonged antibiotic suppression, one must be aware of the potential adverse effects. When they occur, a different antimicrobial agent must be chosen. Resistance of the infecting organism to the antibiotic may occur, thus requiring a change in therapy. Mutated microorganisms are now capable of producing a glycocalyx or slime layer that is impenetrable by antibiotics. This bacterial defense mechanism is responsible for the high rate of failure with antibiotic suppression as well as débridement without component removal. Consequently, antibiotic suppression of an infected total hip arthroplasty should only be reserved for the high risk patient who cannot tolerate surgical removal of the prosthesis or refuses operative treatment. As such, one must be cognizant of less favorable results in this setting.

Depending on the sensitivity of the infecting organism, bactericidal drugs of first choice should be given in high doses for two weeks followed by oral antibiotics for chronic suppressive therapy. Although, ideally, selecting the drug of choice from the large number of antibiotics should not be difficult, several factors limit the selection of the antibiotic, such as the drug resistance of the organism and the general health and tolerance of the patient.

Working in close relation with the infectious disease specialist, all these factors should be thoroughly assessed prior to deciding what antibiotic regimen is to be used, and not infrequently we may have to resort to second-choice antibiotics. If they produce adverse affects, we are forced then to switch to a drug of third choice, narrowing the alternatives even further. The need for careful monitoring of patients on antibiotics should be kept in mind, considering the high doses and prolonged time necessary for adequate treatment. While a combination of three antibiotics acting at different sites on the bacterial metabolism has been recommended, because of the significant toxic potential, we have not used this approach.[99]

Six weeks of intravenous antibiotic therapy can prove difficult, particularly in elderly females with poor veins. The use of a Hickman or Broviac central venous catheter has been beneficial and frees the upper extremities for the use of external support in ambulation.[100]

Surgical Considerations

The treatment of suprafascial subcutaneous wound infections follows the principles of treatment of all surgical wounds. Recovery of the organisms and the establishment of effective antibiotic treatment is of primary importance. Adequate drainage to evacuate loculated hematomata or abscesses is essential and in most cases is followed by primary closure. Secondary closure might be indicated in selected cases of extreme inflammation. For the surgical treatment of deep periprosthetic infections, the patient should be typed and cross-matched for 3 to 4 units of blood. When the acute inflammation is severe, profuse bleeding can be expected, particularly if radical excision and debridement of the inflamed tissues are carried out. Hypotensive epidural anesthesia proves advantageous as the amount of total blood loss, and the corresponding blood replacement are less.

Removal of the prosthetic components and acrylic cement can prove a difficult task, particularly if the septic process is of recent onset. The prosthetic components may not yet be loose and removal of the tight interdigitation between bone and cement demands a laborious, patient, and meticulous technique, if unnecessary loss of bone stock and perforations are to be avoided. In infections of longer duration, the septic process dissects along the bone–cement interface and loosens the components and acrylic cement, facilitating their removal.

While in most instances, adequate exposure is obtained without trochanteric osteotomy, in complex cases a standard or extended trochanteric osteotomy may provide better access to the femur.[101] For these cases, the previously osteotomized greater trochanter is advanced and sutured to the proximal and lateral part of the femur. The proximal shaft can be left outside the acetabulum, resembling a Girdlestone procedure (resection arthroplasty) or introduced into the acetabulum as in the Colonna or Whitman reconstruction (trochanteric arthroplasty). Advantages of the resection arthroplasty usually include less pain and freer range of passive motion. Increased shortening, telescoping, hip instability, and poor muscle control are the main disadvantages. In the trochanteric arthroplasty the opposite is true: usually it is a more stable joint, although it can be painful due to bony contact. The shortening and telescoping are not as severe, but the hip is more prone to stiffness. Considerations such as age, sex, and occupation might influence the choice of the procedure. At The Hospital For Special Surgery, we believe that resection of the superolateral acetabular margin is contraindicated, since it compromises a later prosthetic reconstruction and its value in improving the results of simple removal of the prosthetic component remains to be proved. Following incision, debridement, and removal of the foreign body, including all acrylic cement, if the acute inflammation of the tissues is extreme, the wound should be packed open for 3 to 4 days. A delayed primary closure can then be performed. This approach is safer than a primary closure over the closed suction irrigation. However, we have used it only rarely. Qualitative and quantitative determination of the number of bacteria present in the wound tissue prior to closure has been suggested as a means of determining the best time for closure. Whenever the number of bacteria exceeds the critical level of 10^5/ml tissue, secondary closure is preferred. However, we have not tested the practicality of this principle in our cases.

If the primary wound closure is considered safe (as in most instances in our experience), multi-perforated polyethylene tubes are placed to suction for 24 to 48 hours. The tubes are placed within the femoral shaft and within the acetabulum. The site of exit should be placed anterolaterally, at least 5 cm away from the wound, to reduce the chances of sinus tract formation following removal of the tubes. The lower extremity is kept in balanced suspension with a tibial skeleton traction for about 2 weeks. During this period, physical therapy helps keep these patients both interested and motivated. Active upper and lower muscle setting exercises, gentle range of motion, and deep-breathing exercises are performed under the supervision of a physical therapist. It is advisable to discontinue isolation as soon as the wound is healed in order reduce the possibilities of emotional depression.

Vigorous dorsiflexion of the foot and ankle, pneumatic boots, and prophylactic anticoagulation is indicated to reduce the danger of thromboembolism in view of the long period of recumbence. About 2 weeks after surgery, once acceptable scarring and stability of the hip are obtained, assessed by the push-pull stability of the hip, the skeletal traction is removed and the patient is started on gentle, progressive, active and passive range-of-motion exercises. This is followed by dangling, standing, and partial weight-bearing ambulation with a walker, attended by a physical therapist. Pool therapy can be of particular help. Patients are progressed in their rehabilitation program as tolerated.

The vastus lateralis flap has been recommended for the intractably infected hip with a widely open wound and persistent drainage.[102] Mobilization of the vastus lateralis muscle as a flap can provide adequate definitive closure, cessation of drainage, and a relatively functional extremity.

Debridement Without Component Removal

Operative debridement without component removal, combined with antibiotic treatment, is indicated as the primary form of treatment mainly in the *early postoperative infection* and in the *acute hematogenous infection*, with very recent onset of symptoms. An acute infection within 3 months of implantation, may be treated by a thorough debridement, retention of the components, and antibiotic treatment. Debridement in this setting may be open, with excision of all the necrotic and infected tissue. Complete inspection and subsequent decompression of the pseudocapsule and the surrounding tissues for loculated purulent areas is essential to the success of the debridement, without component removal.

In patients with an *acute hematogenous infection* in whom the onset of symptoms was recent, operative debridement without component removal may also be considered. Criteria to proceed with this treatment plan include: less than a week duration of symptoms, no loosening of the prosthesis, and a positive culture for an organism sensitive to antibiotics. Gustilo et al. reported 74% (26 of 35) success in patients with an *early postoperative infection*, but only 50% (3 of 6) in patients with an *acute hematogenous infection*.[103] They concluded that prompt surgical treatment with intensive debridement and without component removal may be successful in a carefully selected patient population. At our institution, we utilized debridement without component removal for selective patients with an *early postoperative infection* and an *acute hematogenous infection* that is recognized very early.

We have recently studied six cases at our institution in which arthroscopic debridement and profuse irrigation was used to treat an acute hematogenous infected hip arthroplasty. The prostheses were cemented and the patients remained on chronic, suppressive antibiotics. Thus, this technique was not used for treatment, per se, but for assistance with antibiotic suppression. To date, none of the patient's infections have progressed, but the follow-up and study group are limited.

Reinsertion of a Total Hip Prosthesis
Because of the superiority of total hip replacement over resection arthroplasty, attempts have been made to either debride the hip in one stage, removing all foreign material and reconstructing the joint with a total hip prosthesis, or to delay this reconstruction to a second operative session. In either case, massive antibiotic therapy is administered. We have reimplanted total hip prostheses in cases of subacute, latent, or recently arrested hip sepsis, provided the wound was closed and the infecting organism sensitive to antibiotics. Frozen tissue sections at the time of surgery and the macroscopic appearance of the wound should show only mild to moderate inflammation. Gram stain should be negative. All scarred and devitalized tissues should be excised, leaving viable, well-irrigated, healthy tissues.

Adequate preoperative planning is essential in order to have available appropriate prosthetic components to facilitate a satisfactory biomechanical reconstruction, particularly when there is a bone stock deficit. We have carefully selected the patients with latent deep infections in which we have used this procedure. In our view, open wound drainage, pus, resistant organisms or mixed flora, acute inflammation, and granulation tissue all constitute contraindications to one-stage debridement and reconstruction. The presence of a draining wound suggests a severe infection with marked exudate that had to decompress itself spontaneously through drainage. Infections caused by certain resistant single or mixed pathogens are difficult to control, requiring intensive antibacterial therapy, close to toxic levels. Active pus formation implies a continuous process of leukocyte necrosis because of the virulence of the microorganisms. Acute inflammation or the presence of granulation tissue also demonstrates the severity of the infection. The reinsertion of a foreign body would further compromise the situation in these instances. Once clean, dry wound healing has been achieved, a second-stage reconstruction may be considered if other factors are favorable and provided the cellular and humoral immune mechanism is normal.

One-Stage Reconstruction (Primary Exchange)
After debridement and removal of the prosthesis, reimplantation can be performed during the same operative setting.[104–111] This is referred to as a either a one-stage reconstruction or a primary exchange procedure. While the indications of this treatment protocol are controversial, some experienced authors report excellent success.[104–106] In order to consider this treatment option, the patient must meet several of the following criteria: the pathogen must be sensitive to antibiotics, the patient must be healthy and without known risk factors for infection, and the bone and soft tissue must be adequate to assure a good biomechanical reconstruction of the hip. In addition, elderly patients or patients with multiple medical problems who may not be able to tolerate prolonged bed rest and a second procedure are also considered for a one stage reconstruction. Sensitive pathogens include aerobic, gram-positive cocci, methicillin sensitive, oxacillin sensitive, and nonglycocalyx producing organisms. Some examples of such bacteria are specific strains of *Staphylococcus aureus*, coagulase negative *Staphylococcus*, and viridans type *Streptococcus*.

In revision total hip arthroplasty for aseptic loosening of either the acetabular or femoral component, only one of the components may have to be revised. In sharp contrast, a primary exchange for infection mandates the complete removal of all the components, bone cement, wire, and foreign bodies whether the component is well fixed or loose. Therefore, more elaborate and extensive procedures may be indicated in performing a primary exchange, such as the extended trochanteric osteotomy or cortical shaft osteotomy. Because of the complexity of such cases, the surgeon and operating team must be experienced and well prepared for a primary exchange procedure.

The technique of primary exchange arthroplasty was first pioneered by Buchholz and Engelbrecht in 1970 at the Endo-Klinic in Hamburg.[105] Utilizing gentamicin-loaded Palacos R bone cement and no systemic antibiotics, the authors reported a success rate of 73%. Later Carlsson et al. from Sweden performed a multicenter study with primary exchange arthroplasty, gentamicin-loaded Palacos R bone cement, and six months of systemic antibiotics with a success rate of 78%.[112] With greater than 10 year follow-up, Buchholz et al. has published a success rate of 77% after a single primary exchange, and 90% success after subsequent primary exchanges.[104] The authors identified the following causes of failure: gram-negative organisms, group D *Streptococci*, delay in surgery, and inadequate doses of antibiotics in the bone cement.

Two-Stage Reconstruction
At The Hospital for Special Surgery the two-stage reimplantation protocol is considered the gold standard for the treatment of an infected total hip arthroplasty.[14,113,114] The first stage includes removal of the prosthesis, bone cement, and all foreign material, followed by a thorough debridement of the soft tissues.[115] The wound is closed without the insertion of a new

prosthesis. The patient typically has a central venous catheter placed during this procedure with six weeks of postoperative intravenous antibiotics, achieving a minimum bactericidal level of 1:8 dilution at a post-peak level 25% into the time interval between antibiotic doses. In addition, a tibial skeletal traction pin is placed intraoperatively, and the patient is maintained in skeletal traction for approximately 2 weeks. This not only reduces postoperative pain, but also allows interpositional scarring between the acetabulum and the proximal femur. The second stage is usually performed after the six week interval, provided the clinical evolution is uneventful and the wound healing benign, and involves reimplantation of a hybrid total hip arthroplasty with antibiotic loaded acrylic bone cement.

Our success at The Hospital for Special Surgery with the two-stage reimplantation was reported in 1994 with a review of 44 patients (46 hips) with an infected total hip arthroplasty.[14] The initial total hip procedures were performed between 1985 and 1988. Of the 46 infected hips treated with the protocol, 70% (32 hips) were reimplanted with a success rate of 91%. At an average of 40 months after reimplantation infection recurred in only three hips (9%). In two of the three hips, a gram-negative organism was isolated and bactericidal titers of 1:8 were not obtained. Adequate postpeak serum bactericidal titers of 1:8 were obtained in 28 hips and amongst these, there was only one recurrence (4% failure). Interestingly, the presence of retained bone cement after resection arthroplasty in 10 hips was not associated with recurrence of infection.

In the above series of patients 14 hips (30%) were not reimplanted due to: inadequate bone stock, poor soft tissue, intractable skin ulcers, antibiotic resistance to the infecting organism, medical contraindications to further surgery, and poor potential for rehabilitation. All 12 patients with resection arthroplasty required support to ambulate and only 17% (2 of 12 patients) were satisfied. In sharp contrast, only 56% (18 of 32) of the patients with a reimplantation required an assistive device for ambulation, and 90% (29 of 32) were satisfied with their functional result.

During reimplantation, antibiotics should be added to the acrylic cement.[115–121] At our institution we currently utilize heat stable, powdered antibiotics such as tobramycin, depending upon the sensitivity of the infecting organism. The selection of a specific antibiotic according to the sensitivity of the organism is appealing. However, Brien et al. showed erratic elution of vancomycin but better elution when vancomycin is combined with tobramycin.[122] Evaluation of the joint fluid of patients reimplanted with gentamicin-impregnated cement for fixation of prosthesis reveals high levels of gentamicin, approximately seven times higher than those obtained by parenteral administration. The joint fluid levels eluted from gentamicin-impregnated beads is 17 times higher. Serum and urine levels of gentamicin are approximately 10 to 20 times lower, when compared to a control group of patients receiving intravenous gentamicin. No renal or ototoxicity was documented, and none is expected with these low serum and urine levels. The effectiveness of gentamicin in gram-negative infection has been previously documented, and we have demonstrated its efficacy in gram-positive infections, especially staphylococcal, with limited effectiveness against streptococci. Palacos' gentamicin-impregnated cement has good fracture toughness properties, but its penetration to cancellous bone is decreased due to its higher viscosity. This disadvantage appears to be overcome by the new low-viscosity Palacos gentamicin, with improved intrusion characteristics, which also increases the surface area, thus providing higher elution of gentamicin. In reviewing a cohort of patients treated with an uncemented arthroplasty after infection, an 18% recurrence of infection and an 18% rate of loosening was noted, thus further reinforcing the usefulness of antibiotic impregnated cement.[3,4,123]

In comparing primary exchange to the two-stage reimplantation protocol, a review of the literature would suggest that the success rate of primary exchange is approximately 80% if antibiotic impregnated cement is utilized and 70% if it is not. The success rate of the two-stage reimplantation is at least 90%, 10% higher. (Table 53.3). Based upon the above data from our institution and others, we maintain that the two-stage reimplantation protocol is the gold standard in the treatment of the infected total joint arthroplasty, despite the longer durations of treatment and additional cost per patient. The efficacy of any other treatment strategy should be compared to the two-stage reimplantation protocol. A randomized prospective study comparing different techniques could provide the necessary information to alter our current treatment algorithm. Unfortunately, the number of patients treated per year in a given institution is relatively small, and, as such, a multicenter study is needed to assess an alternative treatment or modification of the two-stage reimplantation protocol.

Currently, the two-stage reimplantation protocol is the most accepted treatment of an infected total hip arthroplasty. The protocol includes the removal of the prosthesis, debridement, 6 weeks of postoperative intravenous antibiotics obtaining a minimum post-peak serum bactericidal titer of 1:8 dilution, and reimplantation of a new hybrid prosthesis with antibiotic impregnated cement. The effectiveness of antibiotic impregnated cement has been demonstrated by experimental and clinical studies.[29,104,107,124,125] Contraindications for reimplantation of a new prosthesis after the 6-week interval are inadequate bone stock, poor soft tissue, antibiotic resistance to the infecting organism, medical contraindications to further surgery, and the poor potential for rehabilitation.

Table 53.3 Comparison of one- and two-stage exchanges.

Author	One stage		Two stages	
	No. of hips	Success %	No. of hips	Success %
Cement with antibiotics				
Bucholz et al.	667	77.0		
Lindberg	59	90.0	18	78.0
Murray	13	38.5	22	95.5
Turner et al.	101	86.0		
Wroblewski	102	91.0		
Hope et al.	72	87.5	19	100.0
Elson	235	87.5	61	96.5
Garvin and Salvati et al.	21	90.5	55	92.7
Johnston et al.	24	91.7		
Total	1294	82.2	175	92.5
Cement without antibiotics				
Hunter	55	18.0	10	60.0
Talbott et al.			25	80.0
Cherney and Amstutz	5	80.0	28	64.0
Fitzgerald			111	90.0
Jupiter et al.	18	78.1		
Salvati et al.	31	91.0	28	89.0
Salvati et al.	14	86.0	18	94.5
McDonald et al.			82	86.6
Lieberman and Salvati et al.			32	91.0
Total	123	70.6	334	81.9

The use of antibiotic loaded cement which fills the dead space created at the time of resection arthroplasty has been advocated.[126,127] This technique was originally described by Hovelius and Josefsson with cement beads.[128] Increased doses of antibiotics with significantly greater elution can be used if the cement is not used to stabilize an implant.[129,130] The Prostalac system was developed by Duncan and Masri to fill the dead space with a functional spacer and provide very high elution of local antibiotics after the first stage of a two stage reimplantation.[131–135] In 1993, Duncan and Masri reported on 59 patients treated with this technique noting a simplified reimplantation and only a 6% rate of recurrence.[134,135] While this technique is promising, further study is warranted to verify its success.

Three-Stage Reconstruction
The technique of "three-stage exchange" has been introduced by Fitzgerald et al. for patients with severe bone loss. The initial stage includes removal of the prosthesis, debridement of the soft tissues and bone cement, and postoperative intravenous antibiotic treatment for 4 to 6 weeks. The second stage involves massive bone grafting of large osseous defects to restore the bone integrity. The third stage, after a delay of nine months, entails the insertion of a cementless prosthesis. This technique is quite costly and may require the design of a custom made prosthesis.

Resection Arthroplasty
Excision arthroplasty was first described by White in 1849, and later popularized by Girdlestone who demonstrated that this was an effective procedure at eradicating infection in the hip joint. In 1950, Taylor reported that the results of this operation were satisfactory in elderly patients.[134] He also noted improved results if the acetabular rim was beveled, thus reducing bony impingement.

Unfortunately, the functional outcome was less than satisfactory as noted by several authors.[137] In separate series, Grauer et al. and Canner et al. noted decreased satisfaction in patients with resection arthroplasty.[138,139] The only recent favorable study was that of Marchetti et al. who reported 72% satisfactory results.[140] Problems associated with a resection arthroplasty include difficulty with weight-bearing requiring external support to ambulate, shortening requiring lifts from 3 to 5 cm under the sole and heel, incomplete resolution of pain, and poor active motion.

Patients with an infected total hip arthroplasty that are not suitable for reimplantation should be treated definitively with a resection arthroplasty.[141,142] Such patients include elderly nonambulatory, demented, or uncooperative patients as well as patients at increased risk for reinfection such as intravenous drug abusers and patients with recurrent infections. Other indications for a resection arthroplasty are inadequate bone stock, poor soft tissue, antibiotic resistance to the infecting organism, medical contraindications to further surgery, and the poor potential for rehabilitation.

The Economic Impact of Infected Total Hip Arthroplasty

The treatment of an infected total hip arthroplasty is potentially very expensive, and the utilization of economic resources varies considerably depending upon the treatment protocol.[143–145] In managing a patient with an infected total hip arthroplasty, the ultimate goals are to eradicate the infection and maintain a stable and functional joint. Surgical treatment options such as open debridement, primary exchange, two-stage reconstruction, and three-stage reimplantation each have their associated rates of success and variable costs. For example, debridement with prolonged parenteral antibiotics is usually unsuccessful and costly for the management of deep periprosthetic infection.[130] While a one stage reconstruction for an infected hip arthroplasty is less costly than a two-stage reimplantation, the results, by and large, are not as successful.

Home administration of antibiotics with supportive health care providers is another alternative which can cost between three to four hundred dollars a day. However, this may not provide continuity in dosage and administration, thus preventing the eradication of the periprosthetic infection.[145] Unfortunately, such care is not currently reimbursed for the Medicare patient. Nursing homes in urban areas usually do not have the availability of beds for such type of short term care, and a new diagnostic-related group payment has not been issued to the hospitals for readmission.

Sculco reports that in the state of New York, Medicare reimbursement for the treatment of an infected hip arthroplasty is about $28,000. In contrast, the cost of care for the treatment of an infected total hip arthroplasty averages $58,000. This results in a loss of $30000 to the institution for each infected hip arthroplasty treated.[145] At HSS 80% of the infected total hip replacements treated were implanted elsewhere. Physician reimbursement for this procedure includes the 6 weeks of care and daily visits to the patient. The payment is unreflective of the complexity and potential complications of reimplantation. Referrals to specialized orthopedic institutions results in a monetary loss to the hospital and inadequate reimbursement to the experienced arthroplasty surgeon. Most institutions are currently monitoring such referrals to reduce hospital stay, cost and increase reimbursement.

Conclusion

The management of the infected endoprosthesis at The Hospital for Special Surgery has been based on the time and mode of presentation, virulence, antibiotic sensitivity and bacteriology of the infection, the clinical status of the patient, and the condition of the hip. Early infections have been treated by immediate incision, debridement, and primary closure over closed suction (for 1 to 2 days only). In these early infections, the bone–cement interface is most likely still intact, not yet invaded by the septic process. If recognized early with adequate surgery, there is a chance of salvaging the prosthetic arthroplasty, particularly if the bacterium is highly sensitive to antibiotic therapy.

Late, open, and acute purulent infections have been treated by thorough debridement, including removal of all foreign material, and primary closure over closed-tube suction; and rarely, in badly inflamed cases by open packing, followed a few days later by delayed primary closure over closed-suction. In these cases, reconstruction considerations have been secondary to those of arresting the infection. Although occasionally primary trochanteric reconstructions have been performed, simple resection followed by skeletal traction for 2 weeks have predominated.

Late, closed, subacute infections have also been treated by extensive debridement and removal of all foreign material, followed by a second total hip replacement at the same stage or preferably at a second stage after a minimum interval of 6 weeks. During this period and since 1975, we have used 6 weeks of intravenous antibiotic therapy, producing at least 1:8 post-peak bactericidal serum activity under the supervision of a consultant from the infectious disease division. Inability to obtain 1:8 post-peak bactericidal serum levels, immunodeficiency, frailty of the patient, limited potential for rehabilitation, poor soft tissues, and severe bone loss precluding an adequate biomechanical reconstruction are considered contraindications for reimplantation. Careful preoperative planning prior to reimplantation to obtain a stable and adequate reconstruction is essential. Specific prosthetic components and sophisticated techniques of revision surgery are frequently necessary.

In the majority of patients, routine total hip arthroplasty is a successful operation with highly predictable pain relief and restoration of quasi-normal function. While postoperative complications are quite rare, an infected total hip arthroplasty can be disastrous to both the patient and the surgeon. Fortunately, prompt diagnosis followed by the appropriate treatment may prove successful in the majority of patients. In the current healthcare environment, financial pressure to reduce cost may have a detrimental effect on the successful treatment of an infected total hip arthroplasty. While cost effective modifications of current treatment protocols is rational, one should exercise caution in adopting new protocols until proven success is observed. Reducing the duration of intravenous antibiotic treatment and the abandonment of the two-stage reimplantation protocol for the primary exchange method should proceed with caution.

References

1. Patterson FP, Brown CS. The McKee-Farrar total hip replacement. *J Bone Joint Surg Am*. 1972;53:257–275.
2. Eftekhar NS. *Infection in joint replacement: prevention and management*. St. Louis: CV Mosby, 1984.

3. Fitzgerald RH JR. Infected total hip arthroplasty: diagnosis and treatment. *J Amer Acad Orthop Surg.* 1995;3: 249–262.
4. Wilson MG, Dorr LD. Reimplantation of infected total hip arthroplasties in the absence of antibiotic cement. *J Arthroplasty.* 1989;4:263–269.
5. Anonymous Vital and Health Statistics: National Hospital Discharge Survey—Annual Summary, 1990. 112: 1992. (Abstract)
6. Goodman SB, Schurman DJ. Outcome of infected total hip arthroplasty: an inclusive and consecutive series. *J Arthroplasty.* 1988;3:109–116.
7. Hunter G, Dandy D. The natural history of the patient with an infected hip replacement. *J Bone Joint Surg Br.* 1977;59:293–297.
8. James ETR, Hunter GA, Cameron HU. Total hip revision arthroplasty: does sepsis influence the results. *Clin Orthop.* 1982;170:88–94.
9. Pagano MW, Trousdale RT, Hanssen AD. Patient outcome after reinfection following reimplantation for the infected total hip arthroplasty. *Orthop Trans.* 1996;20:68–69.
10. Wroblewski BM. Revision of infected hip arthroplasty. *J Bone Joint Surg Br.* 1983;65:224–225.
11. Wroblewski BM. One-stage revision of infected cemented total hip arthroplasty. *Clin Orthop.* 1986;211:103–107.
12. Fitzgerald RH Jr, Nolan DR, Ilstrup DM, Van Scoy RE, Coventry MB. Deep wound sepsis following total hip arthroplasty. *J Bone Joint Surg Am.* 1977;59:847–855.
13. Fitzgerald RH Jr, Peterson LFA, Washington JA, Van Scoy RE, Coventry MB. Bacterial colonization of wounds and sepsis in total hip arthroplasty. *J Bone Joint Surg Am.* 1973;55:1242–1251.
14. Lieberman JR, Callaway GH, Salvati EA, et al. Treatment of the infected total hip arthroplasty with a two-stage reimplantation protocol. *Clin Orthop.* 1994;205–212.
15. Tannenbaum DA, Matthews LS, Grady-Benson JC. Infection around joint replacements in patients who have a renal or liver transplantation. *J Bone Joint Surg Am.* 1997;79:36–43.
16. Pisciotta A, Westring D, Deprey C, Walsh B. Mitogenic effect of phytohaemagglutinin at different ages. *Nature.* 1967;215:193–194.
17. Costerton JW, Geesey CG, Cheng KJ. How bacteria stick. *Sci Am.* 1978;238:86–95.
18. Vaudaux PE, Walvogel FA, Morgenthaler JJ, Nydegger UE. Absorption of fibronectin onto polymethylmethacrylate and promotion of *Staphylococcus aureus* adherence. *Infect Immun.* 1984;45:768–774.
19. Gristina AG. Bacterial adherence and the glycocalyx and their role in musculoskeletal infection. *Orth Clin North Am.* 1984;15:517–535.
20. Agins HJ, Alcock NW, Bansal M, Salvati EA, Wilson PD Jr, Pellicci PM, et al. A histologica and quantitative analysis of metallic wear in failed titanium alloy/ultra high molecular weight polyethylene (UHMWPE) total hip replacements. *J Bone Joint Surg Am.* 1988;70:347–356.
21. Ascherl R, Stemberger A, Lechner F. Behandlung der chronischen osteomylitis mit einem kollagen-antibiotica-verbund-vorlaufige mitteilung. *Unfallchirurgie.* 1996;12: 125–127.
22. Rae T. The toxicity of metals used in orthopaedic prostheses: an experimental study using cultured human synovial fibroblasts. *J Bone Joint Surg Br.* 1981;62:435.
23. Gristina AG, Giridhar G, Gabriel BL, Naylor PT, Myrvik QN. Cell biology and molecular mechanisms in artificial device infections. *Int J Artificial Organs.* 1993;16:755–763.
24. Ainskow DAP, Denham RA. The risk of hematogonous infection in total hip replacement. *J Bone Joint Surg Br.* 1984;66:580–582.
25. Inman JN, Gallegos KV, Brause BD, Redecha PB, Christian CL. Clinical and microbial features of prosthetic joint infection. *Am J Med.* 1984;77:47–53.
26. Emerton MA, Crook DW, Cooke PH. Streptococcus-bovis-infected total hip arthroplasty. *J Arthroplasty.* 1995;10:554–555.
27. Small CB, Slater LN, Lowry FD, et al. Group B Streptococcal arthritis in adults. *Am J Med.* 1984;76:367–375.
28. Brause BD. Microbiology of prosthetic joint infection. In *Total hip revision surgery,* Galante JO, Rosenberg AG, Callaghan JJ eds. New York, Raven Press, 1995; 461–468.
29. Garvin KL, Fitzgerald RH JR, Salvati EA, et al. Reconstruction of the infected total hip and knee arthroplasty with gentamicin-impregnated Palacos bone cement. *Instr Course Lect.* 1993;42:293–302.
30. Garvin KL, Hanssen AD. Infection after total hip arthroplasty. *J Bone Joint Surg Am.* 1995;77:1576–1588.
31. Evans RP, Nelson CL. Staged reimplantation of a total hip prosthesis after infection with candida albicans: a report of two cases. *J Bone Joint Surg Am.* 1990;72: 1551–1553.
32. Lim EVA, Stern P. Candida infection after implant arthroplasty: a case report. *J Bone Joint Surg Am.* 1986; 68:143–145.
33. Brown WJ, Microbiology of the infected total joint arthroplasty. *Sem Arthroplasty.* 1994;5:107–113.
34. Gristina AG. Biomaterial-centered infection: microbial adhesion versus tissue integration. *Science.* 1987;237:1588–1595.
35. Gristina AG. Biofilms and chronic bacterial infections. *Clin Microbiol Newsletter.* 1994;16:171–176.
36. Gristina AG. Implant failure and immuno-incompetent fibro-inflammatory zone. *Clin Orthop.* 1994;298:106–118.
37. Gristina AG, Costerton JW. Bacterial adherence to biomaterial and tissue: the significance of its role in clinical sepsis. *J Bone Joint Surg Am.* 1985;67:264–273.
38. Coventry MB. Treatment of infections occurring in total hip surgery. *Orthop Clin North Am.* 1975;6:991–1003.
39. Estrada R, Tsukayama D, Gustilo R. Management of THA infections. A prospective study of 108 cases. *Orthop Trans.* 1993;17:1114–1115.
40. Hughes PW, Salvati EA, Wilson PD, Blumenfeld EL. Treatment of subacute sepsis of the hip by antibiotics and joint replacement: criteria for diagnosis and evaluation of twenty-six cases. *Clin Orthop.* 1979;141:143–157.
41. Burger RR, Basch T, Hopson CN. Implant salvage in infected total knee arthroplasty. *Clin Orthop.* 1991;273:105–112.
42. Bauer TW, Saltarelli MG. Infection vs aseptic loosening in revision arthroplasty: predictive value of frozen section and other laboratory tests. *Orthop Trans.* 1993;17: 1054.
43. Sanzen L, Carlsson AS, Josefsson G, Lindberg LT. Revision operations on infected total hip arthroplasties: two to nine year follow-up study. *Clin Orthop.* 1988;229: 172–187.

44. O'Neill DA, Harris WH. Failed total hip replacement: assessment by plain radiographs, arthrogram, and aspiration of the hip joint. *J Bone Joint Surg Am*. 1984;66:540–546.
45. Nemec B, Matovinovic D, Gulan G, et al. Idiopathic osteolysis of the acetabulum: a case report. *J Bone Joint Surg Br*. 1996;78:666–667.
46. Capello WN, Uri BG, Wellman HN, Ross JA, Stiver PL. Comparison of radiographic and radionuclide hip arthrography in determination of femoral component loosening of hip arthroplasties. *Hip*. 1985:157–168.
47. Johnson JA, Christie MJ, Sandler MP, Parks PF, Homra L, Kaye JJ. Detection of occult infection following total joint arthroplasty using sequential technitium-99m HDP bone scintigraphy and indium-111 WBC imaging. *J Nucl Med*. 1988;29:1347–1353.
48. Rushton N, Coakley AJ, Tudor J, Wraight EP. The value of technetium and galium scanning in assessing pain after total hip replacement. *J Bone Joint Surg Br*. 1983;64:313–318.
49. Maurer AH, Chen DCP, Camargo EE, et al. Utility of three-phase skeletal scintigraphy in suspected osteomyelitis: concise communication. *J Nucl Med*. 1981;22:941.
50. Lieberman JR, Huo MH, Schneider R, Salvati EA, Rodi S. Evaluation of painful hip arthroplasties: are technetium bone scans necessary? *J Bone Joint Surg Br*. 1993;75:475–478.
51. Propst-Proctor SL, Dillingham MF, McDougall IR, Goodwin D. The white blood cell scan in orthopedics. *Clin Orthop*. 1982;168:157–165.
52. Merkel KD, Fitzgerald RH Jr, Brown ML. Scintigraphic examination of total hip arthroplasty: comparison of indium with gallium-technetium in the loose and infected canine arthroplasty. *Hip*. 1984:163–192.
53. Deysine M, Rafkin H, Russell R, et al. The detection of acute experimental osteomyelitis with Ga citrate scannings. *Surg Gynecol Obstet*. 1975;141:40–42.
54. Fehring TK, McAlister JA Jr, Cohen BE, Griffin WL. In: *Total hip revision surgery*. Galante JO, Rosenberg AG, Callaghan JJ. eds. New York: Raven Press, 1995:469–486.
55. Fehring TK, McAlister JA Jr, Cohen BE, Griffin WL. Aspiration and frozen histological section as guides to sepsis in revision total hip arthroplasty. In: *Total hip revision surgery*. Galante JO, Rosenberg AG, Callaghan JJ. eds. New York: Raven Press, 1995.
56. Lachiewicz PF, Rogers GD, Thomason HC. Aspiration of the hip joint before revision total hip arthroplasty. *J Bone Joint Surg Am*. 1996;78:749–754.
57. Mulcahy DM, Fenlon CC, McInerney DP. Aspiration arthrography of the hip joint: its uses and limitations in revision hip surgery. *J Arthroplasty*. 1996;11:64–68.
58. Andrews HL, Arden GP, Hart GM, Owen JW. Deep infection after total hip replacement. *J Bone Joint Surg Br*. 1981;63:53–57.
59. Eftehar NS. Wound infection complicating total hip joint arthroplasty. *Orthop Rev*. 1979;8:49–64.
60. Kreder HJ, Davey JR. Total hip arthroplasty complicated by tuberculous infection. *J Arthroplasty*. 1996;11:111–114.
61. Barrack RL, Harris WH. The value of aspiration of the hip joint before revision total hip arthroplasty. *J Bone Joint Surg Am*. 1993;75:66–76.
62. McCarthy C, Steinberg G, Wyman E, et al. Quantitation of bone resorption of the proximal femur in total hip arthroplasty (abstract). *J Bone Miner Res*. 1990;5:178.
63. Lonner JH, Desai P, Dicesare PE, Steiner G, Zuckerman JD. The reliability of analysis of intraoperative frozen sections for identifying active infection during revision hip or knee arthroplasty. *J Bone Joint Surg*. 1996;78:1553–1558.
64. Feldman DS, Lonner JH, Desai P, Zuckerman JD. The role of intraoperative frozen sections in revision total joint arthroplasty. *J Bone Joint Surg Am*. 1995;77:1807–1813.
65. Frank CJ, Garvin KL, Fox CE, et al. Analysis of the accuracy of preoperative studies in the diagnosis of periprosthetic infection in 105 hip arthroplasty revisions. *Orthop Trans*. 1996;20:68.
66. Balderston RA, Hiller WDB, Ianotti JP. Treatment of the septic hip with total hip arthroplasty. *Clin Orthop*. 1987;221:231–237.
67. Cherney DL, Amstutz HC. Total hip replacement in the previous septic hip. *J Bone Joint Surg Am*. 1983;65:1256–1265.
68. Jupiter JB, Karchmer AW, Lowell JD, Harris WH. Total hip arthroplasty in the treatment of adult hips with current or quiescent sepsis. *J Bone Joint Surg Am*. 1981;63:194–200.
69. Charnley J. *Low-friction arthroplasty of the hip: theory and practice*. New York: Springer-Verlag, 1979.
70. Aglietti P, Salvati EA, Wilson PD, Kutner LJ. Effect of surgical unidirectional filtered air flow unit on wound healing. *Clin Orthop*. 1974;101:99.
71. Lidwell OM, Lowbury EJJ, Whyte W, et al. Effect of ultraclean air in operating rooms on deep sepsis in the joint after total hip or knee replacement: a randomized study. *Br Med J*. (Clin Res Ed). 1982;285:10–14.
72. Salvati EA, Robinson RP, Zeno SM, et al. Infection rates after 3175 total hip and total knee replacements performed with and without a horizontal unidirectional filtered airflow system. *J Bone Joint Surg Am*. 1982;64:525–535.
73. Soave R, Hirsch J, Salvati EA, et al. Comparison of Ceforanide and Cephalothin prophylaxis in patients undergoing total joint arthroplasty. *Orthopedics*. 1986;9:1657–1660.
74. Hill C, Mazas F, Flamant R, Evrard J. Prophylactic Cefazolin versus placebo in total hip replacement. *Lancet*. 1981;8224:795.
75. Sandusky WR. Use of prophylactic antibiotics in surgical patients. *Surg Clin North Am*. 1980;60:83–92.
76. Burke JF. The effective period of preventable antibiotic action in experimental incisions and dermal lesions. *Surgery*. 1961;50:161–168.
77. Coleman DL, Horowitz RI, Andriole VT. Association between serum inhibitory and bactericidal concentration and therapeutic outcome in bacterial endocarditis. *Am J Med*. 1982;73:260–267.
78. Wiggins CE, Nelson CL, Clarke R, Thompson CH. Concentration of antibiotics in normal bone after intravenous injection. *J Bone Joint Surg Am*. 1978;60:93–96.
79. Parker RH, Schmid FR. Antibacterial activity of synovial fluid during therapy for septic arthritis. *Arthritis Rheum*. 1971;14:96–104.
80. Schurman DJ, Hirschman HP, Kajiyama G, Moser K,

Burton DS. Cefazolin concentrations in bone and synovial fluid. *J Bone Joint Surg Am*. 1978;60:359–362.
81. Wilson FC, Worchester NN, Coleman PD, Byrd WE. Antibiotic penetration of experimental bone hematomas. *J Bone Joint Surg Am*. 1971;53:1622–1628.
82. Petty W, Spanier S, Shuster JJ, Silverthorne C. The influence of skeletal implants on incidence of infection: Experiments in a canine model. *J Bone Joint Surg Am*. 1985;67:1236–1244.
83. Petty W. Quantative determination of the effect of antimicrobial irrigating solutions on bacterial contamination of experimental wound. *J Bone Joint Surg Am*. 1985;67: 1236.
84. Fenelon GCC, Von Foerster G, Engelbrecht E. Disarticulation of the hip as a result of failed arthroplasty: A series of 11 cases. *J Bone Joint Surg Br*. 1980;62:441–446.
85. Fitzgerald RH Jr. The infected total hip arthroplasty. Current concepts in treatment. In: *The Hip*, Welch RB ed. St. Louis: CV Mosby, 1984.
86. Fitzgerald RH. Treatment of the infected total hip arthroplasty: indirect exchange arthroplasty. In: *Revision total hip arthroplasty*. pp. 495–508. Galante JO, Rosenberg AG, Callaghan JJ eds. New York: Raven Press, 1995.
87. Fitzgerald RH Jr. Diagnosis and management of the infected hip prosthesis. *Orthopedics*. 1995;18:833–835.
88. Fitzgerald RH Jr. Treatment of the infected total hip arthroplasty. 1996.(Abstract)
89. Masri BA, Salvati EA, Duncan CP. Revision replacement for the infected implant. *Bombay Hosp J*. 1996;38:532–545.
90. Ross AC. Salvage of the infected arthroplasty. *Ann Rheum Dis*. 1992;51:910–913.
91. Thornhill TS. Total joint infection—significance, incidence, risk factors, diagnosis, prophylaxis. 1996. (Abstract)
92. Blomgren G, Lindgren V. Revision Arthroplsaty. 1983, (Abstract); 46.
93. Muller ME. Preservation of the septic total hip replacement versus Girdlestone operation. In: The hip: proceedings of the second scientific meeting of the hip society. Wech RB, ed. St. Louis: CV Mosby, 1974.
94. Murray RP, Bourne MH, Fitzgerald RH. Metachronous infections in patients who have more than one total joint arthroplasty. *J Bone Joint Surg Am*. 1991;73:1469–1474.
95. Wood WB Jr, Smith MR. An experimental analysis of the curvature action of penicillin in acute bacterial infections. I. The relationship of the antimicrobial effect of penicillin. II. The role of phagocytic cells in the process of recovery. III. The effect of suppuration upon the antibacterial action of the drug. *J Exp Med*. 1956;103:487,499,509.
96. Goulet JA, Pellicci PM, Brause BD, Salvati EM. Prolonged suppression of infection in total hip arthroplasty. *J Arthroplasty*. 1988;3:97–102.
97. Drancourt M, Stein A, Argenson JN, et al. Oral rifampin plus ofloxacin for treatment of Staphylococcus-infected orthopedic implants. *Antimicrob Agents Chemother*. 1993; 37:1214–1218.
98. Widmer AF, Gaechter A, Ochsner PE, et al. Antimicrobial treatment of orthopedic implant-related infections with rifampin combinations. *Clin Infect Dis*. 1992;14:1251–1253.
99. Turner RH, Miley GB, Fremont-Smith P. Septic total hip replacement and revision arthroplasty. In: *Revision total hip arthroplasty*. Turner RH, Scheller AD, ed. New York: Grune & Stratton, 1982.
100. Berman AT, Johnson MD III. The use of Hickman catheter in orthopaedic infections. *J Bone Joint Surg Am*. 1985;67: 650–651.
101. Younger TI, Bradford MS, Magnus RE, Paprosky WG. Extended proximal femoral osteotomy. *J Arthroplasty*. 1995;10:329–338.
102. Collins DN, Garvin KL, Nelson CL. The use of the vastus lateralis flap in patients with intractable infection after resection arthroplasty following the use of a hip implant. *J Bone Joint Surg Am*. 1987;69:510.
103. Gustilo RB, Tsukayama D. Treatment of infected cemented total hip arthroplasty with tobramycin beads and delayed revision with a cementless prosthesis and bone grafting. *Orthop Trans*. 1988;12:739.
104. Bucholz HW. Management of deep infection of total hip arthroplasty. *J Bone Joint Surg Br*. 1981;63:342–353.
105. Bucholz HW, Engelbrecht H. Uber die Depotwwirkung einiger Antibitica bei Vermischung mit dem Kunstharz Palacos. *Chirurg*. 1970;41:511–515.
106. Bucholz HW, Engelbrecht H. Erkenntnisse nach wascgel von uber 400 infizierten hugtendoprothesen. *Orthop Praxis*. 1996;12:1117–1123.
107. Elson R, Norman P, Scott I, Stockley I. Exchange cemented joint arthroplasties for deep infection. *J Bone Joint Surg Br*. 1992;74(Suppl III):295.
108. Elson RA. Exchange arthroplasty for infection. Perspectives from the United Kingdom. *Ortho Clin N Am*. 1996;24: 761–767.
109. Gehrke T, VonFoerster G, Frommelt L, Marx A. Elution properties of a gentamicin-clindamycin impregnated bone cement in one stage revision arthroplasty. *Orthop Trans*. 1996;20:68.
110. Raut VV, Siney PD, Wroblewski BM. One-stage revision of total hip arthroplasty for deep infection: long-term followup. *Clin Orthop*. 1995;321:202–207.
111. Salvati EA. Primary exchange of the infected total hip replacement. In: *Revision total hip arthroplasty*, pp. 487–494. Galante JO, Rosenberg AG, Callaghan JJ, ed. New York: Raven Press, 1995.
112. Carlsson AS, Engund A, Gentz C. Radiographic loosening after revision with gentamicin-containing cement for deep infection in total hip arthroplasties. *Clin Orthop*. 1985;194:271–279.
113. Salvati EA, Callaghan JJ, Brause BD, et al. Reimplantation in infection: elution of gentamicin from cement and beads. *Clin Orthop*. 1986;207:83–93.
114. Salvati EA, Chekofsky KM, Brause BD. Reimplantation in infection: a 12 year experience. *Clin Orthop*. 1982;170:62–75.
115. Callaghan JJ, Salvati EA, Brause BD, Rimnac CM, Wright TM. Reimplantation for salvage of the infected hip: Rationale for the use of gentamicin-impregnated cement and beads. 651986. *Hip*. 1985:65–94.
116. McDonald DJ, Fitzgerald RH Jr, Ilstrup DM. Two-stage reconstruction of a total hip arthroplasty because of infection. *J Bone Joint Surg Am*. 1989;71:828–834.
117. Carlsson AS, Joeffson G, Lindberg L. Revision with gentamicin impregnated cement for deep infections in total hip arthroplasty. *J Bone Joint Surg Am*. 1978;60:1059–1064.
118. Eitenmuller J, Schmidt KH, Peters G, et al. Experimental and preliminary clinical experience with absorbable calcium phosphate granules containing an antibiotic or an-

tiseptic for the local treatment of osteomyelitis. *J Hospital Infection.* 1985;6:177–184.
119. Lautenschlager EP, Jacobs JJ, Marshall GW, Meyer PW. Mechanical properties of bone cements containing large doses of antibiotic powder. *J Biomed Mater Res.* 1976;10: 929–938.
120. Lautenschlager EP, Marshall GW, Marks KE, Schwartz J, Nelson CL. Mechanical strength of acrylic bone cements impregnated with antibiotics. *J Biomed Mater Res.* 1976;10: 837–845.
121. Steinbrink K. The case for revision arthroplasty using antibiotic-loaded acrylic cement. *Clin Orthop.* 1990;261:19–22.
122. Brien WW, Salvati EA, Klein R, Brause B, Stern S. Antibiotic impregnated bone cement in total hip arthroplasty. An in vivo comparison of the elution properties of tobramycin and vancomycin. *Clin Orthop.* 1993;296:242–248.
123. Nestor BJ, Hanssen AD, Ferrer-Gonzalez R, Fitzgerald RH Jr. The use of porous prostheses in delayed reconstruction of total hip replacements that have failed because of infection. *J Bone Joint Surg Am.* 1994;76:349–359.
124. Hope P, Kristinsson KG, Norman P, Elson RA. Deep infection of cemented total hip arthroplasty caused by coagulase-negative Staphylococci. *J Bone Joint Surg Br.* 1989; 71:851–855.
125. Murray WR. Use of antibiotic-containing bone cement. *Clin Orthop.* 1984;190:89–95.
126. McLaren AC, Spooner CE. Antibiotic spacer arthroplasty in the staged treatment of infected total joint replacements. *Orthop Trans.* 1996;20:69.
127. Zilkens KW, Casser HR, Ohnsorge J. Treatment of an old infection in a total hip replacement with an interim spacer prosthesis. *Arch Orthop Trauma Surg.* 1990;109:94–96.
128. Hovelius L, Josefsson G. An alternative method for exchange operation of infected arthroplasty. *Acta Orthop Scand.* 1979;50:93–96.
129. Abendschein W. Arthroplasty rounds. Salvage of infected total hip replacement: use of antibiotic/PMMA spacer. *Orthopedics.* 1992;15:228–229.
130. Gerhart TN, Roux RD, Horowitz G, et al. Antibiotic release from experimental biodegradable bone cement. *J Orthop Res.* 1988;6:585–592.
131. Duncan CP, Beauchamp CP. The antibiotic-loaded hip replacement: a valuable tool in the management of the complex infected total hip arthroplasty. *J Bone Joint Surg Br.* 1991;73(Suppl I):115.
132. Duncan CP, Beauchamp CP. Total hip replacement for the management of chronic infection. *J Bone Joint Surg Br.* 1992;74(Suppl III):275.
133. Duncan CP, Beauchamp CP. A temporary antibiotic-loaded joint replacement system for management of complex infections. *Orthop Clin North Am.* 1993;24:751–759.
134. Duncan CP, Masri BA. Antibiotic depots. *J Bone Joint Surg Br.* 1993;75:349–350.
135. Masri BA, Duncan CP, Beauchamp CP. Long-term elution of antibiotics from bone cement: an in vivo study using the PROSTALAC system. *Orthop Trans.* 1996;20:69.
136. Taylor RG. Pseudoarthrosis of the hip joint. *J Bone Joint Surg Br.* 1950;32:161–165.
137. Bourne RB, Hunter GA, Rorabeck CH, Macnab JJ. A six year follow-up of infected total hip replacements managed by Girdlestone's arthroplasty. *J Bone Joint Surg Br.* 1984;66:340–343.
138. Canner CG, Steinberg ME, Heppenstall RB, Balderston R. The infected hip after total hip arthroplasty. *J Bone Joint Surg Am.* 1984;66:1393–1399.
139. Grauer JD, Amstutz HC, O'Caroll PF, Dorey FJ. Resection arthroplasty of the hip. *J Arthroplasty.* 1989;71-A:669–678.
140. Marchetti PG, Toni A, Baldini N, et al. Clinical evaluation of 104 hip resection arthroplasties after removal of a total hip prosthesis. *J Arthroplasty.* 1987;2:37–41.
141. Bittar ES, Petty W. Girdlestone arthroplasty for infected total hip arthroplasty. *Clin Orthop.* 1982;170:83–87.
142. Clegg J. The results of the pseudoarthrosis after removal of an infected total hip prosthesis. *J Bone Joint Surg Br.* 1978;59:298–301.
143. Furnes A, Lie SA, Haveline LI, et al. The economic impact of failures in total hip replacement surgery. *Acta Orthop Scand.* 1996;67:115–121.
144. Sculco TP. The economic impact of infected total joint arthroplasty. *Instr Course Lect.* 1993;42:349–351.
145. Sculco TP. The economic impact of infected joint arthroplasty. *Orthopedics.* 1995;18:871–873.

54
Dislocation Following Total Hip Arthroplasty

John P. McCabe, Paul M. Pellicci, and Eduardo A. Salvati

Reports of complications of total hip arthroplasty and strategies for management have increased in proportion to the accelerated growth of the procedure as a routine orthopedic operation. With the advent of the revision hip surgery era, the occurrence of postoperative hip dislocation has become perhaps the most taxing complication to the arthroplasty surgeon. Dislocation now ranks as the most common clinically apparent complication of hip arthroplasty. The reported incidence has ranged from under 1% to 10% in various clinical series.[1,2] In primary total hip arthroplasty, a 2% to 3% dislocation rate is probably representative of the overall occurrence. With more than 120 000 hip arthroplasties performed annually in the U.S. and accepting a reoperation rate for dislocation of one-third of dislocations, the total number of reoperations performed annually for dislocation is 1200. Experience of a single arthroplasty surgeon with dislocation, however, is usually limited to a small number of cases annually. A thorough understanding of factors involved in dislocation assists in prevention and helps outline the strategy for operative management in the recurrent case. This chapter reviews perioperative factors associated with dislocation and summarizes current approaches to management.

Incidence

By definition, dislocation is present when there is no contact between the two articulating surfaces of a joint. However, a dislocation is part of a spectrum ranging from neck impingement to subluxation before frank dislocation occurs. Instances of impingement/subluxation may be missed whereas, except in rare cases, dislocation is usually quite dramatic with pain and an inability to bear weight, bringing the patient to the immediate attention of the surgeon. Unrecognized dislocation occasionally occurs in the patient with a neurological disorder, senile dementia, or alcoholism. The end point of the problem of hip instability is therefore easier to define and study. A wide variation of reported occurrence of this complication exists in the literature. A review by Morrey of 35 894 procedures reported in 16 studies in the literature between 1973 and 1987 yielded 804 dislocations, suggesting a rate of 2.2%.[3] At the Mayo Clinic, the reported incidence with more than 10 500 total hip arthroplasties is 3.2%.[4] Khan et al. have documented an incidence of 2.1% after 6774 arthroplasties in a multicenter study.[5] The lowest dislocation rate in a large series from one unit has been reported from Wrightington Hospital in England by Etienne, Cupic, and Charnley.[6] The incidence in 8526 low-friction arthroplasties was reduced from 0.8% to 0.4% over the study period. More recently, the same unit has also reported an overall incidence of 0.63% in a review of 14 672 Charnley arthroplasties.[1]

Mechanism

The majority of cases probably occur as a direct effect of initial impingement of the neck of the stem on the rim of the socket. This is followed by the head levering out of the socket to a point of no return, where there is no contact between the two articulating surfaces. The range of motion at which the impingement occurs is a function of the design of the implant with regard to the relative depth of the cup and head-to-neck diameter ratio, as well as the anatomic positioning of the components. Postoperative dislocation generally occurs posteriorly with flexion, adduction, and internal rotation of the hip. Retroversion of the socket and/or stem accentuates this propensity. Anterior dislocation of the hip occurs less commonly with extension, adduction, and external rotation. Excessive anteversion of the socket and/or stem predisposes to anterior dislocation.

Another less common potential mechanism for dislocation is distraction of the joint due to iatrogenic shortening at the time of surgery or loss of muscle tone across the joint that tends to occur with revision cases due to loss of the soft tissue sleeve.

Predisposing Factors

A wide variety of factors have been implicated in the occurrence of postoperative hip dislocation in various series. These can be considered with regard to the patient or the surgery.

Patient Factors
- Age
- Sex
- Height/weight
- Medical history
- Underlying hip condition
- Previous hip surgery

Surgical Factors
- Surgeons experience
- Surgical approach
- Prosthesis design
  Acetabular cup design/degree of head capture
  Femoral component head size
  Head–neck ratio
  Femoral offset
- Component orientation
- Limb length inequality
- Trochanteric nonunion/avulsion

Age

There is no evidence that postoperative hip dislocation is a function of age. The mean age of patients with dislocation tends to match that of the general population undergoing arthroplasty.[6]

Sex

Females are at increased risk of dislocation when compared to males. This female-to-male ratio for dislocation has been documented at 2:1 in various series.[4,5] In the Mayo Clinic experience, this difference was statistically significant ($p < 0.001$) when compared to the control population. In late dislocations, occurring 5 years or more after the surgery, the female predominance was even greater, at 3:1 in one series.[7]

Height and Weight

Although it may be postulated that as a result of increased forces across the joint in taller, more obese patients dislocation may occur more frequently, there is no data to support this assertion. The relative importance of these two variables remains unknown.

Medical History

The prior medical history of the patient with regard to neuromuscular conditions and mental confusion would appear to increase the risk of postoperative dislocation. In one series, conditions including alcoholism, uremic psychosis, senile dementia, cerebral palsy, and muscular dystrophy was present in 22% of patients with a single dislocation and 75% of patients with recurrent dislocations, compared to 14% in a control group.[8] In Amstutz series, 16 of 60 patients (24%) have significant mental confusion or neuromuscular problems.[9]

Underlying Hip Condition

There is somewhat conflicting evidence as to whether the underlying diagnosis affects the rate of hip dislocation. In the Mayo Clinic, Morrey has reported no association with the preexisting hip pathology and this has also been reported by other authors.[3,5] However in a multivariate analysis of 10 500 total hip arthroplasties by Woo and Morrey, a higher postoperative dislocation rate occurred with fracture (8.5%), congenital dislocation (7.5%), and avascular necrosis (4.5%), compared to an overall rate of 2.4%. Rates of dislocation from 0% to 18% have been reported in total hip arthroplasty for femoral neck fractures with a mean of 10% in these studies.[10–18] In a literature review of 601 femoral neck fractures treated by total hip arthroplasty, the total number of dislocations was 61 (10.1%), with 15 (2.5%) occurring more than 4 months after the surgery.[19] The factor thought to be responsible in this fracture group is the significantly greater range of motion found in the postoperative period.[20]

Previous Hip Surgery

Prior surgery is a well recognized predisposing factor for postoperative dislocation.[4,8,21] In the Mayo Clinic series, the incidence of dislocation in patients with prior surgery was 4.8% (173 of 7241 patients), compared to 2.4% (158 of 3259 patients) in patients without prior surgery, and this difference was highly significant ($p < 0.001$). In a report by Williams, the incidence of dislocation was 0.6% in primary cases compared to 20% in revision cases in a total of 32 dislocations following 1280 arthroplasties.[21] Patients with extensive soft tissue dissection or resection of bone were particularly prone to dislocation. In one series of acetabular revisions with metal ring supports, the dislocation rate was 33% (7 of 21).[22] Prior hip surgery is therefore a major risk factor in the postoperative hip dislocation.

Surgeon's Experience

There is no doubt that surgical outcome in general is dependent upon the relative experience of the operating surgeon. In relation to dislocation, the relative importance of a surgeon's experience has not been extensively studied. The yearly incidence of postoperative dislocation at Wrightington Hospital diminished over the ten years from 1966 to 1975, from 0.8% to 0.4%, reflecting the increased experience.[6] Fackler and Poss noted a lower dislocation rate in the surgeons who performed the most arthroplasties.[8] Similiarly, in a study by Lewinnek et al., the most experienced surgeon had a dislocation rate of 0.5% (1 in 190 cases) compared to the overall rate of 3% (9 in 300 cases).[23] A further study of 3199 Charnley total hip arthroplasties in two Swedish centers showed a significantly higher dislocation rate of 8.1% ($p < 0.05$) when performed by surgeons in the first year of training compared with a rate of 3.0% when performed by others.[24] However, the most experienced surgeons and surgeons who performed less than 10 arthroplasties in the series were not shown to have a statistically significant difference in terms of dislocation rate. More recently, a Swedish study of 4230 primary total hip arthroplasties performed using the posterior approach at three centers revealed twice the number of dislocations with inexperienced surgeons.[25] The frequency of dislocation leveled off with increasing numbers of operations and remained constant after approximately 30 cases. For every ten primary cases performed annually, the risk of dislocation decreased by 50%. It therefore appears that experience is an important factor in reducing the incidence of postoperative dislocation.

Surgical Approach

The exact influence of this variable is somewhat controversial and few studies address the issue. Most surgeons or institutions use one approach and are therefore unable to compare the influence of surgical approach on rate of dislocation. A number of studies suggest that the surgical approach is not a significant factor.[5,24,26] Khan et al. found no difference in the risk of dislocation with the lateral anterolateral, and posterior approaches, although the study involved many different designs of prosthesis with no attempt to take other variables into account.[5] Hedlundh et al., studying the Charnley prosthesis, showed that the overall incidence of dislocation with the posterior approach (1361 patients) when compared to the transtrochanteric approach (1838 patients) was similar, but there was a much higher rate of early dislocation (within 2 weeks) with the posterior approach.[24] However, the incidence of early dislocation (within 3 months) in a study of 1016 arthroplasties was not significantly different with the anterolateral (1.3%), direct lateral (0.4%), and posterior approaches (1.9%).[26] Only primary procedures were studied, although the type of prosthetic implants used is not recorded.

Others have found the approach to be a major influence.[4,27,28] Robinson reported no dislocations in 130 primary transtrochanteric arthroplasties, compared to a rate of 7.5% in 160 primary posterior arthroplasties.[27] Roberts et al. reported a dislocation rate of 4% in 100 primary arthroplasties by the posterolateral approach and 1.3% in 75 primary arthroplasties by the anterolateral approach.[28] At the Mayo Clinic, the posterior approach was associated with a significantly higher ($p < 0.01$) dislocation rate than the anterior approach regardless of head size of prosthesis used or whether or not prior surgery was performed.[4] In primary cases, the overall dislocation rate was 5.8% with the posterior approach compared to 2.3% with the anterior approach. A recent analysis of a modified direct lateral approach reported no dislocations in 306 primary cases (0%) and 3 dislocations in 115 revision cases (2.6%).[29] At the author's institution, no dislocations have occurred in a series of 390 patients undergoing a primary total hip replacement by the senior author, utilizing a posterior approach with a 28-mm head prosthesis. This low dislocation rate is probably due to the meticulous soft tissue repair performed, which includes femoral reattachment of the capsule, short external rotators, and gluteus maximus insertion.

Acetabular Cup Design/Degree of Head Capture

The relative contribution of the actual design of the acetabular cup rather than its orientation after insertion remains largely unstudied. Design of the cup in relation to the degree of head capture leads to increasing constraint that is also dependent on the relative head–neck ratio. The use of an elevation to the posterior wall of the acetabular component has been assessed.[6,30] A combination of keeping the socket low in the acetabulum and using a long posterior wall (LPW) cup resulted in a decrease in the dislocation rate from 0.8% in 3820 arthroplasties to 0.4% in 4706 arthroplasties performed after 1972 at Wrightington Hospital.[6] Nicholas et al. in a series of mechanical experiments demonstrated that higher moments are required to dislocate an augmented all-polyethylene or LPW all-polyethylene cup than a standard polyethylene cup.[31] Finite element modeling has also supported the importance of acetabular component design in prevention of dislocation.[32] In the Mayo Clinic experience of 5167 arthroplasties, an elevated-rim acetabular liner used in 2469 cases resulted in a two-year probability of dislocation of 2.19% compared with 3.85% with a standard liner.[30] This favorable outcome with an elevated-rim acetabular liner occurred regardless of the surgical approach used. The angle-bore socket designed for the Charnley prosthesis allows for increased superior and posterior head coverage and has reduced the incidence of dislocation in 400 revision cases from 15% to 2%.[33] Any means used to augment the degree of coverage of the head by the cup may, however, lead to impingement; such impingement may cause earlier loosening of the acetabular component by generating increased torque. This has been thought particularly likely to occur with the development of more constrained implants for revision surgery. However these implants are effective in preventing dislocation with revision surgery and in operative treatment of recurrent dislocation.

Femoral Component Head Size

The theory that a larger head size would result in a lower dislocation rate was the major motivation in many surgeons changing from a Charnley 22.25 mm head size to sizes up to 32 mm. The reasoning was on the basis that a larger head size would need to undergo greater displacement before dislocation would occur. However this has not been borne out in clinical studies of total hip arthroplasty. No strong relationship exists between head size and dislocation. Many of the lowest dislocation rates have been reported with the 22.25-mm head size.[1,34] Dislocation rates of 2% to 5% have been reported with 32 to 35 mm head sizes.[2,8,21,35] Khan et al. found no significant difference in dislocation rates when comparing five different implants.[5] Carlsson and Gentz noted a dislocation rate of 4.8% in 351 implants with a 22-mm head compared to a rate of 3.1% in 194 implants with a 35-mm head.[36] Morris et al. noted a dislocation rate of 3.5% in 313 Charnley implants with a 22-mm head compared to no dislocations in 97 McKee implants with a 41-mm head.[37] In neither study was there a statistically significant difference. Woo and Morrey found no significant difference in the rate of dislocation using 22-mm, 28-mm or 32-mm femoral head sizes in 3353 hip replacements.[4] The surgical approach did not influence the rate of dislocation with these head sizes. Large head size, therefore, does not protect against dislocation in the 22 to 32 mm range.

Head Neck Ratio and Femoral Offset

Apart from a discussion of the contribution of head size to stability, other important variables in the femoral component include the head/neck ratio and the femoral offset. Various prostheses have different ranges of motion before impingement and dislocation occurs.[38,39] This is a function of the head-to-neck diameter ratio. The higher the ratio for a given acetabular cup, the greater the possible range of motion. In an experimental model using a specifically designed apparatus Amstutz et al. demonstrated the effect of head-to-neck diameter ratio for various prostheses on range of motion.[38] This range of motion was also significantly affected by the orientation of the components and the degree of socket wear. Wear of the socket results in a deepened socket, causing the neck to impinge at a smaller range of motion. Chandler et al. confirmed the importance of head–neck ratio and also showed the contribution of neck length, using the same experimental model.[40] Sir John Charnley recognized the importance of a reduced diameter neck in preventing dislocation and, with the introduction of a very tough stainless steel (Ortron, Chas. F. Thackray Ltd), reduced the neck diameter of his prosthesis from 12.5 mm to 10 mm. The head–neck ratio was therefore increased in 1983, from 1.78:1 to 2.25:1, to make it comparable to other prostheses with larger head diameter. However the relative clinical importance of head–neck ratio in preventing dislocation has not been studied in any great detail. The increased risk of dislocation with collar reinforced modular heads that decrease the head–neck ratio, has received some attention.[41]

A decrease in the distance from the tip of the greater trochanter to the center of the femoral head increases the chance of impingement and reduces the tension in the abductors. This change in the femoral offset has been studied by Fackler and Poss and found to be significantly decreased in patients with postoperative dislocation ($p < 0.025$).[8] Increasing the offset by osteotomy of the greater trochanter was associated with a reduced risk of dislocation.[42]

Component Orientation

Malposition of the components has long been recognized as an important factor in dislocation. In particular, correct orientation of the cup is a particularly difficult aspect of technique. This results from the inherent difficulty in reproducibly positioning the patient on the operating table as well as problems with obtaining reliable intraoperative landmarks for cup positioning. It is probably technically easier to orient the cup with the patient in the supine position. In the lateral decubitus position, forward rotation of the pelvis leads to inadvertent anteverted positioning of the cup. In the Mayo clinic series, 5 to 7 degree less anteversion occurs with positioning of the cup using the posterior approach.[4]

Postoperative cup orientation is notoriously difficult to measure radiographically, particularly in relation to version rather than cup abduction.[23,43-48] Attempts have been made to measure the version of the cup from an anteroposterior radiograph using formulas.[23,48] However these techniques are not used as a routine clinically.

In one study by Lewninnek, precise measurement of the orientation of the cup was measured, in nine dislocations out of 300 hip replacements.[23] Anterior dislocation was associated with increased anteversion of the cup, whereas posterior dislocation had no correlation with cup orientation. None of the cups were retroverted more than 4° in the series. A "safe" range of 15+/−10 degrees of anteversion and 40+/−10 degrees of abduction was described by these researchers. The dislocation rate for cups oriented within this range was 1.5%, compared with a rate of 6% if the cup orientation was outside this range ($p < 0.05$). Other researchers have documented malposition of the components as a major cause of dislocation. In Ritter's series, 3 of 7 dislocating hips were adjudged to have component malposition with excessive anteversion of one cup and two femoral components.[2] As with many other studies, the exact orientation of the components in this series is not reported even though malposition is given as a cause of dislocation.[5,34] In the Pellicci and Salvati series, of 14 dislocations, 7 had acetabular malposition.[49] One was too anteverted at 37°, resulting in anterior dislocation. The orientation of the other cups is unspecified. Fackler and Poss found that 44% of 34 patients with dislocation had component malposition compared with 6% in a control group. Excessive femoral anteversion was the most common malposition found. Therefore, in many clinical series malposition of the components is regarded as a major predisposing factor to dislocation.

Limb Length Inequality

Limb length inequality and the associated change in myofascial tension is discussed by many authors as a possible cause of dislocation.[4,6,8,23] However these related factors have not been definitely proven to predispose to dislocation. A number of authors have documented no relationship between leg length and dislocation and have even shown the operated leg to be longer than the contralateral side.[4,8] One study has shown a statistically significant correlation ($p < 0.05$) between shortening of the limb by proximal placement of the implant and dislocation.[36] This finding is in keeping with the Charnley experience, wherein proximal positioning of the pilot hole for the acetabular cup was associated with a 1.2% dislocation rate compared to 0.6% when the pilot hole was more anatomically placed with reference to the teardrop. This remains a factor to be considered, but is of lesser importance than other factors discussed.

Trochanteric Nonunion/Avulsion

Trochanteric osteotomy has declined as an approach for primary total hip replacement. However it is still widely practiced in some revision situations. Nonunion of the trochanter with migration is associated with a much higher risk of dislocation and is an extreme example of loss of myofascial tension. Charnley and Cupic related 28% of 56 dislocations to trochanteric nonunion.[50] Woo and Morrey reported an incidence of dislocation of 17.6% with trochanteric migration of at least 1 cm and 2.8% without migration.[4]

Prevention

A heightened awareness by the arthroplasty surgeon of factors important in causing dislocation allied with meticulous attention to surgical detail should assist in minimizing the risk of dislocation. This process should begin at the preoperative planning stage where a realization of the high risk of dislocation in certain situations such as a patient with multiple prior surgeries, prior dislocation, or neuromuscular problems may dictate a change in the operative plan.

Regardless of the approach used, the surgeon should routinely check the position of the patient on the operating table prior to draping and align the patient in the desired position. We routinely use the lateral decubitus position for the posterolateral approach and secure the patient with pubic, sacral, and posterior thoracic supports. After draping, any alteration of the position of the table or patient should be noted and taken into account when inserting the acetabular component. A wide variety of alignment guides are available to assist in positioning of the acetabular cup. However all techniques depend on the surgeon's estimate, intraoperatively, of the position of the pelvis under the drapes. The true acetabulum is a useful guide for placement of the acetabular component except in patients with severe developmental dysplasia or marked osteophyte formation. The position of the femoral component is somewhat easier to reference with respect to the 90° flexed knee and the lesser and greater trochanters. The acetabular component should at least be placed within the range of the "safe" zone' of $15+/-10°$ of anteversion and $40+/-10°$ of abduction.[23] Neither component should be placed in retroversion. The femoral component should not be anteverted more than 10° and the acetabular component more than about 15°. The acetabular component should not be abducted more than 50°.

Possible dislocation from impingement or distraction is evaluated with trial femoral components in place after trial reduction. The hip is passed through a range of motion from full extension to at least 90° of flexion. Internal and external rotation is assessed in flexion and extension. Straight traction is used to assess relative tissue laxity. Impingement by osteophytes or bony protuberances necessitates excision. At this stage further judgment is required to determine the appropriate neck length and femoral offset for modular components with regard to the preoperative templated plan. Following implantation of the femoral component, a repeat trial reduction is performed. A final decision is made in terms of neck length and femoral offset for modular femoral components. At this stage, the cementless cup offers the advantage of easy exchange of the polyethylene liner to an elevated liner, should the hip be found to dislocate during a functional range of motion. With the original low friction arthroplasty technique, advancement of the greater trochanter, revision, or augmentation of the cemented socket may be the only alternatives after cementing the components.[51]

Attention to detail with regard to repair of tissues divided as part of the approach assists in the prevention of dislocation. Maximizing the surface area for bony apposition and secure fixation are important principles in preventing trochanteric nonunion. This may require additional equipment such as the Wroblewski compression spring device or Dall–Miles clamp and cable system.[1,52] Appropriate soft tissue reconstruction should also be performed for both the direct lateral and posterolateral approaches.

Postoperatively the hip is x-rayed to confirm the located position of the components. A number of measures have been used to decrease the risk of dislocation in the immediate postoperative period. Patients at the Hospital for Special Surgery are immobilized in a Balkan beam bed with balanced suspension slings. At Wrightington Hospital, Charnley used a triangular pillow placed between the legs, preventing marked flexion and adduction. The assistance of experienced staff and patient education in postoperative positioning of the leg are important aspects of care in the prevention of early dislocation.

Treatment

Acute dislocation is usually easily diagnosed by the typical history of acute onset of pain and inability to bear weight, coupled with an examination revealing a malpositioned limb and relative shortness. Examination for movement induces pain and telescoping of the limb with a soft end point is present. The dislocation is confirmed by plain radiographic examination. Posterior dislocation accounts for 75% to 90% of all dislocations, and this direction of the dislocation is strongly influenced by the surgical approach.[4] Patients who present late with dislocation have a higher risk of redislocation (60%) compared with patients who dislocate in the first five weeks following surgery (40%).[8] The overall risk of recurrence is around 33%.[4]

Nonoperative Treatment

Expedient treatment is instituted in the case of an acutely dislocated prosthesis. Closed reduction is possible in over 90% of patients.[8] It may be attempted using either intravenous sedation with morphine or midazolam HCL or with regional or general anesthesia. Image intensification assists the closed reduction by allowing direct visualization of the attempted reduction maneuver and quickly confirming reduction.

Following reduction it is useful to test the limits of stability of the hip in various directions, which also indicates the relative ease whereby a further dislocation may occur. A percutaneous adductor tenotomy may be performed if this muscle group is excessively tight. Occasionally an open reduction is required, although surgery is usually reserved for cases where an obvious cause is present or for recurrence. An argument can be made for elective operative intervention in a patient with an obvious reason for the dislocation such as component malalignment, even after a single dislocation.

This approach is associated with a high rate of success.[57]

With closed reduction, further nonoperative management such as bed rest, cast, or brace should be instituted and tends to be effective in at least two-thirds of cases. In Charnley's experience, just over 20% of cases recurred.[6] Ritter reported that casting for six weeks was successful in 63% of patients.[2] He has also stressed the importance of aspirating the affected hip to remove excess fluid that may be compounding the dislocation as well as outruling infection as a cause.[53] Efthekar used either a spica cast or abduction splint for 4 to 12 weeks in three grossly unstable hips and prevented further dislocation.[34] Spica casting for 6 weeks in another series of 16 patients reported by Williams was successful in all but one patient.[21] Fackler and Poss showed that traction or suspension in bed for 6 weeks following dislocation did not reduce the rate of further dislocation and recommended early ambulation with the patient educated to avoid extremes of leg position.[8] In their series, two patients avoided further dislocation with traction and cast immobilization for 6 or 12 weeks. Fraser and Wroblewski advised bed rest for 3 weeks and external splinting following surgery for recurrent dislocation.[1] Dorr found only 2 recurrent dislocations in 12 patients treated with a brace for 3 months, to give a success rate of 83%.[54] A knee immobilizer to maintain the knee at full extension and thus diminish hip flexion may also be tried.

In summary, early ambulation with the hip protected by an abduction brace or knee immobilizer for three months is a reasonable approach. A spica cast remains less expensive and more readily available, but is probably best reserved for patients who do not follow instructions and may attempt removal of the brace or splint. Occasionally operative intervention is required to reduce the hip. Otherwise, surgery is reserved for recurrent dislocation or where there is an obvious, rectifiable cause for the dislocation. Protection of the hip in bed with an abduction pillow or a short leg cast with an antirotation bar may play a role, particularly in the postoperative patient. All of these approaches require careful supervision of the patient by an experienced physical therapist.

Operative Treatment

The number of patients requiring revision for the complication of dislocation is small, accounting for 1% of patients undergoing primary total hip arthroplasty. Consequently, the experience of any one surgeon in such cases is limited and the literature addressing operative revision is not extensive. The functional impact of recurrent dislocation on the affected patient is significant. These patients tend to walk more slowly, have a diminished single leg support time, and live with a persistent fear of further dislocation.[55] Of revision cases, revision for instability is associated with the least satisfactory clinical results.[56] If revision surgery is undertaken, all the causes of dislocation must be looked for and addressed, if possible, at the time of surgery. Assumptions that a single obvious factor is the cause should not be made. The cause of the dislocation is often multifactorial.

In general, 40% of patients have malorientation of the components and the other 60% are the result of multiple factors.[4,5] Surgical exploration for dislocation may develop into a major revision following thorough intraoperative evaluation. This should be borne in mind when formulating the preoperative plan. Many operative methods have been tried to prevent dislocation, indicating that no one method is universally satisfactory. Fraser and Wroblewski had a 20% failure rate with trochanteric advancement as the revision operation for dislocation.[1] A similar result was found by Kaplan, who reported 5 cases of recurrence (24%) in a series of 21 patients undergoing trochanteric advancement in which the cause of the dislocation was not apparent.[42] In a review of the Mayo Clinic experience of 95 surgical procedures for dislocation, a 70% success rate was achieved when the procedure was performed for detectable causes of dislocation, mainly component malorientation.[57] However, if the cause of the instability was unclear, or if removal of an impingement was the only procedure, the success rate fell to 33% to 50%. The overall failure rate in the series was around 40%, with 10% experiencing resubluxation, 20% redislocation, and 10% requiring a second operation.

Preoperative Plan

All patients in whom nonoperative care has failed should have a thorough evaluation with a broad operative plan developed prior to surgical intervention. Preoperatively, the following procedures should be adhered to.

- A detailed history of the time interval to the first dislocation, the number of dislocations, and the ease with which the dislocation occurred. Dislocation within the first 3 months of surgery is probably associated with soft tissue factors, including altered myofascial tension and immature scar formation. Trochanteric displacement causing diminished myofascial tension, component malposition, or impingement from ostephytes or cement may be obvious mechanical causes. From 4 months, dislocations are more associated with component malposition or problems with the trochanter. Late dislocations, after 5 years, may be associated with acetabular component polyethylene wear altering the range of hip motion or soft tissue stretching, particularly of the pseudocapsule.[58] Surgery in patients with three or more episodes of dislocation is more likely to fail (55%) than if less than this number of dislocations has occurred (28%).[57] This may be due to the fact that patients with no obvious cause for the dislocation experience a greater delay before operative intervention occurs and are therefore likely to form a major part of the multiple dislocation group.
- The direction in which dislocation occurs should be determined from the history, coupled with a review of all radiographs taken with the hip dislocated, if available. Flexion with internal rotation tends to cause posterior dislocation, while extension with external rotation is the main mechanism for anterior dislocation.
- Examination may reveal an increased range of motion, suggestive of soft tissue laxity, particularly in the late case. Restricted abduction may imply reduced femoral offset contributing to dislocation.
- A full x-ray series to include an anteroposterior view of the pelvis, anteroposterior view centered over the hip, as well as direct lateral and frog lateral views. These views allow measurement of component orientation and femoral offset and may indicate potential sources of impingement.
- A full review of the initial operative record should be performed, particularly if the initial surgery occurred at another institution. The implants used and any technical problems encountered at the initial surgery should be noted.
- Examination of the hip under image intensification may assist in further assessment, particularly if the symptoms are subtle and have not resulted in a frank dislocation.
- Aspiration of the hip may be performed, particularly if infection is suspected. Arthrography may demonstrate the presence of a redundant pseudocapsule.
- A full armamentarium of instrumentation should be available to allow for revision of both components in all cases.

Operative Procedure

The goal of surgery for dislocation is to correct the factor or factors responsible for dislocation, thereby preventing a further episode. The operation itself should be performed in a methodical, stepwise fashion aimed at a thorough examination for possible cause of the dislocation. We use a posterolateral approach to the hip unless, as a result of the initial surgery, a nonunion with separation of the greater trochanter exists. This situation usually warrants a transtrochanteric approach with debridement of the osteotomy surfaces of soft tissue and maximizing the surface area for bony apposition for healing of the nonunion. Secure fixation of the trochanter may require additional equipment such as the Wroblewski compression spring device or Dall–Miles clamp and cable system, and is more readily achieved with the leg abducted.[1,52] Grafting of the opposed surfaces, preferably with autogenous bone or with allograft or Grafton, may also aid in healing.

All soft tissue attachments should be preserved or divided in a way that allows repair prior to wound closure. With the posterolateral approach, remnants of the short external rotators are divided close to the femur and tagged with a suture to allow for reattachment to bone. The pseudocapsule is exposed and is often found to be redundant, particularly in more chronic cases. It is divided in a flapwise fashion with the base of the flap on the acetabular side and also tag sutured. As part of the closure, the redundant aspect of this flap may be advanced during reattachment to the femur to aid stability.

Following exposure of the components, orientation, position, and evidence of loosening is then assessed. The hip is dislocated, observing for the direction in which dislocation easily occurs, and for possible factors involved in the dislocation. The cup is inspected for evidence of wear, which may indicate the direction of dislocation and may also mandate replacement. The femoral head should also be inspected for evidence of wear.

With a modular cup, if an augmented polyethylene liner has been used, it may be removed and rotated to see if stability is achieved. Otherwise, the regular liner may be replaced by a trial augmented liner and stability assessed. Impingement may be present from osteophytes or excess bone cement and should be removed. With modular components, improved stability may be achieved by exchange of the femoral head component to allow for improved head–neck ratio and also improve the offset. The head–neck ratio can be improved by increasing head size and changing to an appropriate liner while maintaining a polyethylene thickness of at least 7 to 8 mm. Increasing the neck length will result in an increased offset. A disadvantage of monoblock components is that such changes cannot be made without removal of the complete femoral component. Removal and reorientation of the femoral component is rarely required and it is technically much easier to correct a maloriented acetabular component. A new press-fit acetabular component with an elevated liner should be used. An elevated liner has been shown to improve hip stability.[31–33] Although distal femoral rotational osteotomy has been described for malorientation of the femoral component, it is very rarely necessary.[60]

The approach to cemented, polyethylene cup components such as with low friction arthroplasty, differs somewhat. A well fixed cemented socket may be augmented for posterior dislocation by applying a portion of another socket to its posterolateral aspect with screws.[51] Separate polyethylene stabilizers are now available for this purpose. However failures of this technique have been reported.[21,59] Other alternatives with a cemented polyethylene socket all involve replacement of the component. A replacement cemented socket can be reoriented to a more normal anatomic position. An alternative is to use a cup with a greater amount of head coverage more typical of the normal anatomic arrangement, such as an angle-bore socket, but this requires the manufacture of both right- and left-sided cups.[33]

The older patient with recurrent dislocation, often with poor soft tissue constraint to the hip, presents a particularly difficult challenge. More recently this situation has been addressed with the use of prostheses with a higher degree of constraint.[9,33] Such designs are available with both cemented and cementless cups and usually involve the use of a bipolar stem articulating with a captive polyethylene socket. This degree of constraint may transmit force to the bone–cement or bone–metal interface, predisposing to acetabular component loosening. Increased polyethylene wear is an additional potential problem. Our experience with this approach justifies its use where all other methods have failed or are felt likely to fail, and has resulted in a high rate of success. Another approach involves conversion of the unstable hip to a bipolar arthroplasty. We do not have enough experience of this technique to comment on its efficacy.

Postoperatively, balanced suspension slings or an abduction pillow is used. A hip spica cast or abduction brace may be used. This protection of the hip is normally maintained for 3 months. Careful supervision of the patient by an experienced physical therapist with instruction on avoidance of the mechanism mostly likely to cause dislocation is of paramount importance.

Conclusion

Dislocation is the most common clinically apparent complication of hip arthroplasty. In primary total hip arthroplasty, a 2% to 3% dislocation rate is representative of the overall occurrence. Familiarity with risk factors assists in prevention and dictates aspects requiring further assessment when a dislocation does occur. Previous surgical intervention or avulsion of the greater trochanter is associated with a particularly high risk of dislocation. An augmented acetabular cup reduces the incidence of dislocation. Protection of the hip by bracing should be considered following revision surgery. Most dislocations occur early and can be reduced closed. Postreduction bracing is recommended, usually for a minimum of 3 months. Revision surgery is confined to patients who fail closed reduction, who undergo multiple dislocations, or who show an obvious cause for the dislocation. Preoperative planning is essential and the surgery should be individualized and geared towards addressing the cause in the specific patient. This approach is associated with a higher degree of success. Modularity of the cementless socket facilitates alteration of the position of the polyethylene and exchange to an elevated component during revision surgery. Revision of the femoral component for malorientation is rarely required. A bipolar stem held within a captive polyethylene cup may be used in the patient at high risk for further dislocation. The long-term prognosis with this approach should be guarded.

An understanding of the patient at risk and specific determination of cause during operative intervention remain key aspects of prevention and operative management of this challenging problem.

References

1. Fraser GA, Wroblewski BM. Revision of the Charnley low-friction arthroplasty for recurrent or irreducible dislocation. *J Bone Joint Surg Br.* 1981;63:552–555.
2. Ritter MA. Dislocation and subluxation of the total hip replacement. *Clin Orthop.* 1976;121:92–94.
3. Morrey BF. Instability after total hip arthroplasty. *Ortho Clin North Am.* 1992;23:237–248.
4. Woo RYG, Morrey BF. Dislocations after total hip arthroplasty. *J Bone Joint Surg Am.* 1982;64:1295–1306.
5. Khan MA, Brakenbury PH, Reynolds ISR. Dislocation following total hip replacement. *J Bone Joint Surg Br.* 1981;63:214–218.
6. Etienne A, Cupic Z, Charnley J. Postoperative dislocation after Charnley low-friction arthroplasty. *Clin Orthop.* 1978;132:19–23.
7. Coventry MB. Late dislocations in patients with Charnley total hip arthroplasty. *J Bone Joint Surg Am.* 1985;67:237–248.
8. Fackler CD, Poss R. Dislocation in total hip arthroplasties. *Clin Orthop.* 1980;151:169–178.
9. Amstutz HC, Kody MH. Dislocation and subluxation. In: Amstutz HC, ed. *Hip Arthroplasty.* New York: Churchill Livingstone; 1991:429–447.
10. Coates RL, Armour P. Treatment of subcapital femoral fractures by primary total hip replacement. *Injury.* 1980;11:132–135.
11. Sim FH, Stauffer RN. Management of hip fractures by total hip arthroplasty. *Clin Orthop.* 1980;152:191–197.
12. Cartlidge IJ. Primary total hip replacement for displaced subcapital femoral fractures. *Injury.* 1982;13:249–253.
13. Taine FH, Armour PC. Primary total hip replacement for displaced subcapital fractures of the femur. *J Bone Joint Surg Br.* 1985;67:214–217.
14. Dorr LD, Glousman R, Sew Hoy AL, Vanis R, Chandler R. Treatment of femoral neck fractures with total hip replacement versus cemented and noncemented hemiarthroplasty. *J Arthroplasty.* 1986;1:21–28.
15. Delamarter R, Moreland JR. Treatment of acute femoral neck fractures with total arthroplasty. *Clin Orthop.* 1987;218:68–74.
16. Pun WK, Ip FK, So YC, Chow SP. Treatment of displaced subcapital femoral fractures by primary total hip replacement. *J R Coll Surg Edin.* 1987;32:293–297.
17. Greenough CG, Jones JR. Primary total hip replacement for displaced subcapital fracture of the femur. *J Bone Joint Surg Br.* 1988;70:639–643.
18. Gebhard JS, Amstutz HC, Zinar DM, Dorey FJ. A comparison of total hip arthroplasty and hemiarthroplasty for treatment of acute fracture of the femoral neck. *Clin Orthop.* 1992;282:123–131.
19. Papandrea RF, Froimson MI. Total hip arthroplasty after acute femoral neck fractures. *Am J Orthop.* 1996;15:85–88.
20. Gregory RJH, Gibson MJ, Moran CG. Dislocation after primary arthroplasty for subcapital fracture of the hip. *J Bone Joint Surg Br.* 1991;73:11–12.
21. Williams JF, Gottesman MJ, Mallory TH. Dislocation after total hip arthroplasty. Treatment with an above-knee spica cast. *Clin Orthop.* 1982;171:52–58.
22. Possai KW, Dorr LD, McPherson EJ. Metal ring supports for deficient acetabular bone in total hip replacement. In: *Instructional course lectures of the American Academy of Orthopedic Surgery.* 1996;19:161–169.
23. Lewinnek GE, Lewis JL, Tarr R, Compere CL, Zimmerman JR. Dislocations after total hip-replacement arthroplasties. *J Bone Joint Surg Am.* 1978;60:217–220.
24. Hedlundh U, Hybbinette CH, Fredin H. Influence of surgical approach on dislocations after Charnley hip arthroplasty. *J Arthroplasty.* 1995;10:609–614.
25. Hedlundh U, Ahnfelt L, Hybbinette CH, Weckstrom J, Fredin H. Surgical experience related to dislocations after total hip arthroplasty. *J Bone Joint Surg Br.* 1996;78:206–209.
26. Pace TB. Total hip arthroplasty. Are early dislocations related to the surgical approach. *J Orthop Tech.* 1994;2:173–176.
27. Robinson RP, Robinson HR, Salvati EA. Comparison of transtrochanteric and posterior approaches for total hip replacement. *Clin Orthop.* 1982;147:143–147.
28. Roberts JM, Fu FH, McClain EJ, Ferguson AB. A comparison of posterolateral and anterolateral approaches to total hip arthroplasty. *Clin Orthop.* 1983;187:205–210.
29. Moskal JT, Mann JW. A modified direct lateral approach for primary and revision total hip arthroplasty. A prospective analysis of 453 cases. *J Arthroplasty.* 1996;11:255–266.
30. Cobb TK, Morrey BF, Ilstrup DM. The elevated-rim acetabular liner in total hip arthroplasty. Relationship to postoperative dislocation. *J Bone Joint Surg Am.* 1996;78:80–86.
31. Nicholas RM, Orr JF, Mollan RAB, Calderwood JW, Nixon JR, Watson P. Dislocation of total hip replacements. A comparative study of standard, long posterior wall and augmented acetabular components. *J Bone Joint Surg Br.* 1990;72:418–422.
32. Maxian TA, Brown TD, Pedersen DR, Callaghan JJ. Finite element modeling of dislocation propensity in total hip arthroplasty. Proceedings of the Orthopedic Research Society 42nd annual meeting, Atlanta Georgia. 1996, February 19–22, 259–44.
33. Wroblewski BM. Dislocation. In: Wroblewski BM, ed. *Revision surgery in total hip arthroplasty.* London: Springer-Verlag, 1990:29–46.
34. Eftekhar NS. Dislocation and instability complicating low friction arthroplasty of the hip joint. *Clin Orthop.* 1976;121:120–125.
35. McKee GK, Chen SC. The statistics of the McKee-Farrar

method of total hip replacement. *Clin Orthop.* 1973;95: 26–33.
36. Carlsson AS, Gentz CF. Postoperative dislocation in the Charnley and Brunswick total hip arthroplasty. *Clin Orthop.* 1977;125:177–182.
37. Morris JB, Nicholson OR. Total prosthetic replacement of the hip joint in Auckland. *Clin Orthop.* 1970;72:33–35.
38. Amstutz HC, Lodwig RM, Schurman DJ, Hodgson AG. Range of motion studies for total hip replacements. A comparative study with a new experimental apparatus. *Clin Orthop.* 1975;111:124–130.
39. Amstutz HC, Markolf KL. Design features in total hip replacements. In *The Hip, Proceedings of the second open scientific meeting of The Hip Society.* New York, CV Mosby, 1974;111–114.
40. Chandler DR, Glousman R, Hull D, et al. Prosthetic hip range of motion and impingement. The effects of head and neck geometry. *Clin Orthop.* 1982;166:284–291.
41. Hedlundh U, Carlsson AS. Increased risk of dislocation with collar reinforced modular heads of the Lubinus SP-2 hip prosthesis. *Acta Orthop Scand.* 1996;67(2):204–205.
42. Kaplan SJ, Thomas WH, Poss R. Trochanteric advancement for recurrent dislocation after total hip arthroplasty. *J Arthroplasty.* 1987;2:119–124.
43. McLaren RH. Prosthetic hip angulation. *Radiology.* 1973; 107:705–706.
44. Georgen TG, Resnick D. Evaluation of acetabular anteversion following total hip arthroplasty. Necessity of proper hip centering. *Br J Radiol.* 1975;48:259–260.
45. Ghelman B. Radiographic localization of the acetabular component of a hip prosthesis. *Radiology.* 1979;130: 540–542.
46. Visser JD, Konings JG. A new method for measuring angles after total hip arthroplasty: a study of the acetabular cup and femoral component. *J Bone Joint Surg Br.* 1981;63:556–559.
47. Schneider R, Freiberger RH, Ghelman B, Ranawat CS. Radiologic evaluation of pain and joint prosthesis. *Clin Orthop.* 1982;170:156–168.
48. Ackland MK, Bourne WB, Uhtoff HK. Anteversion of the acetabular cup. Measurement of the angle after total hip replacement. *J Bone Joint Surg Br.* 1986;68:409–413.
49. Pellicci PM, Salvati EA, Robinson AJ. Mechanical failures in total hip replacement requiring reoperation. *J Bone Joint Surg Am.* 1979;61:28–36.
50. Charnley J, Cupic Z. The nine and ten year results of the low friction arthroplasty of the hip. *Clin Orthop.* 1973;95:9–25.
51. Olerud S, Karlstrom G. Recurrent dislocation after total hip replacement. *J Bone Joint Surg Br.* 1985;67:402–405.
52. Dall DM, Miles AW. Reattachment of the greater trochanter. *J Bone Joint Surg Br.* 1983;65:55–59.
53. Ritter MA. A treatment plan for the dislocated total hip arthroplasty. *Clin Orthop.* 1980;153:153–155.
54. Dorr LD, Wolf AW, Chandler R, Conaty JP. Classification and treatment of dislocations of total hip arthroplasty. *Clin Orthop.* 1983;173:151–158.
55. Chandler RW, Dorr LD, Perry J. The functional cost of dislocation following total hip arthroplasty. *Clin Orthop.* 1982;168:168.
56. Kavanagh BF, Illstrup DM, Fitzgerald RH Jr. Revision total hip arthroplasty. *J Bone Joint Surg Am.* 1985;67:517–526.
57. Daly PJ, Morrey BF. Operative correction of the unstable total hip arthroplasty. *J Bone Joint Surg Am.* 1992;74: 1334–1342.
58. Coventry MB. Late dislocations in patients with Charnley total hip arthroplasty. *J Bone Joint Surg Am.* 1985;67: 832–841.
59. Graham GP, Jenkins AI, Mintowt-Czyz W. Recurrent dislocation following hip replacement: Brief report. *J Bone Joint Surg Br.* 1988;70:675.
60. Cohn BT, Krakow KA. Femoral component retroversion treated by supracondylar rotational osteotomy. *Orthopedics.* 1987;10:1057.

55
Prevention of Deep Venous Thromboembolism Following Primary and Revision Hip and Knee Arthroplasty

Jay R. Lieberman

At least 250 000 hip and knee arthroplasties are performed in North America each year.[1] These procedures are effective in relieving pain, increasing mobility and improving the patient's quality of life.[1-3] Patients undergoing hip and knee arthroplasty are at high risk for developing venous thromboembolic disease. Since total joint arthroplasty is usually an elective procedure in relatively healthy individuals, pulmonary embolism may be a devastating complication. The first manifestation of venous thromboembolic disease may be a fatal pulmonary embolism. Therefore, selection of an effective method of prophylaxis is an essential part of the care of these patients.

Despite the completion of a number of well-designed clinical trials that have examined the effectiveness and safety of a variety of thromboprophylactic modalities, the prevention of thromboembolic complications after major hip and knee surgery remains problematic. Newer options for prophylaxis such as low molecular weight heparins and heparinoids have been intensely studied, while other options such as dextran and heparin-dihydroergotamine have been replaced by more efficacious or safer alternatives.[4-9] The selection of thromboprophylaxis regimens and their implementation have been influenced considerably by the pressures of cost-containment and shorter hospital stays. Data on cost-effectiveness is now available to assist with these decisions. At the same time, other important issues and controversies have surfaced, including the optimal duration of prophylaxis, concerns about postdischarge thromboembolic events, the role of screening for silent breakthrough venous thrombosis, and the influence of different methods of anesthesia on rates of deep vein thrombosis.[10]

The focus of this textbook is revision total joint arthroplasty. Unfortunately, limited data are available on prophylaxis to prevent venous thromboembolic disease after revision total joint arthroplasty. However, a number of excellent studies have assessed the efficacy of various prophylaxis regimens after primary hip and knee arthroplasty. We have recently completed two studies at UCLA Medical Center that included revision total hip and knee arthroplasty patients. In this chapter we will review the available data on deep venous thrombosis prophylaxis, cost-effectiveness of thromboprophylaxis, and screening after both primary and revision total joint arthroplasty.

Pathogenesis

A total hip or knee arthroplasty is a potent stimulus for thrombogenesis. The triad of venous stasis, hypercoagulability, and endothelial injury is associated with thrombus formation and is present in the perioperative period in patients undergoing lower extremity arthroplasty. A large proportion of thrombi have been shown to begin intraoperatively.[11,12] Venous stasis occurs in these patients as a result of positioning of the limb during the procedure, localized postoperative swelling and reduced mobility after surgery.[13-18] McNally confirmed dramatic reductions in lower limb venous capacitance and venous outflow after hip arthroplasty.[19] Torsion and complete occlusion of the femoral vein during dislocation of the hip joint and insertion of the prosthesis have also been demonstrated using intraoperative venography.[13,17,20] Finally, knee arthroplasty is performed with a tourniquet on the thigh and the knee flexed for prolonged periods of time.

Injury to the venous endothelium as a result of operative positioning and manipulation, thermal injury from bone cement, and use of a thigh tourniquet may result in foci of vascular damage that provide the nidus for initiation of thrombosis.[13,18,20] The trauma of the procedure itself results in a sustained activation of tissue factor and other clotting factors,[21,22] which then localize at the sites of vascular injury and in the areas of venous stasis. Postoperative reduction in antithrombin III levels[23–26] and inhibition of the endogenous fibrinolytic system may allow continued thrombus growth.[27,28]

Sharrock et al.[12] assayed circulating markers of thrombin generation and fibrinolysis during different stages of total hip arthroplasty in order to determine when the thrombogenic stimulus was at its peak. The total hip arthroplasties were all performed under hypotensive epidural anesthesia. Markers of thrombin generation (prothrombin F1.2, thrombin-antithrombin complexes, and fibrinopeptide A) and fibrinolysis (D-dimer) were assessed at different time points during a total hip arthroplasty. The following time points were assessed: (1) before epidural injection; (2) after insertion of the acetabular component; (3) 90 seconds after trial reduction; (4) after insertion of a cemented or a cementless hip; (5) 90 seconds after final reduction of the hip and (6) 10 minutes later (Fig. 55.1). The prothrombin F1.2, thrombin-antithrombin, fibrinopeptide A, and D-dimer levels were minimally changed by osteotomy of the femoral neck. However, there was marked elevation of these markers after insertion of the femoral components (data points 4 and 5). The levels of fibrinopeptide A and D-dimer were always significantly greater after insertion of a cemented femoral component than a noncemented femoral component.

Epidemiology

Lower extremity arthroplasty presents the greatest risk for the development of venous thromboembolism.[2,14] Without prophylaxis, 40% to 60% of patients undergoing total hip arthroplasty will develop deep vein thrombosis. Of these patients, 15% to 25% develop a proximal deep vein thrombosis, and 0.5% to 2% suffer a fatal pulmonary embolism.[2,24,29–33] Pulmonary embolism is the most common cause of death after a total hip arthroplasty when thromboprophylaxis is not used.[35]

Thromboembolism after a total joint arthroplasty has been associated with considerable cost and morbidity.[36–38] Deep vein thrombosis delays discharge from the hospital by approximately 5 days while pulmonary embolism necessitates an additional 7 days of hospitalization.[39] Inadequate prophylaxis leads to additional diagnostic testing for patients in whom thromboembolism is suspected clinically. Deep vein thrombosis is the most common cause of readmission to the hospital after total hip arthroplasty.[40] Seagroatt et al. reviewed 7547 total hip arthroplasties performed between 1976 and 1985. Of

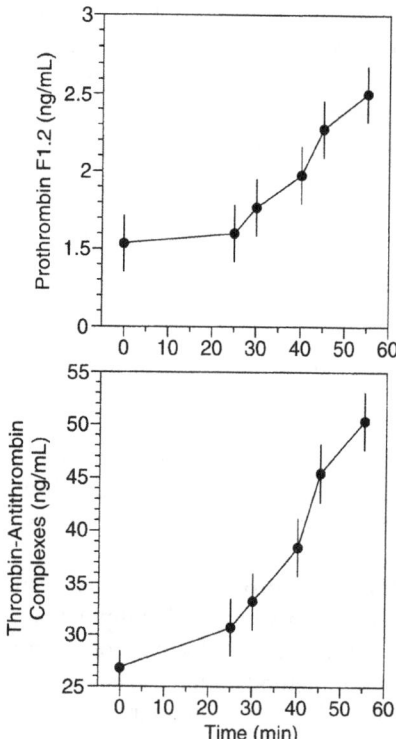
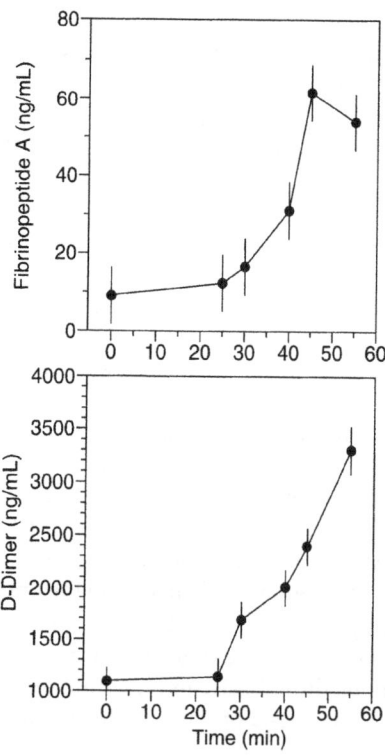

Figure 55.1. The graphs denote the changes in prothrombin F1.2, thrombin-antithrombin complexes, fibrinopeptide A, and D-dimer during total hip arthroplasty with a cemented femoral component. There was no change in the levels of prothrombin F1.2, thrombin-antithrombin A, or D-dimer after insertion of a cementless acetabular component (second data point). These markers increased with the insertion of the cemented femoral components (data points 4 and 5). (Reprinted with permission from Sharrock et al., Thrombogenesis during total hip arthroplasty, Clin Orthop. 1995;319:20.)

the 7547 patients, 208 were readmitted on an emergent basis within 28 days of surgery. Of these readmissions, 54 (26%) were diagnosed with a deep vein thrombosis or a pulmonary embolism. Additionally, proximal venous thrombosis may lead to chronic venous insufficiency that may carry significant long term morbidity and for which no satisfactory treatment exists.[38]

Deep vein thrombosis usually develops locally in the areas of deep flow with frequent initiation at a valve cusp of the soleal, or another vein in the calf. Most distal thrombi are small and clinically insignificant. Proximal, venous thrombosis may also be nonocclusive and asymptomatic. A percentage of proximal thrombi will resolve without clinical sequellae; however; there is a strong association between proximal deep vein thrombosis and pulmonary embolism. Even nonocclusive silent proximal thrombi may result in a symptomatic or a fatal pulmonary embolism.[10,41–43] Furthermore, 20% to 30% of thrombi may develop in the iliofemoral venous segment without originating in the calf.[45]

Thrombosis of the veins in the calf is generally an asymptomatic, self-limiting process that usually resolves spontaneously. Calf thrombi carry a low risk of embolization and chronic venous insufficiency. However, without medical suppression, these thrombi have the potential to propagate substantially increasing the risk of pulmonary embolism. Extension of a distal thrombus may occur more frequently in patients who have had a total joint arthroplasty than in patients with other risk factors.[41–43]

Oishi et al.[42] used duplex ultrasonography to screen 273 consecutive patients who underwent total hip and knee arthroplasty in order to determine the prevalence and clinical course of distal deep vein thrombosis. In this group, 41 patients (15%) developed a distal vein thrombosis. The prevalence of distal deep venous thrombi was significantly higher after total knee arthroplasty (23%) than total hip arthroplasty (9%). Follow-up duplex scans were performed at 7 and 14 days postoperatively on all patients with initially positive scans. Of these patients, 7 (17%) had evidence of proximal propagation by postoperative day 14.

In a retrospective review assessing the efficacy of contrast venography as a screening tool, Pellegrini et al.[43] reported that 4 of 23 patients (17%) with an untreated calf thrombus developed a symptomatic pulmonary embolism. Therefore, distal deep vein thrombosis after total hip arthroplasty has a high potential for proximal thrombus propagation with a concomitant increase in risk for pulmonary embolism. Thus, treatment of calf thrombi probably should include anticoagulation or serial duplex scans to diagnose clot propagation.

Factors associated with the development of venous thromboembolism include: advanced age, prior venous thromboembolism, prolonged immobilization, varicose veins, obesity, and cardiac dysfunction (Table 55.1).

These factors may be present in individuals who undergo a total hip or knee arthroplasty. However, even in the absence of preexisting risk factors, all patients undergoing a total joint arthroplasty are at high risk for deep vein thrombosus or pulmonary embolism; therefore, prophylaxis is mandatory. The mode of prophylaxis that is chosen must be effective, easy to administer and monitor, associated with few side effects or complications, and cost effective. Prophylaxis must be provided for all total hip or knee arthroplasty patients in order to prevent the morbidity associated with a symptomatic deep vein thrombosis or pulmonary embolism.[10,38]

Thromboprophylaxis After Total Hip Arthroplasty

A variety of pharmacological and mechanical approaches have been used to decrease the risk of venous thromboembolism after total hip arthroplasty. The pharmacologic approaches have included aspirin, dextran, warfarin, low- or adjusted-dose heparin and low molecular weight heparins and heparinoids. Mechanical approaches have included early mobilization, graded compression stockings, sequential intermittent pneumatic compression boots, and intermittent plantar compression.

Pharmacological Methods

Warfarin
Warfarin blocks Vitamin K dependent carboxylation of glutamate to gamma-carboxy glutamate (a much stronger chelator of ionic calcium) in the liver, and thereby inactivates the Vitamin K dependent clotting

Table 55.1. Risk factors for venous thromboembolic disease.

Clinical Risk Factors
  Advanced age
  Fractures of the pelvis, hip, femur, or tibia
  Paralysis or prolonged immobility
  Prior venous thromboembolic disease
  Surgery—operations involving the abdomen, pelvis, lower extremities, and abdomen
  Obesity
  Congestive heart failure
  Myocardial infarction
  Stroke
Hemostatic Abnormalities (Hypercoagulable States)
  Antithrombin III deficiency
  Protein C deficiency
  Protein S deficiency
  Dysfibrinogenemia
  Lupus anticoagulant and antiplasphlipid antibodies
  Myeloproliferative disorders
  Heparin-induced thrombocytopenia
  Disorders of plasminogen and plasminogen activation

factors II, VII, IX and X[51] (Fig. 55.2). Warfarin has been used successfully for more than 35 years as prophylaxis following hip surgery.[46–52] Amstutz et al. reviewed 2595 patients at the UCLA Medical Center who received warfarin for an average of 17 days after a total hip arthroplasty.[48] Only 0.46% of patients were diagnosed with a symptomatic pulmonary embolism, and no fatal pulmonary embolic events occurred. One percent (25) of the patients suffered a major bleeding episode. Paiement et al. compared the efficacy of low-dose warfarin (prothrombin time ratio of 1.3 to 1.5 times normal) with intermittent pneumatic compression boots. The overall rate of deep vein thrombosis was 17% (12 patients) and the proximal deep vein thrombosis rate was 7% (5 patients) in the 72 patients that were treated with warfarin. There were no major bleeding complications.[53]

Paiement, et al.[53] evaluated the efficacy and safety of a 12-week low-dose warfarin protocol. Two hundred and sixty-eight patients received low-dose warfarin beginning the night prior to surgery. The pulmonary embolism rate was 1% (2 patients) with no fatal pulmonary emboli, and no pulmonary emboli were diagnosed following discharge from the hospital. Complications included a major bleeding episode in 4% of patients (10 patients).

We recently analyzed 1299 patients who received low-dose warfarin prophylaxis at the UCLA Medical Center after primary or revision total hip arthroplasty performed between 1987 and 1993. Twelve symptomatic pulmonary emboli were diagnosed postoperatively (1.1%). Patients with a prior history of symptomatic venous thromboembolic disease had a significantly increased risk of developing a symptomatic pulmonary embolism after total hip arthroplasty. The incidence of a major bleeding event was 2.3% (32 patients). There was significantly increased risk of developing a postoperative hematoma if the patient's prothrombin time exceeded 17 seconds. The average duration of low-dose warfarin prophylaxis was 15 days. However, 616 patients received an average of 11 days of prophylaxis and only two of these patients developed (0.4%) a symptomatic pulmonary embolism. There was no statistically significant difference in symptomatic pulmonary emboli when comparing 2 weeks versus 3 weeks of prophylaxis. We currently use 2 weeks of low-dose warfarin prophylaxis when this mode of prophylaxis is selected after total hip arthroplasty.[54]

Warfarin prophylaxis is usually initiated with a 10 mg dose either the evening before or the evening of the operation with subsequent doses determined by measurement of the prothrombin time. The target level of anticoagulation is a prothrombin time between 1.3 and 1.5 times the control value. However, the anticoagulant effect associated with a particular prothrombin time has varied considerably among institutions depending on

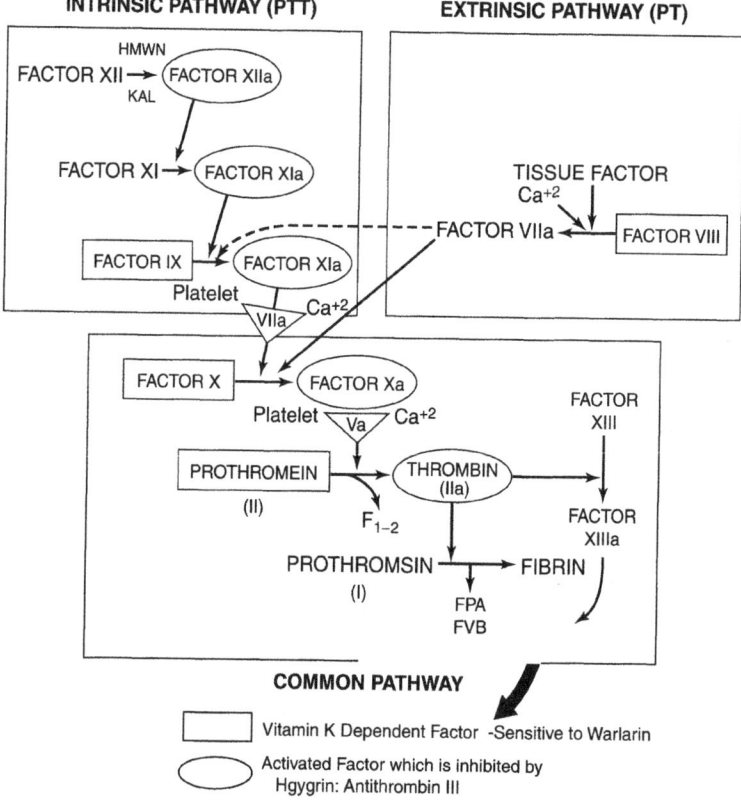

Figure 55.2. The coagulation cascade—intrinsic and extrinsic pathways.

the thromboplastin sensitivity. Therefore the international normalized ratio (INR) has been developed. The international normalized ratio represents a prothrombin time ratio that would have been obtained if the international reference thromboplastin had been used instead of the local reagent. The international normalized ratio is defined as the observed prothrombin time ratio raised to the power of international sensitivity index of the specific thromboplastin used.[45,55] The target INR for total joint arthroplasty is between 1.8 and 2.5. Of note, the international normalized ratio may not be accurate prior to reaching a stable warfarin dose.

The occurrence of deep vein thrombosis is decreased by approximately 60% and proximal venous thrombosis by 70% with warfarin therapy when compared to no prophylaxis.[56] As well as being highly effective, warfarin is inexpensive and easy to administer (oral dosing).[48] However there are several major disadvantages associated with the use of warfarin. There is a 1% to 5% prevalence of major bleeding,[48,53,54,57] and warfarin interacts with a large number of medications.[58] For example, the combination of warfarin and nonsteroidal antiinflammatory agents have been shown to increase the risk of hemorrhagic peptic ulcer by nearly 13-fold in patients 65 years of age and older.[58]

Another disadvantage of warfarin is its delayed onset of action. In our UCLA study, the average patient did not reach a therapeutic level of anticoagulation (prothrombin time of 14 to 17 seconds) for 72 hours. Fifty percent of the patients reached the target level of anticoagulation by postoperative day number three, 69% by postoperative day number four, 85% by postoperative day five, and 92% by postoperative day six. However two of the patients developed an in-hospital symptomatic pulmonary embolism on postoperative day zero and three, respectively. Therefore, when using warfarin prophylaxis the patient may be at an increased risk of developing a symptomatic thromboembolic event during the perioperative period because the patient has not attained the target level of anticoagulation. In addition, with declining duration of hospital stays, approximately 30% of patients would not have reached the target level of anticoagulation if prophylaxis was stopped at the time of discharge. These patients may be at increased risk of developing a symptomatic pulmonary embolism. The low rates of symptomatic pulmonary embolism associated with extended warfarin prophylaxis (2 weeks or more of prophylaxis) suggest that clinically silent early thrombi may be prevented from propagating and causing a symptomatic pulmonary embolism.[48,53,54]

Heparin

Standard unfractionated heparin is a heteogenous mixture of glycosaminoglycans. Heparin contains a unique pentasaccharide which binds antithrombin III with a high affinity. The interaction of heparin with antithrombin III accelerates the ability of heparin to inhibit the coagulation enzymes, thrombin, factor IX, and factor Xa producing its anticoagulant effect. This anticoagulant effect requires the formation of a ternary complex by the binding of a heparin molecule with at least 18 saccharides in length to both thrombin and antithrombin III.[4,5,59]

Standard low-dose heparin (5,000 units subcutaneous twice daily) is relatively ineffective in the prevention of proximal deep vein thrombosis[3,60,61,62] and is, therefore, not used in thromboprophylaxis following total hip arthroplasty. However, adjusted-dose heparin has been utilized based on the assumption that it would be more likely than fixed low-dose heparin to overcome the hypercoagulable state associated with a total hip arthroplasty.[27,62,63] The activated partial thromboplastin time (aPTT), which is a sensitive measure of the inhibitory effects of heparin on thrombin, factor IX, and factor Xa, is used to monitor and adjust the dose of heparin.[59] The first dose of heparin is given 1 to 2 hours preoperatively or within 12 hours of the procedure. Subsequent doses are given every 8 to 12 hours and are adjusted to achieve an aPTT of 1 to 5 seconds more than the upper limit of normal for the hospital laboratory. The blood sample to measure the aPTT must be drawn 4 to 6 hours following the administration of heparin.[10]

Both Leyvraz, et al.[63] and Taberner et al.[33] have shown that adjusted-dose heparin was more effective and was not associated with increased bleeding when compared with low-dose heparin.[33,63] Although adjusted-dose heparin provides effective prophylaxis after total hip arthroplasty, it requires daily laboratory monitoring of the activated partial thromboplastin time.

Low Molecular Weight Heparin

Low molecular weight fractions of commercial heparin are generally prepared by either chemical or enzymatic depolymerization of heparin. The low molecular weight heparins are relatively homogenous in size with molecular weights between 1000 to 10 000 daltons (mean approximately 4500 daltons). Low molecular weight heparins enhance the activity of antithrombin III; however, because of their small size, their primary effect is secondary to the inhibition of factor Xa. Since a minimum chain length of 18 saccharides is required for ternary complex formation (heparin-AT III-thrombin), low molecular weight molecules are able to inhibit factor Xa but not thrombin (Fig. 55.3).[4,5,59]

The low molecular weight heparins produce less bleeding than standard heparin because inhibition of platelet function is reduced, and there is less microvascular permeability than with standard heparin.[4] Other attributes of the low molecular heparins include bioavailability of at least 90% (compared with 30% to 40% for standard heparin); substantially reduced bind-

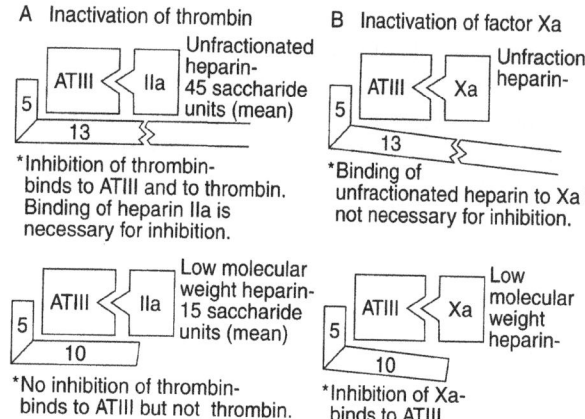

Figure 55.3. A. Inactivation of thrombin. Heparins must bind AT III via the high-affinity pentasaccharide and to thrombin through an additional 13 saccharide units to inactivate thrombin. Low molecular weight heparins which do not contain 18 saccharide units bind to AT III but not to thrombin. B. Inactivation of factor Xa. Heparins bind to AT III via the high-affinity pentasaccharide to inactivate factor Xa. Both standard heparin and low molecular weight heparins can inactivate factor Xa. (Reprinted with permission from Hirsh J, Levine MN. Low molecular weight hep-arin. *Blood* 1992;79(1), 2.)

ing to plasma proteins, vascular endothelium and circulating cells; and a prolonged circulating half-life compared with standard heparin, which allows for once- or twice-a-day dosing. These properties result in limited interindividual variation in the antithrombotic effect. Clinical advantages include the use of the same dose for all patients (or a fixed dose for each patient based on kilograms of body weight), dosing once or twice a day, and no laboratory monitoring.[4] Prophylactic doses of low molecular weight heparin do not increase the activated partial thromboplastin time or the incidence of bleeding complications.[4,64]

Low molecular weight heparins as a class of drugs have been shown to reduce the risk of deep vein thrombosis (proximal and distal) by at least 70% compared with the administration of placebo.[6,7,8,56,65] Turpie et al. compared the efficacy and safety of enoxaparin (50 patients) with those of the placebo (50 patients) after total hip arthroplasty in a randomized clinical trial. The overall rate of deep vein thrombosis in the placebo group was 42% (21 patients) and the proximal thrombus rate was 20% (10 patients). The enoxaparin group had an overall deep vein thrombosis rate of 11% (6 patients) and a proximal clot rate of only 4% (2 patients).[64]

In two randomized trials comparing the low molecular weight heparins, fragmin and enoxaparin, with unfractionated heparin, both Ericksson et al.[66] and Colwell et al.[15] reported a greater efficacy with low molecular weight heparin compared with unfractionated heparin and no increase in the rate of bleeding. Furthermore, in two meta analyses, Nurmohamed et al.[65] and Leizorovicz et al.[7] also noted a decreased overall rate of thrombus formation and decreased bleeding when comparing the low molecular weight heparins with unfractionated heparin after hip surgery.

Hull et al.[51] and the RD Heparin Group[52] have performed direct comparisons between low molecular weight heparins and warfarin. In a double-blind randomized trial, Hull et al. compared tinzaparin, a low molecular weight heparin with low-dose warfarin in 397 patients who had a total hip arthroplasty. The tinzaparin was given once daily in a fixed dose based on kilograms of body weight. The dose of warfarin was adjusted daily to attain a target international normalized ratio between two and three. All patients were screened with a venogram by postoperative day seven. Among the patients who received warfarin, there was a 23% rate of deep vein thrombosis (79 of 340 patients) and a 4% rate of proximal deep vein thrombosis (13 of 340 patients). The overall deep vein thrombosis rate for patients who received tinzaparin was 21% (69 of 332 patients) and the proximal thrombus rate was 5% (16 of 332 patients). Major bleeding episodes were noted in 2% (6 of 397 patients) of patients in the warfarin group and in 3% (11 of 398 patients) in patients that received tinzaparin. The authors concluded that the low molecular weight heparin tinzaparin was as effective as low-dose warfarin in preventing proximal clot formation after total hip arthroplasties. However, there was a significantly increased rate of bleeding in the patients who received the low molecular weight heparin.[51]

Two different doses of RD heparin have been compared with low-dose warfarin in a prospective randomized trial. Patients were randomly assigned to one of the following three groups: (1) 50 antifactor Xa units of RD heparin per kilogram of body weight administered subcutaneously twice daily, (2) 90 antifactor Xa units of RD heparin per kilogram of body weight administered once daily, or (3) 5 milligrams of warfarin preoperatively to prolong the prothrombin time ratio to 1.2 to 1.5. All patients underwent venography to determine the rate of deep venous thrombosis—both symptomatic and asymptomatic. To assess the bleeding associated with the three prophylactic regimens, a blood loss index was calculated. The blood loss index (grams per deciliter) was defined as the preoperative hemoglobin level—the hemoglobin level at discharge + the number of units of blood or packed red blood cells transfused. RD heparin administered twice daily and low dose warfarin were equally safe and effective. In the RD heparin group that received 50 antifactor Xa units twice daily, there was a 7% (12 patients) incidence of overall deep vein thrombosis and a 5% (3 patients) rate of proximal vein thrombosis. In the low-dose warfarin group, 11% (20 patients of 174 patients) developed a deep vein thrombosis and 6% (11 patients) had a proximal thrombus. The blood loss index was equivalent between the RD heparin groups and the low-dose warfarin.[52]

There are considerable differences in the compositions, dosing profiles, and activities of the various low molecular weight heparins. Therefore, additional studies will be required to determine if there is a clinically relevant difference between one low molecular weight heparin versus another. Cost considerations will also be a relevant factor in the determination of the use of these agents by the orthopedic community.

Other Pharmacological Agents
Low-dose warfarin and low molecular weight heparins are unmatched in their safety and efficacy in thromboprophylaxis following total joint arthroplasty. As an alternative anticoagulant, dextran has been shown to provide a moderate reduction in the rate of deep vein thrombosis after joint replacement procedures. However, the use of this agent is limited because of the high risk of complications including volume overloading, hypersensitivity reactions, and bleeding. Additionally, the relatively high cost and the availability of alternatives that offer better thromboprophylaxis dramatically limit the use of dextran following joint arthroplasty.[56,67,68] Aspirin has not been shown to reduce the rate of deep vein thrombosis in most randomized clinical trials, and therefore cannot be recommended at this time as the sole means of prophylaxis after total hip arthroplasty.[56,60,67,69]

Mechanical Methods

Intermittent Pneumatic Compression
Intermittent pneumatic compression boots increase the velocity of venous blood in the extremities, decrease venous stasis, and enhance endogenous fibrinolytic activity.[70,71] The use of these devices is appealing because they do not require laboratory monitoring, there is no potential for bleeding, they are generally well tolerated by patients, and they are relatively inexpensive.

In a number of randomized trials, pneumatic compression boots have been effective in reducing the overall rate of deep vein thrombosis.[50,72] In a randomized, prospective trial, Woolson and Watt studied the efficacy of intermittent pneumatic compression (IPC) alone (76 hips), intermittent pneumatic compression and aspirin (72 hips) and intermittent pneumatic compression and low-dose warfarin (hips). Patients were screened at the time of discharge with either venography on the operated limb or bilateral venous ultrasonography.[59] The frequency of proximal deep vein thrombosis was 12% (9 patients) in the IPC group alone, 10% (7 patients) in the IPC and aspirin group and 9% (6 patients) in the IPC and warfarin group. Although the proximal thrombus rates were similar in all three groups, a significant difference might have been noted if a larger patient population had been analyzed.[50]

Overall rates of thrombus formation are clearly decreased by pneumatic compression devices; however, there is evidence that proximal thrombosis may be refractory to the effects of pneumatic compression devices. In three studies comparing the efficacy of intermittent pneumatic compression with a variety of different regimens, the compression devices provided less protection against proximal deep vein thrombosis.[72,73,74] This issue requires further investigation before pneumatic compression boots can be recommended as a sole means of prophylaxis after total hip arthroplasty.

Intermittent Plantar Compression
Intermittent plantar compression in the foot is another form of mechanical prophylaxis. Flattening of the plantar arch during walking is known to activate a physiologic venous pump in the foot. Phlebographic studies confirmed that the large plantar venous system is rapidly emptied when weight-bearing flattens the plantar arch. A pneumatic device ("foot pump") that fits on to the foot and mimics the hemodynamic effects that occur during normal walking has been utilized as a form of thromboprophylaxis. This device theoretically increases venous return and is not associated with increased risks of bleeding that is seen with pharmacologic prophylaxis.[75,76,77]

Studies comparing intermittent plantar compression to either placebo or a fixed dose of heparin have demonstrated decreased overall thrombosis rates in patients who had intermittent plantar compression as prophylaxis.[76,77] However, larger randomized prospective trials comparing this mechanical device to low-dose warfarin and low molecular weight heparins are needed before intermittent plantar compression can be recommended as the sole means of prophylaxis after total hip arthroplasty.

Compression stockings alone are ineffective in reducing the risk of thromboembolism acceptably and should not be considered as the sole prophylactic agent for patients who have had a hip arthroplasty.[8,56]

Revision Total Hip Arthroplasty

It has been assumed that patients undergoing revision total hip arthroplasty are at a higher risk for developing a deep venous thrombosis than primary hip patients because of increased bleeding, endothelial trauma, and operative time. Unfortunately, there is limited data available and we are not aware of a large randomized trial that compared the efficacy of different prophylaxis regimens after revision total hip arthroplasty.

Our UCLA study[54] included 419 revision total hip arthroplasties (333 patients). The symptomatic pulmonary embolism rate after revision total hip arthroplasty was 0.4% (2 of 418) compared with a symptomatic pulmonary embolism rate of 1.5% (10 of 681) after primary hip arthroplasty. There was no significant difference in the prevalence of symptomatic pulmonary embolism after primary or revision total hip arthroplasty.

In general, we believe that it is essential that prophylaxis in total hip arthroplasty patients be extended beyond hospital discharge and this may be even more important in patients who are not immediately mobilized after revision surgery. We currently recommend 2 weeks of prophylaxis after revision total hip arthroplasty, but a longer duration of prophylaxis may be appropriate particularly in cases that require extensive soft tissue dissections around the proximal femur and pelvis and/or are associated with large postoperative blood loss.

Thromboprophylaxis After Total Knee Arthroplasty

Total knee arthroplasty is associated with deep vein thrombosis even more frequently than hip operations.[51,52,56,78,79,80] Perhaps this is the result of routine use of a thigh tourniquet and flexion of the knee intraoperatively. Studies that have included both groups of patients strongly suggest that those undergoing knee arthroplasty are more resistant to the suppression of venous thrombosis than are patients undergoing hip arthroplasty in response to the same prophylaxis regimen.[41,51,52] Calf vein thrombi have been demonstrated to occur early following knee arthroplasty and they may not be benign. In a study of serial contrast venography, Maynard demonstrated that almost half of the limbs in which a knee arthroplasty had been performed already had venographically-documented deep vein thrombosis (and 8% had popliteal thrombi) within 24 hours of the operation.[81] Furthermore, thrombus propagation was seen in 32% of initially positive limbs despite the use of therapeutic warfarin in all of the patients with deep vein thrombosis documented on the early venograms. At the same time, fatal pulmonary embolism appears to be a very uncommon event following knee arthroplasty.[51,52,82]

Pharmacologic Methods

The optimal pharmacologic prophylaxis for venous thrombosis following total knee arthroplasty remains controversial. The low molecular weight heparins and warfarin have been shown to be effective in reducing the risk of thromboses following total knee arthroplasty.

Low Molecular Weight Heparin
There have been a number of well-done randomized trials comparing the efficacy of the low molecular weight heparins with either placebo or warfarin for prevention of deep vein thrombosis after total knee arthroplasty.[51,52] Leclerc and associates compared the low molecular weight heparin, enoxaparin, to placebo in a double-blind trial of 111 patients undergoing major knee operations (80% with arthroplasty). The risk reduction in total deep vein thrombosis was 71% with enoxaparin ($p < 0.0001$). Proximal vein thrombosis was documented in 19% (12) of the control patients and in none of those who received the low molecular weight heparin ($p < 0.001$). There was no difference in bleeding in the two groups.[85]

Hull and associates[51] performed a randomized, double-blind trial comparing low-dose warfarin with a once-daily, body-weight-adjusted low molecular weight heparin (tinzaparin) in 641 patients undergoing knee arthroplasty. The rates of overall deep vein thrombosis and proximal deep vein thrombosis were 55% (152 of 277 patients) and 12% (34 of 277 patients) in the warfarin patients and 45% (116 of 258 patients) and 8% (20 of 258 patients) in the low molecular weight heparin group. Major bleeding was reported in 0.9% of the warfarin group (3) and in 2.8% (9) of those who received tinzaparin. The efficacy of both interventions was considerably less in these patients than in patients undergoing hip arthroplasty enrolled in the same study.

Two different doses of RD heparin were compared with low-dose warfarin in a prospective randomized trial to determine the efficacy of these regimens in preventing venous thromboembolic disease after total knee arthroplasty.[52] Patients were randomly assigned to one of the following groups: (1) 50 antifactor Xa units of RD heparin per kilogram of body weight administered subcutaneously twice daily, (2) 90 antifactor Xa units of RD heparin per kilogram of body weight administered once daily, or (3) 5 milligrams of warfarin preoperatively to prolong the prothrombin time ratio to 1.2 to 1.5. All patients underwent venography to determine the rate of deep venous thrombosis—both symptomatic and asymptomatic. The blood loss index was used to assess the bleeding associated with the three regimens. Among the 150 patients who received RD heparin 50 antifactor Xa units twice daily, there was a 31% rate of deep vein thrombosis (46 of 150 patients) and a 6% rate of proximal deep vein thrombosis (9 of 150). The overall deep vein thrombosis rate for patients who received warfarin was 51% (75 of 147 patients), and the proximal thrombosis rate was 10% (15 of 147 patients). There was a significant difference in the overall deep vein thrombosis rate ($p = 0.004$) between patients receiving RD heparin twice daily versus those that were treated with warfarin. However, there was no difference between the rates of proximal deep vein thrombosis in either of the three groups. There was a significant increase in the blood loss index in patients that received RD heparin once or twice daily compared with patients who received warfarin.

Leclerc et al.[83] performed a randomized double-blind trial comparing enoxaparin with warfarin in the prevention of venous thromboembolism following total knee arthroplasty. Six hundred and seventy patients were randomly assigned to receive either enoxaparin, 30 mg subcutaneously every 12 hours, or adjusted-dose warfarin (INR 2-3). Deep venous thrombosis occurred in 109 patients (51.7%) in the warfarin group and in 76 (36.9%) of patients in the enoxaparin group ($p = 0.003$). Proximal venous thrombosis occurred in 22 (10.4%) of patients in the warfarin group and in 7 (2.1%) of patients in the enoxaparin group ($p > 0.2$). Bleeding complications occurred in 6 patients (1.8%) in the warfarin group and in 7 patients (2.1%) in the enoxaparin group ($p > 0.2$). The authors concluded that fixed-dose enoxaparin administered following surgery was more effective than adjusted-dose warfarin in reducing the total number of deep venous thromboses. However, there were no significant differences in proximal clot rates. In addition, enoxaparin was not associated with a significantly increased risk of bleeding.

Warfarin
Warfarin blocks Vitamin K dependent carboxylation of glutamate to gamma-carboxy glutamate (a much stronger chelator of ionic calcium) in the liver, and thereby inactivates the Vitamin K dependent clotting factors II, VII, IX, and X[5] (Fig. 55.2). Dosing of warfarin for prophylaxis following total knee replacements is done in the same manner as with total hip replacements. The target INR for total knee arthroplasty is between 1.8 and 2.5. Of note, the international normalized ratio may not be accurate prior to reaching a stable warfarin dose.

We recently evaluated the efficacy of low-dose warfarin in preventing symptomatic pulmonary embolism in 815 primary and revision total knee arthroplasties performed at UCLA Medical Center between 1984 and 1993.[83] Overall, there were a total of 3 symptomatic pulmonary emboli (0.3%) and 8 (1%) symptomatic deep vein thromboses (all distal). There were 2 deaths (0.3%) but neither one was secondary to a pulmonary embolism. Seventeen knees (2.5%) developed a hematoma postoperatively, and 2 of these patients required drainage of the knee.

The average time to attainment of the target level of anticoagulation was 3 days. The average duration of warfarin prophylaxis was 12 days. The three pulmonary emboli occurred on postoperative days 4, 21, and 45, respectively. The patient who developed a symptomatic pulmonary embolism on postoperative day 45 had a history of atrial fibrillation and was still receiving warfarin therapy when the pulmonary embolism was diagnosed. Four hundred and eighty-seven patients in this study received between 8 and 14 days of prophylaxis and none developed a symptomatic pulmonary embolism. Two hundred and ten patients received more than 2 weeks of prophylaxis and no symptomatic pulmonary emboli were diagnosed. There were 131 patients who received 1 week or less of warfarin prophylaxis and one patient developed a symptomatic pulmonary embolism. Thus, the 95% confidence interval for this group of patients was 0.04 to 3.6%. Of course, this one patient may have developed a pulmonary embolism even if she had received 2 weeks of prophylaxis. However, because no symptomatic pulmonary emboli were diagnosed in the 487 patients who received 2 weeks of warfarin prophylaxis, we are presently using 2 weeks of prophylaxis after total knee arthroplasty. Further studies are necessary to determine the appropriate duration of prophylaxis for these patients.

Low-dose warfarin is a safe and effective mode of prophylaxis after total knee arthroplasty. A disadvantage of using warfarin prophylaxis is its delayed onset of action. When using warfarin prophylaxis, the patient may be at an increased risk of developing symptomatic thromboembolic disease during the perioperative period, especially if the target level of anticoagulation has not been attained. Low-dose warfarin prophylaxis has also been associated with a high rate of asymptomatic distal thrombus formation after total knee arthroplasty in a number of different studies.[51,52,85] However, the incidence of symptomatic proximal clots and pulmonary emboli is extremely low. This suggests that the warfarin may prevent silent distal thrombi from propagating and causing a symptomatic pulmonary embolism. Further investigation is required to determine if asymptomatic distal thrombus formation is associated with development of chronic venous insufficiency.

Other Pharmacologic Agents
The use of dextran or low-dose heparin for prophylaxis after total knee arthroplasty has been studied in only a few small trials with discouraging results.[26,80,86] These options cannot be recommended for prophylaxis for deep vein thrombosis. The role of aspirin as a prophylaxis agent remains controversial. Aspirin appears to be effective in the prevention of proximal venous thrombosis formation.[81,87] Further research is clearly necessary to determine the optimal method of preventing venous thromboembolic disease after total knee arthroplasty.

Mechanical Methods

Intermittent Pneumatic Compression
Mechanical methods of prophylaxis would seem to be particularly well suited for patients undergoing knee arthroplasty in view of concerns about the effects of bleeding on postoperative range of motion. Hull and colleagues[30] demonstrated a 90% reduction in the prevalence of deep vein thrombosis (from 66% to 6%) in a trial of patients undergoing major knee procedures randomized to no prophylaxis or intermittent pneumatic compression. Twenty-four percent of the control patients and none of the patients receiving pneumatic com-

pression had proximal thrombi.[88] In a randomized prospective trial, Haas et al.[87] reported that pneumatic compression boots were significantly more effective than aspirin in reducing the overall rate of thrombus formation.

Pneumatic Plantar Compression

Pneumatic plantar compression has been shown to be effective in decreasing the rate of deep venous thrombosis following total knee arthroplasty. A prospective, randomized trial was performed to compare the efficacy of aspirin and pneumatic plantar compression and aspirin alone in the prevention of deep vein thrombosis after total knee arthroplasty. Deep venous thrombosis occurred in 27% (22 of 81 knees) in the pneumatic compression group compared with 59% (49 of 83 knees) in the group that received only aspirin ($p < 0.001$). Proximal thrombosis occurred in 12 patients (14%) who received only aspirin and in no patients who underwent pneumatic plantar compression in conjunction with aspirin therapy. The results of this study suggest that pneumatic plantar compression used in conjunction with aspirin therapy is safe and effective in the prevention of deep venous thrombosis following total knee arthroplasty. Further investigations of this prophylaxis regimen are necessary to confirm the efficacy of this modality.

Continuous Passive Motion

Another potential mechanical method of prophylaxis is the use of a continuous passive motion machine after the total knee arthroplasty. It has been hypothesized that the use of this device would not only maintain motion, but reduce clot formation by stimulating venous flow. In a prospective randomized study, patients who were assigned a continuous passive motion device postoperatively did not experience a reduction in thrombotic events compared with those who were treated without the use of the passive motion machine.[90]

Revision Total Knee Arthroplasty

There is very limited data regarding the incidence of deep vein thrombosis after revision total knee arthroplasty. Since revision procedures are usually longer and are associated with greater blood loss, it has been assumed that such patients are at higher risk for developing a deep vein thrombosis. In addition, we are not aware of any study in the literature that has compared the efficacy of different prophylaxis regimens in a randomized fashion after revision total knee arthroplasty. Various trials have included small numbers of revision patients, but no definitive conclusions could be reached because of the limited data available.

In our UCLA study,[84] there were 157 revision total knee arthroplasties and only one patient developed a symptomatic pulmonary embolism. Therefore, both primary and revision total knee arthroplasties in our institution receive 2 weeks of prophylaxis. However, further studies are necessary to determine if these patients are at increased risk for developing venous thromboembolic disease.

Influences of Anesthesia

Regional anesthetic techniques including spinal and epidural anesthesia have been shown to be associated with a decreased rate of deep vein thrombosis in patients who had a total hip arthroplasty when compared with patients who had arthroplasty performed under general anesthesia.[91-95] Patients in these studies did not receive thromboembolic prophylaxis. The decrease in the formation of thrombi associated with regional anesthesia has been attributed to the sympathetic blockade, with subsequent vasodilatation and an increased blood flow to the lower extremities that occurs with this anesthetic technique. It has been hypothesized that if loss of blood and transfusion requirements could be minimized with the use of hypotensive anesthesia, the tendency for venous thrombosis might be decreased.[12,96-100]

Recently, Sharrock and associates have attempted to test this hypothesis by the use of hypotensive anesthesia in patients undergoing a total hip arthroplasty. In a series of studies, low rates of proximal thrombosis were associated with hypotensive epidural anesthesia. Blood loss and transfusion requirements in these patients were remarkably low compared with those in other studies. Drawbacks to hypotensive anesthesia include the need for considerable anesthetic expertise and routine invasive hemodynamic monitoring. For this reason, routine use of hypotensive epidural anesthesia will likely remain limited to large medical centers.[12,97-100]

These studies suggest that in the absence of medical prophylaxis, patients who have regional anesthesia have a lower overall rate of deep vein thrombosis than those who have general anesthesia. However, the additional benefit of regional anesthesia when combined with an effective medical prophylactic regime has not been determined. A prospective, randomized trial is necessary to answer this question.

Cost Effectiveness

A number of studies in orthopedic surgery have demonstrated that failure to use prophylaxis is expensive, while the routine use of preventive measures is cost effective.[9,101-104] Effective prevention of deep vein thrombosis not only decreases morbidity and mortality, but it may also save health care dollars.

Cost analysis of thromboembolic prophylaxis following total hip arthroplasty has been performed by many investigators. Salzman and Davies[35] estimated that heparin, aspirin, dextran, and warfarin could all be expected to reduce both the rate of thrombosis and the overall cost compared with no prophylaxis. Oster et al. also concluded that each of six possible methods of prophylaxis reduced the rate of death (by 39% to 79%) and cost (from $19.00 to $182.00 per patient), with the most efficacious options resulting in the greatest cost savings.[103] Paiement et al. calculated that compared with clinical surveillance without prophylaxis, routine in-hospital use of warfarin would save the lives of 16 of every 1,000 patients who had a hip arthroplasty and would also decrease the cost of care of these patients by $170 000. According to this theoretical analysis, a combination of low-dose warfarin and screening with ultrasonography before discharge with a continuation of low-dose warfarin for 12 weeks after the procedure on the hip would result in an extremely low rate of fatal pulmonary embolism (less than 1 of every 1,000 patients). In addition, a routine ultrasonography before discharge with this warfarin prophylaxis regimen would result in charges of $50 000 for every life that was saved.[104]

Menzin et al.[106] compared the cost effectiveness of enoxaparin, warfarin, and no prophylaxis in a hypothetical cohort of 10 000 patients undergoing total hip arthroplasty. This study utilized an elaborate decision-analytic model that estimated the expected number of cases of deep venous thrombosis or pulmonary embolism, the expected number of thromboembolic related deaths, and the costs of thromboemboli care (prophylaxis, diagnosis, and treatment) that would result from management with enoxaparin, warfarin, or no postoperative anticoagulation. The results of this study showed that both warfarin and enoxaparin were comparable in overall cost effectiveness and were more cost-effective than no prophylaxis.

Investigations comparing low molecular weight heparins to low-dose warfarin suggest that the low molecular weight heparins may be more cost effective.[37] Prospective studies are necessary to determine the efficacy and cost effectiveness of low molecular heparins compared with other prophylaxis regimens. Any cost effectiveness analysis has definite potential limitations, including uncertainty about many of the assumptions used in the analysis, and the possibility of bias if the study is funded by industry. However, cost effectiveness studies also have potential benefits. These studies encourage consideration of a variety of factors when selecting a mode of prophylaxis rather than just the frequency of deep vein thrombosis and the acquisition cost of the prophylaxis used. They also allow comparison of one intervention, such as thrombus prophylaxis in hip arthroplasty, with other diagnostic, therapeutic, or preventive considerations that are competing for constrained health care resources.[107]

Screening Considerations

In recent years, the length of stay in the hospital after total hip arthroplasty has steadily decreased. Currently, many surgeons are not continuing prophylaxis after discharge because of concerns regarding compliance, bleeding, or the logistics of monitoring. Due to the fact that thromboembolic events occur following postoperative prophylaxis and discharge from the hospital, there has been increased interest in the possible benefits of postoperative screening to detect asymptomatic thrombosis.[108,109] Since clinical findings are unreliable in detection of a deep vein thrombosis,[110] there is concern that a decrease in duration of prophylaxis may not provide adequate protection for patients after total joint arthroplasty.

Screening is designed to detect the patient who is at increased risk for pulmonary embolism; therefore, the screening modality must reliably detect deep vein thrombosis. The goal is to prevent both symptomatic and fatal pulmonary embolism, as well as extensive venous thrombosis. It is well accepted that the major source of pulmonary embolism is a proximal deep vein thrombosis. Screening modalities must be safe, accurate, reproducible, easy to administer, and low in cost. The accuracy of a particular test may vary considerably depending whether the patient is symptomatic or asymptomatic.[111–114] Currently, the modalities that can be considered for screening after elective total hip arthroplasty include: ^{125}I-fibrinogen scanning, doppler sonography, impedance plethysmography, venous ultrasonography, and contrast venography.

Impedance plethysmography and ^{125}I-fibrinogen scanning are not used alone as screening devices because of their limited accuracy in the detection of proximal thrombi after total hip arthroplasty.[32–115] There is also not enough information available on doppler sonography to be recommended as a screening device in asymptomatic patients.

Contrast venography is the "gold standard" for the diagnosis of deep vein thrombosis. Direct visualization of the deep venous system of the lower extremity and direct visible representation of thrombi (Fig. 55.4) is achieved. Venography is able to diagnose distal and proximal thrombosis with equal sensitivity and specificity.[110,116,117] However, venography also routinely detects small thrombi of questionable importance. Limitations of venography for use in routine screening include pain, hypersensitivity reactions to the contrast medium, and thrombosis secondary to the venography itself.[117–119] Contrast venography is not cost effective as a routine screening test.

Venous ultrasonography is a noninvasive diagnostic imaging technique that gives a two dimensional cross-section representation of tissue and a direct visualization of the thrombus. Duplex scanning allows visualization of venous channels and graphic representation of venous flow.[112,120–122] These techniques have been found to be accurate in detection of proximal venous thrombosis in symptomatic patients (Fig. 55.5).[110–112] Several studies have shown that ultrasonography can be used reliably as a screening device.[42,121–124] However, the ability of ultrasonography to detect proximal thrombi accurately in asymptomatic patients after total joint arthroplasty is controversial; therefore, the efficacy of ultrasound as a screening tool remains controversial.[110,120,122,124–126]

Recently Garino et al.[127] assessed the efficacy of ultrasonography as a screening device after both total hip and knee arthroplasty. These authors concluded that the experience of the vascular technician was the essential factor in determining the accuracy of compression ultrasound. It is important that the institution perform a prospective analysis comparing ultrasonography with venography before ultrasonography is used to diagnose asymptomatic proximal thrombi. In addition, intermittent quality assessment is necessary to maintain an effective screening program.

The proper role of postoperative screening for deep vein thrombosis following total joint arthroplasty remains controversial. Some surgeons perform screening just prior to discharge and discontinue anticoagulation prophylaxis if the screening test is negative. Therefore, it is essential that the screening modality accurately detect the presence of asymptomatic proximal thrombi. Our concern is that, although it has been possible to establish effective screening programs in certain centers, expertise may be difficult to establish routinely in all hospitals. Therefore, the discontinuation of prophylaxis at the time of discharge could leave such patients at increased risk for developing a symptomatic pulmonary embolism. It is not clear from the available literature whether screening is necessary or cost-effective. It is safer and more cost-effective to continue prophylaxis af-

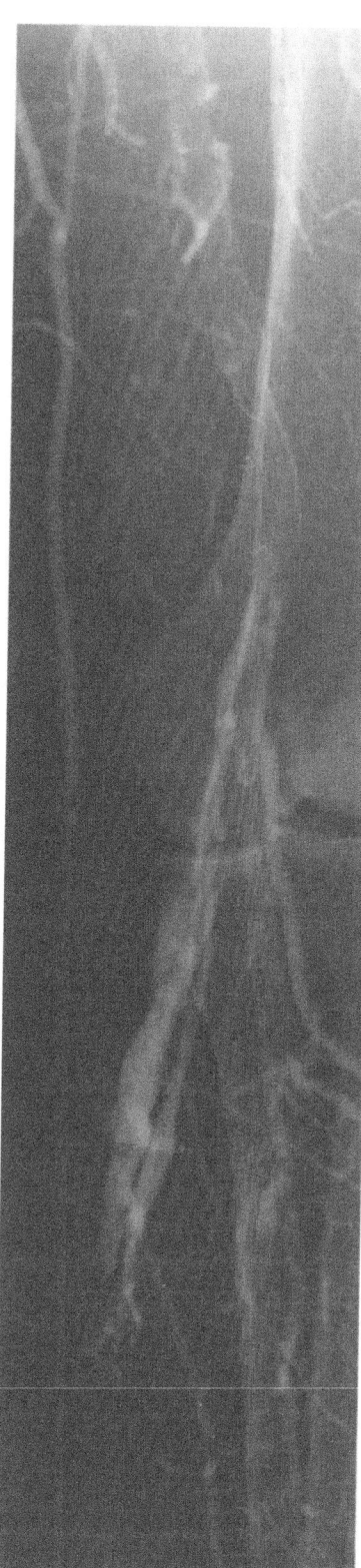

Figure 55.4. A venogram revealing a large thrombus in the popliteal region.

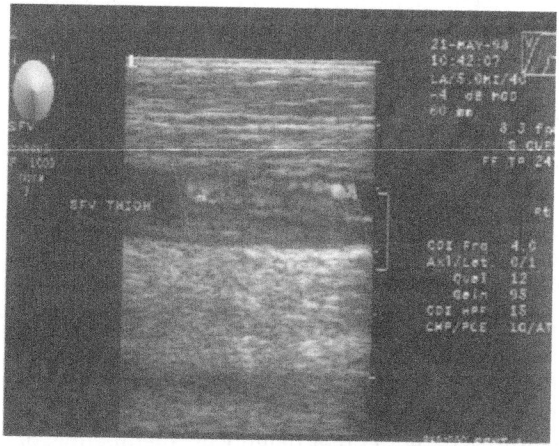

Figure 55.5. An ultrasound of a proximal thrombus.

ter hospital discharge than to rely on an ineffective screening program.

Prophylaxis for the High-Risk Patient

Patients with a history of symptomatic pulmonary embolism or deep vein thrombosis are at increased risk for developing venous thromboembolic disease after total hip arthroplasty. In our UCLA study, there was a significantly increased risk of developing a symptomatic pulmonary embolism after total hip arthroplasty if the patient had a prior symptomatic pulmonary embolism or symptomatic deep vein thrombosis. In our total knee arthroplasty patients, none of the patients with a prior history of symptomatic venous thromboembolic disease developed a symptomatic pulmonary embolism. It would appear that such individuals do not require special prophylaxis regimens, but this data must be confirmed by further studies of a large patient population.

Adjustments in prophylaxis regimens should be considered for patients with prior history of venous thromboembolic disease. Consideration should be given to prolonging the duration of prophylaxis or screening these patients. In addition, prophylaxis regimens that can be started preoperatively or have a rapid onset of action are preferable. Therefore, we recommend that warfarin be given the night before the procedure and in combination with either pneumatic compression boots or plantar compression to provide better protection during the immediate postoperative period. However, the low molecular weight heparins combined with mechanical devices may be even more efficacious because of their rapid onset of action. The duration of prophylaxis should be extended (6 weeks) and a screening test with a duplex scan should be considered prior to stopping prophylaxis. There has been no randomized study in the literature to support this regimen. However, our data suggests that total hip arthroplasty patients with a prior history of symptomatic venous thromboembolic disease require more aggressive prophylaxis.

Recommendations

There is general agreement that patients undergoing total joint arthroplasty are at high risk for developing deep venous thrombosis and pulmonary embolism. Primary prophylaxis with an effective regimen is mandatory in these patients. Although none of the modalities for prophylaxis available today is ideal, there are some that safely protect patients against venous thromboembolic events.

1. *Total hip arthroplasty*—Low molecular weight heparins, low-dose warfarin, and adjusted-dose heparin are all effective in reducing venous thromboembolic events in total hip arthroplasty patients.
2. *Total knee arthroplasty*—Low molecular weight hep-arins, low-dose warfarin, and pneumatic compression boots are effective in reducing the prevalence of pulmonary embolus and proximal clot formation. A number of randomized trials have demonstrated that certain low molecular weight heparins reduce the overall thrombosis rate compared with low-dose warfarin. However, there are no significant differences in proximal clot rates or pulmonary emboli. Plantar pneumatic compression and aspirin also may be effective, but further studies are necessary. Studies are necessary to clearly delineate the risk reduction associated with these various modalities.
3. *Duration of prophylaxis and screening*—The optimal duration of prophylaxis for patients undergoing hip and knee arthroplasty has not yet been determined. Recommendations range from stopping prophylaxis at the onset of patient ambulation to maintaining it for as long as 3 months after the total joint arthroplasty. This issue is especially important because of current trends toward earlier hospital discharge. A number of recent studies have also raised a concern about postdischarge thromboembolic events.[4] Some of the possible options that may be considered to deal with this problem include the use of regimens for prophylaxis that are effective in preventing the onset of thrombosis in the perioperative period, continuation of prophylaxis for a period following hospital discharge, and potentially the use of routine predischarge screening for clinically relevant thrombus formation. There is insufficient data with regard to efficacy and cost effectiveness to make a strong recommendation in support of screening all patients undergoing total joint arthroplasty. It is safer to continue prophylaxis postdischarge then to employ an ineffective screening program.

References

1. Harris WH, Salzman EW, Athanasooulis CA, Waltman AC, DeSanctis RW. Aspirin prophylaxis of venous thromboembolism after total hip replacement. *N Engl J Med.* 1977;297:1246–1249.
2. Laupacis A, Bourne R, Rorabeck C, et al. The effect of elective total hip replacement on health-related quality of life. *J Bone Joint Surg Am.* 1993;75:1619–1626.
3. O'Boyle CA, McGee H, Hickey A, O'Malley K, Joyce CR. Individual quality of life in patients undergoing hip replacement. *Lancet.* 1992;339:1088–1091.
4. Hirsh J, Levine MN. Low molecular weight heparin. *Blood.* 1992;79:1–17.
5. Hirsh J, Dalen JE, Deykin D, Poller L. Oral anticoagulants. Mechanisms of action, clinical effectiveness, and

optimal therapeutic range. *Chest.* 102 (Supplement): 1992;312S–326S.
6. Hoek JA, Nurmohamed MT, Hamelynck KJ, et al. Prevention of deep vein thrombosis following total hip replacement by low molecular weight heparinoid. *Thromb Haemost.* 1992;67:28–32.
7. Leizorovicz A, Haugh MC, Chapuis FR, Samama MM, Boissel JP. Low molecular weight heparin in prevention of preoperative thrombosis. *BMJ.* 1992;305:913–920.
8. Mohr DN, Silverstein MD, Murtaugh PA, Harrison JM. Prophylactic agents for venous thrombosis in elective hip surgery. Meta-analysis of studies using venographic assessment. *Arch Intern Med.* 1883;153:2221–2228.
9. Simonneau G, Leizorovicz A. Prophylactic treatment of post-operative thrombosis: a meta-analysis of the results from trials assessing various methods used in patients undergoing major orthopaedic (hip and knee) surgery. *Clin Trials Metaanal.* 1993;28:177–191.
10. Lieberman JR, Geerts WH. Current Concepts Review. Prevention of venous thromboembolism after total hip and knee arthroplasty. *J Bone Joint Surg Am.* 1994;76:1239–1249.
11. Flanc C, Kakkar VV, Clarke MB. The detection of venous thrombosis of the legs using 125I-labelled fibrinogen. *Br J Surg.* 1968;55:742–747.
12. Sharrock NE, Go G, Harpel PC, et al. Thrombogenesis during total hip arthroplasty. *Clin Orthop.* 1995;319:1–12.
13. Binns M, Pho R. Femoral vein occlusion during hip arthroplasty. *Clin Orthop.* 1990;255:168–172.
14. Clark C, Cotton LT. Blood flow in deep veins of the legs. Recording technique and evaluation of methods to increase flow during operation. *Br J Surg.* 1968;55:211–214.
15. Colwell CW, Spiro TE, Trowbridge AA, et al. Use of enoxaparin, a low-molecular weight heparin, and unfractionated heparin for the prevention of deep venous thrombosis after elective hip replacement. A clinical trial comparing efficacy and safety. *J Bone Joint Surg Am.* 1994;76:3–14.
16. Comerota AJ, Stewart GJ. Operative venous dilation and its relation to postoperative deep venous thrombosis. In: Prevention of venous thromboembolism, pp. 25–49. Goldhaber SZ, ed. New York, Marcel Dekker, 1993.
17. Stamatakis JD, Kakkar VV, Sagar S, et al. Femoral vein thrombosis and total hip replacement. *Br Med J.* 1977;2:223–225.
18. Thomas DP. Venous thrombogenesis. *Ann Rev Med.* 1985;36:39–50.
19. McNally MA, Mollan RAB. [editorial] Venous thromboembolism and orthopaedic surgery. *J Bone Joint Surg Br.* 1993;75:517–519.
20. Planès A, Vochelle N, Fagola M. Total hip replacement and deep vein thrombosis. A venographic and necropsy study. *J Bone Joint Surg Br.* 1990;72:9–13.
21. Bredbacka S, Andreen M, Blomback M, Wykkamn A. Activation of cascade systems by hip arthroplasty. No difference between fixation with and without cement. *Acta Orthop Scand.* 1987;58:231–235.
22. Wilson J, Grant PJ, Davies JA, Boothby M, Gaffney PJ, Prentice CR. The relationship between plasma vasopressin and changes in coagulation and fibrinolysis during hip surgery. *Thromb Res.* 1988;51:439–445.
23. Francis CW, Ricotta JJ, Evarts CM, Marder VJ. Long-term clinical observations and venous functional abnormalities after asymptomatic venous thrombosis following total hip or knee arthroplasty. *Clin Orthop.* 1988;232:271–278.
24. Stulberg BN, Francis CW, Pellegrini VD, et al. Antithrombin III/low-dose heparin in the prevention of deep-vein thrombosis after total knee arthroplasty: A preliminary report. *Clin Orthop.* 1989;248:152–157.
25. Fredin H, Nilsson B, Rosberg B, Tengborn L. Pre- and postoperative levels of antithrombin III with special reference to thromboembolism after total hip replacement. *Thromb Haemost.* 1983;49:158–161.
26. Francis CW, Pellegrini VD, Marder VJ, et al. Prevention of venous thrombosis after total hip arthroplasty. Antithrombin III and low-dose heparin compared with Dextran 40. *J Bone Joint Surg Am.* 1989;71:327–335.
27. D'Angelo A, Kluft C, Verheijen J, et al. Fibrinolytic shut down after surgery: impairment of the balance between tissue-type plasminogen activator and its specific inhibitor. *Eur J Clin Invest.* 1985;15:308–312.
28. Eriksson BI, Eriksson E, Gyzander E, Teger-Nilsson AC, Risberg B. Thrombosis after hip replacement. Relationship to the fibrinolytic system. *Acta Orthop Scand.* 1989;60:159–163.
29. Albrechtsson U, Olsson CG. Thrombotic side effects of lower-limb phlebography. *Lancet* 1976;1:723–724.
30. Hull RD, Delmore TJ, Hirsh J, Gent M, Armstrong P, Lufthouse R, et al. Effectiveness of intermittent/pulsatile elastile stockings for the prevention of calf and thigh vein thrombosis in patients undergoing elective knee surgery. *Thromb Res.* 1979;16:37–45.
31. Hartman JT, Pugh JL, Smith RD, et al. Cyclic sequential compression of the lower limb in prevention of deep venous thrombosis. *J Bone Joint Surg Am.* 1982;64:1059–1062.
32. Cruickshank MK, Levine MN, Hirsh J, et al. An evaluation of impedance plethysmography and 125I-fibrinogen leg scanning in patients following hip surgery. *Thromb Haemost.* 1989;62:830–834.
33. Taberner DA, Poller L, Thomson JM, Lemon G, Weighill FJ. Randomized study of adjusted versus fixed low dose heparin prophylaxis of deep vein thrombosis in hip surgery. *Br J Surg.* 1989;76:933–935.
34. Kraay MJ, Goldberg VM, Herbener TE. Vascular ultrasonography for deep venous thrombosis after total knee arthroplasty. *Clin Orthop.* 1993;286:18–26.
35. Salzman EW, Davies GC. Prophylaxis of venous thromboembolism: analysis of cost effectiveness. *Ann Surg.* 1980;191:207–218.
36. Bergqvist D, Jendteg S, Lindgren B, Matzsch T, Persson U. The economics of general thromboembolic prophylaxis. *World J Surg.* 1988;12:349–355.
37. Bergqvist D, Matsch T. Cost/benefit aspects on thromboprophylaxis. *Haemostasis.* 23 (Supplement 1):1993;15–19.
38. McNally MA, Mollan RAB. Total hip replacement, lower limb blood flow and venous thrombogenesis. *J Bone Joint Surg Br.* 1993;75:640–644.
39. O'Brien BJ, Anderson DR, Goeree R. Cost-effectiveness of enoxaparin versus warfarin prophylaxis against deep-vein thrombosis after total hip replacement. *Canadian Med Assn J.* 1994;150:1083–1090.

40. Seagroatt V, Tan HS, Goldacre M, Bulstrode C, Nugent I, Gill L. Elective total hip replacement: incidence, emergency readmission rate, and postoperative mortality. *BMJ.* 1991;303:1431–1435.
41. Kakkar VV, Howe CT, Flanc C, Clarke MB. Natural history of postoperative deep-vein thrombosis. *Lancet.* 1969;2:230–232.
42. Oishi CS, Grady-Benson JC, Otis SM, Colwell CW, Walker RH. The clinical course of distal deep venous thrombosis after total hip and total knee arthroplasty, as determined with duplex ultrasonography. *J Bone Joint Surg Am.* 1994;76:1658–1663.
43. Pellegrini VP, Clement D, Lush-Elman C, Keller GS, Evarts CM. The natural history of thromboembolic disease following hospital discharge after total hip arthroplasty: the case for routine surveillance. *Clin Orthop.* 1996;333:27–40.
44. Nillius AS, Nylander G. Deep vein thrombosis after total hip replacement: a clinical and phlebographic study. *Br J Surg.* 1979;66:324–326.
45. Hirsh J, Dalen JE, Deykin D, Poller L. Oral anticoagulants. Mechanism of action, clinical effectiveness, and optimal therapeutic range. *Chest.* 1992;102(Suppl):312S–326S.
46. Coventry MB, Noland DR, Beckenbaugh RD. "Delayed" prophylactic anticoagulation: a study of results and complications in 2,012 total hip arthroplasties. *J Bone Joint Surg Am.* 1973;55:1487–1492.
47. Francis CW, Marder VJ, Evarts CM, Yaukoolbodi S. Two-step warfarin therapy. Prevention of postoperative venous thrombosis without excessive bleeding. *JAMA.* 1983;249:374–378.
48. Amstutz HC, Friscia DA, Dorey F, Carney BT. Warfarin prophylaxis to prevent mortality from pulmonary embolism after total hip replacement. *J Bone Joint Surg Am.* 1989;71:321–326.
49. Balderston RA, Graham TS, Booth RE, Rothman RH. The prevention of pulmonary embolism in total hip arthroplasty. Evaluation of low-dose warfarin therapy. *J Arthroplasty.* 1989;4:217–221.
50. Woolson ST, Watt JM. Intermittent pneumatic compression to prevent proximal deep venous thrombosis during and after total hip replacement. A prospective, randomized study of compression alone, compression and aspirin, and compression and low-dose warfarin. *J Bone Joint Surg Am.* 1991;73:507–512.
51. Hull RD, Raskob GE, Gent M, et al. Effectiveness of intermittent pneumatic leg compression for preventing deep vein thrombosis after total hip replacement. *JAMA.* 1990;263:2313–2317.
52. The RD Heparin Arthroplasty Group. RD heparin compared with warfarin for prevention of venous thromboembolic disease following total hip or knee arthroplasty. *J Bone Joint Surg Am.* 1994;76:1174–1185.
53. Paiement GD, Wessinger SJ, Hughes R, Harris WH. Routine use of adjusted low-dose warfarin to prevent venous thromboembolism after total hip replacement. *J Bone Joint Surg Am.* 1993;75:893–898.
54. Lieberman JR, Wollaeger J, Dorey F. The efficacy of low dose warfarin prophylaxis in preventing pulmonary embolism following total hip arthroplasty. *J Bone Joint Surg Am.* 1977;79:319–325.
55. Bussey HI, Force RW, Bianco TM, Leonard AD. Reliance on prothrombin time ratios causes significant errors in anticoagulation therapy. *Arch Intern Med.* 1992;152:278–282.
56. Clagett GP, Anderson FA, Jr, Levine MN, Salzman EW, Wheeler HB. Prevention of venous thromboembolism. *Chest.* 102 (Supplement):1992;391S–407S.
57. Levine MN, Hirsh J, Landefeld S, Raskob G. Hemorrhagic complications of anticoagulant treatment. *Chest.* 102 (Supplement) 1992;352S–363S.
58. Shorr RI, Ray WA, Daugherty JR, Griffin MR. Concurrent use of nonsteroidal anti-inflammatory drugs and oral anticoagulants places elderly persons at high risk for hemorrhagic peptic ulcer disease. *Arch Intern Med.* 1993;153:1665–1670.
59. Becker RC, Ansell J. Antithrombotic therapy. An abbreviated reference for clinicians. *Arch Intern Med.* 1995;155:149–161.
60. Harris WH, Salzman EW, Athanasoulis C, et al. Comparison of warfarin, low-molecular-weight dextran, aspirin and subcutaneous heparin in prevention of venous thromboembolism following total hip replacement. *J Bone Joint Surg Am.* 1974;56:1552–1562.
61. Leyvraz PF, Richard J, Bachmann F, et al. Adjusted versus fixed-dose subcutaneous heparin in the prevention of deep-vein thrombosis after total hip replacement. *N Engl J Med.* 1983;309:954–958.
62. Planès A, Vochelle N, Mazas F, et al. Prevention of postoperative venous thrombosis: a randomized trial comparing unfractionated heparin with low molecular weight heparin in patients undergoing total hip replacement. *Thromb Haemost* 1988;60:407–410.
63. Leyvraz PE, Bachmann F, Hoek J, et al. Prevention of deep vein thrombosis after hip replacement: randomized comparison between unfractionated heparin and low molecular weight heparin. *BMJ.* 1991;303:543–548.
64. Turpie AG, Levine MN, Hirsh J, et al. A randomized controlled trial of a low-molecular-weight heparin (enoxaparin) to prevent deep-vein thrombosis in patients undergoing elective hip surgery. *N Engl J Med.* 1986;315:925–929.
65. Nurmohamed MT, Rosendaal FR, Buller HR, et al. Low-molecular weight heparin versus standard heparin in general and orthopaedic surgery: a meta-analysis. *Lancet.* 1992;340:152–156.
66. Eriksson BI, Kälebo P, Anthmyr BA, et al. Prevention of deep-vein thrombosis and pulmonary embolism after total hip replacement. Comparison of low-molecular-weight heparin and unfractionated heparin. *J Bone Joint Surg Am.* 1991;73:484–493.
67. Harris WH, Athanasoulis CA, Waltman AC, Salzman EW. Prophylaxis of deep-vein thrombosis after total hip replacement. Dextran and external pneumatic compression compared with 1.2 or 0.3 gram of aspirin daily. *J Bone Joint Surg Am.* 1985;67:57–62.
68. Fredin H, Bergqvist D, Cederhold C, Lindblad B, Nyman U. Thromboprophylaxis in hip arthroplasty. Dextran with graded compression or preoperative dextran compared in 150 patients. *Acta Orthop Scand.* 1989;60:678–681.

69. Harris WH, Salzman EW, Athanasoulis CA, Waltman AC, DeSanctis RW. Aspirin prophylaxis of venous thromboembolism after total hip replacement. *N Engl J Med.* 1977;297:1246–1249.
70. Allenby F, Boardman L, Pflug JJ, Calnan JS. Effects of external pneumatic intermittent compression on fibrinolysis in man. *Lancet.* 1973;2:1412–1414.
71. Weitz J, Michelsen J, Gold K, Owen J, Carpenter D. Effects of intermittent pneumatic calf compression on postoperative thrombin and plasmin activity. *Thromb Haemost.* 1986;56:198–201.
72. Bailey JP, Kruger MP, Solano FX, Zajko AB, Rubash HE. Prospective randomized trial of sequential compression devices vs. low-dose warfarin for deep venous thrombosis prophylaxis in total hip arthroplasty. *J Arthroplasty.* 6 (Supplement):1991;S29–S35.
73. Francis CW, Pellegrini VD, Marder VJ, et al. Comparison of warfarin and external pneumatic compression in prevention of venous thrombosis after total hip replacement. *JAMA.* 1992;267:2911–2915.
74. Paiement G, Wessinger SJ, Waltman AC, Harris WH. Low-dose warfarin versus external pneumatic compression for prophylaxis against venous thromboembolism following total hip replacement. *J Arthroplasty.* 1987;2:23–26.
75. Gardner AMN, Fox RH. The venous footpump: influence on tissue perfusion and prevention of venous thrombosis. *Ann Rheum Dis.* 1992;51(10):1173–1178.
76. Fordyce MJF, Ling RSM. A venous foot pump reduces thrombosis after total hip replacement. *J Bone Joint Surg Br.* 1992;74:45–49.
77. Santori FS, Vitullo A, Stopponi M, Santori N, Ghera S. Prophylaxis against deep-vein thrombosis in total hip replacement. Comparison of heparin and foot impulse pump. *J Bone Joint Surg Br.* 1994;76:579–583.
78. McKenna R, Galante J, Bachmann F, et al. Prevention of venous thromboembolism after total knee replacement by high-dose aspirin or intermittent calf and thigh compression. *Br Med J.* 1980;180:514–17.
79. Stringer MD, Steadman CA, Hedges AR, et al. Deep vein thrombosis after elective knee surgery. An incidence study in 312 patients. *J Bone Joint Surg Br.* 1989;71:492–497.
80. Stulberg BN, Insall JN, Williams GW, and Ghelman B. Deep-vein thrombosis following total knee replacement. *J Bone Joint Surg Am.* 1984;66:194–201.
81. Maynard MJ, Sculco TP, Ghelman B. Progression and regression of deep vein thrombosis after total knee arthroplasty. *Clin Orthop.* 1991;273:125–30.
82. Shorr RI, Ray WA, Daugherty JR, Griffin MR. Concurrent use of nonsteroidal anti-inflammatory drugs and oral anticoagulants places elderly persons at high risk for hemorrhagic peptic ulcer disease. *Arch Intern Med.* 153:1665–1670.
83. Lieberman JR, Sung R, Dorey F, et al. The efficacy of low dose warfarin prophylaxis after total knee arthroplasty. *J Arthroplasty.* 1997;12:180.
84. LeClerc JR, Geerts WH, Desjardins L. Prevention of deep vein thrombosis after major knee surgery—a randomized, double-blind trial comparing a low molecular weight heparin fragment (enoxaparin) to placebo. *Thromb Haemostas.* 1992;67:417–423.
85. Leclerc JR, Geerts WH, Desjardins L, et al. Prevention of venous thromboembolism after knee arthroplasty: a randomized, double-blind trial comparing enoxaparin with warfarin. *Ann Int Med.* 1996;124:619–626.
86. Francis CW, Pellegrini VD, Marder VJ. Prevention of venous thrombosis after total hip arthroplasty. Antithrombin III and low-dose heparin compared with Dextran 40. *J Bone Joint Surg Am.* 1989;71:327–335.
87. Haas SB, Insall JN, Scuderi GR, Windsor RE, Ghelman B. Pneumatic sequential-compression boots compared with aspirin prophylaxis of deep-vein thrombosis after total knee arthroplasty. *J Bone Joint Surg Am.* 1990;72:27–31.
88. Hull RD, Raskob GE, Gent M. Effectiveness of intermittent pneumatic leg compression for preventing deep vein thrombosis after total hip replacement. *JAMA.* 1990;263:2313–2317.
89. Westrich GH, Sculco TP. Prophylaxis against deep venous thrombosis after total knee arthroplasty: pneumatic plantar compression and aspirin compared with aspirin alone. *J Bone Joint Surg Am.* 1996;78:826–834.
90. Lynch AF, Bourne RB, Rorabeck CH, Rankin RN, Donald A. Deep-vein thrombosis and continuous passive motion after total knee arthroplasty. *J Bone Joint Surg Am.* 1988;70:11–14.
91. Davis FM, Laurenson VG, Gillespie WJ, et al. Deep vein thrombosis after total hip replacement. A comparison between spinal and general anesthesia. *J Bone Joint Surg Br.* 1989;71:181–185.
92. Modig J, Borg T, Karlstrom G, Maripuu E, Sahlstedt B. Thromboembolism after total hip replacement: role of epidural and general anesthesia. *Anesth and Analg.* 1983;62:174–180.
93. Prins MH, Hirsh J. A comparison of general anesthesia and regional anesthesia as a risk factor for deep vein thrombosis following hip surgery: a critical review. *Thromb Haemost.* 1990;64:497–500.
94. Sculco TP, Ranawat C. The use of spinal anesthesia for total-hip replacement arthroplasty. *J Bone Joint Surg Am.* 1975;57:173–177.
95. Thorburn J, Louden JR, Vallance R. Spinal and general anesthesia in total hip replacement: frequency of deep vein thrombosis. *Br J Anaesth.* 1980;52:1117–1121.
96. Gray DH, Mackie CEF. The effect of blood transfusion on the incidence of deep vein thrombosis. *Aust N Zealand Orthop.* 1989;242:212–231.
97. Lieberman JR, Huo MM, Hanway J, et al. The prevalence of deep venous thrombosis after total hip arthroplasty with hypotensive epidural anesthesia. *J Bone Joint Surg Am.* 1994;76:341–348.
98. Sharrock NE, Mineo RS, Urquhart B. Hemodynamic response to low-dose epinephrine infusion during hypotensive epidural anesthesia for total hip replacement. *Reg Anesth.* 1990;15:295–299.
99. Sharrock NE, Mineo R, Urquhart B. Hemodynamic effects and outcome analysis of hypotensive extradural anesthesia in controlled hypertensive patients undergoing total hip arthroplasty. *Br J Anaesth.* 1991;67:17–25.
100. Sharrock NE, Go G, Mineo R, Harpel PC. The hemodynamic and fibrinolytic response to low dose epinephrine and phenylephrine infusions during total hip replace-

ment under epidural anesthesia. *Thromb Haemost.* 1992;68:436–441.
101. Anderson DR, O'Brien BJ, Levine MN, et al. Efficacy and cost of low-molecular weight heparin compared with standard heparin for the prevention of deep vein thrombosis after total hip arthroplasty. *Ann Intern Med.* 1993;119:1105–1112.
102. Colditz GA. Cost effectiveness. In: *Prevention of venous thromboembolism*, pp 541–576. Goldhaber SZ, ed. New York: Marcel Dekker, 1993.
103. Oster G, Tuden RL, Colditz GA. A cost-effectiveness analysis of prophylaxis against deep-vein thrombosis in major orthopaedic surgery. *JAMA.* 1987;257:203–208.
104. Paiement GP, Wessinger SJ, Harris WH. Cost effectiveness of prophylaxis in total hip replacement. *Am J Surg.* 1991;61:519–524.
105. Salzman EW, Davies GC. Prophylaxis of venous thromboembolism. Analysis of cost effectiveness. *Ann Surg.* 191:207–218, 1980.
106. Menzin J, Colditz GA, Regan MM, Richner RE, Oster G. Cost-effectiveness of enoxaparin vs low-dose warfarin in the prevention of deep-vein thrombosis after total hip replacement surgery. *Arch Int Med.* 1995;155:757–64.
107. Menzin J, Richner R, Huse D, Colditz GA, Oster G. Prevention of deep-vein thrombosis following total hip replacement surgery with enoxaparin versus unfractionated heparin: a pharmacoeconomic evaluation. *Ann Pharmacother.* 1994;28:271–275.
108. Arcelus JI, Caprini JA, Traverso CI. Venous thromboembolism after hospital discharge. *Sem Thromb Hemost.* 19 (Supplement 1):1993;142–146.
109. Trowbridge A, Boese CK, Woodruff B, Brindley HH, Lowry WE, Spiro TE. Incidence of posthospitalization proximal deep venous thrombosis after total hip arthroplasty. A pilot study. *Clin Orthop.* 1994;299:203–208.
110. Leclerc JR, Illescas F, Jarzem P. Diagnosis of deep vein thrombosis. In: *Venous thromboembolic disorders.* pp. 176–228. Leclerc JR. Philadelphia: Lea and Febiger, 1991.
111. Heijboer H, Cate JW, Buller HR. Diagnosis of venous thrombosis. *Sem Thromb Haemost.* 1991;17:259–268.
112. Heijboer H, Buller HR, Lensing AW, et al. A comparison of real-time compression ultrasonography with impedance plethysmography for the diagnosis of deep-vein thrombosis in symptomatic outpatients. *N Engl J Med.* 1993;329:1365–1369.
113. Huisman MV, Buller HR, ten Cate JW, Vreeken J. Serial impedance plethysmography for suspected deep venous thrombosis in outpatients. The Amsterdam General Practitioner Study. *N Engl J Med.* 1986; 314:823–828.
114. Hull RD, Hirsh J, Carter CJ, Jay RM, Ockelford PA, Buller HR, Turpie AG, Powers P, Kinch D, Dodd PE, Gill GJ, Leclerc JR and Lent M. Diagnostic efficacy of impedance plethysmography for clinically suspected deep-vein thrombosis. *Ann Intern Med.* 1985;102:21–28.
115. Paiement G, Wessinger SJ, Waltman AC, Harris WH. Surveillance of deep vein thrombosis in asymptomatic total hip replacement patients. Impedance phlebography and fibrinogen scanning versus roentgenographic phlebography. *Am J Surg.* 1988;155:400–404.
116. Rabinov K, Paulin S. Roentgen diagnosis of venous thrombosis in the leg. *Arch Surg.* 1972;104:134–144.
117. Hoek JA, Lensing AW, Cate JW, et al. The clinical utility of objective diagnostic tests for diagnosing deep vein thrombosis of the leg. *Br J Clin Pract.* 65 (Supplement):1989;26–35.
118. Albrechtsson UJ, Olsson CG. Thrombotic side-effects of lower-limb phlebography. *Lancet.* 1976;1:723–724.
119. Bettmann MA, Paulin S. Leg phlebography: the incidence, nature and modification of undesirable side effects. *Radiology.* 1977;122:101–104.
120. Davidson BL, Elliott CG, Lensing AW, The RD Heparin Arthroplasty Group. Low accuracy of color Doppler ultrasound in the detection of proximal leg vein thrombosis in asymptomatic high-risk patients. *Ann Intern Med.* 1992;117:735–738.
121. Woolson ST, McCrory DW, Walter JF, et al. B-mode ultrasound scanning in the detection of proximal venous thrombosis after total hip replacement. *J Bone Joint Surg Am.* 1990;72:983–987.
122. Woolson ST, Pottorff G. Venous ultrasonography in the detection of proximal vein thrombosis after total knee arthroplasty. *Clin Orthop.* 1991;73:131–135.
123. Grady-Benson JC, Oishi CS, Hanson PB, et al. Postoperative surveillance for deep venous thrombosis with duplex ultrasonography after total knee arthroplasty. *J Bone Joint Surg Am.* 1994;76:1649–1657.
124. Atri M, Herba MJ, Reinhold C, et al. Accuracy of sonography in the evaluation of calf deep vein thrombosis in both postoperative surveillance and symptomatic patients. *AJR Am J Roentgenol.* 1996;166:1361–1367.
125. Ginsberg JS, Caco CC, Brill-Edwards PA, et al. Venous thrombosis in patients who have undergone major hip or knee surgery: detection with compression US and impedance plethysmography. *Radiology.* 1991;181:65–654.
126. Borris LC, Christiansen HM, Lassen MR, Olsen AD, Schott P, the Venous Thrombosis Group. Comparison of real-time B-mode ultrasonography and bilateral ascending phlebography for detection of postoperative deep vein thrombosis following elective hip surgery. *Thromb Haemost.* 1989;61:363–365.
127. Garino JP, Lotke PA, Kitziger KJ, Steinberg ME. Deep venous thrombosis after total joint arthroplasty. The role of compression ultrasonography and the importance of the experience of the technician. *J Bone Joint Surg Am.* 1996, 78:1359–1365.

56
Anesthetic Complications

Michael Smalky and Donald Foster

Airway

In order to prevent intraoperative and postoperative complications from airway management, careful initial evaluation of the airway is mandatory. During the preoperative interview, the anesthesiologist must look at all previous anesthetic records, which might reveal prior difficulties with the patient's airway. Advance warning from surgeons who have elicited such a history during an office visit or witnessed airway management during prior surgery can provide valuable preemptive warning when communicated promptly and *early* to the anesthetic care team. Based on history, physical examination, and review of the records, it is possible to develop an initial plan of action that allows for the safe induction of a general anesthetic if needed. These evaluative steps are no less important even if the primary plan is regional anesthesia.

Many patients presenting for revision total hip arthroplasty have underlying medical conditions that may have progressed since the initial surgery. One such example is rheumatoid arthritis. The patient's airway may have been manageable previously, but disease progression could lead to new profound difficulties in airway management. One should always consider the possibility that airway abnormalities have evolved along with the disease process that led the patient to present for hip replacement.

It is frequently argued that if control of the airway might not be easy to establish, then control of that airway should be achieved prior to commencing surgery. An anesthesiologist faced with a difficult airway needs to have a plan to control that airway, even if the primary technique is a regional anesthetic. Regional techniques are sometimes imperfect, and should any difficulty with the regional arise (such as the inadequacy of a spinal or epidural block), it might be dangerous to then induce general anesthesia with the patient already in the lateral decubitious position.

Fortunately, the last decade has provided anesthesiologists with many new tools to assist in controlling the difficult airway. The American Society of Anesthesiologists (ASA) recently did a closed claim review of airway difficulties, which has led to the current ASA algorithm for management of the recognized and unrecognized difficult airway.[1] This algorithm is not a standard, but rather a guide. It can suggest valuable alternative approaches to the difficult airway, and serves to dissuade the anesthesia care team from persisting with a single failed technique for airway control. Case reports relating catastrophic patient outcomes to repeated failed laryngoscopies (leading to airway edema and inability to ventilate) are far too common. The ASA Difficult Airway Algorithm can provide life-saving strategies in such critical situations.

Another essential element in airway management is the "difficult airway" cart. Located such that it can service a group of anesthetizing locations, the cart contains both commonly and rarely utilized tools for airway control. These include a variety of laryngoscope blades, retrograde wire intubation kits, jet ventilator, pediatric fiberoptic bronchoscope, and tracheotomy kits. The difficult airway cart assures the immediate availability of these items, and provides the anesthesiologist with quick access to equipment necessary for the utilization of alternative airway control techniques.[2]

The following scenarios illustrate just a few tools and approaches:

> The anesthesia care team might commit to a plan for general anesthesia to accompany the primary epidural anesthetic for a patient with a known difficult airway. Once the epidural is placed and noted to be working, the anesthesia care team may then proceed with flexible fiberoptic bronchoscopic intubation of the trachea, utilizing topical local anesthetics and sedation. After anesthetic induction, the patient is then turned to the lateral decubitious position with the airway safely protected.
>
> Another patient receives a spinal anesthetic, and surgery proceeds with the patient in the lateral position. An abnormally high spinal block develops, and the patient's ability to ventilate is compromised. General anesthesia with controlled ventilation is now a requirement. Conventional laryngoscopy with the patient in the lat-

eral position can be exceedingly difficult. An alternative approach may be the insertion of a laryngeal mask airway (LMA) after induction of general anesthesia. Once the LMA is in place, a flexible fiberoptic bronchoscope may be used to guide an endotracheal tube into the trachea through the LMA.[3]

Definitive airway control, without complications, depends on the application of a wide knowledge base combined with practiced techniques. Each technique should be carefully and cautiously applied. Flexible and adaptive approaches, using the ASA Difficult Airway Algorithm as a guide, can lead to airway control safely and rapidly in the most difficult circumstances.

Anemia

Taking a very broad look at the perioperative period, anemia is a complication with a multitude of implications. A primarily preventive approach is needed in any strategy to defeat this complication. When the anesthesiologist enjoys the vigorous support of the surgical department in the application of regional anesthesia for orthopedic surgery, many patients may benefit from reduced intraoperative blood loss.[4,5]

Although the patient, surgeon, and anesthesiologist all have input concerning a particular patient's surgical anesthesia, the patient has the final word. The anesthesiologist's role is to guide the patient in reaching an informed decision concerning the selection of anesthesia. This is accomplished after thorough evaluation of the patient's history and the risk/benefit ratio of various options for anesthesia. Nothing helps set the tone for a balanced view more than a surgical department that fully appreciates and supports the implementation of regional anesthesia wherever possible, consistent with good patient care.

Multiple studies have shown that the administration of regional anesthesia can produce significant beneficial effects. These effects include a relative hypotension, reducing the risk of blood loss in patients undergoing revision hip arthroplasty. The blood pressure almost always goes down with a well-functioning spinal or epidural anesthetic. This decline in blood pressure is a sign recognized by the anesthesiologist that heralds the onset of regional blockade. A well functioning regional anesthetic that raises blood pressure would be remarkable.

Anemia can be reduced by cautious utilization of relative controlled hypotension. Hypotensive anesthesia can be induced by an adequate level of regional anesthesia. Relative controlled hypotension can also be achieved with general anesthesia supplemented with various vasodilating agents. Reductions in intraoperative blood loss increase the probability that autologously donated blood will be adequate to replenish the patient's blood volume, thus maintaining an adequate oxygen-carrying capacity.

If a patient is normally hypertensive, a reduction of 30% from the baseline mean arterial pressure (MAP) can usually be safely induced with regional or general anesthesia. Healthy, nomotensive individuals may sustain reductions of mean arterial pressure (MAP) to the range of 55 to 60 mm Hg before cerebral autoregulation fails.[6] Such severe reductions in MAP are seldom utilized in orthopedic surgery, but are commonly required in neurosurgical procedures such as cerebral aneurysm repair.

Anesthesiologists commonly utilize the MAP readings provided by automated cuff or arterial blood pressure measurements immediately prior to anesthetic induction. If the systolic and diastolic pressures provided by these systems correlate with the patient's recorded preoperative pressures (obtained from the chart or by history), the mean pressure of these readings can be reasonably assumed to be the patient's baseline. A conservative target for controlled hypotension can then be estimated as a 20% reduction from that baseline. A 10% margin of safety is thus obtained, alleviating fear of critical organ hypoperfusion. Careful consideration of each patient's proven or suspected coexisting disease must be accomplished during these procedures, and each plan must be individualized to fit the clinical situation.

Achieving controlled hypotension via various anesthetic regimens means the anesthesia care team can reduce blood loss and allow the patient to perhaps receive only autologous blood during the perioperative period. The risks inherent in homologous transfusion are thus reduced. Any time that blood loss can be minimized, the risk of coagulopathy or dilutional thrombocytopenia can be reduced. Many coagulopathies develop after large volumes of banked blood are transfused in response to hemodilution and loss of coagulation factors. Reduction in total blood loss results in less transfusion, with an accompanying reduction in the development of coagulopathy.

Another complication of anemia is the risk of myocardial ischemia (as addressed elsewhere in this book). The lower limit of hemoglobin (or hematocrit) that an individual patient can tolerate may be addressed. This assessment can be undertaken in conjunction with a patient's primary physician or cardiologist, who may have extensive knowledge of the patient's comorbid disease or past response to anemia. Working together as a team, the surgical and anesthesia physicians can agree on the threshold for hematacrit (or hemoglobin) below which transfusion should be initiated. An ongoing discussion should always take place between the members of the operative team as to the set point and timing of transfusion, whether autologous or homologous blood is used. The recommended lower limits of hemoglobin and hematocrit serving as a trigger for transfusion have varied considerably in the last five years.

Cementing

Cardiac arrest is a dreaded complication associated with the placement of prosthetic joints. Research in the past with animal models implicated the monomer from unpolymerized methyl methacrylate cement. The level of monomer necessary to produce problems in animal models was 20 to 35 times greater than that ever measured in human subjects.[7,8] Currently, few patients receive components as heavily cemented as in the past, if cement is used at all. Current protocols for preparation of cement also seek to have the cement further along in the curing stage after thorough mixing, such that little free monomer exists prior to use of the cement.

In addition, one must keep in mind that patients are more intensely monitored these days with arterial central venous or pulmonary artery (PA) lines. In the past, the vasodilatory effects of general or regional anesthesia led to the patient's vascular space being just full enough to maintain circulation. Catastrophic vascular collapse could then result from a relatively small insult, that is, microemboli consisting of unpolymerized methyl methacrylate, air, or marrow components. With today's practice of more intensive, invasive monitoring, volume status tends to be maximized and maintained in a more ideal range, providing a greater reserve and margin of safety before disastrous decompensation occurs. Invasive monitoring also allows for rapid diagnosis of cardiovascular depression, permitting the institution of ionotropic or vasoconstrictive support required to address the situation. Transesophageal echocardiographic (TEE) monitoring can also allow for the rapid observation of these changes in the patient under general anesthesia. TEE is very sensitive in the detection of air and other microemboli. Placement of the prosthetic component with or without cement can be postulated to produce the release of biologic mediators in addition to monomer, fat, and/or air embolism.[9,10] Vasoactive biological mediators are now known to play a role in many processes that were attributed in the past to other causes. With the discovery of atrial naturetic factor, it has only recently been appreciated that the heart can be an endocrine organ.[11] Perhaps one day new factors from bone marrow will be elucidated. Fortunately, the incidence of disastrous decompensation during cementing is a rare event during current revision total hip arthroplasties. This means that future elucidation of precise mechanisms will most likely come from laboratory studies.

Dislocation

The dislocation of prosthetic hip components is discussed from the surgical perspective elsewhere in this book. It is commonly perceived that the use of epidural analgesia in the postoperative period may lead to dislocation of the prosthetic joint. This is especially worrisome if the choice of local anesthetic infusion establishes muscle relaxation at the intensity of intraoperative surgical anesthesia. Analgesia, however, can be provided without the use of local anesthetics, and therefore without fear of muscle relaxation. Two modalities currently in wide use are intrathecal and peridural narcotics. Intrathecal morphine can be placed in conjunction with a spinal anesthetic, and can provide prolonged analgesia long after the spinal anesthetic "effect" has abated. Peridural morphine has the same long-lasting analgesic action and can be administered via the epidural route prior to epidural catheter removal at the end of surgery.

The use of these spinally-administered narcotics tend to reduce the overall narcotic requirement during the convalescent period. They are especially efficacious when combined with patient-controlled analgesia (PCA). (Other benefits would theoretically include a reduction in postoperative ileus, and certainly a reduction in somnolence.)

Thus, the anesthesiologist can allow the muscle relaxation associated with epidural or spinal local anesthetics to wane at the conclusion of surgery. Pain relief can be continued into the postoperative period utilizing centrally acting narcotics, which have no significant muscle-relaxing effects.

Neurologic Complications

Although neurologic complications have been discussed in depth elsewhere in this book, I will briefly cover items related predominately to the administration of regional anesthesia. One of the dreaded complications of epidural or spinal anesthesia is abscess formation. Epidural abscesses occur with the strikingly low frequency of 1 per 2416 epidurals.[12] In one French study, the incidence was fewer than 1 per 9011 epidural anesthetics in an obstetrical population.[13] The actual incidence in older patients with comorbid disease is perhaps somewhat higher, although no precise figures exist. In the majority of epidural abscesses, there may be a relationship to the length of time the epidural is in place. As with any percutaneous invasive device, the longer the device is indwelling, the higher the chance of infection. If an epidural anesthetic is used for revision total hip arthroplasty, the epidural catheter is usually removed in the immediate postoperative period. Rarely, an epidural catheter is utilized for prolonged postoperative analgesia after revision hip arthroplasty. These catheters should receive the standard regimen of proper nursing and dressing care, with close observation for the development of erythema and purulent drainage.

Signs and symptoms of epidural hematoma or abscess can include loss of sensation or function at levels the epidural anesthetic would ordinarily effect. Impaired spinal cord function, marked by loss of bowel and bladder control, lower extremity weakness or change in sensation, excruciating back pain, spinal root pain, or paralysis are symptoms mandating urgent investigation.[14] These symptoms may be variable and dependent upon the degree of motor and sensory block due to local anesthetics in the epidural infusion. The worst outcomes related to epidural abscess or hematoma are seen in those patients in whom symptoms are ignored and institution of therapy is delayed. If an obvious explanation is not rapidly forthcoming and neurological examination reveals the validity of subjective findings, a prompt imaging study of the epidural site and spine is mandatory. The radiologist can give guidance as to whether emergent CT or MRI scanning is preferable.

In patients with a confirmed epidural abscess or hematoma, prompt neurosurgical evaluation is mandatory. The most significant factor related to poor outcome is *delay* in: recognition, proper evaluation, consultation, imaging, and initiation of therapy (which is often surgical).

Although epidural catheter placement requires routine use of standard sterile techniques, antibiotic prophylaxis is not usually required. *Staphylococcus aureus* is by far the most common organism involved in epidural abscess, and it is generally accepted that careful skin preparation will be adequate for disinfection. Abscess formation due to hematogenous seeding may also occur, although this complication seems to be a far less frequent occurrence. Prophylactic antibiotics are often utilized in instances involving long-term epidural catheter placement (ie, tunneled epidural catheters used for the control of chronic oncologic pain). These patients are often immunocompromised, and such antibiotic use appears to be a sensible approach. Controlled studies concerning antibiotic prophylaxis for epidurals are probably not practical, due to the low frequency of complications and the great numbers of patients required to achieve statistical power.

The use of perioperative anticoagulants has markedly reduced the incidence of deep vein thrombosis (DVT) and pulmonary embolism. A variety of anticoagulation protocols are available, some of which are initiated preoperatively. Some patients arrive in the OR having already received coumadin. The initial preoperative dose may not have significantly modified the patient's coagulation profile and the anesthesiologist can safely proceed with a regional anesthetic.

Subarachnoid and epidural hematoma formation has recently been associated with the use of low molecular weight heparin in the United States. This preparation, widely utilized in Europe, was recently approved by the FDA for DVT prophylaxis in total hip arthroplasty. Used as a fixed dose twice daily, this agent appears to be particularly effective in DVT prevention and has the advantage of eliminating postoperative coagulation testing and dosing adjustment. Due to the fear of neuraxis bleeding complications, many anesthesiologists are reluctant to use regional anesthesia in patients already receiving, or slated to receive, low molecular weight heparin. Some may schedule the placement (and subsequent removal) of epidural catheters to coincide with the nadir of the heparin's effects.[15] A similar approach is successfully employed for major vascular surgery performed under spinal or epidural anesthesia. Any bleeding elicited by the spinal or epidural anesthetic is thought to fully abate via normal clotting mechanisms prior to intravenous heparinization during the vascular surgery.

The anesthesiologist's reluctance to employ regional techniques in any patient with a real or perceived risk of bleeding due to anticoagulation is firmly anchored in the desire to safely and appropriately anesthetize the patient. The application of general anesthesia alone reduces the possibility of spinal compromise due to hematoma formation to the level of risk of spontaneous hematoma. Until the safety of regional anesthesia in patients receiving low molecular weight heparin is firmly established, general anesthesia may be the most commonly employed technique by some anesthesiologists.

The diagnosis and treatment of epidural hematoma is a true emergency, as progressive lower extremity weakness quickly leads to permanent paralysis. Fast recognition of the problem in a patient presenting with severe back pain and new onset paresis requires emergent diagnostic imaging (with CT or MRI), followed by decompression via laminectomy and hematoma evacuation.

Headache Occurring after Regional Anesthetic

Postdural puncture headache (PDPH) is a complication affecting approximately 1% of patients after receipt of a spinal or epidural anesthetic. The headache is usually positional, becoming prominent when the patient sits or stands, and quiescent when supine. Restrictions ordered in the past discouraging ambulation after regional anesthesia are no longer imposed. These constraints on the patient's postoperative mobility have no discernible effect on the incidence of PDPH, and are probably detrimental to convalescence.

The incidence of postdural puncture headache is related to the needle actually making the puncture. Spinal needles with pencil-point (Whitacre) tips appear to be less traumatic than the sharp bevel-tipped (Quincke) variety, and are theoretically able to separate, and not cut, dural fibers. The hole thus formed in the dura may close more readily, preventing a continuous leak of cerebrospinal fluid (CSF). This CSF leak into the epidural space may occasionally require autologous "blood patch" (via epidural injection) for definitive treatment.

Other influences on the incidence of spinal headache, aside from needle tip architecture, are the needle's gauge, the number of attempts to accomplish dural puncture, and the age of the patient. It should be noted that advanced age imparts protection against PDPH, and this fact is especially relevant for the patient presenting for revision total hip arthroplasty. This patient population has a nearly insignificant risk for the development of PDPH, and larger (ie, 22 gauge) spinal needles are advantageous for use here. This needle size allows easy penetration of calcified spinal ligaments, and ensures a successful regional anesthetic. We feel that multiple time-consuming attempts with smaller 25- or 26-gauge needles lead to high failure rates and patient discomfort.

Treatment of PDPH is accomplished with hydration, oral or parenteral analgesics, and increased oral caffeine intake. The administration of an epidural blood patch may be required for refractory cases, but this is rarely seen in an older population.

Peripheral Nerve Injuries

Although neurological injury may occur without obvious cause, most palsies and neuropraxias can be prevented with careful attention to patient positioning. Total hip arthroplasty is performed with the patient in the lateral decubitus position, and neutral, nonstressed well-padded positioning is the key to injury prevention. Patients with peripheral vascular disease, diabetic neuropathy, or cachexia pose additional challenges. The extraordinary efforts needed to check pressure points and peripheral pulses are rewarded by the avoidance of untoward consequences.

Turning an anesthetized patient can be hazardous without adequate personnel. The procedure should be smooth and gentle, guided by the anesthesiologist to assure airway control. A silicone gel chest bolster placed one hand's breadth below the dependent axilla will relieve pressure there and prevent the occurrence of brachial plexus palsy. The liberal use of padding between dependent body surfaces and the OR table is ultimately the best preventive measure to avoid nerve compression. Eyes and ears should be free from pressure and thus vascular compromise.

The pulse oximeter can be used to assure proper circulation by alternating measurements from the dependent to the nondependent upper extremity. Care must be taken to check and recheck pressure points, as surgical manipulation may shift the patient's position.

Intraoperative Monitoring/ Intravenous Access

In practical terms, it is necessary to be sure that the patient has adequate intravenous (IV) access and monitoring lines. Blood loss, despite the utilization of hypotensive anesthetic techniques, may be quite vigorous and/or prolonged. In order to effectively replenish circulating blood volume, at least one and preferably two large-bore peripheral IVs are required. Less commonly, some anesthesiologists utilize 7.5 or 8.5 French peripheral rapid-infusion catheters. If adequate venous access is easily accessible, some will place a second IV only if needed during surgery. It must be remembered, however, that venoconstriction occurs during circulatory depletion, and it may be well to place a second access prior to this occurrence. Frequently, a central venous line is placed which provides a second large-bore IV. It must be remembered, however, that the length of a central venous line directly contributes to resistance to flow. The central venous line is nearly always inferior to peripheral large-bore IVs for volume resuscitation. A pulmonary artery catheter introducer can serve as an excellent large-bore access site, although the introducer is too short to provide accurate central venous pressures. When transduced, the introducer can provide valuable trends concerning volume status.

Many younger, healthier patients undergo revision total hip arthroplasty solely with automated noninvasive blood pressure monitoring. An urgently needed radial arterial line may be placed intraoperatively as needed. When controlled hypotension is planned, arterial pressure monitoring is mandatory. In other patients with significant comorbidity, placement of an arterial line either before or immediately after induction is indicated. Arterial pressure monitoring is absolutely mandatory for prompt and effective response when volume depletion and hypotension are concurrent. This is especially important prior to reaming or femoral component placement, which may lead to embolic phenomena and further cardiovascular insult.

Intravascular volume status can be accurately determined via the measurement of central venous pressure (CVP). At our institution, the anesthesia technical service operates equipment for the rapid determination of hemoglobin, and this information can often be obtained within seconds of sampling. Combined with CVP monitoring, this resource provides us with vital intraoperative "snapshots" of patient condition relating to blood loss and fluid resuscitation.

The central venous pressure can also reflect myocardial performance. Acute rises in CVP, often combined with the sudden development of hypotension, may indicate left ventricular ischemia or right heart decompensation due to emboli with resultant pulmonary hypertension. This rise in CVP may be quite immediate, and can occur well prior to the evolution of ECG changes. Although far from being completely sensitive and specific for cardiopulmonary morbidity during surgery, the CVP provides a valuable clinical indicator of problems in this area. This is especially true when the patient's presurgical left ventricular performance is relatively preserved.

When the patient's preoperative left ventricular function is compromised (ie, ejection fraction less than 40%), we employ a pulmonary artery (PA) catheter to allow fuller, more precise monitoring of cardiac performance. Likewise, any patient with significant "myocardium at risk" as assessed by reversible defects on thallium scan (or assumed via stress echocardiography) is scheduled for PA catheter monitoring. Additional indicators for PA catheter placement include a preoperative creatinine of 2.0 or greater, significant pulmonary compromise (especially pulmonary arterial hypertension), or significant valvular disease.

The PA catheter acts as a multiplier of the anesthesiologist's abilities to accurately assess and correct volume difficulties. Optimization of cardiac output during fluid and blood replacement can be accomplished with careful precision, and inotropic support can be instituted without guesswork. Provided the patient has done well during surgery, we have found that a postoperative intensive care unit stay can be avoided by converting the PA catheter to a central venous line after the patient's stabilization. This is a particularly cost-effective approach, and we are now able to discontinue most PA catheters prior to discharge from the post-anesthesia care unit.

A relatively new modality for monitoring intraoperative cardiac function is transesophageal echocardiography (TEE). In patients receiving regional anesthesia this is unlikely to be used, even though TEE is done solely under sedation and topical anesthesia in the cardiology department. In patients undergoing general, or general plus regional anesthesia, transesophageal echocardiography can be utilized. Numerous studies have been done demonstrating its ability to observe and monitor cardiac function and embolic events during reaming, cementing, and component placement.[9,10,16] The anesthesiologists at our institution have wide experience in the placement and interpretation of intraoperative TEE, and will not hesitate to utilize this resource if circumstances dictate.

In the era of capitation and cost containment, however, the issue of value added versus risk and cost arises. If one is to perform a procedure that carries substantial cost, is it clear that the value added is justifiable in routine revision total hip arthroplasty? There are no studies to support this one way or the other. However, studies have been done in similar fields that can help us arrive at some perspective on this issue. Transesophageal echocardiography has been examined in the sitting neurosurgical patient.[17] TEE detected a patent foramen ovale in four out of six patients, and is a sensitive indicator of air embolism. However, this information did not change the management of anesthesia in these patients. Differences in outcome due to TEE have yet to be demonstrated in these patients.

If we next think about cardiac surgical patients, we suspect the benefit could be much greater. Patients undergoing valve surgery or complex defect repairs are often monitored with TEE, and experience has proven its benefit in interrogating the integrity of new prosthetic valves. In straightforward coronary artery bypass surgery, patients tend only to have central venous lines rather than pulmonary artery lines or even TEE, as intraoperative management is not substantially improved with these modalities.

Thus, some evidence would lead away from the routine utilization of transesophageal echocardiography in the revision total hip arthroplasty patient. TEE could, however, be beneficial in a few selected patients experiencing cardiovascular decompensation with histories of severe, complex comorbid disease. TEE can be placed quickly (even in the lateral decubitus position) in a patient who develops acute difficulties during revision total hip arthroplasty. In patients with sudden decompensation unimproved by management based on data derived from a PA catheter or CVP alone, TEE may permit evaluation of cardiac function and intervention that may be conducive to good outcome. Only future studies will determine definitively whether TEE has a place in routine revision total hip arthroplasty.[18]

Hypothermia

Prevention of hypothermia has always been a great concern of the anesthesia care team. Hypothermia plays an important role in several complications. Core hypothermia to 35.0° C has been demonstrated to increase blood loss during total hip arthroplasty.[19] If the result of hypothermia is increased homologous transfusion, the risk of infection also increases.[20]

Postoperative hypothermia with resultant shivering produces marked increases in cardiac output and oxygen consumption. In patients with compromised oxygenation or cardiac performance, myocardial ischemia can result. Severe hypothermia will induce arrhythmias and ventricular fibrillation.

It is somewhat intuitive that extended intraoperative hypothermia probably leads to an increased infection risk. Biological systems work best within narrow ranges of temperature, and it is logical to assume that the patient's immune system is compromised by low temperatures. No studies exist on the effects of hypothermia on infection rates in revision hip arthroplasty, but a recent study examined these effects in intestinal surgery.[21]

It was noted that relatively mild hypothermia (34.7° C) led to an increased risk of infection there. Should further studies support and expand this finding to other surgeries, it may well be that keeping patients euthermic during revision total hip arthroplasties may prevent some postoperative infection.

In addition, the maintenance of euthermia, or nearly normal core temperature, yields other beneficial effects as well. The effects of muscle relaxants dissipate and are reversed more thoroughly when vigorous efforts are made to protect patients from the cold OR environment. Forced-air warming blankets, intravenous fluid warmers, and the passive humidification of anesthetic gasses all contribute to this effort. These attempts to maintain or return the patient to normal temperature may contribute to subtle but real reductions in the incidence of blood loss, arrhythmias, myocardial ischemia, and infection.

References

1. Caplan RA, Posner KL, Cheney FW. Adverse respiratory events in anesthesia: a closed claims analysis. *Anesthesiology.* 1990;72:828–833.
2. Benumof JL. Management of the difficult adult airway, with special emphasis on awake tracheal intubation. *Anesthesiology.* 1991;75:1087–1110.
3. Pennant JH, White PF. The laryngeal mask airway. Its uses in anesthesiology. *Anesthesiology.* 1993;79:144–163.
4. Sharrock NE, Cazan MG, Hargett MJ, et al. Changes in mortality after total hip and knee arthroplasty over a ten-year period. *Anesth Analg.* 1995;80:242–248.
5. Grosflam JM, Wright EA, Cleary PD, Katz JN. Predictors of blood loss during total hip replacement surgery. *Arthritis Care Res.* 1995;8:167–173.
6. Miller ED. Deliberate hypotension. In: *Anesthesia*, 3rd ed. Miller RD, ed. New York: Churchill Livingstone, 1990: 1347–1367.
7. d'Hollander A, Monteney E, Hooghe L, Camu F, Donkerwolcke M, Brauman H. Cardiovascular effects of methyl methacrylate monomer. *Surg Gynecol Obstet.* 1979;149:61–64.
8. McLaughlin RE, DiFazio C, Hakala M, Abbott B, MacPhail JA, Mack WP, et al. Blood clearance and acute pulmonary toxicity of methyl methacrylate in dogs after simulated arthroplasty and intravenous injection. *J Bone Joint Surg Am.* 1973;55:1621–1628.
9. Ereth MH, Weber JG, Abel MD, Lennon RL, Lewallen DG, Ilstrup DM, et al. Cemented versus noncemented total hip arthroplasty-embolism, hemodynamics and intrapulmonary shunting. *Mayo Clin Proc.* 1992;67:1066–1074.
10. Christie J, Robinson CM, Pell AC, McBirnie J, Burnett R. Transcardiac echo-cardiography during invasive intramedullary procedures. *J Bone Joint Surg Br.* 1995;77:450–455.
11. Gerzer R. Das herz, ein endokrines organ: die entdeckung eines neuen hormons. *Klinische Wochenschrift.* 1985;63:529–536.
12. Brooks K, Pasero C, Hubbard L, Coghlan RH. The risk of infection associated with epidural analgesia. *Infect Control Hosp Epidemiol.* 1995;16:725–726.
13. Palot M, Visseaux H, Botmans C, Pire JC. Epidemiologie des complications de l'analgesie peridurale obstetricale. *Cah Anesthesiol.* 1994;42:229–233.
14. Heusner AP. Non-tuberculous spinal epidural infection. *N Engl J Med.* 1948;239:835–854.
15. Hynson JM, Katz JA, Bueff HU. Epidural hematoma associated with enoxaparin. *Anesth Analg.* 1996;82:1072–1075.
16. Woo R, Minster GJ, Fitzgerald RH Jr, Mason LD, Lucas DR, Smith FE. Pulmonary fat embolism in revision hip arthroplasty. *Clin Orthop.* 1995;319:41–53.
17. Black S, Muzzi DA, Nishimura RA, Cucchiara RF. Preoperative and intraoperative echocardiography to detect right to left shunt in patients undergoing neurosurgical procedures in the sitting position. *Anesthesiology.* 1990;72: 436–438.
18. Propst JW, Siegel LC, Schnittger I, Foppiano L, Goudman SB, Brock-Utne JG. Segmental wall motion abnormalities in patients undergoing total hip replacement: correlations with intraoperative events. *Anesth Analg.* 1993;77:743–745.
19. Schmied H, Kurz A, Sessler DI, Kozek S, Reiter A. Mild hypothermia increases blood loss and transfusion requirements during total hip arthroplasty. *Lancet.* 1996;347: 289–292.
20. Murphy P, Heal JM, Blumberg N. Infection or suspected infection after hip replacement surgery with autologous or homologous blood transfusions. *Transfusion.* 1991;31: 212–217.
21. Kurz A, Sessler DI, Lenhardt R. Perioperative normothermia to reduce the incidence of surgical wound infection and shorten hospitalization. *N Engl J Med.* 1996;334:1209–1215.

57
Cardiac Complications

Gerard A. Sweeney and Charles J. Dow

While the mortality of revision hip arthroplasty (RHA) is reassuringly low (less than 1%), RHA often involves prolonged anesthesia, usually in an elderly population, and the procedure is often accompanied by significant blood loss. Patients are significantly deconditioned in most circumstances, which may increase their risk for coronary artery disease.[1] Pulmonary embolization of cement-bone marrow debris is common, leading to cardiopulmonary stress. In 18 patients undergoing RHA, all patients demonstrated hemodynamic changes involving right ventricular function. These changes were usually small and clinically insignificant, but 4 patients had a greater than 10% decrease in right ventricular ejection fraction and a 10% increase in pulmonary artery systolic pressure. All the patients in this study using transesophageal echocardiography experienced detectable intracardiac emboli during the procedure.[2] Hypotension, hypoxemia, cardiac arrythmias, cardiac arrest, or any combination of these complications characterize bone cement implantation syndrome and fat embolism syndrome. These are rare complications of the procedure and are the result of fat and marrow elements extruded into the venous circulation.

The ischemogenic potential of the procedure increases the risk of cardiovascular complications. Myocardial infarction and cardiovascular complications equal pulmonary embolus as the most common cause of death following hip surgery.[3] This combination of factors necessitates comprehensive preoperative assessment and perioperative management in order to optimize the chance for a successful outcome.

Role of the Cardiovascular Consultant

Although the risks are remarkably low overall, for selected patients undergoing RHA the incidence of complications may be high. It is important to focus on identifying patients in whom complications are more likely to occur. Identifying this high risk group does not necessarily warrant preoperative intervention such as revascularization, as this approach is unproven and carries inherent risk that may be equal to or greater than the risk of the proposed operative procedure. Furthermore, plaque rupture with thrombosis, the cause of acute myocardial infarction, is often secondary to perioperative stress and increased catecholeamine stimulation. Identifying plaques vulnerable to rupture and treating them with percutaneous transluminal angioplasty (PTCA) preoperatively is an approach not justified by available data.

When a patient with known or suspected heart disease requires surgery, the role of the consultant is not simply to "clear" the patient, but to act as an advocate throughout the pre- and perioperative period. The consultant must make a recommendation to proceed with surgery, to postpone surgery and attempt to modify the preexisting morbid condition, or to cancel the procedure.

Preoperative Cardiovascular Risk Assessment

Clinical risk assessment attempts to identify patients at low, intermediate, or high risk for adverse cardiac outcomes (Table 57.1). Patients with high cardiac risk are at increased risk for developing cardiac complications. Certain cardiovascular problems represent absolute contraindications to proceeding with elective RHA. These problems include recent myocardial infarction (less than 3 months), unstable angina, decompensated congestive heart failure, and symptomatic aortic and mitral stenosis.

Relative contraindications include mild CHF, class III angina, and significant arrythmias such as symptomatic ventricular tachycardia, symptomatic complete heart block, and supraventricular arrythmia with poorly controlled ventricular response.

A large proportion of patients presenting for preoperative consultation fall into the more difficult intermediate risk category.[4] Intermediate predictors of risk include mild angina, remote myocardial infarction, history of congestive heart failure, and diabetes mellitus.

Table 57.1. Clinical predictors of increased perioperative cardiovascular risk (myocardial infarction, congestive heart failure, death).

Major
Unstable coronary syndromes
   Recent myocardial infarction* with evidence of important ischemic risk by clinical symptoms or noninvasive study
   Unstable or severe** angina (Canadian Class III or IV) ^
Decompensated congestive heart failure
Significant arrhythmias
   High grade atrioventricular block
   Symptomatic ventricular arrhythmias in the presence of underlying heart disease
   Supraventricular arrhythmias with uncontrolled ventricular rate
Severe valvular disease

Intermediate
Mild angina pectoris (Canadian Class I or II)
Prior myocardial infarction by history or pathological Q waves
Compensated or prior congestive heart failure
Diabetes mellitus

Minor
Advanced age
Abnormal ECG (left ventricular hypertrophy, left bundle branch block, ST-T abnormalities)
Rhythm other than sinus (eg, atrial fibrillation)
Low functional capacity (eg, inability to climb one flight of stairs with a bag of groceries
History of stroke
Uncontrolled systematic hypertension

ECG indicates electrocardiogram.
*The American College of Cardiology National Database Library defines recent MI as greater than 7 days but no less than or equal to 1 month (30 days)
**May include "stable" angina in patients who are unusually sedentary.
^Campeau L. Grading of angina pectoris. *Circulation.* 1976;54:522–523

Minor predictors of risk include advanced age, abnormal electrocardiogram (ECG) rhythm other than sinus, history of stroke, uncontrolled hypertension (diastolic pressure greater than 110), and poor functional capacity.

Perioperative and long-term cardiac risk is increased in patients unable to exercise to meet a 4 metabolic equivalent (MET) level demand during normal daily activity. Climbing a flight of stairs, walking on level ground at 6.4 km/hr, scrubbing a floor, or playing a round of golf equals 4 to 10 METS. Strenuous sports such as swimming and singles tennis exceed 10 METS (Table 57.2).

Many patients presenting for RHA are disabled and severely deconditioned. One study demonstrates a trend for more frequent manifestations of coronary heart disease in patients with severe osteoarthritis compared to age- and sex-matched controls (27% versus 13%; $p > 0.05$).[1] These patients present a special problem in risk stratification.

Patients with intermediate risk predictors, including patients with a functional capacity of less than 4 METS, should undergo further testing. There is evidence that most patients with severe arthritis are capable of maximum symptom limited excercise testing using ergonometric measures (bicycle or arm ergometry). Philbin et al. studied the feasibility and safety of stress testing in a consecutive series of patients with severe arthritis.[5] Arthritic subjects underwent a single-graded, maximal, symptom-limited, cardiopulmonary exercise test using an electronically braked ergometer and a metabolic cart. Subjects were first asked to pedal with their legs; those apparently incapable performed the same task with their arms. Ninety-five percent of subjects were able to perform symptom limited excercise. High rates of achievement of physiologic values indicative of maximal excercise were achieved with both arm and leg tests (age-predicted maximum heart rate $> 80\%$ and mean respiratory gas exchange ratio [RER] $>$ or $= 1.0$). Therefore, ergonometry stress testing may be a viable low cost alternative to dipyridamole-thallium imaging, dobutamine echocardiography, and cardiac catheterization in many patients requiring further risk stratification.

ACC/AHA guidelines[6] suggest the following measures appropriate in the setting of RHA:

1. Revision hip arthroplasty for infection may not allow for preoperative risk evaluation.
2. If the patient has undergone coronary artery bypass

operation in the last 5 years and is asymptomatic without signs of recurrent ischemia, further testing is probably not necessary.
3. If the patient has had coronary risk evaluation in the past 2 years and results were satisfactory and negative, further testing does not need to be repeated.
4. A major clinical predictor of high risk should lead to cancellation of elective surgery.
5. Intermediate risk patients are most likely to benefit from further testing.
6. Patients with intermediate risk and moderate or excellent functional capacity can undergo RHA with acceptable cardiovascular risk.
7. RHA is generally safe for patients with neither major nor intermediate risk factors, with moderate or excellent functional capacity.
8. The results of noninvasive testing can be used to determine further pre- and perioperative management. PTCA and CABG should be performed based only on the merits of the patient's cardiac symptoms and cardiac anatomy, and not to enhance the safety of the surgery.[7]

Maximum utilization of advances in anesthetic technique, intra- and postoperative monitoring are important in minimizing morbidity and mortality in this group of patients.

Management of Specific Preoperative Cardiovascular Conditions

Hypertension

Severe hypertension (diastolic pressure greater than 110 mm Hg) should be controlled prior to elective surgery. Antihypertensive medications should be continued throughout the surgical period with the least possible interruption.

Valvular Heart Disease

Recommendations are identical to those for patients with valvular heart disease in the nonoperative setting.

Significant valvular heart disease, particularly valvular stenosis in the asymptomatic but functionally incapacitated patient, warrants intensive pre- and postoperative monitoring. Every effort should be made to treat heart failure preoperatively. These patients may benefit from perioperative hemodynamic monitoring and adjustment to optimal after load and preload.

There may be a role for percutaneous aortic balloon valvuloplasty in certain patients.[7]

Myocardial Disease

Dilated and hypertrophic cardiomyopathy require careful pre- and perioperative management. Maximizing hemodynamic status with intensive medical therapy is essential. The patient must be hemodynamically compensated prior to the procedure. Careful intraoperative management and postoperative surveillance will help to optimize cardiac performance and prevent complications.

Arrhythmia and Conduction Abnormalities

Symptomatic ventricular arrhythmias need to be addressed and treated as they would be in the nonoperative setting.

First degree heart block, Mobitz type I second degree heart block, asymptomatic bilateral bundle branch

Table 57.2. Estimated energy requirements for various activities.*

1 MET	4 METs
Can you take care of yourself? Eat, dress or use the toilet? Walk indoors around the house? Walk a block or two on level ground at 2–3 mph or 3.2–4.8 km/h? Do light work around the house such as dusting or washing dishes?	Climb a flight of stairs or walk up a hill? Walk on level ground at 4 mph or 6.4 km/h? Run a short distance? Do heavy work around the house such as scrubbing floors or lifting or moving heavy furniture? Participate in moderate recreational activities such as golfing, bowling, dancing, doubles tennis, or throwing a baseball or football?
	>10 METS
	Participate in strenuous sports like swimming, singles tennis, football, basketball, or skiing?

MET indicates metabolic equivalent.
*Adapted from the Duke Activity Status Index and AHA Exercise Standards.

block, or trifascicular block do not require prophylactic pacing. Trifasicular block with a history of unexplained syncope, patients with left bundle branch block who require hemodynamic monitoring, or asymptotic complete heart block may require prophylactic pacing preoperatively.

Atrial fibrillation with the ventricular rate adequately controlled is an acceptable preoperative rhythm.

Permanent Cardiac Pacemakers

Application of electrosurgery provides a high-frequency electrical field that produces electrical voltage on the electrodes of a pacing system. This voltage may be detected within the pacing system and various arrhythmias can be provoked in correlation with the underlying mode of pacing. Proper pacemaker programming can prevent pacing malfunctions due to the electrosurgery application. A consultant should check the pacemaker parameters and function before surgery. Rate-responsive modes should be disabled and a magnet should be available to convert the pacer to the fixed rate mode should that become necessary. Appropriate positioning of the neutral electrode of the electrocautery device in relation to the pacing system may help avoid interference with the pacing system. Implanted defibrillators and antitachycardia devices require special care and consultation with a clinical electrophysiologist for special recommendations and temporary reprogramming. The pacemaker or device should be checked postoperatively to assure appropriate function and parameters.

Prosthetic Heart Valves and Anticoagulation

Anticoagulants continued through the operative period adversely affect hemostasis, and troublesome postoperative bleeding may ensue. Anticoagulants can be temporarily discontinued during the operative period with minimal risk of thrombosis in most cases. In one study[8] no thromboembolic complications occurred in 159 patients with prosthetic valves undergoing 180 noncardiac operations when warfarin was discontinued an average of 2.9 days preoperatively and resumed 2.7 days postoperatively. Katholi et al. did not observe thromboembolic complications in 25 operations on patients with prosthetic aortic valves; however, two such complication occurred in the 10 patients with mitral valve prosthesis when anticoagulants were discontinued for noncardiac surgery.[9]

In patients at low risk for thromboembolism, such as patients with tilting disc aortic valves, anticoagulant therapy may be briefly discontinued 3 to 5 days before RHA and resumed promptly postoperatively. In patients with caged ball prosthetic valves, mechanical mitral valves and atrial fibrillation, or left atrial thrombus, anticoagulation should not be interrupted and heparin may be required preoperatively. Prothrombin time should be restored to within 20% of normal by stopping oral anticoagulants for 3 to 5 days days preoperatively. In patients with prosthesis who are at high risk for thrombosis, heparin should be instituted until about 6 hours prior to surgery. Heparin and oral anticoagulation can be restarted postoperatively when primary hemostasis is established.[10,11,12]

Peroperative Medical Therapy and Intensive Care

There are very few randomized trials of medical therapy before noncardiac surgery to prevent cardiac complications. There is insufficient evidence to draw firm conclusions or make specific recommendations concerning prophylactic antiischemic medications.[6] Previously administered medications should be continued. Patients demonstrating active signs of myocardial ischemia should be treated on an individual basis depending on the specific clinical circumstances.

The pulmonary artery catheter can provide significant information in the perioperative care of the cardiac patient undergoing RHA. There is a role for preoperative invasive monitoring in the patient at increased risk because of significant myocardial or valvular heart disease when optimal compensation is uncertain. Intraoperative and postoperative invasive pressure monitoring is important in the high-risk patient likely to experience great fluid shifts.

Intraoperative transesophageal echocardiography can be extremely useful in certain circumstances such as hypotension; however, there is insufficient data to justify such use on a routine basis.

Postoperative Cardiac Complications

Cardiac complications are relatively infrequent following hip arthroplasty, occurring in 28 (1.7%) of 1684 patients in one large series.[3] These include acute myocardial infarction, acute coronary insufficiency, congestive heart failure, cardiac arrythmias, and cardiac arrest.

Postoperative myocardial infarction peaks on the third postoperative day. The optimal strategy for detecting postoperative infarction has not been developed. In patients with known coronary disease, ECGs at baseline immediately post operatively and on the second and third postoperative day may be the most cost-effective strategy. CK-MB is less specific postoperatively and should be reserved for patients with ECG abnormalities or symptoms or hemodynamic evidence of ischemia. Patients who sustain a perioperative MI or develop evidence of myocardial ischemia should be evaluated carefully, as they are at substantial risk for further ischemic events in the future. Accordingly, they should be evaluated for left ventricular function and for evidence of significant myocardial ischemia on exertion or with pharmacologic stress. Some of these patients would benefit from revascularization with CABG or PTCA. Physicians responsible for the long-term care of the patient should be appraised of any cardiac abnormalities or risk factors identified during the perioperative period.

Postoperative congestive heart failure may be precipitated by myocardial infarction or ischemia, but is more often brought on by excess fluid administration and usually responds to intravenous diuretics. Patients with signs and symptoms of heart failure preoperatively have a high incidence (35%) of postoperative CHF and might benefit from invasive hemodynamic monitoring.

Postoperative arrythmias are often a manifestation of a noncardiac complication such as bleeding, infection, or electrolyte imbalance in a patient with underlying cardiac disease. Management of the arrythmias usually requires recognition and correction of the extracardiac factors. Sinus tachycardia is the most common postoperative rhythm disturbance and may be caused by multiple noncardiac disturbances including pain, hypo- or hypervolemia, fever, anemia, hypoxemia, pulmonary emboli, anxiety, infection, hypotension, or electrolyte abnormalities. In cases of a secondary or compensatory mechanism, treatment should be directed at the underlying cause. Supraventricular tachyarrythmias (atrial fibrillation and atrial tachycardia) were found in 38 of 1210 patients undergoing joint replacement surgery,[13] representing an incidence of 3.1%. The only variables found to be associated with the postoperative development of AF/SVT were a history of atrial fibrillation, increasing age, left anterior hemiblock, and premature atrial beats on the preoperative ECG. In patients over 60 years of age and one or more of these risk factors, the incidence was 18.2%. In patients younger than 60 years of age with none of the identified risk factors, the incidence was 1.9%. Treatment usually consists of underlying noncardiac precipitants and rate control with intravenous beta blockers such as esmolol or calcium channel blockers such as diltiazem. Cardioversion is seldom necessary.

Postoperative hypertension is often precipitated by volume overload, hypoxemia, anxiety, and pain. The main therapeutic approach should concentrate on adequate oxygenation, pain control, and volume control. Nitroprusside may be necessary for immediate control of severe hypertension.

Conclusion

The goal of the cardiovascular consultant in evaluating the patient for RHA should be to focus on identifying low-, intermediate-, and high-risk groups. High-risk patients may have to be cancelled or postponed for further testing. Preoperative hemodynamic monitoring may be indicated in some patients to achieve optimal compensation. Patients at intermediate risk may need further testing according to ACC/AHA guidelines. Low-risk patients and intermediate-risk patients with excellent functional capacity usually do not require further risk stratification with costly noninvasive or invasive testing. Revascularization or cardiac surgery should be recommended for this group of patients based on the merits of the patient's symptoms or cardiac anatomy, and not to improve the safety of RHA.

The cardiovascular consultant should be available for postoperative management considering the significant physiologic stress imposed by large intravascular volume shifts and cement–bone marrow embolization. Convalescence may be complicated by the high incidence of venous thromboembolic disease and the physical demands of rehabilitation in a usually deconditioned and elderly patient.

References

1. Philben EF, Groff GD, Ries MD, Miller TE. Cardiovascular fitness and health in patients with end-stage osteoarthritis. *Arthritis Rheum*. 1995;38(6):799–805.
2. Urban MK, Sheppard R, Gordan MA, Urquhart BL. Right ventricular function during revision total hip arthroplasty. *Anesth Analg*. 1996;82(6):1225–1229.
3. Coventry MB, Beckenbaugh RD, Nolan DR, Ilstrup DM. 2,012 total hip arthroplasties: A study of postoperative course and early complications. *J Bone and Joint Surg Am*. 1974;56:273–284.
4. Blaustein AS. Preoperative and perioperative management of cardiac patients undergoing noncardiac surgery. *Cardiol Clin*. 1995;13(2):149–161.
5. Philben EF, Ries MD, French TS, Feasability of maximal cardiopulmonary exercise testing in patients with end-stage arthritis of the hip and knee prior to total joint arthroplasty. *Chest*. 1995;108(1):174–181.
6. ACC/AHA Task Force, Perioperative Cardiovascular Evaluation Guidelines. *Circulation*. 1996;93:1280–1317.
7. Roth RB, Palacios IF, Block PC. Percutaneous aortic balloon valvuloplasty: its role in the management of patients with aortic stenosis requiring major noncardiac surgery. *J Am Coll Cardiol*. 1989;13:1039–1041.
8. Tinker JH, Tarhan S. Discontinuing antiocoagulant therapy in surgical patients with cardiac valve prostheses. *JAMA*. 1976;239:738.
9. Katholi RE, Nolan SP, McGuire LB. Living with prosthetic heart valve. Subsequent noncardiac operations and the risk of thromboembolism or hemorrhage. *Am Heart J*. 1976;92:162.
10. Goldman L, Wolf M, Braunwald E. *Heart disease a textbook*

of cardiovascular medicine, Braunwald, E., ed. Philadelphia: W.B. Saunders, 1980.
11. White RH, McKittrick T, Hutchinson R, Twitchell J. Temporary discontinuation of warfarin therapy: changes in the international normalized ratio. *Ann Intern Med.* 1995;122(1):40–42.
12. Vongpatanasin W, Hillis LD, Lange RA. Medical progress: prosthetic heart valves. *NEJM.* 1996;335:407–416.
13. Kahn RL, Hargett MJ, Urquhart B, Sharrock NE, Peterson MG. Supraventricular tachyarrythmias during total joint arthroplasty: incidence and risk. *Clin Orthop.* 1993;296:265–269.

58
Broken Femoral Stems

James P. Jamison and St. George Tucker Aufranc

Femoral stem fracture represents a challenging problem in revision total hip arthroplasty. Implant failure also implies a major impact on the patient in terms of loss of function, submission to revision surgery, and rehabilitation. The highest incidence of stem fracture was reported by Martens et al., at 11% with an early design of the Charnley-Müller prosthesis.[1] Later designs had considerably more success. Charnley reported a rate of 0.23% in a review of 6500 cases,[2] while Carlsson showed an incidence of 0.67% with the Charnley prosthesis.[3] Wroblewski noted the incidence of fracture of the Charnley "flat back" prosthesis at a relatively high 1.15%,[4] as compared to Chao and Coventry's review of fracture in various implants at the Mayo Clinic with a more moderate rate of 0.6%.[5]

Etiology of Stem Fracture

The major factors identified as contributing to the etiology of femoral stem fractures may be categorized as clinical, technical, and metallurgic.

Clinical Factors

Clinical factors relating to breakage of the femoral stem are age, weight, height, bone quality, and activity level. Collis reported femoral stem fractures in four patients, all of whom were male, at least 6 feet in height, greater than 200 pounds in weight, and who suffered from back pain and pain or loss of motion in the contralateral hip. Each patient had returned to moderately heavy physical activity following surgery. Collis also cited decreased range of motion in the operated hip as a factor in stem breakage, as it results in increased stresses on the implant.[6] In a study examining possible predisposing factors for stem breakage, Ritter noted a preponderance of males in the fracture group (10 to 4 over females), as compared to a predominance of females in the nonfracture group (108 to 151 over males).[7] The fracture group was also noted to be younger by an average of 7.3 years (52.5 vs. 59.8 years), and heavier by an average of 37.1 pounds (198.5 vs. 160.6 pounds) as compared to the nonfracture group.[7] Similar findings have been noted by other authors.[2,5,8,9]

Technical Factors

Of the technical factors identified, Ritter found varus alignment to be of greatest influence. He noted lack of adequate distal lateral cement support and absence of sufficient proximal medial osseous support secondary to calcar resorption as additional factors in the etiology of femoral stem fracture.[7] The effect of varus positioning and lack of adequate proximal support have been noted by several authors.[4,5,9] Charnley considered calcar resorption to be a leading cause of prosthesis fracture, resulting in defective support for cement proximally and exposing the stem to strong bending stresses as it remains fixed distally. In addition, he noted that failure to remove cancellous bone of poor quality at the level of the calcar could prevent adequate cement contact with stronger cancellous bone, leading to a gap at the bone–cement interface, again resulting in inadequate proximal medial support.[2] Careful cement preparation and insertion are important so as to avoid defects in the cement column.[6] Gruen highlighted the importance of proper cement support for the prosthesis, noting the cantilever bending mode of failure as most common in stem fracture.[10]

Metallurgy and Design

Implant design and composition of metal alloys, as well as flaws at the time of manufacturing, have been recognized as contributing factors in stem breakage, with the goal of more modern implants being to reduce the probability of fracture.[6,8,10,11] Advances in implant design and metallurgic composition have resulted in a decrease in femoral stem fracture due to metal fatigue.[12]

Evaluation of Impending or Existing Fracture

Pain, often referred to the thigh or knee, is usually the first indication of a problem. Onset can be sudden, with or without trauma, or more gradual in nature. Scheller found that pain progressed insidiously in intensity for a 4- to 6-month period before stem fracture was diagnosed in 21 of 29 patients studied. The remainder suffered an acute onset of symptoms directly associated with an identifiable trauma.[13] Discomfort may be greatest when walking or arising from a chair. Reports exist of patients with no symptoms, diagnosed only by radiographs taken for other purposes.[9] Charnley noted a patient who presented with pain seven years after surgery, for whom careful retrospective review of radiographs revealed the presence of a femoral stem fracture three years earlier.[2]

Careful radiographic evaluation is essential as routine follow-up of the total hip arthroplasty patient (Fig. 58.1). Several variables are important in identifying those that may be at risk for stem fracture and in analyzing the cause of failure in those that have fractured. Chao and Coventry reviewed 58 cases of femoral stem fracture and developed a risk index as a predictor and measure of probability of stem failure. The most significant variables involved cement quality at various levels of the stem, particularly medially at the proximal end and laterally at the distal end, porosity and gaps at the cement–bone interface, cancellous bone removal at the calcar and greater trochanter, varus orientation, and nicks on the stem.[5] Excessive remaining cancellous bone is important as it can potentially hinder cement interdigitation if the bone is of poor quality, resulting in inadequate support of the prosthesis proximally.[13] Varus orientation subjects the stem to higher stresses due to the increased moment arm, resulting in an increased bending moment and higher lateral stresses.[13]

Techniques of Stem Removal

A number of techniques for extraction of the broken femoral stem are noted in the literature. Having progressed with advancing technology, these approaches lend the revision hip surgeon several options with which to handle this difficult and often frustrating problem. The methods of fractured stem include use of a cortical window, use of a trephine, removal of all peripheral cement, and use of an extraction device at the fractured surface after drilling.

Cortical Window Techniques

Pellicci et al. discussed the use of a cortical window placed on the anterior cortex of the femur distal to the tip of the stem.[14] Anterior window placement was chosen so as not to compromise the integrity of the lateral femoral cortex where the femur experiences maximal stresses. Via the window a curved Rush rod could be introduced into the medullary canal to aid in removal of the distal cement plug. Once cement had been cleared distally, the same Rush rod could be used to tap out the broken stem. Revision surgery could then be performed using a long-stem prosthesis to span the cortical defect. Alternatively, the window could be placed more proximally at the level of the retained distal fragment. The stem could then be driven proximally with a thin instrument impacting the side of the distal fragment.

Placement of a cortical window just below the level of the implant fracture was favored by Moreland et al.[15] Several reasons for choosing this method versus creating a window distal to the stem or drilling the fractured surface and attaching an extraction device (discussed below) were cited. First, a standard length revision prosthesis can be used in reconstruction, as opposed to the long-stem implant required when placing the window distal to the tip of the broken stem. Second, the technically demanding process of drilling a hole in the fractured proximal end of the retained fragment could be avoided altogether. Machining a hole in the metal surface several centimeters below the canal opening was cited as being time-consuming and difficult. In addition, specialized instruments not readily available at all institutions were required. Finally, if the proximal drilling

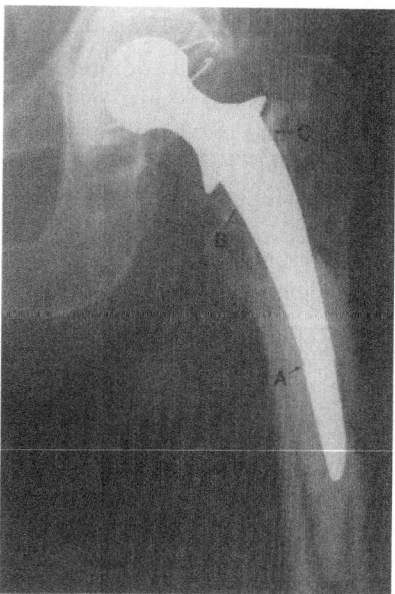

Figure 58.1. A. AP radiograph of a broken femoral stem. Note the varus orientation and the fracture line. B. Cement support for the prosthesis is minimal both proximal-medial and distal-lateral, with lateral cortical hypertrophy. C. The lateral gap at the proximal cement-prosthesis interface indicates motion prior to fracture and further collapse into varus.

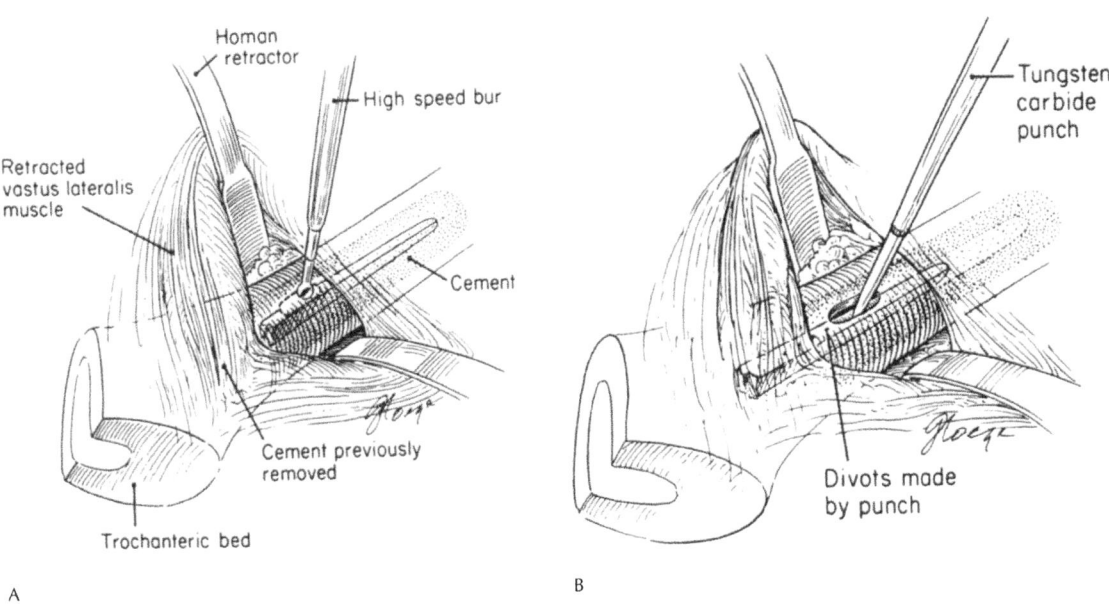

Figure 58.2. A. A window measuring 4 × 20 mm with a high-speed burr through the anterior cortex and cement to expose metal. B. A carbide punch is used first to indent the stem; it is then tilted to drive the stem cephalad with a mallet. (From Moreland J, Marder R, and Anspach W,[15] by permission of Clinical Orthopedics and Related Research)

technique failed, the cortical window approach provided a dependable alternative. Despite having the disadvantage of weakening the femur, the authors preferred the window technique for its simplicity and dependability.[15]

Their procedure of windowing the femur just distal to the fracture surface of the stem was described using a lateral transtrochanteric approach. After dislocation, the proximal stem fragment is removed and osteotomes are used to clear away cement down to the level of the fractured metal. A ruler or other reference guide is used to measure the distance from the canal opening to the broken surface, and a point on the anterior cortex just distal to the broken surface is marked for the window. Excessive trauma to the overlying vastus lateralis muscle is avoided by exposing the cortex via a small incision with the aid of two narrow Homan retractors (Fig. 58.2A). With this exposure a window measuring 4 mm in width by 10 mm in length is made with a high-speed burr through anterior cortex and cement to expose metal. A carbide punch is used first to indent the stem to gain purchase, then tilted with the tip pointed cephalad to drive the stem proximally with a mallet (Fig. 58.2B). A metal drilling burr can be used to indent the stem if the carbide tip is not sufficient for this purpose. As the stem is driven out, the steps of indenting the stem and driving it proximally are repeated progressively as the more distal portions of the stem move into the window, until the stem can be removed easily at the femoral canal opening. At this point, the cortical window provides light and visualization for the removal of distal cement. Stem removal was usually achieved in five to ten minutes.[15]

The success of this technique in ten cases of broken femoral stems was described by Moreland et al., five of which followed failure of the proximal drilling technique described by Harris (see below).[15,16] Windows were repaired by bone grafting, revision completed in most cases with a stem of standard length, and patients returned to full weight-bearing after two months. There were no complications due to the window at one to four year follow-up.[15]

A similar technique was outlined by Amstutz et al.[17] A minor variation was in the recommended size of the window, 5 mm by 15 mm. They noted the advantage of needing only a standard length revision stem as opposed to the long stem required with the distal window method. In addition, they illustrated how starting with a window distal to the tip of the prosthesis could result potentially in the need for a much larger window. As the stem is pushed proximally, the tip becomes more difficult to reach as it moves away from the window, making it necessary to extend the window proximally for access. This problem is avoided by exposing the prosthesis near the fractured proximal surface. They preferred this approach over drilling the proximal end of the stem, made difficult by a narrow canal, a distal fracture, a stepped fracture surface, harder metals, and the need for specialized instruments and technical skill.

Trephine Techniques

A different method of extraction of broken femoral stems involve the use of a trephine. Collis and Dubrul described such a technique using a trephine sized to fit the diameter of the stem. Once the loose proximal piece is removed, any remaining cement down to the fractured stem surface is cleared away. To facilitate seating and alignment of the trephine, an additional 1 mm of cement distal to the fractured surface must also be cleared. The proper trephine size is chosen by comparing the distal fractured end of the proximal stem fragment to a set of trephines of different diameters, selecting the size which just clears the stem. Careful sizing is important to prevent excessive loss of bone stock. The appropriate trephine is then applied to a powered reamer and placed into the femoral canal to align with the remaining stem fragment (Fig. 58.3A). As the trephine advances, the stem serves to guide it down the canal. Both heat and friction disrupt the cement, necessitating copious irrigation to prevent thermal injury to the bone.[18]

Once the trephine stops and cools, the cement repolymerizes inside it, making the stem adherent to its internal surface. It can then be easily removed. In the event of a stem too long for available trephines, a curved stem, or a stem with its distal tip directly against cortical bone, two options are available. First, a slaphammer can be attached to aid in extraction. Second, a collet instrumentation system can be clamped on to the proximal end of the stem to facilitate removal (Figure 58.3B). This technique was used successfully to remove 25 broken stems and can be applied both to cemented and to porous ingrowth stems. The authors cited the difficulty of drilling the proximal end of the broken stem, further complicated by work-hardening, as well as the resistance of newer super alloy metals and the complication of creating metal chips in the canal as reasons to avoid Harris' drilling technique (see below).[16] In addition the trephine was felt to cause little to no injury to the surrounding cortex, unlike the cortical window approach. Also, use of a trephine is applicable to stems of different geometrical designs, is not hampered by fenestrations in the stem filled with bone or cement, and can be completed in a relatively short operating time, decreasing blood loss.[18] Of note, however, no mention was made of metal debris created by the trephine against the stem, especially in the case of the porous coated noncemented implant.

Amstutz et al. also listed the trephine approach as an option for stem removal, noting that the cortical window and carbide punch method does not apply to porous ingrowth stems. They mentioned the importance of careful sizing and orientation of the trephine as crucial to avoid accidental cortical perforation.[17]

Cement Removal Techniques

A third procedure for removal of broken femoral stems involves removal of all peripheral cement around the retained distal fragment, allowing it to be removed from the femoral canal with a grasping instrument. Stillwell et al. cited this method using the Midas Rex instruments with the long, thin TU-10 dissecting tool.[19] Positioning of the instrument and progress of the bit through the cement mantle is monitored by biplanar fluoroscopy intraoperatively. Though noted as an improved method to avoid weakening the femur with a cortical window, the limitation of the extremely narrow femoral canal that prevents passage of the bit was identified, risking perforation of the femoral cortex.

Metal Drilling / Extraction Techniques

The fourth category in techniques of fractured femoral stem removal involves several variations of a common idea: drilling of the exposed proximal fractured end of the retained fragment and attaching an extraction device for removal. This concept has been documented by several authors.

Pellicci briefly mentioned drilling and tapping of the distal fragment with attachment of an *ad hoc* extractor for removal of the retained stem portion.[14]

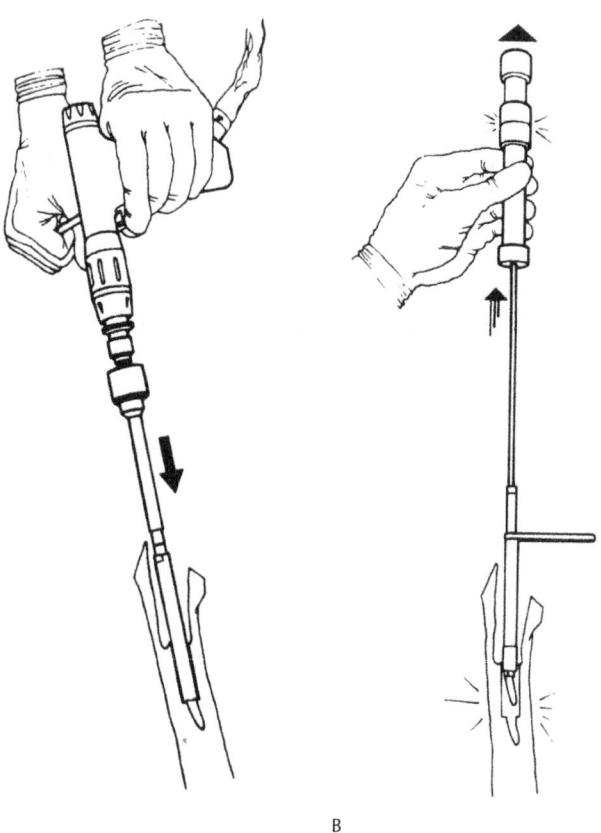

Figure 58.3. A. The appropriately sized trephine is used to disrupt the cement. B. If necessary, a collet instrumentation system can be clamped on the proximal end of the stem to facilitate removal. (From Collis D, Dubrul W,[18] by permission of Contemporary Orthopedics)

Wroblewski described an approach that entails marking the fractured surface and drilling a hole into which is screwed a sliding extractor. Once exposure, dislocation, and removal of the proximal fragment and cement have been achieved, a cannulated guide is used with a punch to indent the fractured surface, marking the site for drilling. However, as the guide is not self-centering, care must be taken not to place the mark eccentrically. The punch is felt necessary due to the probable work-hardening of the fractured surface, making penetration by a drill alone more difficult and prone to sliding off the metal surface, risking damage to or perforation of the cortex. The stem is then drilled to a depth of 1 cm via the cannulated guide. Finally, the stem extractor with sliding hammer is attached at the hole via a left-handed thread for implant removal. Thirty-five fractured stems were extracted successfully by this method.[20]

Mollan et al. described a similar yet more involved process of broken stem removal requiring the use of a mold of the femoral component as a guide.[21] This approach evolved from the authors' desire to eliminate the problems of maintaining correct drill alignment within the femoral canal and to prevent drill "whipping" while trying to penetrate the rough, hardened, often irregular or sloped fractured surface. These problems were addressed by using a rubber guide molded to the exact dimensions of the component with a longitudinal cannulation. Following removal of the proximal fragment at surgery, it is set against the matching rubber mold drill guide as a reference for length. The guide is then cut slightly shorter than the proximal fragment and the distal portion of the mold is discarded. The proximal piece of the guide is then inserted into the proximal femur, automatically oriented into proper alignment by the proximal cement column. Cutting it shorter than the proximal stem fragment allows for circulation of cooling irrigation during drilling. A carbide burr is then used to abrade a centering mark on the fractured surface to aid in preventing wandering of the drill bit. Once marked, a 3.2 mm armor-piercing drill is inserted via the rubber guide for initial drilling to a depth of 12 to 15 mm, then widened to 4 mm with a second drill to facilitate tapping. A 3/16-inch diameter tap is used next to prepare for the threaded extractor which is screwed into the hole for component removal with a sliding hammer.

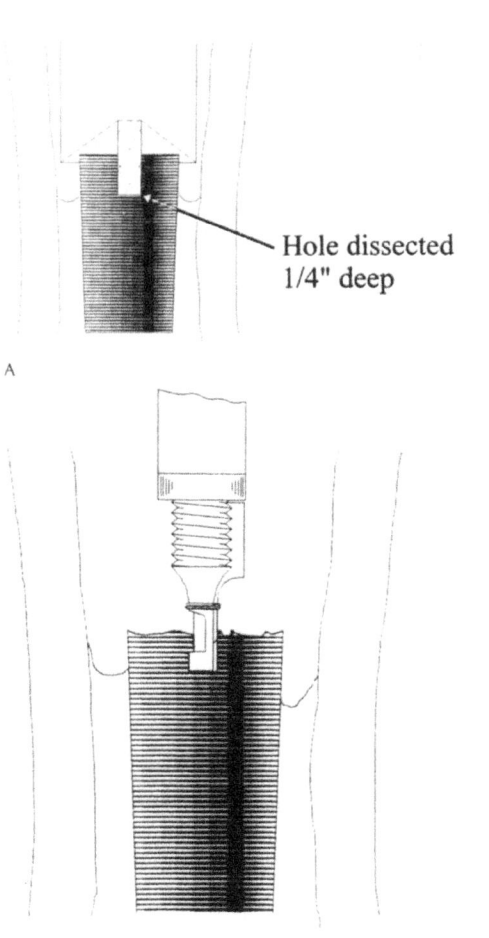

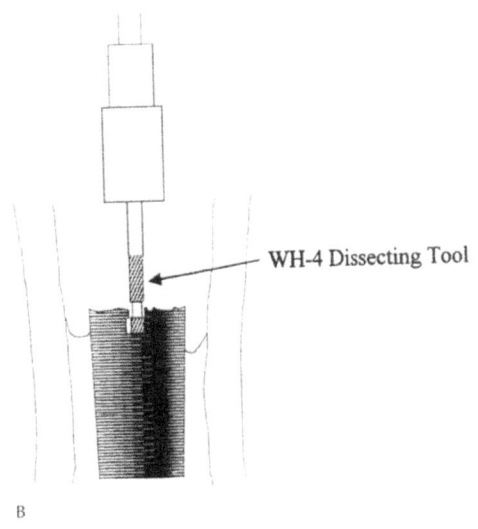

Figure 58.4. A. The WH-3 end-cutting bit drills a smooth cylindrical hole in the fractured surface of the retained distal portion of the fracture stem. B. The WH-4 side-cutting bit drills an undercut in the cylindrical hole. C. The extractor consists of a toe that is inserted into the undercut and a wedge that is engaged to stabilize the toe into the undercut. The extractor and the stem are then removed as a unit with a slap hammer. (By permission of Midas Rex Institute, Inc., Fort Worth, Texas)

The authors preferred using a burr over a punch to mark the starting point for drilling, suggesting that a punch only caused further work-hardening of the fractured surface. Similarly, an armor-piercing drill was favored over a standard drill, which produces more heat and blunts more readily, thereby also causing further work-hardening of the surface. The molded rubber guides were felt to provide correct alignment for drilling of the fractured surfaces at all levels of the stem. In addition, they noted the benefit of having a stock supply of rubber molds for all implants and sizes commonly used at one's institution to be ready for emergency situations.[21] The limitations of this technique are obvious, however, especially at referral institutions where fractured stems of a variety of shapes and dimensions may be encountered. In addition, no mention was made of disruption of the proximal cement column caused by the mobile proximal fragment, which would make firm positioning of the rubber mold difficult if not impossible.

Harris introduced use of the Midas Rex instruments for fractured femoral stem extraction, facilitated by undercutting the drilled hole for attachment of a special extraction tool. After obtaining adequate exposure and cement removal from the proximal femur, cement must be removed from around the proximal end of the retained stem portion with the AM-10 or TU-10 cutting tools to allow proper positioning of the drill guide. A specifically designed drill guide with depth gauge is used with the WH-3 end-cutting bit to drill a hole ¼ inch deep into the fractured surface (Figure 58.4A). The drill guide fills the medullary canal, stabilizing the drill and preventing the tip from wandering until the hole is started.

The WH-4 side cutting dissecting tool is then inserted to undercut the hole, allowing application of the extractor (Figure 58.4B). The extractor consists of a toe that is inserted into the undercut and a wedge that is engaged to stabilize the toe into the undercut (Figure 58.4C). Once firmly seated, a slap hammer is attached to the extractor for removal of the distal stem fragment. Harris noted the importance of maintaining proper alignment while drilling to prevent formation of an oblique hole and possible perforation of the cortex. Also, copious irrigation is required for cooling and clearing metal debris from the canal. Harris' initial report of this technique illustrated success in seven cases and failure in one, in which the drilled hole was elliptical in shape due to wandering of the drill bit. The extractor toe could not be utilized and the stem was removed via a cortical window.[16]

Conclusion

The fractured femoral stem presents a difficult challenge to the revision total hip surgeon. An understanding of the etiology of this complication has led to the development of newer alloys and designs of femoral implants that have reduced but not completely eliminated the problem.[12] In addition, improved surgical and cementing techniques have helped to decrease the incidence of stem fracture.[4] Recognizing the clinical and radiographic presentation of the fractured femoral stem is the first step in proper management. This chapter outlines the various approaches to extraction of the retained distal fragment. The technique most suitable must be individualized to the particular case and to the expertise of the operating surgeon. Knowledge of more than one technique is beneficial in the event of failure of the initial approach. A firm grasp of the problem and its management should direct the surgeon toward successful treatment of this complication in revision total hip arthroplasty.

References

1. Martens M, Aernoudt E, de Meester P, et al. Factors in the mechanical failure of the femoral component in total hip prostheses. *Acta Orthop Scand.* 1974;45:693–710.
2. Charnley J. Fracture of femoral prostheses in total hip replacement. A clinical study. *Clin Orthop.* 1975;111:105–120.
3. Carlsson A, Gentz C, Stenport J. Fracture of the femoral prosthesis in total hip replacement according to Charnley. *Acta Orthop Scand.* 1977;48:650–655.
4. Wroblewski B. Fractured stem in total hip replacement. *Acta Orthop Scand.* 1982;53:279–284.
5. Chao E, Coventry M. Fracture of the femoral component after total hip replacement. An analysis of fifty-eight cases. *J Bone Joint Surg Am.* 1981;63:1078–1094.
6. Collis D. Femoral stem failure in total hip replacement. *J Bone Joint Surg Am.* 1977;59:1033–1041.
7. Ritter M, Campbell E. An evaluation of Trapezoidal-28 femoral stem fractures. *Clin Orthop.* 1986;212:237–244.
8. Marmor L, Gruen T. Stem fractures of extra-heavy cobra femoral hip prostheses. Report of two cases. *Clin Orthop.* 1984;190:148–153.
9. Callaghan J, Pellicci P, Salvati E, et al. Fracture of the femoral component. Analysis of failure and long-term follow-up of revision. *Orthop Clin North Am.* 1988;19:637–647.
10. Gruen T, McNeice G, Amstutz H. "Modes of failure" of cemented stem-type femoral components. A radiographic analysis of loosening. *Clin Orthop.* 1979;141:17–27.
11. Galante J. Causes of fracture of the femoral component in total hip replacement. *J Bone Joint Surg Am.* 1980;62:670–673.
12. Galante J. Metals used in orthopaedic surgery. In: Asher M, Gartland J, Lovell W, et al., eds. *Orthopaedic knowledge update I: Home study syllabus.* Chicago: American Academy of Orthopaedic Surgeons, 1984:89–98.
13. Scheller A, Mitchell S, Barber F. Femoral component fracture in revision hip arthroplasty. In: Turner R, Scheller A, eds. *Revision total hip arthroplasty.* New York: Grune & Stratton, 1982:147–179.
14. Pellicci P, Salvati E, Robinson H. Mechanical failures in to-

tal hip replacement requiring reoperation. *J Bone Joint Surg Am.* 1979;61:29–36.
15. Moreland J, Marder R, Anspach W. The window technique for the removal of broken femoral stems in total hip replacement. *Clin Orthop.* 1986;212:245–249.
16. Harris W, White R, Mitchel S, et al. A new technique for removal of broken femoral stems in total hip replacement. A technical note. *J Bone Joint Surg Am.* 1981;63:843–845.
17. Amstutz H, Luetzow W, Moreland J. Revision of femoral component: cemented and cementless. In: Amstutz H, ed. *Hip arthroplasty.* New York: Churchill Livingstone, 1991:829–854.
18. Collis D, Dubrul W. Removal of fractured prosthetic components from the medullary cavities: a new technique. *Contemp Orthop.* 1984;8:61–65.
19. Stillwell W, Barber F, Mitchell S. Instrumentation for total hip arthroplasty. In: Stillwell W, ed. *The art of total hip arthroplasty.* Orlando: Grune & Stratton, 1987:97–122.
20. Wroblewski B. A method of management of the fractured stem in total hip replacement. *Clin Orthop.* 1979;141:71–73.
21. Mollan R, Watters P, Luney W, et al. New technique for removal of broken femoral stems in THR. *Orthop Rev.* 1983;12:77–80.

59
Surgical Complications in Revision Arthroplasty

Steven J. Camer

In spite of recent advances in anethestic management and volume replacement, revision hip arthroplasty continues to frequently involve prolonged anesthesia with significant blood loss and replacement.[1] Furthermore, revision hip surgery is often performed on elderly patients who are more susceptible to diseases that can present as acute nonorthopedic surgical emergencies. The diagnosis of these surgical emergencies can often be difficult in the postrevision period unless the orthopedic surgeon has a high index of suspicion. The danger of metastatic infection of the hip prosthesis from a septic focus to the implant must always be kept in mind. In addition, the proximity of the operative field to other intrapelvic structures (rectum, bladder, and iliofemoral vessels) has caused some unique problems that the general surgeon can help solve.

Surgical Abdominal Complications in the Postrevision Period

Preoperative Evaluation

As previously implied, postoperative surgical patients are subject to the full range of abdominal surgical catastrophes. A review of all of them is beyond the scope of this discussion. In many cases a careful history taken at admission, will show symptoms that will alert the examiner to potential causes of acute abdominal disease in the postrevision period. Appropriate preoperative studies could then be ordered. Thus, patients with diseases such as cholelithiasis, peptic ulcer, or diverticulitis can be identified before they undergo hip surgery. Judgment as to whether the abdominal problem should be treated prior to subjecting the patient to revision arthroplasty would properly be rendered at this time. Prophylaxis of abdominal complications is the best and safest treatment, especially when compared to the consequences of joint sepsis.[2–5]

Acute Complications of Peptic Ulcer Disease

Quiescent peptic ulcers, both gastric and duodenal, are sometimes reactivated during the stress of major nonabdominal surgery, with perforation or bleeding as the first indication. The increasing use of endoscopy has also shown us that damage to the gastric mucosa can occur early in stressed patients, and if not adequately treated can lead to erosive gastritis with life-threatening hemorrhage. We have found the first 3 or 4 days after orthopedic surgery to be the most dangerous period for these complications. Some etiologic factors predisposing patients to the complications of acute peptic ulcer disease can be elicited preoperatively. Smoking, nonsteroidal antiinflammatory drugs (NSAID) use, and *Helicobactyer pylori* infection have been increasingly implicated. Steroids, along with NSAIDs, also have a well-deserved reputation for reactivating dormant ulcer disease or allowing new ulcers to develop, as well as decreasing host resistance to infection. A history of steroid or NSAID therapy in a rheumatoid patient must be kept in mind when evaluating for abdominal pain in the postrevision period.[6,7] Aspirin, still often used in the therapy of arthritis patients, is another ulcerogenic factor.

Perforated Ulcer

The physical signs and diagnostic features of peritonitis secondary to perforated peptic ulcer are well known. They can be masked significantly in patients on steroid medication.[8] On plain upright x-ray of the abdomen, the presence of free air can aid in the diagnosis, but this is not a consistent finding. Abdominal computerized tomography (CT) scan with oral contrast, now routinely available on an emergency basis, can show extravasation of contrast consistent with a perforated peptic ulcer (Fig. 59.1). It should be emphasized, however, that in the presence of peritonitis one should not delay surgical therapy for an unreasonable time in order to

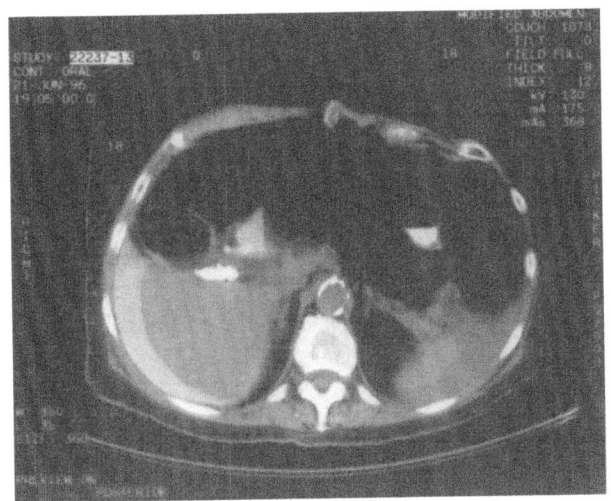

Figure 59.1. Computed tomography scan illustrating massive leakage of contrast from perforated duodenal ulcer in a patient on steroids 6 days after revision arthroplasty.

"clinch" the diagnosis. Although the initial efflux from a perforated ulcer may be sterile, as the disease progresses colonization takes place from oral intestinal tract flora and the stage is set for intra-abdominal abscess, placing the patient and prosthesis at high risk.[9] In some cases perforation can occur and the perforation can then seal with a localized peritonitis, which can be quite evanescent. In patients with a known ulcer, this can be misinterpreted as acute exacerbation and lead the examiner away from the true sequence of events.[10] Hours later, recurrence of the perforation can occur with shock and full-blown peritonitis. Thus, repeated examinations at short intervals is indicated to allow early surgery to minimize contamination of the peritoneum. Finally, especially in elderly patients and those on high-dose steroid medications, symptoms and signs may be minimal or nonexistent. Abdominal distention may be the only sign and may be confused with postoperative ileus.

If the perforated ulcer is acute with no previous history, simple closure of the perforation is sufficient.[11,12] If chronic ulcer disease is present and there is no long-standing soilage of the peritoneal cavity or preoperative shock, definitive surgery such as proximal gastric vagotomy in addition to closure, or vagotomy and pyloroplasty may be considered.[13,14] The decision to embark on a definitive ulcer operation as opposed to the speedier alternative or simple closure of the perforation requires mature surgical judgment and assessment of the abdomen at the time of operation.[15-19]

Bleeding Peptic Ulcer

Hemorrhage occurs in about 35% of patients with duodenal ulcer and is a leading cause of death in those patients.[20,21,15] Therefore, the orthopedic surgeon should be sensitized to this complication since early endoscopy and involvement of the surgical team is essential. Endoscopy will confirm the diagnosis and identify factors predictive of rebleeding or of the necessity for surgery. At endoscopy, initial therapy for the control of bleeding can be done with electrocautery, laser, or sclerosis. In patients who have failed medical therapy, surgery is required and should be undertaken promptly before prolonged transfusion with bank blood or prolonged existence of a low flow state. In unstable patients, suture of the bleeding point, vagotomy, and pyloroplasty are acceptable but associated with a 15% to 30% rate of rebleeding.[20] Thus vagotomy and antrectomy should be considered in the stable patient.

Stress Erosive Gastritis

Like patients who undergo extended operation and/or trauma, the revision hip patient is a potential candidate for extensive hemorrhage from stress erosive gastritis.[22] In elderly patients, the prevalence of this complication also arises with the necessity for mechanical ventilation or the presence of sepsis. The diagnosis is made by endoscopy and characteristically several sites of bleeding are identified and often cannot be treated by endoscopic therapy. The best treatment for hemorrhage from acute stress gastritis is prevention, which is aimed at reducing acid production (antacid and H_2 blocking agents) or protecting gastric mucosa (sucralfate misoprostol).[23,21] Some form of prophylaxis is appropriate in elderly or immunocompromised patients undergoing revision hip anthroplasty.[24,25]

Acute Cholecystitis Following Joint Replacement Surgery

Since Glenn's report in 1947, acute cholecystitis as a specific entity following surgery in areas remote from the biliary system has received increasing attention in the literature.[26,27] Some series since then also implicate severe trauma or prolonged low flow state as an antecedent factor in the development of a particularly fulminating cholecystitis with a relatively high mortality[28,29] if it is undiagnosed or inadequately treated. An observed increased incidence of such cholecystitis in patients after joint replacement first prompted a review of our experience at the New England Baptist Hospital that has since been updated.

This type of acute cholecystitis is most common in older patient groups, especially after the sixth decade. It does not exhibit gender predominance and there is a higher incidence of acalculus cholecystitis than would be expected in this older age group. We noted 18 cases of acalculus cholecystitis in our updated series of 47 patients.

One of the significant features observed both in our patients and in the literature is the onset of symptoms after resumption of the intake of food after a postoperative period of starvation. It has been postulated that during absent or limited oral intake the gallbladder may fail to empy for 2 or 3 days. Under these conditions bile stasis, increased viscosity, and sludge formation cause obstruction of the cystic duct in patients with and without stones. Acute inflammation can then follow, with mucosal injury and thrombosis of blood vessels in the seromuscular layer of the gallbladder. Culture of aspirated bile early on is positive in 38% of patients and increases as the necrosis takes place. The time interval between resumption of full oral intake and the onset of symptoms appears to be more important than the interval between orthopedic operation and the attack of cholecystitis. In our series the initial episode occurred most commonly between the third and seventh day after revision surgery. Another possible etiologic factor in these patients is the almost universal use of narcotic drugs. Most narcotics cause increased tonicity of biliary sphincters and can also retard gallbladder emptying.

The diagnosis of cholecystitis can be rendered more difficult by postoperative fever, ileus and incisional pain. Further, the symptoms are often initially quite mild and can progress rapidly so that repeated clinical examination at short intervals is necessary. Over half our patients complained of pain in the right upper quadrant of the abdomen or epigastrium with associated nausea and vomiting. Fever and abdominal tenderness was present in over 75% of patients. Laboratory studies are not significantly helpful in aiding diagnosis. The white blood count was not elevated or slightly elevated in half of the patients. Liver function tests were abnormal in only a few patients. The serum amylase was elevated in only 4 of 47 patients. This test, however,

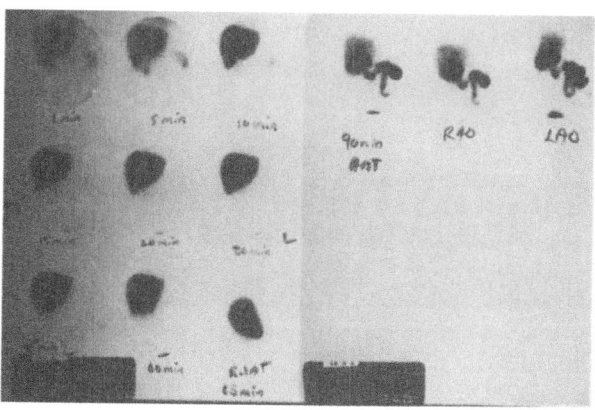

Figure 59.3. Normal hepatic diacetic acid scan demonstrating good filling of the gallbladder and bile ducts in a patient with paralytic ileus and right upper quadrant tenderness, three days after revision hip surgery.

should always be performed to help rule out pancreatitis, the presence of which may significantly change the management. Noninvasive radiologic studies are of significant benefit in making the diagnosis. Gallstones can almost always be demonstrated by ultrasonography, which also images the biliary ductal system. Ultrasonography can also show thickening and edema of the gallbladder wall and pericholecystic fluid (Fig. 59.2) both indications of gallbladder inflammation. Radionuclide hepatic aminodiacetic acid (HIDA) scanning can assess for cystic duct obstruction, which is present most of the time in both calculous and acalculous acute cholecystitis (Fig. 59.3 and 59.4). Both of these

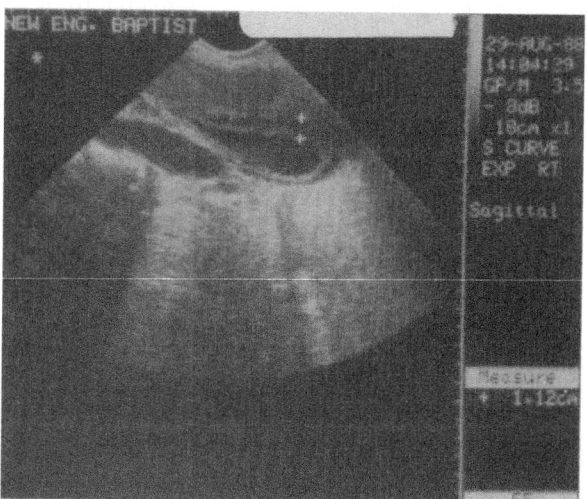

Figure 59.2. Gallbladder ultrasound illustrating edema of gallbladder wall and pericholecystic fluid consistent with acute cholecystitis.

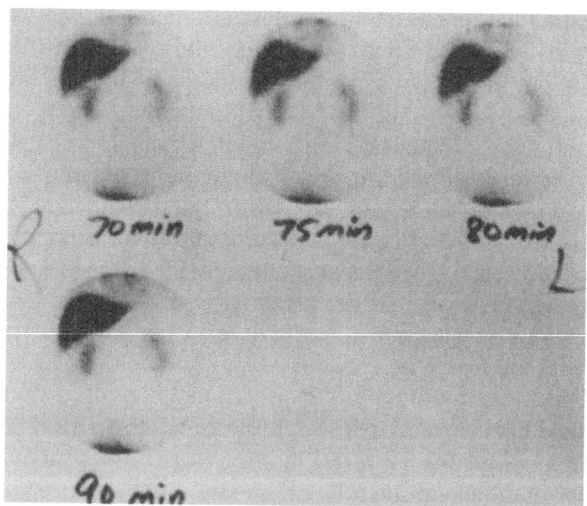

Figure 59.4. Abnormal hepatic diacetic acid scan in a patient 7 days after hip replacement with fever, ileus, right upper quadrant tenderness. The gallbladder fails to take up the isotope. At surgery acute inflammation and dilatation of the gallbladder with an impacted stone obstructing the cystic duct.

studies can be performed with minimal discomfort to the postoperative hip patient.

Once the diagnosis is made, emergent or urgent surgery is required. Cholecystectomy should be performed as soon as the disease is recognized to avoid the complications of gangrene, empyema with abscess, or perforation with biliary peritonitis. Simple drainage of the gallbladder either surgically or percutaneously in the radiology suite should be reserved for only the sickest patients because of its disadvantage of leaving a septic focus behind with subsequent possible seeding of the prosthesis. Although open surgical management is considered by many to be the safest way of managing patients with severe cholecystitis, there is a strong case for an increasing trend towards laparoscopic management.

As general surgeons gain more experience and confidence in the arena of elective laparascopic cholecystectomy, we have in the last five years used laparoscopy initially in almost all patients, at least as a diagnostic inspection. In the presence of established gangrene and perforation, the operation can quickly be converted to open management. If laparoscopic cholecystectomy can be safely performed, however, there are undoubted advantages over open surgery with the prompt resumption of rehabilitation activity for the postoperative hip patient. Because of the observed increased incidence of this complication and the high stakes involved, we recommend that ultrasonography be performed in all patients who have a history of biliary symptoms and that the gallbladder be laparoscopically removed prior to the performance of the orthopedic procedure whenever it is in a diseased state. A normal preoperative sonogram, of course, does not rule out the diagnosis in the postoperative period because the patient may develop acalculous cholecystitis.[30]

Intestinal Obstruction

Mechanical obstruction of the small or large bowel may occur at any time. The symptoms of abdominal distention, cramps, vomiting, and obstipation are well known. Predisposing factors such as hernias, previous surgery leading to intra-abdominal adhesions, or a history of intestinal obstruction should alert one to the possible existence of mechanical intestinal obstruction in the postoperative hip revision period. Small hernias, both ventral and inguinal, may be difficult to diagnose, particularly in obese or supine immobilized patients. Irreducible or symptomatic hernias should be repaired prior to arthroplasty. Patients with partial small bowel obstruction and patients with the potential for reversibility, such as patients with adhesions as a result of a previous abdominal operation, may undergo a trial of nonoperative therapy. Physical examination and abdominal x-ray should be repeated at least every 12 hours, and worsening findings or failure to improve mandate operative treatment. In patients who have not had previous abdominal surgery, the most common causes of intestinal obstruction are conditions that are not reversible and must be surgically corrected as soon as possible. If a diagnosis is not definite, one may initiate NG decompression and follow-up with a small bowel contrast study if the diagnosis is still in doubt. In patients with complete obstruction, closed loop obstruction, or incarcerated external hernia, prompt surgery after fluid resuscitation is mandatory to avoid the development of gangrene and perforation, both of which have grave consequences for the patient and the hip prosthesis.[31,32]

More common problems in the postrevision period are acute gastric dilatation and functional obstruction (paralytic ileus). Acute gastric dilatation can present quite dramatically with massive vomiting without nausea. In the supine immobilized patient, such vomiting can lead to aspiration and immediate death. Massive gastric dilatation can also cause cardiovascular collapse, which can mimic coronary thrombosis or pulmonary embolism. The early warning signs of acute gastric dilatation are an unexplained rise in pulse rate, belching, hiccups, or epigastric distention. On observation of these signs, prompt nasogastric tube aspiration of the stomach is rewarded with large volumes of air and fluid, which can be both diagnostic and lifesaving.

Patients with sliding hiatus hernia are particularly prone to regurgitation and aspiration in the recumbent position. The postoperative hip patient with hiatus hernia, narcotized, and possibly in traction is at high risk for the development of these complications. In patients with known sliding hiatus hernia, nasogastric decompression and intermittent suction should be instituted during the operation, along with the administration of H_2 blockers, and maintained during the immediate postoperative period until the patient is alert and can be elevated in bed.

Paralytic ileus refers to a functional large and small bowel obstruction without a mechanical component. It occurs in the postoperative period and can be initiated by retroperitoneal bleeding, as is often present in revision arthroplasty. Anesthesia and the administration of analgesic drugs, particularly the opiates, may also contribute to postoperative paralytic ileus.[33] The differentiation between paralytic ileus and mechanical obstruction may be quite difficult and becomes moreso as the ileus is longstanding. The degree of distention may be greater in paralytic ileus, and the distention is usually painless. The most helpful immediate study is a flat film of the abdomen, which will show diffuse dilatation of the entire small and large intestine in paralytic ileus and distal collapse of the intestine in mechanical obstruction (Figs. 59.5 and 59.6). It should be emphasized that a portable film at the bedside is usually not of good enough quality to make the above distinction, and the

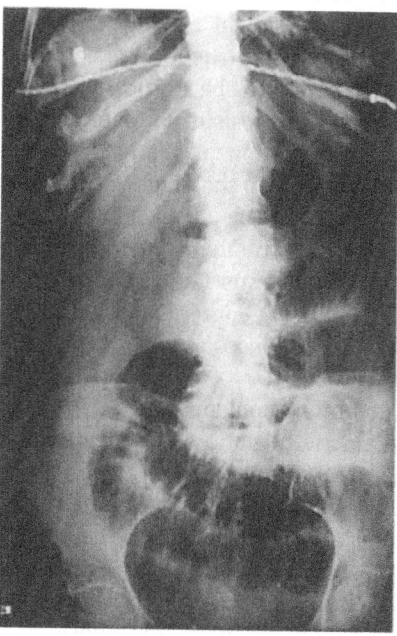

Figure 59.5. Flat plate of a patient with mechanical obstruction of the small intestine. There is an absence of gas in the large intestine. Note the ladder-like arrangement of distended small bowel. The abnormal distention is confined to the center of the abdomen.

ness, and leukocytosis is unusual unless present from a secondary source. The etiology of this potential lethal condition is unknown, and is probably caused by multiple factors. However, the final common path may be parasympathetic stimulation of the distal colon with spasm. Colonic distention, if it is truly massive, can put the intestine, especially the cecum, at risk. The measurement of cecal diameter is therefore crucial in determining a diagnostic and therapeutic strategy for this condition. Plain abdominal films can be used to assess the diameter of the cecum, and one would usually not see small bowel distention or air fluid levels (Fig. 59.7). Other conditions such as sigmoid or cecal volvulus, mesenteric ischemia, fecal impaction, or toxic megacolon must be ruled out, either by contrast enema or endoscopy.[34] Nasogastric suction, correction of fluid and electrolytic imbalance, cessation of oral intake, and serial physical examinations should be employed once mechanical obstruction has been excluded and one should rectify possible pharmacologic causes contributing to ileus. A rectal tube can be used, but must be inserted carefully to avoid bleeding and perforation. In many cases the tube will become occluded quite rapidly and provide the patient with minimal relief. If the cecum is 8 cm. or larger, daily abdominal films should be scruti-

patient should be transferred to the radiology suite for optimal imaging. An upright or decubitus film, if possible, will also help in the differential diagnosis because it will show air fluid level interfaces, which are more common in mechanical obstruction. Once the diagnosis of paralytic ileus is established, nasogastric aspiration and careful attention to fluid and electrolyte balance, particularly potassium replacement, is mandatory if the ileus is to resolve. One must guard against premature removal of the nasogastric tube and too early institution of oral intake, these conditions may lead to vomiting and aspiration in the recumbent position. In some cases, if the ileus is prolonged, total parenteral nutrition for a period of time may be necessary.

Oglivies syndrome (colonic pseudo-obstruction) is a variant of paralytic ileus that deserves special mention. It presents as a clinical obstruction of the colon without a mechanical cause and has been increasingly recognized in postoperative patients after various procedures, including orthopedic procedures. The patients present with acute or increasing abdominal distention, typically with little or no associated pain. Passage of flatus and/or stool may continue. Massive distention can occur, with pressure on the diaphragm causing respiratory compromise, and the typical symptoms of obstruction such as colicky pain, nausea, vomiting, and fever are often not present. Physical examination may show impressive distention but with minimal tender-

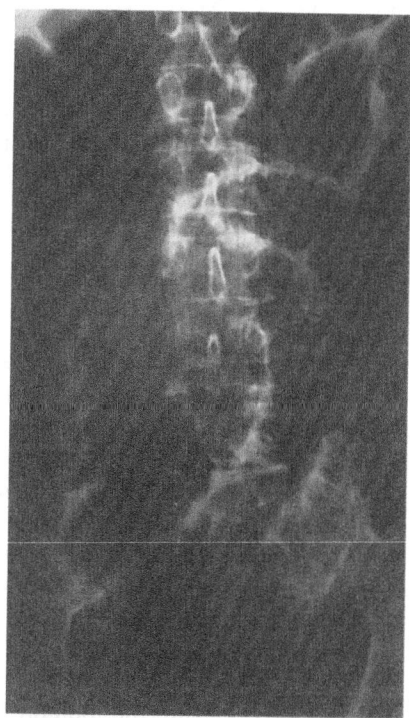

Figure 59.6. Flat plate of a patient with paralytic ileus. Paralytic ileus was present with both dilated colon and small intestine. Small bowel loops are more randomly arranged than in mechanical obstruction and the abnormal loops are scattered throughout the abdomen.

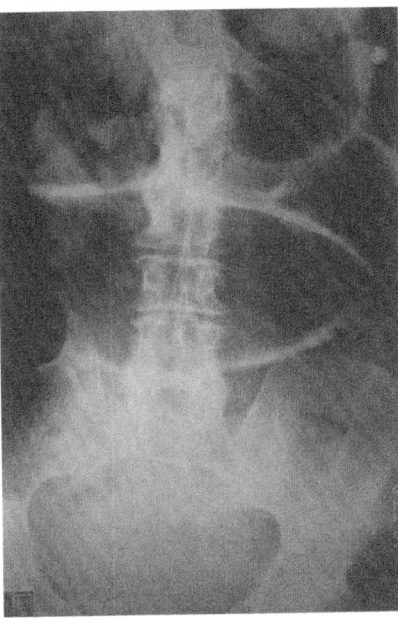

Figure 59.7. Massive cecal dilatation consistent with Ogilvies syndrome. This patient responded to colonoscopy with eventual decompression. No evidence of mechanical obstruction was found.

nized, and if no improvement is noted colonoscopy should be undertaken as an emergency procedure. Colonoscopic decompression performed carefully by an experienced endoscopist can be used to decompress the colon, and a long intestinal tube may be passed along with the scope and left in place after removal of the colonoscope.[35] Radiographic examination can be used to reassess successful colonoscopy. In the majority of patients (80% to 90%) colonoscopic decompression is successful, but almost half of the patients may require repeat colonoscopies if serial flat plates demonstrate reaccumulation of air. If the cecal diameter approaches 12 cm. or peritoneal signs supervene, or if the surgeon believes that perforation is imminent, surgical intervention may be needed. Ileocecal resection with ileostomy and mucous fistula can be performed if there is a vascular embarrassment to the cecum, or a tube cecostomy with a large bore tube can also be done.[36,37] In our experience, however, colonoscopy, if performed in a timely fashion, has been successful in treating these patients.

Complications of Anticoagulation Therapy

In patients on anticoagulant therapy, bleeding and hematoma formation may mimic acute surgical conditions. Bleeding into the mesentery of the small bowel, for example, can cause hematoma with small bowel obstruction. Retroperitoneal hemorrhage can lead to paralytic ileus. A hematoma may form in the rectus abdominus sheath secondary to straining and coughing and can resemble a strangulating internal hernia or lead to signs of tenderness mimicking peritonitis. A patient history of anticoagulant therapy along with a drop in hematocrit should alert one to the possible presence of these complications in the face of these symptoms. Administration of vitamin K and possibly fresh frozen plasma and cessation of the anticoagulant medication is the obvious treatment. However, in some cases surgical exploration may be necessary to relieve obstruction, rule out peritonitis, or drain a compressing hematoma. In such cases, if anticoagulant therapy is indicated but undesirable, alternative modes of treatment such as insertion of a vena cava filter should be considered to protect the patient from pulmonary embolus.

Diverticulitis

Diverticulitis, most frequently of the sigmoid colon, is the most common colonic disease affecting elderly patients and presents a real challenge in diagnosis and management in the postoperative hip patient. Diverticulitis is an inflammation resulting from a perforation of a colonic diverticulum. The condition can be very localized or it can be a more diffuse, intense process, and the nature of management depends on the exact extent of the problem.[38,39] It is difficult to specify the exact surgical management of diverticulitis because the spectrum of disease is so broad. It can vary from a small pericolic abscess confined to the mesentery, which will respond quickly to antibiotic therapy, to perforation with generalized peritonitis which can, especially in immunocompromised or elderly patients, come on very quickly.[40] Computed tomographic (CT) scan can delineate with considerable accuracy the stage of the inflammation (Fig. 59.8), but it should be noted that if the inflammation occurs in the setting of a postoperative hip patient, the surgeon should be aggressive about resecting the diseased segment. If resolution of abdominal tenderness, fever, and white count do not occur after 12 to 24 hours, the safest and most expeditious procedure in this setting would be resection of the sigmoid colon with creation of a temporary stoma. Long-term broad-spectrum antibiotic therapy would then follow with reconstitution of the gastrointestinal tract after the patient has completely recovered.

Technical Complications of Hip Surgery

In the course of the performance of hip arthroplasty, damage to the external iliac artery or the common femoral artery and its branches may result.[41,2,1] These injuries may present as hemorrhage, ischemia, or the development of a false aneurysm.[42,43] Previous authors have emphasized the anatomic proximity of the exter-

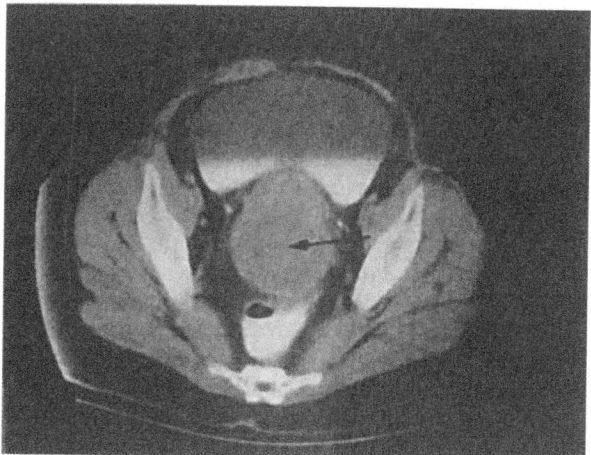

Figure 59.8. Computed tomographic (CT) scan of patient 4 days after knee replacement, showing diverticulitis with pelvic abscess (*arrow*) anterior to the rectum and posterior to the uterus and bladder.

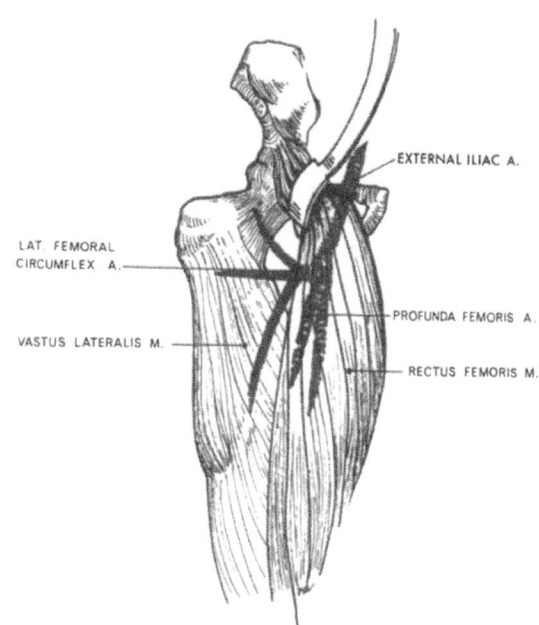

Figure 59.10. The common femoral or the lateral femoral circumflex artery can be injured as a result of vigorous retraction during lateral approach to the hip joint.

nal iliac and common femoral arteries to the hip joint.[41]

Injury to the external iliac artery can be caused by direct instrumental trauma during preparation of the acetabulum or subsequently by exothermic reaction of extruded methyl methacrylate cement[44] (Fig. 59.9). Injury to the common femoral artery and its branches can be caused by too vigorous retraction of the hip capsule, as well as by exothermic reaction from extruded cement[45] (Fig. 59.10). Disruption, false aneurysm formation, and rupture of atherosclerotic plaque with immediate occlusion and ischemia have all been described.[45,5] Careful clinical assessment of preoperative vascular status should be part of the routine workup of every patient upon whom hip revision arthroplasty is planned in order to assess postoperative changes. Thus, all pulses should be palpated and recorded in the admission history and physical for back reference if necessary. Patients who have a clinical history suggestive of lower extremity ischemia should be referred for noninvasive vascular studies, including Doppler vascular imaging. Knowledge of the anatomic relationship of the vessels to the hip joint is of extreme importance. Patients who are known to have intrapelvic cement protrusions should have routine imaging studies to ascertain the exact location of the external iliac vessels in relationship to the cement. Thus CT scanning, vascular ultrasound studies, and even venography may be necessary to ascertain the exact location of the external iliac vessel's relationship to the cement. Any compression of the iliac vein may contribute to venous stasis and increase the possibility of embolic complications. Imaging studies will also provide a road map for the revision surgeon and will forewarn the surgeon of the possibility of intra-operative laceration of the iliac vessels during cement removal. Cement removal by retroperitoneal approach (as discussed below) may be more satisfactory and safer than transacetabular removal.

The proximity of the iliac artery and vein to the acetabulum must also be kept in mind during the operative preparation of this structure. Gouging of the acetabulum can cause direct trauma to the iliac vessels. They can also be damaged by the exothermic reaction of extruded cement especially in patients with major medial acetabular defects (Fig. 59.9). The course of the

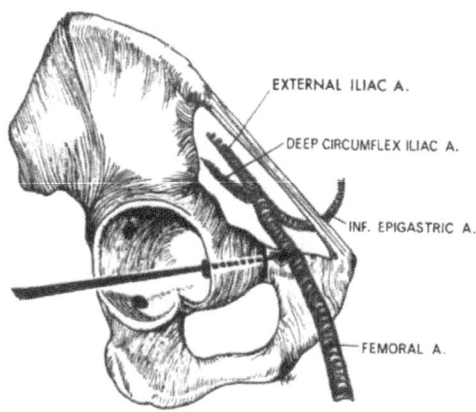

Figure 59.9. Relationship of the iliac artery to the acetabulum is illustrated. Mechanical injury or injury by exothermic reaction of cement can occur.

59. Surgical Complications

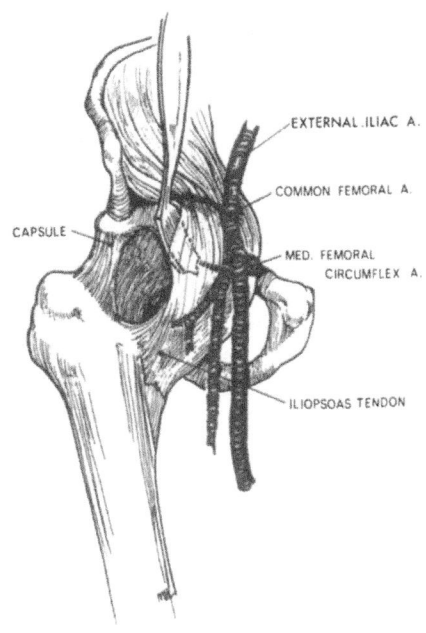

Figure 59.11. The acetabular branch of the medial femoral circumflex artery can also be injured by hip capsule retraction.

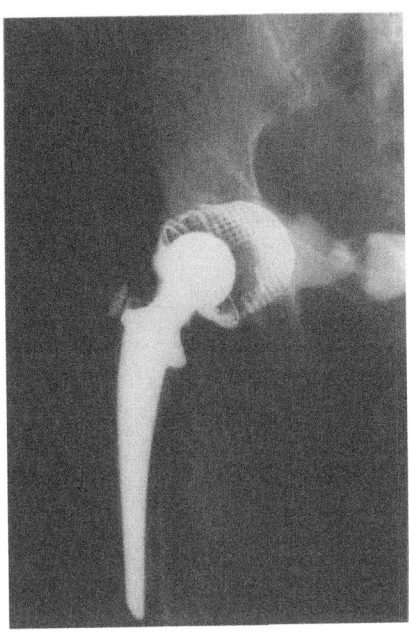

Figure 59.12. A 60-year-old patient with cement extrusion. Arthrographic study shows communication with the urinary bladder. Retroperitoneal approach was utilized to remove the cement and repair the bladder. The revision arthroplasty was done 10 weeks later after intravenous antibiotic therapy.

common femoral artery and its branches must always be kept in mind when placing retractors in the region of the rectus femoris and vastus lateralis muscles. The atherosclerotic vessels of the elderly patient undergoing hip arthroplasty are particularly prone to injury (Figs. 59.10 and 59.11). If vascular injury is suspected because of massive intra-operative or postoperative hemorrhage, hematoma formation, or ischemia, the assistance of a vascular surgeon should be obtained immediately. Angiography may be of value in delineating an arterial injury, and in some cases injection of autogenous clot or procoagulant material may be done at angiography to provide both diagnosis and therapy.

Cement Extrusion

Extrusion of cement from the acetabular defect into the pelvic retroperitoneal space can cause impingement on other structures in addition to the arteries. We have seen erosion into the urinary bladder with arthrovesical fistula in two cases (Fig. 59.12). We have also seen impingement on the rectum and vagina with a palpable mass on digital examination (Fig. 59.13 and 59.14). During the orthopedic procedure, repair of acetabular defects, care in placement of the cement, and protection of the soft tissue from exothermic reaction should minimize extrusion and damage to intrapelvic structures. If the extruded intrapelvic cement is causing symptoms or if one fears possible gradual erosion, removal of the cement is indicated. Cement removal is also indicated if revision arthroplasty is contemplated. We have used a retroperitoneal approach through a low inguinal incision with splitting of the muscles and careful identification of the ureter and the great vessels without violating the peritoneum (Fig. 59.15). The cement mass was invariably surrounded by a pseudocapsule. Incision of the iliac muscle allows the extruded cement to be ex-

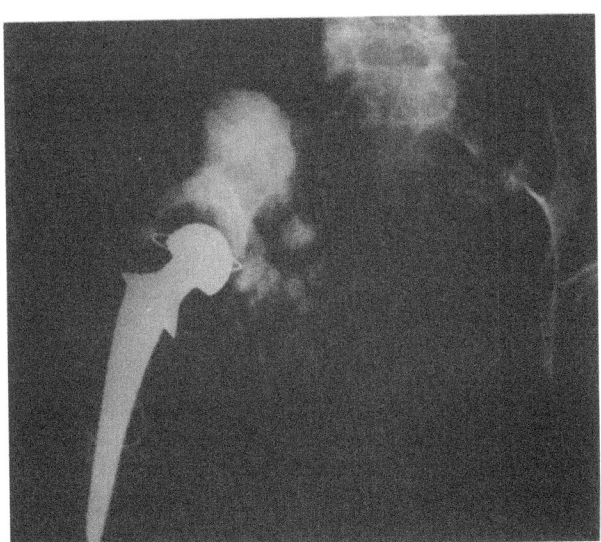

Figure 59.13. Intrapelvic cement collection in a 58-year-old female with groin pain and edema of the right lower extremity. The cement could be palpated rectally and vaginally.

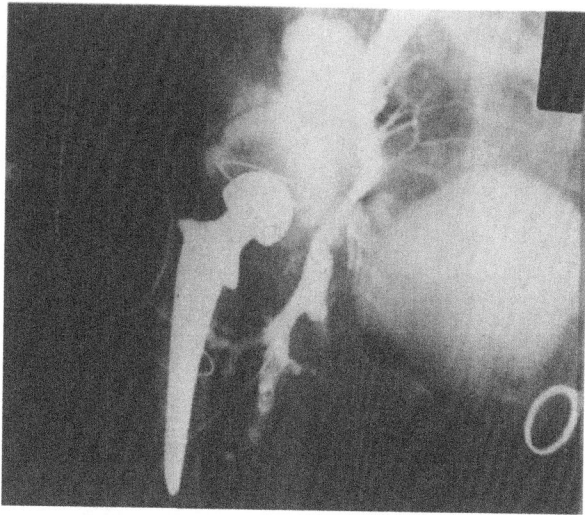

Figure 59.14. Venogram in the same patient. The cement is partially surrounding and narrowing the iliac vein.

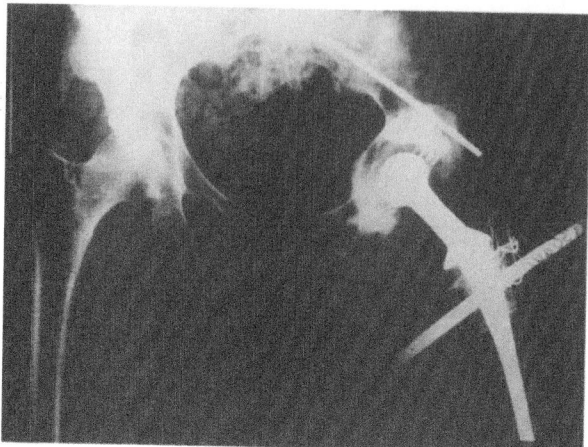

Figure 59.16. A Kirschner wire has penetrated the pelvic wall and was thought to be lying partially within the abdominal cavity. Removal was made through a lower midline laparotomy. No vascular intestinal injury had occurred. Withdrawal through the hip joint should not be done since this may infect the orthopedic field if the wire has penetrated the intestinal tract or bladder.

posed. While protecting the great vessels and ureter, the cement can be freed laterally by drill and osteotome and removed without harming adjacent structures. Earlier in our experience when removing cement in combination with revision arthroplasty, the cement was removed at the first stage and the transarticular surgery was done at a second stage. But in our last twelve cases we have done both procedures at the same stage with equivalent good results.

Instrument Perforation

Instrument perforation of the pelvis and into the abdominal cavity and urinary bladder has also been noted (Fig. 59.16). Immediate and thorough exploration of the abdomen, identification and repair of any urologic, intestinal or vascular injury is mandatory. We do not recommend a policy of "watchful waiting" since the grave consequences of infection of the prosthesis with an intestinal or a bladder perforation must be avoided.

Conclusion

The prevention, diagnosis, and management of general surgical complications continue to be an important part of the complete management of the revision hip arthroplasty patient. Only by maintaining a high index of suspicion and an acute awareness of these complications may they be detected and promptly treated.

References

1. Muller ME. Total hip prostheses. *Clin Orthop*. 1970;72:46–68.
2. Coventry MB, Beckenbaugh RD, Nolan DR, Ilstrup DM. 2012 total hip arthroplasties. A study of postoperative course and early complications. *J Bone Joint Surg. Am.* 1974;56:273–284.
3. Green DL. Complications of total hip replacement. *South Med J*. 1976;69:1559–1564.
4. NIH Consensus Conference. Therapeutic endoscopy and bleeding ulcers. March 1989;7:1–7.
5. Torgerson WR: Three-year experience with total hip replacement. *Clin Orthop*. 1973;95:151–157.
6. Roseman PL, Econmav SG: Treatment of complications of gastroduodenal "steroid ulcers." *Arch Surg*. 1965;90:488–492.

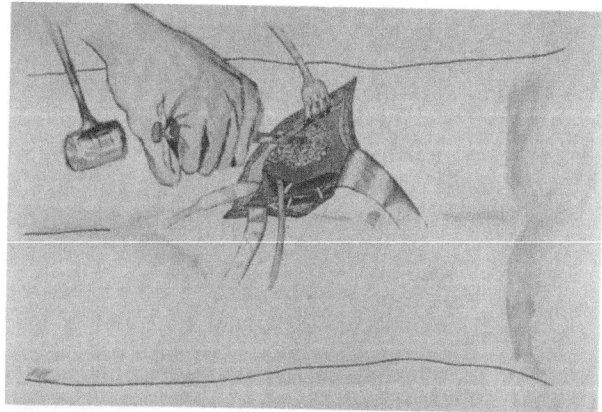

Figure 59.15. Retroperitoneal approach to the hip joint through a left low groin incision with separation of the muscles and mobilization of the peritoneum and ureter medially. The iliac artery and vein are dissected away and protected as the cement is removed through this approach.

7. Sawyers JL, Herrington JL, Mulkerin JL, et al. Acute perforated duodenal ulcer. *Arch Surg.* 1975;110:527–534.
8. ReMine WH, McIlrath DC. Bowel perforation in steroid treated patients. *Am Surg.* 1980;192:581–583.
9. Rees JR, Shan KG, Thorbjarnson B. Perforated duodenal ulcer. *Am J Surg.* 1970;120:775–779.
10. Singer HA, Vaughan RT. Treatment of the forme fruste type of perforated peptic ulcer. *Surg Gynecol Obstet.* 1932;54:945–948.
11. Berne CJ, Mikkelsen WP. Management of perforated peptic ulcer. *Surgery.* 1958;44:591–598.
12. Mikal S, Morrison WR. Acute perforated peptic ulcer: criteria for operation and analysis of 500 Cases. *N Engl J Med.* 1952;247:119–125.
13. Booth RAD, Williams JA. Mortality of perforated duodenal ulcer treated by simple suture. *Br J Surg.* 1971;58:421–424.
14. Emmett JM, Williams HL. Gastric resection: A definitive treatment for perforated peptic ulcer. *Am Surg.* 1957;23:993–996.
15. Cohen MM. Treatment and mortality of perforated peptic ulcer: a survey of 852 cases. *Can Med Assoc J.* 1971;105:263–266.
16. Gray JG, Roberts AK. Definitive emergency treatment of perforated duodenal ulcer. *Surg Gynecol Obstet.* 1976;1:143–146.
17. Heberer G, Teichmann RK. Recurrence after proximal gastric vagotomy for gastric pyloric and prepyloric ulcers. *World J Surg.* 1987;11:283–287.
18. Jordan GL Jr, Angel RT, DeBakey ME. Acute gastroduodenal perforation: comparative study of treatment with simple closure, subtotal gastrectomy and hemi-gastrectomy and vagotomy. *Arch Surg.* 1966;92:449–456.
19. Kirkpatrick JR. The role of definitive surgery in the management of perforated duodenal ulcer disease. *Arch Surg.* 1975;110:1016–1020.
20. Branicki FJ, Boey J, Fok PH, Pritchett W, Fan ST, Lai CT, et al. Bleeding duodenal ulcer; a prospective evaluation of risk factors for rebleeding and death. *Ann Surg.* 1990;211:411–418.
21. Christensen A, Bousfield R, Chistiansen J. Incidence of perforated and bleeding peptic ulcers before and after the introduction of H_2 receptor antagonists. *Ann Surg.* 1988;207:4–6.
22. Miller TA, Tornwall MS, Moody FG. Stress erosive gastritis. *Curr Probl Surg.* 1991;28:459–509.
23. Allen A, Flemstrom G, Garner A, Kivilaakso E. Gastroduodenal mucosa protection. *Physiol Rev.* 1993;73:823–857.
24. Cook DJ, Fuller HD, Guyatt GH, Marshall JC, Leasa D, Hau R, et al. Risk factors for gastrointestinal bleeding in critically ill patients. *N Engl J Med.* 1994;330:377–381.
25. Fabian TC, Boucher BA, Croce MA, et al. Pneumonia and stress ulceration in severely injured patients—a prospective evaluation of the effects of stress ulcer prophylaxis. *Arch Surg.* 1993;128:185–192.
26. Glenn F. Acute cholecystitis following the surgical treatment of unrelated disease. *Ann Surg.* 1947;126:477–483.
27. Glenn F, Wartz GE. Acute cholecystitis following the surgical treatment of unrelated diseases. *Surg Gynecol Obstet.* 1956;102:145–153.
28. Hoffmann E. Acute gangrenous cholecystitis secondary to trauma. *Am J Surg.* 1956;91:288–292.
29. Robertson RD. Noncalculous acute cholecystitis following surgery, trauma, and illness. *Am Surg.* 1970;36:610–614.
30. Winegarner FG, Jackson GF. Post-traumatic acalculous cholecystitis. A highly lethal complication. *J Trauma.* 1971;116:567–569.
31. Waldron GW, Hampton JM. Intestinal obstruction: A half century comparative analysis. *Ann Surg.* 1961;153:839–846.
32. Welch CE. *Intestinal Obstruction.* Chicago, Year Book Publishers, 1958.
33. Cappell MS, Simon T. Colonic toxicity of administered medications and chemicals. *Am J Gastroenterol.* 1993;88:1684–1689.
34. Ballantyne GH, Brandner MD, Beart RW Jr, Ilstrup DM. Volvulus of the colon: incidence and mortality. *Ann Surg.* 1985;202:830–892.
35. Brothers TE, Strodel WE, Eckhauser FE. Endoscopy in colonic volvulus. *Ann Surg.* 1987;206:1–4.
36. Fry RD, Fleshman JW, Kodner IJ. Abdominal colectomy with ileorectal anastomosis. *South Med J.* 1984;77:711–714.
37. Sloyer AF, Panella VS, Demas BE, Shike M, Lightdale CJ, Winawer SJ, et al. Ogilvie's syndrome. Successful management without colonoscopy. *Dig Dis Sci.* 1988;33:1391–1396.
38. Fleshman JW. Initial evaluation and treatment of acute diverticulitis. Standards Task Force Parameters (in press).
39. Gordon PH. Diverticular disease of the colon. In: Gordon PH, Nivatvongs S, eds. *Principles and practice of surgery for the colon, rectum and anus.* St. Louis: Quality Medical Publishing, 1992:739–798.
40. Sackier JM. Colonic surgery for acute conditions: perforated diverticular disease. In: Fielding LP, Goldberg SM, eds. *Rob and Smith's operative surgery: Surgery of the colon, rectum and anus.* 5 ed. Oxford, UK: Butterworth-Heinemann, 1993.
41. Aust JC, Bredenberg CE, Murry PG. Mechanisms of arterial injuries associated with total hip replacement. *Arch Surg.* 1965;116:345–523.
42. Dameron TB. False aneurysm of femoral profundus artery resulting from fixation device. *J Bone Joint Surg. Am.* 1964;46:577–580.
43. Dorr LD, Conaty JP, Kohl R, Harvey JP Jr. False aneurysm of the femoral artery following total hip surgery. *J Bone Joint Surg. Am.* 1974;56:1059–1062.
44. Scullin JP, Nelson CL, Bever GB: False aneurysm of the left external iliac artery following total hip arthroplasty. *Clin Orthop.* 1975;113:145–149.
45. Salama R, Stavorosky MM, Itellin A. Femoral artery injury complicating total hip replacement. *Clin Orthop.* 1972;85:143–144.

60
Genitourinary Complications

Gary P. Kearney and Christopher J. Doyle

Genitourinary complications may complicate total hip arthroplasty and threaten successful joint replacement. Underlying urological disease, intraoperative events, and unexpected postoperative complications may each require special management in the patient undergoing total hip arthroplasty. These events pose a special hazard to the patient in this stressful setting and have the potential for significant morbidity in the elderly population. Urological consultation is required by elderly patients at a rate twenty times that of the younger population. Awareness of the common urological problems that may arise in the perioperative period is a valuable asset to the orthopedic surgeon. In this chapter we will examine the urological disorders and circumstances relevant to this population. We stress the factors important in preoperative assessment, intraoperative protocol, and postoperative management in order to avoid compromise of this organ system.

The common problems encountered by patients differ markedly according to sex in the age group most commonly undergoing total arthroplasty. In men, prostatic obstruction and malignancy are common problems, resulting in frequent difficulty with urinary retention and catheter passage. In women, problems with infection and incontinence predominate, leading to potentially serious infectious complications or annoying problems in postoperative management. Both sexes are vulnerable to sudden stone-related renal colic, or to catastrophic intraoperative injury to the urinary and reproductive systems. Awareness of these underlying considerations should permeate encounters with these patients during the operative experience.

While a complete review of urological assessment and management in these patients is beyond the scope of this chapter, we hope to enhance the reader's ability to appreciate and assess difficulties they may encounter.

Preoperative Evaluation
Preoperative Evaluation of the Male Patient

The common problems that may affect male patients undergoing total hip arthroplasty are: (1) postoperative urinary retention; (2) urethral trauma due to traumatic or difficult catheterization; (3) iatrogenic urinary infection due to urethral catheterization; and (4) the discovery of other urological conditions such as renal calculi or genitourinary malignancy, necessitating urological procedures that are potentially morbid in the postarthroplasty setting. Preoperative assessment should be tailored to detect these underlying areas of potential difficulty in order to avoid compromising the primary procedure.

Key Points in the History

A careful history of obstructive symptoms, such as hesitancy, decreased caliber of stream, nocturia, poor urinary flow, intermittency, and difficulty voiding should be elicited from the patient. These symptoms suggest that bladder outlet obstruction may be present[1] which may predispose the patient to problems of postoperative retention, urinary infection, or difficult urethral catheterization.[2]

A past history of radical prostatectomy, transurethral resection of the prostate (TURP) for obstructive disease, urethral trauma, or previous surgery for urethral stricture disease should raise suspicion of the possibility of either persistent obstruction or a scarred, tortuous urethra. These procedures cause characteristic changes in the course of the urethra. Radical prostatectomy requires an anastamosis of the bladder to the urethra just proximal to the membranous urethra. The resultant channel is often placed more anteriorly than the usual anatomic structure. Scar tissue or surgical distortion may result at this point, leading to frequent difficulties with passage of catheters, even though an adequate lumen exists. A similar difficulty may result from transurethral prostatectomy.[3] In this situation, resection of tissue from the floor (posterior aspect) of the prostatic fossa may cause a posterior lip at the bladder neck. Standard urethral catheters may pass below the raised edge of tissue, failing to enter the bladder. Urethral stricture surgery, even when successful in relieving symptoms, can result in either wide caliber narrowing or tortuous, fixed areas which may complicate catheter passage. In such cases, urethral abnormalities may be significant enough to complicate urethra management even though the patients may not be symptomatic. Many orthopedic surgeons are all too familiar with the scenario that results when such problems are not appreciated preoperatively. Vigorous and unsuccessful attempts at catheterization result in delay of surgery, false passages, and gram negative septicemia, and risk of infection to the joint replacement may result.

Patients should be questioned regarding the occurrence of hematuria, dysuria, and flank pain. Patients with a history of prostate cancer in first-degree relatives, in successive generations, or arising in men less than 60 years of age should invoke laboratory evaluation and careful attention to appropriate aspects of the physical examination.

Physical Examination

Examination should screen for signs of inflammation, anatomic obstruction, or malignancy. The flanks and upper abdomen should be examined for signs of mass or tenderness; the abdomen for bladder distention, the genitalia for phimosis, meatal stenosis, urethral fibrosis; and the prostate for nodularity, size, and tenderness. Suspicious findings should lead to laboratory or radiologic investigation.

Laboratory Evaluation

Simple laboratory evaluation (urinalysis, urine culture, and creatinine level) effectively screens for most important urological disorders, especially acute problems which affect the timing of arthroplasty. Further testing can be performed when indicated by the initial screening studies, history, or physical examination.

Prostatic enlargement, nodularity, or history of prostate cancer, surgery, or significant voiding symptoms should be evaluated by a Prostate Specific Antigen level (PSA).[4-6]

Hematuria (greater than 5 RBCs/HPF) evaluation should include a careful microscopic examination of the urinary sediment for the presence of red cell casts, as well as chemical testing for the presence of proteinuria. A urine cytology should be obtained in addition to suitable imaging studies of the upper urinary tracts, the kidneys, and ureters.

Symptoms of infection such as dysuria, frequency, malodorous or cloudy urine, or a history of frequent or asymptomatic past infections should be evaluated by standard bacterial culture.[7]

Preoperative Urological Consultation

Urological consultation should be obtained to address significant questions that arise from the preoperative evaluation. In many cases laboratory abnormalities are minor in nature, explained by obvious self-limited processes, or so familiar to experienced examiners that they can clearly be shown to be unimportant. However, invasive evaluation of the urological organs does entail some risk of disseminating infection, and all reasonable efforts to evaluate findings or solve problems should be completed before major joint reconstruction. The general evaluation of the problems that are likely to arise in preoperative evaluation are summarized below.

Catheterization Problems

Patients with symptoms suggesting significant outflow obstruction should undergo urine flow measurement and either flexible cystoscopy or retrograde urethrography if critical obstruction is documented. If either flow rates are acceptable or no symptoms are present, then invasive preoperative assessment can be deferred.[8] If difficult catheterization is expected, the operating room will need to have available the equipment needed in such circumstances: Filiforms and followers, a variety of catheters including Council tip and Coude tip models, and a flexible cytoscope (with an Amplatz dilator set). This last combination has become the method of choice. The flexible cystoscope is introduced into the urethra and a guide wire is passed through the stricture. Over an appropriate wire the Amplatz set of dilators can be passed, dilating the narrowed segment. Advantages of this method include reliability, brevity, and minimization of urethral trauma since the crucial location of the narrowed channel is accomplished under direct vision.

Hematuria

Hematuria may herald stone disease, malignancy, infection, or medical renal disease. Initial studies should consist of urine analysis for protein and casts, serum testing for sedimentation rate and creatinine, and urine cytology. New methods of detecting occult bladder tumors using molecular biological methods (eg, Urinary NMP22) show promise but have no established place within evaluation algorithms yet.[9] If no clear source is established, subsequent testing should include an anatomic study of the upper tracts and a cystoscopic examination of the bladder. Controversy rages within urology as to the best way to radiographically examine the upper tracts (ie, ultrasound, intravenous pyelography, computed tomography, or retrograde pyelography). However, a general principle is that the evaluation as a whole should include studies that examine all areas of the urinary tract. Therefore, ultrasound plus a retrograde pyelogram, an intravenous polygram (IVP) alone, or a computerized tomography (CT) scan with and without contrast should be performed. Recently ultrasound alone has become an acceptable isolated screening study of the upper tracts in low-risk patients. It should be noted that none of the radiological studies has been shown to adequately substitute for cystoscopy in the evaluation of the bladder, and this visual examination can now routinely be performed with virtually no anesthesia in almost all patients using a fiberoptic cystoscope.

Possible Retention

Severe voiding systems suggesting outflow obstruction or bladder atony should be evaluated and quantified by measurement of urine flow and categorized by the American Urological Symptom Questionnaire.[10] In most cases, evaluation of the upper urinary tract is not needed. If severe impairment of outflow is present, then treatment should be considered, consisting of medical treatment, usually by alpha adrenergic blocking agents (Terazosin or Doxazosin) or by surgical removal of obstructing prostatic tissue.[8,11] No criteria exist to accurately predict which patients will develop retention after major orthopedic surgery. In general, patients who experience the most severe actual obstruction preoperatively will be the most likely to develop retention, and the least likely to recover voiding function quickly. These patients will be faced with the need for postarthroplasty TURP, with its attendant risk of infection, stress, and prolongation of hospitalization.[12]

Nephrolithiasis

Flank pain, hematuria, or patient history may evoke concern about possible renal or ureteral calculi. The diagnostic study of choice is computed tomography of the kidneys and ureters performed without oral or intravenous contrast. This study is most useful when performed with either thin sections or using a spiral technique. Both of these techniques depict the entire renal and ureteral length. Even stones less than 1 mm reliably stand out dramatically on this study, and a negative result is definitive, ruling out renal or ureteral stones. Phleboliths can mimic distal ureteral calculi on CT, as is the case on intravenous pyelography, and in some cases intravenous contrast is needed to evaluate this possibility. The specifically tailored "CT for Stone" is a limited study, focused on a single problem. It is not a complete evaluation of the kidneys or the GI tract, and is not reliable in the evaluation or renal masses or inflammatory disorders.

In general, ureteral calculi should be treated prior to total hip arthroplasty because of the high likelihood that significant symptoms will disrupt recovery or require invasive evaluation in the near future. Usually upper tract stones can be fragmented by extracorporeal lithotripsy[13] and allowed to pass, while lower tract stones can be extracted cystoscopically,[14,15] or treated by ESWL.[16] Open removal is rarely necessary where contemporary equipment is available.

If the stones are less than 4 mm in diameter, it is reasonable to expect that the patient would pass the stone successfully with time and conservative management. Infected stones (magnesium ammonium phosphate or struvite) should be removed prior to joint replacement surgery since the stones themselves are infected and complete stone removal is necessary to cure infection.

Infection

The great majority of urinary infections resolve quickly after appropriate therapy and are not associated with significant abnormalities of the urinary tract.[17] These patients do not require urological assessment. While it is often said that men should be assessed urologically for any infection, in reality, if no other signs of urinary dysfunction are present, the yield of such evaluations is low. Only when an infection seems part of a recurring process that is likely to continue postoperatively, or is resistant to standard treatment, should urological help be sought.

In women, recurring or isolated infections clinically confined to the lower urinary tract can be adequately evaluated by careful physical exam and history. Upper tract studies are not usually needed if there is no history of flank pain, fever, or systemic prostatitis to indicate the occurrence of pyelonephritis. The examiner should try to establish a lack of neurological dysfunction, intrapelvic pathology of the digestive or reproductive systems, and to verify normal bladder emptying. The most common cause of infection is bowel flora that ascends the urethra. Major risk factors are sexual intercourse, use of diaphragms for contraception, atrophic vaginitis, and a recent antecedent infection. Management is by use of prophylactic antibiotics.[18,19,20]

In men, impaired bladder emptying and chronic prostatitis contribute to infection. Measures to improve emptying or suppress prostatic colonization may be useful.[21]

In both sexes, persistent, recurring, or resistant infection with a single organism, or involvement of the kidneys, indicates a need for assessment of the entire urinary tract, usually initially by ultrasound. When recurrent pyelonephritis occurs, a voiding study to rule out vesico-ureteral reflux is imperative. Vesico-enteric fistulas are uncommon, but important sources of repeated urinary infection and their presence should be conclusively ruled out by CT in appropriate cases.

Sterilization of the urinary tract should be carried out prior to any joint replacement surgery and consideration for long-term suppressive therapy in patients with a history of urinary tract infection after joint replacement surgery should be strongly considered, (ie, 1 tablet of Bactrim or Ciprofloxacin at bedtime). The risk of infecting a total joint replacement, and the morbidity associated with this, far outweigh the disadvantages of long-term antibiotic use.[1,3]

Management of Urologic Problems Post-Joint Replacement Surgery

Urinary Retention

Male Patients: Postoperative urinary retention commonly occurs after major surgery, caused by many reversible factors not specifically related to the anatomy and function of the urological organs.

Pain, sedatives, anxiety, and restricted body posture markedly impair the efficiency of detrussor contraction and bladder outlet relaxation. In addition, several medications possess specifically anticholinergic properties (antihistamines, psychotropics, spasmolytics, and decongestants) that directly interfere with bladder emptying. Severe constipation, commonly a byproduct of postoperative narcotic-based analgesia, may impair bladder emptying by a reflex mechanism. Occasionally overdistention caused by unrecognized perioperative retention may stretch detrussor fibers beyond their tolerable functional length and result in muscle dysfunction of variable duration.[22] When appropriately recognized and corrected, these factors will abate and usually allow a return to normal voiding.

In certain patients, normal voidings will not resume because of uncorrectable anatomic or neurologic factors. In the great majority of such patients, the history indicates the likelihood of the presence of such factors (see Preoperative evaluation). The most common of these are bladder outlet obstruction due to benign prostatic hypertrophy or bladder neck contracture that is congenital or related to prior surgery, or bladder muscle dysfunction due to diabetic myopathy or chronic overdistention due to outlet obstruction or to end-motor neuron dysfunction. This last may be associated with radical pelvic surgery, spinal root injury, or radiation-induced damage.

In most patients undergoing hip arthroplasty who require catheterization because of a need for fluid monitoring or bladder drainage indicated by the magnitude or length of surgery, the catheter should be removed as soon as the patient is fully alert and cooperative. Occasionally the patient may not void successfully. If the patient has no history of antecedent voiding symptoms, a repeat voiding trial may be administered in 24 to 48 hours, depending on the patient's general condition. However, in patients with a history of nocturia, decreased caliber of stream, or known urological conditions, it is usually best to defer a voiding trial until the patient is able to stand to void with a minimum of assistance.[23]

Occasionally intermittent bladder catheterization is utilized when it is felt that return of normal bladder function is imminent or when the bladder dysfunction is felt likely to be permanently uncorrectable—usually when chronic retention was known to be present preoperatively. While this has been shown to be the superior method of bladder management in ambulatory outpatients—associated with fewer septic complications and better preservation of the upper tracts—it is often a problematic form of approach in older male patients. Previous urethral or prostatic surgery, bed position, and patient anxiety increase the difficulty of catheterization in patients after total hip arthroplasty.

In a patient who fails a voiding trial, we favor an additional period of catheter drainage as an outpatient, followed by a subsequent voiding trial with alphasympatholytic agents, such as Terazosin or Doxazosin to relax the internal sphincter. For the patient who fails this voiding trial, transurethral prostate surgery should be considered.

Recently-introduced treatments for bladder outlet obstruction such as radiofrequency ablation (TUNA)[24] or microwave thermotherapy (Prostatron)[25] or the use of laser energy to ablate prostatic tissue may be shown to have some role in the management of patients suffering from urinary retention.[26] Currently they remain unproven as treatments for complete retention and should be reserved for management of symptoms of outlet obstruction, not complete retention. In certain high-risk patients, placement of intraprostatic metal stents may have some role, although the long-term risk of infection in these patients is not clarified as yet. Reversible hormonal therapy such as Ketoconazole or luteinizing hormone (LHRH) agonist treatment are effective methods of decreasing prostatic size and relieving retention; however they work slowly and require a delay of 4 to 12 weeks before they have sufficient effect to reliably relieve retention. Their effect will last only weeks to months beyond their continued use, and retention will recur unless anatomic correction is effected. Transurethral prostatectomy is the treatment of choice in such patients. Recent modifications have considerably improved the safety and efficacy of this procedure. Postoperative hospitalization time and intraoperative blood loss have been markedly reduced using modified electrosurgical techniques.[27,28] This should be considered once the patient has recovered from his joint replacement surgery. Appropriate antibiotics are essential in the patient undergoing subsequent transurethral surgery.[29,30]

Kidney and Bladder Stones

Although in some occasions nephrolithiasis may be detected preoperatively because of symptoms or screening studies (see Preoperative Evaluation), occasionally renal colic develops in the immediate postoperative period. The first priority is to establish the etiology of the symptom by imaging study to be certain that surgical injury to the urinary tract has not occurred. This evaluation is discussed elsewhere in this chapter (see Radiological Imaging of Urological Injury). When colic or ureteral obstruction is found to be caused by a renal or ureteral calculus, management is guided by standard urological principles, placing particular emphasis on the importance of avoiding urinary infection. Unnecessary instrumentation should be avoided, but obstruction associated with infection should be relieved immediately to prevent systemic sepsis. In general, fever, persistent vomiting impairing hydration, and intolerable pain are indications for prompt investigation. Large stones that are unlikely to pass spontaneously are also commonly treated without "trials of passage."

When immediate decompression of an obstructed collecting system is required, the two possible approaches are cystoscopic retrograde stone extraction with stent placement or antegrade percutaneous nephrostomny. The cystoscopic approach has the advantage of very likely removing the stone and resulting in immediate resolution of the crisis, but requires anesthesia.[14,15] Percutaneous decompression can be performed under local anesthesia in the radiological suite and is a highly reliable means of draining a septic collecting system. Tube occlusion or malfunction can be carefully monitored. This is the treatment of choice in acutely septic patients.

As discussed earlier, urinary calculi in all positions of the urinary tract can be treated by extracorporeal lithotripsy, open surgical removal, or endoscopic approaches or dissolution therapy. Individual treatment in arthroplasty patients often is guided by concerns about general patient stability (fluid balance, postoperative anemia, impaired GI function, for example), as well as the specific details of the urological problem. In general, the main factors that influence the decision are stone size, position, composition, the presence or absence of sepsis, and any unusual anatomic details that may be present (eg, solitary kidney, duplicate collecting system, ureteral tortuosity).

Necessary anatomic and functional information are best provided by kidneys-ureter-bladder x-ray, CT scan, and functional studies such as intravenous pyelography (IVP).

Scrotal Abnormality

General Principles
In the postoperative setting, acute scrotal enlargement commonly arises. This may be caused by benign, self-limited processes, or it may signal important pathological events. Occasionally careful examination reveals long-standing findings of no acute importance. In most cases the distinction can be made on the basis of physical examination and ultrasonography.

Scrotal enlargement is caused by a process affecting the scrotal skin, such as cellulitis or monilial dermatitis; or involving the subcutaneous tissues, such as infiltrating extravascular fluid or blood; or affecting the intrascrotal organs, the testes, and epididymides, such as torsion, infection, or trauma. Distinguishing which layer is affected is the key to diagnosis.

The scrotal skin is usually delicate, rugated, and slightly darker than surrounding abdominal or thigh skin. When pinched, a thin fold is created. It is not normally translucent or shiny. In the presence of skin infection, it develops blanching erythema and becomes thick and tender. In most cases when the skin is the primary tissue affected by a process, the amount of scrotal enlargement is modest. When these features are apparent, examination should search for a portal of entry such as nearby folliculitis, paraphimosis, or monilial dermatitis. Treatment is either topical, as in cases with uncomplicated fungal eruptions, or systemic, as in cases of cellulitis.

Most scrotal enlargement noted after total hip arthroplasty is caused by infiltration of extracellular fluid from the incision and sites of tissue injury around medially to the lax and easily distended scrotal compartment. The scrotum can become massively enlarged, two or three times is usual size. In this situation the scrotal skin remains pale and becomes clear and translucent without thickening. Thumb printing of the tissue can be appreciated, and the testes can be palpated as normally mobile and without enlargement within the thickened surrounding cakelike tissue. Usually very little tenderness is present and the tissues may feel cool to the touch. The surrounding thigh and lower abdomen exhibit similar, if less spectacular, tissue changes, and this is often the feature that makes the diagnosis certain. If the testes can be palpated and are normal, no confirmatory studies are necessary. No specific treatment other than scrotal elevation on towels or by use of an athletic supporter is needed. When blood infiltrates into the wall, the skin remains delicate and thin and becomes discolored by the blood pigments, exhibiting nonblanching discoloration. Again the surrounding region is often the key to diagnosis. In some cases the distinction between hematoma and scrotal wall necrosis (Fourniers Gangrene) can be difficult.[31] Usually the latter is marked severe induration of the skin with blistering and loss of skin sensation associated with fever and severe toxicity. It is a rare development in the immediate postoperative setting and most commonly occurs in diabetic patients.

The Testes and Epididymides
Acute enlargement of the scrotal contents can be caused by infection, ischemia, or trauma. Usually infection spreads to these structures through the vas deferens, involving the spermatic cord and the tail of the epididymis to a substantial degree. Ischemia caused by torsion of

the spermatic cord is unusual in adult patients, and affects both the testesticular and epididymal tissues. The management of these processes is very different: Infection is treated by antibiotics, ischemia by immediate exploration, and trauma by surgical repair. Although the latter two diagnoses are very rare in the postarthroplasty setting, accurate diagnosis does affect management dramatically. Examination reveals thin, erythematous skin, mild edema of the subcutaneous tissue, and painful enlargement of the testes and epididymides. Often discrete outlines of the organs themselves are obscured by inflammatory reaction, and tenderness/pain may be so marked that examination is severely limited. Accumulation of reactive fluid or blood within the tunica vaginalis can further impair diagnosis by physical examination.

Scrotal ultrasound is of great use in this setting. The size, outline, and echotexture of the testes are usually crisply depicted. The relative enlargement of the testes and the epididymis can be shown, often clarifying the location and nature of the pathologic process. Blood flow within the testes can be demonstrated by doppler analysis; while this examination alone does not absolutely rule out the presence of torsion, the information it yields, coupled with the history and examination, is often conclusive and accurate.

In addition, multiple benign scrotal abnormalities, heretofore unrecognized in a patient, can be detected in the postoperative setting. Accurate identification may enable the patient to avoid unnecessary diagnostic studies and anxiety.

Hydroceles result from increase in the volume of peritisticular fluid retained within the tunical vaginalis. The usual balance between fluid secretion and absorption is abnormal, resulting in expansion of the fluid-filled space around the testes. These may feel soft, in which case the testicular outline is discernible, or tense, in which case the testicle and epididymis cannot be appreciated.

Spermatoceles represent soft cystic structures that arise from the epididymis. They may contain sperm and often develop as a multilobular aggregate of variably sized cysts. Since they develop beside the testes, the testicle itself can often be palpated. The cysts are benign, rarely interfere with fertility, and may recur after surgical correction and new "daughter cysts" develop beside the site of a previously excised lesion.

Both of these cystic entities can be accurately diagnosed by physical examination, often using a light source to "transilluminate" the fluid-filled mass. The cystic lesion glows dramatically when in contact with the light source, distinguishing it from solid lesions. Examination should define all scrotal structure, rule out the presence of solid lesions or the presence of a hernia, and characterize the testicular texture and outline. A hydrocele can mask a testes tumor. Scrotal ultrasound is a highly useful and definitive modality in this setting.

Hydroceles and spermatoceles do not require any treatment unless they become symptomatic or cosmetically unacceptable.

A variocele represents dilation of an internal spermatic vein near the testes in the scrotum. This is notable on examination as a mass of tortuous venous channels usually located behind or above the testes. In the upright position, it fills with blood traveling retrograde down into the scrotum. It decompresses in the supine position and can be distinguished from an enlarged irregular epididymis by this maneuver. Although associated with infertility in 10% to 15% of patients, it is of no clinical significance to the orthopedic surgeon performing joint replacement and requires no treatment.[32]

Phimosis or the inability to retract the foreskin can complicate cleansing of the glans prior to catheter placement and may make placement more difficult, but emergency circumcision or performance of a dorsal slit is rarely necessary in this setting.

Paraphymosis (the foreskin has been retracted with the glans exposed, resulting in bleeding to massive edema of the glans and the prepuce distal to a phimotic ring) can occur with a catheter in place, especially if the foreskin is left retracted after catheter placement. Immediate correction is imperative to avoid necrosis of the glans and prepuce, but can be difficult. Usually manual compression of the glans penis and retraction of the foreskin can be carried out without anesthesia, but placement of a penile block, and occasionally incision of the phimotic band that prevents reduction, may be necessary. Prompt recognition of the condition is important. A shiny, edematous, exposed glans in a patient who has not been circumcised should elicit a prompt response.

Intraoperative Urogenital Injury During Total Hip Arthroplasty

General Principles

During total hip arthroplasty, perforation of the medial cortex of the ischium in the acetabular region can lead to damage to the ureter, bladder, or other intrapelvic organs.[2,33,34] The extent of injury may involve direct laceration of these structures, compression by hematoma, or later entrapment by secondary scar. Hemorrhage, immediate urinary extravasation, or remote obstruction may result. Awareness of these possibilities and prompt diagnosis are essential to avoid subsequent damage. In general these problems can be readily corrected by securing effective urinary drainage or by direct repair.

Direct laceration of retroperitoneal structures is exceedingly rare, and the most dramatic presentation will usually involve immediate vascular compromise and extensive intraoperative bleeding. Acute decompensation or hypotension requires immediate fluid resuscitation, prompt wound closure or packing, and patient repositioning for a midline incision and immediate exploratory laparotomy to establish vascular control. In most cases immediate consultation with appropriate surgical subspecialists should be sought. Injury to the genitourinary tracts is best managed by a urological surgeon. If during this exploration ureteral or bladder disruption are noted, these structures should be repaired or managed expeditiously as appropriate to the clinical setting. The mechanisms of injury to the different structures will be considered separately.

Bladder Injury

The most common mechanism of bladder injury is laceration by bone fragments created by manipulation of the pelvic girdle. This results in partial or full thickness injury of the bladder walls.[10] Since the origin of injurious force is from the lateral, retroperitoneal surface of the bladder, it is highly likely that this resultant injury will be to a retroperitoneal surface of the vessel as well. Usually a penetrating injury will not lead to a large devascularized flap of bladder wall. The possibility of a bone fragment remaining within the bladder lumen or near the laceration must be considered. The tissue is usually healthy enough to heal without formal repair,[35] but the possibility of a sequestrum that would complicate healing is high.

Other possible types of injury are far less common. Direct shredding of the intrapelvic structures by surgical instruments is exceedingly rare. Likewise, dome injuries caused by overdistention or compromise of vascular supply to the bladder wall are unusual; the shearing type of injury seen in pelvic fracture, in which the bladder is torn extensively at the sites of its attachments to the pelvic ring, are seldom seem. As a result, urethral disruption above the membranous diaphragm is not a consideration in the management of these cases.

In short, the bladder injury sustained during the course of total hip arthroplasty is most often a focal laceration of healthy tissue adjacent to an open bone and near a freshly placed prosthesis. The lesion is most often on a retroperitoneal surface of the bladder and possibly could include a bone fragment. These essential factors dictate the management approach.

Management of Bladder Injury

Successful management of bladder disruption requires attainment of several key elements: complete diversion of urine from the open site; secure apposition of healthy tissues; the absence of infection, foreign body or functional barrier to healing; and maintenance of adequate vascular supply and general health of the patient.[36] A common additional and often cited factor is the site of injury, whether intraperitoneal or extraperitoneal. Formerly all extraperitoneal injuries were managed in closed fashion, and all intraperitoneal injuries were managed by open repair. It is currently believed that the site of injury is not so important per se as was once held. Careful assessment of the local tissue character, the likelihood of a bone fragment or other structure acting as a barrier to healing, the presence of regional sepsis, and the general health and constitution of the patient are important factors in selecting the optimal approach.

Intraoperative Situations

Once a bladder injury has been appreciated in the course of an emergency exploration and the patient has been stabilized, repair of the injury can usually be performed expeditiously. The bladder wound should be carefully inspected to ascertain the viability of surrounding bladder wall and the location of the injury with respect to the ureteral orifices and the bladder neck. The lesion should be debrided carefully, avoiding trauma to the crucial landmarks. Ureteral stents can be placed by an opening in the bladder wall. The laceration can then be closed with a running closure and a drain can be left in place.

Extraperitoneal hematomas, in general, should not be opened. Many bladder repairs can be performed through the peritoneal surfaces of the bladder. In general bladder lacerations are much more easily appreciated and precisely closed from inside the bladder. This route should be considered, even when the bladder injury is thought to be located very distally from preoperative studies. In the setting of an adjacent disruption of the surrounding bone, the perivesical space will be extremely difficult to negotiate, and damage to the obterator nerve, infection of an adjacent hematoma, or additional ureteral injury may result from poorly conceived attempts to traverse this space. The best plan is to enter the retroperitoneal cavity and open the bladder and repair the distal damage from within.

Bladder injuries occurring with blunt pelvic trauma can be managed nonoperatively and will close in 1 to 6 weeks. However, the possibility of a penetrating one segment is very high in the setting of surgical disruption of the pelvic bone. This will compromise healing and may lead to permanent sinus infection. Either computerized tomography or cystoscopy must exclude the presence of a sequestrum. CT examination of the bladder is often difficult to interpret because the bladder and prostate are angled anteriorly, not perpendicular to the plane of the tomographic images. Partial voluming can confound interpretation. In many cases direct visual examination of the bladder cavity is the simplest and most certain means to exclude sequestrum.

The Mechanism of Ureteral Injury

In the rare cases that require immediate exploration because of either hemodynamic instability or the clear recognition that intrapelvic injury has been incurred, the ipsilateral ureter should be identified and its continuity verified. If ureteral injury is recognized, repair usually can be successful and should be attempted immediately.

Ureteral Injury: Repair

A complete discussion of the techniques of ureteral reconstruction is beyond the scope of this chapter, but a review of the general concepts is appropriate here.

Severe ureteral damage may consist of direct destruction of the ureteral tissue, creating a gap between segments of viable ureter.[7,37,38] It may consist of a simple perforation of the ureter without tissue loss, or it may consist of a partial thickness injury in which continuity is not lost, but the damage is severe enough so that significant scar will accrue during the healing phase, possibly causing fibrotic narrowing and resultant obstruction.

In most cases ureteral injury will heal spontaneously if ureteral continuity can be established and protected by passing a ureteral stent across the damaged segment.[39] These devices are made of flexible plastic or silicon and fashioned with a pigtail or J-shaped curve at both ends to prevent migration. Multiple side holes allow free passage of urine within, alongside, and in and out of the lumen of the catheters. They are extremely effective in maintaining a patent lumen despite extrinsic compression or intramural edema and preventing urine from flowing out through perforations in the ureteral wall. Renal function and ureteral healing are greatly facilitated.

Ureteral stents can be placed retrograde by a cystoscopic procedure, antegrade by a percutaneous approach, or at the time of an open surgical exploration.

Ureteral repair should utilize viable tissue, avoid tension on the repair, minimize the chance of extravasation through the repaired site by stenting or proximal decompression, and be performed in such a way as to minimize the chance of stone formation and infection. Other tissue characteristics such as prior radiation exposure or steroid use must be considered, and the status of the contralateral renal unit must also be understood as fully as possible. Any reconstructive approach that jeopardizes the function of the opposite unit must be critically scrutinized, especially if there is any history of malignancy or stone disease on the injured side that might spread to the unaffected unit.

The site of injury should be carefully exposed and the quality of the tissue appraised critically and debrided until healthy tissue remains. A tension-free reconstruction should then be performed. In the simplest cases involving only a short portion of the mid-ureter, and end-to-end anastamosis will suffice. In the region of the distal ureteral, a reimplantation is often the treatment because of the ease with which the well vascularized bladder wall can be brought up to meet the lower ureter. This anastamosis is readily performed and reliable. In the proximal ureter the kidney can often be mobilized and brought down to compensate for lost ureteral length. In any of these reconstructions an isolated segment of ileum or stomach tissue can be fashioned into a conduit if the ureteral gap cannot be bridged after mobilization of the kidney and ureters. Transureteroureterostomy is a reliable technique in selected cases in which stone disease, malignancy, and poor healing prospects are not present.

Radiological Imaging of Urological Injury

Immediate gross hematuria may immediately herald urological trauma. Other common signs are abdominal pain, distention, or voiding dysfunction. Oliguria may signal bladder injury; however, ureteral injury most often is not associated with oliguria because urine production from the contralateral kidney will continue at an accelerated rate, concealing signs of the injury. Acute peritoneal signs and early postoperative ascites also signal the need for evaluation of the urinary system.

General Principles

When urological injury is suspected, on the basis of physical examination, hematuria, or the radiological findings of extensive intrapelvic fluid or obvious bony disruption, prompt radiological evaluation should be undertaken (Fig. 60.1). No single radiological test approaches are suitable to different situations. The special applications of the major different studies to this setting will now be reviewed briefly.

Abdominal CT Scan

Abdominal/pelvic CT has become the standard evaluation of traumatic, urological injury.[40] Examination with orally administered and without intravenous contrast should be carried out. Continuity of renal cortex, the anatomy of the intrarenal collecting system, ureter, and bladder are best seen on this single study.

The presence of metal-backed cups or other metallic implants will result in considerable "scatter" artifact, which often makes the CT scan much less valuable than the plain anteroposterior radiograph (Fig. 60.2).

In addition, if bladder injury is suspected, a cystogram should be performed (see below). This single study provides much or all of the information previously obtained from intravenous pyelography and stress cystography. The urological organs are beautifully seen in cross-section traveling coaxially with the CT table. "Spiral" CT has been shown to evaluate the entire ureteral length with unsurpassed accuracy. This technique obtains information from the entire abdomen during a single breathhold, eliminating artifact and slip

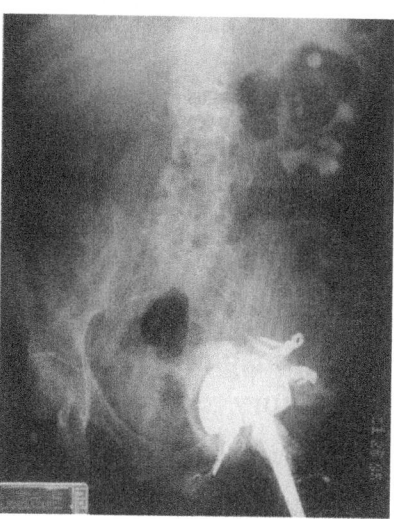

Figure 60.1. *Protrusio Acetabuli Prosthetica.* After a complex reconstruction this patient exhibits a dramatic intrapelvic complex of bone, cement and components. No ureteral injury was incurred but subsequent revision would risk major visceral injury.

areas due to respiration. The bladder, prostate, and male urethra travel from posterior to anterior and are less well seen; however the dome and lateral walls of the bladder do show up very nicely. The CT may show wall thickening extravesical contrast or actual wall disruption. The bony pelvis is also shown in detailed fashion, and the position and orientation of bony spicules and intactness of the medial cortex of the pelvis can stand out dramatically.

Soft tissue and bone windows can be used to scrutinize specific tissues to clarify questionable areas.

Cystography

Although computed tomography does give two-dimensional, cross-sectional views of the bladder, so that the presence of contrast "behind" the bladder is more easily seen than on conventional urography, experience has shown that bladder distention remains a crucial component in evaluating possible bladder disruption.[41] The bladder should be distended to a volume of approximately 400 cc. This can be accomplished either by injection of an intravenous agent with its accompanying diuresis or by direct infusion into the bladder through a ureteral catheter. Post-drainage views are more crucial than conventional cystography.

Cystography is a simple, inexpensive, and rapid way to evaluate bladder trauma. It can be performed either in the Intensive Care Unit or in the Radiology Department. Through an in-dwelling catheter, the bladder should be distended to at least 400 cc. Oblique views and a drainage film should be obtained; these studies will yield highly accurate information.

Intravenous Urography

Intravenous urography is less commonly used with the development of contrast tomography; however, occasionally emergency intraoperative evaluation is imperative and an IVP may be of crucial importance.

Intraoperative Technique

The patient should be positioned supine. As much instrumentation as possible should be removed from the patient's abdomen and the examination should survey the field of the obstruction. A high dose of contrast should be utilized since often opacification will be poor due to either hypotension or ongoing diuresis.

Detailed views of the anatomy are often very difficult to obtain under these circumstances, and subtle extravasation cannot be confirmed with certainty. The goal is often to conserve renal function and this goal can usually be met if adequate contrast is administered.

Radioisotope Scanning

Radioisotope scanning is rarely utilized in the emergency setting or in the immediate management of urological trauma. The principal indication is to assess renal function. Radionucleotide scanning is then needed to evaluate the lateralization of renal function. The study does not yield precise facial resolution and is widely felt to be inaccurate in assessing traumatic bladder injury or ureteral disruption. Although this may be considered in cases of contrast allergy, CT scanning, computerized tomography without contrast, or retrograde cystoscopy/pyelography are often more useful and yield more precise and accurate information. The relative component overall renal function contributes by a single kidney.

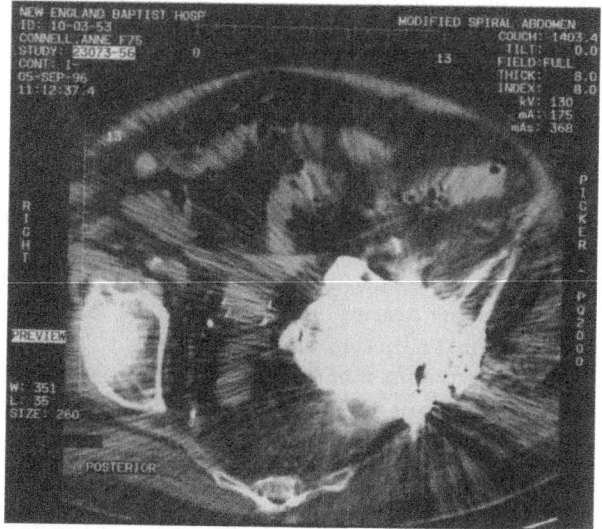

Figure 60.2. Computerized tomography of the same patient shows extensive artifact due to scatter of the x-ray caused by metal.

Retrograde Pyelography

Retrograde pyelography yields the most certain and precise evaluation of the distal ureter. Combined with ureteroscopy, this is the most definitive means of evaluating distal-ureteral obstruction or discontinuity. On tomography or cystography, contrast may infiltrate between tissue planes and among tissue planes in the pelvis so widely that the precise origin of the extravasated material cannot ascertained.

Direct inspection of the bladder wall and selective ureteral injection is definitive.

Percutaneous Nephrostomy

In the critically ill patient, stabilization is of crucial importance and percutaneous nephrostomy is the treatment of choice in the immediate setting to establish drainage and to facilitate further investigation.

Using either contrast or with fluoroscopy or ultrasonography, the location of the intrarenal urinary collecting system is established. A needle is introduced through the flank into the collecting system. The most effective of these involves a fixed coil formed by a thread that prevents the coil from unraveling. This prevents catheter dislodgment during respiratory excursions.

Once percutaneous access has been established, the kidney will usually drain well and leakage of urine into the peritoneum will stop. Antegrade ureterography and stent passage can be performed through the renal access at a later time.

References

1. Irvine R, Johnson BL, Jr, Amstutz HC. The relationship of genitourinary tract procedures and deep sepsis after total hip replacements. *Surg Gynecol Obstet.* 1974;139:701–706.
2. Lowell JD, Davies JA, Bennett AH. Bladder fistula following total hip replacement using self-curing acrylic. *Clin Orthop.* 1975;3:131–133.
3. Pitfield J, Saxton HM. Urinary tract complications of total hip replacement. *Clin Radiol.* 1981;32:429–430.
4. Carter HB, Partin AW, Osterling JE, et al. The use of prostate specific antigen in the management of patients with prostate cancer: The Johns Hopkins Experience. In: Catalona WJ, Coffey DS, Karr JP, eds. *Clinical aspects of prostate cancer. Assessment of new diagnostic and management procedures.* New York, Elsevier, 1989;247–251.
5. Catalona WJ, Smith DS, Ratliff TL, Dopps KM, Coplen DE, Yuan JJ, et al. Measurement of prostate specific antigen in serum as a screening test for prostate cancer. *N Engl J Med.* 1991;324:1156–1161.
6. Carter HB, Pearson JD, Wacliwew X, Metter EJ, Guess HA, Walsh PC. PSA variability in men with BPH. *J Urol.* 1994;151:101A.
7. Solomon MH, MacGregor RJ. Ureterocutaneous fistula following hip surgery. *J Urol.* 1980;124:427–428.
8. Ball AJ, Feneley RCL, Abraqms PH. The natural history of untreated prostatism. *Br J Urol.* 1981;53:613–616.
9. Soloway M, Briggman J, Carpinito G, Chodak GW, Church PA, Lamm DL, et al. Use of a new tumor marker, urinary NPM22, in the detection of occult or rapidly recurring transitional cell carcinoma of the urinary tract following surgical treatment. *J Urol.* 1996;156:363–367.
10. Madsen PO, Iverson P. A point system for selecting operative candidates, In: Hinman F Jr, ed. *Benign prostatic hypertrophy.* New York, Springer-Verlag, 1983;763.
11. Boyarsky S, Jones G, Paulson DF, Prout GR Jr. A new look at bladder neck obstruction by the Food and Drug Administration: Guidelines for investigation of benign prostatic hypertrophy. *Trans Am Assoc Genitourin Surg.* 1976;68:29–38.
12. Mebust WK, Holtgrewe HL, Cockett AT, Peters PC. Transurethral prostatectomy: Immediate and postoperative complications. A cooperative study of thirteen participating institutions evaluating 3,885 patients. *J Urol.* 1989;141:243–248.
13. Chaussy C, Schuller J, Schmiedt E, Brandl H, Jocham D, Liedl B. Extracorporeal shock wave lithotripsy (ESWL) for treatment of urolithiasis. *Urology.* 1984;23:(5 Spec No):59–66.
14. Willscher MK, Conway JF, Babayan RK, Morrisseau P, Sant GR, Bertagnoll A. Safety and efficacy of electrohydraulic lithotripsy by ureteroscopy. *J Urol.* 1988;140:957–958.
15. Dretler SP. Laser lithotripsy: A review of 20 years of research and clinical applications. *Laser Surg Med.* 1988;8:341–356.
16. Jenkins AD: ESWL of ureteral stones below the pelvic brim. *Problems in Urology.* 1987;1:641.
17. Hooten TM, Stamm WE. Management of acute uncomplicated urinary tract infections in adults. *Med Clin North Am.* 1991;75:339–357.
18. Stapleton A, Latham RH, Johnson C, Stamm WE. Postcoital antimicrobial prophylaxis for recurrent urinary tract infection. A randomized, double-blind, placebo controlled trial. *JAMA.* 1990;264:703–706.
19. Scherz HC, Parsons CL. Prophylactic antibiotics in urology. *Urol Clin NA.* 1987;14:265–271.
20. Johnson JR, Stamm WE. Urinary tract infections in women: diagnosis and treatment. *Ann Intern Med.* 1989;111:906–917.
21. Stamm WE, Hooton TM. Management of urinary tract infections in adults. *N Engl J Med.* 1993;329:1328–1334.
22. Ritter MA, Faris PM, Keating EM. Urinary tract catheterization protocols following total joint arthroplasty. *Orthopedics.* 1989;12:1085–1087.
23. Ritter MA, Faris PM, Keating EM. Urinary tract catheterization protocols following total joint arthroplasty. Center for Hip and Knee Surgery, Mooresville, Ind & Indiana Medical School, August 1989, Vol 12/No 8.
24. Meier AH, Weil EH, van Waalwijk van Doorn ES, Verhaegh GT, Janknegt RA. Transurethral radio-frequency heating or thermotherapy for benign prostate hypertrophy: a prospective trial on 65 consecutive cases. *Eur Urol.* 1992;22:39–43.
25. Blute ML, Tomera KM, Hellerstein DK. Transurethral microwave thermotherapy: an alternative for the treatment of BPH. One year clinical results of the Prostatron study group. *J Urol.* 1993;149:143A.

26. Walsh, Patrick C, Retik A, Stamey TA, Vaughan ED. *Minimally invasive management of benign prostatic hyperplasia. Campbell's Urology* 6th ed. PC Walsh, ed. Philadelphia: Saunders;1992.
27. Patel A, Fuchs GJ, Gutierrez-Aceves J, Ryan T. Prostate heating patterns comparing electrosurgical transurethral resection and vaporization: a prospective randomized study. *J Urol.* 1997;157:169–172.
28. Narayan P, Tewari A, Schalow E, Leidich R, Aboseif S, Cascione C. Transurethral evaporation of the prostate for treatment of benign prostatic hyperplasia: results in 168 patients with up to 12 months of followup. *J Urol.* 1997;157:1309–1312.
29. Fincke BG, Friedland G. Prevention and management of infections in the catherized patient. *Urol Clin North Am.* 1976;3:313–321.
30. Garibaldi RA, Burke JP, Dickman ML, Smith CB. Factors predisposing to bateriuria during indwelling urethral catheterization. *N Engl J Med.* 1974;291:215–219.
31. Cohen MS. Fournier's gangrene. *AUA Update Series.* 1986;5(6).
32. Belker AM. The varicocele and male infertility. *Urol Clin North Am.* 1981;8:41–51.
33. Ray B, Baron TE, Bombeck CT. Bladder and ureteral displacement complication of total replacement hip arthroplasty. *Urology.* 1979;13:554–556.
34. Schneider HJ, Mufti GR. Vesico-acetabular fistula after total hip replacement. *Br J Urol.* 1993;71:754–755.
35. Salvatierra O Jr, Rigdon WO, Norrus DM, Brady TW. Vietnam experience in 252 urological war injuries. *J Urol.* 1969;101:615–620.
36. Corriere JN Jr, Sandler CM. Mechanics of injury, patterns of extravasation and management of extraperitoneal bladder rupture due to blunt trauma. *J Urol.* 1988;139:43.
37. Mattingly RF, Borkowf HI. Acute operative injury to the lower urinary tract. *Clin Obstet Gynecol.* 1978;5:123–149.
38. Fry DE, Milholen L, Harbrecht PJ: Iatrogenic ureteral injury: Options in management. *Arch Surg.* 1983;188:454–457.
39. Zinman LM, Libertino JA, Roth RA: Management of operative ureteral injury. *Urol.* 1978;12:290–303.
40. Bretan PN, McAninch JW, Federle MP, Jeffrey RB Jr. Computerized tomographic staging of renal trauma: 85 consecutive cases. *J Urol.* 1986;136:561–565.
41. Lis L, Cohen Allen J. CT Cystography in the evaluation of bladder trauma. *J Comp Assist Tomog.* 1990;14:386–389.

61
Postoperative Wound Problems

Leonard B. Miller

General Principles

There are a number of important considerations in the management of the soft tissues overlying the hip joint, especially in the revisional arthroplasty patient. Prevention is better than cure and in reoperative joint surgery, where there may be scarred and deficient periarticular tissues. Anticipation of postoperative wound problems is essential. To avoid this, corrective measures need to be taken both pre- and intraoperatively. For example, incisions need to be designed through old scars to avoid further devascularization. Various manifestations of scarring, for example, depressed scars, multiple scars, and scar contractures, all need to be addressed preoperatively. Areas of tightness or soft tissue deficiency can be replaced or augmented with local tissue flaps. At all costs the mobility and thickness of the tissues overlying the joint prosthesis must be maintained and tension on the incision line avoided. Significant scar contractures of the hip joint can be released and the soft tissue deficiency replaced with a fair-sized myocutaneous flap, also allowing a lengthening procedure on the hip to be performed (Fig. 61.1).

In situations where the previous incisional scars are too thinned out or depressed, increasing the risk of postoperative wound breakdown, these scars can be excised preoperatively, advancing the local tissues and creating a more stable incision line closure.

Usually in cases of trauma where multiple procedures have been performed on the hip and femur, there may be adjacent areas of recurrent wound breakdown and/or osteomyelitis with unstable scarring and infection. These areas should be eradicated preoperatively and usually do best with aggressive debridement and local or regional muscle flap procedures (Fig. 61.2).

Salvage of the Exposed Joint Prosthesis

Not enough attention has been paid to the expeditious management of the early postoperative wound, where limited incision line breakdown and or drainage may occur. This may indicate an early exposure of the prosthesis to the outside via even a small communation through the skin. The underlying fascia and capsule may not be fully intact, and before a periprosthetic infection develops a local soft tissue reconstruction (muscle flap) may be indicated in order to salvage the arthroplasty. Continuity of the soft tissue layers needs to be reestablished without tension, wound edges debrided, and appropriate antibiotic coverage implemented. There is little documentation in the literature regarding such occurrences, appropriate management, and outcome. In situations where this treatment fails or where reimplantation was not performed and the wound continues to drain, a resection arthroplasty or girdlestone procedure is performed.

Management of the Nonhealing Girdlestone Arthroplasty Defect

With an increasing number of total hip arthroplasty operations and therefore secondary procedures being performed annually in the United States, there is also an increasing number of infections. Conventional treatment of the infected total hip arthroplasty has been the removal of the prosthesis and cement with closure over drains. More effective antibiotic therapy is probably responsible for keeping the incidence of nonhealing wounds at an acceptable rate. Some surgeons favor immediate reimplantation after a period of wound care and intravenous antibiotics. The patient may continue to function well in this situation, but once again there is the possibility for recurrent infection and drainage creating a chronically debilitating hip wound. This unfavorable result is due in part, especially in secondary hip arthroplasties, to the noncollapsibility of the surrounding tissues, which consist of poorly vascularized scar tissue. The plastic surgeon is usually consulted at this stage. Following an aggressive debridement procedure to remove all the nonviable tissue (including bone), chronic granulation tissue, and scar tissue, the enlarged defect is filled with one of a variety of muscle transpo-

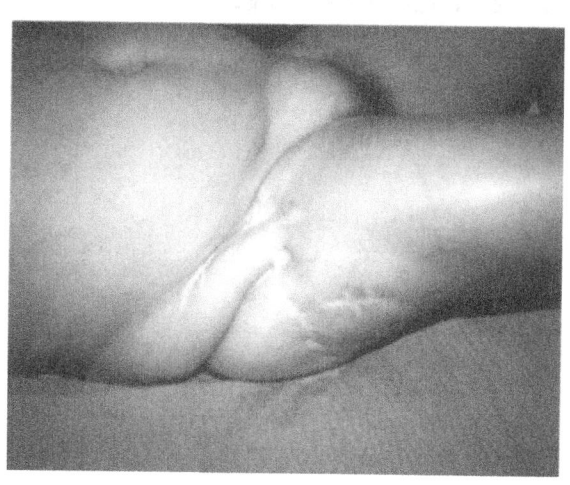
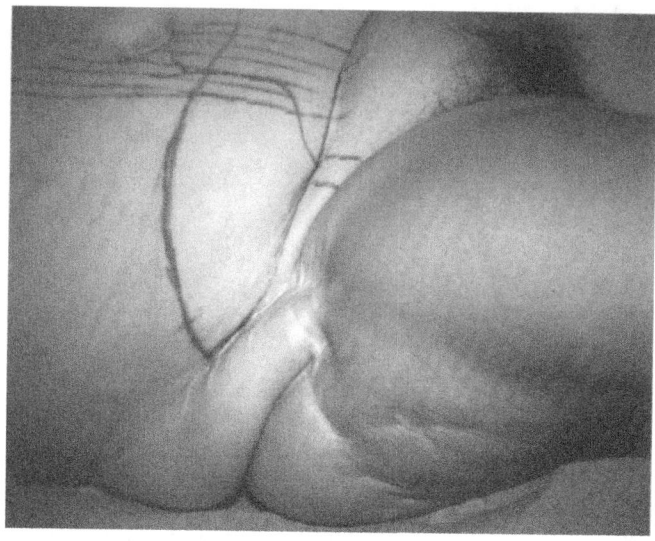
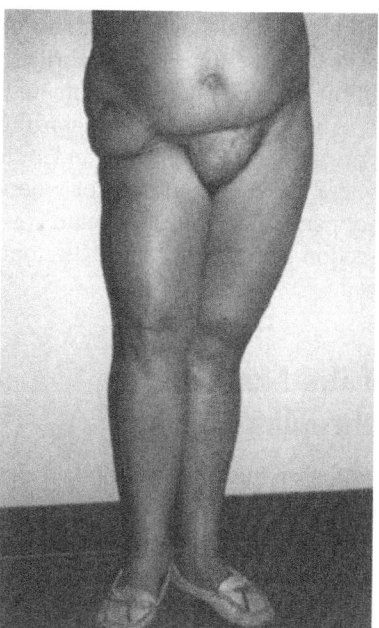
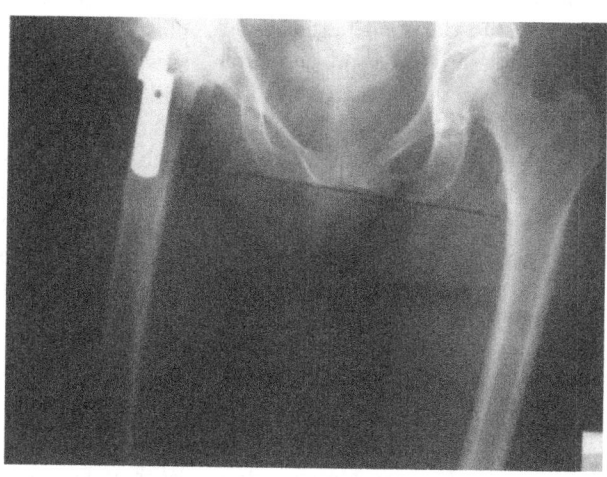

Figure 61.1. A. Scar contracture right hip status post multiple hip procedures. B. Design of inferiorly based rectus abdominis myocutaneous flap. C. Healed flap. D. Pre-op radiograph following muscle reconstruction. (See color insert.)

sition flaps (Fig. 61.3). Reimplantation of the hip prosthesis can then be considered 6 to 12 months later.

Methods of Soft Tissue Reconstruction

Most often, a regional muscle flap is transposed to manage a complex wound problem around the hip joint. The rectus femoris, vastus lateralis, and tensor fascia lata have been the three muscles most frequently used.[1-6] However, use of those muscle groups may result in some functional loss or instability; the inferiorly based rectus abdominus muscle is gaining more popularity because it has a wide arc of rotation and does not involve sacrifice or local muscle tissue.[7]

In some institutions, the rectus femoris and vastus lateralis muscle flaps are still used frequently to cover or fill the hip joint.[1] In secondary hip arthroplasty, however, these muscles may be too scarred down or atrophic from previous procedures. This is where a more distant muscle (the inferiorly based rectus abdominus muscle) may be preferable. The rectus abdominis muscle can be passed preperitoneally or above the inguinal ligament into the hip area. It also has the advantage of carrying a fairly sizable skin island with it. If these muscle groups are not available, other considerations are the use of a posterior thigh fascia cutaneous flap based on the gluteus medial muscle or a free microvascular tissue transfer. With early incision, breakdown and exposure of the prosthesis expeditious management is indicated, probably with the transposition of a muscle flap to allow for rapid healing, control of infection, and stable closure.

The presence of depressed, contracted, or unreliable scar tissue can be managed by a number of local procedures, for example advancement skin flaps, rotational fasciocutaneous flaps, or microvascular free tissue transfer of skin fascial flaps.

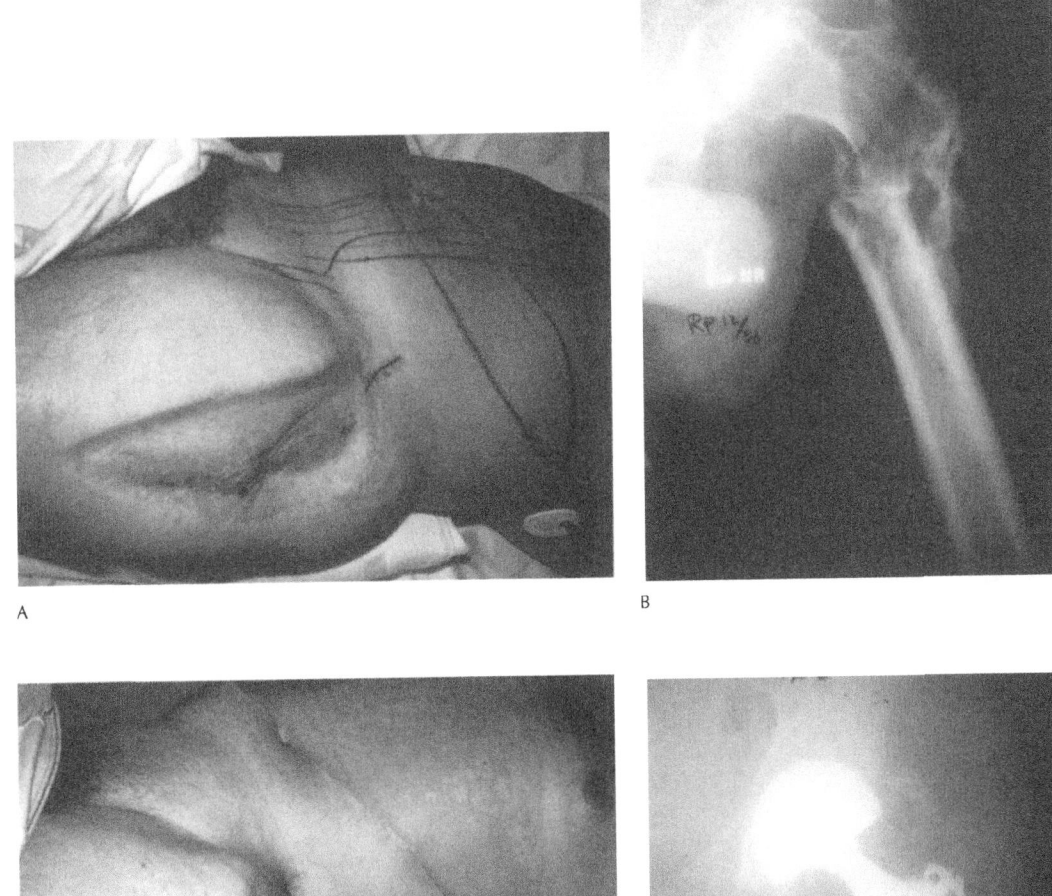

Figure 61.2. A. Traumatic wound left hip. B. Osteomyelitis at fracture site. C. Inferiorly based rectus abdominis myocutaneous flap following debridement. D. Total hip arthroplasty after muscle reconstruction. (See color insert.)

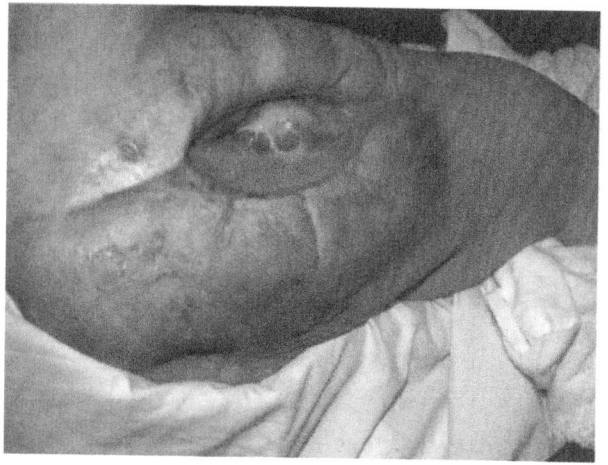
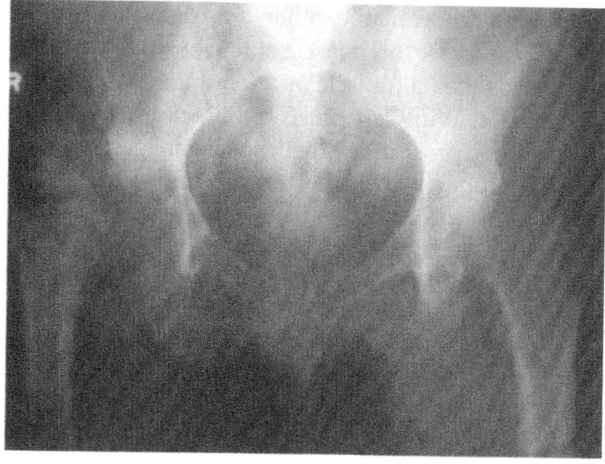
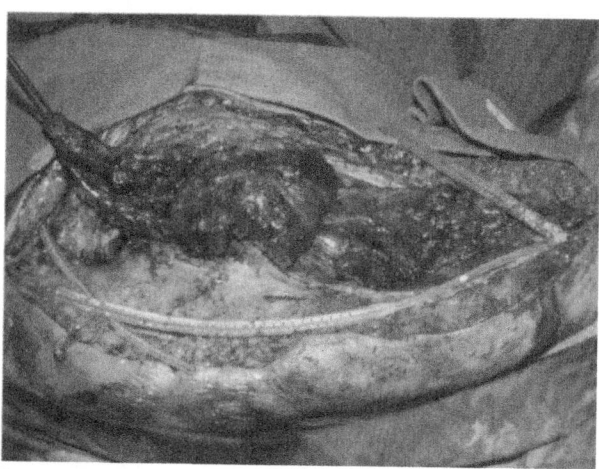
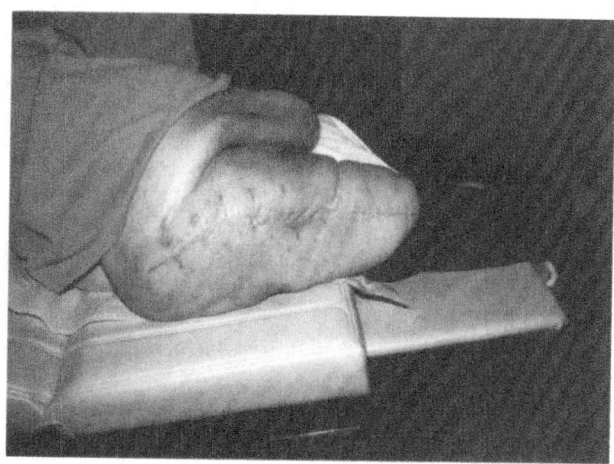
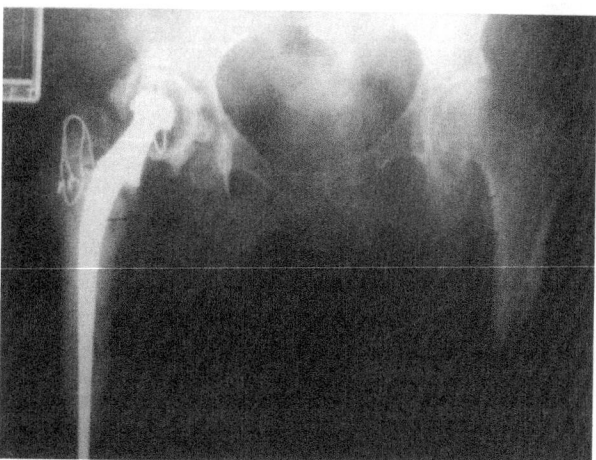

Figure 61.3. A. Infected girdlestone hip wound. B. Radiograph of hip. C. Vastus lateralis muscle flap. D. Healed wound 6 months later. E. Hip arthroplasty following muscle reconstruction. (See color insert.)

References

1. Meland NB, Arnold PG, Weiss HC. Management of the recalcitrant total-hip arthroplasty wound. *Plast Reconstr Surg.* 1991;88:681.
2. Ger R, Adar N. The management of chronic cavities in the region of the hip joint. *J Bone Joint Surg Am.* 1973;55:758.
3. Arnold PG, Witake DJ. Management of failed total hip arthroplasty with muscle flaps. *Ann Plast Surg.* 1983;11:474.
4. Collins DN, Garion KL, Nabon CL. The use of the vastus lateralis flap in patients with intractable infections after resection arthroplasty following the use of a hip implant. *J Bone Joint Surg.* 1987;69:510.
5. McGraw JB, Arnold PG. *Atlas of muscle and muscolocutaneous flaps.* Norfolk, VA: Hampton Press, 1986.
6. Pederson WC. Coverage of hips, pelvis, and femur. *Orth Clin N Am* 1993;24:3.
7. Windle BH, Stroup RT Jr, Beckenstein MS. The inferiorly based rectus abdominus island flap for the treatment of complex hip wounds. *Plast Recon Surg J.* 1996; July.

62
Heterotopic Ossification

Douglas E. Padgett

Prior to the advent of total hip arthroplasty, degenerative disease of the hip was a progressive, disabling condition that led to a life of pain, stiffness, and loss of function. This crippling condition often resulted in patients living a life confined or at least dependent upon the support of others for the performance of activities of daily living. The outlook for many of these patients was, indeed, bleak. The development of the modern total hip arthroplasty has surely been a godsend to many. In the words of Dr. Mark Coventry, "No orthopedic procedure of this century has captured the imagination of both the medical profession and the lay public as has total arthroplasty of the hip".[1]

The success of total hip arthroplasty can be measured by surgeon and patient alike. The main features of a successful total hip arthroplasty can be summarized as relief of pain, return to function, and restoration of motion.[2] Mobility, or the loss thereof, is one of the first manifestations of hip disease that patients often notice. Difficulty in ascending or descending stairs, difficulty in bending, or the problem of simply putting on ones shoes or socks is often one of the initial complaints that a patient will state upon presentation to the physician. When these functional losses are due to degenerative disease of the hip and total hip arthroplasty is proposed, the patient and the surgeon both anticipate a return of these functional activities.

Unfortunately, restoration of motion and function following total hip arthroplasty is difficult to predict. While surgical technique has advanced in the past decade, resulting in more predictable implant fixation, certain complications of total hip arthroplasty persist. These include instability, limb length inequality, nerve palsy, and—perhaps the most annoying of all—postoperative total hip complications: heterotopic ossification. The formation of ectopic bone in the soft tissues about the hip following hip arthroplasty can, unfortunately, lead to pain, stiffness, and an overall decrease in the function of an otherwise well-performed arthroplasty.[3] When heterotopic ossification becomes clinically significant, patient satisfaction is greatly diminished and often can strain the physician–patient relationship.

In this chapter, the topic of heterotopic ossification about the hip will be discussed in detail. The proposed biology and mechanism of ectopic bone formation will be examined and the clinical sequelae of heterotopic ossification described. In addition to describing the various classification schemes, incidence and a description of the at-risk groups will be given. Finally, examination of the various treatment methods as well as prophylactic regimens currently used to prevent heterotopic ossification will be given.

Biology of Heterotopic Ossification

The mechanism of formation of ectopic bone following total hip arthroplasty has been the subject of great debates for decades. The factors that allow soft tissues to ossify are, unfortunately, poorly understood. The phenomena of soft tissue ossification is readily apparent in three clinical entities: (1) myositis ossificans progressiva, a congenital disorder resulting in the formation of ectopic ossification in the soft tissues of children; (2) traumatic myositis ossificans circumscripta, observed following local trauma, yielding ossification of muscle or other soft tissue; and (3) atraumatic myositis ossificans circumscripta, a condition resulting in the formation of ectopic ossification following injuries to the central nervous system, burns, and even polio.[4] The unique feature of all these clinical entities is the formation of bone in the soft tissues of muscle, fascia, or other connective tissue adjacent to a joint structure. The histologic picture at maturity demonstrates the presence of Haversian systems and well organized lamellar bone structure. While the term *myositis* is used to describe the phenomena, it is in fact not really a manifestation of a chronic inflammatory condition at all, with little histologic evidence to support chronic inflammation as an etiology.[5] Some have suggested that heterotopic ossification is solely the result of local trauma leading to the release of bone debris or local osteogenic cells that are responsible for the observed development of mature bone. However, if this were true, then the observation of massive ectopic bone following either trauma to the central nervous system or following major burn in the absence of any local insult would be difficult to explain. It is these seeming inconsistencies in the expression of ectopic bone formation that perplexed clinicians for many decades.

It was the work of Chalmers et al.[6] that gave perhaps the greatest insight into the phenomena of ectopic bone formation. For many years, investigators had observed that certain tissues had the capacity to induce the formation of bone when transplanted to orthotopic sites. These tissues included gall bladder epithelium, epithelium of the urinary tract, as well as human amnion tissue. This observation persists whether the tissue is devitalized or not, reinforcing the notion of inducing capable tissue. Ironically, devitalized allograft bone tissue was found to have little inducing capability.[7] However, in addition to the type of transplanted tissue, the site into which the tissue was transplanted appeared to have influence on the ultimate development of ectopic bone: muscle and fascia appeared favorable sites for bone formation while kidney, liver, and spleen did not.[8] Chalmers and coworkers designed a series of experiments to determine what factors were responsible for the development of ectopic bone employing a rabbit model. Using differing presumed inducing agents (decalcified rib, fascia, or frozen homograft bone) implanted in differing milieus (muscle, liver, spleen, or kidney), the authors were able to observe vastly differing responses to implants as measured by ectopic bone formation.[6] Fascia alone could not induce bone formation regardless of site of transplantation; decalcified bone was a highly effective inducing agent, especially when combined with fascia. There was clearly differing osteogenic induction capacity for different tissues at different sites. Based upon their unique set of experiments, these authors were able to postulate the requisites for the formation of ectopic bone, namely, an inducing stimulus, the presence of cells capable of being induced along osteoblastic cell lines, and a local environment that is able to support bone formation. These three factors form the basis for understanding the biology of heterotopic bone formation.

Unfortunately, much of the detail of this proposed schema remains unclear. While an inducing stimulus appears necessary, the exact nature of this stimulus is unknown. Whether due to a specific paracrine factor such as fibroblast growth factor or insulin-like growth factor or a combination of factors, induction appears too dependent upon their presence. What role the local tissue environment plays is also unclear. The fact remains that muscle and fascia appear to be the ideal milieu for the development of ectopic bone. Whether there is a release of local tissue factors such as prostaglandins that could maximize production of bone matrix is also unknown. Finally, what about the cell line of origin? Where do the bone precursor cells arise? It has been suggested that pleuripotential cells in the local environment liberated at the time of local tissue trauma or injury are induced along osteoblastic/chondroblastic cell lines, resulting in formation of mature bone.[9] Unfortunately, this does not explain the observation of atraumatic myositis ossificans with no specific local injury. The hypothesis of distant migration of pleuripotential stem cells into the local area perhaps in response to the inducing agent, as well as local concentrations of prostaglandin then undergoing transformation into osteoblastic cell lines, appears a plausible explanation. To date, none of these theories has been shown to be correct. However, the concept of (1) cells capable of transformation, (2) an inducing stimulus, and (3) a local environment suitable for ossification appear to be the prerequisites for the formation of heterotopic bone.

Clinical Presentation of Heterotopic Ossification

Heterotopic ossification following total hip arthroplasty is, unfortunately, often recognized only after radiographic features are apparent. By the time of radiographic confirmation of diagnosis, treatment and certainly prophylactic regimens are no longer effective. As will be discussed later in this chapter, the identification of high-risk groups in whom prophylaxis against heterotopic bone is most warranted should be the surgeon's top priority. Some clinical features of the complication that are apparent during the early postoperative period might alert the clinician to the possible onset of the formation of heterotopic bone.

It has been reported that within the first two to three weeks following total hip arthroplasty, an increase in local tenderness, muscle spasm, and mild rest pain may be noted. The distinction between incipient heterotopic bone and "normal" postoperative pain is, unfortunately, quite difficult to make. Most patients assume that the increased pain experienced is due to progression of the rehabilitative process. Early heterotopic bone may be associated with a low-grade temperature although, again, this is a very nonspecific finding. This constellation of clinical findings is not pathognomonic for heterotopic ossification, and the differential diagnosis may include infection as well as deep vein thrombosis.[4]

While restriction of hip motion eventually becomes the salient feature of heterotopic ossification, there has been no correlation between initial early postoperative decrease in range of hip motion and late development of heterotopic ossification (HO). However, in patients in whom clinically significant HO develops by 4 weeks postoperatively, restriction of hip motion is noted. This is especially true of hip flexion and rotation. It is not uncommon for muscle spasm to occur during this period.[10]

Unfortunately, laboratory studies are of little value in differentiating the disease process at this early stage. While the level of preoperative serum alkaline phosphatase directly correlated with the extent of postoperative heterotopic bone in those patients developing HO, serum alkaline phosphatase alone is *not* predicative of at-risk patients.[11] Changes in white blood cell count, erythrocyte sedimentation rate, and serum calcium have demonstrated no relationship to the ultimate development of HO. To summarize, laboratory analysis is of little value in determining the presence of developing HO following total hip arthroplasty.

The radiographic appearance of HO is confirmatory of the diagnosis. The degree of ossification observed is temporally related to the surgery itself. Within the first 4 to 6 weeks following surgery, a haze of calcification is visible, often outlining the eventual extent of the ectopic bone formation. As the process of ectopic bone formation progresses, the development of mature lamellar bone follows, which is evidenced radiographically by increasing density and opacification.[4] The radiographic extent of heterotopic ossification is usually complete by 6 months.[3]

The histologic appearance of heterotopic ossification is dependent upon the timing of examination. The initial stages of the process demonstrate vascular connective tissue with apparent proliferation of presumed undifferentiated mesenchymal cells. It is not uncommon to observe some nuclear pleomorphism in addition to the presence of occasional mitoses. As the process matures, osteoblastic differentiation of the mesenchymal cells is seen, with the subsequent formation of osteoid and or woven bone trabeculae.

Occasional zones of cartilage in various stages of differentiation and endochondral ossification may be present, especially at the periphery of the disease process. As the weeks into months progress, formation into mature lamellar bone with established Haversian systems occurs.[5]

Classification Schemes

While HO following total hip arthroplasty may be suspected on clinical grounds, the diagnosis is confirmed radiographically. As will be discussed later, the incidence of the disease process varies greatly, but in addition, the clinical significance also varies greatly. That is, some patients have little loss of mobility, while others are profoundly affected with restriction of motion. It is the unpredictable clinical nature of the process that led investigators to avoid using a clinical rating scale and to develop a more reproducible and hopefully accurate radiographic rating system for the presence and extent of HO.

One of the first systems developed to help quantify and classify HO following total hip arthroplasty was developed by Brooker et al.[3] The *Brooker classification* was based on the author's observation of the pattern of ectopic bone formed during analysis of 100 consecutive total hip arthroplasties. Anteroposterior radiographs of the hip were standardized and analyzed for degree of ectopic bone at a minimum of 6 months following surgery. Heterotopic ossification was graded as follows:

Class I: Islands of bone within the soft tissue about the hip

Class II: Bone spurs extending from the pelvis or proximal femur leaving at least 1 cm between opposing surfaces

Class III: Bone spurs extending from either pelvis and or proximal femur, but with less than 1 cm between opposing bone surfaces

Class IV: Apparent bone ankylosis

Based upon this initial work, Brooker and investigators noted that classes I, II, and III did not seem to have a major adverse effect upon outcome following total hip arthroplasty. However, when class IV, bone ankylosis, occurred, there was a decrease in the overall hip function and hip score, due primarily to loss of motion.

Modifications of this classification scheme have been proposed, including that of Maclennan, who added a class 0 rating to signify the absence of any ectopic bone formation in the soft tissues.[12]

The advantage of the system devised by Brooker is that it is relatively simple and appears to correlate well with the clinical picture of overall hip function.

The disadvantage of the system of Brooker is that it is based solely upon anteroposterior radiographs, that is, a two-dimensional picture of an obvious three-dimensional problem. In addition, it does not quantify the amount of bone formed within each class. However, despite these limitations, the system of Brooker remains the most widely used system for classifying ectopic bone formation following total hip arthroplasty.

In an attempt to better quantify the amount of heterotopic bone formed about the hip, Parkinson et al.[13] formulated a modification of the Brooker scheme. The authors divided the region about the hip into thirds and attempted to determine total area of involvement of the ectopic bone. It was the authors' contention that this type of classification would produce a closer correlation between grade of heterotopic bone and the functional effect it would impose. This subclassification (Fig. 62.1) was defined as follows:

Sub-class A: 0 to 33% of the area involved

Sub-class B: 34 to 66% of the area involved

Sub-class C: 67 to 100% of the area involved

While the use of the Parkinson modification appears logical in an attempt to better correlate extent of radi-

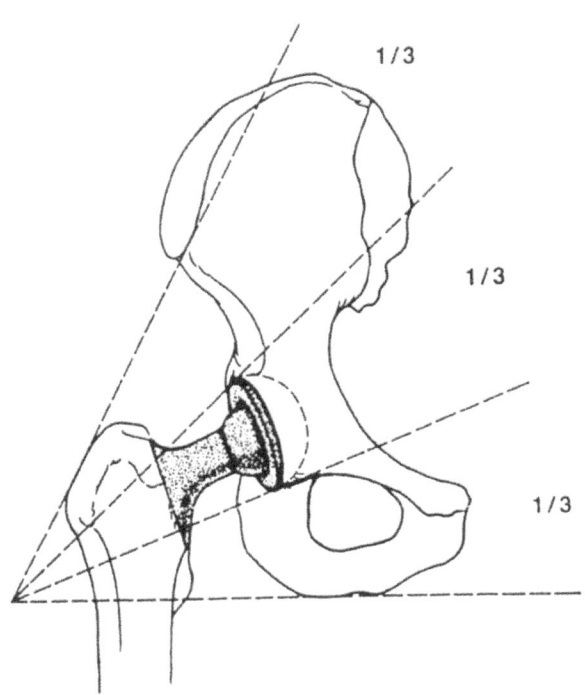

Figure 62.1. Schematic of extent of heterotopic bone formation as identified on the anteroposterior radiograph (Reprinted with permission from Parkinson et al. *Hip*, 1982, 211–227).

ographic heterotopic ossification and functional outcome, verification of this scheme has not confirmed; for this reason, most surgeons today continue to utilize the original Brooker scheme for the description of heterotopic ossification following total hip arthroplasty.

Occurrence of Heterotopic Ossification

Incidence

The reported incidence of HO following total hip arthroplasty has ranged from as low as 5% to as high as 81% following revision hip surgery.[3,14,15] With such a wide range of occurrence, it is often difficult for the clinician to estimate the patient's real risk for encountering this complication. However, some basic guidelines are apparent in understanding two main features of HO: (1) the incidence of this complication varies greatly and is probably multifactorial in origin, and (2) once extensive HO has formed, the only known treatment is surgical excision.[16] Therefore, an understanding of the incidence and the groups at risk for development of heterotopic bone is mandatory if the surgeon wishes to minimize the risk of his/her patients to this complication and, as will be seen, effectively institute prophylactic treatment.

The observation of HO following total hip arthroplasty was recognized by Charnley in his review of the results of the original low-friction arthroplasty.[17] In this original series of total hip arthroplasties on hips with no prior history of surgery, an incidence of 5% was noted. It was reported that the clinical significance of the heterotopic bone was felt to be minimal. Wilson et al. found ectopic bone formation following primary total hip arthroplasty in 30% of their patients, noting some restriction of motion in patients.[18] Finally, Bisla et al.[19] demonstrated an incidence of ectopic bone formation of 61% in patients undergoing total hip arthroplasty due to ankylosing spondylitis. While the grading technique of each of these authors was different, it was clear that the incidence of ectopic bone formation appears to vary widely. With such a wide degree of expression, it became apparent that ectopic bone formation was probably multifactorial in origin, and identification of groups that appeared to be at highest risk for development was essential.

Risk Factors

In reviewing the available literature, several factors appear to influence the development of HO following total hip arthroplasty. These include sex of patient, underlying diagnosis of the patient, surgical approach utilized, method of fixation, primary versus revision surgery, length of surgery, and the presence of ipsilateral or contralateral heterotopic bone.[14,20–23]

Gender

The effect of gender upon the development of heterotopic bone is somewhat controversial, for it is often inherently tied in with the patient's diagnosis; that is, more males tend to have hypertrophic osteoarthritis than do their female counterparts. Ritter was one of the first to suggest that male gender may be linked as a risk factor for HO. In their experience, the authors noted that males were twice as likely to develop ectopic bone following hip arthroplasty as were females.[20] This finding was consistent with the observations of Delee[14] and that of Morrey.[21]

Diagnosis

Blasingame and coworkers were among the first to recognize that not only gender but diagnosis might play a predictive role in identifying at-risk individuals for the formation of ectopic bone.[22] Specifically, these authors noted that the presence of spinal osteophytes appeared to correlate well with the development of HO. The presence of bridging spinal osteophytes along three or more vertebrae seen preoperatively was associated with a greater than 50% incidence of ectopic bone formation following hip arthroplasty. These authors concluded that active hypertrophic osteoarthritis as well as diffuse idiopathic skeletal hyperostosis (DISH syndrome) are predisposing conditions for the development of HO following total hip arthroplasty.[22] This is especially true in bilateral hip disease. Ritter was able to demonstrate a significant increase in the incidence of HO in cases where bilateral hip arthroplasty was performed.[20]

Another diagnosis often associated with an increased incidence of HO is ankylosing spondylitis. The association of extensive heterotopic bone after hip arthroplasty in patients with ankylosing spondylitis was originally reported by Bisla et al.[19] These authors noted an incidence of 62% of heterotopic bone, with 9 of 23 hips demonstrating class III or IV. It was concluded from these results that patients with ankylosing spondylitis are at high risk for the development of clinically significant HO following total hip arthroplasty. It should be noted that, in the majority of these cases, a trochanteric osteotomy was performed to facilitate exposure; what role this may have played in the development of HO is unclear. Other authors have questioned whether ankylosing spondylitis predisposes patients to HO. Kjaersgaard-Andersen has been unable to confirm that the diagnosis of spondylitis alone is responsible for the increase rate of observed heterotopic bone.[23] Despite these reservations, most surgeons today consider ankylosing spondylitis a relative risk for postoperative HO and treatment decisions regarding prophylaxis are based accordingly.

Surgical Approach
The effect of surgical approach upon the development of HO following total hip arthroplasty has been widely debated for decades. The literature is replete with studies that seem to implicate certain approaches, specifically the transtrochanteric approach and the anterolateral approach, with a higher incidence of HO. Bischoff et al., reporting on the results of uncemented total hip arthroplasties performed with either an anterolateral or posterior approach, found that the anterolateral approach was associated with a 26.5% incidence of clinically significant HO, compared to only 11% in the group in whom the posterior approach was employed. It was felt that the posterior approach is less invasive to the abductor musculature and the relative lack of trauma to this region is responsible for the low rate of heterotopic bone.[24] These findings were echoed by Pai et al., who demonstrated that the anterolateral approach using the Liverpool modification (the anterior gluteus medius is detached with a sliver of bone) was associated with a 42% incidence of heterotopic bone.[25] While it may be proposed that the partial osteotomy be implicated in the development of the ectopic bone, patients in whom a transtrochanteric approach was utilized in this series did not have any increased incidence of HO.

The effect of trochanteric osteotomy upon the development of ectopic bone following total hip arthroplasty remains unclear. Errico et al. have shown an increased incidence of HO in patients undergoing hip arthroplasty using the transtrochanteric approach.[26] Morrey and coworkers from the Mayo Clinic compared the effect of three differing approaches (anterolateral, posterior and transtrochanteric) upon the development of ectopic bone and could demonstrate no significant difference among groups.[21] In a prospective randomized study comparing the transtrochanteric approach to the anterolateral approach of Harding, Horwitz et al. could not demonstrate any functional difference between patients at one year follow-up. However, the incidence of HO in the anterolateral group was 45% compared with only 20% in the osteotomy group. These authors suggest that the anterolateral approach may be more invasive to the abductor muscle plane and set the stage for the development of HO. In this study, the functional significance of the heterotopic bone was minimal.[27] While firm conclusions are difficult to draw, it appears that the literature suggests a slightly higher risk for the development of HO following hip arthroplasty using the anterolateral approach, but the clinical significance of this appears minimal.

Method of Fixation
With the advent of cementless hip arthroplasty, many surgeons noted an apparent increase in perioperative blood loss. When compared with cemented femoral fixation, which utilizes acrylic for fixation as a seal of the upper femur, cementless fixation can be associated with extrusion of blood and marrow elements during and after stem insertion. The clinical significance of this in terms of the development of heterotopic bone occurrence was first studied by Maloney et al.[28] Using a matched set of patients in whom either a cemented femoral component or a noncemented, porous femoral component was used in conjunction with a noncemented porous acetabular component, the authors noted a significant increase in the rate of HO in the noncemented group. Of particular concern was the observation of class III or IV HO in 38% of the noncemented group, while only 13% of the cemented femoral components demonstrated class III or IV HO. The noncemented implant utilized was a diffusion-bonded mesh-padded noncircumferentially proximally-coated implant. These authors concluded that the use of cementless femoral reconstruction is associated with an increased risk for the development of clinically significant HO following total hip replacement (THR). Other authors have shown that noncemented femoral fixation is itself not a risk for the development of HO. Bischoff et al. demonstrated an overall incidence of 8% class III or IV HO following noncemented total hip arthroplasty with a proximal circumferential coated porous implant. These authors suggest that the use of a circumferential coated implant may decrease the occurrence of heterotopic bone formation by providing a better seal to the extrusion of marrow and blood elements from the proximal femur.[24]

Prior Surgery
It has been postulated that the risk of HO following revision hip arthroplasty is greater than that of primary

surgery (Pai et al.)[25] This is certainly true when heterotopic bone was noted following the index procedure. However, in cases where previous HO was not present, revision surgery appears to be associated with an overall general increase risk of ectopic bone.[29] It appears that the increase in ectopic bone may be due to the additional soft tissue dissection that accompanies revision surgery, the longer duration of surgery, and the greater degree of blood loss during revision arthroplasty.

Presence of Existing Ectopic Bone
Perhaps the best predictor of risk of postoperative ectopic bone formation is the presence of heterotopic bone in either the contralateral or ipsilateral hip preoperatively. Ritter was one of the first to observe the effect of prior ectopic bone. In a consecutive series of patients undergoing reoperation upon hips with established ectopic bone, all patients subsequently developed ectopic bone in the ipsilateral hip to the same degree as observed after the index arthroplasty.[20] Additionally, when ectopic bone is present in the contralateral hip following hip arthroplasty, the risk of ectopic bone formation in the ipsilateral hip appears as high as 90%.[14] Of all the risk factors, the presence of preexisting ectopic bone formation following total hip arthroplasty is the best predictor for postoperative occurrence (Fig. 62.2).

Risk Classification
Based upon observations of the development of HO following total hip arthroplasty, Ayers et al. developed a risk classification scheme to assess the relative risk.[30] The risks are classified from I through IV, with class IV being at the greatest risk for the development of heterotopic bone.

Class I: A diagnosis of hypertrophic osteoarthritis, ankylosing spondylitis, or diffuse idiopathic skeletal hyperostosis with no prior heterotopic bone

Class II: The occurrence of contralateral hip heterotopic bone

Class III: The presence of ipsilateral heterotopic bone following prior surgery

Class IV: The presence of prior ipsilateral HO resulting in ankylosis

Utilizing these risk classes, the surgeon can be guided as to the possibility of postoperative ectopic bone formation and whether prophylactic treatment is warranted.

Treatment and Prevention of Heterotopic Ossification

Treatment of Established HO

The only known treatment for established HO is surgical excision. The use of physical modalities such as physical therapy, hot or cold packs, or medicinal therapies has never proven to be of benefit in either decreasing the amount of ectopic bone mass or improving lost function predictably. Warren and Brooker[16] reported their experience with excision of heterotopic bone after total hip arthroplasty. Their series included 12 patients in whom either class III or IV heterotopic bone had occurred, resulting in significant limitations of motion. The authors used a protocol of aggressive surgical excision of ectopic bone mass, postoperative

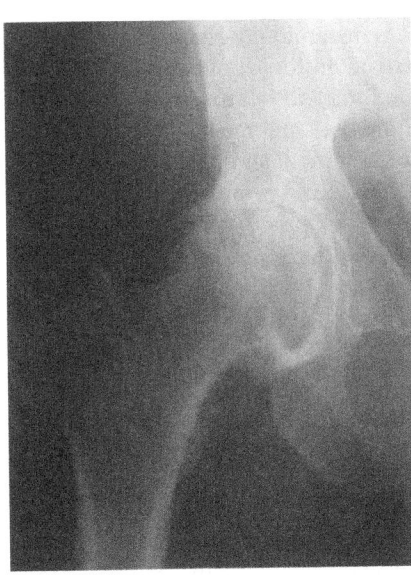
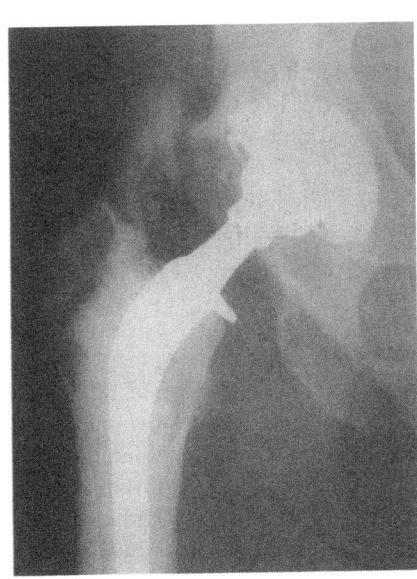

Figure 62.2. A. Preoperative AP radiograph of a patient in whom class III heterotopic bone had developed on the contralateral hip following total hip arthroplasty. No form of prophylaxis was administered. B. Six-month postoperative radiograph of the same patient with clinical evidence of restricted motion and radiographic evidence of class III heterotopic ossification.

A   B

ionizing radiation, and rapid mobilization with physical therapy. In this series, all patients experienced significant improvement of function as measured by range of motion and increase in ambulation. Two patients had recurrence of heterotopic ossification (Class II), with only one being symptomatic and that patient considered a failure. These results suggest that surgical management of severe HO can be successful but does require a second surgical procedure and is certainly associated with some morbidity and risk for recurrence. Based upon this, it is apparent that prophylactic preventive measures against the formation of heterotopic bone is rational.

Prophylaxis Against HO

Since the observation of the phenomena of ectopic bone formation following total hip arthroplasty, there have been many attempts at identifying effective means of prophylaxis. It had been proposed that the interposition of free autogenous fat in the region about the hip following arthroplasty would fill the apparent void and diminish the amount and intensity of postoperative scar as well as the possibility of ectopic bone formation. Riska and Michelsson were among the first to propose the use of fat transplantation specifically for this purpose. In their group of six patients in whom ectopic bone had formed following index arthroplasty, free fat was transplanted to the region around the prosthetic femoral neck. At follow-up, while motion had improved, radiographic evidence of ectopic bone recurrence was found in four of the six.[31] While these results suggest some clinical effect, it is difficult to assess the overall efficacy of this procedure in such a small series of patients.

The use of chemical prophylaxis directed toward the prevention of ectopic bone has always appeared attractive. One of the first class of medications proposed as an effective agent against ectopic bone formation were chelating agents such as diphosphonates. As a class of drugs, chelating agents inhibit the mineralization of deposited bone matrix (osteoid). They have shown proven efficacy in the treatment of certain diseases such as Paget's disease. Initial reports using diphosphonates appeared encouraging. However, following the termination of drug treatment, rapid bone mineralization occurred and ectopic bone formation appeared to the same degree as if no form of prophylaxis had been employed.[32,33] Unfortunately, this treatment scheme failed to adequately address the formation of ectopic osteoid matrix and merely delayed the final steps in mineralization of bone matrix. Discontinuance of use could be predictably associated with bone formation. Unfortunately, chronic diphosphonate usage is not a reasonable alternative. It has been demonstrated that the long-term use of diphosphonates can lead to osteomalacia.[33] Furthermore, the concomitant use of oral diphosphonates in the setting of cementless hip implants has been shown to lead to a significant decrease in the extent of bone ingrowth and may compromise long-term fixation.[34] For these reasons, chelating agents such as diphosphonates are no longer used as prophylactic agents against ectopic bone formation following total hip arthroplasty.

It is important to remember the requisites for ectopic bone formation as outlined by Chalmers: (1) pluripotential cells capable of being induced, (2) an inducing or transforming stimulus, and (3) a local environment suitable for ossification.[6] Any effective prophylactic scheme must be directed at one of these three conditions. Current strategies at reducing the incidence of HO have been aimed at (1) reducing the environment suitable for induction and transformation of pluripotential cells or at (2) reducing the viability of the pluripotential cells capable of being induced. Both of these measures attempt to arrest heterotopic bone formation prior to the formation of osteoid matrix rather than simply inhibiting the final phase of mineralization.

The use of nonsteroidal antiinflammatory drugs (NSAIDs) as effective prophylaxis against heterotopic ossification is based on the ability of these drugs to inhibit prostaglandin synthesis. It is felt that prostaglandin inhibition decreases the overall inflammatory response following surgery.[23,35,36] Ectopic bone is inhibited by two proposed mechanisms with NSAID use. There is an overall decrease in the cellular response to the surgery and therefore perhaps a decrease in the number of pluripotential cells available for induction. In addition, by decreasing prostaglandin synthesis, the local humoral stimulus for induction is decreased. By inhibiting cellular induction, there is no formation of osteoid matrix; therefore, once treatment is discontinued, late formation of ectopic bone does not occur. However, it seems reasonable that some initial period of NSAID usage is required to effectively mitigate the inflammatory response prior to termination of the drug.

Many different nonsteroidal agents have been used as means to prevent heterotopic bone. These include the use of aspirin, naproxyn, and—the most popular of all—indomethacin. Ritter was among the first to note the beneficial effects of indomethacin administered postoperatively. In a retrospective review of 81 hips felt to be at high risk for the development of HO, 90% of his patients developed no ectopic bone following surgery and the remaining 10% developed only Brooker class I.[37] Clear efficacy was demonstrated by Schmidt et al., who performed a randomized, double-blind study to evaluate indomethacin as a prophylactic agent. In their series, patients were randomized to either 6 weeks of indomethacin or placebo. At a minimum of one year follow-up, none of the patients in the indomethacin group had developed class II or greater heterotopic bone. However, in the placebo group, 30 patients developed class II HO and 18, class III. The patients with class III ectopic bone formation demonstrated significant reduction in movement of the hip.[36] It is clear from this work that indomethacin use for 6 weeks following total hip arthroplasty can lead to a significant reduction in the risk of postoperative HO.

The advantages of NSAID therapy is that it is inexpensive, easy to prescribe, and in general, a relatively safe therapeutic modality. Unfortunately, while the use of NSAIDs appears a rationale approach to prophylaxis, there are several limitations. As a systemic treatment for a local process, there are several comorbid conditions such as peptic ulcer disease, renal dysfunction, and hepatic insufficiency may preclude their use. Cella et al. demonstrated an almost 30% incidence of gastrointestinal symptoms associated with his patients on indomethacin resulting in an inability to fully complete the recommended six-week course of treatment.[35] The optimal duration of therapy with NSAIDs for effective prophylaxis to occur remains unclear. Additional concerns have been raised regarding the concomitant use of NSAIDs and the implantation of noncemented, porous hip components. Trancik has demonstrated a significant reduction in bone ingrowth into porous coated implants in a rabbit model treated with therapeutic doses of NSAIDs.[38] The clinical significance of this reduction in biologic fixation in humans is unknown at this time.

Due to some of the aforementioned concerns, the use of ionizing radiation as a modality has increased in popularity. Ionizing radiation prophylaxis is directed at the cell rather than altering the inducing stimulus. Ionizing radiation appears to interfere with the processing of nuclear deoxyribonucleic acid during cell division and inhibits the transformation of pluripotential cells.[12] Coventry and Scanlon were among the first to utilize radiation as a means to prevent ectopic bone formation after surgery. Their original scheme recommended a dose of 2000 centigray given in divided doses over a 10 days. Radiation was initiated at a mean of 6.5 days following surgery. While some frank failures of therapy were noted, the authors were encouraged with the results.[39] In a later study, Ayers et al.[30] from Rochester demonstrated the effectiveness of 1000 centigray over a 5-day period. In the series of 45 hips felt to be at high risk for the development of HO, only two hips developed significant heterotopic bone: one class II and one class III. Radiation in both of these patients was initiated on postoperative day 7 or greater. Based upon their experience, the authors recommended that treatment be initiated prior to postoperative day 4.

Three issues remain unclear with the use of ionizing radiation for prophylaxis: (1) the dose of radiation required, (2) the timing of radiation, (3) adverse effects and long-term concerns over the use of ionizing radiation.

The recommended dose of radiation that effectively prevents the formation of ectopic bone has steadily declined in the past decade. Pelligrini has demonstrated efficacy in using single-dose administration with 800 centigray with a 94% success rate in preventing clinically significant HO in a series of high-risk patients.[40] Healey, using 700 centigray in a single dose, demonstrated 97% success in preventing HO in a series of high-risk patients.[41] Hedley also employed single-dose 600 centigray with excellent clinical results.[42] In a prospective randomized series evaluating the use of 500 centigray versus 1000 centigray in prevention of HO in high-risk patients, Padgett et al.[29] were unable to demonstrate any difference between the two treatment groups. Based on their findings, the authors suggest that 500 centigray is an effective dose of radiation in pre-

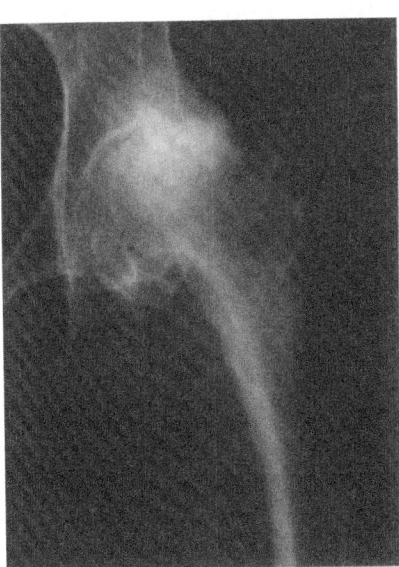
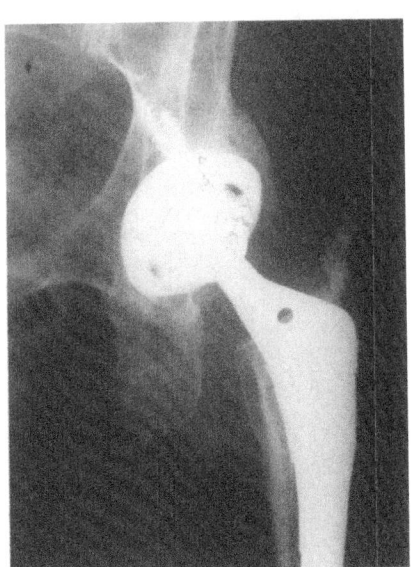

Figure 62.3. A. Preoperative anteroposterior radiograph of a 45-year-old male with hypertrophic osteoarthritis of hip. Patient felt to be at high risk for the development of heterotopic ossification. B. Following single-dose administration of 500 centigray radiation, there is no evidence of heterotopic ossification. The use of cerrobend blocking effectively shielded the regions of porous pads from the effect of the radiation.

venting the occurrence of postoperative HO following total hip arthroplasty (Fig. 62.3). While multiple dosing schedules have been used in the past, single-dose treatments have the benefit of limiting the amount of time patients require going to the radiation therapy suite as well, freeing up time in the radiation suite for treatment of conditions more dependent on radiation therapy such as neoplastic diseases. It appears that single-dose therapy is the most expedient method of delivery of radiation at this time.

The timing of radiation to discourage the development of HO has become apparent over the past decade. Ayers et al. were clearly able to delineate the adverse effect of delaying radiation treatment beyond 7 days, and their data suggests that optimal therapy requires initiation within 72 to 96 hours following surgery. Recent data from Pellegrini et al.[43] have shown efficacy in the use of preoperative radiation in discouraging the formation of ectopic bone formation. In a prospective, randomized series, the authors employed single-dose 800 centigray treatment 1 to 6 hours prior to total hip arthroplasty in a selected group of patients at high risk for the development of HO and compared these results to a group receiving traditional postoperative radiation. The authors were unable to demonstrate any difference in the incidence of ectopic bone formation between these two groups. This data also seems to support the contention that the cells responsible for ectopic bone formation following total hip arthroplasty are derived locally rather than being the result of distant migration.

While radiation therapy is generally well tolerated, there are some adverse effects. In many clinical series employing the use of radiation, occasional patient complaints of skin warmth and mild burning are noted.[30,40]

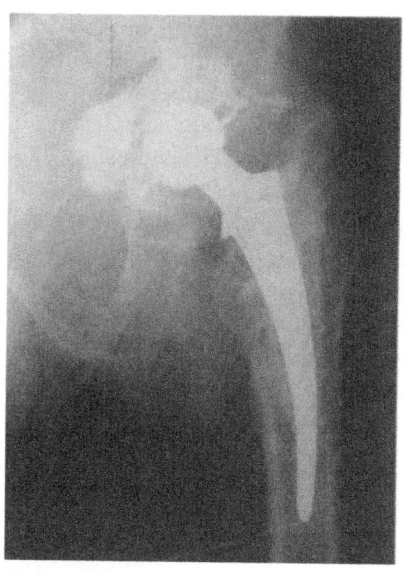
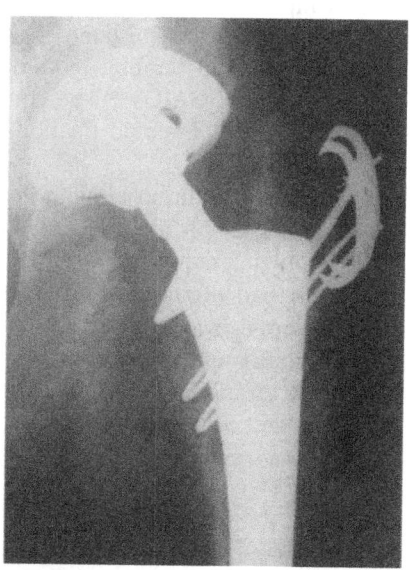
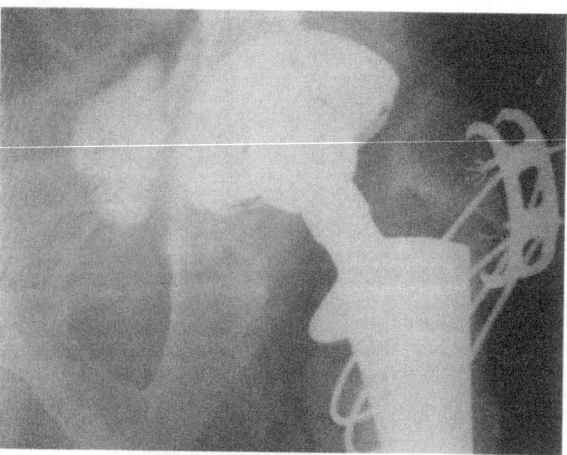

Figure 62.4. A. Preoperative radiograph of patient with aseptic loosening of total hip arthroplasty and evidence of class II heterotopic ossification. B. Following reconstruction with a cementless acetabular and femoral components, the patient received 700 centigray radiation. The region of the greater trochanter was not shielded during radiation administration. At 6 weeks, trochanteric fixation appears adequate. C. At 4 months postoperative, trochanteric migration and nonunion is apparent. Reoperation with supplemental autologous bone graft and cable fixation was necessary in order to restore abductor function.

However, these are often transitory and have no long-term significance. More problematic is the effect that radiation has upon the healing of trochanteric osteotomies in cases where such techniques are used. The risk of trochanteric nonunion (Fig. 62.4) or migration has been shown in several series and is presumed to be related directly to the inhibitory effect that radiation has upon the osteoblastic cell line.[30,40,41,42] An additional concern is the inhibitory effect of radiation upon the strength of fixation of porous coated implants. Sumner et al.[44] demonstrated significant initial decrease in the fixation strength and extent of bone ingrowth of canine humeri exposed to 1000 centigray radiation. In this study, radiation therapy with 500 centigray had no significant effect. Due to these concerns over the inhibitory effect of radiation upon osteotomy healing and biologic fixation, the use of selective shielding with cerrobend blocking is recommended. The cerrobend shield effectively limits radiation exposure to the unblocked regions. While its use may be associated with some extrafield ossification frequently along the trochanteric ridge, it is rarely associated with symptoms.[40]

Many surgeons have raised concerns regarding the use of radiation therapy, a potentially malignant inducing agent in the treatment of a nonmalignant condition. Reports of tumor induction by ionizing radiation in low doses are few. Kim et al.[45] reported that there was no evidence of tumor induction in any patient receiving less than 3000 centigray. However, Ron et al.[46] reported several cases of neural tumors arising after treatment of tinea capitis with doses of 1000 to 2000 centigray with latency periods of up to 24 years. Given this long latency period, efforts to find the minimal effective and safe dose of radiation for the prevention of heterotopic ossification appear justified.

Conclusions

Heterotopic ossification is a commonly occurring complication following total hip arthroplasty. For most patients, it has little clinical significance, but in selected patients in whom ectopic bone formation has a propensity, significant limitation of motion and function can occur. While the only known treatment of established heterotopic bone is surgical excision, identification of patients felt to be at high risk appears warranted to initiate prophylaxis against HO. Currently utilized effective forms of prophylaxis include the use of nonsteroidal antiinflammatory drugs or the use of external beam ionizing radiation. In the properly selected patient believed to be at high risk for the development of heterotopic bone following hip arthroplasty, prophylaxis can effectively minimize the risk of ectopic bone and ensure improved hip function following surgery.

References

1. Coventry MB. Historical perspective of hip arthroplasty. In Morrey BF, ed. *Joint replacement arthroplasty*. Churchill-Livingstone, New York, 1993.
2. Harris, WH. Traumatic arthritis of the hip after dislocation and acetabular fractures: Treatment by mold arthroplasty. An end-result study using a new method of result evaluation. *J Bone Joint Surg Am*. 1969;51:737–755.
3. Brooker AF, Bowerman JW, Robinson RA, Riley LH. Ectopic ossification following total hip replacement. Incidence and a method of classification. *J Bone Joint Surg Am*. 1973;55:1629–1632.
4. Hamblen DL. Ectopic ossification. In: Ling RSM, ed. *Complications of total hip replacement*. London, England: Churchill Livingstone: 1984;100–109.
5. Schajowicz F. *Tumors and tumorlike lesions of bone and joints*. New York: Springer-Verlag; 1981.
6. Chalmers J, Gray DH, Rush J. Observations on the induction of bone in soft tissue. *J Bone Joint Surg Br*. 1975;57:36–45.
7. Urist MR, McLean JFC. Ostogenic potency and new-bone formation by induction in transplants to the anterior chamber of the eye. *J Bone Joint Surg Am*. 1952;34:443–470.
8. Huggins CB, Sammett JF. Function of the gall bladder epithelium as an osteogenic stimulus and the physiological differentiation of connective tissue. *J Exper Med*. 1933;58:393–400.
9. Puzas JE, Reynolds PR. Basic science concepts related to the formation of heterotopic bone after total hip arthroplasty. *Semin Arthroplasty*. 1992;3:147–155.
10. Pedersen NW, Kristensen SS, Schmidt SA, Pedersen P, Kjaersgaard-Andersen P. Factors associated with heterotopic bone formation following total hip replacement. *Arch Orthop Trauma Surg*. 1989;108:92–95.
11. Mollan RAB. Serum alkaline phosphatase in heterotopic para-articular ossification after total hip replacement. *J Bone Joint Surg Br*. 1979;61:432–434.
12. MacLennan I, Keys HM, Evarts CM, Rubin P. Usefulness of postoperative hip irradiation in the prevention of heterotopic bone formation in a high risk group of patients. *Int J Radiat Oncol Biol Phys*. 1984;10:49–53.
13. Parkinson JR, Evarts CM, Hubbard LF. Radiation therapy in the prevention of heterotopic ossification after total hip arthroplasty. In: *The hip: Proceedings of the 10th open scientific meeting of the hip society*, St. Louis: CV Mosby, 1982.
14. Delee J, Ferrari A, Charnley J. Ectopic bone formation following low friction arthroplasty of the hip. *Clin Orthop*. 1976;121:53–59.
15. Healey WL, Lo TCM, Pfeiffer BA, Wasilewski SA. Radiotherapy in the prevention of heterotopic ossification after total hip arthroplasty. *Complications Orthop*. Spring, 1992;207–210.
16. Warren SB, Brooker AF. Excision of heterotopic bone followed by irradiation after total hip arthroplasty. *J Bone Joint Surg Am*. 1992;74:201–210.
17. Charnley J, Cupic Z. The nine and ten year results of the low-friction arthroplasty of the hip. *Clin Orthop*. 1973;95:9–25.
18. Wilson PD Jr, Amstutz HC, Czerniecki A. Total hip replacement with fixation by acrylic cement. *J Bone Joint Surg*

Am. 1972;54:207–236.
19. Bisla RS, Ranawat CS, Inglis AE. Total hip replacement in patients with ankylosing spondylitis with involvement of the hip. *J Bone Joint Surg Am.* 1976;58:233–238.
20. Ritter MA, Vaughan RB. Ectopic ossification after total hip arthroplasty: Predisposing factors, frequency, and effect on results. *J Bone Joint Surg Am.* 1977;59:345–351.
21. Morrey BF, Adams RA, Cabenela ME. Comparison of heterotopic bone after anterolateral, transtrochanteric, and posterior approaches for total hip arthroplasty. *Clin Orthop.* 1984;188:160–167.
22. Blasingame JP, Resnick D, Coutts RD, Danzig LA. Extensive spinal osteophytes as a risk factor for heterotopic bone formation after total hip arthroplasty. *Clin Orthop.* 1981;161:191–197.
23. Kjaersgaard-Andersen P, Hougaard K, Linde F, Christiansen SE, Jensen J. Heterotopic bone formation after total hip arthroplasty in patients with primary or secondary coxarthrosis. *Orthopedics.* 1990;13:1211–1217.
24. Bischoff R, Dunlap J, Carpenter L, Demouy E, Barrack RL. Heterotopic ossification following uncemented total hip arthroplasty: effect of the operative approach. *J Arthroplasty.* 1994;9:641–644.
25. Pai VS. Heterotopic ossification in total hip arthroplasty: the influence of approach. *J Arthroplasty.* 1994;9:199–202.
26. Errico TJ, Fetto JF, Waugh TR. Heterotopic ossification: incidence and relation to trochanteric osteotomy in 100 total hip arthroplasties. *Clin Orthop.* 1984;190:138–142.
27. Horwitz B, Rockowitz N, Goll S, et al. A prospective randomized comparison of two surgical approaches to total hip arthroplasty. *Clin Orthop.* 1993;291:154–163.
28. Maloney WJ, Krushell RJ, Jasty M, Harris WH. Incidence of heterotopic ossification after total hip replacement: the effect of the type of fixation of the femoral component. *J Bone Joint Surg Am.* 1991;73:191–193.
29. Padgett DE, Cummings M, Rosenberg AG, et al. The efficacy of 500 centigray radiation in the prevention of heterotopic ossification after total hip arthroplasty. Transactions of the annual meeting of the American Academy of Orthopaedic Surgeons. San Francisco, CA, February, 1993.
30. Ayers DC, Evarts CM, Parkinson JR. The prevention of heterotopic ossification in high-risk patients by low dose radiation therapy after total hip arthroplasty. *J Bone Joint Surg Am.* 1986;68:1423–1430.
31. Riska EB, Michelsson JD. Treatment of para-articular ossification after total hip replacement by excision and use of free fat transplants. *Acta Orthop Scand.* 1979;50:751–754.
32. Plasmans CMT, Kuypers W, Slooff TJ. The effect of ethane-1-hydroxy-1,1-diphosphonic acid (EHDP) on matrix induced ectopic bone formation. *Clin Orthop.* 1978;132:233–243.
33. Thomas BJ, Amstutz HC. Results of the administration of diphosphonate for the prevention of heterotopic ossification after total hip arthroplasty. *J Bone Joint Surg Am.* 1985;67:400–403.
34. Rivero DP, Skipor AK, Urban RM, Galante JO. Effect of disodium etidronate (EHDP) on bone ingrowth in a porous material. *Clin Orthop.* 1987;215:279–286.
35. Cella JP, Salvati EA, Sculco TP. Indomethacin for the prevention of heterotopic ossification following total hip arthroplasty. Effectiveness, contraindications, and adverse effects. *J Arthroplasty.* 1988;3:229–234.
36. Schmidt SA, Kjaersgaard-Andersen P, Pedersen NW, Kristensen SS, Pedersen P, Nielsen JB. The use of indomethacine to prevent the formation of heterotopic bone after total hip replacement. A randomized, double-blind clinical trial. *J Bone Joint Surg Am.* 1988;70:834–838.
37. Ritter MA, Sieber JM. Prophylactic indomethacine for the prevention of heterotopic bone formation following total hip arthroplasty. *Clin Orthop.* 1985;196:217–225.
38. Trancik T. The effect of piroxicam, meclofenamate, and prostaglandin F-2 alpha on bone ingrowth into a porous coated implant. *Semin Arthroplasty.* 1992;3:178–182.
39. Coventry MB, Scanlon PW. The use of radiation to discourage ectopic bone. A nine year study in surgery about the hip. *J Bone Joint Surg Am.* 1981;63:201–208.
40. Pellegrini VD, Konski AA, Gastel JA, Rubin P, Evarts CM. Prevention of heterotopic ossification with irradiation after total hip arthroplasty: radiation therapy with a single dose of eight hundred centrigray administered to a limited field. *J Bone Joint Surg Am.* 1992;74:186–200.
41. Healey WL, Lo T, Pfeifer BA, Wasilewski SA. Single dose radiation therapy for prevention of heterotopic ossification after total hip arthroplasty. *J Arthroplasty.* 1990;5:369–375.
42. Hedley AK, Mead LP, Hendren DH. The prevention of heterotopic bone formation following total hip arthroplasty using 600 rad in a single dose. *J Arthroplasty.* 1989;4:319–325.
43. Pellegrini VD, Gregoritch SJ. Preoperative irradiation for prevention of heterotopic ossification following total hip arthroplasty. *J Bone Joint Surg Am.* 1996;78:870–881.
44. Sumner DR, Turner TM, Pierson RH, et al. Effects of radiation on fixation of non-cemented porous-coated implants in a canine model. *J Bone Joint Surg Am.* 1990;72:1527–1533.
45. Kim JH, Chu FC, Woodward HQ, et al. Radiation induced soft tissue and bone sarcomas. *Radiology.* 1978;129:501–508.
46. Ron E, Modan B, Boice JD, et al. Tumors of the brain and nervous system after radiotherapy in childhood. *N Engl J Med.* 1988;319:1033–1039.

Part 6
Special Considerations

Benjamin E. Bierbaum

The contents of this part draw attention to the wide dimension of diagnoses and complicating issues that frequently present in revision hip surgery. These chapters emphasize the importance of a multidisciplinary approach to the evaluation and total management of patients who are candidates for another hip operation. Some of the special considerations are iatrogenically produced. The majority are related to infectious, metabolic, neuromuscular, moral, or genetic causes. Nowhere in the field of orthopedic surgery does the interaction between the multiple disciplines of medicine come into play better than in those interactions, evaluating and preparing patients for additional surgery.

In the management of patients with metastatic disease, the timely intervention of revision surgery for the prevention of morbidity and prevention of impending fractures is paramount in the decision-making process. The presence of metal implants from prior surgery complicates the diagnostic evaluation, both by the lack of penetration of x-rays through the metallic components and the scatter that is seen on CT and MR evaluations.

We have not included a separate chapter on metabolic bone disease because the authors feel that the individual considerations are too specific for a general outline of management of revisions in metabolic states. This is best addressed in works on primary hip replacement, where the concepts and algorithms for management of metabolic bone disease in the primary carry onto revision surgery.

In reference to fusion takedown and creation of a moving joint, the expectations, lifestyle, and demands of the individual must be addressed. Nowhere in revision surgery is the coordination of expectations on the part of patient and surgeon alike more defined than in the situation where a stable, painless nonarticulation is replaced with a moving, potentially weak, and potentially symptomatic joint. On the other hand, the pleasures of being able to sit comfortably and correctly and to get in and out of structures, chairs, and awkward places are not noted in hip evaluation assessments. Therefore, a different set of standards needs to be created in assessing the overall value of this kind of surgery.

The role of perioperative radiation in the management of heterotopic ossification is well covered. What isn't known at this time is that the potential for increased bleeding at the time of surgery and the type of scar formed if preoperative radiation is used. The long-term effects of minimal radiation, particularly of sequential operations in which sequential miniradiation doses are administered, are also not known.

A note does need to be made about the patient who has had radiation for malignancy. Such radiation renders the skeleton in the region of the radiation to an incentive state similar to Charcot joints. The creation of an arthroplasty or revision arthroplasty in these conditions is mentioned only to advise avoidance of arthroplasty when the bony tissues have received significant doses of radiation. Reconstruction in such cases—whether used in combination with bone grafting, cement, or cementless fixation—is likely to lead to early mechanical failure because of the Charcot quality of sensory receptors. As tempting as it is to try to reconstruct a surgery in the postradiation state, disaster is likely and mechanical failure will undoubtedly ensue.

A cautionary note also needs to be added for reconstructive surgery in neuromuscular conditions where there is essentially no muscle control about the hip. As tempting as it is to try to build constrained construct as a substitute for ligamentous and muscular stability of the hip joint, this type of construct is not likely to succeed. Revision surgery for special considerations, as in primary arthroplasty, requires careful planning, reasonable expectations, honest evaluation of likely outcomes, and a sound—not heroic—application of surgical principles. Even though the temptation to offer surgical help in the most difficult situation is tempting, the ultimate decision not to operate may be the soundest advice that can be given.

63
Total Hip Replacement Following Prior Surgeries

Michael H. Huo, Peter R. Jay, and Robert L. Buly

Total hip replacement has been applied to salvage failures of previous hip surgeries. When total hip replacement is performed for failed previous hip surgeries other than an index total hip replacement, it is generally termed a *conversion hip replacement*. The various etiologies may include:

1. Failure of internal fixation of previous hip fracture
2. Failure of hemiarthroplasty
3. Failure of surface replacement
4. Failure of previous femoral osteotomy
5. Failure of previous arthrodesis or ankylosis of the hip

Different technical challenges, considerations for implant selection, clinical results, and complications are present for these various situations. This chapter will focus on discussions about conversion surgery following previous hip fractures and following previous fractures of the acetabulum. Moreover, a section will focus on the discussion of femoral osteotomies as an adjunct surgical technique in conversion or revision hip replacement surgery.

Total Hip Replacement After Failure of Surgical Treatment of Fracture of The Hip

Indications

It is estimated that over 250 000 fractures of the hip occur each year in the United States.[1,2] The mainstay of surgical treatment of the majority of femoral intertrochanteric and neck fractures remains anatomic reduction with internal fixation.[1,2] These surgeries, unfortunately, have not been uniformly successful. On average, failure rate due to nonunion following internal fixation of femoral neck fractures has been reported to be approximately 33%, especially if the fracture was initially displaced.[1,2] The incidence of femoral head osteonecrosis has been reported in the literature to be approximately 16%.[3] Although the incidence of nonunion has been reduced to 4%[4] with improved surgical techniques, incidence of osteonecrosis has remained at 25.7% for the same series of patients. Overall failure rate for intertrochanteric hip fractures treated by internal fixation has been reported in the range of 4% to 12%,[1,2] with malrotation, nonunion, and loss of fixation being the primary modes of failure (Fig. 63.1).

Total hip replacement has been applied for the salvage of failed treatment of hip fractures with internal fixation in nearly 70% of the cases.[3] Various technical difficulties may be encountered during conversion surgery. These technical challenges may not only predispose patients to increased morbidity during the perioperative period, but also may compromise the clinical results and durability of the hip replacement.

Hemiarthroplasty of the hip using endoprostheses or bipolar prostheses has most frequently been applied to the treatment of acute displaced femoral neck fractures. On occasion, they have been used as the primary mode of treatment for patients with osteoarthritis or femoral head osteonecrosis with the hope of preserving acetabular bone stock for future reconstructions.[5-7] Discussion in this section will focus only on conversion surgery for failure of a primary hemiarthroplasty reconstruction, and will not address the special situation of failure of a hemiarthroplasty used for revision of a previous total hip replacement.[8]

The most common indication for considering conversion surgery following previous hemiarthroplasty is pain. Pain can result from loosening of the femoral stem,[9] erosion of the acetabulum,[10,11] combination of the two, disassembly,[12] wear,[13] or sepsis. One of the most commonly encountered clinical situations is the need for conversion surgery due to erosion of the acetabular cartilage following index hemiarthroplasty surgery. Whittaker et al. were among the first to report 64% incidence of loss of acetabular cartilage with a 24% in-

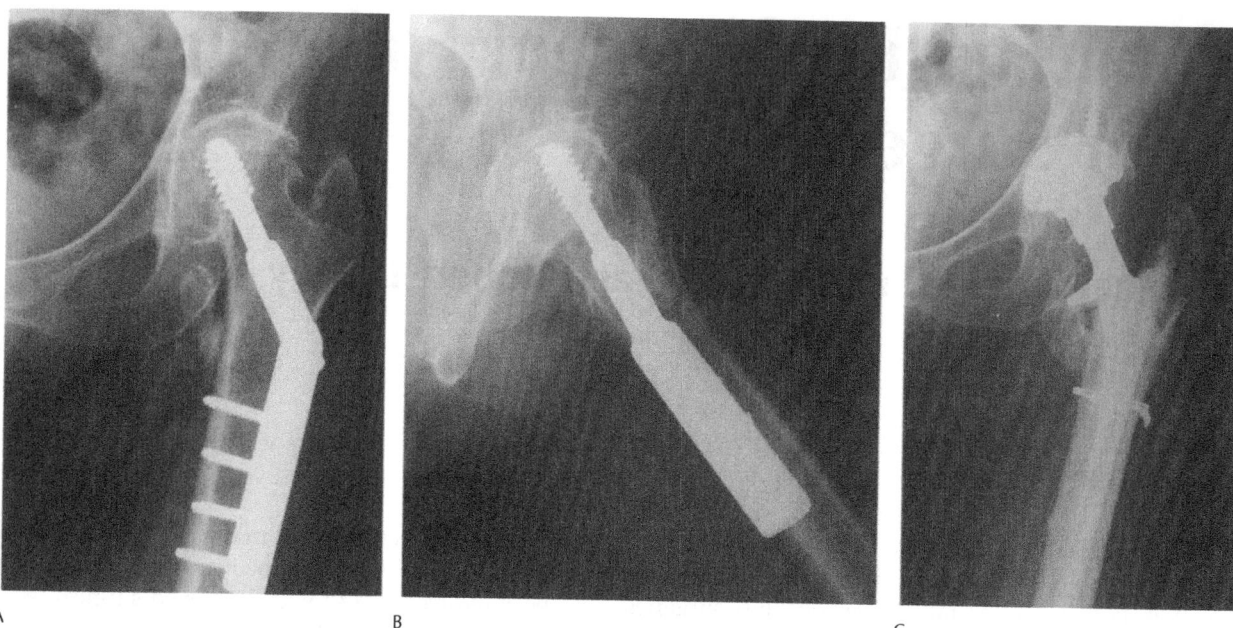

Figure 63.1. A. Anterior-posterior radiograph of a healed intertrochanteric fracture that was initially treated with a sliding hip compression screw. B. Lateral radiograph demonstrating protrusion of the screw into the hip joint space. C. Anterior-posterior radiograph demonstrating conversion hip replacement using hybrid fixation at 3 years follow-up. A medium-length stem was selected to bypass the cortical defects from the screws.

dence of development of protrusio at 15 years following hemiarthroplasty surgery.[14] Kofod and Kofod reported 37% incidence of conversion to total hip replacement within the first two years following hemiarthroplasty using the Austin-Moore prosthesis in 106 patients with femoral neck fractures.[15] The most significant finding ($p < 0.001$) was that presence of acetabular degeneration was four times greater in patients who underwent conversion surgery than in those who did not. A common feature among patients who required conversion surgery was that they were predominantly younger and more active. Dalldorf et al. recently reported evidence of acetabular cartilage degeneration using histology of biopsied specimens during conversion surgery in patients who had previously undergone hemiarthroplasty surgery.[10] They found significant differences in the histology of the cartilage when compared to a group of control patients who were undergoing primary replacement surgeries for femoral neck fractures. The degree of cartilage degeneration was significantly related to the duration of articulation against the metallic implant. There was no difference whether it was a unipolar or a bipolar prosthesis.

Technique

Conversion surgery for failed internal fixation of femoral neck and intertrochanteric hip fractures will be considered separately since there are different technical issues in each case. In general, surgical exposure, acetabular preparation, and selection of cup designs are similar to routine primary total hip replacements. The subchondral bone of the acetabulum may be very soft due to disuse osteoporosis, and care should be taken while reaming so as not to violate the central or the posterior wall of the acetabulum, which can compromise the fixation of the cup.

Failure of Femoral Neck Fractures

The most frequently encountered internal fixation devices are multiple screws or pins. They are usually easily removed, and femoral neck osteotomy can be performed at the appropriate level. In rare occasions, the screw heads may be buried below the lateral cortex. Moran described a technique to remove these buried screws in a retrograde fashion.[16] The remaining calcar is rarely deficient, and a standard femoral stem design can be used with or without cement using the same principles as for primary total hip replacements. The screw or pin holes can be plugged by hand or by using the removed screws themselves to facilitate pressurization of the cement if cement fixation is selected. These small cortical defects can either be left alone or grafted using bone from the femoral head.[17]

Failure of Intertrochanteric Hip Fractures

Conversion surgery for failed internal fixation of intertrochanteric hip fractures is generally more difficult than conversion surgery for failed femoral neck fractures. Several special anatomical considerations must be appreciated: (1) there is often medial displacement of the shaft in relation to the femoral neck; (2) malrotation of the fracture can further distort the proximal femoral geometry; (3) the calcar is often deficient to a level below the lesser trochanter; (4) and the greater trochanteric fragment may not yet have healed, thus necessitating supplemental fixation using multiple wires or a cable system. Breakage of cortical screws of the side plate in hip compression screw/plate devices is occasionally a problem. These broken screws may interfere with reaming and broaching of the femoral canal. These issues can be addressed either by overdrilling the lateral cortex and removing the screws or by cutting the intramedullary portion of the screws using a high-speed burr.

The distorted proximal femoral anatomy usually does not pose a formidable technical challenge, especially if cement fixation of the stem is selected. The stem selected must offer sufficient length to bypass the most distal cortical defect.[18] Significant proximal calcar bone deficiency can be addressed by using a calcar-replacement stem design. Leg length can be addressed using modular femoral head components. Restoration of soft tissue tension and femoral offset can be addressed with the modular neck lengths of the prosthesis, a stem design that offers greater offset, and/or advancement of the greater trochanteric fragment. Patterson et al. described a technique of plugging the cortical defects from the screws by using the screws themselves while pressurizing cement during insertion of the stem.[17] This technique allows only for plugging of the lateral cortex. This will maximize the pressurization effect and minimize cement extrusion, which has been reported to result in stress fracture of the femur.[19] The authors have generally found that the soft tissues on the medial side are not disturbed by surgical dissection, and can most often keep cement extrusion to a minimum.

Occasionally, a stem design for insertion without cement may be desirable for a particular case. The distorted femoral geometry may compromise the surgeon's ability to achieve maximal fit-and-fill of the canal. Furthermore, there is the risk of perforations or fractures since one of the fundamental principal surgical techniques in inserting stems without cement is to obtain maximal cortical contact. The surgeon may consider using modular stem designs that can allow for fitting the proximal and distal femoral geometry separately. In addition, corrective osteotomy may be necessary if there is significant deformity. These issues will be discussed later in the section on femoral osteotomy.

Technical challenges of conversion total hip replacement of a previous hemiarthroplasty are very similar to those of revision surgery of a failed total hip replacement. Preoperative workup should be able to determine with some certainty whether only acetabular reconstruction is necessary, or if stem revision is also necessary. Implant selection should be based on the same criteria as for routine revision hip replacement surgery using templates. Surgical approach should be based on the individual surgeon's preference, previous surgical incisions, and the specific requirements of each case. The transtrochanteric approach may especially be more practical if only acetabular reconstruction is necessary in the presence of a fixed-head stem. This will allow for more versatility in restoring soft-tissue tension with advancement of the trochanter.

Removal of the stem with a unipolar component such as an Austin-Moore endoprosthesis is usually necessary due to stem loosening or acetabular erosion. Some newer designs have offered modular unipolar components. Exchange to a regular femoral head component with the appropriate taper and neck length will allow for retaining the original stem if only acetabular reconstruction is necessary. In cases with a bipolar component, the shell can be removed without removing the stem in monolithic designs. The femoral head component in modular systems can be removed to better expose the acetabulum. The femoral stem must be carefully examined for stability and orientation. If the stem is to remain in situ, the neck taper junction or the femoral head itself must be protected from abrasion during retraction.

Acetabular reconstruction is similar to primary total hip replacement. In some cases, subchondral bone of the acetabulum can be extremely weak, especially in elderly patients with previous femoral neck fractures. Careful attention in reaming, as in the case of conversion surgery for failed internal fixation of hip fractures described earlier, should be given. Acetabular cups inserted with cement may be best in cases with osteoporotic bone. In some of these conversions, sclerosis of the subchondral bone is present, which presents an obstacle to optimal cement–bone interface. Cups inserted without cement with or without adjunct screw fixation may be preferred. Bone grafting may be necessary if significant protrusion of the acetabulum is present. Deficiency of the acetabulum is generally mild and major structural graft is usually not necessary. However, on occasion erosion of the acetabular bone stock may be severe enough to even consider the use of reinforcement rings or cages along with bone grafting.

If the femoral stem is to be removed, the same principles and techniques in removing cemented or cementless stems in a previous total hip replacement should be followed. Femoral reconstruction is similar to routine femoral revision surgery. It is unnecessary to use a longer stem unless the femoral cortex is violated either from stem removal or the loosening process itself. If the stem is to remain in situ, areas of osteolysis in the proximal femoral zones should be grafted using autograft or allograft.

Results

In general, the clinical results of conversion total hip replacements for the failure of internal fixation of previous hip fractures are satisfactory overall. The reported series, however, have indicated inferior results to routine primary hip replacements. In one of the earliest series, Turner and Wroblewski[20] reported satisfactory pain relief, joint motion, and walking ability in nearly 90% of the 205 patients who underwent conversion surgery for late complications of femoral neck fractures. The major complications in this series were superficial (7.8%) and late deep infections (3.9%). Fixation loosening occurred in 3.4% at an unspecified follow-up interval. These cases were studied with early cementing techniques and implant designs. Stambough et al.[21] reported a series of 27 conversions for failed internal fixation of hip fractures. Complications with the trochanteric osteotomy and malpositioning of the stem each occurred in 26% of the hips. There was a 3.7% rate of revision for aseptic loosening at a mean follow-up of 6.3 years. More importantly, the authors observed radiographic loosening in 33% of the cups and 22.2% of the stems. There was no incidence of sepsis in this series.

In another study, Mehlhoff et al.[22] compared the results of conversion surgery for failed femoral neck and intertrochanteric hip fractures separately. The mean operating time was 143 minutes for the femoral neck fracture groups and 170 minutes for the intertrochanteric hip fracture group. The mean estimated blood loss was 960 mL and 1216 mL, respectively. These were in contrast to a mean operating time of 125 minutes and estimated blood loss of 730 ml in a group of patients undergoing routine primary total hip replacements at the same institution. The overall clinical results were generally satisfactory. Better results were realized in the femoral neck fracture group. Dislocation occurred in none of the femoral neck fracture patients, but did occur in 23% of those who underwent conversion surgery for failed intertrochanteric hip fractures. Franzen et al.[23] reported specifically on the incidence of mechanical failures of conversion total hip replacements done with cement for failed internal fixation of femoral neck fractures in 84 patients at 6 to 12 years follow-up. Revision surgery was necessary in 9 patients: 4 for recurrent dislocation, 2 each for infection and loosening, and 1 for fracture of the stem. There were 42 surviving hips at final follow-up, among whom 6 stems (14.3%) were radiographically loose while none of the cups was loose. Survivorship analysis demonstrated an overall 2.5 times greater risk of failure of the conversion hip replacements than routine primary total hip replacements done at the same institution over the same time interval.

Results of conversion surgery done for failed hemiarthroplasty have been reported to parallel routine revision total hip replacement surgery with similar rates of complications. Dupont and Charnley[24] were among the first to report the clinical results of conversion hip replacements after previous hip surgeries. The series included 217 conversion surgeries. Previous surgeries included 121 femoral osteotomies, 51 endoprostheses, and 45 various other diagnoses, including arthrodesis, pseudoarthrosis, and failed cup arthroplasties. Satisfactory pain relief was achieved in 96% of the 51 conversions for failed endoprostheses. Hip motion was good to excellent in 96% as well. Length of follow-up was not specified. The major complication was infection (3.7%). Most importantly, 23.6% had positive bacterial cultures from the hip joint at the time of conversion surgery. Similarly, Turner and Wroblewski[20] reported infection to be the major problem (3.9%) in their series of 205 conversions for late complications of femoral neck fractures. Forty-five of the procedures were done for previous hemiarthroplasties.

Amstutz and Smith[25] reported the results of 41 conversions using early cementing techniques for failed hemiarthroplasties at a mean follow-up of 3 years. The mean interval between initial hemiarthroplasty and the conversion procedure was 5.5 years. Overall satisfactory clinical results were achieved in nearly all patients. They specifically focused upon the discussion of femoral loosening. Radiographic evidence of suboptimal fixation of the stem was present in 13 (31.7%) cases, with 6 being progressive. They concluded that a previous femoral hemiarthroplasty even without cement could significantly compromise the quality of bone–cement interface at conversion surgery. Sarmiento and Gerard[26] reported another series of 95 conversions following failed hemiarthroplasties. The mean operating time was 2.3 hours, and nearly 2000 mL of blood loss occurred during surgery. Mean follow-up was 2.8 years. Satisfactory clinical results were achieved in over 95% of the patients. Loosening was evident in six (6.3%) stems and one cup. The major complication was dislocation with a 5.5% rate, which was similar to many early reported series of revision total hip replacements done with cement.[27] Improved cementing techniques developed over the past two decades probably would offer better results today.[28]

Stambough et al.[21] reported on a series of 140 conversions with 32 having been done for failure of hemiarthroplasties. The mean follow-up was 8 years with a minimum of 4 years. Loosening of the stems was evident in 22% by radiographic criteria. Loosening of the cups was present in 34%. Revision surgery was necessary in 2 cases (6.3%) in this subgroup. In addition, trochanteric complications occurred in 28.5%. However, overall clinical improvement was consistently satisfactory. Llinas et al.[29] reported results of a series of 120 conversions, with 99 for failed hemiarthroplasties and 21 for failed mold arthroplasties. The mean follow-up was 7.6 years. The results were presented using survivorship analysis. Moreover, these results were compared to those of routine primary total hip replacements. The probability of cup survival was better in the group of conversion surgeries than for primary hip replacements. In contrast, the femoral stems in the conversion group were at significantly greater ($p < 0.001$) risk of cement fracture, cement-bone radiolucencies, and progressive loosening. The overall revision rate was 6%.

Conclusion

Conversion total hip replacements for the failure of either internal fixation of previous hip fractures or hemiarthroplasty can be expected to provide excellent pain relief and improvement of overall function. The technical difficulties are generally few for those failures from previous internal fixation surgeries, especially for femoral neck fractures. In contrast, conversion reconstruction for failure of fixation of intertrochanteric hip fractures can be technically demanding, and can be associated with greater perioperative complications. The technical challenges for conversion surgery done for failure of hemiarthroplasty are similar to routine revision total hip replacement surgery. In general, durability of the conversion total hip replacements has been reported to be inferior to that of uncomplicated total hip replacements Some of the reported data could be due partly to older surgical techniques and selection of implants. Improved results may be expected with current surgical techniques.

Total Hip Replacement Following Previous Femoral Osteotomy

Indications

The advancement of prosthetic arthroplasties over the past three decades has led to a significant decrease in the use of joint-sparing procedures such as proximal femoral osteotomy. The clinical success of well-performed proximal femoral osteotomies, even in properly selected patients, has been estimated to be approximately only 50% at 10 years.[30] Total hip replacement has become an accepted salvage option for patients whose clinical conditions have deteriorated following previous proximal femoral osteotomies. The most common indication for conversion surgery is increasing pain and loss of function. Nonunion of the osteotomy is another indication.

Technique

The technical challenges of total hip replacement in the presence of a previous proximal femoral osteotomy can be formidable due to the distorted anatomy. The complication rate has been reported to be greater than primary surgery.[31,32] Moreover, the clinical results and durability have been less predictable than primary replacements.[31,32,33]

The surgical approach selected is partially determined by the surgeon's preference, and in part by previous surgical incisions. The transtrochanteric approach in general would offer the greatest versatility in reaming and broaching the femoral canal in the presence of deformities, thus minimizing the risks of perforations and fractures.

Preparation of the acetabulum is similar to routine primary surgery. Many of the osteotomies have been performed in patients with dysplasia of the hip. Acetabular dysplasia, therefore, is frequently present. The principles and techniques used in such situations should be followed. The majority of cases can be successfully reconstructed using porous-coated cups inserted without cement. On occasion cups with smaller outer diameters are necessary due to acetabular dysplasia. It may be more appropriate to consider using femoral head components of smaller diameters (such as 22 mm or 26 mm), or using an all-polyethylene cup inserted with cement, in order to maximize the polyethylene thickness.

The major technical challenge lies in the femoral reconstruction in the presence of deformed geometry and previous hardware. Some authors have suggested removing the hardware as a separate procedure prior to conversion total hip replacement.[31] This would allow for healing of any cortical defects from the hardware, which can result as stress-risers with the possible complication of fractures. It is perhaps not necessary if the principles outlined above in the section of conversion surgery for failed internal fixation devices are followed in terms of modification of cementing techniques and implant selection.[17,18]

Similar to what has been described for the case of failed internal fixation of an intertrochanteric fracture, the deformed femoral geometry is often not a significant limitation if cement fixation of the stem is selected. The deformed proximal femur, however, can be a problem for maximizing the fit-and-fill of a cementless stem since most of such designs are straight in geometry. On occasion, a corrective femoral osteotomy may be necessary.[34-38] Various techniques for corrective osteotomy have been described. The general principles are: making the osteotomy at the level of the greatest deformity; correcting both axial and rotational components of the malalignment; removing as little bone as possible in order to minimize shortening; providing secure fixation of the osteotomy; and selecting a stem design that is sufficiently long to bypass the osteotomy to prevent periprosthetic fractures.

Custom-designed stems can be used in some cases, although they are not routinely necessary, especially if corrective osteotomy is performed as a part of the conversion total hip replacement. The limitation of any custom-designed stem is that only one size is manufactured. Moreover, the instrumentation used to prepare the canal for the custom-designed stem may be limited as well. Another option is to use modular designs such as the S-ROM system (Johnson & Johnson, Rayhnam, MA), which offers the versatility of separately maximizing proximal and distal fit of the femoral canal. This may allow for adequate femoral reconstruction without a corrective osteotomy. Regardless of which stem design is selected, attention must be given to restoring leg length, abductor offset, and soft-tissue tension.

Techniques for Femoral Osteotomy

Optimal fit and subsequent successful biologic stabilization of the femoral component can be greatly compromised in situations such as angular deformities in hip dysplasia, revision surgery, previous peritrochanteric osteotomies, malunion of previous proximal femoral di-

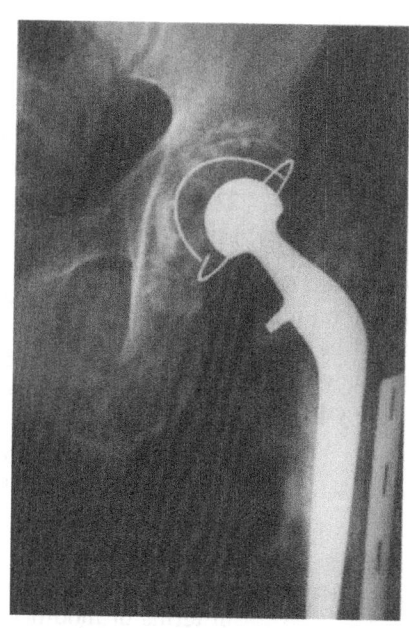
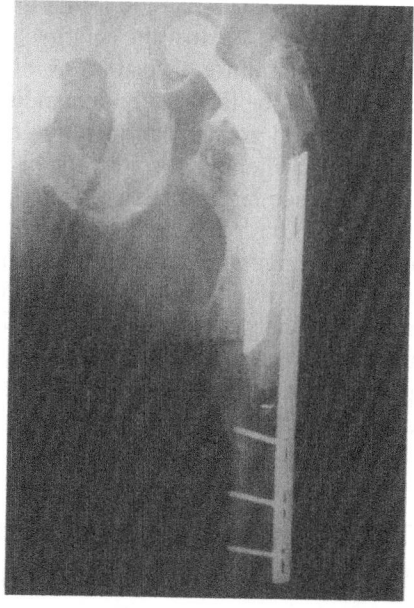
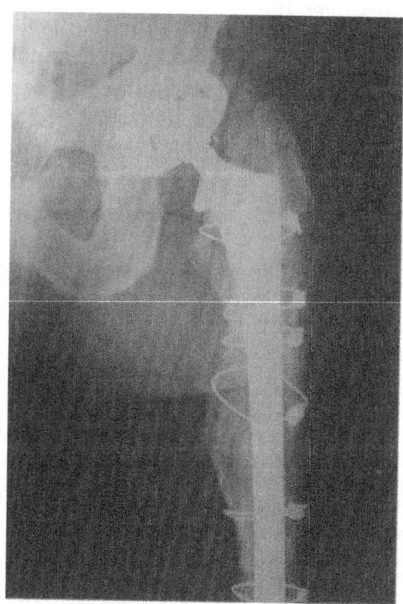
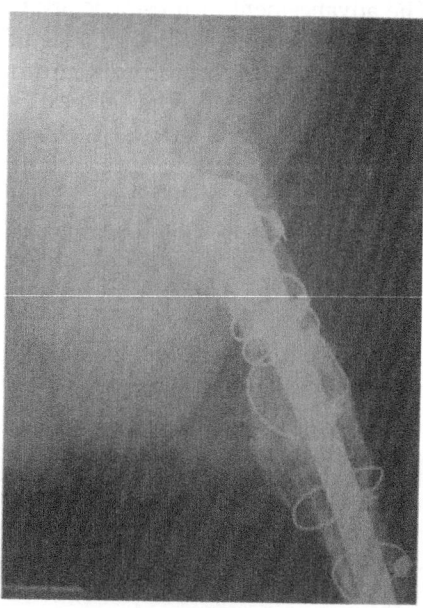

Figure 63.2. A. Anterior-posterior radiograph demonstrating loosening of both components along with significant osteolysis in femoral zones 5 and 7. B. Anterior-posterior radiograph of the femur demonstrating the presence of a previous plate used for fixation of the femur fracture 20 years prior. C. Anterior-posterior radiograph demonstrating revision hip replacement performed using the extended femoral osteotomy technique with long-stem extensively porous-coated stem. The osteotomy has healed completely, and fixation of the stem has remained stable. D. Lateral radiograph of the femur demonstrating healed osteotomy. Note also regression of the osteolysis lesions that were not grafted at the time of revision surgery. The osteotomy perhaps allowed for thorough debridement of the lesions, and the healing process of the ostetomy may have contributed to the observed regression of these lesions.

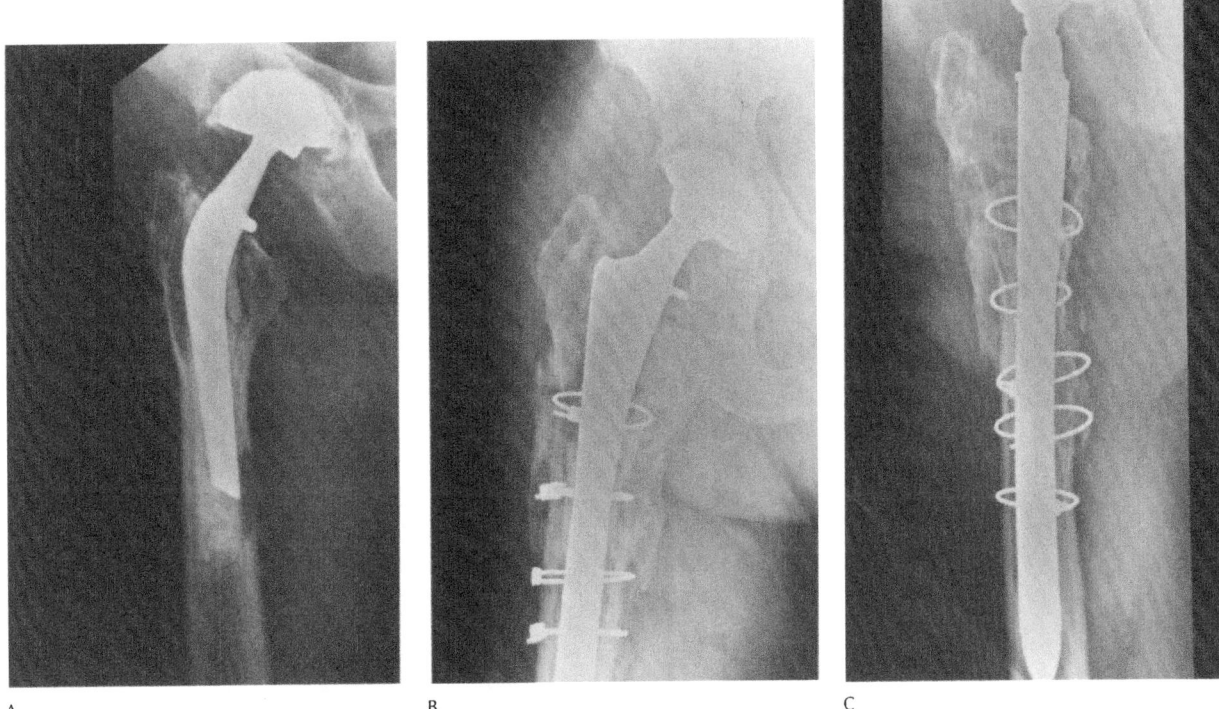

Figure 63.3. A. Anterior-posterior radiograph demonstrating significant femoral osteolysis with loosening of the components. B. Anterior-posterior radiograph demonstrating a stable fixation at one year following revision surgery using the extended femoral osteotomy, and a long-stem prosthesis with extensive porous coating. The osteotomy has healed completely with improved bone stock in the proximal femur. C. Lateral radiograph of the reconstruction.

aphyseal fractures, cortical defects from previous surgery or created during surgery, or retained bone cement in revision situations. Occasionally realignment of the proximal femur is necessary to optimize fit and stability of the femoral prosthesis.

Two specific reported surgical techniques will be discussed in this section. The first technique involves the use of an *oblique femoral osteotomy* described by Huo et al.[37] The proposed advantages of an oblique osteotomy include: (1) ease to perform; (2) presence of extensive cortical contact between the fragments, thus providing theoretically greater rotational stability than a transverse or wedge-shaped osteotomy; and (3) reported good clinical efficacy in a series of 26 hips.[37] The original technique was developed with the use of a modified anterior surgical approach to the hip.[39] This technique can also be easily applied using either the posterior or anterolateral surgical approach. Trochanteric osteotomy is not recommended in conjunction with this technique.

The level of the osteotomy is determined by assessing the preoperative radiographs. It should always be at the apex of the greatest deformity in those cases with distorted anatomy. In selected cases with a fractured stem and thinned distal cortex, the osteotomy is generally performed at zone 4 of the femur. The direction of the osteotomy is determined by the deformity and the curvature of the femur. In most cases, the osteotomy is performed from a superolateral toward an inferomedial direction (Fig. 63.4). Muscle attachment was left intact on the cut fragments as much as possible to preserve vascular supply for healing. Once the osteotomy has been completed, the femoral canal is widely accessible for cement or stem removal in revision situations. Reaming of the canal can then be done in a retrograde and antegrade fashion through the osteotomy, similar to open femoral rodding techniques. The fragments are then reduced with multiple 16-gauge cobalt-chromium wires in a cerclage fashion. Provisional stabilization of the osteotomy is further supplemented with bone clamps. The proximal metaphysis is then sequentially broached using proper instrumentation. The selected femoral stem is impacted into the canal, and the wires are tightened to their final tension to securely fix the osteotomy. Bone grafting using either autograft from the resected femoral head in primary surgery cases, or al-

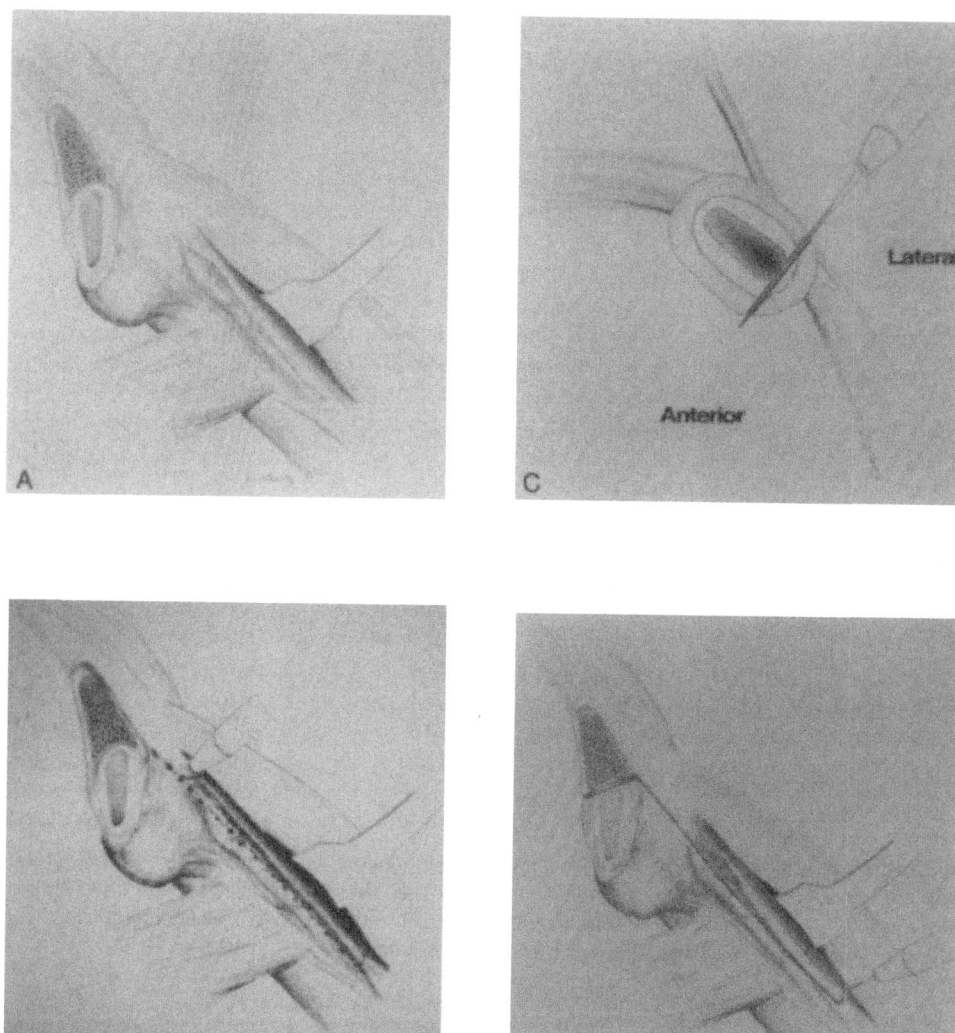

Figure 63.4. Surgical technique of the extended proximal femoral osteotomy. A. Posterolateral view of the femur, with the anterior retractor holding the vastus lateralis anteriorly and the soft tissue dissected off the linea aspera. B. The posterior extent of the osteotomy is marked with multiple perforations with the pencil burr. C. Cross-section of the proximal femur. The pencil burr is being directed from posterolateral to anterolateral to perforate the anterior cortex. This allows the osteotomy to involve the posterolateral one third of the proximal femur. D. The posterior osteotomy line is completed by connecting the multiple perforation sites posteriorly. The distal extent is then completed with the pencil burr as shown. The proximoanterior cortex osteotomy has been completed with an oscillating saw in the region of the trochanter. E. The wide osteotomes are then passed from posterior to anterior to crack open the anterior cortex through the previously made perforations. The osteotomy is then levered open with the osteotomes, as a single unit, to prevent cracking of the fragment. F. The osteotomy fragment is retracted anteriorly. The proximal cement mantle is now easily removed with an offset osteotome as shown. An alternative is to use a high-speed barrel burr. Note the cerclage wire distally to protect the intact femur. G. The osteotomy allows direct access to the distal cement plug. The drill can now be placed through the center of the plug on both the anteroposterior and lateral views, decreasing the risk of cortical perforation. The plug is removed in 1- to 2-cm segments by drilling, then removing with a tap. H. The osteotomy allows direct canal access for placement of the extensively porous-coated femoral prosthesis. Again note the cerclage wire distal to the osteotomy to protect the intact femur. I. The osteotomy fragment is shaped to allow intimate contact with the femoral prosthesis. The fragment is held in place with multiple cables, which also allows some collapsing of the proximal femur around the prosthesis. (Reprinted by permission of *The Journal of Arthroplasty*, Vol. 10, No. 3, June 1995, pp. 332–333.)

63. Prior Surgeries

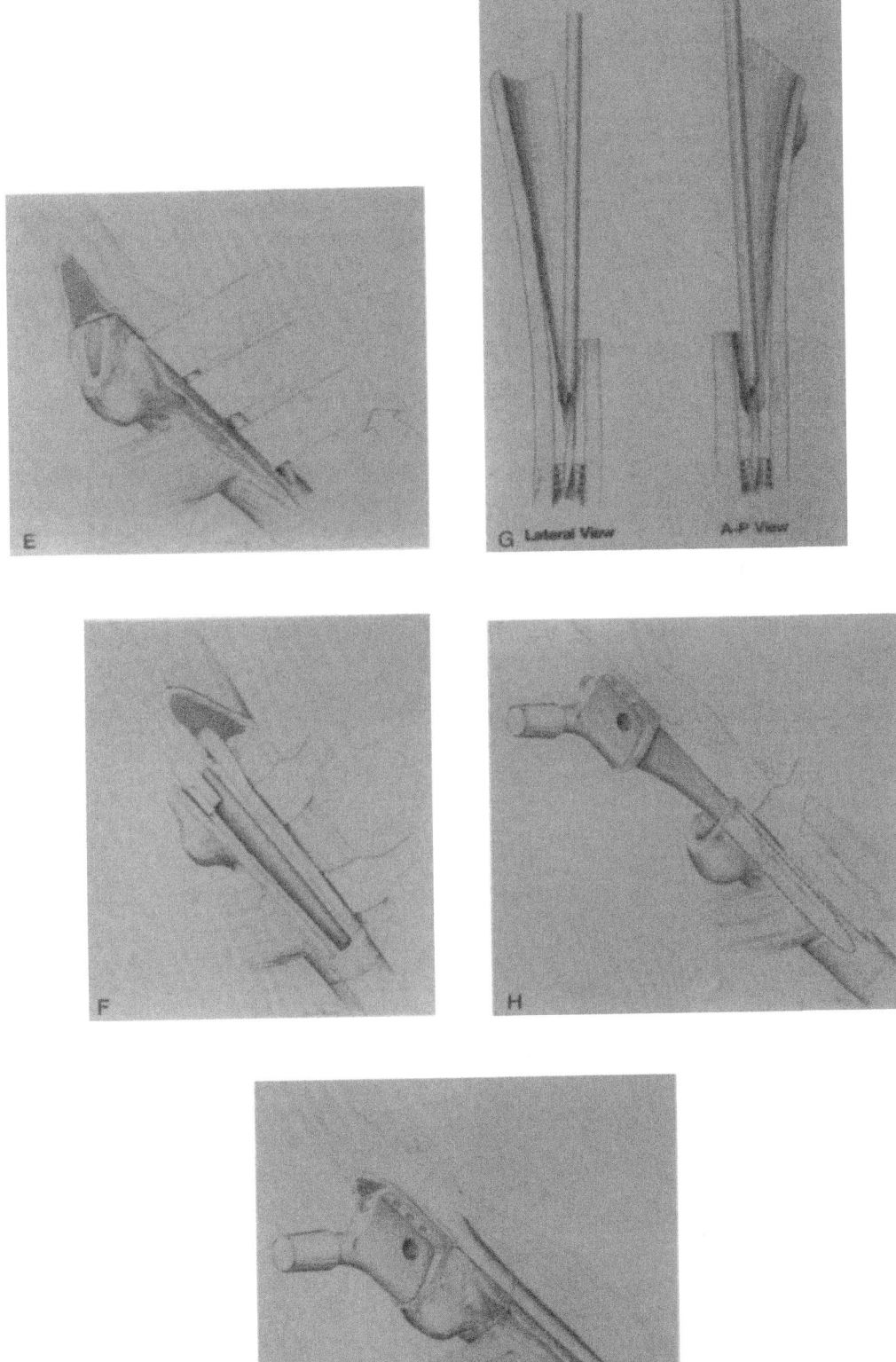

Figure 63.4. Continued.

lograft in revision cases, can then be done around the osteotomy to enhance healing.

Huo et al. reported the results of using this surgical technique in 26 cases.[37] The mean operation time was 182 minutes with a mean estimated blood loss of 700 mL. The mean proximal level of the osteotomy was at 41 mm below the lesser trochanter, with a mean length of the osteotomy of 96 mm. The mean follow-up was 49 months with a minimum of 3 years. One nonunion of the osteotomy occurred and revision surgery was done at 44 months after the index procedure. Failure occurred in 3 hips due to stem loosening. Good to excellent clinical results were observed in 81% of the surviving hips. There was no incidence of significant shortening, axial or rotational malalignment of the osteotomy, or leg length inequality.

The second technique involves the use of an *extended proximal femoral osteotomy* originally proposed by Paprosky.[40] This technique was developed primarily to address the technical challenges of revision total hip replacement, in particular removal of distally fixed cemented and cementless femoral components. The advantages of this technique include: (1) wide exposure of the femoral canal, (2) preservation of soft tissue attachment to the proximal femur, (3) minimization of the risk of placing the stem in varus position, and (4) allowance of the bony fragments to conform to the stem inserted to provide maximal contact with the surface of the prosthesis for stability and biologic fixation (Fig. 63.2).

The original surgical technique was developed using the posterior surgical approach. It has also bee applied using the anterolateral surgical approach. The osteotomy can be performed before or after hip dislocation. It can also be performed before or after removal of the original stem. The vastus lateralis muscle is dissected along its posterior border at the linea aspera and is retracted anteriorly. Multiple perforations are made using high-speed burr to mark the extend of the osteotomy along the posterior 1/3 of the proximal femur. These holes are then connected once the osteotomy is outlined. The osteotomized fragment has the majority of the vastus lateralis still attached to it, and is retracted anteriorly to expose the entire lateral aspect of the femoral canal. Preservation of soft tissue attachments to the fragments would better allow for healing of the osteotomy, and restoration of bone stock (Fig. 63.3). Preparation of the canal can then be done using standard surgical techniques based upon the implant system selected. Shaping of the osteotomy fragment can be done in some cases to allow for maximal intimate contact with the new stem after reduction and fixation using either multiple wires or cables (Fig. 63.4). This in some cases can even be thought of as "closure osteotomy," especially in cases where the proximal femur has become patulous from the loosening process. This would maximize initial fixation of the new stem, thus allowing for successful biologic stabilization.

Younger et al. reported overall uniform successful clinical outcome in a series of 20 cases.[40] The mean length of the osteotomy was 165 mm (range 80 to 160 mm). The mean follow-up was relatively short at 18 months. Subsidence of the stem less than 2 mm was observed in 2 hips. No revision was necessary during the follow-up period.

The authors for both studies recommended protected weight-bearing for 8 to 12 weeks to allow for stabilization of the osteotomy. One of the most commonly encountered perioperative complications was dislocation, which reflected the extensive nature of the procedures.

Results

Total hip replacements done for the failure of proximal femoral osteotomy have in general been reported to involve longer operating time and more blood loss than primary surgery. Ferguson et al.[31] reported on the experience with a large series of 215 conversion surgeries for failed femoral osteotomies. The mean operating time was 171 minutes, mean estimated blood loss was 1340 mL, and the mean blood transfusion requirement was 3.3 units. Moreover, the mean hospital stay was 17 days for that series. Similarly, Souminen et al.[32] reported mean operating time of 142 minutes, and a mean estimated blood loss of 1680 mL in a series of 42 hip replacements following previous femoral osteotomies.

Dupont and Charnley[24] first reported on 121 hip replacements for failed femoral osteotomies. Clinically satisfactory results were achieved in 87% of the patients at short-term follow-up. Benke et al.[41] reported on 105 hip replacements for failed femoral osteotomies. Overall clinical success was 82%. There were, however, an infection rate of 8.6% and a complication rate of 17% due to technical difficulties. Soballe et al.[33] reported on 112 hip replacements for failed osteotomies, and compared the results to a series of routine primary total hip replacements. Mean follow-up was 4.7 years. Satisfactory results were maintained in nearly 90% of the patients. There was no difference when compared to the routine hip replacement patients. In fact, there was less malpositioning of the stem and fewer mechanical failures in the conversion group. There were 6 (5.4%) fractures in the conversion group, with 4 involving the greater trochanter and only 2 involving the femoral shaft. They reported no incidence of infection. Nagi and Dhillon[42] reported 93% clinical success in 15 cases of hip replacements for failed McMurray femoral osteotomy. There was no deep infection, but superficial infection occurred in 2 (13.3%) cases. Radiographic loosening of either component however was evident in 27% at a mean follow-up of 5.3 years.

The success and durability of total hip replacements after femoral osteotomies have not been confirmed by other studies, especially with longer follow-up. Ferguson et al.[31] reported the results at a mean follow-up of 10 years. There were technical problems at surgery in 23%, with a total perioperative complication rate of 11.8%. Deep infection occurred in 2.3%, and trochanteric nonunion occurred in 6.7%, both of which were higher than the incidences for routine primary total hip replacements done at the same institution over the study period. More importantly, 18.1% of the hips required revision, with a rate of 14.9% for aseptic failures. Moreover, radiographic loosening was evident in 30.9% of the stems and 19.8% of the cups at final follow-up. Survivorship analysis further demonstrated 20.6% probability of failure of the hip replacement at 10 years, and 33% failure probability at 15 years. Shinar and Harris (personal communication) recently reported the long-term follow-up results of 19 cemented total hip replacements following proximal femoral osteotomies. The mean follow-up was 15.5 years. Second-generation cementing techniques were used in all cases. Revision for aseptic loosening was 10.5%, with additional 10.5% rate of radiographic loosening. The overall mechanical failure rate for the stem was therefore 21.2%. The mechanical failure rate for the cups was, however, 47.4%. All 4 hips with mechanical failure of the stem had significant proximal femoral deformity, which could have contributed to the suboptimal fixation.

Conclusion

Total hip replacement surgery for failed femoral osteotomies can be technically challenging. Selection of stem design should be carefully considered to meet the limitations of distorted femoral geometry. Short-term clinical and radiographic results have matched those of routine primary total hip replacements. Medium- to long-term results, however, have been less satisfactory. Two primary modes of failure reported in the literature are loosening and infection. Loosening may be improved with contemporary cementing techniques and prosthetic designs. Infection may be improved with careful preoperative work-up, intraoperative cultures and histology examination of the periarticular tissues, and possibly approaching those cases with suspected sepsis using a two-stage protocol.

Total Hip Replacement Following Previous Fracture of the Acetabulum

Indication

Fractures of the acetabulum are serious and uncommon orthopedic injuries. Many of these fractures may potentially result in late complications including posttraumatic arthritis, osteonecrosis of the femoral head, and chondrolysis, which can all contribute to pain and deterioration of hip function. These complications can occur with or without initial surgical treatment of the fracture. The overall incidence of late degenerative changes of the hip following acetabular fractures in earlier reports has been in the range of 12% to 57%. Even with the advances of using open reduction and internal fixation in treating these fractures, Mayo recently reported an overall incidence of 14% posttraumatic arthritis of the hip in 163 acetabular fractures treated by contemporary open reduction techniques.[43]

Total hip replacement can be used as a salvage option for the failure of previous internal fixation of fractures of the acetabulum. There have been only a few reported series in the literature.[44-46] Application of this treatment option in this particular clinical setting is expected to increase with increasing age of the patients with this injury, and increased use of surgical treatment for fractures of the acetabulum over the past two decades (Fig. 63.5).

Techniques

The major technical challenge in performing hip replacement surgery in patients with previous fractures of the acetabulum is in the acetabular reconstruction. However, on occasion, there could have been associated fractures of the proximal femur or subsequent proximal femoral osteotomy done for salvage purpose, thus creating similar types of anatomical technical problems as have been previously described in this chapter.

The surgical approach should be determined by the surgeon's preference and by the previous incision(s). In general, trochanteric osteotomy offers the greatest exposure of both the anterior and posterior columns of the acetabulum. It also offers the advantage of restoring soft-tissue tension and improving the offset for the abductors by distal and lateral advancement of the trochanter during reattachment. Moreover, the transtrochanteric approach also allows for resection of any periacetabular heterotopic bone that has formed from the previous surgery.

Hardware from previous surgery should be removed whenever possible. The most frequently used hardware for internal fixation of fractures of the acetabulum are the standard implants from the AO group, which are made of stainless steel. These implants can in theory pose a problem of galvanic corrosion, especially if a cup made of titanium alloy is inserted. The hardware may present as an obstacle for proper reaming of the acetabulum, and may prevent full seating of the cup. In some cases, complete removal of all the hardware may not be necessary if it does not prevent proper reconstruction of the acetabulum and seating of the cup. In some cases, the surgical dissection necessary to remove

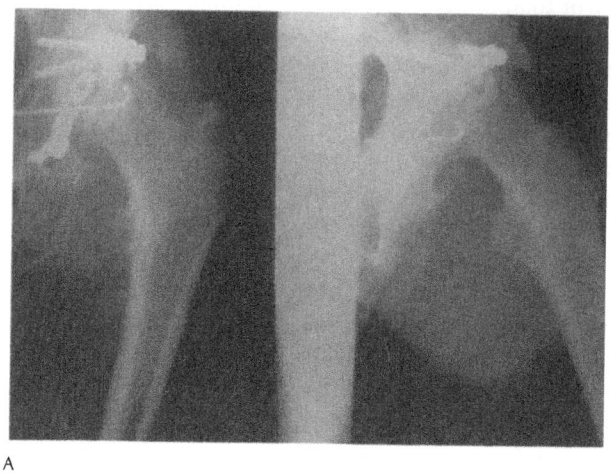
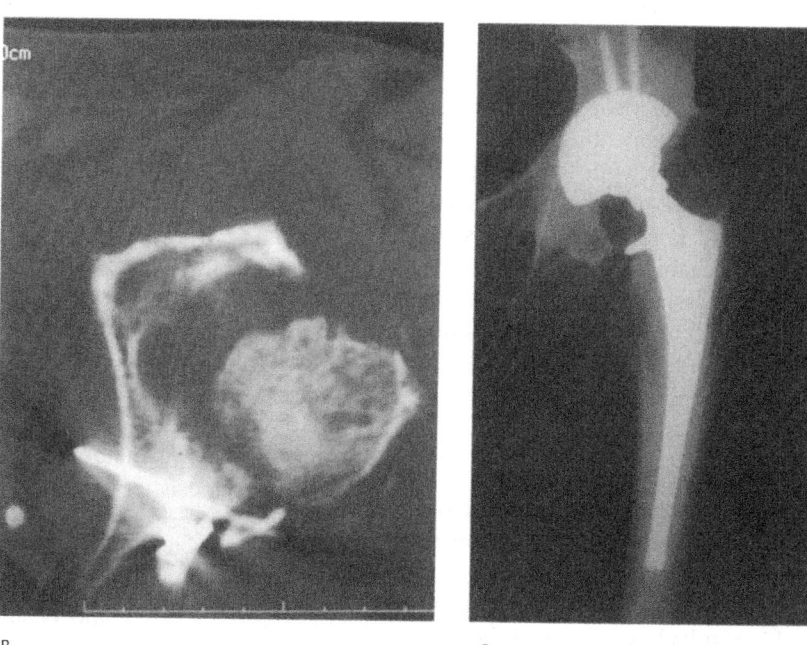

Figure 63.5. A. Anterior-posterior and lateral radiographs of the hip demonstrating proximal subluxation of the femoral head following attempted open reduction and internal fixation of an acetabular fracture. B. Axial computerized tomography scan demonstrating subluxation of the femoral head with hardware in the posterior wall. C. Anterior-posterior radiograph demonstrating conversion hip replacement using hybrid fixation at 5 years of follow-up.

all the hardware may be so extensive that it may significantly lengthen the operating time and blood loss. Therefore, the surgeon must assess each case individually and accordingly.

The acetabular fossa is often distorted and is very sclerotic. The same principles of acetabular reconstruction for routine hip replacement surgery should be followed. The goal is to prepare the fossa to allow for placement of the cup as inferiorly and medially as possible. On occasion, the medial wall may require bone grafting for protrusio deformity. Such grafting can be done using autograft from the resected femoral head. Similarly,

any other contained cystic defects can be addressed with morselized autograft. In some cases, the posterior wall and column may be deficient from the original injury and surgery. Structural bone allograft along with pelvic reconstruction plates may be needed to restore the bone stock of the posterior column in order to achieve adequate fixation of the acetabular cup. Hemispherical cups with porous coating can generally be used, especially if inserted with adjunct screws. For cases that require major structural segmental allograft bone supplementation, a cup inserted with cement may occasionally be preferred. An acetabular reinforcement ring or antiprotrusio cage may even be necessary as adjunct measures to acetabular reconstruction (Fig. 63.6). Femoral reconstruction is usually similar to routine primary surgery. Care should be taken to ensure increased femoral offset to minimize impingement and dislocation after surgery.

Results

In general, the clinical outcome of hip replacements done in patients with previous fractures of the acetabulum has been reported to be satisfactory. The major limitation observed in these few series has been the durability of fixation of the prostheses, in particular fixation of the cup. Romness and Lewallen[46] reported the data of hip replacements done with cement following fractures of the acetabulum. The revision rate for the stem was similar to that for a matched group of primary total hip replacements done for osteoarthritis at the same institution. On the contrary, the revision and loosening rates for the cups were fourfold higher than those in the osteoarthritis patients. Their data demonstrated cup revision rate of 14%, and loosening rate of 49% at medium-term follow-up. One of the major risk factors identified by Romness and Lewallen was young age in patients in whom revision or loosening were observed.

Karpos and Christie[47] reported the results of 15 hip replacements done without cement following fractures of the acetabulum. Morselized bone graft was used in 47%, while structural bone graft was necessary in 40% of the cases. All cups were semispherical with porous coating, and were inserted with supplemental screws.

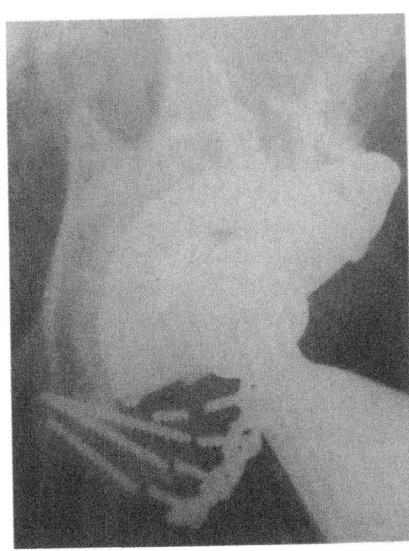

Figure 63.6. Anterior-posterior radiograph of the hip demonstrating reconstruction of the acetabulum with pelvic reinforcement cage along with retention of the previous hardware.

The mean follow-up was 68 months. There was one cup revision for malpositioning and recurrent dislocations. Possible radiographic cup loosening was observed in 27% of the hips. Huo et al.[48] recently reported the results of 21 hip replacements done without cement in patients with previous fractures of the acetabulum. Previous surgery was done in only 7 cases. The mean follow-up was 58 months (range 36 to 100 months). Good to excellent clinical results were achieved and maintained in 95% of the patients. There has been no cup revision. Radiographic cup loosening was observed in 4 hips (19%). All 4 cups that were judged to be loose in that series were of the Mittelmeier design, a smooth, truncated, and macro-threaded design. None of the cups with a hemispherical design and porous-coating was loose. Radiographic evaluation demonstrated high placement of the reconstructed hip center in 4 hips. Lateral placement of the hip center was evident in 7 hips. These findings reflected the distorted anatomy of the acetabulum. There was, however, no correlation between suboptimal placement of the cups and the patterns or treatments of the initial acetabular fracture. Moreover, there was no correlation between suboptimal placement of the cups and the incidence of cup loosening. Morselized autograft from the resected femoral head was used in 6 hips (28%).

One stem in this series was revised for periprosthetic femur fracture from a fall 6 months following the index surgery. Five additional stems were judged to be radiographically loose among the remaining 20 hips. Four of these stems offered no porous coating. In contrast, stable stem fixation was observed in 94% of the stems with porous coating surface texture. There was no case of osteolysis observed in the pelvis, whereas 2 cases of femoral osteolysis was seen at 87 and 64 months of follow-up, respectively.

Conclusion

Total hip replacement in patients with previous fractures of the acetabulum can be technically challenging due to the deformed anatomy, retained hardware, sclerotic acetabular subchondral bone, presence of heterotopic bone, and distorted soft tissues. Clinical outcome has generally been successful. Durability of fixation of the prostheses has been the major limitation in this patient population at medium-term follow-up. Cementless fixation of the cup appears to be superior to cement fixation in reported series. Cement fixation of the stem offers similar durability as total hip replacements done in routine osteoarthritic patients. Modern cement techniques should offer even better durability of stem fixation. Cementless fixation for the stem has had similar limited success as in other high-risk patient populations. This has especially been true if nonporous stems are used.

Conclusion

Total hip replacement is an excellent option in the salvage of failure of previous hip surgeries. The technical challenges in most cases are deformed anatomy, distorted soft tissues, deficiency of the bone stock, retained hardwares, and in some cases unrecognized low-grade sepsis from previous surgeries. Selection of mode of fixation of either the cup or the stem should be based on similar criteria as used for routine total hip replacements. Cementless fixation has been shown to be more durable, especially in hips with previous acetabular fractures. Cement fixation of the stem using contemporary techniques can offer excellent durability. Corrective osteotomy of the femur may be necessary in patients with previous femoral osteotomies, especially if cementless fixation is selected for the stem. Selection of a stem with sufficient length to bypass all the potential stress risers should be made to avoid periprosthetic fractures. Excellent short- to medium-term clinical outcome can be expected in majority of the patients following total hip replacement surgery if these fundamental principles are followed.

References

1. Koval KJ, Zuckerman JD. Hip fractures: I. Overview and evaluation and treatment of femoral-neck fractures. *J Am Acad Orthop Surg.* 1994;2:141–149.
2. Koval KJ, Zuckerman JD. Hip fractures: II. Evaluation and treatment of intertrochanteric fractures. *J Am Acad Orthop Surg.* 1994;2:150–156.
3. Lu-Yao GL, Keller RB, Littenberg B, Wennberg JE. Outcomes after displaced fractures of the femoral neck. A meta-analysis of one hundred and six published reports. *J Bone Joint Surg Am.* 1994;76:15–25.
4. Asnis SE, Wanek-Sgaglione L. Intracapsular fractures of the femoral neck. Results of cannulated screw fixation. *J Bone Joint Surg Am.* 1994;76:1793–1803.
5. Bateman JE, Berenji AR, Bayne O, Greyson ND. Long-term results of bipolar arthroplasty in osteoarthritis of the hip. *Clin Orthop.* 1990;251:54–66.
6. McConville OR, Bowman AJ Jr, Kilfoyle RM, McConville JF, Mayo RA. Bipolar hemiarthroplasty in degenerative arthritis of the hip: 100 consecutive cases. *Clin Orthop.* 1990;251:67–74.
7. Prieskorn D, Burton P, Page BJ 2d, Swienckoski J. Bipolar hemiarthroplasty for primary osteoarthritis of the hip. *Orthopedics.* 1994;17:1105–1111.
8. Brien WW, Bruce WJ, Salvati EA, Wilson PD Jr, Pellicci PM. Acetabular reconstruction with a bipolar prosthesis and morseled bone grafts. *J Bone Joint Surg Am.* 1990;72:1230–1235.
9. Nilson LT, Stromqvist BN, Thorngren KG. Secondary arthroplasty for complications of femoral neck fracture. *J Bone Joint Surg Br.* 1989;71:777–781.
10. Dalldorf PG, Banas MP, Hicks DG, Pellegrini VD Jr. Rate of degeneration of human acetabular cartilage after hemiarthroplasty. *J Bone Joint Surg Am.* 1995;77:877–882.
11. Vazquez-Vela E, Vazquez-Vela G. Acetabular reaction to the Bateman bipolar prosthesis. *Clin Orthop.* 1990;251:87–91.
12. Barmada R, Mess D. Bateman hemiarthroplasty component disassembly. A report of three cases of high-density polyethylene failure. *Clin Orthop.* 1987;224:147–149.
13. Messieh M, Mattingly DA, Turner RH, Scott R, Fox J, Slater J. Wear debris from bipolar femoral neck-cup impingement. A cause of femoral stem loosening. *J Arthroplasty.* 1994;9:89–93.
14. Whittaker RP, Abeshaus MM, Scholl HW, Chung SM. Fifteen years' experience with metallic endoprosthetic replacement of the femoral head for femoral neck fractures. *J Trauma.* 1972;12:799–806.
15. Kofod H, Kofod J. Moore prosthesis in the treatment of fresh femoral neck fractures. A critical review with special attention to secondary acetabular degeneration. *Injury.* 1983;14:531–540.
16. Moran MC. A technique for removal of cannulated screws with buried heads from the femoral neck in the course of total hip replacement. *J Bone Joint Surg Am.* 1992;74:1245–1246.
17. Patterson BM, Salvati EA, Huo MH: Total hip arthroplasty for complications of intertrochanteric fracture. A technical note. *J Bone Joint Surg Am.* 1990;72:776–777.
18. Panjabi MM, Trumble T, Hult JE, Southwick WO. Effect of femoral stem length on stress raisers associated with revision hip arthroplasty. *J Orthop Res.* 1985;3:447–455.
19. Eschenroeder HC Jr, Krackow KA. Late onset femoral stress fracture associated with extruded cement following hip arthroplasty. *Clin Orthop.* 1988;236:210–213.
20. Turner A, Wroblewski BM. Charnley low-friction arthroplasty for the treatment of hips with late complications of femoral neck fractures. *Clin Orthop.* 1984;185:126–130.
21. Stambough JL, Balderston RA, Booth RE Jr, Rothman RH, Cohn JC. Conversion total hip replacement. Review of 140 hips with greater than 6-year follow-up study. *J Arthroplasty.* 1986;1:261–269.
22. Mehlhoff T, Landon GC, Tullos HS. Total hip arthroplasty following failed internal fixation of hip fractures. *Clin Orthop.* 1991;269:32–37.
23. Franzen H, Nilsson LT, Stromqvist B, Johnsson R, Herrlin K. Secondary total hip replacement after fractures of the femoral neck. *J Bone Joint Surg Br.* 1990;72:784–787.
24. Dupont JA, Charnley J. Low-friction arthroplasty of the hip for the failures of previous operations. *J Bone Joint Surg Br.* 1972;54:77–87.
25. Amstutz HC, Smith RK. Total hip replacement following failed femoral hemiarthroplasty. *J Bone Joint Surg Am.* 1979;61:1161–1166.
26. Sarmiento A, Gerard FM. Total hip arthroplasty for failed endoprostheses. *Clin Orthop.* 1978;137:112–117.
27. Callaghan JJ. Results and experiences with cemented revision total hip arthroplasty. *Inst Course Lect.* 1991;40:185–187.
28. Estok DM 2d, Harris WH. Long-term results of cemented femoral revision surgery using second generation techniques. An average 11.7-year follow-up evaluation. *Clin Orthop.* 1994;299:190–202.
29. Llinas A, Sarmiento A, Ebramzadeh E, Gogan WJ, McKellop HA. Total hip replacement after failed hemi-

arthroplasty or mould arthroplasty. Comparison of results with those of primary replacements. *J Bone Joint Surg Br.* 1991;73:902–907.
30. Miegel RE, Harris WH. Medial-displacement intertrochanteric osteotomy in the treatment of osteoarthritis of the hip. *J Bone Joint Surg Am.* 1984;66:878–887.
31. Ferguson GM, Cabanella ME, Ilstrup DM. Total hip arthroplasty after failed intertrochanteric osteotomy. *J Bone Joint Surg Br.* 1994;76:252–257.
32. Suominen S, Antti-Poika I, Santavirta S, Konttinen YT, Honkanen V, Lindholm TS. Total hip replacement after intertrochanteric osteotomy. *Orthopedics.* 1991;14:253–257.
33. Soballe K, Boll KL, Kofod S, Severinsen B, Kristensen SS. Total hip replacement after medial-displacement osteotomy of the proximal part of the femur. *J Bone Joint Surg Am.* 1989;71:692–697.
34. DeCoster TA, Incavo S, Frymoyer JW, Howe J. Hip arthroplasty after biplanar femoral osteotomy. *J Arthroplasty.* 1989;4:79–86.
35. Glassman AH, Engh CA, Bobyn JD. Proximal femoral osteotomy as an adjunct in cementless revision total hip arthroplasty. *J Arthroplasty.* 1987;2:47–63.
36. Holtgrewe JL, Hungerford DS: Primary and revision total hip replacement without cement and with associated femoral osteotomy. *J Bone Joint Surg Am.* 1989;71:1487–1495.
37. Huo MH, Zatorski LE, Keggi KJ. Oblique femoral osteotomy in cementless total hip arthroplasty. Prospective consecutive series with a 3-year minimum follow-up period. *J Arthroplasty.* 1995;10:319–327.
38. Paavilainen T, Hoikka V, Solonen KA. Cementless total replacement for severely dysplastic or dislocated hips. *J Bone Joint Surg Br.* 1990;72:205–211.
39. Light TR, Keggi KJ. Anterior approach to hip arthroplasty. *Clin Orthop.* 1980;152:255–260.
40. Younger TI, Bradford MS, Magnus RE, Paparosky WG. Extended proximal femoral osteotomy. A new technique for femoral revision arthroplasty. *J Arthroplasty.* 1995;10:329–338.
41. Benke GJ, Baker AS, Dounis E. Total hip replacement after upper femoral osteotomy. A clinical review. *J Bone Joint Surg Br.* 1982;64:570–571.
42. Nagi ON, Dhillon MS. Total hip arthroplasty after McMurray's osteotomy. *J Arthroplasty.* 1991;6 Suppl:S17–S22.
43. Mayo KA. Open reduction and internal fixation of fractures of the acetabulum. Results in 163 fractures. *Clin Orthop.* 1994;305:31–37.
44. Coventry MB. The treatment of fracture-dislocation of the hip by total hip arthroplasty. *J Bone Joint Surg Am.* 1974;56:1128–1134.
45. Harris WH. Traumatic arthritis of the hip after dislocation and acetabular fractures: treatment by mold arthroplasty. *J Bone Joint Surg Am.* 1969;51:737–755.
46. Romness DW, Lewallen DG. Total hip arthroplasty after fracture of the acetabulum. Longterm results. *J Bone Joint Surg Br.* 1990;72:761–764.
47. Karpos PAG, Christie MJ. THA following acetabular fracture using cementless acetabular components: 4 to 8 year results. Presented at the Annual Meeting of the American Association of Hip and Knee Surgeons. Dallas. October,1995.
48. Huo MH, Solberg BD, Zatorski LE, Keggi KJ. Total hip replacements done without cement after acetabular fractures. A 3- to 8-year follow-up study. *J Arthroplasty.* 1997;12:219–220.

64
Leg Length Inequality Following Total Hip Replacement

José A. Rodriguez and Chitranjan S. Ranawat

Most patients who undergo total hip replacement for arthrosis can expect dramatic improvement in their preoperative hip pain. However, leg length discrepancy following total hip replacement can result in significantly impaired postoperative function and persistent pain. Although surgical techniques for hip replacement continue to improve, leg length discrepancy following total hip replacement remains a source of frustration for patients and surgeons alike.

Early studies that evaluated leg length following hip arthroplasty have demonstrated a notable inconsistency in restoring leg lengths. In 1978, Williamson and Reckling published a study of 144 patients undergoing total hip replacement in whom the average postoperative leg length was 1.6 cm longer, with 27% of patients sufficiently symptomatic to require a contralateral shoe lift.[1] Similarly, in 1983 Rand and Ilstrup reported on a series of hips in which 50% were lengthened by over 1 cm.[2] Turula et al. found an average of 9 mm of lengthening in unilateral cases and 12 mm in bilateral cases. Ten of these patients had discrepancies exceeding 14 mm and a marked limp.[3]

Anatomic Leg Length Inequality

An actual or anatomic leg length inequality exists when the objective lengths of the legs are measurably different. Minor leg length inequality due to anatomic asymmetry is quite common in the general population. Discrepancies of up to 2 cm have been noted in two-thirds of army recruits subjected to routine radiography.[4] Minor developmental length discrepancies such as these are readily compensated for by pelvic tilt.

Post-operative leg length discrepancies are less tolerable if there is lateral decompensation of the spine with a lowering of the pelvis on the short side, often resulting in a short leg limp and a sense of pelvic imbalance (Fig. 64.1). In this way, any limitation in lumbar motion, such as may result from spondylosis, will accentuate this sense of imbalance. In addition, in some studies leg length discrepancy has been associated with low back pain, which may improve with corrective measures.[5,6]

Edeen et al. have reported on a series of patients undergoing total hip replacement in whom the average postoperative actual inequality was 9.7 mm. Thirty-two percent of these patients were aware of the inequality, and over half required a corrective contralateral shoe lift. The magnitude of the discrepancy in this study correlated well with abnormal gait, use of a cane, and the need for a shoe lift.[7]

Techniques of accurate preoperative templating, anatomic component geometry, and intraoperative assessment have diminished the prevalence of inadvertent lengthening of the limb by reproducing the normal anatomical relationships.[8] McGee and Scott described using a bent Steinman pin impacted into the ilium and pointing toward the trochanter as a means to compare intraoperative leg lengths.[9] Woolsen and Harris described a device that is bolted to the ilium, with a preoperative measurement made onto the greater trochanter, which is then compared to the postimplantation measurement.[10] Using this technique along with preoperative templating, Woolsen achieved a postoperative lengthening of <6 mm in 89% of patients undergoing total hip replacement.[11]

Jasty et al. used a similar caliper technique in a consecutive series of 85 primary total hip replacements. Clinical measures as well as scanograms were used to assess leg lengths. Forty-three of the 85 hips were lengthened by 0 to 5 mm, and 40 were lengthened by 5 to 40 mm, while 2 hips were slightly shorter. On postoperative measurement, 11 hips (13%) were clinically longer by more than 5 mm compared to the contralateral side, but only 2 required the use of a contralateral shoe lift.[12]

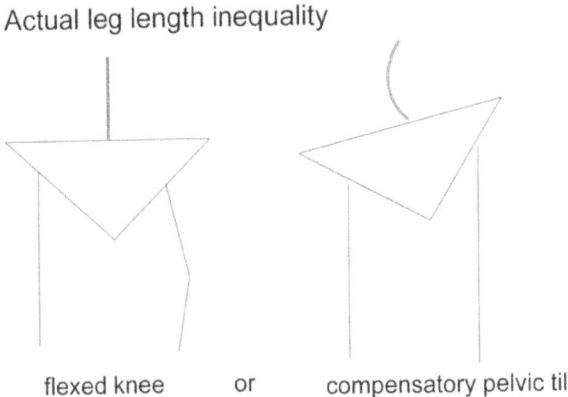

Figure 64.1. Illustration of actual or anatomic leg length inequality.

For many years we have utilized preoperative templating of the distance between the lesser trochanter and the center of rotation of the femoral head on the pelvis radiograph of both hips, and compared these measurements to the intraoperative finding prior to osteotomy of the femoral neck as a guide to reestablishing leg length.[13] Given the loss of cartilage involved in the arthritic process, we generally seek to add 3 to 5 mm to the preoperative length of the leg, in the absence of deformity or excessive soft tissue laxity.

The reproducibility of this technique has been evaluated in a consecutive series of 100 cemented total hip replacements.[14] In this study 72 hips were lengthened by 0 to 5 mm, 20 hips were lengthened by 6 to 10 mm, and 7 were lengthened 11 to 18 mm. Two patients required the use of a contralateral shoe lift due to a sense of imbalance. More recently, we have adopted an additional technique of measuring from a fixed point on the ischial ramus to the greater trochanter using a perpendicular Steinman pin. We are currently studying the reproducibility of this technique.

Functional Leg Length Inequality

A sense of leg length discrepancy after total hip replacement can usually be broken down into two components.[15] The actual or true leg length inequality is caused by lengthening of the prosthetic head–neck distance. The apparent or functional leg length inequality (FLLI) describes the amount that is attributable to other factors, such as the tightness of the anterolateral soft tissues about the hip and/or degenerative disease with scoliosis of the lumbar spine causing obliquity of the pelvis.

The incidence and causes of functional leg length inequality are not well described. Most surgeons perform total hip replacement with a goal of reestablishing leg length and optimizing soft tissue tension around the hip to maximize stability. The soft tissue tension can be considered to have a horizontal and a vertical component, both of which should be reestablished and balanced with hip replacement (Fig. 64.2). In cases in which the horizontal component of the soft tissue tension is exceeded (offset increased), a painful stretching of the contracted anterior and lateral structures may result.

Ireland described the functional leg length inequality in children with pelvic obliquity.[16] Functional leg length inequality after total hip replacement may similarly be caused by degenerative disease of the lumbar spine with structural scoliosis and pelvic tilt. In these cases the limitation in the mobility of the spine makes the patient more sensitive to alterations in the length and kinematics of the hip joint due to their inability to compensate for these changes.

Pelvic obliquity may result from soft tissue tightness in the structures that cross the hip joint, joining the pelvis to the femur. These include the anterior capsule with the capsular insertion of the iliacus muscle, the rectus femoris muscle and its origins, the psoas muscle and tendon, the tensor fascia lata, the gluteus minimus muscle, and the gluteus medius muscle. Pelvic obliquity that results from abduction contracture of the hip will lead to a sense of lengthening on the affected side. Similar lengthening can occur with contralateral adduction contracture without soft tissue contracture on the affected side.[17,18]

Preoperative flexion contracture similarly affects the lordotic position of the pelvis and lumbar spine (Fig. 64.3). This may predispose to functional leg length inequality if the anterior capsule remains tight after reconstruction, thereby limiting abduction and external rotation. Conversely, if the anterior capsule is appropriately released and a flexion contracture persists in the contralateral hip, the pelvis is tilted to the contralateral side, also resulting in a feeling of imbalance.

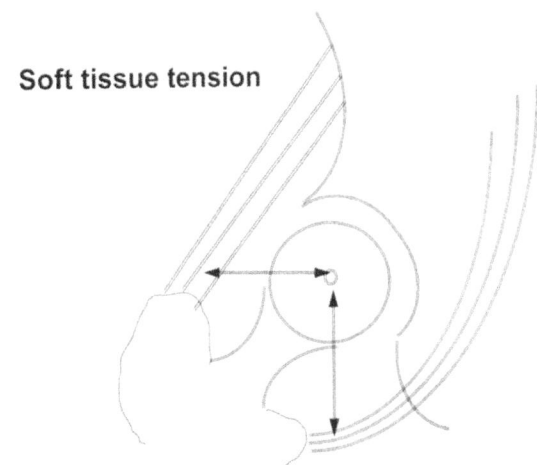

Figure 64.2. Vertical and horizontal components of periarticular soft tissue tension.

The diagnosis of functional limb length inequality is usually apparent when viewing the patient standing. The patient complains of a sense of imbalance and leg lengthening. The pain may be in the groin or laterally in the abductor mechanism. Pain in the lower back or along the iliac crest may also be present. The knee is slightly flexed while the pelvis is tilted downwards on the affected side due to the contracture of the lateral and/or anterior structures. This position differs from that of an actual inequality, where the pelvis is level or tilted away from the affected side (Fig. 64.4). The patient's sensation of inequality will far exceed the radiographic measurements, and the gait appears awkward and painful. Examining the movement of the hip will reveal the abduction or abduction-flexion contracture. The patient is usually quite unhappy.

There are many techniques for measuring leg length inequality, but they all suffer from lack of reproducibility. Since the functional disability associated with leg length inequality is related to the sense of pelvic imbalance, it makes sense to measure the discrepancy in a way that best relieves that sense of imbalance, which is the graduated blocks test. Progressively larger wooden blocks are placed under the shorter leg until a sense of pelvic balance is restored (Fig. 64.5).

In a review of 100 consecutive total hip replacements performed at our center, 14% of cases were noted to have pelvic obliquity 1 month postoperatively.[18] These were usually hips with dysplasia and preoperative shortening (10 hips). All 14 of these patients had gradual resolution of the FLLI between 3 and 6 months postoperatively with stretching exercises. These can be considered transient functional leg length inequalities.

We have noted persistent functional leg length inequality in approximately one in 300 total hip replacements performed at our center. Nine patients have been identified in the last 15 years with persistent functional inequality.[19] Persistent functional leg length inequality

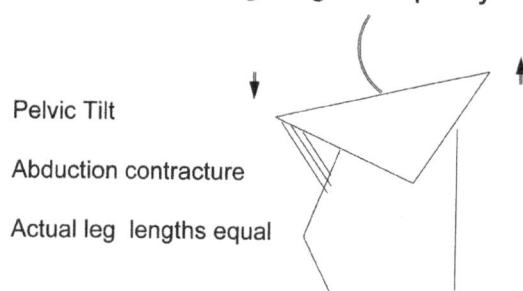

Figure 64.4. Illustration of functional leg length inequality.

is noted following total hip replacement usually in females who are of short stature (less than 5'6"); it is also noted in (1) patients with varus alignment of the femoral neck, with or without flexion contracture, and small bony dimensions or (2) patients with protrusio deformity and flexion contracture with limited range of motion (Fig. 64.6). All of these patients had degenerative spondylosis of the lumbar spine.

Treatment

The treatment of leg length inequality following total hip replacement should be based on the severity of the symptoms that it causes. Anatomic lengthening of up to 5 mm is rarely noticeable. Most patients over 5 feet 6 inches in height can tolerate 5 to 7 mm of leg length inequality without discomfort. The patients in this group who feel unbalanced generally achieve symptomatic relief with the use of a contralateral shoe lift. Inequalities that exceed 10 mm may not achieve symptomatic relief with shoe lift alone, particularly if there is a component of functional leg length inequality as well. In rare instances these patients may fare better with elective prosthetic shortening. In these cases the surgeon should be prepared to perform a trochanteric advancement to improve the soft tissue stability, which may be compromised by prosthetic shortening.

Most patients with functional leg length inequality have gradual improvement in their symptoms with appropriate physical therapy to help stretch the tight soft-tissue structures, and thereby relieve the pelvic obliquity.[1] This type of transient FLLI commonly occurs in dysplastic hips with associated valgus and antetorsion. When the arthritis results in a flexion-abduction contracture, reconstruction with most standard implants will increase the offset of this typically valgus femoral neck (Fig. 64.7). A small increase in the actual length (ie, 5 mm) may produce a significant functional inequality if the soft tissue structures are left too tight. In these patients the sensation of inequality usually resolves in the

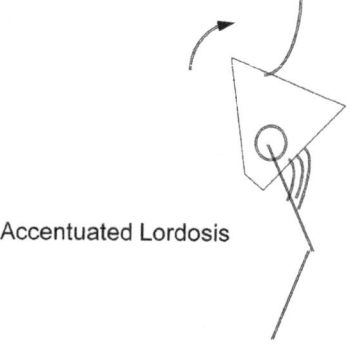

Figure 64.3. Effect of flexion contracture on pelvic imbalance.

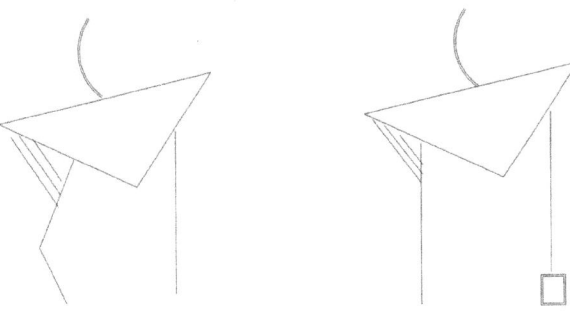

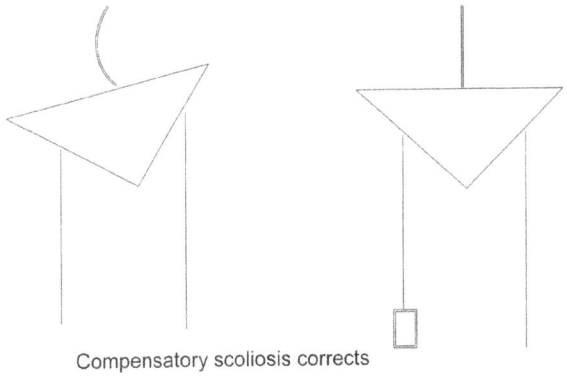

Figure 64.5. A. and B. Effect of shoe lift on anatomic and functional leg length inequality.

months following arthroplasty with appropriate physical therapy.

The exercises we advocate are stretching of the anterior structures by lying prone and hyperextending the lumbar spine and hips by pushing the torso up on the arms. The affected leg can be safely crossed behind the other leg in this extended position with the pelvis held fixed, to further stretch the tight lateral structures of the hip. In addition, standard pelvic tilt exercises, bringing the affected hip into a neutral to slightly adducted position will address the tight lateral structures.

After 4 to 6 months of conservative treatment with physical therapy, one should be able to assess the progress or improvement in the pelvic obliquity. Patients who do not achieve a symptomatic improvement with physical therapy may benefit from surgical release of the tight soft tissue structures. During such an operation, attention should be paid to correct any anatomical inequality that exists.

With an anatomic inequality of less than 5 mm and persistent FLLI, simple soft tissue release should be suf-

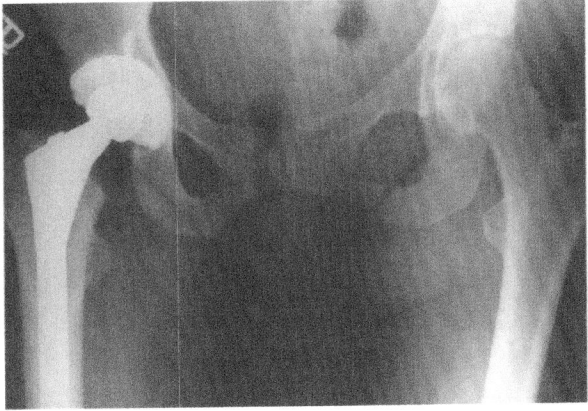

Figure 64.6. Anteroposterior views of the pelvis in a 45-year-old patient with protrusio deformity with inflammatory arthritis associated with a varus femoral neck and a flexion contracture. Postoperatively she had 4 mm of actual leg lengthening, but 14 mm of functional leg lengthening based on pelvic tilt. With physical therapy this has improved partially after 8 months, and she uses a lift of 6 mm in the contralateral shoe.

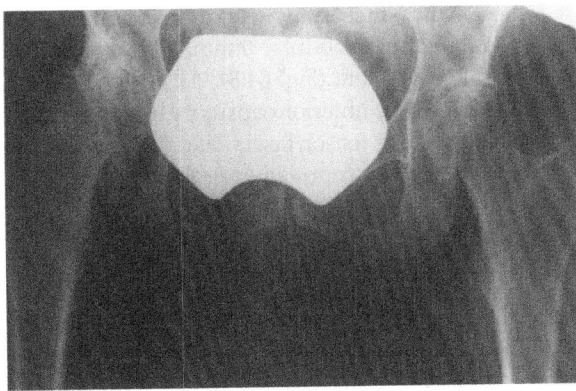

Figure 64.7. Anteroposterior pelvis radiograph of a hip with dysplasia and coxa valga.

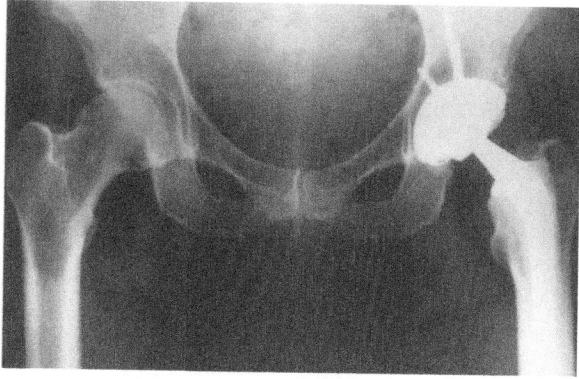

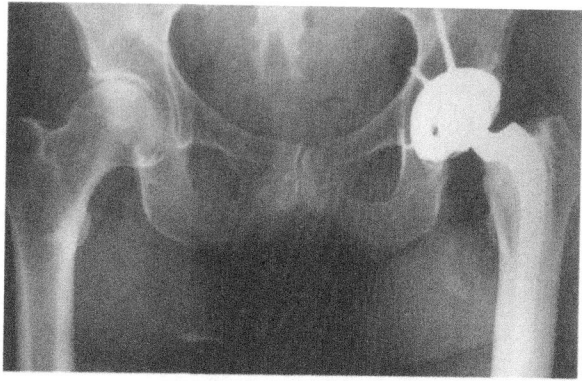

Figure 64.8. A. Anteroposterior views of the pelvis in a 67-year-old woman with persistent functional leg length inequality of 18 mm in the face of an actual leg length inequality of 3 mm and pain associated joint stiffness. B. After circumferential release of the capsule and pericapsular scar tissue, she underwent prosthetic shortening of 5 mm utilizing a custom femoral component. Postoperativley she had complete resolution of her pain and felt well balanced, although her anatomic measurement was 3 to 4 mm shorter on the previously lengthened side.

ficient to improve symptoms. Infrequently, the offset of the femoral component may need to be diminished, either by exchanging a modular femoral head or a different femoral component (Fig. 64.8). All structures about the hip, such as the anterior capsule, gluteus minimus, rectus femoris, and tensor fascia lata, should be tested for tightness and appropriately released.

Technique for Prevention

While performing a primary total hip replacement through a posterior exposure, the surgeon should seek to reproduce the normal anatomy in terms of neck length, offset, and socket position while assuring proper balance of the soft tissue envelope. As noted above, the preoperative length can be marked and compared to the postimplantation length prior to applying the modular head. A small increase in the neck length may help with stability, but every attempt should be made not to increase the leg length by more than 1 to 7 mm.

Once the reconstructed hip is reduced, the soft tissues should be routinely checked for tightness. The tensor fascia lata and rectus femoris muscles can be checked with the Ober test. The gluteus minimus can be directly palpated beneath the medius, and released if necessary. The anterior capsule can be palpated with the hip in full extension and external rotation. If the capsule feels tight, like a cord, or if the hip will not externally rotate enough for the posterior trochanter to come within 1 fingerbreadth from the ischial tuberosity, then surgical release of the anterior capsule is advisable.

Conclusion

Residual leg length inequality following total hip replacement can be a source of profound discomfort and pain. Advances in surgical technique have improved our precision in measuring and reestablishing leg length. Attention should be paid to the tightness of the periarticular soft tissue sleeve intraoperatively, particularly when the anatomy and offset are being altered. Although small increases (5 mm) in leg length are readily tolerated, larger amounts will often produce symptoms, particularly in patients with established spondylosis and degenerative scoliosis.

Many cases of symptomatic leg length inequality will resolve with time, but some will persist. The use of a contralateral shoe lift will successfully address the symptoms of FLLI in most patients. Rarely, additional surgery will be required to address anatomic discrepancies or excessively taut soft tissues. Most importantly, with careful preoperative planning and intraoperative measurement, length inequalities are avoidable in most patients.

References

1. Williamson JA, Reckling FW. Limb length discrepancy and related problems following total hip replacement *Clin Orthop*. 1978;134:135–138.
2. Rand JA, Ilstrup DM. Comparison of Charnley and T-28 total hip arthroplasty. *Clin Orthop*. 1983;180:201–205.
3. Turula KB, Freiberg O, Lindholm TS, et al. Leg length inequality after total hip arthroplasty *Clin Orthop*. 1986;202:163–168.
4. Rush WA, Steiner AJ. A study of lower extremity length inequality. *AJR*. 1956;56:619.
5. Friberg O. Clinical symptoms and biomechanics of lumbar spine and hip joint in leg length inequality. *Spine*. 1983;8:643–651.
6. Tjernstrom B, Rehnberg L. Back pain and arthralgia before

and after leg lengthening. *Acta Orthop Scand.* 1994;65:328–332.
7. Edeen J, Sharkey PF, Alexander H. Clinical significance of leg length inequality after total hip arthroplasty. *Am J Orthop.* 1995;24:347–351.
8. Müller ME. M E Müller straight stem total hip replacement system, Protek Ltd. Manual. Berne, Switzerland, 1982.
9. McGee JMJ, Scott JHS. A simple method of obtaining equal leg length in total hip arthroplasty. *Clin Orthop.* 1985;194:269–270.
10. Woolsen ST, Harris WH. A method of intraoperative limb length measurement in total hip arthroplasty. *Clin Orthop.* 1985;195:207–210.
11. Woolsen ST. Leg length equalization during toal hip replacement. *Orthopedics.* 1990;13:17–21.
12. Jasty M, Webster W, Harris WH. Management of limb length inequality during total hip replacement. *Clin Orthop.* 1995;333:165–171.
13. Ranawat CS. Preoperative planning of total hip arthroplasty. In: Dorr LD, ed. *Revision of total hip and knee.* Baltimore: University Park Press, 1984:1–7.
14. Miyasaka K, Romeo L, Rodriguez JA, Ranawat CS. Cemented total hip replacement, a study of reproducibility. Proceedings of the Closed Meeting of the Hip Society., September 12, 1997, New York.
15. Abraham WD, Dimon JH. Leg length discrepancy in total hip replacement. *Orthop Clin North Am.* 1992;23:201–209.
16. Ireland J, Kessel L. Hip adduction/abduction deformity and apparent leg-length inequality. *Clin Orthop.* 1980;153:156–157.
17. Wagner H. Pelvic tilt and leg length correction *Orthopäde.* 1990;19:273–277.
18. Love BRT, Wright K. Leg length discrepancy after total hip replacement. *J Bone Joint Surg Br.* 1983;65:103–107.
19. Ranawat CS, Rodriguez JA. Functional leg length inequality following total hip replacement. *J Arthroplasty.* 1998;13.

65
Metastatic Disease of the Hip

Stephen M. Horowitz and Arnold T. Berman

It has been reported that 90% of all patients dying of malignancies have skeletal metastases. Of the metastatic lesions, roughly 10% are found in the hip.[1,2] Metastases to bone most frequently arise from breast, prostate, lung, renal, and thyroid carcinomas. The tumor that metastasizes to the hip with the greatest frequency is carcinoma of the breast. An incidence of from 5% to 75% of metastatic lesions of the hip have been reported to have originated from breast tissue.[3-7] Ten percent of patients with disseminated breast cancer, and 1.4% of all breast cancer patients, will ultimately sustain a pathologic fracture of the hip.[7] Approximately 40% of patients with pathologic fractures survive 6 months postfracture, and 30% survive for more than one year.[8] In a recent study, patient survival following surgery for impending or pathologic fractures about the hip ranged from 1 to 42 months, with a median of 7 months and a mean of 12.5 months.[12]

Pathologic fractures or impending pathologic fractures in the region of the hip is a problem that all orthopedic surgeons will encounter during the course of their careers. Breast, lung, prostate, thyroid, and renal carcinoma are the most common primary tumors to metastasize to bone. The spine and pelvis are the sites most often affected, accounting for about 70% of cases. Metastasis to the area of the hip may occur in approximately 10% of all cases.

Evaluation

When it has been established that metastatic disease is present, the patient should be questioned regarding the severity of pain and what activities increase the level of discomfort. Lesions that are small and minimally symptomatic can often be treated with radiation therapy, protected weight-bearing, and careful observation. Questions at the time of the initial evaluation should include the need for assistive devices such as a cane or walker, and the distance the patient can walk before having to stop to rest.

The radiographic evaluation should include plain radiographs that visualize the hip, pelvis, and femur. A recent bone scan is recommended to assess for other areas in the skeleton that may also be at risk for pathologic fractures. A bone scan that shows multiple lesions is also evidence that the lesion in the hip is metastatic and not a new primary. In certain instances, such as with multiple myeloma, the bone scan may not reveal lesions associated with skeletal destruction. In addition, the patient may be too uncomfortable to tolerate lying supine in the nuclear medicine suite while the bone scan is being performed. In those instances, a skeletal survey may be more useful. Further diagnostic studies in the form of a computed tomography scan (CT) or magnetic resonance imaging (MRI) to evaluate the amount of bony destruction in acetabular lesions is also recommended.

Guidelines for internal fixation of impending fractures that have been proposed are based upon the evaluation of plain radiographs.[9] Lesions at significant risk for causing a pathologic fracture are those that (1) are greater than 2.5 cm in diameter, (2) have destroyed 50% of the cortex, or (3) are painful despite treatment with radiation. Added to these guidelines for lesions about the hip include the presence of an avulsion fracture of the lesser trochanter. These are currently the most commonly used criteria for determining which fractures are in need of internal fixation.

Patients who present with lesions that do not meet the criteria for internal fixation should be referred to a radiation oncologist for consideration of radiation therapy. These patients need to be followed by the orthopedic surgeon during and after their radiation treatments. An increase in the amount of bone destruction or a lesion that remains or becomes symptomatic despite radiation may be an indication for operative intervention. In addition, the weight-bearing status of these patients needs to be monitored by the orthopedic surgeon. The majority of these patients need to be partial weight-bearing for at least 6 weeks, and usually until there is evidence that their lesion(s) have healed. If the patient undergoes surgery, the weight-bearing status also has to be carefully monitored by the orthopedic surgeon. Most patients are made partial-weight bearing for a period of at least 6 weeks following the procedure.

If a patient sustains a fracture through a lesion, the treatment is internal fixation or prosthetic replacement similar to that used for impending fractures. If the fracture occurs through a lesion that has been irradiated and the patient has a relatively long projected survival, strong consideration should be given to prosthetic replacement. This is because these patients may have a nonunion of their fracture, and if they survive long enough, they could experience failure of their internal fixation. It is always preferable to fix impending fractures prophylactically so that the patient can avoid the discomfort and morbidity associated with having a pathologic fracture.

Treatment

The use of polymethylmethacrylate cement (PMMA) as an adjunct to internal fixation in cases in which a large amount of bone is lost as a result of metastatic disease around the hip is a technique used by a majority of surgeons. Harrington reported on 375 cases where his technique was to excise the lesion and all inadequate bone stock, then to perform internal fixation or to insert an appropriate prosthetic replacement and reinforce it with PMMA.[9] He claimed a 94% ambulation rate postoperatively and asserted that the presence of the PMMA did not interfere with the rate of union or with radiation therapy.

In the 1970s, Zickel reported on 35 pathological fractures and 11 impending fractures in the subtrochanteric region treated with an intramedullary device.[5] He did not use PMMA and did not attempt tumor excision or perform bone grafting. It was found that those patients with an impending fracture ambulated sooner and survived longer than those who presented with a complete fracture. Operating time and blood loss were not significantly different for the two groups.

In 1980, Lane reported on the use of endoprosthetic replacement, or total hip prostheses, for pathologic fractures or impending fractures of the hip.[7] Impending fractures as determined by the size of the lesion and amount of pain experienced by the patient and a life expectancy of more than one month was an indication for surgical intervention. Good to excellent results were reported with regard to relief of pain in all patients treated with either an Austin-Moore endoprosthesis (cemented or uncemented) or a total hip replacement.

In 1981, Harrington reported on the use of total hip prostheses in patients with acetabular lesions.[10] A number of these patients had lost so much acetabular bone that a conventional prosthesis would not provide sufficient support. Harrington designed a larger acetabular component that would distribute the mechanical load to areas of more uninvolved bone.

Techniques

Prior to surgery, all patients should have a thorough preoperative evaluation that includes radiographs of the hip, pelvis, entire femur, recent bone scan, and also an MRI or CT scan of the pelvis in patients with acetabular lesions.[11] All patients receive preoperative medical clearance and an attempt is made to communicate directly with the patient's medical oncologist. Individuals who have a highly vascular lesion such as metastatic renal carcinoma are treated with arterial embolization prior to surgery to decrease intraoperative blood loss.

Acetabulum

It is recommended that patients with a pathologic fracture or impending fracture of the acetabulum be preoperatively evaluated with an MRI or CT scan so that the extent of bone destruction can be more accurately assessed.[11] Patients with relatively small to moderate amounts of bone destruction can frequently be treated with a protrusio ring alone or in combination with an acetabular cup (Fig. 65.1).

Harrington has subdivided patients with acetabular involvement into four groups based on the location of the lesion, extent of involvement, and the technique required to accomplish the acetabular reconstruction.[10] In class I, the lateral cortices, superior, and medial parts of the acetabulum were structurally intact. These patients were treated by conventional total hip arthroplasty with mesh frequently placed along the medial part of the acetabular wall for reinforcement. In class II, the medial part of the wall was deficient. These patients were treated with a protrusio ring. In class III, the lateral cortices and superior part of the wall were deficient. The patients in this group were treated with steinmann pins directed along the medullary canal of the ilium, in addition to the protrusio ring and acetabular prosthetic component. In class IV, patients who had only a solitary metastasis in the acetabular area underwent an en bloc resection.

In patients who undergo hip replacement with a protrusio cup, postoperative care is similar to that for a hip replacement for nonmetastatic disease.[11] This involves dislocation precautions and partial weight-bearing for 6 weeks postoperatively. In cases of very extensive bone loss, some consideration should be given to treating the patient nonoperatively or with a girdlestone procedure because of the unreliability of internal fixation.

In a recent series, there were no dislocations in patients treated with a protrusio cup. One patient required a second procedure for progression of a lesion proximal in the pelvis.[12]

Some surgeons use morselized allograft to pack the defect left in the acetabulum prior to cementation of the acetabular component. This provides a surface with the potential for healing and restoration of bone, and also

Figure 65.1. A. Lytic lesion in acetabulum. B. Anti-protrusio device placed for lesion in acetabulum. (Illustrations reproduced with permission of Clinical Orthopaedics and Related Research.)

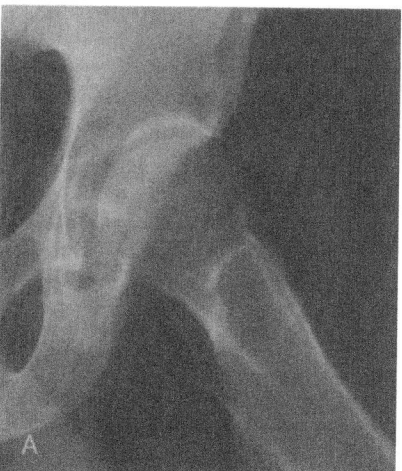
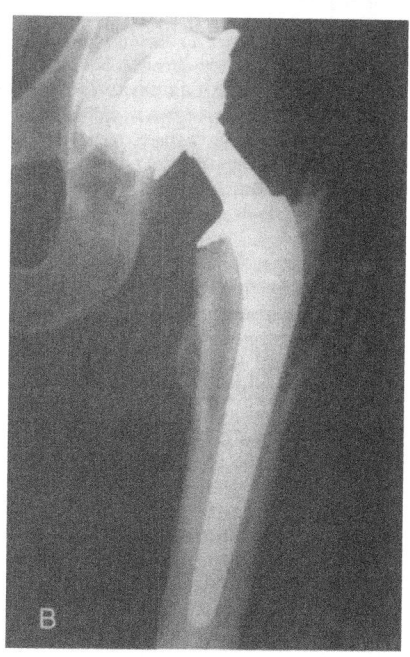

prevents cement extrusion into the pelvis. The role of allograft in treating acetabular defects is not as significant in patients with metastatic disease as it is in patients with arthritis or nonmalignant conditions. This is because the decreased life expectancy in patients with metastatic disease and the use of radiation therapy and chemotherapy make it unlikely that this allograft will ever heal and restore the prior bone architecture.

Femoral Head and Neck

It is recommended by the authors that impending and complete fractures of the femoral head and neck be treated by cemented hemiarthroplasty because progression of these lesions may result in failure of internal fixation. A common error in the treatment of pathologic fractures in the femoral head and neck is a lack of appreciation of distal lesions. This may result in unrecognized perforation while preparing the femoral canal and placing the stem of the prosthesis through this perforation. In addition, a stem that ends just proximal to a lesion may cause a stress-riser leading to later fracture. Therefore, it is recommended that all patients have radiographs taken of their entire femur before undergoing this procedure. In patients who have only proximal disease, a long-stem component can frequently bypass these lesions. If there is a large lesion in the supracondylar area, it may be necessary to place a fixation device, such as a supracondylar screw and side plate, to avoid a stress-riser and possible fracture around the tip of the prosthesis.

In a recent series, bipolar replacement was successful in patients without acetabular involvement, with all reporting improvements in their level of comfort and ambulatory ability.[12]

Postoperatively, patients who undergo bipolar hemiarthroplasty for metastatic disease are treated in a way similar to patients who undergo this procedure for other conditions. This involves dislocation precautions and partial weight-bearing for 6 weeks following surgery.

Intertrochanteric Fractures

Impending or complete fractures in the intertrochanteric area with a minimal amount of bone destruction can usually be treated with a screw and side plate device. This is often performed with adjunctive bone cement to assist in fixation of the lag screw or proximal screw in the plate. This type of fixation is especially advantageous in individuals who present with a solitary lesion in the intertrochanteric area that is suspected of being a metastasis, but who have no known primary and no other lesions on bone scan. The lesion can be partially excised and sent to pathology for a tissue diagnosis. Because the direct lateral approach is usually used for biopsy of these lesions, if the lesion should turn out to be a primary, an unsalvageable situation has not been created. If a sarcoma is encountered on the frozen section, surgery should stop unless this situation has been considered preoperatively and en block resection planned. A biopsy should be performed as a separate procedure on any lesion strongly suspected of being a sarcoma.

In a recent study, the use of a screw and side plate device was effective in treating patients with intertrochanteric lesions. When fixation was believed to

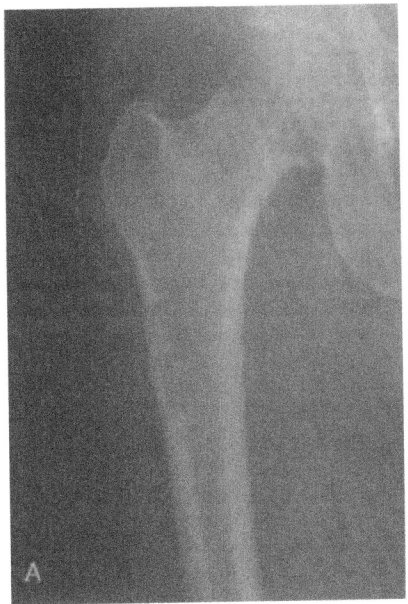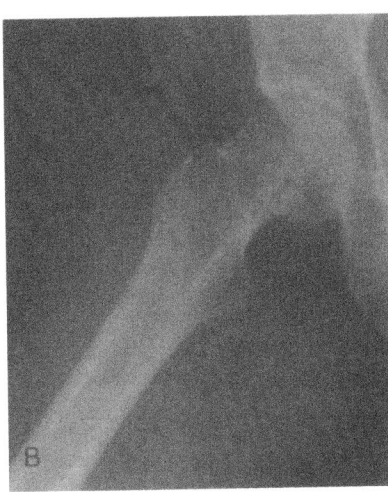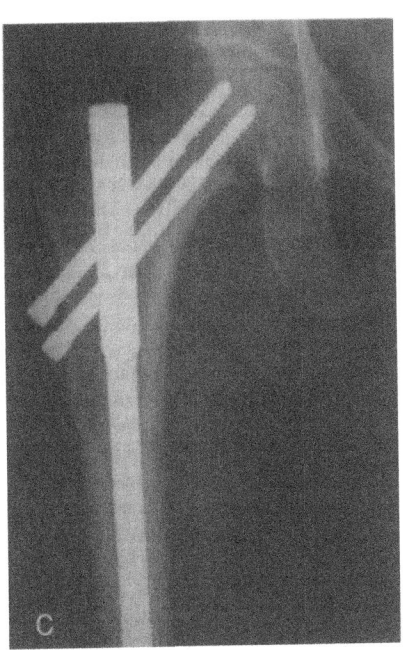

Figure 65.2. Preoperative radiographs (A, B) of lesion in subtrochanteric region of the right femur. C. Postoperative radiograph after placement of femoral Recon intramedullary nail. (Illustration reproduced with permission of Clinical Orthopedics and Related Research.)

be inadequate due to the size or location of the lesion, this fixation was augmented with PMMA.[12]

The disadvantage of using the screw and side plate for these fractures is the significant stress placed on the device during ambulation that may cause it to eventually fail if the patient becomes a long-term survivor. Progression of the tumor may also interfere with fixation, especially if it is relatively radioresistant. In addition, in patients who have radiation therapy in this area and survive for a relatively long period of time, the end of the plate may cause a stress riser on bone that is weakened from the radiation and may eventually cause a fracture at the distal aspect of the plate.

For patients who have extensive destruction in the intertrochanteric area with a complete or impending fracture, it is recommended that a long-stem hip prosthesis or a proximal femoral replacement be used. We have had good success with the latter. Proximal femoral replacement prostheses are available in an off-the-shelf format from a variety of manufacturers. The femoral component is usually combined with a bipolar head. The use of the bipolar head reduces the risk of dislocation that would be encountered with a separate acetabular component.

Postoperatively, patients who are treated with a compression screw and side plate do not require dislocation precautions, and have their weight-bearing status progressed depending upon the extent of bone loss and stability of fixation. Patients who undergo proximal femoral replacement are maintained in a hip abduction brace with a knee-foot-ankle orthosis extension for 6 to 8 weeks postoperatively to decrease the risk of dislocation.

Subtrochanteric Fractures

In patients with obvious metastatic disease, we recommend intramedullary fixation with screws placed along the femoral neck.[11] This device is biomechanically superior to the screw and side plate and is believed to have a lower probability of mechanical failure. In the past, the Zickel nail (Howmedica, Rutherford, NJ) was the "gold standard" for this type of fixation. Currently, most manufacturers who produce trauma instrumentation offer "reconstruction" nails. In most of these devices, two screws are directed up the femoral neck, and the nail can be locked distally. Recently, Synthese Inc. (Paoli, PA) has introduced an unreamed femoral nail that utilizes a spiral blade rather than screw fixation in the femoral head and neck. The advantage of this device is that it can be inserted without reaming, which makes the surgery faster. In addition, the angle of the blade to the nail can be changed, which gives the surgeon more flexibility.

In the majority of these cases, we recommend locking the rod both proximally and distally because of the low incidence of complications associated with placing the distal screws and the potential for loss of stability if

Table 65.1. Patient profile.

Patient number	Age (years)	Primary diagnosis	Site	Procedure
1	59	Breast	L IT	ORIF
2	80	Renal	L IT	ORIF
3	47	Breast	L IT	ORIF
4	57	Poor Diff Ca.[2]	L IT	ORIF
5	65	Renal	L ST	ORIF
6	50	Breast	R IT	ORIF
7	50	Breast	L acet, FN, IT	Protrusio THA
8	69	NH Lymphoma[3]	L acetabulum	Protrusio THA
9	67	Palate	R acetabulum	Protrusio THA
9	69	Palate	R acetabulum	Pins, plates
10	53	Renal	L acetabulum	Protrusio THA
11	56	Renal	L acetabulum	Protrusio THA
12	54	Breast	L FN	Bipolar
13	33	Renal	L FH, FN	Bipolar
14	53	Breast	R FH, FN[1]	Bipolar
15	83	Breast	L FN[1]	Bipolar
16	74	Breast	L FN[1]	Bipolar
17	73	Renal	L FN[1]	Bipolar
18	64	Breast	R FN[1]	Bipolar[4]
19	62	Breast	R ST, FN	Recon rod
20	42	Breast	L ST, FN, femur	Recon rod
21	59	Myeloma	R prox femur	Recon rod
22	50	Lung	L FN, ST	Recon rod
23	43	Myeloma	L femur (ST)	Recon rod[5]
24	41	Breast	L femur/pelvis	Recon rod
16	77	Breast	R FN, ST	Recon rod
25	54	Breast	L FN, femur	Recon rod[6]
18	64	Breast	L ST	Recon rod
26	52	Breast	R ST	Recon rod
27	68	Plasmacytoma	L Femur ST	Recon rod
28	53	Renal	R Femur ST	Recon rod
29	70	Transitional	R prox femur[7]	Prox fem repl

L = left; R = right; IT = intertrochanteric; ST = subtrochanteric; FN = femoral neck; FH = femoral head; recon = reconstruction; THA = total hip arthroplasty; ORIF = open reduction internal fixation; 1 = pathologic fracture present; 2 = poorly differentiated carcinoma; 3 = non-Hodgkin's lymphoma; 4 = additional placement of supracondylar plate for distal femoral lesion; 5 = partial iliectomy for pelvic lesion; 6 = Recon rod augmented with screws; 7 = proximal femoral replacement.

they are not used (Fig. 65.2). We use only bone cement in cases in which loss of bone makes the screw fixation tenuous. In those cases, a ¼-inch drill bit is used to make portals in the bone both proximal and distal to the screws. The area is first irrigated with saline, and then the PMMA is inserted using a syringe so that if flows around the rod and the screws.

Postoperatively, these patients do not require dislocation precautions. Their weight-bearing status is progressed depending upon the extent of bone loss and sta-

Table 65.2. Average estimated blood loss, operative time, length of stay, and survival for each procedure.

Procedure	Estimated blood loss	Operative time (minutes)	Length of stay (days)
Screw, sideplate	600 (200–1000)	123 (80–165)	7 (6–8)
Protrusio total hip arthroplasty	1800 (800–4000)	168 (150–195)	10.5 (8–13)
Bipolar	900 (400–2000)	155 (130–180)	13.4 (7–19)
Recon nail	620 (200–1500)	183 (135–210)	8.6 (4–14)

Values are expressed as the mean with the range for each procedure in parentheses. Because a single proximal femoral replacement was performed, this procedure is not included in the table.

Table 65.3. Preoperative and postoperative pain and ambulation.

Patient number	Preoperative ambulation	Postoperative ambulation	Preoperative pain	Postoperative pain	Postoperative radiation therapy
1	Walker	Walker	Severe	Occasional	Yes
2	nwb	pwb	Occasional	Occasional, less	
3	Normal	Normal	None	None	Yes
4	nwb	Walker	Moderate	None	Yes
5	Crutches	No device	Moderate	Mild	Yes
6	Cane	fwb	Moderate	None	
7	Walker	Walker	Severe	None	Yes
8	Wheelchair	Walker	Moderate	None	Yes
9	Cane	Cane	Moderate	None	
9	Cane	Cane	Moderate	None	
10	Normal	Normal	Moderate	None	Yes
11	Crutches	Cane	Moderate	None	Yes
12	Crutches	Walker	Severe	None	
13	Bedridden	Crutches	Moderate	None	Yes
14	Crutches	No device	Moderate	None	
15	Walker	Cane	Moderate	None	
16	Bedridden	Walker	Moderate	None	
17	Normal	Normal	Moderate	None	
18	Bedridden	Walker	Severe	Minimal	
19	Bedridden	Walker	Severe	Moderate	
20	Crutches	Crutches	Moderate	None	
21	pwb	No device	Mild	Minimal	Yes
22	Crutches	No device	Moderate	Mild	
23	Cane	No device	Moderate	Mild	
24	Cane	Crutches	Severe	None	Yes
16	Bedridden	Walker	Moderate	None	
25	Walker	Walker	Moderate	Mild	Yes
18	Bedridden	Walker	Severe	Minimal	
26	Limited distance	No device	Mild	None	Yes
27	Limited distance	No device	Moderate	None	Yes
28	nwb	Crutches	Severe	None	Yes
29	Bedridden	Transfers	Severe	Moderate	

nwb = nonweight-bearing; pwb = partial weight-bearing; fwb = full weight-bearing.

bility of fixation. Most patients are full weight-bearing or ambulatory with a cane 6 to 12 weeks postoperatively.

In a recent study, 11 patients were treated with this device for lesions about the hip. There were no failure of fixation and no perioperative complications. The results compared favorably with the results of acute nonpathologic fractures treated with the reconstruction nail.[12]

Following surgery, patients are referred for consideration of radiation therapy. In patients who have not received radiation preoperatively, radiation in the postoperative period may be helpful in slowing progression of a lesion, which may ultimately lead to disruption of the internal fixation. Townsend has demonstrated a causal relationship between the use of postoperative radiation therapy and surgery leading to a better outcome versus surgery alone. His study demonstrated a five times greater probability of attaining maximal use of the extremity and a decreased need for a second surgery in the surgery-plus-postoperative-radiation-therapy versus the surgery-alone group. We favor postoperative rather than preoperative radiation therapy whenever it is likely that internal fixation will need to be used. This is, in part, because of the interference with fracture healing when preoperative radiation therapy is used.

Conclusion

In summary, the patient who presents with a metastatic lesion about the hip is first evaluated using a careful history, physical exam, and diagnostic studies. Depending on the results of these studies, the treatment can be nonoperative or operative. Nonoperative treatment usually consists of radiation therapy, protected weight-bearing, and close observation. Operative treatment is either internal fixation or prosthetic replacement, depending on the location of the lesion.

The results of internal fixation of impending and complete pathologic fractures about the hip secondary to metastatic disease has continued to improve with time. In a recent study the results of internal fixation for lesions about the hip were similar to those for the same operative procedures performed for nonmetastatic conditions.[12] This study of 29 patients treated at Allegheny University Hospital showed patient profiles (Table 65.1), operative data (Table 65.2), and successful pain relief (Table 65.3) similar to other studies in the literature.[3–7]

In conclusion, lesions in the area of the hip secondary to metastatic disease continue to present challenging problems for the orthopedic surgeon. With the advent of improved medical therapies for many types of cancer has come not only an increase in life expectancy, but also an increased opportunity for symptomatic metastatic lesions of bone to appear. An improved understanding of which patients are at risk for fracture, in association with advances in internal fixation, has enabled the orthopedic surgeon to provide the patient with metastatic disease an increased level of comfort and mobility.

References

1. Bonarigo BC, Rubin P. Nonunion of pathologic fracture after radiation therapy. *Radiology.* 1967;88:889–898.
2. Bonarigo BC, Rubin P. Nonunion of pathologic fracture after radiation therapy. *Radiology.* April 1981; 653–664.
3. Habermann ET, Sachs R, Stern RE, Hirsch DM, Anderson WJ Jr. The pathology and treatment of metastatic disease of the femur. *Clin Orthop.* 1982;169:70–82.
4. Parrish FF, Murray JA. Surgical treatment for secondary neoplastic fractures. *J Bone Joint Surg Am.* 1970;52:665–686.
5. Zickel RE, Mouradian WH. Intramedullary fixation of pathological fractures and lesions of the subtrochanteric region of the femur. *J Bone Joint Surg Am.* 1976;58:1061–1066.
6. Levy RN, Sherry HS, Siffert RS. Surgical management of metastatic disease of bone at the hip. *Clin Orthop.* 1982;169:62–69.
7. Lane JM, Sculco TP, Zolan S. Treatment of pathological fractures of the hip by endoprosthetic replacement. *J Bone Joint Surg Am.* 1980;62:954–959.
8. Marcove RC, Yang DJ. Survival times after treatment of pathologic fractures. *Cancer.* 1967;20:2154–2158.
9. Harrington KD, Sim FH, Enis JE, Johnston JO, Dick HM, Gristina AG. The use of methylmethacrylate as an adjunct in internal fixation of pathological fractures. *J Bone Joint Surg Am.* 1976;58:1047–1055.
10. Harrington KD. The managment of acetabular insufficiency secondary to metastatic malignant disease. *J Bone Joint Surg Am.* 1981;63:653–664.
11. Horowitz SM. The management of pathological hip fractures. *Operative Techniques in Orthopaedics.* 4 (2): 1994;122–129.
12. Algan SM, Horowitz SM. Surgical treatment of pathologic hip lesions in patients with metastatic disease. *Clin Orthop.* 1996;332:223–231.

66
Conversion of Girdlestone Arthroplasty to Total Hip Replacement

Eric Masterson, Bassam A. Masri, and Clive P. Duncan

Girdlestone arthroplasty is currently used as a generic term to describe any surgical procedure about the hip joint, either primary or secondary, that involves excision of the femoral head and neck and results in a pseudarthrosis of the joint. The most common indication for the procedure in contemporary Western practice is as a definitive or interval operation for the management of an infected hip prosthesis.[1-6] Less common indications include septic arthritis,[7] aseptic loosening of a hip prosthesis where further reconstruction is not considered,[8] cerebral palsy or other chronic neurologic conditions with chronic hip dislocation and, rarely, certain tumor resections in the region of the hip joint. Prior to the emergence of total hip replacement as the treatment of choice for advanced degenerative arthritis of the hip joint, satisfactory results were reported following management by joint resection, especially in cases with markedly reduced joint mobility and fixed contractures.[9] In countries with limited medical facilities and funding, resection arthroplasty remains a treatment option, albeit not ideal, for femoral neck fractures and degenerative hip joint disease.[10]

Girdlestone first reported on resection of the hip joint for the management of tuberculosis of the joint in 1928.[11] Fifteen years later, he published a detailed report of the procedure, which he advocated for the management of pyogenic infection of the hip joint, both primary and secondary to gunshot injuries.[12] His experience in the management of the latter stemmed from his years as a director of the orthopedic division of an Oxford army hospital during the first World War.

It is instructive to read the details of the operative technique advocated by Girdlestone. He used a long transverse incision above the greater trochanter with wide elliptical excision of the distal abductors and greater trochanter. This was followed by joint capsulectomy, excision of the femoral head and neck, and excision of the superolateral acetabular rim. The wound was left widely open and allowed to granulate, and full closure usually took several months. In chronically infected cases with ankylosis of the hip joint, he recommended preservation of the femoral head with wide excision of infected soft tissues about the hip joint via a lateral and, if necessary, an additional medial incision.

Conversion of a classical Girdlestone arthroplasty to a total hip replacement would be difficult or impossible in the absence of any abductor mechanism and with a major segmental acetabular deficiency. Fortunately, the majority of hip pseudarthroses that the reconstructive surgeon will see in current practice will not have undergone so extensive a resection. Recent authors have stressed the importance of maximal preservation of femoral bone stock[5] and of making every effort to preserve the abductor muscles.[13]

Nonetheless, the conversion of a Girdlestone arthroplasty to a total hip replacement has been described as "one of the great challenges in adult reconstructive surgery."[14] These procedures demand comprehensive preoperative clinical evaluation as well as detailed laboratory and radiological investigations. The surgeon should be thoroughly familiar with reconstructive techniques about the hip joint and must ensure that the appropriate armamentarium of instruments and implants is available. The occasional revision hip surgeon should consider referral of such cases to a surgeon with a special interest in revision hip arthroplasty. The ensuing sections will outline the indications for conversion, preoperative workup and intraoperative considerations.

Indications and Contraindications for Girdlestone Conversion

Patients with a definitive Girdlestone arthroplasty may be dissatisfied with the result for one or more of the following reasons: walking difficulties, limb length inequality, pain, persistent infection, poor medical condition, high risk of recurrent infection, unreconstructable bone stock deficiency, abductor mechanism problems, or neuromuscular disorders.

Walking Difficulties

There is broad agreement that walking with a resection arthroplasty of the hip is both ungainly and difficult. Waters et al. performed a detailed analysis of walking patterns and energy expenditure in a series of patients with hip joint resections at an average of 1.2 years postoperatively.[15] Of the nine patients examined, seven required bilateral crutches, one a walker, and only one patient could walk without an assistive device. They demonstrated a substantial reduction in walking velocity, cadence, and stride length, while energy expenditure per meter walked, as measured by oxygen consumption, was more than twice normal values.

Clinical reviews point out the Trendelenberg test is always positive and that a prominent abductor lurch may be expected in the absence of a fixed fulcrum for abductor muscle function. Patients almost always require the use of walking aids such as walking frames, crutches, or canes, and two canes or crutches are more likely to be required than one. This may cause particular difficulties for patients with systemic arthropathy and extensive upper limb involvement.

In a review of 22 patients who had undergone excision arthroplasty for an infected hip prosthesis, McElwaine and Colville found that only one patient could walk better than before the original hip replacement.[6] Nine patients had maintained their previous levels of activity, but the remainder were either bedridden or were restricted to walking a few yards indoors. Clegg reviewed 29 patients with a pseudarthrosis after removal of an infected total hip prosthesis and also demonstrated that, in general, they walked more poorly than prior to the initial hip replacement surgery.[4] This is likely to be a source of dissatisfaction and a reason for seeking conversion to a hip replacement.

Limb Length Inequality

All reports agree that substantial shortening of the limb is a constant feature of a Girdlestone procedure. Shortening may range from 3 to 11 centimeters, but is most typically in the 4–6 cm range. There is no evidence that the practice of prolonged postoperative traction influences the final leg length,[1,3] although a correlation has been described with the level of femoral resection.[5] There is also no objective evidence that an ischial-bearing caliper has any influence on the ultimate leg length, and most patients find these devices too cumbersome and uncomfortable to wear.

Limb shortening further contributes to walking difficulty and may also cause problems with scoliosis secondary to an oblique pelvis. It is most commonly managed by a prescription for a shoe raise, but the degree of shortening is usually such that the raise cannot be concealed within the shoe and an external raise is required. This is often cosmetically unacceptable, especially in female patients, and may be an additional reason for seeking conversion to a hip replacement.

Figures 66.1 and 66.2 show an example of an infected total hip arthroplasty that was initially managed by excision arthroplasty. This resulted in considerable pain relief and the infection was successfully eradicated. Nonetheless, the patient was reluctant to accept the marked shortening of the limb and a poor gait pattern. Figure 66.3 shows successful restoration of leg length following reimplantation with a total hip arthroplasty. The patient's gait was also substantially improved.

Pain

Relief of pain and eradication of infection are cited as the principal reasons for performing a Girdlestone arthroplasty. Reviews of the procedure report that patients usually experience a reduction in pain lev-

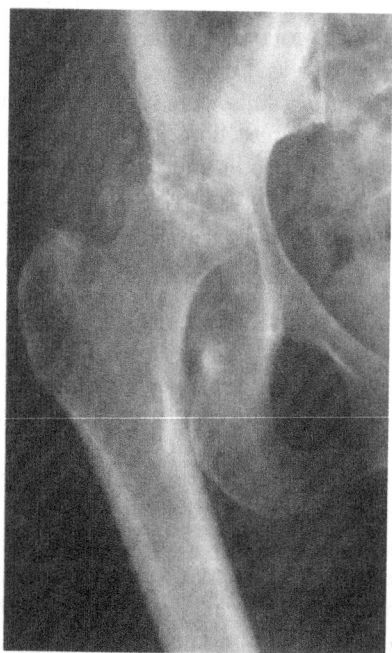

Figure 66.1. A thirty-year-old female intravenous drug abuser with primary septic arthritis of the hip. The organism was *Staphylococcus aureus*, methcillin resistant.

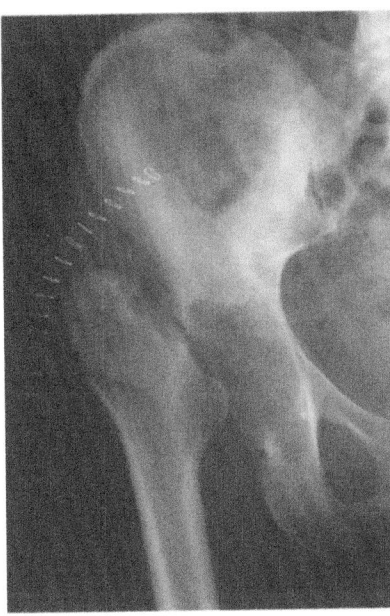

Figure 66.2. The same patient as in Figure 66.1. Treatment by excision arthroplasty. This patient will not be considered for reimplantation.

els,[1,3–6,16,17] although a small number will continue to have significant discomfort and seek revision surgery primarily for this reason. Occasionally, painful articulation between the proximal femur and the outer table of the ileum or between the lesser trochanter and the ischium may be identified by diagnostic injections of local anesthetic under fluoroscopic control. In procedures performed because of infection, ongoing pain may be an indication of failure to eradicate sepsis.

Persistent Infection

A chronically discharging sinus tract following a resection arthroplasty suggests the presence of retained foreign material (most commonly cement) or an unrecognized sequestrum. Some authors have emphasized the importance of removing all cement when removing a hip prosthesis for sepsis,[4] while others[1,18] have not found this to be routinely necessary. Identification of retained cement may be extremely difficult if it is radiolucent, and magnetic resonance imaging may have a role in these cases. Plain radiography may reveal the presence of chronic osteomyelitis with an involucrum surrounding an infected sequestrum. Elimination of infection by radical debridement of retained material and sequestrum should be regarded as a mandatory initial procedure prior to considering reimplantation. This initial exploration will also be helpful in assessing the requirements for any future reconstruction.

Whereas there are a number of reasons for considering conversion of a long-standing hip pseudarthrosis to a total hip replacement, there are also several situations in which it may be more prudent to encourage the patient to accept the limitations. These contraindications are not written in stone and will vary depending on the individual surgeon and the risks a patient is prepared to take. However, the following discussion provides some guidelines as to which patients may be better managed nonoperatively.

Poor Medical Condition

Many patients with resection arthroplasties are elderly and some of them will have significant cardiopulmonary disease. These patients represent a significant potential perioperative morbidity. In addition, restriction of walking distance in this group may be secondary to their medical condition and, in the absence of significant pain, little purpose will have been served by the revision procedure.

High Risk of Recurrent Infection

Even in the absence of documented residual infection in the resected hip joint, there are some patients who are at high risk of secondarily infecting their new hip prosthesis. The obvious example is the patient with rheumatoid arthritis who is on long-term maintenance steroid therapy and who has one or more other chronically infected joint replacements still in situ. Other sources of infection that predispose to infection of the new implant include chronic or recurrent urinary tract

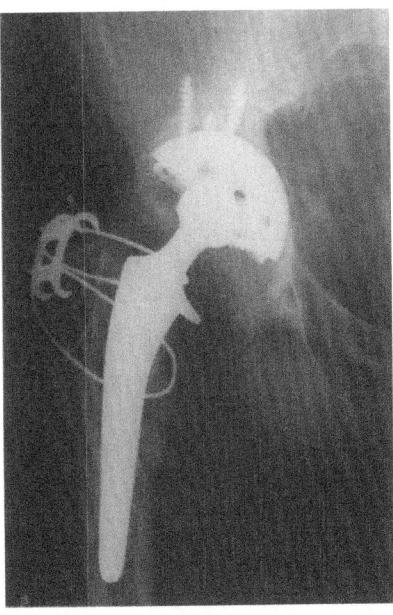

Figure 66.3. A sixty-year-old male patient with chronic periprosthetic infection. The organism was *Staphylococcus epidermidis*.

infections, chronic venous incompetence with varicose ulceration, recurrent episodes of streptococcal cellulitis, dental sepsis, or a focus of chronic osteomyelitis. One particular patient population that is at high risk of secondarily infecting their implant is intravenous drug abusers; it is the policy at our center not to reimplant any patient with a recent history of such abuse (Fig. 66.4 and 66.5). Another patient population in which it may be wise to avoid reimplantation is organ transplant recipients on immunosuppressive medications.

Unreconstructable Bone Stock Deficiency

Some patients will have come to resection arthroplasty following numerous surgical interventions, the cumulative effect of which will have been a serious diminution in available bone stock. Reconstruction may be possible only with the use of extensive structural allografts or with tumor-type prostheses, and such interventions may not always be appropriate.[8,17]

Abductor Mechanism Problems

Patients with absent or deficient abductor muscles as a result of previous surgery have a substantial risk of postoperative dislocation following reimplantation. It may be safer not to replace a stable pseudarthrosis with an unstable total hip replacement. This is especially true of patients who are unlikely to cooperate fully with postoperative bracing or other restrictions.

Neuromuscular Disorders

Patients with poorly functioning abductor muscles or spastic adductors as a result of conditions such as po-

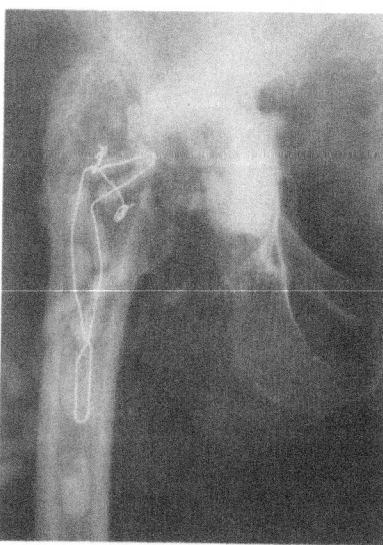

Figure 66.4. Same patient as in Figure 66.3 following excision arthroplasty and insertion of antibiotic-loaded cement beads.

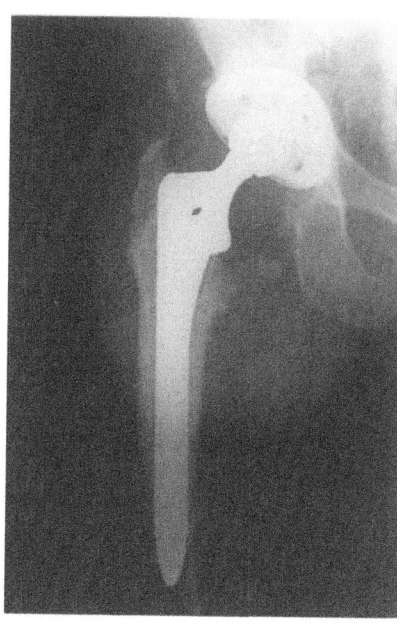

Figure 66.5. Same patient as in Figures 66.3 and 66.4 following reimplantation with a total hip arthroplasty.

liomyelitis, cerebral palsy, or previous cerebrovascular accident with residual neurological deficit have a substantial risk of postoperative dislocation. Extensive release of spastic or unopposed muscle groups may leave the patient without adequate motors to permit effective hip function.

Preoperative Evaluation

The purpose of the preoperative assessment is to ensure that the conversion procedure is appropriate to the general condition of the patient, to rule out ongoing sepsis, and to assess the available bone and soft tissues so that the reconstruction can be accurately planned. The salient aspects of this preoperative workup may be considered under a number of headings.

Original Records

If the Girdlestone arthroplasty was performed elsewhere, every effort should be made to retrieve a copy of the original hospital records. This should include the reasons the procedure was performed, the presurgical patient function, culture and sensitivity reports where appropriate, and a copy of the operative procedure indicating the surgical approach used, the quality of the bone stock, and the condition of the abductor muscles.

History

Inquiries should be made regarding general health and the presence of any medical conditions or allergies.

Sometimes the Girdlestone arthroplasty will have been performed as a definitive procedure because of concerns regarding the health of the patients and the ability to withstand the rigors of reimplantation. In these cases, a medical opinion is appropriate.

Efforts should be made to rule out any of the contraindications to reimplantation outlined in the previous section. A comprehensive history of the events surrounding the original resection should be documented. This should include the indications for the procedure, the postoperative course, wound healing problems or persistent drainage, and antibiotic usage. Note should be made of any other ongoing sources of sepsis remote from the hip that would require management prior to reimplantation. With regard to current problems, the Harris hip score is an appropriate means of assessing levels of pain, function, and walking ability.

Most patients fall into one of two categories. The first is resection arthroplasties that were performed relatively recently and were intended as the first stage in a two-stage exchange for sepsis. The second group underwent a Girdlestone arthroplasty many years previously for any of a number of indications and has functioned for years without a hip joint. It is particularly important to ascertain the exact reasons that these patients are now seeking possible conversion.

Physical Examination

This should include both a general physical assessment and an examination directed at the hip joint. In the general assessment of the patient, respiratory and cardiovascular examination should be included with a search for remote sources of sepsis and an assessment of any other ongoing medical conditions. Examination of the hip joint should include an assessment of upper limb function to determine the ability to use walking aids and an examination of spinal movement and stability. Attention should be paid to the location of previous surgical incisions, true and apparent leg length discrepancies, the presence of palpable abductor muscle activity, and the range of movement of the pseudarthrosis. This should be followed by a comprehensive neurovascular examination of the lower limbs.

Hematology

We perform an erythrocyte sedimentation rate, a C-reactive protein measurement, and a peripheral leukocyte count on all patients undergoing complex revision hip surgery. In our experience, the sedimentation rate is rarely normal in the presence of ongoing sepsis. This concurs with the experience of Feldman et al.[19] However, Tsukayama et al. were able to demonstrate an elevated sedimentation rate in only 63% of 106 infections following total hip arthroplasty.[20]

We also find the C-reactive protein measurements to be reliable and to have the advantage of more rapid return to normal following eradication of infection.[21] Peripheral leukocyte counts may occasionally be elevated but are usually not helpful in the diagnosis of ongoing sepsis. They can, however, be useful occasionally useful in indicating the presence of significant sepsis remote from the hip joint.

Aspiration and Biopsy

In cases in which the Girdlestone arthroplasty was performed for noninfected reasons, we do not routinely aspirate the pseudarthrosis preoperatively. Aspiration is indicated if the original procedure was performed for infection or if the original indication is unknown, especially if the sedimentation rate or C-reactive protein are elevated. It is imperative that the patient not have taken a course of antibiotics in the 4 weeks prior to the aspiration because this diminishes the likelihood of a positive culture.

Aspiration and biopsy of a hip joint pseudarthrosis present certain technical difficulties. The acetabulum and femoral shaft may be filled with fibrous tissue and localization of a fluid-containing pseudarthrosis may be difficult. Swan et al. have described a technique for aspiration of the hip in patients treated with Girdlestone arthroplasty.[22] The needle is introduced anteriorly at a point midway between the greater and lesser trochanters under fluoroscopic control and directed towards the pseudarthrosis, taking care to avoid the femoral neurovascular structures. This is more cranial than the usual approach for hip aspiration because of the missing femoral head and neck. A small amount of contrast material may be used to identify what is generally a linear pseudarthrosis roughly paralleling the acetabular margins. In cases of infection where cables, cement, or other foreign material has been left in situ, it may be appropriate to base the aspiration on the foreign material. It is our routine to additionally use a synovial biopsy needle such as the Westcott needle (Becton Dickinson and Company, Franklin Lakes, NJ) to obtain a tissue sample for culture in each case. If inadequate material is available for bacteriologic study, consideration should be given to core needle biopsies of the bone adjacent to the pseudarthrosis.

Radiography

Preoperative radiographic assessment aims to precisely define the available bone stock and to measure leg length discrepancies. Special investigations are rarely necessary to define the soft tissues, identify radiolucent cement, or identify ongoing sepsis.

Initial evaluation should be with plain radiography. An anteroposterior view of the pelvis as well as anteroposterior and lateral views of the full femur are mandatory. In addition, it is our practice to perform Judet views of the pelvis in each case.[23] We find that this provides useful information regarding the integrity of the anterior and posterior columns, which cannot be visualized on the anteroposterior view alone.

Usually the true shortening of the limb can be assessed by measuring proximal migration of the lesser trochanter relative to the pelvis on the anteroposterior view. However, it is advisable to perform scanograms of both lower limbs in uncertain cases. Examples include inability to identify the lesser trochanter due to bone loss and leg length discrepancy secondary to causes other than the resection arthroplasty. The scanograms have the added advantage of permitting a screening radiographic assessment of the knees and ankles. Care should be taken to take into account any apparent leg length discrepancy secondary to fixed spinal or pelvic deformities. In such cases it is more important to try to correct the apparent rather than the real leg length discrepancy.

We do not routinely request computerized tomography of the hip pseudarthrosis. In selected cases it may, however, provide useful information regarding the available bone stock in the acetabular roof, anterior and posterior columns, and proximal femur. It also allows the formatting of 3D reconstructions of the pelvis and proximal femur, which may facilitate preoperative planning to unusually complex cases. If necessary, the 3D reconstructions can be used to create equal models of the pelvis using computer-assisted design and manufacture (CAD-CAM) technology. Another rare indication for the use of computerized tomography in these patients is to measure leg lengths on the initial scout films because this is somewhat more accurate than scanography.

Magnetic resonance imaging (MRI) allows very accurate definition of soft tissues and may provide useful preoperative information regarding the presence, location, and condition of the abductor muscles in cases where the original operation report is unavailable. This modality is extremely sensitive to tissue edema, and interpretation in the postoperative period may be difficult. Other uses for MRI include identification of the sciatic nerve, visualization of any fluid collections, and determination of the extent of any retained radiolucent cement.[24]

Isotope bone scanning and radioisotope-labeled white cell scanning are rarely indicated, as the presence of sepsis will generally be indicated by other modalities. They may, very rarely, play a role in identifying a focus of residual sepsis remote from the pseudarthrosis. They are also occasionally useful as a confirmatory tool in cases in which clinical suspicion of residual sepsis is high and in which it has not been possible to obtain positive cultures.

Preoperative Templating

Prior to any surgical intervention, it is imperative that the surgeon know what instrumentation and implants will be required and ensure that these tools are readily available. Nowhere is this more important than in revision hip arthroplasty. Conversion of a Girdlestone arthroplasty to a total hip replacement may necessitate reconstruction of major cavitary and segmental deficiencies of both the femur and acetabulum and restoration of substantial limb length.

Templating should begin with reference to the acetabulum on the anteroposterior radiograph. Other views, as well as any special investigations, should be readily available. The position of the original true acetabulum should be determined and an assessment should be made of any bony deficiency centrally or superolaterally. Columnar deficiencies are better visualized on the Judet views or on a CT scan. A superolateral segmental deficiency will commonly be present in long-standing Girdlestone arthroplasties, as excision of the superolateral rim was part of the original description and was emphasized by others.[9] In these cases the surgical options include proximal and medial placement of the component, acceptance of some component overhang and, finally, allograft reconstruction. These techniques are discussed in more detail in the relevant chapters of this text. Major columnar deficiencies may also require allograft reconstruction with or without reconstruction cages and, once again, it is important to emphasize the preoperative recognition of such possibilities.

When a decision has been reached regarding the anticipated position of the acetabulum, the estimated future position of the center of the acetabulum should be marked on the radiograph. A second mark should then be placed as many centimeters proximal to the first mark as the leg is short. This second mark now indicates the ideal position of the femoral head with reference to the femur if complete correction of leg length discrepancy is to be achieved. The femoral component templates should now be superimposed on the radiograph with the center of the femoral head overlying this second mark. This may, of course, have to be modified in light of the intraoperative findings, such as soft tissue contractures or excessive sciatic nerve tension.

The femur may also have any of a range of segmental and cavitary deficiencies from removal of old implants or sequestrae. Angular deformities from previous abduction osteotomies may be present, as osteotomies were sometimes performed to reduce apparent leg length discrepancy secondary to fixed adduction.[25] The deficiencies may necessitate osteotomy or design of a customized implant as part of the reconstructive strategy. Cavitary deficiencies may require management by long-stemmed cemented or uncemented components or by impaction allografting techniques, with or without supplementary cortical onlay allografts. Segmental deficiencies may also necessitate the use of cortical onlay allografts. Severely ectatic proximal femora may require allograft or prosthetic replacement of the proximal femur. Again, the importance of ensuring availability of the necessary equipment is emphasized.

Timing of Revision Surgery

The appropriate timing of the conversion procedure depends on the original indication for the Girdlestone arthroplasty. In cases of periprosthetic infection where the excision was the first operation of a planned two-stage exchange, patients should receive 6 weeks of intravenous antibiotics. There is evidence that in the absence of antibiotic-loaded bone cement, the administration of systemic antibiotics for less than 28 days is associated with a higher recurrence rate.[26] How soon the reimplantation should be done following cessation of antibiotic therapy is controversial and should be based on clinical, hematologic, and radiologic indices more than any fixed formula. Our practice in two-stage exchange procedures is to reaspirate the joint 6 weeks following cessation of antibiotic therapy and to proceed with implantation of a definitive prosthesis if this is negative. Factors that will delay reimplantation include a persistently elevated sedimentation rate without obvious cause that is not showing signs of returning toward normal, recurrent local infection or a positive repeat aspiration culture, poor wound healing with prolonged wound drainage, poor patient compliance with antibiotic therapy, decubitus ulcers, and poor general medical condition with limited rehabilitation potential. Reimplantation may not be appropriate in patients with poor general health, dementia, a history of substance abuse, or in the immunocompromised host.

The timing of conversion of hip joint resection to total hip replacement is less critical in cases that were performed for reasons other than sepsis. Limb shortening, instability, and poor walking ability may make patients reluctant to accept a permanent Girdlestone arthroplasty and may lead to requests for early conversion. Ahlgren et al., in a review of 27 patients with Girdlestone arthroplasties, found that gait, walking distance, and range of movement improved gradually over a one-year period postoperatively.[1] However, other reports have not demonstrated any improvement with time,[2,5] and in the appropriate patient who is dissatisfied with the hip pseudarthrosis, it is probably better to proceed with reimplantation rather than wait for possible minor improvements in function and walking ability that may occur with time.

Surgical Procedure

Surgical Approach

Before deciding on a surgical approach, the following aspects of the reconstruction should be considered:

- The femur is typically medialized and may also be in fixed adduction. This results in a narrow soft tissue interval between the femur and the pelvis.
- The femur has usually migrated proximally by 4 to 6 cm and substantial lengthening will be required. This necessitates extensive mobilization of the proximal femur and good exposure of the sciatic nerve. It also militates against stable reduction and fixation of a classic trochanteric osteotomy.
- Wide exposure of the acetabulum is always required to permit identification of its proper location as well as reconstruction of segmental or cavity defects.
- Extensive exposure of the proximal femur is frequently required to allow reconstruction of bone deficiencies with cables or cortical strut allografts or to correct angular deformities from old osteotomies.
- The condition of the abductor mechanism is highly variable. The abductor muscles may be intact or may have been excised or interposed between the bone ends and replaced by scar tissue. The greater trochanter may be in continuity with the femur or it may be attached only by fibrous tissue or may even be absent.

Based on the above observations, we find that the anterolateral Hardinge-type approach to the joint is usually inadequate. We generally expose the hip by a posterior incision, using as much of any old healed incisions as is practical. When basing any incisions on the greater trochanter, it is important to remember the extent to which that structure has migrated proximally. Occasionally a recalcitrant wound following removal of a hip prosthesis will have been managed by local or free muscle flaps.[27,28] In these situations any incisions should be planned in consultation with a plastic surgeon so that transection of a vascular pedicle and subsequent wound slough may be avoided. The sciatic nerve is carefully exposed and the condition of the abductor muscles and greater trochanter are assessed. If the abductors are absent or deficient, we attempt to preserve a tether of scar tissue to act as a static stabilizer of the joint replacement. At this stage we generally expose the proximal femur via a trochanteric slide. If a trochanteric nonunion exists, it is utilized. Otherwise a shallow trochanteric osteotomy is performed from behind and the trochanter is elevated anteriorly in continuity with the abductors and vastus lateralis as described by Glasmann et al.[29] This approach has the advantages of providing extensive exposure of the proximal femur and acetabulum while minimizing the risk of wide trochanteric separation postoperatively should the fixation wires or cables fail.

Occasionally, no identifiable greater trochanter is present. In this situation a soft tissue envelope consisting of the gluteal abductors and vasti in continuity is elevated forward in the manner similar to that described by McFarland and Osborne.[30] A modification of this approach, coined the *vastus slide*, may be considered.[31] In contrast to both of these descriptions, we routinely carefully develop the interval between the gluteus minimus and the pelvis, thereby preserving this muscle as part of the soft tissue flap.

Cement Beads

If antibiotic-impregnated cement beads are present, they should be carefully removed as part of the surgical exposure. Care should be taken to identify the entire chain of beads, and an assessment of the preoperative radiographs may prove helpful in locating chains embedded in scar tissue. The chains should be removed by gentle straight traction in the line in which they were inserted combined with careful dissection of the intervening soft tissues. Failure to do so may have potentially disastrous consequences such as vascular or neurological injury. Fiddian et al. (1984) reported injury to a femoral vein from attempted bead chain removal that ultimately resulted in an amputation.[32]

Intraoperative Specimens and Antibiotics

Unlike a primary hip arthroplasty, antibiotics should not be administered preoperatively. They should be withheld until three appropriate tissue specimens for culture and sensitivity are obtained during surgical exposure of the pseudarthrosis. This increases the likelihood of obtaining a positive result in the presence of low-grade infection. The use of three separate intraoperative specimens reduces the chance of a false positive result from contamination, as contamination is unlikely to be present in all three tissue cultures. Once the specimens have been obtained, the appropriate intravenous antibiotic may be administered. In revision of Girdlestone arthroplasties performed for infection, the antibiotic should be appropriate to the original infecting organism. Prophylaxis in cases with no history of sepsis is most commonly achieved with a first generation cephalosporin.

We have not found intraoperative gram stain to be useful in diagnosing infection and have abandoned its use. This is in accordance with other reports.[33]

In contrast, frozen section has been reported as both sensitive and specific in identifying infection.[19] Infection is likely when more than five polymorphonuclear leukocytes are found per high-power field in at least five distinct fields. We have found this technique helpful in choosing between repeat debridement and reimplantation in borderline cases, although we suspect that it may be somewhat interpreter-dependent. In the hands of an experienced musculoskeletal pathologist, however, we have found this technique to have a sensitivity of 0.81 and a specificity of 0.95 at our center.[21]

Technical Factors in Achieving Leg Lengthening

A number of important factors need to be considered in any attempt to restore limb length during conversion of a resection arthroplasty to total hip replacement. These include methods of mobilizing the proximal femur, identification of the true acetabulum, preservation of a functional abductor mechanism, and avoidance of sciatic nerve injury.

Following the initial surgical exposure, the proximal femur must be comprehensively released from a mass of dense scar tissue. This involves gradually lifting the proximal femur out of the wound while the enveloping scar tissue is divided with scalpel or cautery close to bone. Particular attention must be paid to the scar tissue retaining the medial aspect of the proximal femur. The iliopsoas tendon should always be released, both because it is frequently involved in scar and because the muscle itself will have contracted, thus contributing to shortening, fixed flexion, and fixed external rotation. Ensure preoperatively that the patient has a functional rectus femoris to permit active hip flexion in the absence of iliopsoas.

When the femur has been adequately mobilized, it may be retracted anteriorly or posteriorly, providing access to the acetabulum. Working with sharp dissection, the bony margins of the true acetabulum are defined and redundant scar tissue is excised. Care is taken to avoid damage to the sciatic nerve and superior gluteal bundle as they exit the pelvis through the greater sciatic notch. Attention must also be paid to any bone deficiencies in the medial wall or anterior column that will predispose to injury of pelvic organs or iliac vessels. Continue to work distally until an inferior retractor can be placed in the obturator foramen or cotyloid notch of the ischium, thus defining the inferior margin of the true acetabulum. Failure to identify this may result in a high center of rotation of the hip replacement.

Management of the abductors in these cases can be difficult. On one hand, a trochanteric osteotomy optimizes surgical exposure, while on the other, reduction and stable fixation of the trochanter following a substantial lengthening may be difficult to achieve and may predispose to failure of the fixation devices with a high trochanteric avulsion and compromised joint stability. Several maneuvers may be helpful. First, the functional continuity of the abductors and vastus lateralis can be maintained by preserving the aponeurosis overlying the greater trochanter. Thus use of the trochanteric slide helps to prevent severe trochanteric migration. Second, it is reasonable to accept some fixed abduction of the hip joint; it is our experience that the fixed deformity disappears with time. Avoidance of overenthusiastic physiotherapy and the occasional use of an abduction brace when fixation of the greater trochanter is suboptimal are recommended. In some cases where substantial lengthening has been achieved, reduction of the hip may be impossible without an extreme fixed abduction deformity. In these cases, we first ensure that any remaining scar tissue is removed from the deep surface of the abductors. If this does not help, we then mobilize the abductors by blunt subperiosteal elevation off the outer table of the pelvis. It may be necessary to mobilize them very extensively as far proximally as the iliac crest, thus allowing them to slide and at the same time rotate on the pivot of the superior gluteal bundle. This procedure is not necessary frequently and is not a benign one, as it may be associated with extensive hematoma formation in the dead space that has been created and may also predispose to heterotopic bone formation.

The final issue of importance when lengthening the limb is the avoidance of a sciatic nerve palsy. This may occur due to direct injury during dissection, retraction or, more commonly, as a result of stretching of the nerve, especially when it is tethered by scar tissue. Other rare causes of sciatic nerve injury include entrapment during reattachment of the greater trochanter,[34,35] migration of broken trochanteric wires,[36] and bleeding following surgery.[37] The true incidence of direct injury to the sciatic nerve during dissection is unknown, as the majority of postoperative palsies are presumed to be secondary to traction injury and are often not reexplored.

There is no clear consensus in the literature as to how much lengthening may safely be achieved. Edwards et al.[38] reported an average leg lengthening of 2.7 cm associated with postoperative peroneal nerve palsy and an average of 4.4 cm associated with sciatic nerve palsy. They recommended that lengthening be limited to 4 cm in order to minimize the risk of sciatic nerve palsy. Nercessian et al.[39] reported on 1284 hip replacements, of which 66 were lengthened from 2 to 5.8 cm. The only nerve palsy in this group was a single partial sciatic nerve palsy from a direct laceration, and no injuries secondary to lengthening could be identified. They point out that percentage of lengthening was more important than absolute lengthening and suggest that lengthening of up to 10.2% of the length of the femur is safe.

Regardless of the etiology, several authors point to the increased incidence of nerve palsy in revision procedures.[40-42] A number of steps may be taken to reduce the risk of damage to the sciatic nerve. First, as the sciatic nerve is frequently embedded in dense scar tissue from previous procedures, it is our practice in this situation to identify the nerve distally in virgin tissues and carefully mobilize it proximally as far as the sciatic notch. This avoids the risk of tethering of the nerve by scar tissue following lengthening. Second, we are meticulously careful about our placement of retractors behind the posterior lip of the acetabulum. Third, following reduction of the trial components, the sciatic nerve is routinely assessed clinically for tension. If the nerve is a little taut with the knee in full extension but becomes lax with the knee flexed, we may accept the situation and nurse the patient postoperatively with some pillows behind the knee. If, however, the nerve remains taut with the knee flexed, we retrial the components with less lengthening. This may necessitate resection of the proximal femur.

A number of authors have described the use of somatosensory evoked potential monitoring of the sciatic nerve during surgery for acetabular fractures and have found the technique useful.[43-46] However, there have been no studies to show that this technique is effective in the prevention of sciatic nerve injury in total hip arthroplasty. To the contrary, the evidence available to date suggests that monitoring of the sciatic nerve using somatosensory evoked potentials has no influence on the rate of sciatic nerve injury following total hip arthroplasty.[47,48]

An alternative possibility in assessing the sciatic nerve intraoperatively is to wake the patient briefly after the trial components have been inserted and the hip reduced. This so-called *wake-up test* has been used in surgical correction of spinal deformity.[49] It requires close cooperation of the anaesthetist, who should be informed in advance that an intraoperative wake-up test will be required. Once confirmation of satisfactory nerve function has been obtained, the patient is rapidly reanaesthetised. It is unusual for the patient to recall the event postoperatively with the use of modern anaesthetic agents that have a potent amnesic effect. Nevertheless, it is wise to inform the patient ahead of time that this maneuver may be necessary, but will be painless.

Reconstructive Options

Following adequate surgical exposure and mobilization of tissues, the reconstructive surgeon may face any of the full gamut of acetabular or femoral bone deficiencies. In the context of conversion of a classic Girdlestone arthroplasty, the most likely acetabular deficiency will be a superolateral rim defect due to beveling of the acetabulum at the time of the index procedure. Minor defects may be managed by accepting some component overhang or by proximal and medial placement of the component. Major defects may necessitate the use of structural allograft. These techniques are dealt with elsewhere in this textbook. In cases where there is a deficient abductor mechanism, it may be appropriate to consider the use of a bipolar hemiarthroplasty or a constrained socket in order to reduce the risk of postoperative dislocation.

Any of the full range of bone deficiencies may also be found on the femoral side. Attention is directed to the appropriate chapters in this text. However, two specific aspects of the femoral reconstruction are worthy of note. First, the degree of lengthening achieved will be determined by tension on the sciatic nerve. If this tension is excessive, the surgeon may need to resect some of the proximal femur. Second, patients may occasionally present with a long-standing abduction osteotomy. This brings into consideration the need to remove old fixation devices and the use of intraoperative corrective osteotomies or customized femoral stems.

If the original resection arthroplasty was performed for the control of infection, consideration should be given to the use of implants fixed with antibiotic-loaded cement. The use of uncemented components in the second stage of a two-stage exchange procedure for sepsis has been associated with a higher rate of recurrent infection.[50]

Postoperative Management

Postoperative management is determined largely by the extent and nature of the reconstruction and will, therefore, need to be individualized for each case. Some specific points are worth emphasizing:

- We routinely continue intravenous antibiotics for 5 days postoperatively and then discontinue the antibiotics when the 5-day culture report is confirmed as negative for all three specimens obtained intraoperatively. A single positive report may be ignored as being most likely secondary to contamination. Two or three positive reports with the same organism are an indication of persistent sepsis. In this situation, appropriate intravenous antibiotic therapy should be continued for 6 weeks and the patient's course carefully monitored.[20] In doubtful cases, careful review of the synovial histology can prove helpful.
- The postoperative neurological status of the limb should be carefully assessed. Partial nerve palsies usually recover, while the prognosis for a full sciatic nerve palsy is poor. In the absence of an obvious abnormality on the radiograph such as a misplaced screw, wire, or bolus of cement, there is little to be gained by early reexploration. If, however, there is concern about possible excessive tension on the sciatic nerve and a palsy is recognized immediately postoperatively, there may be a role for returning the patient to the operating theater and purposely dislocating the hip joint by closed means with the aid of a brief anesthetic. The patient can then be observed postoperatively and, if the nerve recovers promptly, can be placed on gradually increasing skeletal traction for a period of time followed by a closed reduction when the acute insult to the nerve has passed.
- The condition of the abductor mechanism will determine the appropriateness or otherwise of active abduction exercises or the use of a brace postoperatively to allow trochanteric healing or to prevent early dislocation.
- The range of movement of the hip is usually less than is typically achieved in a primary hip arthroplasty.
- It is best to delay the issuing of any new prescriptions for shoe raises until after the acute postoperative period, when the patient is mobilizing satisfactorily.

Conclusions

Girdlestone arthroplasty as a definitive procedure for an infected hip prosthesis, aseptic loosening, or other indication provides reasonable levels of pain relief and infection control, but results in a short limb with poor walking ability. Conversion to a total hip replacement is usually technically feasible but requires careful preoperative patient selection and planning, as well as considerable experience in adult hip reconstruction techniques. Major intraoperative considerations include the restoration of leg length, avoidance of sciatic nerve injury, and maintenance of an effective abductor mechanism. Identification and management of residual sepsis prior to revision surgery is of paramount importance. Finally, careful preoperative planning should make every effort to identify bone deficiency so that the necessary tools and techniques are available to reconstruct significant defects and achieve stable fixation of the components.

References

1. Ahlgren S-A, Gudmundsson G, Bartholdsson E. Function after removal of a septic total hip prosthesis. A survey of 27 girdlestone hips. *Acta Orthop Scand*. 1980;51:541–545.
2. Bittar ES, Petty W. Girdlestone arthroplasty for infected total hip arthroplasty. *Clin Orthop*. 1982;170:83–87.
3. Bourne RB, Hunter GA, Rorabeck CH, Macnab, JJ. A six-year follow-up of infected total hip replacements managed by Girdlestone's arthroplasty. *J Bone Joint Surg Br*. 1984;66: 340–343.
4. Clegg J. The Results of the pseudarthrosis after removal of an infected total hip prosthesis. *J Bone Joint Surg Br*. 1977;59:298–301.
5. Grauer DJ, Amstutz HC, O'Carroll PF, Dorey FJ. Resection arthroplasty of the hip. *J Bone Joint Surg Am*. 1989;71:669–678.
6. McElwaine JP, Colville J. Excision arthroplasty for infected total hip replacements. *J Bone Joint Surg Br*. 1984;66: 168–171.
7. Klein N, Moore T, Capen D, Green S. Sepsis of the hip in paraplegic patients. *J Bone Joint Surg Am*. 1988;70:839–843.
8. Harris WH, White RE Jr. Resection arthroplasty for nonseptic failure of total hip arthroplasty. *Clin Orthop*. 1982;171:62–67.

9. Taylor RG. Pseudarthrosis of the hip joint. *J Bone Joint Surg Br.* 1950;32:161–165.
10. Sharma S, Gobalakrishnan L, Yadav SS. Girdlestone arthroplasty. *Int Surg.* 1982;67:547–550.
11. Girdlestone GR. Arthrodesis and other operations for tuberculosis of the hip. In: *The Robert Jones birthday volume.* London: Oxford University Press, 1928:347.
12. Girdlestone GR. Acute pyogenic arthritis of the hip, an operation giving free access and effective drainage. *Lancet.* 1943;1:419.
13. Hanssen AD, Mariani EM, Kavanagh BF, Coventry MB. Resection arthroplasty (Girdlestone procedure), nerve palsies, limb length inequality, and osteolysis following total hip arthroplasty. In: Morrey BF, ed. *Joint replacement arthroplasty.* New York: Churchill Livingstone, 1991, 891–905.
14. Berman AT, Mazur D. Conversion of resection arthroplasty to total hip replacement. *Orthopedics.* 1994;17:1155–1158.
15. Waters RL, Perry J, Conaty P, Lunsford B, O'Meara P. The energy cost of walking with arthritis of the hip and knee. *Clin Orthop.* 1987;214:278–284.
16. DeLaat EAT, Van der List JJJ, Van Horn JR, Sloof TJJH. Girdlestone's pseudarthrosis after removal of a total hip prosthesis; a retrospective study of 40 patients. *Acta Orthop Belg.* 1991;57:109–113.
17. Renvall S, Einola S. Girdlestone operation. An acceptable alternative in the case of unreconstructable hip arthroplasty. *Annales Chirurgiae et Gynecologiae* 1990;79:165–167.
18. Lieberman JR, Callaway GH, Salvati EA, Pellicci PM, Brause BD. Treatment of the infected total hip arthroplasty with a two-stage reimplantation protocol. *Clin Orthop.* 1994;301:205–212.
19. Feldman DS, Lonner JH, Desai P, Zuckerman JD. The role of intraoperative frozen sections in revision total joint arthroplasty. *J Bone Joint Surg Am.* 1995;77:1807–1813.
20. Tsukayama DT, Estrada R, Gustilo R. Infection after total hip arthroplasty. A study of the treatment of one hundred and six infections. *J Bone Joint Surg Am.* 1996;78:512–523.
21. Spangehl MJ, Duncan CP, O'Connell JX, Masri BA. Prospective analysis of preoperative and intraoperative studies for the diagnosis of infection in 210 consecutive revision total hip arthroplasties. Presented at the 1997 annual meeting of the American Academy of Orthopaedic Surgeons, San Francisco, CA, February, 1997.
22. Swan JS, Braunstein EM, Capello W. Aspiration of the hip in patients treated with Girdlestone arthroplasty. *Am J Radiol.* 1991;156:454–546.
23. Judet R, Judet J, Letournel E. Fractures of the acetabulum: classification and surgical approaches for open reduction: preliminary report. *J Bone Joint Surg Am.* 1964;46:1615–1646.
24. Fehrman DA, McBeath AA, DeSmet AA, Tuite MJ. Imaging barium-free bone cement. *Am J Orthop.* 1996;25:172–174.
25. Milch H. The resection-angulation operation for hip-joint disabilities. *J Bone Joint Surg Am.* 1955;37-A:669–717.
26. McDonald DJ, Fitzgerald RH Jr., Ilstrup DM. Two-stage reconstruction of a total hip arthroplasty because of infection. *J Bone Joint Surg Am.* 1989;71:828–834.
27. Collins DN, Garvin KL, Nelson CL. The use of the vastus lateralis flap in patients with intractable infection after resection arthroplasty following the use of a hip implant. *J Bone Joint Surg Am.* 1987;69:510–516.
28. Meland NB, Arnold PG, Weiss HC. Management of the racalcitrant total-hip arthroplasty wound. *Plast Recon Surg.* 1991;88:681–685.
29. Glassman AH, Engh CA, Bobyn JD. A technique of extensile exposure for total hip arthroplasty. *J Arthroplasty.* 1987;2:11–21.
30. McFarland B, Osborne G. Approach to the hip: A suggested improvement on Kocher's method. *J Bone Joint Surg Br.* 1954;36:364–367.
31. Head WC, Mallory TH, Berklacich FM, Dennis DA, Emerson RH, Wapner KL. Extensile exposure of the hip for revision arthroplasty. *J Arthroplasty.* 1987;2(4):265–273.
32. Fiddian NJ, Sudlow RA, Browett JP. Ruptured femoral vein. A complication of the use of gentamicin beads in an infected excision arthroplasty of the hip. *J Bone Joint Surg Br.* 1984;66:493–494.
33. Brause BD. Infections associated with prosthetic joints. *Clin Rheum Dis.* 1986;12:523–536.
34. Mallory TH. Sciatic nerve entrapment secondary to trochanteric wiring following total hip arthroplasty. A case report. *Clin Orthop.* 1983;180:198–200.
35. Ritter MA, Carlson SR. Sciatic nerve injury in total hip arthroplasty. *Orthop Rev.* 1983;12:117.
36. Asnis SE, Hanley S, Shelton PD. Sciatic neuropathy secondary to migration of trochanteric wire following total hip arthroplasty. *Clin Orthop.* 1985;196:226–228.
37. Fleming RE, Michelson CB, Stinchfield FE. Sciatic paralysis: a complication of bleeding following hip surgery. *J Bone Joint Surg Am.* 1979;61:37–39.
38. Edwards BN, Tullos HS, Noble PC. Contributory factors and etiology of sciatic nerve palsy in total hip arthroplasty. *Clin Orthop.* 1987;218:136–141.
39. Nercessian O, Piccoluga F, Eftekhar NS. Postoperative sciatic and femoral nerve palsy with reference to leg lengthening and medialization/lateralization of the hip joint following total hip arthroplasty. *Clin Orthop.* 1994;304:165–171.
40. Navarro RA, Schmalzried TP, Amstutz HC, Dorey FJ. Surgical approach and nerve palsy in total hip arthroplasty. *J Arthroplasty.* 1995;10:1–5.
41. Nercessian OA, Macaulay W, Stinchfield FE. Peripheral neuropathies following total hip arthroplasty. *J Arthroplasty.* 1994;9:645–651.
42. Amstutz HC, Ma SM, Jinnah RH, Mai L. Revision of aseptic loose total hip arthroplasties. *Clin Orthop.* 1982;170:21–33.
43. Calder HB, Mast J, Johnstone C. Intraoperative evoked potential monitoring in acetabular surgery. *Clin Orthop.* 1994;305:160–167.
44. Helfet DL, Koval KJ, Hissa EA, Patterson S, DiPasquale T, Sanders R. Intraoperative somatosensory evoked potential monitoring during acute pelvic fracture surgery. *J Orthop Trauma.* 1995;9:28–34.
45. Helfet DL, Schmeling GJ. Somatosensory evoked potential monitoring in the surgical treatment of acute, dis-

placed acetabular fractures. Results of a prospective study. *Clin Orthop.* 1994;301:213–220.
46. Vrahas M, Gordon RG, Mears DC, Krieger D, Sclabassi RJ. Intraoperative somatosensory evoked potential monitoring of pelvic and acetabular fractures. *J Orthop Trauma.* 1992;6:50–58.
47. Black DL, Reckling FW, Porter SS. Somatosensory-evoked potential monitored during total hip arthroplasty. *Clin Orthop.* 1992;262:170–177.
48. Porter SS, Black DL, Reckling FW, Mason J. Intraoperative cortical somatosensory evoked potentials for detection of sciatic neuropathy during total hip arthroplasty. *J Clin Anesth.* 1989;1:170–176.
49. Dorgan JC, Abbott TR, Bentley G. Intra-operative awakening to monitor spinal cord function during scoliosis surgery. Description of the technique and report of four cases. *J Bone Joint Surg Br.* 1984;66:716–719.
50. Nestor BJ, Hanssen AD, Ferrer-Gonzalez R, Fitzgerald RH Jr. The use of porous prostheses in delayed reconstruction of total hip replacements that have failed because of infection. *J Bone Joint Surg.* 1994;76:349–359.

67
Conversion of the Fused Hip to Total Hip Arthroplasty

Benjamin E. Bierbaum and Russell G. Tigges

Total hip arthroplasty is the current treatment of choice for many hip diseases. With the increasing availability and success of total hip arthroplasty and the concomitant treatment of TB infection, and better management of childhood hip problems, the number of surgical arthrodeses of the hip has declined. A limited number of hip fusions are still performed today for posttraumatic arthritis, unilateral osteoarthritis in the young, or as end-stage treatment for an infected hip. Unilateral hip arthrodesis can provide a stable, painless limb for ambulation and function. This was a common surgical treatment prior to the advent of hip arthroplasty.

Patients with many years of excellent results from hip arthrodesis may develop related symptoms in other musculoskeletal areas. Callahan et al.[1] found 60% of hip fusions developed low back pain at an average of 25 years postarthrodesis. A similar percentage developed ipsilateral knee pain an average of 23 years postfusion. Ipsilateral knee instability was also found in 80% of the fused hip patients. Pain in the contralateral hip was found in 25% of people, developing an average of 20 years after hip fusion.

Position of the fused hip plays an important role in the long-term outcome. Patients may develop spontaneous hip ankylosis after a hip infection or following traumatic injury. Abnormal positions of fusion can lead to severe functional disability. Most orthopedists agree that the ideal position of fusion for the hip is 30° to 40° flexion, 0° to 5° of external rotation, and 0° to 5° of adduction. Callahan et al.[1] found a hip fused in abduction tended to have a greater risk for degenerative changes in the lower back and ipsilateral knee. Gore et al.[2] evaluated the walking patterns of men with unilateral hip fusions. They found that absent hip motion is compensated for by increased transverse and sagittal rotation of the pelvis, increased motion of the contralateral hip, and increased flexion of the knee throughout the stance phase on the fused side. These findings correlate with the clinical degenerative changes seen in the long-term studies by Callahan et al.[1] and Sponseller et al.,[3] where the most commonly reported related pain was in the lower back, ipsilateral knee, and contralateral hip.

Indications

Conversion of a well functioning hip fusion to a total hip arthroplasty is a difficult procedure and should not be performed without strong indications. The most common indications for conversion arthroplasty are listed in Table 67.1.[4-11]

Low back pain is the most common musculoskeletal complaint in people with unilateral hip fusion.[1,3] This pain may result from malposition of the fusion or may be due to the increased stresses and motion placed on it by the fused hip.[2] Ipsilateral knee pain and/or instability results from the abnormal walking patterns of the limb.[2] Increased flexion of the knee during stance phase and the resultant varus or valgus strain resulting from the fixed hip position may lead to instability and/or degeneration. Contralateral hip pain results from the increased motion and forces transmitted through it. With the current success of hip arthroplasty, a primary hip replacement on the contralateral hip is the better choice of treatment when compared with the difficult surgery and functional results of conversion arthroplasty. A painful pseudoarthrosis of an attempted hip fusion is a strong indication for conversion arthroplasty. A careful evaluation of the pseudoarthrosis must be done to be certain that infection is not the primary cause of the pain.

Not infrequently an old childhood infection or severe intra-articular hip trauma results in a spontaneous fusion. These fusions may stabilize in an awkward position, and may necessitate conversion to hip arthroplasty to allow the person to have adequate mobility and function. These may be more satisfactorily approached through corrective osteotomy of the femur.

Table 67.1. Indications for conversion of hip fusion to THA

Low back pain
Ipsilateral knee pain or instability
Contralateral hip pain
Painful pseudo-arthrosis of the hip fusion
Malpositioned hip fusion

All patients with a recent or remote history of infection need to be evaluated for latent infection. A baseline sedimentation rate and meticulous evaluation of the soft tissue is of critical importance in evaluation of elimination of the infection. Identification of prior organisms, antibiotic susceptibilities including dilution, and prior antibiotic treatment all assist in patient evaluation.

Preoperative Planning

One of the most important aspects of a conversion arthroplasty is preoperative planning. Evaluation of the patient includes the measurement of true and apparent leg lengths, functional musculature—especially abductors and gluteus maximus—and flexibility of the lumbar spine and lumbosacral junction. It may be difficult to palpate the contraction of the gluteus medius in the fused hip. If there is any suspicion of denervation or functional quality of the abductors, an EMG may be warranted. The lack of any functioning abductors may be a relative contraindication to perform conversion arthroplasty. Denervation or simple disruption of the abductors may have occurred during previous operations. Reconstruction of the absent abductors has been described by several different techniques,[12–15] though all have their own risks and limitations. Use of a constrained acetabular component and selective positioning of the acetabular component to enhance stability or adapt to leg length difference in fixed pelvic obliquity and muscle imbalance is critical.

Templating of the preoperative radiographs allows for determination of the necessary implants and tools to be available during the procedure. It also allows determination of the true anatomic hip center, where the acetabulum should be placed, and the location of the femoral osteotomy. Careful preoperative evaluation of neurovascular status is imperative to compare pre- and postoperative changes if present.

Technique

The patient is placed in the lateral decubitus position. Prior incisions need to be respected and utilized if appropriate. Debridement of superficial and deep scar will improve flexibility and enhance the cosmetic appearance. A transtrochanteric approach may enhance visualization of the femoral-acetabular junction and allow for proper tension of the abductors. An in situ osteotomy is then performed just distal to the pelvic rim (Fig. 67.1). A second osteotomy is performed distal to the first, close to where the final femoral neck cut will be.[16] This allows removal of the bone fragment and easier visualization and manipulation of the proximal femur.

The acetabulum is addressed first. A small reamer is placed at the desired level of the acetabular component halfway in the midline between the anterior and posterior columns. The attachment of the straight head of the rectus femoris muscle at the anterior inferior iliac spine (AIIS) is a key landmark and is often present in spite of prior infection and multiple operations. This anatomical point is the key to position of the superior rim of the bony acetabulum. The anterior and posterior columns are exposed, palpated, and visualized to confirm the position of the reamer. If there is any uncertainty as to the exact placement, a K-wire may be drilled into the lateral aspect of the pelvis and an anteroposterior (AP) pelvic radiograph taken to check the placement of the site to be prepared. Reaming is then performed medial and cephalad until the medial wall is encountered and a sufficient lateral and posterior supporting wall is created. Progressive reaming up in size to fit a cup between the columns is then performed. An ingrowth cup is ideally placed at 40° abduction and 20° to 30° anteversion. Variations for short leg and pelvic obliquity are necessary to achieve implant stability. Screw augmentation is usually necessary because of the marked osteopenia.

The femur is then prepared for cementless or cemented component fixation. A trial reduction is per-

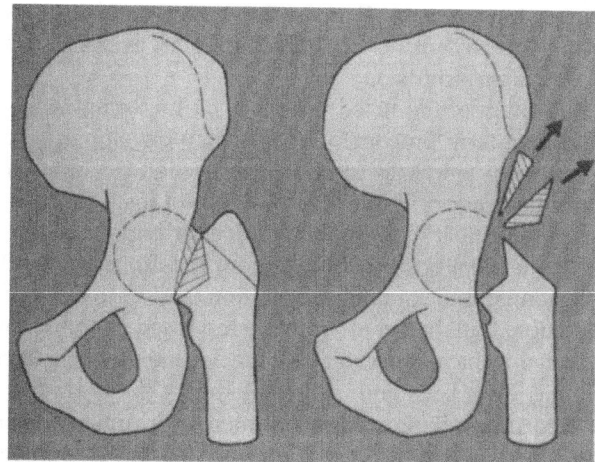

Figure 67.1. After a transtrochanteric approach is used, an in situ osteotomy is performed just distal to the pelvic rim. A second osteotomy is done distal to this and the bone fragment is removed to allow easier visualization and manipulation of the proximal femur.

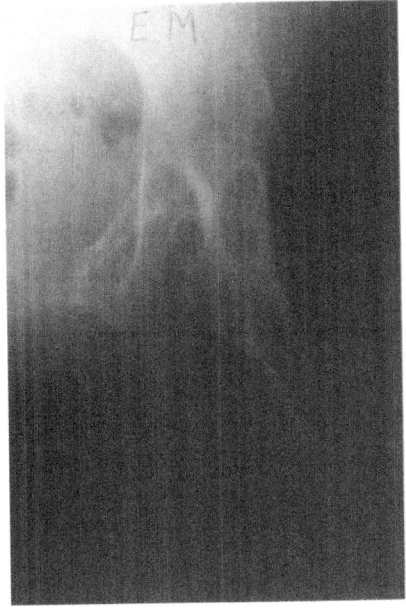 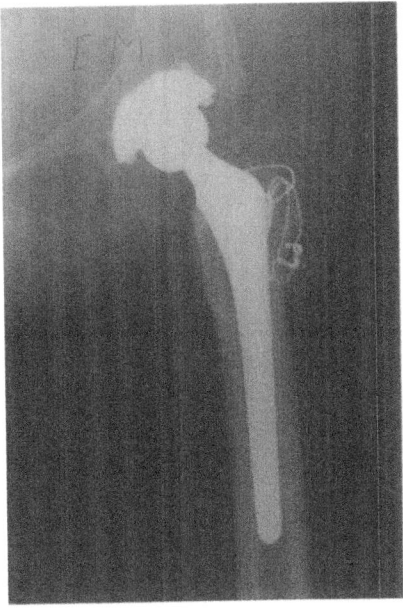

Figure 67.2. EM is a 50-year-old female, status post childhood TB infection of the left hip and fusion at age 13. She is status post left total knee arthroplasty and right total hip arthroplasty, but persisted with low back pain. A. Preoperative radiograph displaying solid fusion. B. She underwent conversion of left hip fusion to total hip arthroplasty. Four year follow-up showed a Hospital For Special Surgery score of 92.

formed and proper leg length and soft tissue tension is attained. Final components are inserted and the trochanter is reattached with wires or cable grip to the lateral femoral shaft under appropriate tension. The common tendency is to overlengthen a short femur at the expense of enhanced motion. The authors have long believed a shorter limb with increased abduction and flexion is a better compromise than true leg length equality.

Postoperative care includes out-of-bed on postoperative day one if leg control is achieved. Partial weight-bearing is encouraged for 6 weeks to allow for bone and soft tissue healing. Active abduction is avoided during this time to protect the trochanteric attachment. Active abduction strengthening is begun at 6 weeks. Active DVT prophylaxis is instituted. Perioperative single-dose radiation or postoperative Indomethacin is used to prevent heterotopic ossification in patients who have demonstrated prior ossification. Figures 67.2 and 67.3 demonstrate two cases of hip fusion conversion.

Results

Several reports of conversion hip arthroplasty appear in the literature.[4-11] All of these series show similar results. Pain relief in the back, ipsilateral knee, and contralateral hip is commonly achieved provided that significant degenerative joint disease is not present. Back pain associated with ankylosing spondylitis will not be helped by takedown of the hip fusion.[7] Degenerative changes in the ipsilateral knee or contralateral hip may require operative replacement of these joints to fully relieve their symptoms.[4]

Range of motion after conversion arthroplasty can be expected to be considerably less than the motion after primary THA.[6,10] This limitation results from contracted scar from previous surgery or contracted, inactive muscles and tissues. Attempts at limb lengthening to equalize length may also adversely tighten the soft tissues. Multiple soft tissue releases to optimize motion may be needed, including psoas release, iliotibial band release, and percutaneous adductor tenotomy.

Muscle strength is slow to recover in ankylosed hips after surgery, but has been shown to increase for 2 or more years after conversion arthroplasty.[10]

Long-term results in conversion arthroplasty show increased risk of failure in surgical versus spontaneous fusions and in patients less than 30 years old at the time of THA.[9] Strathy and Fitzgerald showed a 48% failure rate in conversion of a surgical fusion versus a 5% failure rate in conversion of spontaneous fusions at 10 year follow-up. They reported that the length of time the hip had been fused had no effect on the failure rate of the subsequent THA.

Conclusion

Conversion of a hip arthrodesis to a total hip replacement is a technically demanding procedure. Careful preoperative planning for the surgery, thorough examination of the patient, and realistic education of the patient are all important factors to optimize patient and surgeon satisfaction after surgery. The real benefit of arthrodesis conversion is achieving hip flexibility. This allows for normal sitting posture, ease of dressing shoes and stockings, ready access to automobiles and theater

Figure 67.3. CN is a 37-year-old female, status post left hip arthrodesis at age 27 for acetabular trauma. A. She presented for conversion total hip arthroplasty secondary to low back pain and contralateral hip pain. B. She presented at 6 month follow-up with trochanteric pain and weakness with evidence of trochanteric nonunion. C. She remained mildly symptomatic for 2 years until she presented with increasing groin pain and evidence of acetabular loosening. D. She underwent acetabular revision and reattachment of the trochanter during her last visit.

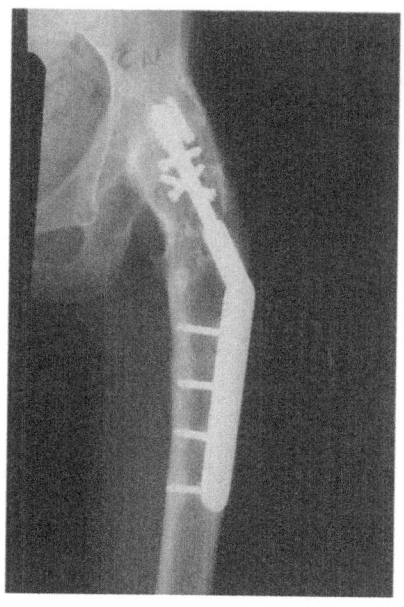

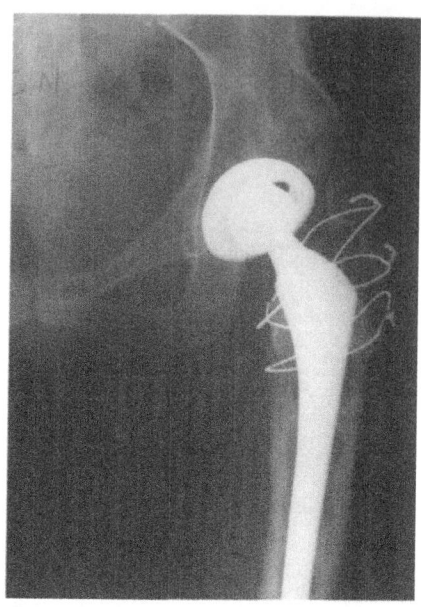

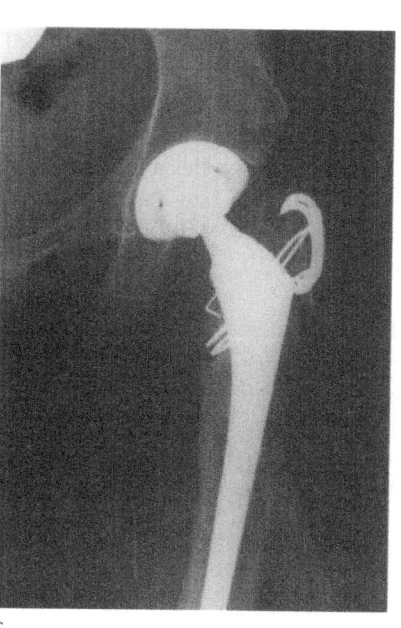

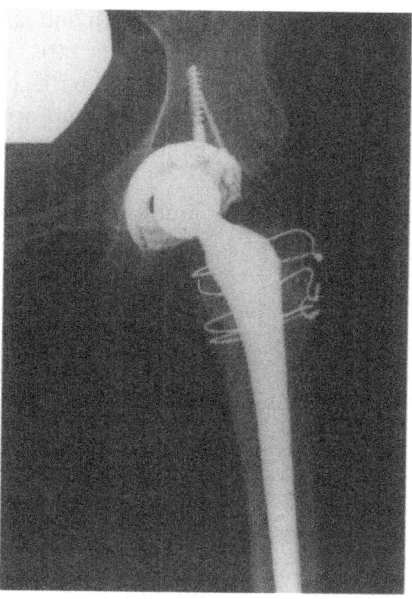

type seats, and ease of strain on the back and knee. The tradeoff is substituting a stable, painless pelvic-femoral nonarticulation to a weaker, painful hip replacement that may require a cane for support in walking. The benefit to the patient is not a high score on a hip evaluation scale (which is unlikely because of potential pain and weakness), but the flexibility in ambulation that can lead to a more normal life.

References

1. Callaghan JJ, Brand RA, Pedersen DR. Hip arthrodesis: a long-term follow-up. *J Bone Joint Surg Am*. 1985;67(9):1328–1335.
2. Gore DR, Murray MP, Sepic SB, Gardner GM. Walking patterns of men with unilateral surgical hip fusion. *J Bone Joint Surg Am*. 1975;57(6):759–765.

3. Sponseller PD, McBeath AA, Perpich M. Hip arthrodesis in young patients: a long-term follow-up study. *J Bone Joint Surg Am*. 1984;66(6):853–859.
4. Brewster RC, Coventry MB, Johnson EW Jr. Conversion of the arthrodesed hip to a total hip arthroplasty. *J Bone Joint Surg Am*. 1975;57(1):27–30.
5. Amstutz HC, Sakai DN. Total joint replacement for ankylosed hips: indications, technique, and preliminary results. *J Bone Joint Surg Am*. 1975;57(5):619–625.
6. Hardinge K, Williams D, Etienne A, MacKenzie D, Charnley J. Conversion of fused hips to low friction arthroplasty. *J Bone Joint Surg Br*. 1977;59(4):385–392.
7. Lubahn JD, Evarts CM, Feltner JB. Conversion of ankylosed hips to total hip arthroplasty. *Clin Orthop*. 1980;153:146–152.
8. Hardinge K, Murphy JCM, Frenyo S. Conversion of hip fusion to Charnley low-friction arthroplasty. *Clin Orthop*. 1986;211:173–179.
9. Strathy GM, Fitzgerald RH. Total hip arthroplasty in the ankylosed hip: a ten-year follow-up. *J Bone Joint Surg Am*. 1988;70(7):963–966.
10. Kilgus DJ, Amstutz HC, Wolgin MA, Dorey FJ. Joint replacement for ankylosed hips. *J Bone Joint Surg Am*. 1990;72(1):45–54.
11. Reikeras O, Bjerkreim I, Gundersson R. Total hip arthroplasty for arthrodesed hips. 5- to 13-year results. *J Arthroplasty*. 1995;10(4):529–531.
12. Besser MIB. A muscle transfer to replace absent abductors in the conversion of a fused hip to a total hip arthroplasty. *Clin Orthop*. 1980;173–174.
13. Mustard WT. Iliopsoas transfer for weakness of the hip abductors. A preliminary report. *J Bone Joint Surg Am*. 1952:34(3):647.
14. Sherrard WJW. Posterior iliopsoas transplantation in the treatment of paralytic dislocation of the hip. *J Bone Joint Surg Br*. 1964;46:426.
15. Thomas LI, Thompson TC, Straub LR. Transplantation of the external oblique muscle for abductor paralysis. *J Bone Joint Surg Am*. 1950;32(1):207.

68
Motor Deficits

Russell G. Cohen and Aaron G. Rosenberg

Since the inception of total joint replacements in 1959 by Sir John Charnley, surgeons have cited numerous factors relating to their success and failure. While articles addressing implant design, methods of fixation, and surgical techniques have abounded in the orthopedic literature, one facet has received little attention as a general category. Motor weakness of the supporting musculature around a total hip arthroplasty and how it affects the results of surgery is mentioned only sporadically. It is typically discussed in conjunction with other more common problems associated with these complex reconstructions, and not as a separate entity. Motor deficits can arise for a number of reasons, particularly in the revision setting where prior surgery may leave muscles denervated or the trochanter displaced from its anatomic position (Fig. 68.1A).

Strength of the periarticular musculature is vital to ensure stability of the hip and restore the patient's gait to as near normal as possible. A number of diagnoses exist that can alter the patient's strength and ultimately the result of surgery. In instances where the problem exists preoperatively, careful planning can prevent disastrous results that may otherwise be encountered. Quite frequently, however, the weakness arises out of a surgical complication and needs to be addressed postoperatively to prevent premature failure of the reconstruction.

The subject of motor weakness can best be divided into two categories: (1) problems that can be identified preoperatively and (2) factors related to the technical aspects of surgery. Preoperative weakness may be noted with neurologic problems such as hemiplegia, post-polio syndrome, cerebral palsy, myelomeningocele, spinal stenosis, and spinal cord injury. Other diagnoses recognized preoperatively that can be accompanied by weakness include neuropathic joints and entities that present with alteration of the normal resting length of muscle (developmental dysplasia of the hip, coxa vara, and arthroplasty after Girdlestone or arthrodesis).

Weakness more commonly arises out of a complication related to either surgical technique or postoperative complications. These may be secondary to the surgical approach used, use of trochanteric osteotomy and union of the osteotomy, restoration of soft tissue tensioning, and damage to the musculature or muscular attachments during surgery.[1-10] These issues have been addressed more frequently in the literature and can be reviewed in greater detail.

While the literature remains devoid of an organized approach to motor weakness about total hip arthroplasty, it is important for the revision hip surgeon to understand the implications, causes, and solutions to the problems presented by this subset of patients. Early recognition of these problems and careful preoperative planning will assist both the patient and surgeon in attaining a successful result.

Implications of Motor Weakness

Instability and dislocation after total hip arthroplasty (THA) have been cited in numerous publications since the earliest articles relating to hip replacement surgery, and they continue to be a dilemma for even the most skilled surgeons.[11-20] Motor weakness is one of several potential causes of hip instability and dislocation. It needs to be recognized preoperatively, dealt with intraoperatively, and specifically addressed during the rehabilitation of the surgical patient. However, once the problem of weakness is known to exist, there is not always an easy way to compensate for the problem, as is the case in patients with primary neuromuscular involvement. However, if discovered preoperatively, there are means to compensate for the weakness that can prevent recurrent dislocation.

Hip instability resulting in dislocation is a well recognized complication of both primary and revision hip arthroplasty. After reviewing 35 000 cases in the literature through 1987, Morrey[4] found the incidence to be 2.2%, with a similar incidence in the Mayo Clinic study.[21] While preoperative diagnosis has not been found to correlate with the development of dislocation, numerous factors relating to dislocation have been noted, including femoral offset, component malposi-

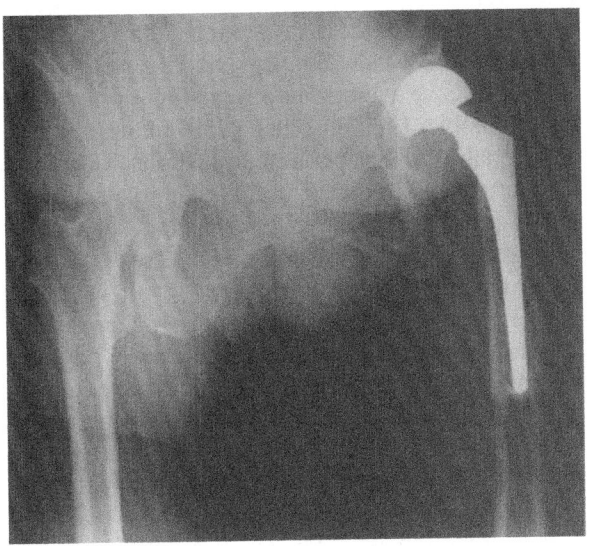 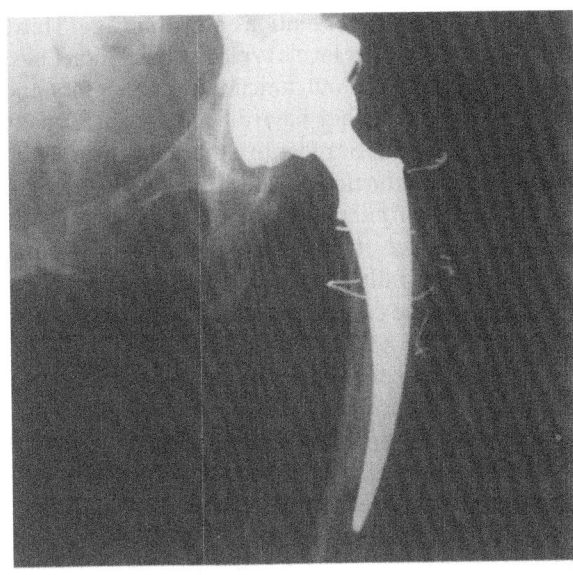

Figure 68.1. A. Radiograph of a patient with a bipolar arthroplasty, now with resorbtion of the greater trochanter. B. Patient with rheumatoid arthritis and prior revision hip arthroplasty, now with ununited, proximally migrated, and painful greater trochanter.

tion, surgical approach, and femoral component head size.[4] However, most reviews address only such common diagnoses as osteoarthritis, rheumatoid arthritis, avascular necrosis, and congenital hip dysplasia. Few articles exist that address comorbid neuromuscular conditions (Parkinson's, post-stroke, cerebral palsy (CP)), post-arthrodesis and post-Girdlestone arthroplasty, as well as coxa vara and other associated deformities and their specific correlation with the development of hip instability.

A second problem relating to post-arthroplasty weakness around the hip is the development of a limp. This most often relates to abductor weakness and may result in an abductor lurch or Trendelenburg gait due to the inability to fully support the hemipelvis during single leg stance.[22] This produces a noticeable limp that may ultimately affect the degree of patient satisfaction. Several surgical factors are discussed in greater detail below that contribute to the development of abductor weakness.

Causes of Motor Weakness

Preoperative Factors

Several neurological disorders exist that may ultimately progress to total hip arthroplasty or may be seen in conjunction with degenerative arthritis of the hip. Patients with hemiplegia resulting from a cerebrovascular insult may develop degenerative joint disease. The two diagnoses are not codependent, but since both typically occur in the aging population, they may be present concurrently. Similarly, patients with cerebral palsy may develop arthritic hips as a result of long-standing hip dysplasia or dislocation.[23,24] In both populations, the abductors and extensors are preferentially weaker than the adductors and flexors. This leads to a flexion deformity with scissoring of the legs and generally requires adductor tenotomies as well as extensive capsular release during surgery.

Treating cerebral palsy patients with hip arthritis is a complicated issue. However, the literature supports treating them with hip arthroplasty to alleviate pain and maximize their care and function.[23,24] Root et al. reported his 6-year follow up of fifteen patients treated with total hip replacement. Thirteen of fifteen were painfree and functioning at a level consistent with their degree of involvement, with only two requiring revision.[24] He later reported the 10-year survivorship of the prostheses in these patients to be 86%.

Recognizing these results, performing hip arthroplasty in CP patients remains a viable option. However, recognizing the muscle imbalances around the hip with relative abductor weakness, one can carefully plan the approach and implant design to avoid complications related to the muscle imbalances. Use of the anterolateral approach with preservation of the posterior capsule adds stability to these patients, who may spend more time sitting than the average total hip patient.

Myelomeningocele patients have varying needs for surgery about the hip, depending on the level of the neural defect.[25] The mid-lumbar levels have the highest incidence of dislocation in childhood and usually have the greatest need for intervention at a young age. Third, fourth, and fifth lumbar levels typically have intact flexors and adductors without functioning abductors and extensors. As a result, they have the greatest propensity to dislocate over time. Surgery to correct this usually involves an open reduction, capsulorrhaphy, or derotational osteotomy on either the femoral or acetabular side of the joint. The age at which the diagnosis of dislocation is made can influence the procedure that is performed, and it is the unrecognized dislocations that may ultimately develop osteoarthritis of the hip.

While total hip arthroplasty in this population of patients has not been reported many patients will maintain some degree of sensation, and in those patients left dislocated or subluxed, hip degeneration and pain may become an issue later in life. Adult reconstructive surgery requires not only joint replacement, but muscle balancing as well if problems with instability and dislocation are to be avoided.

It does not occur infrequently that patients with spinal stenosis have concomitant hip arthritis. These patients tend to become deconditioned from the inability to ambulate, not only from their hip pathology, but from the neurogenic claudication as well. Unless their stenosis is a mid to high lumbar level with associated myelopathy or neuropathy, the hip musculature is not generally weakened. However, a complete neurological exam and preoperative evaluation of the supporting muscles needs to be performed so that if deficits do exist, they can be addressed at the time of surgery and during the postoperative rehabilitation.

Other conditions such as post-polio syndrome and the spinal cord injury patient occasionally present with hip arthritis. Although no literature exists on outcome and management of these patients undergoing hip replacement surgery, management presents similar problems. Recognizing the diagnosis and associated lack of muscle support preoperatively will enable the surgeon to modify the technique and choice of components in an effort to avoid chronic instability.

Another group of patients who create a challenge to the reconstructive surgeon are patients who have previously undergone arthrodesis. These include patients with surgical arthrodesis and those with spontaneous ankylosis, such as in ankylosing spondylitis. In either case, the patients lose muscle strength as a result of disuse, sometimes for more than 20 years. Surgically ankylosed hips may have significant abnormality or loss of the trochanter as a result of the technique used for the arthrodesis, and the abductors are often damaged during surgery.

The early results of hip arthroplasty in these patients seemed favorable, with few problems at early follow-up. In separate studies, both Lubahn and Brewster reported good results after takedown of a hip fusion and conversion to a total hip arthroplasty.[26,27] Complication rates were acceptable, and 50% of patients did not require an assistive device for ambulation at one year follow-up. However, Strathy and Fitzgerald reported their results at average 10-year follow-up to be much less favorable. They reported a 25% failure rate and an additional 11% with poor clinical results. Most failures were attributed to mechanical loosening, with an additional group developing deep infections. Only one was revised for recurrent dislocation.[10] These results would imply that, while these patients initially do well, altered mechanics and weakness of the supporting musculature may lead to earlier failure than in a control population.

More recently, Reikeras et al. reported on 46 patients at a mean of 8 years following conversion of an arthrodesed hip to a joint replacement, citing seven failures that required revision. While no patients required assistive devices for ambulation prior to conversion, 34 patients required assistive devices at follow-up and the group as a whole had a mean abductor score of 3 (scale of 0 to 5).[28] Patients were generally satisfied with the added mobility, but the results are not as good as primary arthroplasties and patients have additional needs to compensate for the weakened musculature around the reconstruction.

Developmental dysplasia of the hip occurs in another group of patients with altered mechanics about the hip.[29,30] The diagnosis is known preoperatively, and testing of the musculature can be performed. Besides the problem of compromised abductors, several other issues need to be addressed in these patients. Transtrochanteric osteotomy has frequently been used to aid in exposure of the acetabulum. This, too, may predispose to weakening of the abductors, particularly if nonunion occurs. The center of rotation of the hip is not always in the usual location and results in altered mechanics and forces around the hip. Linde reported a cumulative survivorship of 89% after 10 years, but a significantly higher failure rate when the acetabulum was placed high (42% versus 13%) rather than low.[31] One may not always have the luxury of placing the acetabulum in the original position, and in these cases the long-term results may be compromised.

Operative and Postoperative Factors

Surgical Approach

The surgical approach to the hip has long been discussed regarding its contribution to the development of instability around a total hip replacement. Three standard approaches to hip—anterolateral (Hardinge), transtrochanteric (trochanteric osteotomy), and posterior (Kocher-Langenbach)—have all been critically evaluated regarding the incidence of instability and dislocation. While each technique has numerous modifications, there is a general consensus that the posterior approach has the highest incidence of dislocation.

Robinson found a significant difference in the dislocation rate between hips exposed through a posterior approach compared to the trochanteric osteotomy group. He found a lower incidence of dislocation in subjects who underwent trochanteric osteotomy compared to a posterior approach (0 vs. 7.5%).[9] Other studies have found similar findings, including the Mayo report of a 2.3% dislocation rate using an anterior approach in comparison to 5.8% using the posterior approach.[21] Roberts found a threefold increase in dislocation using the posterior approach compared to the anterior approach.[8] None of the studies, however, critically analyzed the specific reasons for this difference.

An important factor contributing to instability is the effect of the approach on the surrounding muscles. The posterior approach, while protecting muscle innervation, detaches all the short external rotators and frequently the main hip extensor, the gluteus maximus. The replacement of healthy, contractile muscle posterior to the joint with scar tissue that is unable to respond to changing loads may contribute to higher instability rates seen with this approach.

On the other hand, the anterolateral approach is not without its complications. This technique involves detachment of the anterior fibers of the gluteus medius and minimus. Splitting the fibers of the gluteus medius proximally jeopardizes the inferior branch of the superior gluteal nerve, potentially leaving the muscle flap denervated. Baker performed nine cadaveric dissections of the superior gluteal nerve and found it to course from 3 to 5 cm proximal to the anterior edge of the trochanter.[32] Excessive splitting of the muscle proximally risks denervation and potentially leaves this portion of the muscle without contractile ability.

Another concern is reattachment of the anterior fibers of the gluteus medius and minimus to the greater trochanter. This potentially weakens the abductors and may result in a limp or instability around the hip.[6] In the same study by Baker, ten hips approached through an anterolateral exposure demonstrated abductor denervation at 10 weeks, and 56% continued to have a positive Trendelenburg sign at 12 months.[32] Minns et al. compared patients who underwent an anterolateral approach using his technique to those undergoing trochanteric osteotomy. They found that his method was safe and effective, and no difference was found in strength testing of the abductors.[3] The posterior approach is typically used for revision surgery, and recognizing the hazards of dissecting through altered anatomy is imperative. The muscles are more susceptible to injury due to the extensive stripping required for exposure, as are the nerves, which may be in altered positions. They are equally susceptible to injury during the lengthening of a shortened limb, as is typically the case during these difficult reconstructions. However, in both primary and revision surgery, variability in surgeon technique may account for the substantial differences in complications reported. Recognizing the potential hazards of a given approach is important when deciding on a preferred approach to the hip and no technique is free of complications.

The concern of trochanteric osteotomy and its relationship to the development of instability remains a controversial subject. Where there is union of the trochanter without proximal migration beyond 2 cm,[21] this technique aids greatly in exposure without compromising muscle strength.[1,3,5] However, today most surgeons have given up the technique of transtrochanteric osteotomy except in more complex cases where exposure is not adequate without its use. The main concern over such a technique is the high number of nonunions associated with repair of the small fragment.[33] Variations of that technique such as the trochanteric slide where the soft tissue sleeve is kept in continuity with the bony fragment, and the use of the extended trochanteric osteotomy, are both excellent alternatives to separation of the proximal trochanteric fragment from the remaining femur.

A number of factors have been measured to determine whether the presence of a nonunion affects gait, pain, hip stability, and functional outcome. Ritter found a higher incidence of pain associated with nonunion and a greater ability to walk in the presence of a well united fragment.[7] Robinson's article, previously mentioned, found trochanteric osteotomy to be safe and effective with no dislocations using that technique. Fraser and Wroblewski, on the other hand, cited loss of the abductor mechanism as a major factor contributing to dislocation following trochanteric osteotomy, not only from nonunion of the fragment, but also as a result of the approach.[34]

A controversy arises when discussing the effects of trochanteric nonunion on the function of the THR. When the trochanter migrates proximally, allowing the abductor lever arm to shorten, instability and dislocation become a problem for the patient. While some authors feel that migration of more than 15 mm results in abductor weakness,[35] most feel that greater than 20 mm of migration leads to functional impairment.[36-39] Patients with more than 1 cm of separation will usually demonstrate a Trendelenburg sign[38] (Fig. 68.1B).

Although the effect of releasing the trochanter for exposure of the hip is desirable in select cases, its contribution to developing motor weakness is not universally accepted. Murray et al. performed a controlled study of 82 cases, half undergoing THR by trochanteric osteotomy and the other half by anterior approach described by Muller. At 2-year follow-up, there was no difference to muscle kinesiologic testing between the two groups of patients.[5] Borja et al., in a similar study, found no difference in isometric and isokinetic measurements between those undergoing trochanteric osteotomy and a posterolateral approach.[1] The argument, therefore, remains to be settled whether trochanteric osteotomy or nonunion thereof plays a significant role in the development of weakness and hip instability following arthroplasty.

Soft Tissue Tensioning

The success of hip arthroplasty depends to some degree on the ability to balance the soft tissues around the joint, particularly in revision surgery, where the normal tissue architecture has been altered. Restoring normal length to the extremity, achieving the desirable degree of offset, and finding the center of rotation of the femoral head relative to the revised acetabulum is more complex in this setting. However achieving these parameters is crucial to the success of revision surgery.

Every muscle has an optimum resting length and tension that maximizes its efficiency during contraction. An overstretched muscle will not have overlap between the thick and thin myofilaments within the sarcomere, whereas a muscle that is overly shortened will have abutment of thick bands between adjacent sarcomeres.[40] Similarly, a muscle that has improper innervation will undergo changes at the neuromuscular junction and muscular atrophy, resulting in alterations of the contractile properties of skeletal muscle and the efficiency of their function.

Failure to restore adequate tension of the soft tissues around the hip has two deleterious effects. The first relates to stability of the reconstruction and the subsequent increased risk of dislocation. While many authors have addressed the issue, no consensus exists that restoring limb length alone affects hip stability. Morrey found that in a series of unstable hips, the limb was 1.6 mm longer than the nonoperated control.[4] Coventry reported similar findings, with 75% of 32 patients being equal in length. Only 25% had a shorter limb on the unstable side.[13] Carlsson and Gentz, however, found a statistically significant correlation with limb shortening and dislocation.[11] Kristiansen et al. made the observation that the unstable hip was slightly more proximal than the control group, but the numbers were not statistically significant.[16]

The distance from the center of the femoral head to the greater trochanter is referred to as the *offset of the prosthesis*; while it does not add length to the extremity, it provides clearance of the trochanter from impinging on the acetabulum by bringing the trochanter laterally and maximizes the efficiency of the abductors. As a result, it also affects the amount of force generated by the muscles and the dynamic stabilizing elements across the joint. The amount of offset in any given patient is highly variable, and restoring this offset is an important goal of hip reconstruction. In the revision setting where the femoral component has loosened and subsided within the femur, the offset is lost and the result is inadequate abductor function preoperatively. Patients with coxa vara, on the other hand, have a greater degree of offset to begin with, and choosing an appropriate prosthesis to match this offset is critical. Failure to do so will leave the abductors relatively loose and inefficient, increasing the likelihood of limp, instability, and dislocation postoperatively.

In Poss' study of offset in a population of patients with unstable hips, he found a strong correlation with a shorter distance from the tip of the trochanter to the center of the femoral head in patients with unstable hips.[15] They demonstrated the importance of both lateralization and distal advancement of the trochanter in order to restore the efficiency of the abductor mechanism.

In the revision setting and certain primary situations, the degree of offset is limited from the outset. Patients with protrusio acetabulae, for example, have a shortened acetabular-trochanteric distance (ATD), and consequently lose the efficiency of the abductors to some degree. Adding offset by appropriate prosthesis selection adds tension to the muscles, improves the abductor lever arm, and at the same time provides clearance of the trochanter from the pelvis. In revision settings where the cup has eroded into the pelvis and migrated proximally, restoration of offset during surgery provides the same advantage in optimizing the clinical result.

Resection arthroplasty (Girdlestone procedure) is most commonly performed for sepsis and subsequent removal of the implants in an effort to eradicate the infection. However there are instances where it is done for aseptic reasons such as cerebral palsy, multiple failures of hip arthroplasty, fractures in debilitated patients, and neuropathic joints. In patients who have undergone a Girdlestone procedure, conversion to an arthroplasty remains a viable option, assuming the underlying problem has been resolved.

In these cases the soft tissues have frequently shortened, become fibrotic, and undergone significant atrophy to result in supporting muscle that is compromised. Such cases require careful attention to restoration of offset, orientation of the components, and diligent postoperative rehabilitation in order to minimize postoperative fatigueability, limp, and dislocation.

Treatment of Motor Weakness

The development of instability and dislocation resulting from motor weakness is a challenging problem, often not easily resolved. However, recognizing the potential complications associated with periarticular muscle weakness and planning accordingly may help alleviate some of these difficulties. There is really no literature to guide the surgeon in these circumstances, but avoiding certain situations that can accentuate the problem may reduce the potential for complications. Such measures include use of an anterior approach where possible, meticulous closure of the posterior structures when feasible, selection of a prosthesis with adequate offset, and restoration of limb lengths. These goals are really no different from routine primary arthroplasties, but the margin for error in the subset of patients is so narrow that extra attention to these details is vital if one is to avoid potentially catastrophic results.

Dorr et al. classified dislocations into three categories: Type I includes positional dislocations; Type II, soft tissue imbalance; and Type III, component malposition.[41] Type I patients can most often be treated with closed reduction; in the rare instance that it's not successful, an open reduction is performed. This was necessary in 17% of Dorr's patients. Those in group III required reoperation for multiple dislocations 77% of the time. This usually required reorientation of either the femoral or acetabular component. Patients in group II had a reoperative rate of 46%, and 15% of these hips ultimately went on to resection arthroplasty.

The treatment plan should follow a logical sequence, as it should in any patient who dislocates following total hip replacement. A closed reduction is performed and the patient is placed in either an abduction brace or hip spica cast for a period of time and then allowed to resume usual activities. In patients with known abductor weakness, physical therapy should be added as an adjunct following bracing to strengthen the abductors and extensors. This is particularly helpful in patients who have been converted from an arthrodesis or Girdlestone to a total hip replacement. In fact, therapy should routinely be instituted following surgery, and not after the complication has occurred.

For patients who have weakness in a limp but not recurrent dislocations, the use of a cane potentially avoids long-term complications with wear of the prosthesis. By using a cane, the forces across the hip joint can be reduced and abnormal wear patterns can be avoided.

For patients in whom recurrent dislocation develops, several options exist. The first is use of a hip spica cast for a 6-week period while allowing the periarticular soft tissues to heal. Mallory et al. reported on the use of an above-knee hip spica cast following dislocation and had only 1 redislocation out of 16 patients.[20] For those who experience recurrent dislocations, a permanent brace to maintain reduction and function of the hip is also a reasonable option. For patients in whom surgery is not advisable for medical reasons, the brace may provide stability to the hip and allow them to resume limited activities without the need for additional surgery. However, patients are generally dissatisfied with the brace because it is cumbersome to wear, and difficult to apply and restricts activities.

Where trochanteric nonunion is believed to be the cause of recurrent dislocation, surgical options are available when nonoperative treatment has failed. An attempt should be made to attain union of the trochanter in the normal anatomic position. This is not always easy to accomplish because the ununited fragment is frequently a shell of thin cortical bone and the bone on which it lies is typically less than ideal. Nonetheless, numerous fixation devices are available to hold the fragment in place while an attempt at union is made; monofilament wires in an array of orientations, the Volz bolt, wire mesh, braided cables, and cable grip systems are a few of the devices that have been used to secure the trochanter. On rare occasion, particularly in the revision setting, releasing the origin of the abductors from the ilium is necessary to allow sufficient distal transfer of the trochanter to prevent excessive tension on the repair. This requires a subperiosteal dissection of the abductors off the ilium to their origin at the iliac crest. Electrocautery is used to aid in the dissection, and careful avoidance of the superior gluteal neurovascular bundle as it courses anteriorly from the sciatic notch is imperative. A separate incision along the iliac crest may be necessary to release the abductors from their origin. The use of a postoperative spica cast with the leg held in abduction for 6 weeks is also recommended to allow the muscle to scar down to its new bed.

In cases where the instability is due to improper soft tissue tensioning around the joint, trochanteric advancement is one option to restore the appropriate ten-

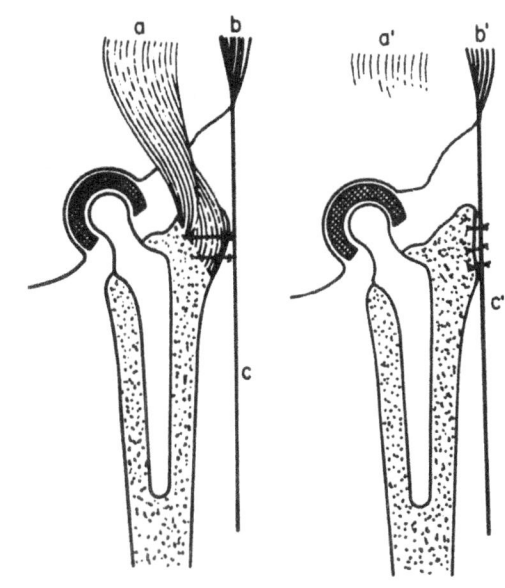

Figure 68.2. (*Left*) Diagram showing the original operation: a, abductor muscles; b, tensor fascia lata; c, fascia lata. (*Right*) Diagram showing the revision operation: a', remnant of abductor muscles; b', tensor fascia lata; c', attached fascia lata. (From Besser M, by permission *Clin Orthop*.)

sion. The trochanter is osteotomized and advanced distally in order to restore myofascial tension to the periarticular abductor sleeve. Eklund performed such a procedure in 21 patients for recurrent dislocation and stabilized 17 patients with this procedure alone. Three others required additional operations to become stable, while the fourth patient underwent resection of the components.[42] Kaplan and Poss had similar success in 17 of 21 patients and felt such a procedure is indicated where other factors such as component malposition and impingement have been ruled out.[15]

Another option that is gaining popularity is the use of a constrained capture cup mechanism. This cup allows the acetabular component to be fixed to the pelvis, unlike the bipolar prosthesis, and yet have a constrained interface within the cup. This affords stability to the reconstruction through a greater range of motion but adds additional stresses on the acetabular prosthesis–bone interface. No long-term studies have been reported to date, but a recent article by Lombardi, Mallory, and others using the S-ROM constraining acetabular insert showed a reduction in dislocation rate for revision cases from 19% to 4.5%. Their follow-up period was 30 months and as yet they have not noted a significantly higher loosening rate. Five of the 50 patients had redislocated an additional 8 times, 1 due to improper neck length and the others because of underlying neurologic problems.[43] While this technique remains an option, it does not always solve the problem definitively and the long-term results are not yet known.

Less common solutions to the problems of instability around the hip due to muscle weakness include muscle transfers and soft tissue slings. Besser reported on use of the tensor fascia lata sling to the bed of the greater trochanter in order to provide stability to the hip (Figure 68.2). He reported this operation in a patient who was converted from an arthrodesis and had poor abductor function from the long-term immobility. He tenodesed the tensor fascia to the bed of the greater trochanter to allow the proximal portion to function as an abductor. The patient's hip remained stable 2 years postoperatively.[44]

Enneking describes another method to either replace or augment absent or deficient abductors in the tumor setting. This method can also be applied to revision patients who may need additional means to compensate for weakness resulting from prior reconstructive surgery. A 5-cm-wide strip of tensor fasica is peeled from distal in the thigh to the level of the trochanter and kept in continuity with its proximal extension. After the surgery is completed, with the leg held in abduction, this strip is reattached to its bed and acts as an abductor sling through the tensor fascia lata. The limb is then maintained in spica cast where the soft tissues heal.[45]

On rare occasions, we have used the gluteus maximus as a sling that is rotated anteriorly and sutured to fascia lata, transferring the pull of the deficient abductors to the fascia lata. This technique adds an additional option to the revision surgeon, who may otherwise be left with an unstable reconstruction despite judicious use of all other options.

Finally, a rare situation may arise whereby the hip cannot be stabilized by any of the aforementioned methods and conversion to a Girdlestone is the only feasible option. While this limits the patient in many ways, it is a solution that affords the patient peace of mind and enables them to move forward in their lives without the constant fear of the hip dislocating without warning.

In summary, for patients undergoing revision surgery and in certain primary settings where the abductor mechanism is either weakened or deficient, careful planning and early recognition of such a situation is vital to the success of hip reconstruction. The surgeon may change the operative approach, select an appropriate prosthesis, or change the postoperative protocol to achieve a stable reconstruction without recurrent instability or dislocation. While these optional results may not always occur, recognizing these unique conditions will hopefully prevent avoidable complications and allow both the patient and surgeon to enjoy a successful surgical outcome.

References

1. Borja F, Latta L, Stinchfield F, Obreron L. Abductor performance in total hip arthroplasty with and without trochanteric osteotomy. *Clin Orthop.* 1985;197:181–190.
2. Eftekhar N. *Total hip arthroplasty*. St. Louis: Mosby Publishing; 1993.
3. Minns RJ, Crawford B, Porter M, et al. Muscle strength following total hip replacement. *J Arthroplasty.* 1993;8:625–627.
4. Morrey BF. Instability after total hip replacement. *Orthop Clin North Am.* 1992;23:237–247.
5. Murray MP, Gore DR, Brewer BJ, Gardner GM, Sepic SB. Comparison of Müller total hip replacement with and without trochanteric osteotomy. *Acta Orthop Scand.* 1981;52:345–352.
6. Obrant K, Ringsberg K, Sanzen L. Decreased abduction strength after charnley hip replacement without trochanteric osteotomy. *Acta Orthop Scand.* 1989;60:305–307.
7. Ritter M, Groe T, Stringer E. Functional significance of nonunion of the greater trochanter. *Clin Orthop.* 1981;159:177–182.
8. Roberts J, Fu F, McClain E, Ferguson AB Jr. A comparison of the dislocated hip and anterolateral approach to total hip arthroplasty. *Clin Orthop.* 1984;187:205–210.
9. Robinson RP, Robinson HJ Jr, Salvati EA. Comparison of the transtrochanteric and posterior approaches for total hip replacement. *Clin Orthop.* 1980;147:143.
10. Strathy G, Fitzgerald R. Total hip arthroplasty in the ankylosed hip. *J Bone Joint Surg Am.* 1988;70:963–966.
11. Carlsson A, Gentz C. Postoperative dislocation in the Charnley and Brunswick total hip arthroplasty. *Clin Orthop.* 1977;125:177–182.

12. Charnley J, Cupic Z. Internal Publication No. 46, Center for Hip Surgery, Wrightington Hospital: England, 1974.
13. Coventry M. Late dislocations in patients with Charnley total hip arthroplasty. *J Bone Joint Surg Am.* 1985;67:832–841.
14. Fackler CD, Poss R. Dislocation in total hip arthroplasty. *Clin Orthop.* 1980;151:169–178.
15. Kaplan S, Thomas W, Poss R. Trochanteric advancement for recurrent dislocation after total hip replacement. *J Arthroplasty.* 1987;2:119–124.
16. Kristiansen B, Jorgensen L, Holmich P. Dislocation following total hip arthroplasty. *Arch Orthop Trauma Surg.* 1985;103:375–377.
17. Lindberg H, Carlsson A, Gentz C, Pettersson H. Recurrent and non-recurrent dislocation following total hip arthroplasty. *Acta Orthop Scand.* 1982;53:947–952.
18. McCollum D, Gray W. Dislocation after total hip arthroplasty. *Clin Orthop.* 1990;261:159–170.
19. Vicar A, Coleman C. A comparison of the anterolateral, transtrochanteric, and posterior surgical approaches in primary total hip arthroplasty. *Clin Orthop.* 1984;188:153–159.
20. Williams J, Gottesman M, Mallory T. Dislocation after total hip arthroplasty. *Clin Orthop.* 1982;171:53–58.
21. Woo R, Morrey B. Dislocations after total hip arthroplasty. *J Bone Joint Surg Am.* 1982;64:1295–1306.
22. McLeish RD, Charnley J. Abduction forces in the one legged stance. *J Biomech.* 1970;3:191–209.
23. Bully R, Huo M, Root L, Binzer T, Wilson PD Jr. Total hip arthroplasty in cerebral palsy. *Clin Orthop.* 1993;296:148–153.
24. Root L, Goss J, Mendes J. Treatment of painful hip in cerebral palsy by total hip arthroplasty or hip arthrodesis. *J Bone Joint Surg Am.* 1986;68:590–598.
25. Benton L, Salvati E, Root L. Reconstructive surgery in the myelomenigocele hip. *Clin Orthop.* 1975;110:261–268.
26. Brewster R, Coventry M, Johnson E. Conversion of the arthrodesed hip to a total hip arthroplasty. *J Bone Joint Surg Am.* 1975;57:27–30.
27. Lubahn J, Evarts M, Feltner J. Conversion of ankylosed hips to total hip arthroplasty. *Clin Orthop.* 1980;153:147–152.
28. Reikeras O, Bjerkheim I, Gundersson R. Total hip arthroplasty for arthrodesed hips. *J Arthroplasty.* 1995;10:529–531.
29. Crowe J, Mani J, Ranawat C. Total hip replacement in congenital dislocation and dysplasia of the hip. *J Bone Joint Surg Am.* 1979;61:15–23.
30. Herold HZ. Congenital dislocation of the hip treated by total hip arthroplasty. *Clin Orthop.* 1989;242:195–200.
31. Linde F, Jensen J. Socket loosening in arthroplasty for congenital dislocation of the hip. *Acta Orthop Scand.* 1988;59:254–257.
32. Baker AS, Bitounis VC. Abductor function after total hip replacement. *J Bone Joint Surg Br.* 1989;71:47–50.
33. Glassman AH. Complications of trochanteric osteotomy. *Orthop Clin North Am.* 1992;23:321–333.
34. Fraser GA, Wroblewski BM. Revision of the Charnley low-friction arthroplasty. *J Bone Joint Surg Br.* 1991;63:552–555.
35. Boardman K, Bocco F, Charnley J. An evaluation method of trochanteric fixation using three wires in the Charnley low-friction arthroplasty. *Clin Orthop.* 1978;132:31–38.
36. Amstutz H, Maki S. Complications of trochanteric osteotomy in total hip replacement. *J Bone Joint Surg Am.* 1978;60:214–216.
37. Amstutz HC, Mai LL, Schmidt I. Results of interlocking wire trochanteric reattachment and technique refinements to prevent complications following total hip arthroplasty. *Clin Orthop.* 1984;183:82–89.
38. Johnston RC. Clinical follow up of total hip replacement. *Clin Orthop.* 1973;95:118–126.
39. Nutton R, Checketts R. The effects of trochanteric osteotomy of abductor power. *J Bone Joint Surg Br.* 1984;64:180–183.
40. Simon S. Anatomy, physiology and mechanics of skeletal muscle. In: *Orthopedic Basic Science.* Am Acad Orthop Surg. 1994;106.
41. Dorr LD, Wolf AW, Chandler R, Conaty JP. Classification and treatment of dislocation of total hip arthroplasty. *Clin Orthop.* 1983;173:151–158.
42. Ecklund A. Trochanteric osteotomy for recurrent dislocation of total hip arthroplasty. *J Arthroplasty.* 1993;8:629–632.
43. Lombardi V, Mallory T, Kraus T, Vaughn B. Preliminary report on the S-ROM constraining acetabular insert. *Orthop.* 1991;14:297–303.
44. Besser MI. A muscle transfer to replace absent abductors in the conversion of a fused hip to a total hip arthroplasty. *Clin Orthop.* 1982;162:173–174.
45. Enneking WF. *Musculoskeletal tumor surgery.* New York: Churchill Livingstone. 1983;559.

69
Fractures after Total Hip Replacement

Mitchell H. Geiger, Merrill A. Ritter, John B. Meding, and Philip M. Faris

The treatment of a femur fracture in a total hip patient is one of the most challenging situations the total hip surgeon may encounter. The most critical factor in determining the best treatment method is the stability of the hip prosthesis.[1-9] Other considerations include the level of the fracture, the fracture pattern, the general health of the patient, and the functional goals of the patient. Whether operative or nonoperative treatment is chosen, poor functional results are likely to occur when a prosthesis is left loose at the time of fracture treatment.[1-9] In this situation, the most consistent satisfactory results have been obtained by fracture stabilization with a well-fixed revision long-stem femoral prosthesis.[1,4,5,6,10,11]

Periprosthetic Femoral Fracture Classification

Periprosthetic femur fractures can be classified by the region of the femur at which the fracture occurred.[1,10,11,12] Proximal fractures occur at the level of the prosthesis, middle fractures occur about the level of the prosthetic tip, and distal fractures occur below the prosthesis. Kelley reviewed seven different classifications of periprosthetic femur fractures and concluded that none adequately predicted treatment outcome because they failed to include fracture pattern, fracture stability or displacement, and prosthesis loosening along with the fracture level. Proximal and middle region fractures are strongly associated with prosthesis loosening, although loosening may not occur until after the fracture has healed.[2,3,4,9,10,13,14] Therefore any proximal or middle region periprosthetic fracture should raise a high index of suspicion of eventual prosthesis loosening. Fractures distal to the prosthesis, while not associated with prosthesis loosening, are still a challenge to treat and avoid complications.[2,3,10,15]

Treatment

Nonoperative Treatment

Nonoperative treatment of fractures about a hip prosthesis involves restricted weight-bearing, traction, a spica cast, or a fracture brace, depending on the clinical circumstances.[2,3,4,7,8,10,13] Table 69.1 summarizes the results of six studies that included nonoperative treatment of periprosthetic femur fractures. These studies show that nonoperative treatment usually produces fracture healing, but complications are common. For example, Johansson et al.[4] observed fracture healing in 9 of 10 periprosthetic femur fractures treated nonoperatively; however, satisfactory results occurred in only 2 patients. Malunion, nonunion, and prosthesis loosening led to secondary operative procedures. McElfresh and Coventry[13] noted that in 4 of 6 patients with periprosthetic femur fractures treated nonoperatively, secondary operative procedures were required. Two studies that classified the prosthesis as loose or well-fixed at the time of fracture noted that, when nonoperative treatment was used in patients with a loose prosthesis, the results were unsatisfactory. In one study by Jensen et al.[3] unsatisfactory results occurred in 7 of 11 patients; and in another by Beals et al.,[10] unsatisfactory results occurred in five of five patients.

On the other hand, results of closed treatment for fractures associated with well-fixed hip prostheses vary with the level at which the fracture occurred.[1,2,4,10] Femur fractures that occur distal to a prosthesis may do well with closed treatment. Cooke et al.[2] reported satisfactory results in all 20 of the femur fractures that were distal to the prosthesis and treated closed, while Beals et al.[10] found satisfactory results in 7 of 7 distal femur fractures with ipsilateral hip prosthesis treated closed. Femur fractures that occur at the level of the prosthetic stem or at the prosthetic stem tip had variable results.

Table 69.1. Results of nonoperative treatment in the management of femur fractures about THRs.

Author (ref) year	n	Type	Satisfactory results	% Healed	Comp
Beals et al.[10] 1996	5	Loose Prosthesis	0/5		A
	11	fixed prosthesis		89%	
		FX about prosthesis	3/3		
		FX about tip of prosthesis	5/8		
		FX distal to prosthesis	7/7		
Bethea et al.[1] 1982	6	FX about prosthesis	1/6	6/6	B
	7	FX about tip of prosthesis	3/7	4/7	C
Cooke et al.[2] 1988	6	FX about fixed prosthesis	1/6	6/6	D
	12	FX about tip of prosthesis	5/12	8/10	E
	20	FX distal to prosthesis	20/20	20/20	F
Jenson et al.[3] 1988	11	FX about loose prosthesis	4/11	10/11	G
	26	FX about fixed prosthesis	13/26	24/24	H
Johansson et al.[4] 1981	2	FX about prosthesis	1/2	2/2	I
	7	FX about tip of prosthesis	0/7	6/7	J
	1	FX distal to prosthesis	1/1	1/1	K
Scott et al.[7] 1982	2	FX about tip of prosthesis	1/2	2/2	L
	2	FX distal to prosthesis	2/2	2/2	M

Complications: A: 45% malunion, 11% nonunion, 19% prosthesis loosening. B: 4/6 painful prosthesis loosening, 1/6 malunion. C: 3/7 nonunions, 1/7 painful loose prosthesis. D: 5/6 prosthesis loosening. E: 2/12 death, 3/12 nonunion, 2/12 malunion. F: none. G: 1/11 nonunion, 2/11 painful loosening. H: 2/26 death, 1/24 prosthesis loosening. I: 1/2 prosthesis loosening. J: 7/7 prosthesis loose preop, painful after fx healing, 2/7 malunion, 1/7 nonunion. K: none. L: 1/2 malunion. M: none

Johansson et al.[4] had only 1 of 9 satisfactory results, Bethea et al[1] had 4 of 13 satisfactory results, Cooke et al.[2] had 5 of 18 satisfactory results, Jensen et al.[3] had 13 of 24 satisfactory results, and Beals et al.[10] had 8 of 11 satisfactory results following nonoperative treatment of fractures either about the prosthetic stem or the stem tip. Complications may include malunion, delayed union, prosthesis loosening, bed sores, and death.[2,4,8,10,13,16]

There are several specific indications when nonoperative management may be the most appropriate form of treatment for a hip arthroplasty patient with a periprosthetic fracture. Often nondisplaced fractures that occur or are noted postoperatively are treated with restricted weight-bearing.[2,10] However, when a nondisplaced periprosthetic fracture is treated this way, a functionally unsatisfactory result may be expected if prosthesis loosening is noted by the time bony healing has occurred.[1,2,4,10] Occasionally during fracture healing, a loose uncemented femoral prosthesis will subside into a stable position and allow for a satisfactory result.[10] Frail health may create a significant risk to surgical treatment, but long periods of bed rest may create an equal danger to the patient.[10,11,12] Finally, if traction or casting cannot produce acceptable fracture alignment, a malunion or nonunion may necessitate surgery on the patient after all.

Operative Treatment

Open reduction and internal fixation (ORIF) of femur fractures about a hip prosthesis has been advocated by several surgeons claiming satisfactory results.[9,14,15] Table 69.2 summarizes the results of seven studies that included ORIF for the management of periprosthetic femur fractures. The fact that ORIF may refer to one of several surgical techniques makes comparison of results difficult. Techniques used to fix these fractures include AO plate and screw fixation, interfragmentary screw fixation, cerclage fixation, cortical bone graft struts and cerclage fixation, and Ogden or Dall-Miles plate fixation.[3,4,9,10,14,15] Some of the listed studies used only one method of fixation but were vague on describing the fracture pattern, while others used many techniques without specifying the indications for each technique. Despite these limitations, conclusions can certainly be made about the effectiveness of ORIF of periprosthetic femur fractures. Femur fractures associated with loose femoral prostheses do less well than fractures associated with well-fixed prostheses when treated by ORIF.[3,9,10,14] Jensen et al.[3] had only 4 of 11 satisfactory results after treatment of femur fractures associated with a loose femoral prosthesis by ORIF. In contrast, Jensen et al.[3] had 30 of 44 satisfactory results after treatment of femur fractures associated with a well-fixed femoral prosthesis by ORIF. Satisfactory results were obtained by Seroki et al.[16] in 7 of 10 periprosthetic femur fractures treated by ORIF with an AO 4.5 broad DC plate and screws. A minimum of 8 cortices fixation proximal and distal to the fracture were obtained in addition to lag screw fixation when possible. Screws were placed anterior or posterior to the prosthesis. Two failures due to prosthesis loosening and one failure due to fracture nonunion required revision with long-stem femoral prosthesis. Wang et al.[8] had satisfactory results in 5 of 6 periprosthetic femur fractures treated with Ogden plates. The one failure was due to prosthesis loosening and was successfully treated by revision with a long-stem femoral prosthesis. Zenni et al.[14] had satisfactory results in 15 of 19 periprosthetic femur fractures treated with an Ogden plate. Complications included nonunions and a second fracture distal to the plate. After multiple surgeries, Zenni et al.[14] had 17 of 19 satisfactory results. Beals et al.[10] had 7 of 13 satisfactory results with ORIF treatment. Jensen et al.[3] recommended against performing a staged ORIF with implant extraction followed by second stage reimplantation after healing based on the unsatisfactory results obtained in a series of 6 patients.

In summary, when a loose prosthesis is left in place without revision, ORIF of a periprosthetic femur fractures has an unacceptably low success rate. The variable results seen in the literature with ORIF imply that adequate stabilization of the fracture is critical. Figure 69.1 demonstrates a postoperative femur fracture treated by ORIF that progressed to malunion. Although concern has been raised regarding the need to avoid periosteal devitalization, in view of the fact that the endosteal blood flow has already been disrupted by the intramedullary prosthesis, fracture stabilization must be obtained.[17] Some have also recommended the routine use of cancellous bone graft to enhance healing.[6,18] In addition, cortical allograft struts fixed with cerclage wires appear to be an effective means of increasing femoral bone mass along with fracture stabilization.

Importance of Long-Stem Prostheses

Without a question the most consistent satisfactory results in the treatment of periprosthetic femur fracture utilize long-stem femoral revision.[1,3,4,5,10,11] Table 69.3 reviews the current literature regarding results of long-stem revision for periprosthetic femur fractures. Kelley[6] points out that when a long-stem prosthesis is used as an intramedullary fixation device, the combined nonunion, refracture, and revision rate is only 12% to 20%. Indeed, 20 of 92 long-stem revision cases we reviewed in the literature demonstrated unsatisfactory results. Beals et al.[10] reviewed 17 femur fractures with a loose prosthesis treated by femoral revision and fracture stabilization. This produced good or excellent results in 14 of 17 patients, although it is not clear that long-stem revision was performed in all revision cases. In contrast nonoperative treatment in a group of 5 patients with a loose prosthesis resulted in poor results in all 5 patients. Cemented revisions were found to do far less well than noncemented revisions. The nonunion rate was 31% for cemented and 3% for uncemented revisions. The rate of postrevision prosthesis loosening was 38% in the cemented revisions and 7% in the uncemented revisions, with an additional 18%

Table 69.2. Results of ORIF in the management of femur fractures about THRs.

Author (ref) year	n	Type	Satisfactory results	% Healed	Comp
Beals et al.[10] 1996	5	Loose prosthesis	0/0		
	11	Fixed prosthesis		83–90%	A
		FX about prosthesis	2/2		
		FX about tip of prosthesis	2/6		
		FX distal to prosthesis	2/6		
Bethea et al.[1] 1982	1	FX about prosthesis	1/1	1/1	B
	2	FX about tip of prosthesis	0/2	2/2	C
Jensen et al.[3] 1988	12	Loose prosthesis			
		Uncemented prosthesis	6/7	7/7	D
		Cemented	2/5		E
	46	Fixed prosthesis	30/46	35/44	F
Johansson et al.[4] 1981	1	FX distal to prosthesis	1/1	1/1	G
Seroki et al.[16] 1992	10	FX at or distal to prosthesis	7/10	9/10	H
Wang et al.[8] 1985	6	FX level unspecified	5/6	6/6	I
Zenni et al.[14] 1988	10	FX about prosthesis			
	9	FX distal to prosthesis	15/19	16/19	J

Complications: A: 17% nonunion with interfragmentary fixation (IF), 10% nonunion with plate fixation (PF), 0% malunion with IF, 7% malunion with PF, 33% new fracture with IF, 13% new fracture PF, 50% loose or painful prosthesis with IF, 13% loose prosthesis with PF. B: none. C: 2/2 painful loose prostheses preoperative had pain postoperative, but because of poor health, functional goals were limited. D: 1/7 loosening. E: 3/5 refracture or nonunion. F: 2 deaths, 9 nonunions, 4 refractures, 1 late prosthesis loosening. G: none. H: 2 prosthesis loosening later required revision, 1 nonunion. I: loose prosthesis noted at surgery required later revision. J: 3/19 nonunions, 1 new fracture.

Figure 69.1 This 86-year-old man underwent revision THR using an impaction bone grafting technique with a collarless, polished, tapered stem (A, preoperative and B, postoperative). Note cerclage wire placed about midshaft of the femur to reinforce mechanically weak bone. No fracture was noted at surgery. C. Twelve months postoperative he fell and sustained a transverse fracture through osteoporotic bone. The fracture was stabilized using an Ogden plate, with screws and cerclage bands. D. The stem was judged to be stable at the time of surgery. The fixation failed. E. Fortunately, the fracture healed, although in varus deformity. Two years postsurgery, he is painfree and ambulating.

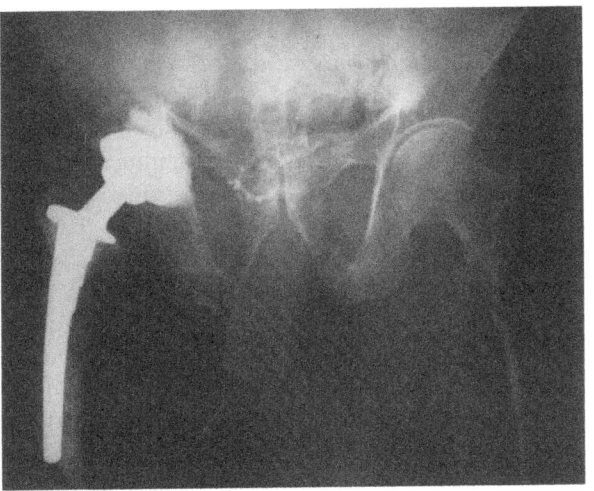
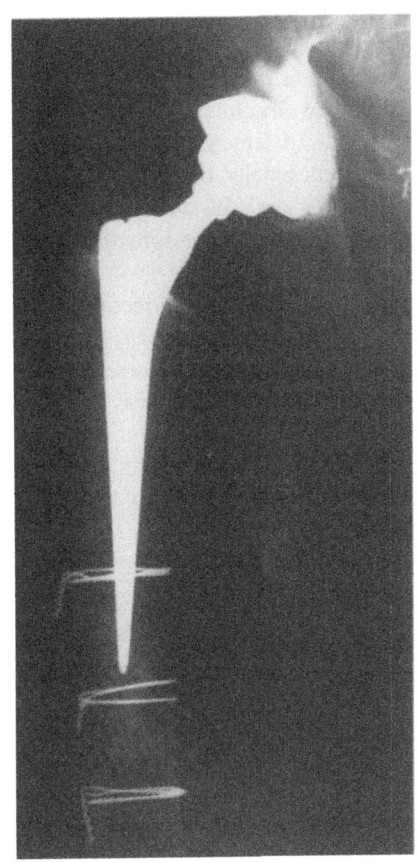
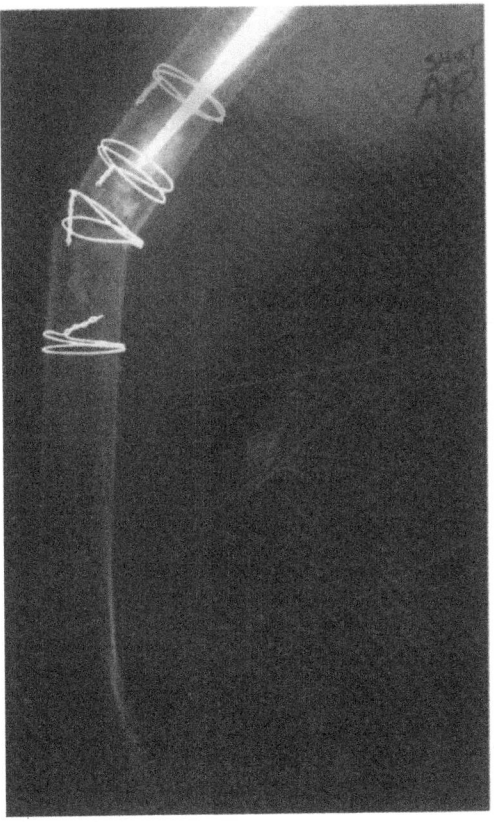
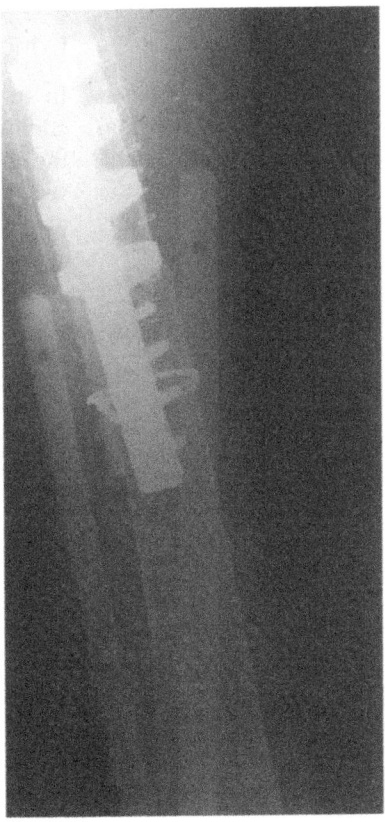
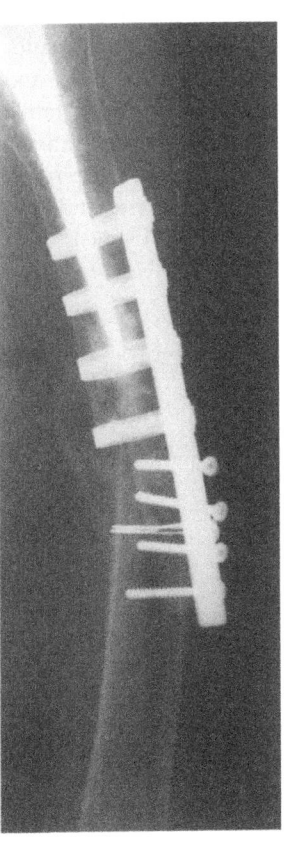

of uncemented revisions undergoing stable subsidence. Although failure of fracture fixation was not noted in either cemented or uncemented revisions, a new fracture occurred in 15% of cemented revisions and 7% of uncemented revisions. Finally, the rate of sepsis was 8% for cemented revisions and 3% for uncemented revisions.[10] Fredin et al.[11] reviewed 6 periprosthetic femur fractures stabilized with a long-stem revision, and all 6 had satisfactory results. In contrast, nonoperative management of periprosthetic femur fractures was successful only in a stress fracture and failed in 3 cases. The hospital stay of patients treated nonoperatively was 3.6 times longer than those treated with revision to a long-stem prosthesis.

Bethea et al.[1] found that revision to a long-stem prosthesis uniformly allowed fracture healing. Fifteen of 16 fractures treated with long-stem revision had satisfactory results. The single failure in treatment with a long-stem prosthesis was due to cementing the distal fragment with the fracture in distraction. Of 6 fractures proximal to the prosthetic tip treated nonoperatively, 5 fractures healed, but 3 required stem revision due to pain and prosthetic loosening. Jensen et al.[3] also found that the best results for the treatment of a periprosthetic femur fracture associated with a loose prosthesis were attained after revision to a long-stem prosthesis, while traction was equally effective to long-stem revision when the prosthesis was well fixed. Kavanagh[5] recommended that, if a periprosthetic fracture occurs about a loose prosthesis, revision with a long-stem prosthesis provides the best results. In addition, cortical allograft bone, cerclage wires, and plates may be helpful in providing maximum stability. Kelly[6] noted that revision rates after nonoperative treatment of fractures proximal to the prosthetic tip result in subsequent revision in 50% to 100% of cases and a nonunion rate for fractures at the tip of the prosthesis of 25% to 42%. Kelly[6] recommends extramedullary augmentation of long-stem prosthetic intramedullary fixation any time stability is questioned. Figure 69.2 demonstrates a periprosthetic femur fracture treated successfully by revision to a long-stem prosthesis with extramedullary augmentation.

Although revision about hip fractures with a long-stem prosthesis can be performed with or without cement,[1,3,4,10,11] there are a number of drawbacks to the use of cement in this setting. First, long-stem cemented prostheses do less well in the revision fracture situation than do long-stem uncemented prostheses, as noted in the study by Beals et al.[10] Second, extrusion of cement through the fracture site can interfere with fracture healing and result in soft tissue irritation.[10,19] Third, the presence of cement in the distal femur complicates future revisions. Fourth, cementing the prosthesis not only prevents dynamic compression at the fracture site, but care must also be taken to avoid fixing the prosthesis with the fracture in distraction.[1] Finally, Dohmae et al.[20] have shown that the shear strength at the cement–bone interface in a cemented revision femur is only 20% of the shear strength of a primary cemented prosthesis. This is apparently due to the loss of the interdigitating bone microstructure. Even more striking, the shear strength of a second revision is only 6.8% of a primary cemented femoral implant.[20] Thus the use of a cement prosthesis in revision periprosthesis fracture surgery appears to be less desirable.[10,20,21]

Conclusion

In summary, several studies have found that the best clinical results in the treatment of a loosened hip prosthesis associated with a femur fracture utilize prosthesis revision and fracture fixation with a noncemented long-stem femoral component that bypasses the fracture

Table 69.3. Results of revision THA in the management of femur fractures about THRs.

Author (ref) year	n	Type	Satisfactory results	% Healed	Comp
Beals et al.[10] 1996	17	Loose prosthesis	13/17		A
	11	Fixed prosthesis		(69% cement)	
		FX about prosthesis	2/2	(97% uncemented)	
		FX about tip of prosthesis	11/16		
		FX distal to prosthesis	0		
Bethea et al.[1] 1982	10	FX about prosthesis	10/10	15/16	B
	6	FX distal to prosthesis	5/6		
Fredin et al.[11] 1987	6	FX about prosthesis or tip	6/6	6/6	C
Jenson et al.[3] 1988	16	Loose prosthesis	11/16	NA	D
	11	Fixed prosthesis	12/16	NA	

Complications: A: Uncemented Rev. 3% nonunion, 7% new fracture, 7% loosening, 3% sepsis, 7% shortening; Cemented Rev. 31% nonunion, 15% new fracture, 38% loosening, 8% sepsis, 8% dislocation. B: 1/16 nonunion due to cementation in distraction. C: none. D: Not available (NA)

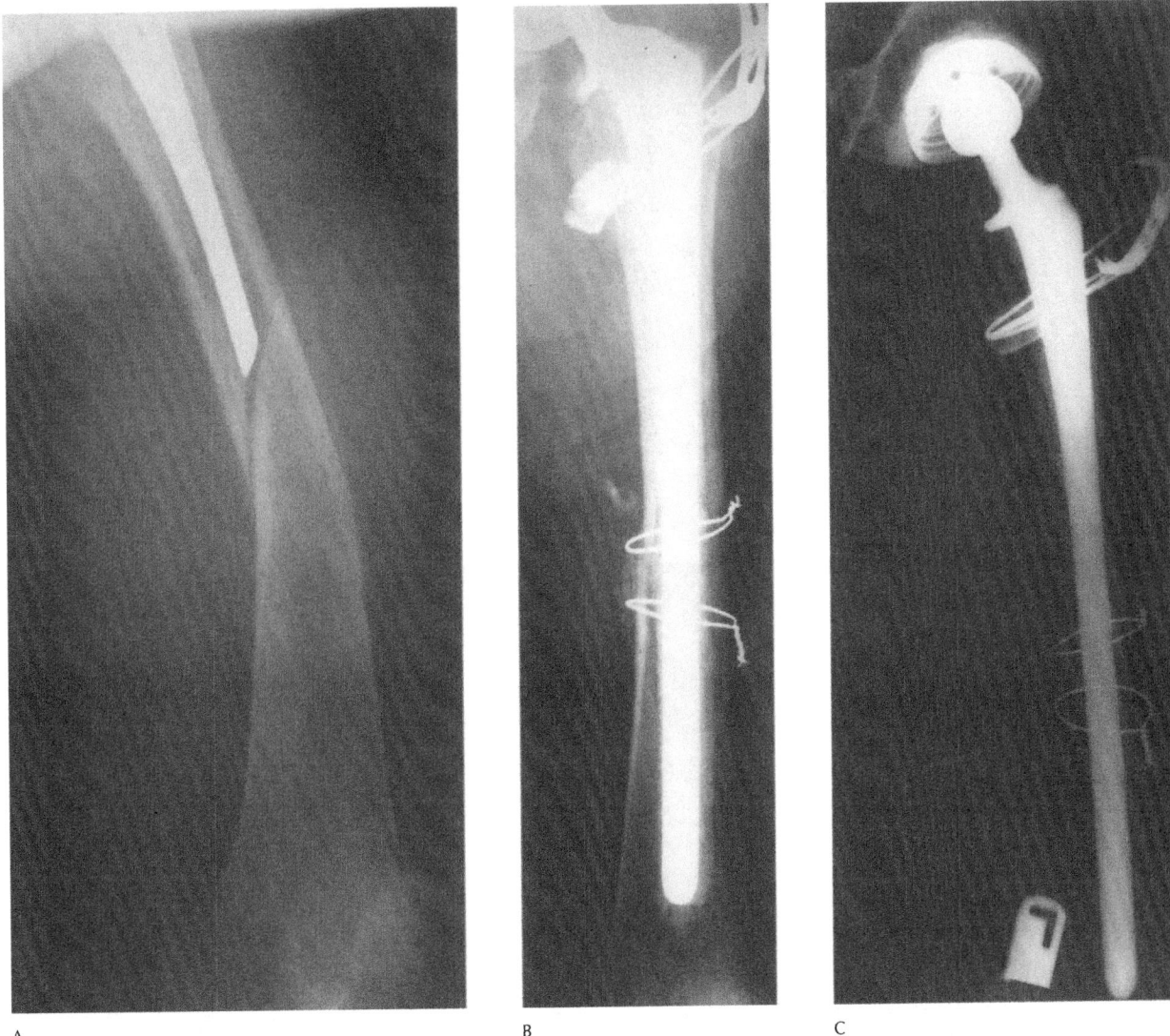

Figure 69.2 A. This 74-year-old man, a nursing home patient, presented with a femur fracture distal to the tip of a press-fit Austin Moore prosthesis, 4 months after being treated for a femoral neck fracture. B. He underwent prosthesis revision and fracture fixation with a cemented long-stem prosthesis. C. At 16 months follow-up he was ambulating with a walker.

site by at least two diameters of the femur.[1,3,4,10,11,19,22] Occasionally structural stability must be attained with extramedullary augmentation.[6] Femur fractures occurring in association with a well-fixed prosthesis may be treated by ORIF.[1,3,4,9,10,14,15] Satisfactory results can be anticipated if standard principles of fracture stabilization are attended to. Supplementary bone graft is advised. However, late loosening of the prosthesis may require further operative intervention.[3,9,10,14] Finally, in many nondisplaced fractures, restricted weight-bearing or operative intervention with cerclage permits fracture healing and a satisfactory outcome if component stability is attained.[2,10] The use of traction or spica casts to treat periprosthetic fractures has a role, but complications such as malunion, nonunion, prosthesis loosening, bed sores and death are common.[2,4,10]

Periprosthetic Acetabular Fractures

The literature is sparse on the topic of postoperative periprosthetic acetabular fractures. McElfresh et al.[19] described a displaced acetabular fracture about a cemented acetabular component that failed. The authors found the hip to be septic, which they presumed occurred prior to the injury. The loose component was unsalvageable and

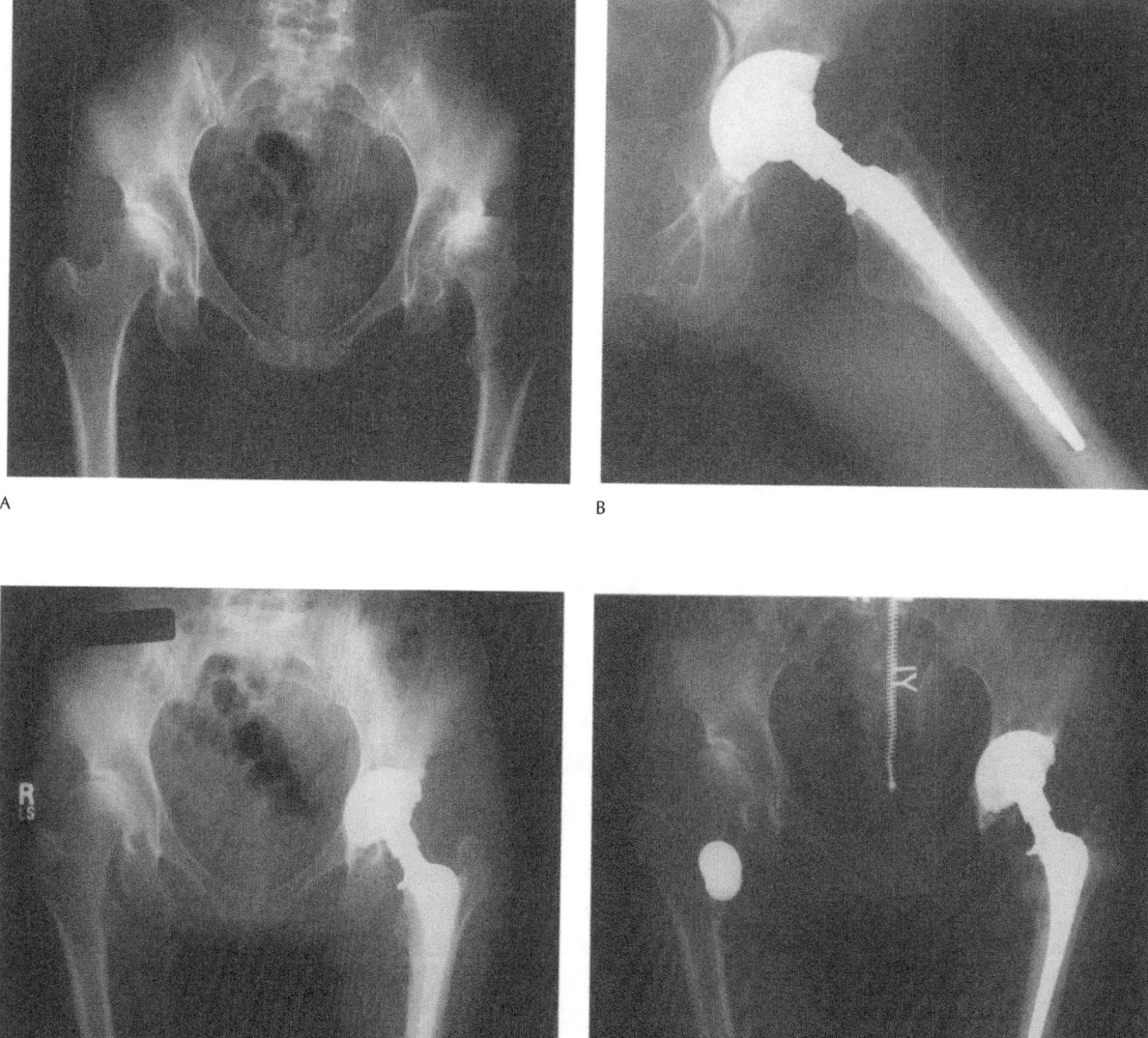

Figure 69.3 This 54-year-old female underwent a hybrid THA for arthritis associated with developmental dysplasia of the hip. B. Oblique pelvis x-rays obtained postoperative day 2 after the patient fell out of bed demonstrate a displaced acetabular fracture. C. Note that the extent of fracture displacement could not be appreciated on AP pelvis x-ray. D. The fracture healed with restricted weight-bearing. At 12 months follow up the patient is ambulating painfree and there is no evidence for acetabular component loosening.

an excisional arthroplasty was performed. Miller,[15] Ranawat et al.,[23] and Dandy[24] have described other cases of medial wall periprosthetic acetabular erosion resulting in fracture. Kim et al.[9] have demonstrated that intraoperative acetabular fractures may be common when oversized press-fit acetabular components are inserted. They also demonstrated that some fractures are difficult to identify on x-ray. We noted one case of a displaced acetabular fracture about a press-fit acetabular component after the patient fell on postoperative day 2. This fracture was successfully treated with restricted weight-bearing (Fig. 69.3). On the other hand, Romness et al.[22] have noted that total hip replacements performed for arthritis following an acetabular fracture have an unusually high rate of acetabular component loosening. Periprosthetic acetabular fractures should be approached with a high index of suspicion for acetabular component loosening. Component stability, fracture pattern, as well as the functional demands and general health of the patient help dictate the most appropriate approach to periprosthetic fracture care.

References

1. Bethea JS III, DeAndrade JR, Fleming LL, Lindenbaum SD, Welch RB. Proximal femoral fractures following total hip arthroplasty. *Clin Orthop.* 1982;170:95–106.
2. Cooke PH, Newman JH. Fractures of the femur in relation to cemented hip prostheses. *J Bone Joint Surg Br.* 1988;70:386–389.
3. Jenson JS, Barfod G, Hansen D, Larsen E, Linde F, Menck H, et al. Femoral shaft fracture after hip arthroplasty. *Acta Orthop Scand.* 1988;59:9–13.
4. Johansson JE, McBroom R, Barrington TW, Hunter GA. Fracture of the ipsilateral femur in patients with total hip replacement. *J Bone Joint Surg Am.* 1981;63:1435–1442.
5. Kavanagh BF. Femoral fractures associated with total hip arthroplasty. *Orthop Clin North Am.* 1982;23:249–257.
6. Kelley SS. Periprosthetic femoral fractures. *J Am Acad Orthop Surg.* 1994;2:164–172.
7. Scott RD, Turner RH, Leitzes SM, Aufranc OE: Femoral fractures in conjunction with total hip replacement. *J Bone Joint Surg Am.* 1975;57:494–501.
8. Wang GJ, Miller TO, Stamp WG. Femoral fracture following hip arthroplasty. *J Bone Joint Surg Am.* 1985;67:956–958.
9. Kim YS, Callaghan JJ, Ahn PB, Brown TD. Fractures of the acetabulum during insertion of an oversized hemispherical component. *J Bone Joint Surg Am.* 1995;77:111–117.
10. Beals RK, Tower SS. Periprosthetic fractures of the femur. *Clin Orthop.* 1996;327:238–246.
11. Fredin HO, Lindberg H, Carlsson AS. Femoral fracture following hip arthroplasty. *Acta Orthop Scand.* 1987;58:20–22.
12. Booth RE, Balderston RA, Rothman RH. *Total Hip Arthroplasty.* Philadelphia: WB Saunders, 1988.
13. Missakian JL, Rand JA. Fracture of the femoral shaft adjacent to long stem femoral components of total hip arthroplasty: report of seven cases. *Orthopedics.* 1993;16:149–152.
14. Zenni EJ Jr, Pomeroy DL, Caudle RJ. Ogden plate and other fixations for fractures complicating femoral endoprostheses. *Clin Orthop.* 1988;231:83–90.
15. Miller AJ. Late fractures of the acetabulum after total hip replacement. *J Bone Joint Surg Br.* 1972;54:600–606.
16. Serocki JH, Chandler RW, Dorr LD: Treatment of fractures about hip prostheses with compression plating. *J Arthroplasty.* 1992;7:129–135.
17. Petty W. *Total joint replacement. Total hip arthroplasty: complications.* Philadelphia: W.B. Saunders Company, 1991;291–299.
18. Scott RD, Schilz JP, et al. Femoral fracture and revision arthroplasty. In: Turner RH, Scheller AD, ed. *Revision total hip.* New York: Grune & Stratton; 1982:133–145.
19. McElfresh EC, Coventry MB. Femoral and pelvic fractures after total hip arthroplasty. *J Bone Joint Surg Am.* 1974;56:483–492.
20. Dohmae Y, Bechtold JE, Sherman RE, Puno RM, Gustilo RB. Reduction in cement-bone interface shear strength between primary and revision arthroplasty. *Clin Orthop.* 1988;236:214–220.
21. Hungerford DS, Jones LC. The rationale of cementless revision of cemented arthroplasty failures. *Clin Orthop.* 1988;235:12–24.
22. Romness DW, Lewallen DG. Total hip arthroplasty after fracture of the acetabulum. *J Bone Joint Surg Br.* 1990;72:761–764.
23. Ranawat CS, Greenberg R. Tripartite fracture of the acetabulum after total hip arthroplasty: a case report. *Clin Orthop.* 1981;155:48–51.
24. Dandy DJ, Theodorou BC. The management of local complications of total hip replacement by the McKee-Farrar technique. *J Bone Joint Surg Br.* 1975;57:30–35.

70
Protrusio Acetabuli

Michael J. Chmell and Richard D. Scott

Protrusio acetabuli is the migration of the femoral head along the femoral neck axis, medially and proximally, through the medial acetabular wall into the pelvis. This deformity results from excessive stresses upon the medial cortical bone of the acetabulum. Successful reconstruction of protrusio requires reestablishment of the hip center of rotation to its anatomic position, restoration of medial acetabular bone loss, and redirection of stresses away from the medial wall of the acetabulum toward its intact periphery.

Definition and Etiology

Medial and proximal migration of the femoral head into the pelvis has been termed *protrusio acetabuli*. Radiographically this is noted as migration of the femoral head medial to Kohler's line (ilioischial line) on an anteroposterior view of the pelvis.[1,2,3]

Many etiologies for this type of deformity exist. It may be associated with inflammatory arthritis, with over 14% of patients with rheumatoid arthritis involving the hips demonstrating acetabular protrusion.[4] Other forms of inflammatory arthritis, including juvenile rheumatoid arthritis and ankylosing spondylitis, are sometimes associated with protrusio acetabuli. Metabolic and mechanical disorders of bone may also lead to acetabular protrusion. Among these diagnoses are rickets, osteomalacia, osteogenesis imperfecta, and Paget's disease.[2,5,6,7]

In a series of 182 patients with protrusio acetabuli undergoing primary total hip arthroplasty, Sotelo-Garza noted that 18.7% had rheumatoid arthritis and 4.4% had Paget's disease.[5] The remaining 75% of the patients were diagnosed as having idiopathic protrusio. It is likely that the majority of these patients had osteoarthritis with primarily medial femoral head migration, as is noted in roughly 20% of cases with osteoarthritis.[8]

Osteoarthritis thus represents the most common underlying diagnosis in patients with protrusio who undergo total hip arthroplasty and should not be confused with patients having primary protrusio acetabuli. These patients are typically females over the age of 40 with bilateral, often symmetric, progression of protrusio as a primary deformity leading to restriction of motion, degenerative changes, and increasing pain.[9] Finally, protrusio may be caused by an acute traumatic event or the resultant deformity following acetabular trauma such as a central fracture dislocation of the hip.

A common pathway is responsible for this deformity's development and progression regardless of the specific patient diagnosis. Forces exceeding the bone's endurance limit are transmitted to the medial wall of the acetabulum, resulting in stress fracture, medial femoral head migration, and bony remodelling. This phenomenon is seen radiographically as progressive medial and proximal migration of the femoral head along the femoral neck axis relative to the ilioischial line, often with the laying down of new bone on the inner surface of the pelvis. In severe cases the medially-directed loads may ultimately exceed the bone's remodelling capacity, resulting in fragmentation and a bony defect. This process may continue until contact of the greater trochanter with the pelvis presents further migration.

In any disorder in which bone mass or strength is compromised for any reason, such as steroid induced osteopenia, metabolic bone disease, or Paget's disease, this process may be initiated under physiologic loading conditions. At the other extreme are cases of trauma, in which the medial wall acutely fails due to excessive force acting upon normal bone. In the majority of patients with acetabular protrusio and osteoarthritis, the deformity likely results from a combination of increased medially directed loads secondary to alterations in normal hip biomechanics due to peripheral osteophyte formation, altered motion, and articular cartilage loss, combined with variable degrees of diminished bone mass and strength due to age-related osteoporosis.

Patient Evaluation and Preoperative Planning

In evaluating a candidate for total hip arthroplasty with protrusio acetabuli, consideration must first be given to the potential causes for the deformity, as these may impact upon the patient's general health, anesthetic management, long-term functional status, and prosthetic durability. An assessment should initially be made as to the degree of deformity present, the status of bone stock, and the potential means of restoring normal hip biomechanics.

The distance the femoral head migrates medially perpendicular to Kohler's line can be measured on a standard anteroposterior pelvic radiograph and provides a simple method of quantitating the magnitude and progression of acetabular protrusio.[3] Similarly, an increase in the center-edge angle of Wiberg can be followed radiographically.

Edelstein has described an alternative radiographic method using the ilioischial line and the acetabular line.[1,2] The acetabular line is the laterally concave medial cortical wall of the acetabulum as visualized on an anteroposterior pelvic radiograph. In males, the acetabular line has been found, on average, to be 2 mm lateral to the ilioischial, line whereas in females the acetabular line is 1 mm medial to the ilioischial line. Using this method, protrusio acetabuli is said to be present in males when the acetabular line is 3 mm or more medial to the ilioischial line and 6 mm or more medial in females. These measurements can be used to document and follow the degree of severity of protrusio.

In planning for total hip arthroplasty in patients with protrusio, an assessment must next be made as to the quality and quantity of pelvic bone stock and as to the presence of any additional deformity that could compromise the reconstruction. Because the prime deforming forces in acetabular protrusion are along the axis of the femoral neck, the resulting deformity is usually a contained medial and proximal defect. In this situation a standard battery of pelvic and hip radiographs will suffice to confirm an intact acetabular rim and columns. In special circumstances where additional defects or deformity are suspected or are present, evaluation should include Judet views of the pelvis and computed tomography. This is of particular importance in posttraumatic deformity in order to adequately define the entire injury complex.

In evaluating these imaging studies, the main assessment to be made is whether adequate peripheral bone contact can be achieved utilizing a hemispherical acetabular component such that initial stability of the prosthesis will result. Conversely, if such contact and stability cannot be accomplished due to a superior or columnar deficiency, this other deformity should become the primary focus of attention. Planning would then proceed toward dealing with this deformity first, followed by reconstruction of the protrusio defect, as will be described.

Finally, attention must still be given to the femoral side of the hip joint. Because the protrusio deformity often has a component of proximal migration as well as medial migration, restoration of the acetabulum to an anatomic position will result in relative lengthening of the extremity following arthroplasty. This fact must be incorporated into the planning for femoral arthroplasty in terms of neck resection level and prosthetic neck length for equalization of leg lengths. Also, femoral head/trochanteric offset must be maintained in order to optimize abductor strength, stability, and prosthetic range of motion.[10]

Surgical Reconstruction

Treatment Rationale

Individuals with acetabular protrusio come to total hip arthroplasty with the primary goal of pain relief. Although this goal is readily attainable initially, maintaining this status on a long-term basis via durable fixation of the acetabulum can be a problem. As has been noted, acetabular protrusion results from, and progresses due to, an imbalance between medially directed loads and the strength and remodelling capacity of the medial acetabular wall. Thus, additional goals when reconstructing a protrusio defect must include a transfer of loads to the intact peripheral portions of the acetabulum with restoration of the medial bony defect in order to provide lasting acetabular fixation.

Johnston has calculated that medial, inferior, and anterior placement of a prosthetic acetabulum will minimize prosthetic loads due to shortening of the body weight's lever arm and lengthening of the musculotendinous lever arms across the hip joint.[11] This theoretical analysis, however, is not generally applicable to protruded hips because the existing medial bony insufficiency may be inadequate to withstand these loads. Further, Crowninshield has studied acetabular protrusio using finite element analysis and has found that medial placement of the acetabulum results in increased medial cortical stresses when compared to lateral anatomic placement of the cup.[12] Thus, the acetabular component of a total hip replacement should be restored to an anatomic position such that forces will be directed to the ilium, ischium, and pubis, and away from the medial cortical wall.

Treatment Methods

Initial series of total hip replacements in cases of acetabular protrusion utilized cemented all-polyethylene acetabuli. Historically a variety of methods and materials, including medial cup placement, excess cement, wire mesh, and bone grafting, have been utilized to address the medial bony deficiency present in protrusio acetabuli.[5,6,7,13,14,15]

Ranawat reported on 35 total hip arthroplasties done in patients with rheumatoid arthritis and protrusio acetabuli utilizing cemented all-polyethylene cups without wire mesh or medial bone graft support.[15] At an average follow-up of 4.3 years, it was noted that in the 18 hips in which the acetabulum was restored to within 5 mm of its anatomic position, no loosening or progression of bone/cement radiolucencies occurred. In 16 of 17 hips in which anatomic cup placement was not achieved, however, complete bone/cement demarcation was present radiographically. This is consistent with Crowninshield's findings as to the role of lateral, or anatomic, cup placement in decreasing stress levels borne by the medial acetabular wall following arthroplasty in hips with acetabular protrusio.

Wire mesh has been utilized as a means to reinforce the medial cement in cases of acetabular protrusion in an attempt to provide enhanced cement strength medially, as well as to facilitate cup positioning. Good results have been achieved in cases of protrusio with mild degrees of deformity using this technique. Jasty, however, has reported generally unsatisfactory results in terms of acetabular component loosening in cases with medial cortical defects of a centimeter or more, and has advocated the use of alternative techniques when performing arthroplasty in hips with acetabular protrusion.[6] Theoretically the use of wire mesh to provide increased medial cement strength may seem appealing. Failures when implanting cemented all-polyethylene cups for acetabular protrusio, however, generally result due to loosening at the bone/cement interface and cup migration rather than cement fracture. Increased cement strength and stiffness, therefore, should not necessarily improve on this, and main in fact cause poorer long-term fixation due to increased stress transmission to the bone–cement interface.

Bone grafting has also been utilized to provide an initial medial buttress at the time of cemented acetabular arthroplasty in order to restore the hip center to an anatomic location.[13,14,15] The potential for healing of this graft with restoration of medial acetabular bone stock is an additional benefit of this technique. Mendes has demonstrated the potential for bone grafts to heal beneath a layer of polymethylmethacrylate cement in both a dog model and in the clinical use of bone grafts to support cemented all-polyethylene acetabular components in cases of protrusio acetabuli.[14] Hirst, likewise, reported on 61 hips with protrusio treated in this manner. At an average follow-up of over 4 years, there were no cases of recurrence of deformity and all grafts healed radiographically.[7]

Although bone graft has the capacity to heal beneath a cemented cup, the problem of persistent excessive medially directed forces in this situation is addressed only partially via lateral cup placement. Redirection of loads toward the intact portions of the pelvis is also desirable, but cannot be achieved with a cemented all-polyethylene cup. One means aimed at solving this problem is a variety of metal antiprotrusio shells, or cages.[16–19] Each of the varied designs of these devices incorporates flanges that rest on the external acetabular margins with the goal of force transmission to the intact ilium, ischium, and pubis. Such shells may either be cemented in place overlying the grafted acetabulum, or be fixed to the pelvis with screws. A polyethylene acetabular insert is then cemented into the metal shell.

Finite element analysis has demonstrated that the use of these anti-protrusio cups significantly decreases medial cortical bone stresses following arthroplasty when compared to an all-polyethylene acetabular component, even when each is placed in an anatomic position.[12] Several authors have reported excellent midterm clinical results using these devices with bone grafting in both primary and revision procedures to reconstruct protrusio defects.[16,18,19] Bone grafts appear radiographically to heal to the surrounding pelvis, as has been noted when using cemented acetabular cups. The long-term durability of fixation of the uncemented nonporous metal shell to the pelvis in these cases deserves continued follow-up.

A final alternative method for reconstructing a protrusio defect is the use of a bipolar hemiarthroplasty rather than a fixed socket acetabular component. When employing this technique, the acetabulum is reamed sequentially until its outer rim is engaged circumferentially. The protrusio defect is then filled with cancellous bone graft, which is reamed in reverse utilizing the final reamer that achieved rim contact in order to shape and compact the graft. Theoretically this technique transmits forces to the intact rim of the acetabulum, allows biological reconstruction of the bony defect, and avoids the issue of long-term acetabular loosening. The disadvantage of this method is the potential for recurrence of the deformity. Wilson has reported on the use of this technique in 22 hips with protrusio acetabuli followed for a mean of 54 months following bipolar hemiarthroplasty. Clinically, all hips demonstrated excellent results at follow-up. Five of the 22, however, exhibited greater than 3 mm of cup migration radiographically.[20,21] Additional follow-up of a larger population of such patients may provide information as to the role of bipolar hemiarthroplasty in the management of acetabular protrusion.

Current Treatment Recommendations

In the treatment of acetabular protrusio the hip center must be restored to its normal lateral position, medial stresses must be diminished, and the protrusio defect must be reconstituted. Currently most surgeons favor the use of a metal-backed porous-coated hemispherical acetabulum that is press-fit in an anatomic position via rim contact, with medial bone grafting in order to achieve these goals.

The hip is approached as per surgeon preference, the femoral neck is osteotomized, and the acetabulum is exposed. Great care must be taken to avoid femoral shaft fracture when dislocating the hip because the femoral head is often ankylosed to or captured by the acetabulum. It is often prudent to osteotomize the femoral neck in situ before dislocating. If necessary the protruded ankylosed head can be extracted by sectioning it into smaller pieces. The acetabulum is sequentially reamed in order to provide peripheral contact sufficient to achieve immediate acetabular component stability. The size of the final reamer is noted. The acetabulum does not need to be deepened, but a bleeding cancellous bony bed for graft placement is preferable to encourage healing of the graft to host bone. This graft placement is achieved by light reaming with an undersized reamer or the use of currettes or small drill holes.

All cartilage and sclerotic cortical bone is removed from the osteotomized femoral head. If there is a structural defect in the medial wall of the acetabulum, slices of the femoral head measuring about 2 mm in thickness are placed in the depths of the acetabulum in order to provide some initial mechanical support for subsequent bone graft placement. The remainder of the femoral head is morselized, gradually packed within the acetabulum, and reamed in reverse to pressurize and shape the graft (Fig. 70.1). In this manner a medial wall and hemispherical acetabulum is gradually developed. This process should be performed slowly, with the building up of layers of impacted cancellous bone, rather than all bone graft being added at once to the acetabulum. In this fashion the graft can be packed much more densely to form a more stable construct. If insufficient bone is available using the patient's femoral head, the iliac crest or curetted bone from the femoral canal may be obtained additionally. In general, fresh frozen

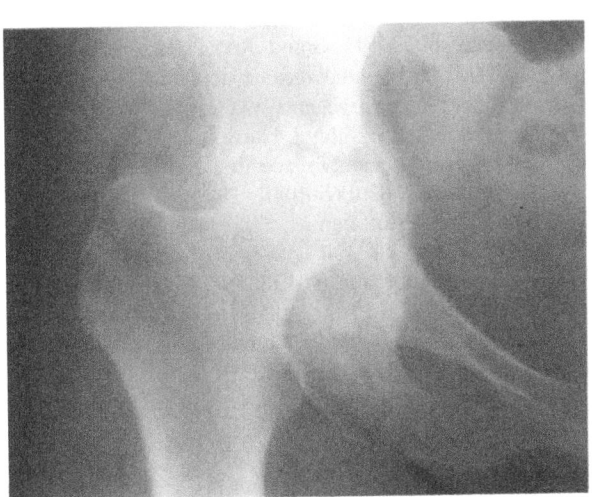
A

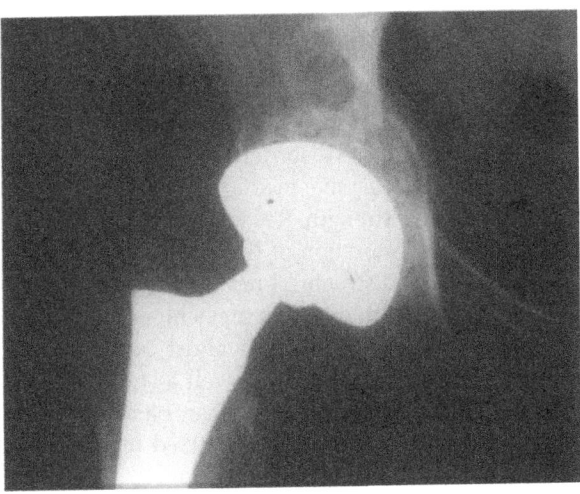
B

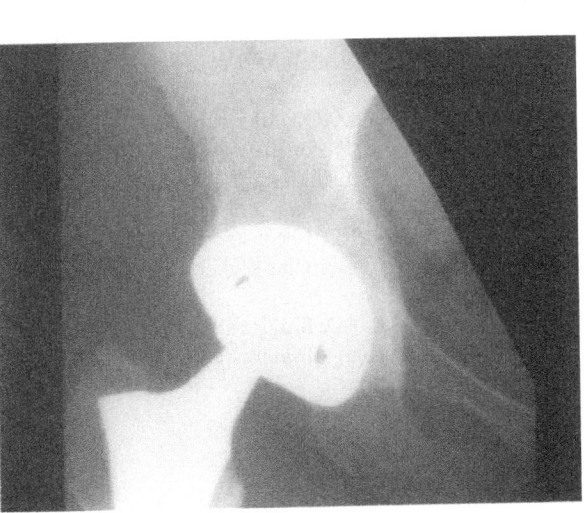
C

Figure 70.1. A. A preoperative radiograph in a 45-year-old female patient with rheumatoid arthritis demonstrates acetabular protrusion as well as cystic changes involving the superior acetabulum. B. Femoral head autograft was utilized to reconstruct the protrusio defect as described in the text, and was also used to fill the superior cyst, as seen on an immediate postoperative radiograph. C. At 3 months following surgery, excellent healing of the bone graft has occurred, maintaining the acetabular component in an anatomic position.

femoral head allografts are used rather than iliac crest graft in this situation as these patients' iliac crests often are poor sources of bone graft, and harvesting the graft can increase operative morbidity. Once the acetabular defect has been reconstituted with graft, an appropriate size metal-backed hemispherical cup is impacted in place and hip arthroplasty proceeds in a routine fashion. The size chosen is usually 2 mm larger than the final acetabular reamer used to achieve rim contact. Ancillary screw fixation is avoided if possible.

As has been noted, use of this technique is supported in terms of the need to restore the hip to its anatomic location as well as the need for bone grafting to reconstruct the medial protrusio defect. In addition, finite element analysis has demonstrated that a metal-backed hemispherical acetabulum reduces medial cortical stresses in much the same manner as has been noted for the antiprotrusio type devices.[12] Additionally, the biologic fixation achieved with a porous-coated acetabular component may provide the greatest possibility for successful long-term fixation, although no data is currently available to prove this assertion.

Conclusion

Various underlying disorders may result in protrusio acetabuli. Each of these disorders leads to a worsening deformity due to excessive medial acetabular loads relative to the bone's strength. Reconstruction of protrusio defects requires restoration of the anatomic position of the acetabulum and structural reconstitution of the medial bony defect, both of which are achieved with bone grafting. Medial cortical stresses must be reduced to achieve and maintain fixation as well as to prevent recurrent deformity. This reduction can be achieved via implantation of a peripherally well-fixed metal-backed porous acetabular component.

References

1. Armbruster TG, Guerra J, Resnick D, Goergen TG, Feingold ML, Niwayama G, et al. The adult hip: an anatomic study. I. The bony landmarks. *Radiology*. 1978;128:1–10.
2. Edelstein G, Murphy WA. Protrusio acetabuli: Radiographic appearance in arthritis and other conditions. *Arthritis Rheum*. 1983;26:1511–1516.
3. Hubbard MJ. The measurement of progression in protrusio acetabuli. *Am J Roentgenol Radium Ther Nucl Med*. 1969;106:506–508.
4. Hastings DE, Parker SM. Protrusio acetabuli in rheumatoid arthritis. *Clin Orthop*. 1975;108:76–83.
5. Sotelo-Garza A, Charnley J. The results of Charnley arthroplasty of the hip performed for protrusio acetabuli. *Clin Orthop*. 1978;132:12–18.
6. Jasty M, Harris WH. Results of total hip reconstruction using acetabular mesh in patients with central acetabular deficiency. *Clin Orthop*. 1988;142–149.
7. Hirst P, Esser M, Murphy JC, Hardinge K. Bone grafting for protrusio acetabuli during total hip replacement: a review of the Wrightington method in 61 hips. *J Bone Joint Surg Br*. 1987;69:229–233.
8. Resnick D. Patterns of migration of the femoral head in osteoarthritis of the hip. *Am J Roentgenol Radium Ther Nucl Med*. 1975;124:62–74.
9. Alexander C. The aetiology of primary protrusio acetabuli. *Br J Radiol*. 1965;38:567–580.
10. McGrory BJ, Morrey BF, Cahalan TD, An KN, Cabanela ME. Effect of femoral offset on range of motion and abductor muscle strength after total hip arthroplasty. *J Bone Joint Surg Br*. 1995;77:865–869.
11. Johnston RC, Brand RA, Crowninshield RD. Reconstruction of the hip: a mathematical approach to determine optimum geometric relationships. *J Bone Joint Surg Am*. 1979;61:639–652.
12. Crowninshield RD, Brand RA, Pedersen DR. A stress analysis of acetabular reconstruction in protrusio acetabuli. *J Bone Joint Surg Am*. 1983;65:495–499.
13. McCollum DE, Nunley J, Harrelson JM. Bone-grafting in total hip replacement for acetabular protrusion. *J Bone Joint Surg Am*. 1980;62:1065–1073.
14. Mendes DG, Roffman M, Silbermann M. Reconstruction of the acetabular wall with bone graft in arthroplasty of the hip. *Clin Orthop*. 1984;186:29–37.
15. Ranawat CS, Dorr LD, Inglis AE. Total hip arthroplasty in protrusio acetabuli of rheumatoid arthritis. *J Bone Joint Surg Am*. 1980;62:1059–1065.
16. Berry DJ, Muller ME. Revision arthroplasty using an antiprotrusio cage for massive acetabular bone deficiency. *J Bone Joint Surg Br*. 1992;74:711–715.
17. Oh I, Harris WH. Design concepts, indications, and surgical technique for use of the protrusio shell. *Clin Orthop*. 1982;162:175–184.
18. Rosson J, Schatzker J. The use of reinforcement rings to reconstruct deficient acetabula. *J Bone Joint Surg Br*. 1992;74:716–720.
19. Zehntner MK, Ganz R. Midterm results (5.5–10 years) of acetabular allograft reconstruction with the acetabular reinforcement ring during total hip revision. *J Arthroplasty*. 1994;9:469–479.
20. Wilson MG, Scott RD. Reconstruction of the deficient acetabulum using the bipolar socket. *Clin Orthop*. 1990;251:126–131.
21. Wilson MG, Scott RD. Bipolar socket in protrusio acetabuli: 3–6 year study. *J Arthroplasty*. 1993;8:405–411.

Part 7
Making Revision Hip Surgery Work

Joseph C. McCarthy and James V. Bono

This section deals with the future of revision total hip replacement. Over the last 30 years, great strides have been made in total hip replacement surgery. Each advance in technology or technique has introduced new problems and complications. The field of revision hip replacement surgery has had to adapt to the trends of primary hip surgery and to the stream of new complications that follow.

In an effort to control spending on medical care, we have been forced to examine how we plan care and manage costs. Hip replacement surgery can no longer be viewed as a purely surgical exercise. The surgical procedure plays only a part in the surgical event. Preoperative and postoperative care receive as much emphasis as the surgical procedure. Current efforts to maximize efficiency in revision total hip surgery are a result of imposed restrictions and critical self-examination. Our own experience at the New England Baptist Hospital is chronicled in the first chapter of this section. Over the last ten years, our institution has provided the highest volume of revision hip surgery in the Western Hemisphere. From 1984 through 1994, the average operating room case time has decreased from 5 hours, 30 minutes to 4 hours, 20 minutes, with similar decrease in blood loss during surgery (2800 cc to 1200 cc), and length of stay (26 days to 8.6 days). Further decreases in length of stay have continued to the present time, when patients are discharged typically on postop day 5. The interdisciplinary approach utilized at the New England Baptist Hospital is essential in maximizing efficiency while ensuring continued quality outcomes.

As hospital lengths of stay continue to decrease, preoperative patient preparation becomes increasingly important. Our appreciation of the importance of preoperative patient education is paying off. At the New England Baptist Hospital, a preoperative teaching class is available and recommended for all patients. In these classes, our physical therapy and nursing departments educate the patient on what to expect before, during, and after surgery so that they may be better prepared. Patients' expectations fall into line with the clinical pathways to provide a seamless, efficient continuum of care.

The use of outcome studies in total hip replacement surgery has just recently become appreciated. Outcome research enables clinicians and administrators to determine if the end justifies the means. We are indebted to those investigators providing quality orthopedic outcomes research who have validated the claim that hip replacement surgery improves health-related quality of life. If we are to continue to provide the highest quality care for our patients, we also must continue to document the effectiveness of our treatments using the validated outcome instruments.

Advances in total hip designs and materials have been a driving force in the evolution of hip replacement surgery. The goals of implant longevity, biological compatibility, and enhanced patient function drive the field of orthopedic biomechanics. The use of finite element analysis allows new ideas to be tested analytically prior to clinical trials and has become an invaluable tool to address clinical problems such as thigh pain following cementless total hip arthroplasty or cement cracking and debonding at the distal tip of the femoral component, which may play a role in the initiation of stem loosening. Advances in Co-Cr-Mo and titanium implant alloys, along with a better understanding of ultrahigh molecular weight polyethylene, offer hope that new materials and bearing surfaces will provide enhanced implant durability.

The final chapter of this section discusses removal of cement in total hip revision surgery using a robot. The ability to quickly and safely remove long cement columns in revision hip surgery using a CT guided robotic arm is quite appealing. The experience at the New England Baptist Hospital with the ROBODOC computer-integrated system for primary hip replacement procedures has been quite successful and has set the foundation for the revision application of this technology. The complexity of femoral revision surgery lends itself to robotic machining to remove old cement and prepare the new cavity. We look forward to developing ROBODOC as a valuable tool in revision hip surgery as we enter the 21st century.

71
Maximizing Efficiency in Revision Total Hip Surgery

Joseph C. McCarthy and Nancy L. Hiltz

Health care delivery is changing rapidly. With the federal health budget outpacing the consumer price index and a progressively aging population, the health care team has to confront and overcome great challenges. Despite rising patient medical acuity and diminishing resources, the health care team needs to maintain quality outcomes while providing cost-effective care. The well-informed patients often have increased expectations and the goal to remain more active and mobile throughout their life. Nowhere is this formidable challenge more evident than in revision total hip replacement.

In 1996, 532,532 total joint arthroplasties were performed in the United States at a cost of more than $300 million.[1] Of these total numbers, 265,203 were total hip replacements.[2] This number has more than doubled since the early 1980s. The number of revision hip surgeries has also increased during this time due to implant loosening, sepsis, and polyethylene wear with osteolysis. New technology, prosthetic design changes, and improved surgical techniques have diminished the risks associated with the operation as well as positively affected outcomes. But the work does not stop there. In school, physicians are taught pathophysiology and treatment of disease, however they now must know how to institute and carry out a treatment plan in the most cost effective and timely manner.

The federal government first became involved in trying to control spending on medical care in the early 1970s. From 1975 through 1987, Medicare spending for physicians' services grew at twice the Gross Domestic Product (GDP).[3] In 1985, Medicare established the Prospective Payment System (PPS) and Diagnosis Related Groups (DRG). The PPS not only changed the way in which care was paid for, but also forced us to examine how we plan care and manage costs. Despite this, expenditures continued to grow at 12% annually.[4] Next, the Physician Payment Review Commission (PPRC) was introduced to reform Medicare reimbursement to surgeons. The commission's conclusions were presented in the HSAIO Report that established the Resource Based Relative Value Scale (RBRVS) as a way to determine physician reimbursement. The scale identifies a formula for each procedure for reimbursement that includes total work, relative practice overhead, and the added cost associated with being a specialist.[5]

During the 1980s cost containment became the primary method used to reduce hospital costs. The strategy was to eliminate unnecessary hospital days and shift as much inpatient care as possible to an outpatient setting.

In 1991, Schwartz and Mendelson evaluated the effect of these cost containment methods on admissions and length of stay during the 1980s.[6] The findings suggested a significant reduction in hospital costs due to a reduced inpatient stay. However, they felt that once inappropriate inpatient stays had been reduced, other areas would need to be examined in order to maintain cost savings.

Sommers et al., in 1990, demonstrated that clinician-directed cost management can significantly decrease costs.[7] They documented the cost savings realized by decreasing unnecessary lab procedures and reducing operating room time on a population undergoing total hip surgery.

More recently, Barber and Healy reported in 1993 on hospital cost of total hip arthroplasty during the 1980s.[8] They documented how costs were controlled in the 1980s primarily by decreasing length of stay. They recommend that, in the 1990s, the focus of cost containment measures must be on controlling the costs of prosthetics, personnel, and other supplies.

Revision Hip Surgery: The New England Baptist Experience

The New England Baptist Hospital has a long history of performing revision hip surgery. Our high volume service has enabled us to be responsive to the changing health care environment.

In an effort to examine our practice patterns, we began by taking a look at the past 13 years of revision hip surgery. We examined our strategies for the operating room and patient care delivery to see how it has evolved. We have found that, despite the complexities and challenges, revision hip surgery can be done in a revenue-effective manner.

We began by looking at our historical data. We examined 1984, 1989, and 1994 to review practice patterns and determine how they had changed. The data collected included the number of cases performed, length of stay, implant selection, use of bone graft, operating room time, surgical approach, blood loss, blood transfusions, cost, complications, rehabilitation programs, and discharge planning.

In 1984, we performed 145 revision total hip surgeries. This was the year that Medicare began the DRG system of prospective payments. During this time patients were admitted to the hospital 2 to 3 days prior to surgery. All preoperative preparation occurred in this time frame, including lab work, chest and hip x-rays, and hip aspirations. Many consultant physicians were involved in the patient's care and the patient frequently had medical interventions performed under the same admission (ie, cardiac catheterization, chlolecystectomy).

In the operating room the average OR time was 5.5 hours. Blood loss during surgery averaged 2800 cc. The prostheses were most often cemented long stems. There was extensive use of bone grafting. Trochanteric osteotomy was routine, and reattachment was performed with a three-wire technique.

The postoperative course included extended bedrest (2 to 3 weeks) and skeletal traction was often utilized, especially when bone grafting was done. Patients began ambulation late in their postoperative course. The average length of stay was 26.1 days. The disposition was most often home with home health services.

Five years later, in 1989, we saw some changes. During this period we performed 218 revision hip cases. The prescreening process was evolving and being streamlined. The preoperative stay was down to 1 day. The majority of testing and consults were still conducted during this period. Hip aspiration continued to be performed under general anesthesia. Autologous blood donation was encouraged, but less than 2 units per patient were obtained on an average.

In the operating room (OR) the average case time was down—4 hours 40 minutes. This was due in part to better OR planning and also reflected the increase in surgical expertise among physicians and OR staff. Blood loss, too, was decreasing (an average of 1800 cc). The trochanteric slide osteotomy as a surgical approach supplanted the conventional trochanteric osteotomy. Use of the Dall-Miles cable grip improved healing of the trochanter. Porous-coated long stems were now used for femoral fixation.

The postoperative course was also undergoing changes. Patients were being mobilized more quickly. The average time of bedrest was reduced to 1 to 2 weeks. There was less use of skeletal traction. Dispositions were split between home and rehabilitation facilities. Patients requiring more time to work on their rehabilitation program were being transferred to extended care facilities for additional time. These combined changes in practice brought the average length of stay to 13.7 days.

The next five-year time span saw the most pronounced changes. The number of cases continued to grow to 247 cases in the 1994 calendar year. Patient preoperative stay had been eliminated. Patients were now being admitted on the day of surgery. The prescreening testing was done during a 5-hour visit to the pre-admission screening unit that could occur any time within a month of surgery. During this visit patients received preoperative education, testing, x-rays, and consults. We were beginning to see primary care physicians performing preoperative clearance on their patients. The hospital accelerated an active autologous donation program. Hip aspirations were now being performed only on selected cases and they, too, could be performed within a month of surgery as an outpatient.

In the operating room the average case time had dropped to 4 hours 20 minutes. The prosthesis of choice was a modular cementless stem that reduced the need for extensive bone grafting. With a greater prosthetic inventory, structural bulk grafts were greatly supplanted by use of onlay and morselized graft. The Dall clip was still utilized for trochanteric reattachment. Blood loss had decreased to an average of 1200 cc.

Postoperatively, patients were participating in early ambulation often by the second postoperative day. Patients continued to be split on discharge destinations between home and a rehabilitation unit. Active discharge planning was started earlier in the patient's stay. We saw a drop in length of stay to 8.6 days.

Operative Costs

As we examined our practice patterns, we uncovered some hidden costs in doing revision hip surgery that we had been less aware of prior to this review. When reading this, it is important to recognize that practitioners have differing practice patterns and hospitals have varying cost-to-charge structures. In addition, each uncovered cost must be examined for its cost/benefit ratio. We cite the following as examples for review. One of the major costs is for OR supplies. For the trochanteric reattachment, wires may cost $5 to $6 versus Dall cables, which cost $600. In the area of bone grafting, a distal femoral bone graft often costs 400% what a femoral head bone graft costs. When used for equivalent bone deficiencies, there is little evidence to suggest that one outlasts the other. On the prosthetic side, a ceramic femoral head may cost 200% to 300% of the price of a cobalt-chrome head. The use of cement can have hidden costs because one must take into account not only the price of the cement, but also the cement plug, bowl, gun, irrigation, and the additional operating time for acrylic setting. All of these examples illustrate the need to examine practice patterns and costs so that you, the health care team, can make informed decisions in this day of cost containment.

Orthopedic Collaborative Practice Model

Following our review, our goal remained the same: to coordinate care among physicians, nursing staff, therapy staff, and hospital administration to meet fixed reimbursement demands while ensuring quality patient care. We strive to maintain quality patient outcomes in a cost-effective manner. To meet this goal, the process of examining practice patterns and forces in health care that affect practice has to be ongoing. We have learned that it can be done. We have put together an interdisciplinary team that includes physicians, administrators, case managers, OR personnel, nurses, and therapists to ensure this process improvement. Being a high-volume center has also enabled us to provide specialty equipment, expertise among personnel, a blood management program, and diverse prosthetic inventory. All of these factors contribute to successful and high-quality outcomes.

In the last three years, we have further refined our program in the following ways. At the physician's office visit when the decision for surgery is made, the physician schedules surgery and at the same time indicates a clinical pathway that serves to guide the patient's hospitalization. This process is decided after discussion with the patient. We encourage the patient to become an active participant in all planning. The pathways are geared to discharge home or to a rehabilitation facility. Armed with that information, the patient is then seen in our prescreening unit. Our comprehensive prescreening visit includes a thorough medical history and physical, anesthesia consultation, preoperative teaching, physical therapy evaluation, and meeting with a member of the case management team. We have seen a rise in the primary care physician's role with preoperative health screening.

The physical therapist reviews the physician's plan and assesses the patient's rehabilitation potential. In addition the therapist reviews the postoperative rehabilitation program, begins exercise instruction, and initiates gait training. During this visit, a social worker from the case management department also meets with the patient to review the discharge plan. The social worker looks at insurance benefits, home situation, and social supports to ensure that the tentative discharge plan is right for the patient. This enables the postoperative course to be smooth for the patient. It also allows the patient, family, and friends to do any of the necessary planning *in advance*. Included in this preparation is the signing of advanced directives, which enables patients to give direction to the care they would receive in the event of a catastrophic event.

Patient education is an instrumental component of our program. It is an ongoing process beginning in the physician's office when patients receive a booklet entitled "A Guide to Total Hip Surgery" as well as a video that follows a patient through total hip surgery and recovery. Patients and families are encouraged to attend the total joint education class taught by an interdisciplinary team (nurse, physical therapist, and social worker). The class provides an overview of the surgery and postoperative course. We encourage families and friends who may be involved in the patient's care to participate. This helps to set realistic expectations for the surgery, hospitalization, and the weeks following until a patient returns to his physician for his postoperative visit. It has helped to alleviate the patient's anxieties by providing him with information and an opportunity to have his questions and concerns addressed.

During the acute hospitalization, interdisciplinary clinical paths are used to guide the patient care. Clinical pathways are an interdisciplinary plan of care that assist in coordinating resources and directing activity to outcome achievement. The case management service, along with the attending physician, oversees the pathways to ensure coordinated care for the patients. The paths are reviewed concurrently and retrospectively to identify variances and rectify inefficiencies in patient care delivery. The retrospective variance analysis allows identification of system issues that may be barriers to goal achievement.

A key part of the postoperative course is the rehabilitation program, which begins ambulation the first day after surgery. We are able to offer our patients physical therapy twice a day, 7 days a week. This has greatly impacted our ability to prepare patients in a timely manner for discharge home or early transfer to a rehabilitation facility when appropriate.

In the OR we have begun a system of demand matching for prosthetic choices. The criteria assess the individual's activity level, demands to be placed on the prosthesis, and bone quality. The physician matches those criteria to the best prosthetic choice for that patient. In addition, the greater array of implant choices now available enables the prosthesis to be matched to case complexity and has reduced the need for bone grafts. The OR has worked on expediting admission to the OR so cases begin at the designated times. The expertise of the surgical team and the anesthesia department also enhances the efficient use of OR time. We are utilizing autologous donations, direct donors, and cell saver for blood salvage. At this time we are also exploring the use of auto transfusion devices and erythropoietin.

The volume of orthopedic surgery performed at our institution has provided value-added services to our patients. The expertise of surgeons, OR personnel, physical therapists, nursing staff, the specialty equipment, blood management program, and diverse prosthetic inventory all enable us to provide the highest quality care to our patients.

But we cannot stop here. Health care continues to undergo change. We must stay abreast of changes to ensure our continued quality outcomes. One recent program was developed to address the increased number of patients being discharged to home care. It was our goal to provide a seamless continuum of care for our patients. The challenge was to maintain the same quality of care in a setting apart from the hospital. We developed a preferred provider network of home care agencies that have agreed to adopt our rehabilitation protocols and work closely with our physicians and discharge planners to provide a seamless transition from acute care to home. We are tracking outcome information on goal achievement and patient satisfaction to ensure that this happens.

Despite all of these changes in the revision total hip surgery, the experience continues to be a successful endeavor. First and foremost in this experience is the patient. We exist to meet their needs, alleviate their concerns, and fulfill their aspirations in the most effective, timely, caring, and cost-effective manner possible. The feedback from our program continues to encourage us that we are accomplishing these goals.

References

1. Orthopedic Network News. *1997 Hip and Knee Implant Review.* Vol. 8, No. 3, July 1997.
2. Orthopedic Network News. *1997 Hip and Knee Implant Review.* Vol. 8, No. 3, July 1997.
3. Hsaio WC, Braun P, Dunn D, et al. Resource-based relative values. *JAMA.* 1988;260:2347–2353.
4. Becker ER, Dunn D, Hsaio WC. Relative cost differences among physicians' specialty practices. *JAMA.* 1988;260: 2397–2402.
5. Hsaio WC, Braun P, Yntema D, et al. Estimating physicians' work for a resource based relative value scale. *N Engl J Med.* 1988;319:835–841.
6. Schwartz WB, Mendelson DN. Hospital cost containment in the 1980s: hard lessons learned and prospects for the 1990s. *N Engl J Med.* 1991;324:1037–1042.
7. Sommers LS, Schurman DJ, Jamison JQ, et al. Clinican-directed hospital cost management for total hip arthroplasty patients. *Clin Orthop.* 1990;258:168–175.
8. Barber TC, Healy WL. The hospital cost of total hip arthroplasty. *J Bone Joint Surg Am.* 1993;75:321–325.

72
Physical Rehabilitation

Donna Dinardo

Patients who undergo revision total hip surgery at New England Baptist Hospital are referred by the attending surgeon to the pre-admission screening unit where a team approach to preoperative patient assessment, education, and discharge planning is utilized. The patient is progressed postoperatively by the health care team using surgeon-approved Clinical Pathways that document the patient's daily activity and compliance with clinical outcomes. However, it continues to be our philosophy that "a program of rehabilitation be established for revision arthroplasty patients that is directed not only at the restoration of function in the immediate postoperative period, but also at establishing a life-long set of habits to protect the hip."[1]

As hospital lengths of stay continue to decrease, it is critical to develop the most complete picture possible of the patient and his support system preoperatively so as to formulate the best clinical opinion of the patient's ability to understand and to participate in the rehabilitation program. The patient must be routed from the acute care setting as soon as medically stable, into the best alternative setting. Since the insurance provided will determine that setting, the patient must become familiar preoperatively with his benefit package so that postoperative decisions are better understood. The physical therapist must design each patient's program to achieve realistic goals within the allotted acute care timeframe, preparing the patient to function safely in that alternative setting. In the near future, patients will receive a copy of a general Clinical Pathway preoperatively, to become more familiar with daily expectations. This will also allow the patient to be a more active participant in the health care team walk rounds, as he will have an individualized summary of each day's progress.

Preoperative Evaluation

At the time of the preadmission screening unit visit, the physical therapist performs a physical assessment of the patient with emphasis on the strength, range of motion, and presence of any deformity such as a leg length discrepancy and gait deviation caused by the affected joint. This information becomes the basis of the postoperative exercise and gait training program. The patient is instructed in and given a written illustrated preoperative exercise program, including joint precaution information, to begin at home as an introduction to postoperative exercises. The patient is expected to demonstrate the exercises independently at this time. An upper extremity strengthening exercise program is also added, when necessary, to improve upper extremity strength for postoperative activities such as bed mobility, transfers, and crutch walking. Even if the patient has had previous experience with crutches, a review of partial weight-bearing is essential as it is important for the patient to fully understand that the bone, hip prosthesis, hip musculature, and trochanter if an osteotomy is performed must be protected during the postoperative recovery period.

It is important to discuss discharge planning relative to where the patient will go upon hospital discharge as well as to understand the physical[3] layout of the home to which the patient will ultimately return. A barrier-free environment is the goal, and items such as scatter rugs may present a hazard to a patient on crutches. Stairs may also present a barrier, and the patient could be advised to spend as much time as possible on the main floor of his two-story home to minimize stair climbing, for example, as long as there is an accessible bathroom and a safe place for the patient to rest on that level of the home. A safe place to rest does not usually include a recliner chair or a pullout sofa but in our philosophy means a bed. The patient is also advised to use an armchair such as a captain's chair, the seat height of which should measure at least 18 inches off the floor. Various chair heights may be discussed based upon the patient's height and other factors that would affect the safety of chair transfers.

Short-term inpatient rehabilitation is discussed as an option, as well as the possibility of continued convalescence at the home of a family member or friend prior to returning to the patient's own home. Especially important for the patient who lives alone is the necessity to request and to arrange assistance for many household and personal activities from family members and friends. In many cases some assistance may be available from an outside agency providing services in the patient's community. The social worker is available in the preadmission screening unit to assist the patient in these and other discharge matters.

The restrictions further emphasize our philosophy as explained in this paragraph from the original work on this subject:

> The patient should be made to understand that the time spent recovering from revision hip surgery is not merely an inconvenience, but a vital contribution to the success and long-term survival of the revision arthroplasty. He or she should be discouraged from feeling "free" to use or abuse the affected hip, on the assumption that repeated revision hip surgery is always available. The patient is encouraged to examine his or her life style and to make necessary adjustments to a specific set of guidelines, including the use of external support, first in the form of crutches, and ultimately a cane.[1]

A nutritional consult can be made if the patient has a weight problem that will complicate his or her recovery from revision hip surgery. The dietitian will educate the patient and family member or friend in weight reduction as well as in determining that the patient's protein intake is adequate during the postoperative healing process.

Financial concerns can be a source of additional stress for this patient population, especially if the patient is the family provider or has incomplete/inadequate insurance coverage after repeated hospitalizations and procedures. Frequently this patient must face the reality of not being able to return to his previous occupation either because of the physical requirements of the job or because of the restrictions placed upon him by the surgeon. Additional input may be required from the surgeon to request modified duty if the patient is to return to the present job; Social Service may also be able to provide the patient with information concerning alternative job training programs.

If it is known that the patient is having a Girdlestone procedure in which all prosthetic components and infected tissue are removed and are unable to be replaced at this time, balanced suspension with skeletal traction must be reviewed with the patient. Another reason that a Girdlestone procedure would be performed is for a mechanical reason such as inadequate bone stock or fracture. Proper alignment of the affected limb is stressed in the event that reimplantation of a hip prosthesis is planned at some future date. This patient must also be advised that there will be a leg length difference postoperatively and that a lift will be added to the shoe of the operated leg. Pin care will be reviewed by the nurse.

A hospital bed with a Balkan frame, balanced suspension, and side handles is used postoperatively. The patient is instructed in the use of this equipment so that he understands its use relative to proper bed mobility and out-of-bed transfers. The balanced suspension is used to maintain proper hip alignment, to facilitate nursing care, and to allow the patient to initiate gentle hip and knee motion postoperatively. To minimize the chance of dislocation of the newly operated hip and to provide patient comfort, the patient is moved into the bed and balanced suspension from the operating table.

To further stress the importance of his active participation in his recovery, the patient is encouraged to bring a family member or friend when attending a preoperative hip class. This class is coordinated by an orthopedic nurse and physical therapist with input from a social worker. During this group session, the anatomy of the hip as well as a general description of the surgery are reviewed. The nurse will continue with a description of the usual patient experience on the day of surgery beginning in the admitting department through the post-anesthesia care unit and transfer into the inpatient unit. The therapist will review in detail the specific daily progression of the inpatient rehabilitation program, including goals to be achieved prior to discharge home from the acute setting or rehabilitation center. These goals generally include a good understanding of joint precautions and necessary lifestyle changes, independence with bed and bathroom transfers, independence with home exercise program, and independence and safety with crutches on level surfaces and stairs. The role of the occupational therapist in providing instruction to meet the goals of independence with self-care and lower extremity dressing activities is reviewed during this session. The patient is advised to bring loose, comfortable clothing and a pair of sturdy shoes or sneakers to the hospital for use during occupational therapy as well as during the postoperative recovery phase.

Group interaction and questions are encouraged during this two-hour informal patient education session. The patient must be listened to and feel that he is taken seriously as "the patient's fears, thoughts and questions are never trivial to him".[2] Upon completion of the preadmission screening visit and attendance at this class, the patient must understand that he is an active member, indeed the most important member, of the health care team.

Postoperative Rehabilitation

The patient will be on bed rest with the operated limb in balanced suspension until the first postoperative day, but the surgeon may order a longer period of immobilization should it be deemed necessary. During the time that the balanced suspension is being used, proper alignment must be maintained with neurovascular and skin integrity status being assessed frequently. The patient is taught to use the bed controls to position the bed for comfort, as elevation of the head and knees of the bed may decrease hip and back muscle spasms. Flat time is also encouraged, especially if the patient had a flexion deformity preoperatively. The bedside table, overbed table, and other items needed by the patient should be placed on the operated side of the bed within close reach in order to promote abduction and to minimize extremes of passive rotation of the operated hip. It is good practice to review with the patient what movement is necessary and how one will assist the patient moving rather than lifting the unprepared patient. If the patient initiates the movement and the caregiver supports the operated limb, there is less of a load on the patient's muscles, decreasing antagonistic contraction as well as pain. The result will be a less fearful, more trusting and cooperative patient.

The patient should be encouraged to perform deep breathing and coughing exercises, including the use of an incentive spirometer, to help clear the lungs of the postanesthesia gases and to raise secretions. Ankle dorsi and plantar flexion exercises are performed to prevent circulatory complications by imitating the pumping action that occurs with walking. The patient will also have lower leg external compression sleeves on and will wear knee-high surgical elastic stockings during the postoperative recovery.

The patient will perform other exercises previously instructed such as quadriceps and gluteal setting, internal and external rotation, the "hula" or alternate hip hiking, and the Thomas stretch if a preoperative flexion deformity was present. When the balanced suspension is removed, a knee sling or pulley type apparatus is placed on the operated limb to begin gentle range of motion exercises. The patient will next dangle on the edge of the bed, preferably on the operative side, to decrease trochanteric strain, especially if an osteotomy was performed at the time of the revision. Another day-one postoperative activity is standing at the bedside if comfort and endurance permit. Standing and stretching at the bedside begin with a walker that provides maximum stability. The patient is to bear partial weight on the operated leg and will perform bilateral toe raises with the knees in full extension and marching in place, which helps both circulation and proprioception to the extremity.

During the first three days postoperatively, gait training continues with the walker, and chair and bathroom transfers are instructed. Since chair selection depends upon the patient's height, control of the operated leg, and general overall physical ability, an armchair is preferred for comfort, stability, and ease of transfer. For taller or less able patients such as someone with weak upper extremities, the chair could be raised on blocks or the seat raised with bed pillows so that the patient will be in a semi-erect position before raising his body weight off the chair. The toilet height should be assessed in the similar fashion with the general principle being that the patient uses the unoperated leg to lift himself from a seated position. During the recovery period, as the operated leg becomes less painful and stronger, the patient will begin to use both legs for sit-to-stand activity. The patient must be reminded to sit for short periods of time and to keep the legs abducted, especially while performing seated range of motion exercises.

Patients on a rehabilitation pathway will be discharged by postoperative day four to an impatient facility for additional strengthening exercises, gait training with crutches, and compliance with expected patient outcomes. Patients on a home pathway will continue physical therapy in the acute care setting and be discharged home by postoperative day six.

Usually by postoperative day three or four, the patient has sufficient leg control, good balance, and endurance to initiate three-point partial weight-bearing with crutches. The goal of gait training is that when the patient is independently ambulating a functional distance, the crutches could hypothetically be removed and the patient would exhibit a normal gait pattern. The patient must understand that partial weight-bearing with external support of crutches reduces the load across the revision hip joint and minimizes abductor muscle activity, reducing the stress on the trochanteric osteotomy. If the patient has an abduction contracture or has had distal advancement of the trochanter, the patient will describe the operated leg as feeling too long. Intensive gait training and a program of active-assisted abduction exercises should correct this problem, if the surgeon feels that it is not due to a fixed anatomical problem and that trochanteric fixation will allow such exercise. If the leg length difference cannot be corrected through an exercise program, a heel lift can be added to the heel of the shorter side. If the heel lift is greater than half an inch, a lift should also be added to the sole of the shoe, tapered to match the normal pitch of the shoe. The patient must also be taught a heel strike–toe off gait with the operated leg, taking equal length steps, maintaining an erect posture, and keeping the knee straight with the foot flat on the floor in the stance phase of gait.

When the patient ambulates safely with crutches on level surfaces, the patient is instructed in stair climbing. The patient will bear most of his weight on the unoperated leg and the crutches or crutches and hand rail. Going upstairs is done by leading with the unoperated leg, bringing the operated leg up to the same step while leaning on the crutches, which are then brought up to the same step. Going downstairs is the reverse process: leading with the crutches, the operated leg down onto the same step, and finally the unoperated leg down to the same step. The patient may be instructed in sidelying and pronelying, keeping the operated leg in abduction, prior to hospital discharge.

The patient who undergoes a Girdlestone procedure will remain on bedrest with the operated leg in balanced suspension and skeletal traction for a length of time determined by the surgeon. Due to the constant pull of the skeletal traction at the foot of the bed, the patient's bed should be kept in Trendelenberg position to prevent the patient from being pulled down into the bed. To the same end, the patient should also keep the knee gatch of the bed in slight flexion. When the patient is allowed out of bed activity, the skeletal traction is detached for short periods of time each day to allow participation in therapy and then replaced when the patient returns to bed. Time out of skeletal traction is increased daily as the patient's out-of-bed activity and therapy program is advanced. The skeletal traction pin is usually removed the day prior to discharge and could be in place for up to 6 weeks after surgery. This patient may be more acutely ill and generally more debilitated than the routine revision total hip patient. This patient could also be receiving intravenous antibiotic therapy for up to 6 weeks after surgery and then be on oral antibiotics for a length of time determined by the infectious disease physician.

Discharge Planning and Follow-Up

When the patient is able to meet the goals established preoperatively and as the rehabilitation program progresses, he is ready for discharge. Written home exercise and activity guidelines are reviewed with the patient, as well as the family member or friend whenever possible. The patient is given a copy with both his and the therapist's signatures; the agency providing the home therapy receives a copy; and a third copy is kept in the patient's medical record. This is done to be sure that everyone involved in the patient's care has the identical surgeon-approved guidelines, to be followed without additions unless further permission is obtained from the surgeon, until the first postoperative follow-up appointment.

With the surgeon's approval, the patient may include pool swimming as part of the recovery program if the pool has steps with a handrail to allow descent into the pool with crutches until buoyancy unloads the joint. The patient is instructed to avoid unnecessary bending, lifting, and unsupported weight-bearing, performing as many activities as possible, such as showering, in the seated position. Prolonged periods of sitting should be discouraged, as the hip muscles may become stiff or a flexion deformity or stasis edema may occur. After a maximum sitting time of 60 minutes, the patient should stand with crutches and perform stretching exercises before taking a walk. Other adjustments that must be made include putting frequently used items in convenient, easily accessible places, especially in the kitchen, bathroom, and bedroom. Unless advised by the surgeon, hip mobility and comfort should determine when the patient is able to resume sexual activity as the less aggressive partner. Driving is not advised until the surgeon gives permission. The patient will be instructed in progression to full weight-bearing with both crutches over a period of time determined by the surgeon regarding such things as trochanteric fixation, strength of the hip musculature, especially the abductors and the integrity of any bone grafting that was done at the time of revision surgery. When the patient has a negative Trendelenburg test in standing, the surgeon may progress the patient to use of a single crutch or cane used on the unoperated side.

Prior to discharge, the patient must know the schedule for his initial follow-up appointment with the surgeon. The patient must understand the importance of these visits to monitor the progress and compliance with established ground rules. The patient must know that members of the health care team, including the surgeon, encourage and expect to be notified when questions or problems arise during the recovery period. If the patient feels that the team is genuinely interested in a positive outcome, the patient will believe that it is possible and worth the time and effort that must be devoted to a successful recovery.

References

1. Aufranc OE, Harris JM, McKay SJ, Dinardo DM. Rehabilitation in hip arthroplasty. In: *Revision total hip arthroplasty*. Turner RH, Sheller AD Jr., eds. New York: Grune and Stratton; 1982:379–380.
2. Stillwell WT. *The art of total hip arthroplasty*. Orlando, Fla.: Grune & Stratton; 1987.
3. Lichtenstein R, Semaan S, Marmar EC. Development and impact of a hospital-based perioperative patient education program in a joint replacement center. *Orthop Nurs*. 1993; 12:17–25, 46.

73
Outcome Studies

Richard Iorio and William L. Healy

Outcomes research, which focuses on patient outcome and patient satisfaction after medical intervention, has become a popular method of analyzing the clinical results of orthopedic operations during the last decade. Outcomes research is not new. The focus of clinical research in orthopedic surgery has changed from physician measures of the result of care to patient evaluations of the outcome of care. In orthopedic outcomes research, perceptions of patients are used to evaluate the success or failure of orthopedic interventions. Evaluations of pain, quality of life, function, satisfaction, social and emotional well-being, as measured by patients, are critical elements of outcomes-based research.[1] Outcomes-based research is different from traditional clinical research, which evaluates results of physical examination, radiographic examination, and laboratory examination, as measured by health care professionals.

Outcomes research enables clinical investigators to determine appropriate levels of operative intervention, reduce variation in orthopedic practice patterns, improve the quality of intervention, and eliminate physician uncertainty concerning appropriateness of the intervention. Orthopaedists have been slow to accept patient-oriented, quality-of-life type data. One objection has been that these data are subjective and inadequate for scientific interpretation. However, reproducible, valid instruments have been developed for patient-oriented outcome evaluation that focuses on function and patient satisfaction. These outcome measures have been validated, and they are more reproducible than traditional measures of process, such as radiographic interpretation, range of motion, and physician interpretation of pain and function.[2]

Total hip arthroplasty (THA) is a predictably successful surgical procedure, and THA patients are well suited to process-oriented measurement and patient-oriented outcomes measurement. Traditional clinical research has been used to carefully evaluate the results of THA over the last 30 years. However, several unresolved and contentious issues regarding THA may be answered with outcomes research: the impact of volume effects, technology, and cost, as well as the appropriate rate of and timing of THA intervention.

Historical Perspective

During the last three decades, THA has been studied in detail with traditional clinical research instruments dependent upon physician-defined parameters of success. Many of these studies have been dependent upon nonstandardized terminology, variable sample sizes, variable length of follow-up time, and invalid clinical information. Little attention was focused on patient satisfaction or quality of life following THA.

Several clinical THA grading systems have been developed to express physician evaluation of success after THA. In 1954, Merle d'Aubigné and Postel[3] described a system of grading the functional capacity of a hip joint. Pain, mobility, and walking ability are expressed on three different six-point scales and reported separately or as an aggregate. Charnley[4] modified the scale and simplified the reporting of the mobility score. Charnley also introduced stratification of comorbidities by ranking patients into three categories: patients with unilateral disease, patients with bilateral disease, and patients with other diseases that may affect their function. Charnley[4] recognized that functional outcome would be negatively affected by increasing the number of comorbidities.

In the United States, Larson[5] introduced a 100-point scale based on pain (35), function (35), motion (10), deformity (10), and gait (10). Harris[6] modified Larson's scale and assigned pain (44), function (47), range of motion (5), and absence of deformity (4) to a 100-point scale. Harris emphasized function, which was devalued in Larson's scale. On the other hand, motion is undervalued in the Harris score. Both scores express patient results as one number, thus limiting the ability to profile individual patients.[6]

In an attempt to better evaluate the potential survival of a THA implant, the Mayo hip score was developed. This clinical (80 points) and radiologic (20 points) assessment score was developed to improve the accuracy and validity of reporting of long-term results of THA. The Mayo hip score deducted points for painless, asymptomatic, fully functional hips with early signs of radiologic loosening. In order to include a radiologic score in the 100-point scale, the measurement of hip motion was omitted. The Mayo hip score was criticized for a lack of consensus concerning the definition of radiologic loosening.[7]

Bryant et al.[8] evaluated and compared 13 different clinical hip scores and 19 variables of hip function to identify which scores and/or variables best represented functional outcome. The essential variables for measurement of clinical success were walking distance, hip flexion, and pain. Measurement of any more than these three variables was found to add little additional information about the outcome of hip arthroplasty. These authors stated that combining the scores was arbitrary, and they suggested that the individual scores be expressed separately for maximal assessment value.[8]

The inherent weaknesses of the traditional clinical THA hip scores were recognized by the American Academy of Orthopedic Surgeons (AAOS), and an attempt was made to standardize terminology, nomenclature, and method of reporting the results of THA. Consensus functional, radiographic, and patient satisfaction information was developed by a committee composed of representatives of the Société Internationale de Chirurgie Orthopédique et de Traumatologie (S.I.C.O.T.), the Hip Society, and the AAOS Outcome Evaluation Committee.[9] The consensus committee outlined which variables may be important for long-term follow-up of THA operations, but no guidelines were offered as to how to implement these variables into an evaluation system.

Subsequent to the Consensus Hip Committee report, the AAOS convened a task force on outcome studies to evaluate patient measures of pain, function, and health in addition to the conventional physician-derived measurements of impairment. Where possible, valid, reliable, sensitive instruments were included to standardize data collection for THA. Follow-up data collection was recommended at regular intervals. By standardizing the systematic evaluation of THA and applying outcomes assessment techniques, it is hoped that the process and the results of medical and operative care of these patients will be improved.[10]

Outcome assessment is an integral component of orthopedic research in 1997. The AAOS is committed to creating a national musculoskeletal outcomes data base to create normative statistics that can be used as a baseline to assess outcomes in a local practice compared with national standards. The concept of a national hip registry is not new. Scandinavian countries have a long-term experience with this tool. A national hip registry in the United States that includes patient-oriented outcome assessment and the standardized measures of outcome will demonstrate the significant improvements in quality of life provided to patients with THA. Outcome information regarding THA will be important for government agencies and third-party payers who control the health care system reimbursement and access to THA.[11]

Methodology

The development of small area analysis by Wennberg and Gittelsohn[12] permitted the study of health care utilization on the basis of population. With the use of hospital discharge data bases and computer analysis, per capita rates of medical and surgical care for patients was determined for hospitals and physicians as well as service areas. A wide variation was found in utilization rates of many types of medical care despite controlling for potential confounding variables, such as age, sex, and surgical treatment.[12] These variations have been found in almost all areas of elective orthopedic procedures, whereas hip fracture and polytrauma show almost no variation.[13]

Geographically, the intervention rate associated with THA varies by a factor of 1.9, and no consensus exists as to what an appropriate rate of intervention for THA should be. The establishment of Patient Outcome Research Teams (PORTs) by the Agency for Health Policy and Research (AHPR) is an attempt by the Federal Government to use outcomes data to develop guidelines for medical practice and to evaluate the effectiveness of medical intervention. The need for cost effectiveness, clinical utility, and third party payer evaluation of providers is driving this movement.[2]

Ideal outcomes research users randomized clinical trials exclusively to analyze treatment and outcome variables. The randomized clinical trial (RCT) involves a prospective cohort with concurrent controls and represents the gold standard of scientific clinical study. RCTs minimize bias and confounding variables, but they are expensive to perform and are difficult to implement with surgical procedures when the quality of the results are measured over many years.

In THA, the introduction of new technologies, the evaluation of surgical techniques, and the evolution of better instrumentation discourage the use of RCTs. In 1988, Gross[14] found that few, if any, methodologically sound studies existed before his study. He called for carefully controlled clinical trials before the widespread introduction of new technology or techniques for THA.

Meta-analysis is an outcomes tool that aggregates clinical study results to draw conclusions concerning clinical effectiveness. Meta-analysis compares the results of several smaller methodologically sound studies with one larger cohort to look at treatment and outcome variables. Meta-analysis was designed for use with RCTs, but it has been modified for use with prospective cohort trials. Studies included in a meta-analysis must have similar inclusion criteria and similar analysis of outcome to be effective. The paucity of methodologically sound studies in the orthopedic literature limits the usefulness of meta-analysis at this time in orthopedics. Meta-analysis is time-consuming and expensive, but it can give a reasonable summary of the current status of knowledge in a specific discipline.[2,15]

A meta-analysis of 130 patient-outcome studies concerning total knee arthroplasty (TKA) was performed to provide estimates of patient outcome and to examine variation in outcome as a result of patient and implant characteristics. The reporting style of the articles severely constrained the ability of the authors to explain the variability of outcome or generalize their conclusions. TKA was found to be safe and effective for the patients included in the analysis.[16]

Large data bases have also been employed to evaluate outcomes of THA. The difficulty with extrapolating clinically relevant information from these data bases, for example, Agency of Health Care Administration and Medicare, is a reflection of the gross nature of the information. Large data bases are usually constituted for financial purposes and rarely are compatible with detailed clinical research. Outcomes research can be performed in a limited way with these data bases as long as the clinical scope is narrow. Utilization variation, cost, demographics, length of stay, rehospitalization, complications, and in-hospital mortality rates are some of the information that can be retrieved from these data bases. However, case severity, patient perception, and functional outcome are not available from these data bases.[2,17]

The establishment of statistically and methodologically sound data from THA outcome studies extrapolated from large cohorts of patients permits precise meaningful analyses of difficult clinical problems. Decision analysis permits the rigorous examination of statistical results and translates these results into clinical probabilities. Because decision analysis has become more sophisticated and computerized, sensitivity analyses can be performed over several dimensions simultaneously and thus produce clinically relevant measures of utility. In this way, outcomes can be given relative weights, and patients and physicians can make better informed decisions concerning treatment options and the probability of good outcomes.[2,18]

Variation in THA practice patterns may be reduced as THA outcome information is developed. Patients who are given good clinical data comparing the outcomes of various treatment options can, in conjunction with the physician, make better informed choices. This concept of shared decision making is an attempt to narrow practice variation by permitting the patient to participate in decisions that will affect the outcome. Where these decisions have no clear-cut clinical solution, well-informed patient preferences have been shown to increase the value of treatment by increasing patient satisfaction with the ultimate outcome.[19]

Cost-effectiveness analysis is an increasingly important method of outcomes assessment for orthopedic interventions. Cost-effectiveness analysis can be used to set priorities for funding health care programs. These priorities are measured by comparing the cost and clinical outcomes between two different treatment methods. If an intervention resulted in improved outcome but cost more or used more resources, a cost-effectiveness ratio is calculated, thus measuring the incremental increase in outcome with the increased cost of that outcome. In an era of scarce resources, demonstrating the utility of an intervention on a cost-effectiveness basis is critical for the intervention's survival.[20]

Quality of outcome data affects the measurement and usefulness of cost-effectiveness analysis. Life expectancy is a useful measurement of outcome, but it is not especially meaningful where THA is considered. Utility is a quantitative method of determining the preference of a patient for a certain health status. Cost utility studies generally use quality adjusted life years (QALY) as a unit of measurement for life expectancy. The treatment cost, increased life expectancy (utility, quality of life), and adjusted utility (QAL expectancy) can be combined into calculations of incremental cost effectiveness, incremental cost utility, and incremental cost-benefit ratios. These measures are being used to evaluate the net health benefit of a particular intervention or a given population with limited health care resources.[20]

Outcome Instruments

In the past, health assessment measures regarding THA have been dominated by instruments dependent upon physician-derived data. However, recently, assessment of patient function after THA has been studied with data obtained from patient questionnaires. The AAOS Consensus Committee on Hip Evaluation developed a standardized nomenclature of data collection that exhaustively covers the physician-derived portion of outcome assessment (eg, physical examination, radiographic examination, complications). A consensus concerning patient-oriented outcome questionnaires has not been achieved. Several generalized measures of health are self-administered and measure function and quality of life. As a practical guide, these questionnaires should be valid, reproducible, sensitive, short, and applicable to arthritis and THA. To meet these criteria, the instrument must measure what it is supposed to measure (validity), reproduce similar responses when the clinical condition has not changed appreciably (reproducibility), and change appreciably when the clinical condition has changed appreciably (sensitivity).[2]

Outcome-research instruments can be divided into two classifications: general health instruments and disease-specific instruments. Patient-oriented instruments, which focus on general health, are useful because of their availability across all disease states. Disease-specific instruments are less common because of the difficulty and expense of creating specific instruments that are valid. These instruments are critical to outcomes research because they enable assessment of patient function and comparison between studies. General health status includes quality-of-life measures of social and emotional well being in addition to physical parameters.

General health outcome instruments, which have been validated and proven to be reproducible, include the Medical Outcomes Study Short Form 36 (SF-36) Health Status Survey,[21] the Index of Well Being (IWB),[22] the Sickness Impact Profile (SIP),[23] and the Nottingham Health Profile (NHP).[24] No one of these instruments is optimal for measurement of THA outcomes. However, when combined with a disease-specific instrument, these tools permit a measure of quality-of-life impairment across social, emotional, physical, and pain scales while controlling for overall health status.

Disease-specific outcome instruments used for THA evaluation include the Western Ontario at McMaster University Osteoarthritis Index (WOMAC),[25] the Cornell Hip Rating Questionnaire (CHRQ),[26] the Functional Status Index (FSI),[27] the Health Assessment Questionnaire (HAQ),[28] the Arthritis Impact Measurement Scales (AIMS),[29] the six minute walk,[46] and the Functional Milestones Scale (FMS).[30] Two other instruments are currently being validated for widespread application within orthopedics. The AAOS Consensus Committee on the Hip has developed a THA outcome evaluation questionnaire as a follow-up to the standardized clinical and radiologic evaluation form.[31] The Musculoskeletal Functional Assessment (MFA) is being developed to evaluate the broad range of patients with musculoskeletal disorders of the extremities that are commonly seen in clinical practice.[32]

In order to document the results of THA properly, traditional physician-derived measures will be combined with patient-derived measures of outcome. The task force on outcome studies of the AAOS has recommended a combination of a generalized health status instrument with a disease-specific instrument to create a comprehensive system for the evaluation of the results of THA.[30]

Among the validated global health measures available for implementation, the SF-36 is the most popular instrument and represents a compromise between comprehensiveness and brevity.[21] The SF-36 has 36 multiple-choice questions aggregated into eight subscales. These subscales measure physical function, emotional function, social function, bodily pain, vitality, general health perception, physical limitations, and emotional limitations. In addition, a one-item subjective assessment of general health status is given. The SF-36 takes a patient 8 to 10 minutes to complete. The psychometric properties of the SF-36 have been tested extensively, and it has been used as an instrument by several PORTs.[21]

More extensive health status instruments have not been found to be more responsive or more sensitive than the brief health status measures for THA investigation. The SIP has been used widely in THA research since the 1970s. It is responsive to the impact of THA on quality-of-life improvement. The SIP consists of 136 questions and takes 15 to 35 minutes to complete. The SIP has 12 subscales, and a global score is calculated from the weighted sum of all items.[32] The IWB is not self-administered and is complicated, lengthy, and cumbersome to employ. Correlation of the IWB with other instruments is low.[33]

Disease-specific and general health instruments measure two distinct but important aspects of patients' health. In a comparison of the SF-36 and the disease-specific WOMAC for the measurement of outcomes after TKA, Hawker et al.[34] demonstrated that the WOMAC is more sensitive in detecting disease-related disabilities than the generalized instrument. Although the SF-36 demonstrates sensitivity toward disease-specific disability, the magnitude of the change is not large enough to be detected in small sample sizes. However, the SF-36 distinguishes comorbidities at different levels of general health status, which the WOMAC could not detect. This study supported the inclusion of both a disease-specific and a generic measure of health status in outcome studies and in particular studies of the elderly in whom comorbidity is common.[34] A similar study by Bombardier et al.[35] demonstrated that the distribution of scores on the three dimensions common to both instruments (pain, physical function, and overall score) showed consistently higher scores on the WOMAC than on the SF-36, indicating less disability from arthritis than from conditions after surgery in an elderly population. The WOMAC discriminated better among subjects with varying severity of knee problems, whereas the SF-36 discriminated better among patients with differing levels of reported health status and comorbidity.[35]

The Cornell Hip Rating Scale, which consists of 14 items related to hip arthritis, has also been validated for disease-specific analysis. The instrument has been shown to be responsive and detects relatively small differences in improvement after THA. Other disease-specific instruments, such as the AIMS, the FSI, and the HAQ, have been well established for reproducibility and validity. However, the responsiveness of these instruments has been questioned.[26–29] In the assessment of patients who had a THA, the AIMS performed best for the two subscales of mobility and pain. The Index of Well Being, which has been used to calculate QALY for economic comparisons, was less responsive than the Cornell instrument.[33] The six minute walk measures the distance covered by a patient using whatever aids are necessary while walking up and down a 30 meter corridor. This allows objective comparison of walking ability but does not take into account comorbidities.[46]

Two other disease-specific instruments require widespread testing in THA before universal adoption can be recommended. The AAOS Consensus Committee instrument was validated in a small population and approved for use with a traditional measure and a health status instrument, such as the SF-36.[30] The MFA is an extensive, disease-specific tool for the orthopedic researcher, which has been validated for use throughout the musculoskeletal system. Specific studies with THA have yet to be published. The instrument is intended to be used in research studies and asks patients to assess their function on 100 items. It takes about 15 minutes to complete. A shorter instrument, which could be used for more widespread purposes, is being developed.[31]

Outcome Studies in THA

The development of national musculoskeletal data bases by the Committee on Musculoskeletal Specialty Societies (COMSS) and the AAOS permits high-quality, outcome-based studies with cross-sectional validity to be performed throughout the United States and perhaps the world. However, this type of research is expensive, it requires time and personnel, and it may not be possible in an average orthopedic practice.[36] Orthopedic surgeons need to evaluate the reports of traditional clinical research and outcomes research in order to decide the future of orthopedic research and assessment.

Clinical research detects small changes in patient function or clinical results made by variations in technique. When small differences in techniques are aggregated, the measured outcome can be improved. Significant results may be obtained from small sample sizes.[36] Outcomes research requires a different philosophy. Minor variations in technique usually do not affect outcomes significantly. Large sample sizes are necessary to provide meaningful results. A difference must be seen between assessment and research. Research is expensive and difficult.[36] Office practice can easily be altered to measure patient satisfaction and assessment of physical performance with short, valid instruments. Assessment of this type should be widespread and will help the office-based orthopaedist to document the high quality of work generally performed in this country. Research, however, requires a much more extensive and rigorous commitment to data gathering. To accrue the large numbers of patients necessary to produce meaningful outcome data, a large-scale concerted, national effort must be undertaken.

In outcomes research, collection methods vary with the complexity of the project. Depending on the length of the outcome instrument, the flow of an orthopedic office may be slowed. If at all possible, patients should fill out these forms before the visit, either in the office or through the mail. The data collection system may either be paper or electronic. Computerization makes analysis of data much easier. Forms can be conventional or scannable or the instrument may be included on a touch-screen format. Any method that involves nonscannable paper creates a secondary problem of data entry for analysis and is labor intensive and expensive. Predesigned, off-the-shelf, commercially available, turnkey products are the most efficient design. Individual designs can be tailored to your needs but are labor intensive and expensive. Several commercially available systems are available through the AAOS.

Patient and physician privacy are concerns with any computerized national data base. Who will see the data? Is it anonymous? Will it be used for individual bench marking, procedure authorization, or institutional characterization? Clearly, patients and physicians are concerned with the anonymity of the data, and these issues must be resolved before participation will be universal.

From 1960 through 1986, only four papers in the English orthopedic literature reported prospective studies of THA, and these four papers had grave deficiencies in design.[14] Since that time, the outcomes research movement has sought to correct this deficiency. In 1987, Wennberg et al[37] published their study of hospital utilization rates comparing New Haven and Boston. A discharge data base, which included nonfederal, short-term, general, and selective speciality hospitals, from 1982 was analyzed. The populations were adjusted for out-of-area admissions to make the populations comparable. Utilization rates were based on hospital discharges and days and were adjusted for age and sex using 1980 census information. One conclusion of the study was that admission rates for THA and TKA were substantially higher in Boston than in New Haven. No explanation was given for this difference, and no inference was made as to whether the Boston rate was too high or the New Haven rate was too low.[37] A similar study showed the same small area of variations over four geographic areas of Maine.[38]

Liang et al.[39] performed a prospective cost-effectiveness analysis 6 months following THA in selected consecutive patients with osteoarthritis. The conclusion of this study showed that, although the operation improves function and diminishes pain, health care cost savings associated with these outcomes are small in the first 6 months after surgery. Because the majority of the patients are not working, earnings were judged not to be a fair or relevant measure of benefit. Further studies were suggested to determine the effects of other medical and surgical options on outcomes and also on the value our society as a whole places on relief of pain and improved quality of life.[40] Other early cost-effectiveness studies have dealt with the issues of dental prophylaxis in total joint arthroplasty (TJA), rheumatoid patients, and work-related disabilities in patients undergoing TJA.[39,41,42]

Wiklund and Romanus[43] addressed the issue of quality of life before and after THA in patients who had osteoarthrosis of the hip. Functional assessments were performed with the Charnley modification of the Merle d'Aubigné scale, and the patients assessed quality of life before and 1 year after THA using the NHP. Statistically significant improvement was observed regarding pain, energy, sleep, and social isolation. There was a significant reduction in the frequency of health-related problems relating to housework, hobbies, social life, sexual function, and family history. Quality of life after THA was in close agreement with that of a healthy reference group of similar age and sex distribution. The conclusion was that quality of life after THA has improved considerably.[43]

Using more sophisticated quality of life measures, O'Boyle et al.[44] applied the schedule for the evaluation of individual quality of life derived from judgment analysis techniques to a measurement of the patient's level of function in five self-nominated facets of life and the relative weight or importance attached to these areas. The use of individualized value systems assumes that the quality-of-life indicators will be relevant to the assessed patient. The McMaster Health Index questionnaire was also used as an adjunct to measure health status. Health status in individually measured quality of life was increased significantly after THA when measured by this method.[44]

Laupacis, Bourne, Rorabeck et al.[45] have been the foremost providers of quality orthopedic outcomes research in the 1990s. In 1993, a study of the effect of THA on the health-related quality of life of patients who had osteoarthrosis was examined as part of a randomized, controlled trial comparing femoral head prostheses, which were performed with or without cement. The health-related quality of life was assessed with the use of the Harris Hip Score, the Merle d'Aubigné hip score, the SIP, the WOMAC, the McMaster-Toronto Arthritis Patient Preference Disability Questionnaire (MACTAR), and the time trade-off technique as a measure of utility. Patients took the 6-minute walk test as well.[46]

The study from London, Ontario, demonstrates great improvement in physical function, social interaction, and overall health that occurs after THA, as well as the feasibility of the performance of randomized trials to compare two types of hip implants. Preoperative analysis of patients undergoing THA shows that they have severe pain and that advanced osteoarthritis greatly affects physical activity, social interaction, and overall health. The improvement in health-related quality of life after THA is rapid and substantial, and it affects all aspects of well being. The improvement in well being was substantially better than that seen for patients who have end-stage renal disease with corrected anemia on hemodialysis.[46]

This same group of authors[45] looked at the cost effectiveness of cemented versus cementless THA as well as a calculation of cost per quality of life year. This also was a randomized control trial. No difference in cost was seen in the initial hospitalization when the cementless and cemented groups were compared. Clearly, revision percentage will be the ultimate determinant of cost, but only long-term follow-up study will provide this information. The cost per QALY gained was $27,139.00 This figure was an improvement over the medical treatment of hypertension, estrogen therapy for postmenopausal women, and hemodialysis.[45]

Ritter et al.[47] looked at quality of life after THA and TKA using the SF-36 in a prospective fashion. The results indicated that THA and TKA significantly improved the functional status and quality of life among patients with osteoarthritis.[47] McGuigan et al.[48] looked at the SF-36 prospectively in a more detailed fashion. A highly significant improvement was seen comparing preoperative with postoperative scores at 2 years for physical function, social function, physical role function, emotional role function, mental health, energy, and pain. Despite a significant change in health status, no change was seen in health perception. The conclusion of the study was that the poor ability of the SF-36 to predict postoperative improvement on an individual basis makes the instrument inappropriate to be used alone to determine treatment selection.[48]

A community hospital-based, prospective study[49] measuring the success of THA and TKA as a factor of case selection and public policy was performed in 1995. The authors used the SF-36 and other physician-derived scoring systems for analysis. Patient-defined success was related closely to post-treatment physical function and bodily pain. Patient ratings of success are also in line with physician-derived clinical scores. Success of THA is related to the change from pretreatment function. Although patient ratings of success are generally consistent with other outcome measures, their relationship to patient expectations, satisfaction, and attribution needs to be better defined before these instruments can be used for performance monitoring and case selection.[49]

Outcome Studies in Revision THA

Well-constructed, randomized, controlled studies that reflect current trends in outcomes research are not available in revision THA. Small sample sizes, elderly patient populations, vastly differing uses of technology, and nonstandardized reporting of the degree of difficulty of the cases contribute to the paucity of available outcome studies in revision THA.

The construction of a national hip registry with compatible data bases using validated instruments will permit multicenter collated data studies to be constructed and provide outcome information heretofore unavailable. Additionally, multicenter, randomized, clinical trials can be performed that may provide answers to some of the hotly debated topics in revision THA: how long a stem, cemented versus noncemented, and bone graft versus custom implant. These unresolved issues remain to be explored through the establishment of a national hip registry.

Significance of the Outcomes Research

Wide variations exist in the patterns of orthopedic practice in the United States. Elective THA surgery performed for a wide range of diagnoses follows this variable practice pattern.[38] Lavernia and Guzman[17] have shown a volume-outcomes relationship for physicians and hospitals performing THA. Physicians and hospitals with low volumes of THA cases had significantly higher mortality rates, costs, and hospital length of stay than physicians and hospitals with high volumes of THA cases. This information was generated from patient discharge information without regard for case severity.

Variations in practice are also associated with variations in information. For example, revision THA is coded as "a complication of an orthopedic device." This is not an accurate description of revision THA, and this coding practice can be detrimental to surgeons who perform a large number of revision procedures.[17] Outcomes research can aid the surgeon performing THA by evaluating and influencing the quality of the arthroplasty literature, by manipulating large data base information for the development of prospective trials, by providing patients with feedback concerning success and complication rates, and by creating the information base for true clinical shared decision making, thus reducing unwanted variation. It is imperative that orthopedic surgeons control the quality of these data so that well-reasoned choices are made about the role of THA in the care of patients with arthritis. If the orthopedic profession does not accept these challenges and put forth solutions, third parties, such as government agencies and insurance companies, will present solutions.

Some health care planners have predicted that, by the end of this decade, 90% of Americans will receive their medical care through a managed care arrangement. The inherent conflict of interest present in the capitation reimbursement systems demands an outcomes-based physician-reimbursement system to deal with the conflicts that surround managed care.[50] Patient satisfaction or consumer satisfaction is generally the sum of the outcome minus the expectation. Outcomes research will allow orthopedic surgeons and hospitals to document patient satisfaction with THA.

To accomplish these goals, universal collection of outcome data will be necessary. The current movement in Medicare funding toward the "Center of Excellence" concept illustrates why even the smallest joint replacement practice should collect outcome data. In the future, if a surgeon wishes to reserve the privilege of performing procedures, such as THA, the surgeon may be required to demonstrate good outcomes. If data are not collected, the surgeon may not be approved to perform the procedure or be reimbursed for the procedure.

It is not clear whether all orthopedic surgeons need to track outcomes for purposes of evaluating the outcome of orthopedic interventions. In fact, the cost required for all orthopedic surgeons to track outcomes suggests that outcomes research should be limited to an appropriate sampling of orthopedic practices. However, all orthopedic surgeons should become familiar with outcomes research so that they may be able to participate in outcomes tracking when and if it is necessary.

On a more global scale, as orthopedic surgeons seek to preserve their position as the highest quality providers of musculoskeletal care, they must document the effectiveness of orthopedic treatment methods. Based on traditional clinical results research, THA is one of the most successful medical innovations of the past 30 years. It has been shown to be cost effective, and patient satisfaction is high. Orthopedic surgeons must now confirm the success of THA with validated instruments among large populations of patients and in varied practice settings. Outcomes research permits orthopedic surgeons to attain this goal.

References

1. Keller RB. Outcomes research in orthopaedics. *J Am Assoc Orthop Surg.* 1993;1:122–129.
2. Rudicel SA. Outcomes assessment. In: Kasser JR, ed. *Orthopaedic knowledge update.* American Academy of Orthopaedic Surgeons, 1996:85–88.
3. Merle d'Aubigné R, Postel M. Functional results of hip arthroplasty with acrylic prosthesis. *J Bone Joint Surg Am.* 1954;36:451–475.
4. Charnley J. The long-term results of low-friction arthroplasty of the hip performed as a primary intervention. *J Bone Joint Surg Br.* 1972;54:61–76.
5. Larson CB. Rating scale for hip disabilities. *Clin Orthop.* 1963;31:85–93.

6. Harris WH. Traumatic arthritis of the hip after dislocation and acetabular fractures: treatment by mold arthroplasty. An end-result study using a new method of result evaluation. *J Bone Joint Surg Am.* 1969;51:737–755.
7. Kavanagh BF, Fitzgerald RH Jr. Clinical and roentgenographic assessment of total hip arthroplasty: a new hip score. *Clin Orthop.* 1985;193:133–140.
8. Bryant MJ, Kernohan WG, Nixon JR, Mollan RA. A statistical analysis of hip scores. *J Bone Joint Surg Br.* 1993;75:705–709.
9. Johnston RC, Fitzgerald RH Jr, Harris WH, et al. Clinical and radiographic evaluation of total hip replacement: a standard system of terminology for reporting results. *J Bone Joint Surg Am.* 1990;72:161–168.
10. Liang MH, Katz JN, Phillips C, Sledge C, Cats-Baril W. Total hip arthroplasty outcome evaluation form of the American Association of Orthopaedic Surgeons Task Force on Outcome Studies. *J Bone Joint Surg Am.* 1991;73:639–646.
11. Fitzgerald RH, Callaghan JJ, Colwell CW, Skinner HB. Symposiums: The National Hip Registry: a new resource for measuring and improving the quality of health care. *Contemp Orthop.* 1995;31:127–136.
12. Wennberg J, Gittelsohn A. Variations in medical care among small areas. *Sci Am.* 1982;246:120–134.
13. Keller RB, Rudicel SA, Liang MH. Outcomes research in orthopaedics. *AAOS Instruc Course Lect.* 1993;43;699–711.
14. Gross M. A critique of the methodologies used in clinical studies of hip-joint arthroplasty published in the English-language orthopaedic literature. *J Bone Joint Surg Am.* 1988;70:1369–1376.
15. L'Abbé KA, Detsky AS, O'Rourke K. Meta-analysis in clinical research. *Ann Intern Med.* 1987;107:224–237.
16. Callahan CM, Drake BG, Heck DA, Dittus RS. Patient outcomes following tricompartmental total knee replacement: a meta-analysis. *JAMA.* 1994;271:1349–1357.
17. Lavernia CJ, Guzman JF. Relationship of surgical volume to short-term mortality, morbidity, and hospital charges in arthroplasty. *J Arthroplasty.* 1995;10:133–140.
18. Kassirer JP, Moskowitz AJ, Lau J, Paulker SG. Decision analysis: a progress report. *Ann Intern Med.* 1987;106:275–291.
19. Weinstein JN. Shared decision making. Outcomes and effectiveness in musculoskeletal research and practice. American Academy of Orthopaedic Surgeons Symposium #363, October 1996.
20. Detsky AS, Naglie G. A clinician's guide to cost-effectiveness analysis. *Ann Intern Med.* 1990;113:147–154.
21. Ware JE Jr, Sherbourne CD. The MOS 36 item short form health survey (SF-36). 1. Conceptual framework and item selection. *Med Care.* 1992;30:473–483.
22. Kaplan RM, Bush JW, Berry CC. Health status: types of validity in the index of well-being. *Health Serv Res.* 1976;11:478–507.
23. Bergner M, Bobbitt RA, Pollard WE, Martin DP, Gilson BS. The sickness impact profile: validation of a health status measure. *Med Care.* 1976;14:57–67.
24. Hunt SM, McEwen J, McKenna SP. Measuring health status: a new tool for clinicians and epidemiologists. *J R Coll Gen Pract.* 1985;35:185–188.
25. Bellamy N, Buchanan WW, Goldsmith CH, Campbell J, Stih L. Validation study of WOMAC: a health status instrument for measuring clinically important patient relevant outcomes following total hip or knee arthroplasty in osteoarthritis. *J Orthop Rheumatol.* 1988;1:95–108.
26. Johanson NA, Charlson ME, Szatrowski TP, Ranawat CS. A self-administered hip-rating questionnaire for the assessment of outcome after total hip replacement. *J Bone Joint Surg Am.* 1992;74:587–597.
27. Jette AM. Functional Status Index: reliability of a chronic disease evaluation instrument. *Arch Phys Med Rehab.* 1980;61:395–401.
28. Fries JF, Spitz P, Kraines G, Holman HR. Measurement of patient outcome in arthritis. *Arthritis Rheum.* 1980;23:137–145.
29. Meenan RF, Gertman PM, Mason JH. Measuring health status in arthritis: the arthritis impact measurement scales. *Arthritis Rheum.* 1980;23:146–152.
30. Kroll M, Ganz S, Backus S, Benick R, MacKenzie C, Harris L. A tool for measuring functional outcomes after total hip arthroplasty. *Arthritis Care Res.* 1994;7:78–84.
31. Martin DP, Engelberg R, Agel J, Snapp D, Swiontkowski MF. Development of a musculoskeletal extremity health status instrument: the Musculoskeletal Function Assessment instrument. *J Orthop Res.* 1996;14:173–181.
32. Katz JN, Larson MG, Phillips CB, Fossel AH, Liang MH. Comparative measurement sensitivity of short and longer health status instruments. *Med Care.* 1992;30:917–925.
33. Liang MH, Fossel AH, Larson MG. Comparison of five health status instruments for orthopedic evaluation. *Med Care.* 1990;28:632–642.
34. Hawker G, Melfi C, Paul J, Green R, Bombardier C. Comparison of a generic (SF-36) in a disease specific (WOMAC) (Western Ontario and McMaster Universities Osteoarthritis Index) instrument in the measurement of outcomes after knee replacement surgery. *J Rheumatol.* 1995;22:1193–1196.
35. Bombardier C, Melfi C, Paul J, et al. Comparison of a generic and a disease-specific measure of pain and physical function after knee replacement surgery. *Med Care.* 1995;33:AS131–AS144.
36. Noalo DL. Office based assessment: how to process, transfer and secure data. Outcomes and effectiveness in musculoskeletal research and practice. American Academy of Orthopaedic Surgery Symposium, October 1996.
37. Wennberg JE, Freeman JL, Culp WJ. Are hospital services rationed in New Haven or over-utilized in Boston? *Lancet.* 1987;1:1185–1189.
38. Keller RB, Soule DN, Wennberg JE, Hanley DF. Dealing with geographic variations in the use of hospitals: the experience of the Maine Medical Assessment Foundation Orthopaedic Study Group. *J Bone Joint Surg Am.* 1990;72:1286–1293.
39. Liang MH, Larson M, Thompson M, Eaton H, McNamara E, Katz R, Taylor J. Costs and outcomes in rheumatoid arthritis and osteoarthritis. *Arthritis Rheum.* 1984;27:522–529.
40. Liang MH, Cullen KE, Larson MG, et al. Cost-effectiveness of total joint arthroplasty in osteoarthritis. *Arthritis Rheum.* 1986;29:937–943.
41. Tsevat J, Durand-Zaleski I, Pauker SG. Cost-effectiveness of antibiotic prophylaxis for dental procedures in patients

with artificial joints. *Am J Public Health.* 1989;79:3739–3743.
42. Nevitt MC, Epstein WV, Masem M, Murray WR. Work disability before and after total hip arthroplasty: assessment of effectiveness in reducing disability. *Arthritis Rheum.* 1984;27:410–421.
43. Wiklund I, Romanus B. A comparison of quality of life before and after arthroplasty in patients who had arthrosis of the hip joint. *J Bone Joint Surg Am.* 1991;73:765–769.
44. O'Boyle CA, McGee H, Hickey A, O'Malley K, Joyce CR. Individual quality of life in patients undergoing hip replacement. *Lancet.* 1992;339:1088–1091.
45. Laupacis A, Bourne R, Rorabeck C, et al. Costs of elective total hip arthroplasty during the first year: cemented versus noncemented. *J Arthroplasty.* 1994;9:481–487.
46. Laupacis A, Bourne R, Rorabeck C, et al. The effect of elective total hip replacement on health-related quality of life. *J Bone Joint Surg Am.* 1993;75:1619–1626.
47. Ritter MA, Albohm MJ, Keating EM, Faris PM, Meding JB. Comparative outcomes of total joint arthroplasty. *J Arthroplasty.* 1995;10:737–741.
48. McGuigan FX, Hozack WJ, Moriarity L, Emg K, Rothman RH. Predicting quality-of-life outcomes following total joint arthroplasty: limitations of the SF-36 Health Status Questionnaire. *J Arthroplasty.* 1995;10:742–747.
49. Bayley KB, London MR, Grunkmeier GL, Lansky DJ. Measuring the success of treatment in patient terms. *Med Care.* 1995;33(4 Suppl):AS226–AS235.
50. Michaels RM, Sanderson-Austin J. Outcomes based physician reimbursement: a solution for dealing with conflicts of interest in managed care. *Group Pract J.* 1996;45:16–23.

74
Looking Forward: Implant Research

Harold Aberman, Michael Bushelow, Larry Gustavson, Cas Stark, D.C. Sun, Aiguo Wang, and Kathy Wang

Use of Finite Element Analysis in the Development of Total Hip Arthroplasty Femoral Components

The finite element method for solution of structural analysis problems can simply be stated as a method in which highly complex geometric problems are transformed from a differential equation approach to an algebraic problem. Complex geometries or systems are broken into smaller building blocks or finite elements. Simple algebraic equations defining these building blocks are assembled into a series of simultaneous equations and solved using a high speed computer. Figure 74.1 shows a typical finite element model of a total hip arthroplasty femoral component implanted in a human femur.

The concept of breaking complex geometries into smaller regions for analysis was first proposed by a mathematician by the name of R. Courant in 1943. Development of the concept into what is now known as the finite element method (FEM) or finite element analysis (FEA) occurred within the aircraft industry during the mid to late 1950s. The lag between the original concept and development of FEA into a useful tool for structural analyses was probably because computers of the size and speed necessary to solve the large number of simultaneous algebraic equations were not available.[1]

The use of the FEM in orthopedic biomechanics can be traced back to 1972. Articles by Brekelmans et al.[2] and Rybicki et al.[3] show the development of 2-D plane stress models of the human femur. An excellent review of the early use of FEA in the orthopedic biomechanics field was presented in a 1983 article by Huiskes and Chao.[4] The article does an excellent job of describing the early FEA work performed in the area of orthopedic biomechanics, as well as discussing the limitations of the method.

Initial use of the finite element method in orthopedics was generally restricted to the academic arena. There, the computer resources and dedicated personnel necessary to generate the complex finite element models were located. In the early to mid 1980s, the exponential growth in computer speed and the similar decrease in the cost of the computer itself made the use of the finite element analysis more cost effective. Analyses that needed large, costly main frame computer resources could now easily be handled by relatively inexpensive engineering workstations and high end personal computers. Additionally, the introductions of graphical user interfaces, automatic mesh generators, FEA/CAD translators, and improvements in solver technology have significantly increased the user friendliness of commercial FEA software packages. These advances in both hardware and software capabilities have made FEA an everyday tool in the design and development of orthopedic devices.

While the FEM is now readily available as a tool in the design of orthopedic implants, it should be noted that the tool should be used by personnel trained in both stress analysis and in the use of the individual finite element code. As quoted from an article by Baumgartner and Kensinger, ". . . the computer is the automation of Murphy's Law: with it an engineer can make more mistakes, faster, with greater magnitude, and more confidence than ever before!!"[5]

That being said, the FEM has proven to be an extremely useful tool in the development of recent total hip arthroplasty components. When properly used, FEA allows the design team to investigate specific design features and evaluate their effect on multiple variables including but not limited to stress shielding, thigh pain, cement stresses, component strength, and so on. To better demonstrate the capabilities of the FEM, examples of analyses performed in the development of two new cementless and one new cemented total hip will be reviewed. Specifically, the application of FEA techniques to the reduction of thigh pain in cementless components and reduction of distal cement stress in cemented components will be demonstrated.

Thigh pain is a problem in all cementless hip designs, occurring in stems fabricated from both Co-Cr and titanium alloys.[6-9] The exact etiology of thigh pain in well-fixed devices is not well understood. Recent reports have

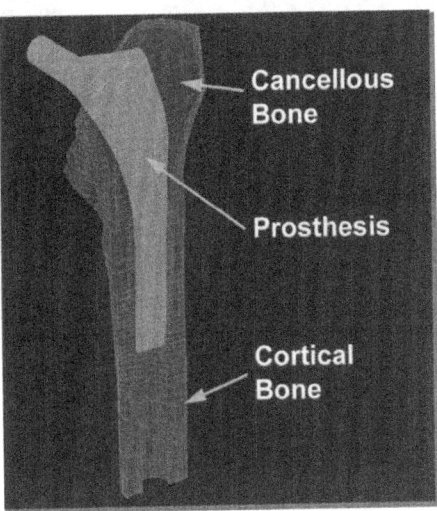

Figure 74.1. Typical finite element model of a prosthesis implanted in a bone. The model has been cross-sectioned along the M/L plane to allow viewing of the position of the implant in the femur.

indicated that stiffness mismatch between the distal femoral component and distal femur is a key factor in the occurrence of midthigh pain in patients with otherwise clinically successful arthroplasties. Skinner et al.[10] reviewed one hundred consecutive uncemented hip arthroplasties at one year follow-up. The results of their study comparing the flexural rigidity of the bone to the prosthesis indicated a trend towards reduced thigh pain with decreased flexural rigidity of the prosthesis. Cameron et al.[11] presented the results of a multi-center study on various stem designs. Their results for the S-ROM component, where a solid vs. coronal split device were compared showed a significant reduction in the incidence of the thigh pain with more flexible coronal split design. Hungerford and coworkers (Hungerford et al.[12] and Franks et al.[13]) reviewed a study group of 45 patients, less than 45 years of age, with a minimum three year follow-up. Their results indicated that a mismatch in the bending rigidity of the prosthesis to bone correlated to thigh pain. Dujovne et al.[14] compared stiffness characteristics of human femoral to several commercially available prostheses. The results of this study indicate that larger implants, greater than 15 mm in diameter, are significantly stiffer than the human femora.

In an effort to correlate the relationship between distal stem stiffness and thigh pain, a detailed three-dimensional finite element model of a femoral component implanted in a femur was developed (Fig. 74.1). A perfect fit of the prosthesis in the diaphysis and full bone ingrowth into the porous coated region was assumed. The porous coating covered the proximal one-third region of the stem. Frictionless contact was modeled between the distal stem and the inner cortex of the bone.

The effect of distal stem stiffness on bone stresses was evaluated by changing geometry of the distal end and stem material. Loads simulating walking and stair climbing were placed on the model.

Results of the analyses indicated that the reaction force between the distal tip and the inner cortex is concentrated over a short distance. Reducing the distal stiffness of the implant decreased the reaction force and the maximum and minimum principal stresses at the distal tip of the implant. Additionally, the analyses indicated that the resultant load on the bone at the distal tip of the implant acted at an angle 20° to 25° anterior to the lateral side for the walking load case and 34° to 43° anterior to the lateral side for stair climbing load case. The direction of the resultant load is an indication of the direction that stem flexibility should be oriented.

Considering the FEA results and clinical findings reported above, a system of straight and anatomical cobalt-chromium (Co-Cr) femoral components with reduced distal stiffness were designed. The reduction in stiffness was achieved by modifying the distal geometry of the components by the addition of flutes and a distal split. Symmetrical flutes and a coronal slot were developed for the straight designs and rotated flutes and a slot were developed for the anatomical designs. Finite element analysis and optimization techniques were used to modify the distal geometry of the components to meet the design goals of maximum flexibility within a specified strength limit.

Stiffness results for the straight and anatomic stems are shown in Fig. 74.2. The figure shows a comparison of distal stem stiffness results for a 12 mm through 18

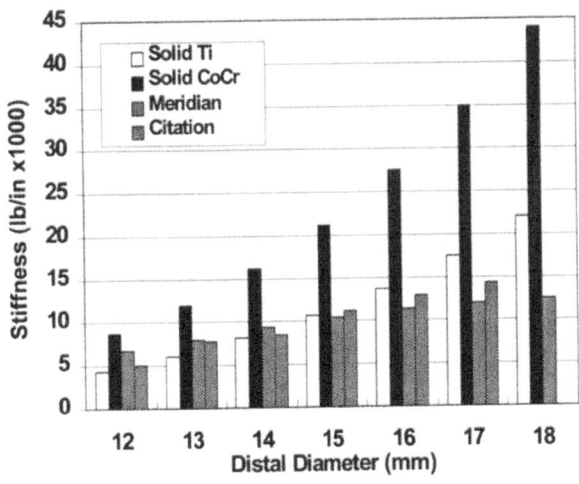

Figure 74.2. Results of stiffness analyses for the straight (Meridian ST) and anatomic (Citation AT) Co-Cr stems with distal flutes and splits. Data on solid cylindrical Co-Cr and Ti-6Al-4V are presented for comparison. Note that the optimized fluted and slotted stems have distal stiffnesses in the range of a 12 to 13 mm solid Co-Cr stem.

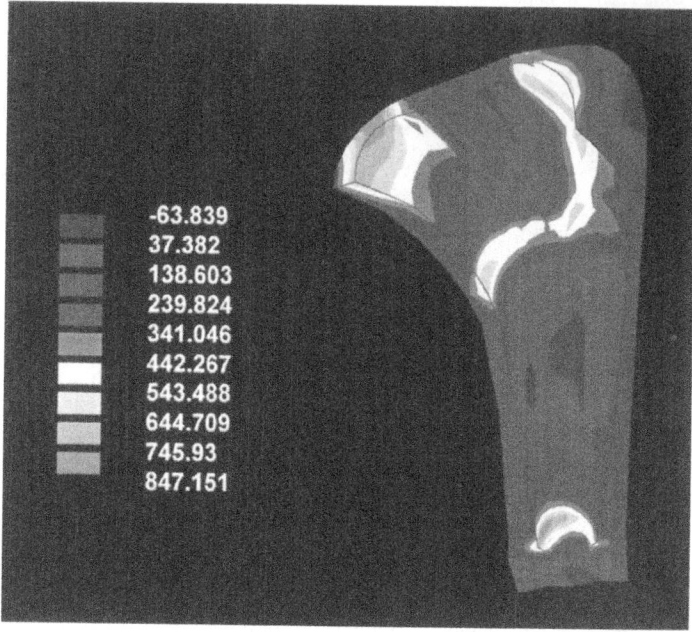

Figure 74.3. Finite element model and result showing location of maximum principal stress in the region of the distal tip of a femoral component. The bone and prosthesis have been removed and the cement mantle has been cross-sectioned along the M/L plane. (See color insert.)

mm solid circular Co-Cr and Ti-6Al-4V alloy stems against distal stiffness values for the fluted/slotted straight and anatomical femoral components of similar diameter. From this figure it can be seen that the modified femoral component's stiffness range from just below that of a solid circular 12 mm Co-Cr stem to that of a solid circular 13 mm Co-Cr stem.

It is generally believed that cement is the weak link in cemented total hip arthroplasty. Autopsy studies have shown that cement cracking and cement debonding at the distal tip of the femoral component may play a key role in the initiation of stem loosening.[15] Additionally, many experimental and theoretical analyses have indicated that high cement strains/stresses exist at the distal tip of a femoral component under physiological loading conditions.[16,17]

In order to investigate the affect of distal tip design on cement stresses a detailed finite element model of a prosthesis implanted with bone cement in a bone was developed. Initial analyses were performed to determine the overall effect of cement mantle thickness on cement stresses. As in other studies, the maximum principal stress occurred in the region of the distal tip of the implant (Fig. 74.3, see color insert). Results from these analyses indicated that reduction of the stiffness of the distal stem would lead to reduced stresses at the distal tip of the implant.

Further studies were performed to look at the effect of specific distal stem designs on distal cement stresses. The designs investigated included a cylindrical geometry, a tapered geometry, a tapered plus flutes geometry, and a tapered plus flutes with hemispherical tip geometry (Fig. 74.4). Analyses were performed with the femoral component perfectly bonded to the cement mantle and with the femoral component debonded from the cement mantle over the distal one third of the component. Load cases representing normal level walking loads and rising from a chair were applied to the models.

Results of the perfectly bonded analyses indicated, as in the initial study, that increased flexibility reduced distal cement mantle stresses. Review of the debonded analyses results, however, indicated that flutes acted as a stress concentration and significantly increased the stress magnitude if cement debonding occurred. Modifying the geometry to a tapered-fluted design with a hemispherical tip brought the stresses back into the range seen for the bonded cases.

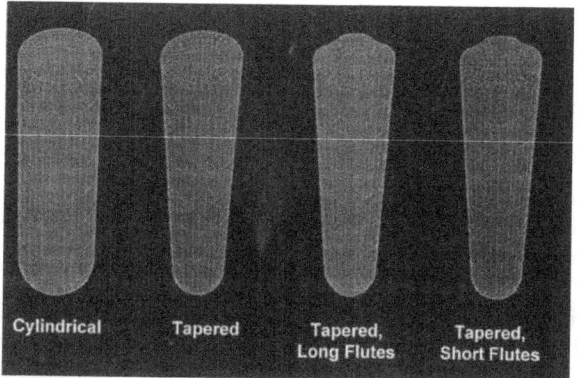

Figure 74.4. Finite element model representations of the distal geometries of the stems analyzed.

The FEA technique, as demonstrated above, is a powerful tool. Figure 74.5 shows the final designs of the stems that have been developed due in part to the finite element analyses described above. It should be noted that, in addition to the finite element analyses, significant experimental and laboratory work was performed to insure the biomechanical function of these devices and that they meet the need of the end user, the orthopedic surgeon.

What the future of this technique will bring is hard to predict. FEA models that take into account the effects of stress shielding and predict adaptive bone remodeling and models that look at the effect of cemented stem design on interface stress and predict cement-stem interface debonding have been and are continually being developed.[18,19] Use of quantitative tools, such as DEXA that measure bone morphological changes, should improve our understanding of the bone remodeling process and allow for the development of more predictive bone remodeling theorems. Increases in computer speed, will allow for larger and more detailed models of the femur to be developed. All of this coupled together may allow FEM to be developed that will predict the long-term outcome of individual implant designs.

Advances in Cobalt-Chromium-Molybdenum and Titanium Implant Alloys

Forged Co-Cr-Mo alloy and Ti-6Al-4V alloys first saw widespread use in the United States in the mid-1970s for total hip stem manufacturing.[20] The forged Co-Cr-Mo alloy represented an improvement over the cast al-

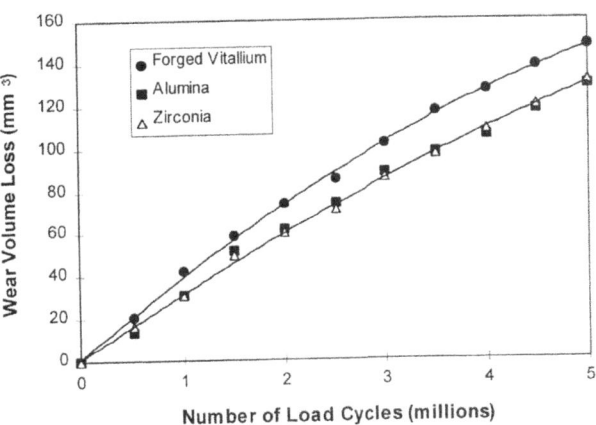

Figure 74.6. Hip simulator wear of gamma irradiated UHMWPE cups against Co-Cr-Mo, Alumina, and Zirconia modular femoral heads.

loy, while Ti-6Al-4V provided greater strength than commercially pure (CP) titanium. Initially both were applied in cemented stem designs. In monolithic designs, Ti-6Al-4V proved to have unacceptable wear properties against polyethylene and questions arose with regard to the compatibility of the more flexible titanium alloy stem with cemented fixation.[21] Forged Co-Cr-Mo alloy has since emerged as a preferred material for cemented stems, while titanium alloys have been widely used in noncemented press-fit and porous coated stem designs.

Co-Cr-Mo alloys have also been used extensively in articulating surfaces of endoprostheses and total joint designs. Current modular total hip designs employ the alloy in the forged or wrought conditions to take advantage of its high hardness and fine grain microstructure. Recent hip simulator wear studies have shown these forged Co-Cr-Mo heads to perform exceptionally well, with wear rates against polyethylene approaching those reported for ceramic heads (Fig. 74.6).

Forging imparts increased strength to cast alloys by refining the grain structure and imparting "cold work" to the alloy crystal structure, which improves the material's ability to resist deformation. When properly performed, the forging of Co-Cr-Mo alloy raises tensile and fatigue strengths significantly above those of the cast alloy. The forged alloy develops an extremely fine grained microstructure well suited to resist the bending loads imposed on a hip stem (Fig. 74.7). Because of its exceptional strength, forged Co-Cr-Mo alloy permits stem design options which reduce cement stresses, while maintaining good stem strength.[22]

The introduction of porous coated Co-Cr-Mo hip stem designs in the 1980s, prompted a move back to the cast alloy, primarily due to the detrimental effects porous coating processing has on the mechanical strength of the forged alloy. Porous coatings created by

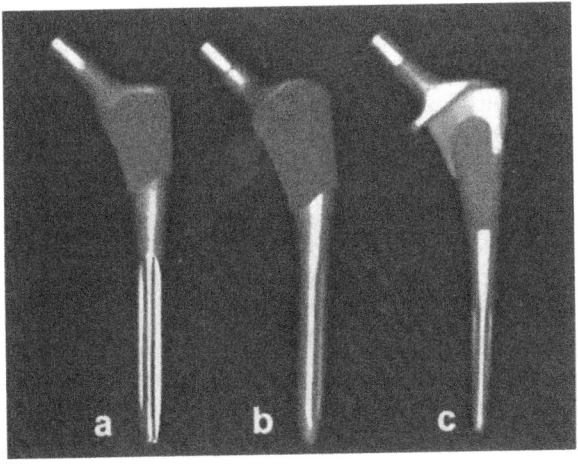

Figure 74.5. Photographs of final design of femoral components based upon FEA results: A. Meridian ST, B. Citation AT, and C. Definition PM femoral components.

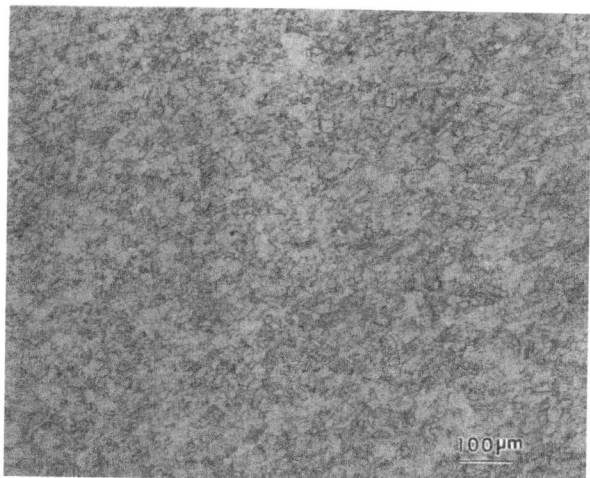

Figure 74.7. A forged Co-Cr-Mo alloy grain structure (100×).

Table 74.1. Effect of sintering temperature on Co-Cr-Mo alloy.

Alloy	Smooth rotating beam fatigue strength (MPa)	
	Before sintering	After sintering
Cast Co-Cr-Mo	500 ± 15	380 ± 15
Forged Co-Cr-Mo	775 ± 15	320 ± 15

sintered beads require processing at elevated temperatures to achieve bonding between the coating particles. When a sintered coating is applied to a forged hip stem, the temperatures involved serve to anneal the forged Co-Cr-Mo alloy, cause excessive grain growth in the alloy microstructure, and effectively lower the strength of the forged alloy to below that of a casting (Fig. 74.8). The cast Co-Cr-Mo alloy is less affected by the sintering temperature, particularly when porous coating is followed by hot isostatic pressing (HIP) (Table 74.1). For this reason, sintered porous coated Co-Cr-Mo hip stems have historically been produced using the cast alloy.

Gas Atomized Dispersion Strengthened Co-Cr-Mo Alloy

A variation on the forged Co-Cr-Mo alloy, developed by Howmedica, addresses the loss of fatigue strength caused by exposure to the porous coating sintering temperature. Utilizing powder metallurgy and a technology known as oxide dispersion strengthening, a forged alloy microstructure was created which resists the annealing effects of the sintering thermal cycle. Modeled after technology utilized in the aerospace industry to increase high temperature strength of jet engine components,[23] the Howmedica process utilizes the gas atomization process to produce Co-Cr-Mo alloy powder in which a uniform dispersion of sub-microscopic oxide particles is created. The atomized powder is consolidated to form bar stock, which is then used to produce a forged hip stem (Fig. 74.9). The forged stem is finished and porous coated in the conventional manner.

The advantage of the gas atomized dispersion strengthened (GADS) alloy appears following exposure to the sintering thermal cycle. Unlike a conventional forged Co-Cr-Mo alloy which loses strength and its fine grain structure following porous coating sintering, the dispersion strengthened alloy retains a fine grain structure and high fatigue strength after the high temperature exposure (Fig. 74.10). The difference lies in the stabilizing effects of the dispersion particles, which "pin" the alloy's microstructural grain boundaries to prevent grain growth at the elevated temperature. The result is a retained fine grain structure that imparts a fatigue strength close to that of the original forged alloy (Table 74.2). Utilization of this GADS Co-Cr-Mo alloy increases the design safety of small porous coated hip stems while permitting design options such as distal sitting to improve stem flexibility.

Titanium Alloys: Beta Titanium

Since its introduction in the 1950s, the use of titanium in orthopedics has principally been in the form of commercially pure grade (CP titanium) and Ti-6Al-4V alloy. Both of these materials were originally developed for military or industrial applications and later adopted for medical devices.[24] In the 1980s, two variations of Ti-6Al-4V alloy, Ti-6Al-7Nb and Ti-5Al-2.5Fe, were introduced in which vanadium was replaced to address concerns over vanadium biocompatibility. The alloys are metallurgically similar to Ti-6Al-4V, being alpha-beta alloys, which exhibit a two phase metallurgical structure of alpha and beta titanium.

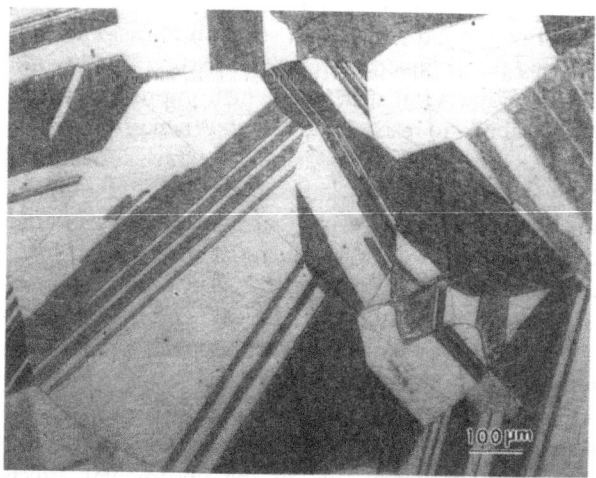

Figure 74.8. Forged Co-Cr-Mo alloy microstructure following porous coating sintering (100×).

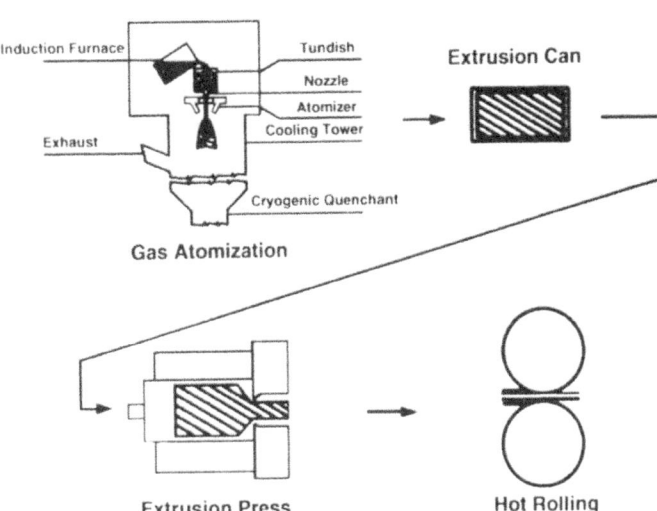

Figure 74.9. GADS alloy process schematic.

Pure titanium exists in two crystallographic forms, or phases, depending upon temperature. Alpha titanium exists in a hexagonal close-packed (hcp) crystal structure below 882°C and transforms to the body-centered cubic (bcc) beta titanium above this temperature. Through elemental additions that elevate or lower the transformation (transus) temperature and strengthen the alpha and beta phases, combined with heat treating and thermomechanical processing, to alter the amount and form of the alpha and beta phases, titanium alloys with distinct metallurgical properties are created.

Certain elements, such as aluminum, oxygen and nitrogen, are soluble in the alpha phase. They strengthen alpha titanium and elevate the alpha-beta transformation temperature. Other elements, such as vanadium, molybdenum, zirconium, niobium and iron, help strengthen and stabilize the beta phase and prevent formation of the alpha phase on cooling through the transformation temperature range.[25]

Alpha-beta alloys, primarily Ti-6Al-4V, have for years been the sole titanium alloys used in orthopedics. Recently attention has been directed toward the potential beta titanium alloys offer, particularly for noncemented hip stem applications. Beta alloys can be processed to higher strength levels and exhibit better notched properties and toughness than alpha-beta alloys. They can be designed to contain more biologically acceptable alloying elements, for example, Zr, Mo, Nb, Fe and can be processed to achieve a significantly lower elastic modulus, for increased stem flexibility. Through appropriate metallurgical processing, beta titanium alloys with elastic modulus approaching those of some composite systems can be achieved, providing a conservative alternative to composites for improving hip stem flexibility.[26]

One beta titanium alloy that has been approved for use in implants and is now being applied commercially in noncemented hip stems is Ti-12Mo-6Zr-2Fe (TMZF). In the annealed condition, TMZF exhibits a single-phase beta titanium microstructure (Fig. 74.11). The alloy is 25% more flexible than Ti-6Al-4V with a 20% higher yield strength. Smooth fatigue properties are comparable to Ti-6Al-4V, while notched properties are improved (Table 74.3). TMZF exhibits the same excellent corrosion resistance as Ti-6Al-4V (Fig. 74.12) but has demon-

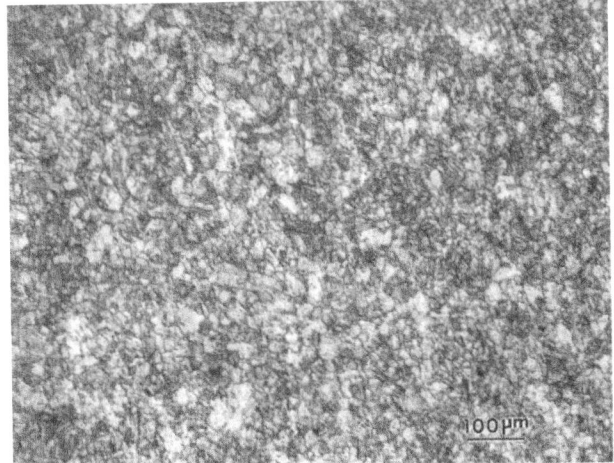

Figure 74.10. Forged GADS alloy microstructure following porous coating sintering (100×).

Table 74.2. Fatigue strength of GADS Co-Cr-Mo vs forged Co-Cr-Mo

	Smooth rotating beam fatigue strength (MPa)	
Alloy	Before sintering	After sintering
GADS Co-Cr-Mo	775 ± 15	605 ± 15
Forged Co-Cr-Mo	775 ± 15	320 ± 15

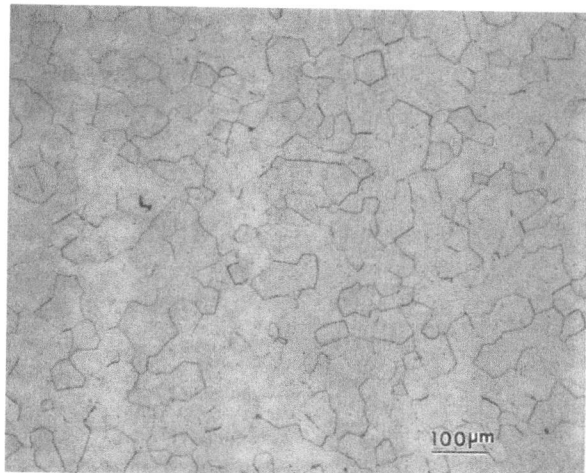

Figure 74.11. Annealed TMZF beta titanium alloy microstructure (100×).

strated improved abrasion resistance in pin on disc wear tests against a bone cement counterface.[27]

The safety of TMZF alloy was tested in a series of assays based on the Tripartite Agreement, ASTM recommendations. Where appropriate, Ti-6Al-4V was the concurrent control. This battery of safety studies showed there was no difference in the biocompatibility of either TMZF or Ti-6Al-4V alloys (Table 74.4).

To determine if there was any difference in the tissue reaction to particulates of these materials, in vivo and in vitro studies were conducted. The particles used in these studies were <37 microns with average diameters of 27.0 microns for the Ti-6Al-4V alloy and 23.5 microns for the TMZF alloy. All particles were produced by gas atomization and sieved to separate the desired size fraction. By using the same methodology to produce the particles, the only variable for the study was the alloy composition and not the particle shape or size. The size range used examined the ability for the particles of either alloy to stimulate cells from either surface or internal means.

In Vitro Particulate Assay
The objective of this study was to analyze the capability of particulate debris from potential implant materials (TMZF and Ti-6Al-4V) to affect the release of PGE_2, IL-1 and IL-6 by human peripheral blood macrophages in an in vitro cell culture system. Synovial cells from pa-

tients with rheumatoid arthritis retrieved at total joint arthroplasty were also used for this study since this disease may affect the response of these cells to particulate materials. At concentrations ranging from 10^6 to 10^3 total particles, the peripheral blood macrophages and synovial cells did not response to either the TMZF or Ti-6Al-4V alloys. Neither particle induced release of cellular mediators that are known to induce bone resorption.[28]

In Vivo Particulate Assay
A slight modification of the animal model used by Goodman et al. was used to investigate the in vivo response by bone and bone marrow to 10^6 particles of TMZF or Ti-6Al-4V alloy after 8 and 16 weeks implantation. Undecalcified histology of the implantation sites showed that there was no difference in the bone or bone marrow response to TMZF particles to Ti-6Al-4V particles compared to each other or controls implanted with the carrier (hyaluronic acid) alone at either time period.[29]

Advances in Ultra High Molecular Weight Polyethylene Technology

Background

Oxidation resulting from the gamma radiation sterilization of ultra high molecular weight polyethylene (UHMWPE) can in time lead to mechanical and chemical changes in the UHMWPE.[30-32] These changes in turn may influence the wear performance of UHMWPE, leading to the generation of particulate wear debris having the potential to cause osteolysis. In order to prevent radiation induced oxidation from occurring, a patented manufacturing process[33] was developed. In this procedure, finished UHMWPE components are packaged in

Table 74.3. Fatigue strength of TMZF vs Ti-6Al-4V

Alloy	Rotating beam fatigue strength (MPa)	
	Smooth	Notched ($k_t = 1.6$)
TMZF	585	410
Ti-6Al-4V	585	280

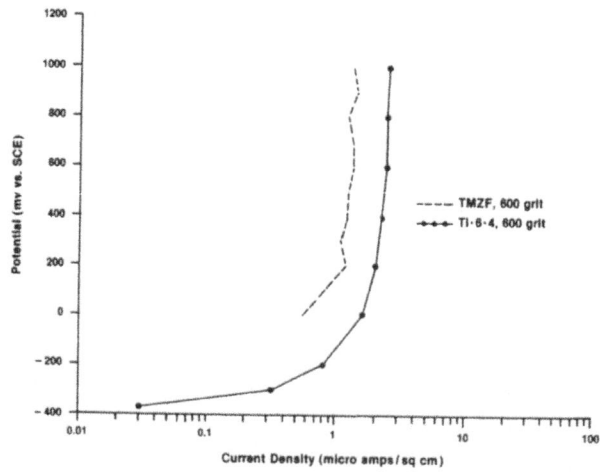

Figure 74.12. Anodic polarization corrosion results for TMZF and Ti-6Al-4V alloys.

Table 74.4. Results of safety test.

Safety test	Test material	Control material	Result
Agar overlay assay (ASTM F-898)			
(a) Direct contact	TMZF	Plastic	Passed
(b) Saline extract	TMZF	Extractant	Passed
Colony Suppression Assay	TMZF	Ti-6Al-4V	Passed
USP intracutaneous toxicity test (ASTM F-749)			
(a) Saline extract	TMZF	Extractant	Passed
(b) Cottonseed oil extract	TMZF	Extractant	Passed
USP mouse systemic test (ASTM F-750)			
(a) Saline extract	TMZF		Passed
(b) Cottonseed oil extract	TMZF		Passed
In vitro hemolysis in rabbit, whole blood			
(a) Direct contact	TMZF	Ti-6Al-4V	Passed
(b) Saline extract	TMZF	Ti-6Al-4V	Passed
Guinea pig sensitization (maximization)	TMZF	Ti-6Al-4V	Passed
Ames salmonella/reverse mutation assay	TMZF	Ti-6Al-4V	Passed
90-day muscle implant study in the rabbit	TMZF	Ti-6Al-4V	Passed

an inert environment prior to radiation sterilization. After irradiation, the packaged component is subjected to a low temperature heating step that results in the virtual elimination of the free radicals generated in the UHMWPE by the gamma radiation. The mechanism of free radical elimination leads to crosslinking in the UHMWPE, creating a three-dimensional molecular network in the polymer that can have a positive influence on wear behavior.

Oxidation of UHMWPE

The examination of shelf-aged, nonimplanted, sterile UHMWPE components can provide information as to the effects of oxidation on the material. The appearance of a subsurface white band in UHMWPE acetabular cups that is observed when a component is sectioned has been reported in the literature.[34–36] This white band is ascribed to radiation induced oxidation over time and radiation sterilization. The band is also associated with changes in the mechanical and chemical properties of the UHMWPE. Figures 74.13 and 74.14 show sections cut from nonimplanted acetabular component and tibial components. These were commercial products made by a compression molding process. In each case a subsurface white band is seen following the contour of the component. This white band is a region associated with high oxidation.

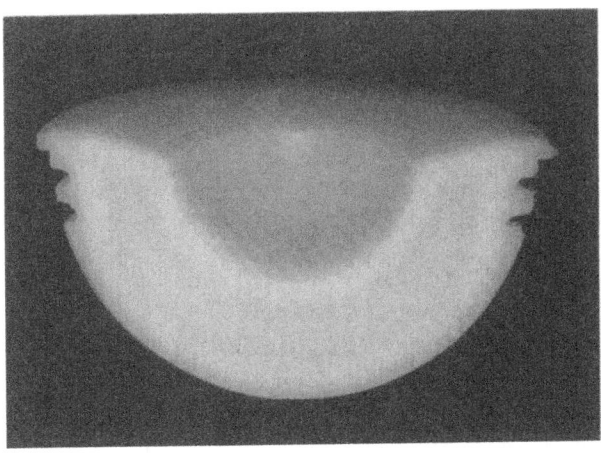

Figure 74.13. Section cut from molded acetabular component, never implanted.

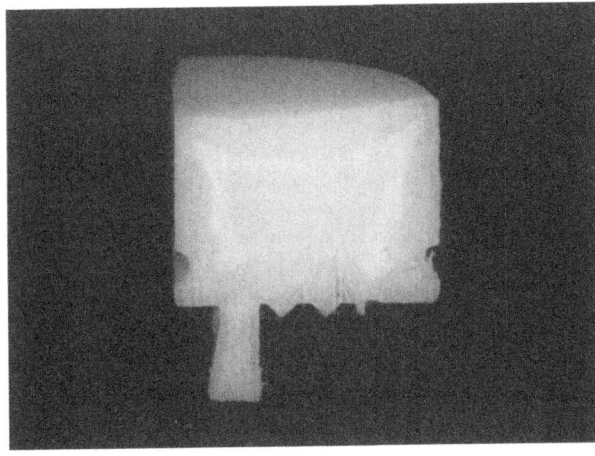

Figure 74.14. Section cut from molded tibial component, never implanted.

Figure 74.15. The FTIR oxidation index as a function of shelf aging time for air-irradiated UHMWPE.

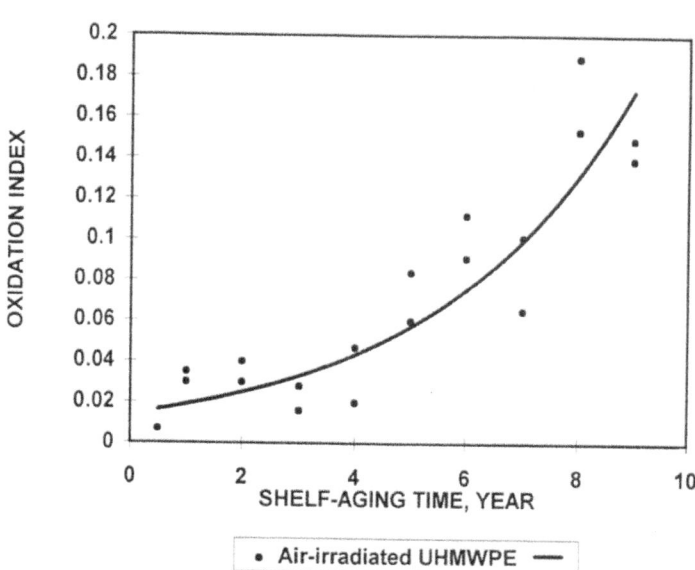

The chemical change resulting from oxidation can be measured by Fourier Transform Infra-red Spectroscopy (FTIR). The oxidation index (OI) obtained from analysis of the spectrum is defined as the ratio of the peak areas between 1650 and 1750 cm^{-1} (carbonyl peaks) and a reference peak at 1468 cm^{-1} (methyl/methylene peak). The greater the index value, the greater the chemical change. Figure 74.15 plots the oxidation index as a function of shelf aging time for several UHMWPE components. Up to 5 years, little change in index value is seen. Beyond that point the effect of aging becomes more pronounced.

The oxidation mechanism results from the free radicals that are formed by the breakage of mainly C-H bonds and, to a lesser extent, C-C bonds in the UHMWPE during gamma irradiation.[37] Figure 74.16 and 74.17 depict the process when UHMWPE is irradiated in air. Figure 74.16 shows the ordered crystalline regions connected by amorphous tie molecules. After irradiation in air, (Fig. 74.17), the free radicals will react with oxygen in the air and in the UHMWPE to initiate a series of oxidation reactions resulting in the formation of ketones, aldehydes, esters, carboxylic acid, or C-C bonds. This can result in weak bonds, chain scission or free radical reactions with one another other to form chemical crosslinks. These oxidation reactions can take place during irradiation, during shelf-aging, or potentially in vivo, but the latter to a lesser extent.[38]

Figure 74.16. Schematic of the molecular structure of UHMWPE before gamma irradiation in air. Ordered crystalline regions are connected by tie molecules. Some physical chain entanglements in the tie molecules are shown.

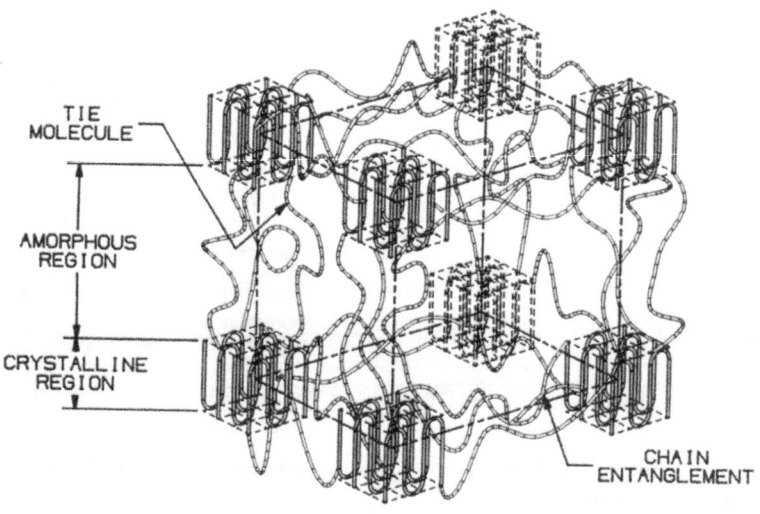

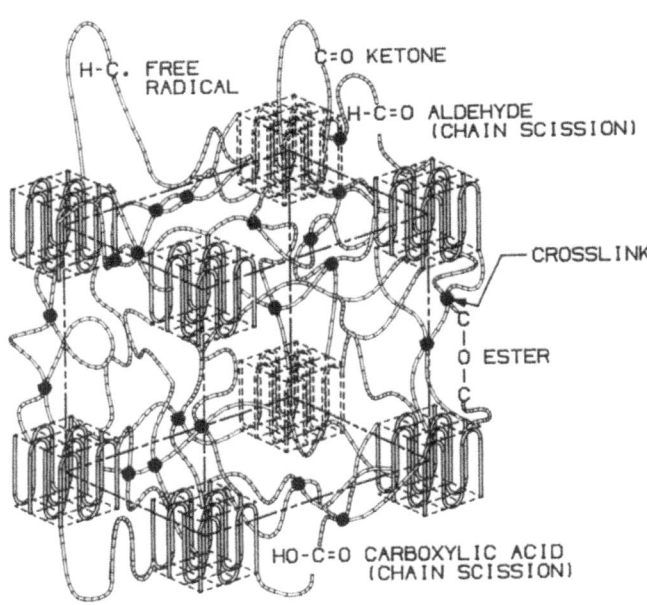

Figure 74.17. Schematic of the molecular structure of UHMWPE after gamma radiation in air. Free radicals are formed. Chemical crosslinks can be formed as well as various oxidation products such as ketones, esters, aldehydes, and acids.

Oxidation Prevention

Oxidation was shown previously to be a long term process. In order to study oxidation in a reasonable timeframe, an accelerated aging test protocol was developed. The method consists of heating the UHMWPE from room temperature to 80°C at 0.6°C/min. in air, followed by holding the material at 80°C for a period of time.[39] Table 74.5 lists some of the changes that can be induced in the UHMWPE by aging the material for 23 days at 80°C, simulating approximately 8 years of shelf aging. More vigorous accelerated aging methods have been described[40,41] that either increase the oxygen exposure level to 5 atmospheres pressure or extend the aging period. These methods will cause oxidation to take place, but to such an extent to be considered overly aggressive or unrealistic. Even unirradiated UHMWPE would be markedly effected by such exposure.

Inert Packaging

Irradiation in an inert atmosphere was one of the first methods proposed to combat oxidation. This involves packaging the UHMWPE components in an inert gas atmosphere (nitrogen, argon) or vacuum prior to gamma irradiation. Since no oxygen is present during irradiation, free radicals will combine with other neighboring free radicals to form crosslinks (Fig. 74.18). The crosslinking reaction will continue after irradiation, but at a slow rate at room temperature. Some uncombined free radicals are still present in UHMWPE even after several years of post-irradiation aging.[42] During shelf storage, oxygen can leak into the package and react with uncombined free radicals to cause oxidation. Oxidation may also occur in vivo, although to as lesser extent, between uncombined free radicals and oxidants. Therefore, irradiation in an inert atmosphere or under vacuum can eliminate short-term oxidation, but cannot prevent oxidation in the long-term.

Nonradiation Sterilization

Alternative methods such as ethylene oxide sterilization or gas plasma sterilization have also been proposed to address oxidation. In these cases, since the UHMWPE is not exposed to radiation, no free radicals are formed and hence no oxidation occurs. Recalling Figure 75.16, after such treatment the unirradiated UHMWPE will contain relatively few physical crosslinks and no chemical crosslinks. This will impact on the wear behavior, as will be discussed later.

Table 74.5. Effect of accelerated aging on UHMWPE properties.

Process/property	Unaged	23-day/80°C aging
FTIR oxidation index		
Unirradiated	~0	~0
Air irradiated	0.02	0.11
Extent of crosslinking, %		
Unirradiated	10%	—
Air irradiated	46%	—
Low m.w. fraction, %		
Air irradiated	28%	47%
Ultimate tensile strength, psi		
Unirradiated	7762	6714
Air irradiated	6500	3200
Compressive creep, %		
Unirradated	1.2	1.2
Air irradiated	0.8	0.75
Izod impact strength, ft-lb/in²		
Air irradiated	48	33

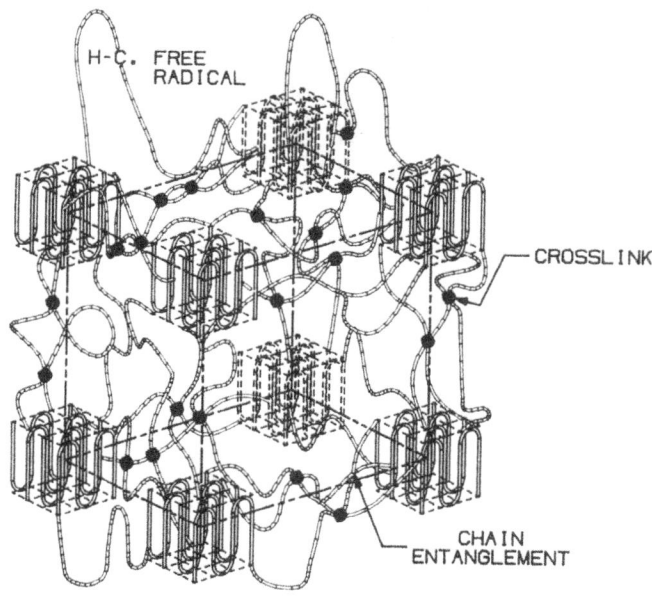

Figure 74.18. Schematic of the molecular structure of UHMWPE after gamma irradiation in an inert atmosphere. Free radicals are formed, some of which can remain long term. Some chemical crosslinks are formed.

Stabilization

This new process consist of three steps, namely the packaging of the UHMWPE component in an inert environment (nitrogen), exposure to gamma irradiation and finally stabilization after irradiation. The inert atmosphere in the packaging prevents oxidation during irradiation. During the stabilization step, the package containing the irradiated UHMWPE component is held at a slightly elevated temperature for a sufficient time to crosslink all the reactive free radicals (typically 50°C for 144 hours). Figure 74.19 shows the post-stabilization structure. After stabilization, oxidation will not occur in UHMWPE when the component is reexposed to oxygen since the free radicals were eliminated. Not only are short-term and long-term oxidation avoided, but crosslinking, resulting from the stabilization process, also leads to improvements in wear resistance and creep resistance. These benefits are best explained by a three-dimensional molecular network created by crosslinking which resists mechanical deformation under multi-axial loading conditions. This increased level of crosslinking that occurs between tie molecules (Fig. 74.19) is not sufficient to cause loss of ductility. Recall that ethylene oxide (EtO) or gas plasma sterilization, unlike gamma irradiation, do not generate free radicals and therefore cannot cause an increase in crosslinking.

Wear Behavior

Hip simulator testing is the best and most accurate means of assessing the in vitro wear performance of UHMWPE. Due to its multi-directional motion and physiological loading nature, the simulator can reproduce wear rates, wear patterns, and wear debris seen clinically.

Figure 74.20 describes the results after 5 million cycles on the MTS hip simulator (MTS Corporation, Eden Prairie, Minnesota) for unaged UHMWPE specimens. Nonsterilized UHMWPE shows the highest wear, approaching a total wear volume of 700 mm^3. The ethylene oxide sterilized UHMWPE is similar to the nonsterile material, showing a wear volume in excess of 650 mm^3. These values are over three times greater than the stabilized gamma irradiated UHMWPE or conventional air irradiated UHMWPE. The reasons for the poorer wear performance for both the unirradiated and the eth-

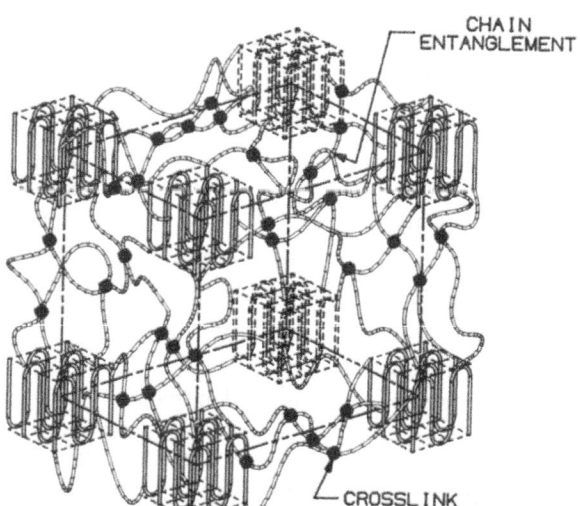

Figure 74.19. Schematic of the molecular structure of UHMWPE after gamma irradiation in an inert package and stabilization. Free radicals are eliminated. The level of chemical crosslinks is increased.

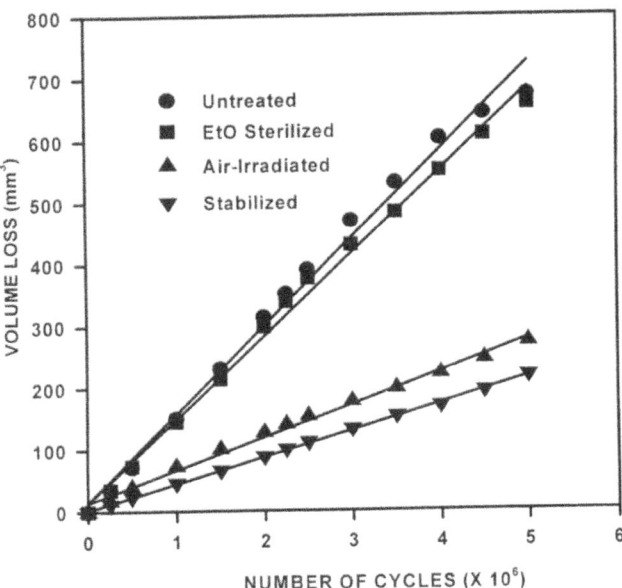

Figure 74.20. Hip simulator wear data, unaged, for UHMWPE cups nonirradiated, gamma irradiated in air, ethylene oxide sterilized and gamma irradiated/stabilized. Nonirradiated (untreated) and ethylene oxide sterilized UHMWPE have over three times greater wear than air irradiated or stabilized UHMWPE.

ylene oxide sterilized UHMWPE has to do with the molecular structure of the material. The amount of insoluble gel component of the material, related to the crosslinking level, can be assessed by a hot solvent extraction procedure as described in ASTM D2756-90. Figure 74.21 shows that the higher the measured gel content, the better the wear performance of the UHMWPE. Stabilized UHMWPE, with the highest gel content, shows the lowest wear because its more highly crosslinked molecular structure has a greater resistance to multi-directional stresses imposed by the hip simulator. Other researchers have also confirmed that EtO sterilization results in poorer hip simulator wear.[43–45]

The effect of the accelerated aging protocol on wear is seen in Figure 74.22. The material being gamma irradiated in air exhibits about six times more wear than the stabilized specimen after 1.5 million cycles in the simulator.

Conclusions

The stabilization process for UHMWPE can minimize both short term and long term oxidation by reducing

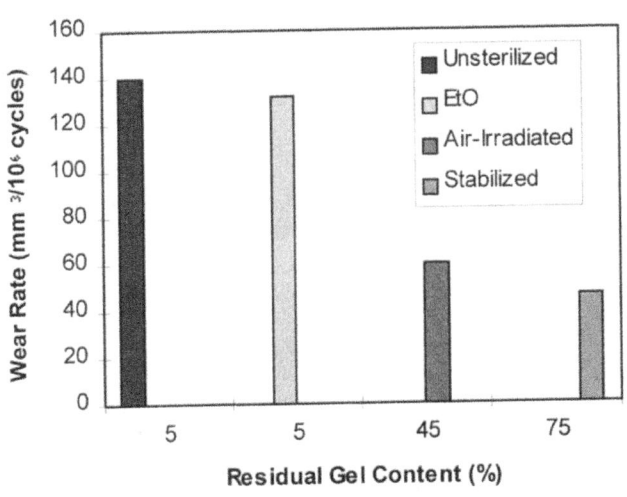

Figure 74.21. Comparison of the hip simulator wear rate of UHMWPE unirradiated, gamma irradiated in air, ethylene oxide sterilized, and gamma irradiated/stabilized as a function of gel content. Low gel content UHMWPE (unirradiated or ethylene oxide sterilized) shows greater wear rates than high gel content UHMWPE (air irradiated or stabilized).

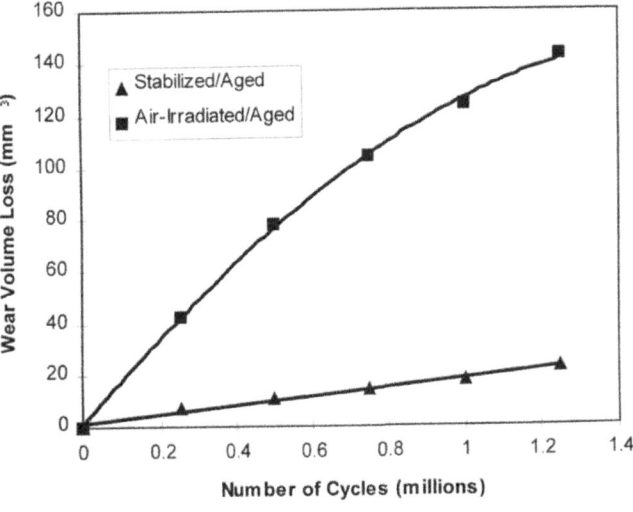

Figure 74.22. Hip simulator data comparing UHMWPE gamma irradiated in air and gamma irradiated/stabilized after aging in air at 80°C for 23 days. Aging causes the air irradiated UHMWPE to have sixfold greater wear than stabilized UHMWPE.

the free radical level in the material through a crosslinking reaction. This leads to an improved chemical stability and to a retention of mechanical properties over time. The enhanced level of crosslinking also increases the wear resistance of the UHMWPE in hip simulator wear testing. Non-ionizing sterilization methods such as ethylene oxide or gas plasma do not increase crosslinking and do not improve the wear resistance.

References

1. Barron GE. *What every engineer should know about finite element analysis 1*; Brauer R, ed. Marcel Dekker: New York, 1988.
2. Brekelmans WAM, Poort HW, Slooff TJJH. A new method to analyze the mechanical behavior of skeletal parts. *Acta Orthop Scand*. 1972;43:301–317.
3. Rybicki EF, Simonen FA, Weis EB. On the mathematical analysis of stress in the human femur. *J Biomechanics*. 1972;5:203–215.
4. Huiskes R, Chao EYS. A survey of finite element analysis in orthopedic biomechanics: the first decade. *J Biomechanics*. 1983;16:385–409.
5. Buamgartner M, Kensinger S. Re-engineering engineering: facing reality. *Computer Aided Eng*. 1997;May:80.
6. de Nies F, Fidler MW. The Harris-Galante cementless femoral component: poor results in 57 hips followed for 3 years. *Acta Orthop Scand*. 1996;67:122–124.
7. Engh CA, Bobyn JD, Glassman AH. Porous-coated hip replacement: the factors governing bone ingrowth, stress shielding, and clinical results. *J Bone Joint Surg Br*. 1987;69:45–55.
8. Callaghan JJ, Dysart SH, Savory CG. The uncemented porous-coated anatomic total hip prosthesis: two-year results of a prospective consecutive series. *J Bone Joint Surg Am*. 1988;70:337–345.
9. Haddad RJ, Cook SD, Brinker MR. A comparison of three varieties of noncemented porous-coated hip replacement. *J Bone Joint Surg Br*. 1990;72:2–8.
10. Skinner HB, Curlin FJ. Decreased pain with lower flexural rigidity of uncemented femoral prostheses. *Orthopaedics*. 1990;13:1223–1228.
11. Cameron HU, Trick L, Shepard B, Turnbull A, Noiles D, McTighe T. An international multi-center study on thigh pain in total hip replacements, Scientific Exhibit, 1990 AAOS, New Orleans, LA, 1990.
12. Hungerford DS, Jones LC. The rationale for cementless total hip replacement. *Orthop Clin North Am*. 1993;24:617–626.
13. Franks E, Mont MA, Maar DC, Jones LC, Hungerford DS. Thigh pain as related to bending rigidity of the femoral prosthesis and bone. Proc. 38th ORS, 1992;296.
14. Dujovne AR, Bobyn JD, Krygier JJ, Miller JE, Brooks CE. Mechanical compatibility of noncemented hip prostheses with the human femur. *J Arthroplasty*. 1993;8:7–22.
15. Jasty M, Maloney WJ, Bragdon CR. The initiation of failure in cemented femoral components of hip arthroplasties. *J Bone Joint Surg Br*. 1991;73:551–558.
16. O'Conner DO, Burke DW, Sedlack RC, Harris WH. Peak cement strains in cemented femoral total hip. Proc. 37th ORS, 1991;220.
17. Estok DM III, Orr TE, Harris WH. Factors affecting cement strains near the tip of a cemented femoral component. *J Arthroplasty*. 1997;12:40–48.
18. Weinans H, Huiskes R, Grootenboer HJ. Effects of fit and bonding characteristics of femoral stems on adaptive bone remodeling. *J Biomech Eng*. 1994;116:393–400.
19. Zhen L, Ebramzadeh E, McKellop H, Sarmiento A. Stable partial debonding of the cement interfaces indicated by a finite element model of total hip prosthesis. *J Orthop Res*. 1996;14:238–244.
20. Semlitsch M, Panic B. 15 years of experience with test criteria for fracture-proof anchorage stems of artificial hip joints. In: Buchhorn G, Willen H-G, eds. *Technical principles, design and safety of joint implants*. Kirkland, Wash.: Hogrefe & Huber, 1994:23–36.
21. Dobbs HS, Scales JT. Behavior of commercially pure titanium and Ti-6Al-4V in orthopaedic implants. *ASTM-STP*. 1983;796:173–186.
22. Kelly W, Bushelow M, Dudasik M, et al. Distal design of a cemented femoral hip stem component. Fifth World Biomaterials Congress Transactions; 1996:668.
23. Benjamin JS. Mechanical alloying—a perspective. In: Arzt E, Schultz L, ed. *New materials by mechanical alloying techniques*. Deutsche Gesellschaft fur Metallkunde e.V., 1989:3–18.
24. Farthing TW. The development of titanium and its alloys. *Clin Materials*. 1987;2:15–32.
25. Titanium Alloys Handbook MCIC-HB-02, MCIC 1972.
26. Steinemann SG, Beta-titanium alloy for surgical implants. In: Froes FH, Caplan I, eds. *Titanium '92 science and technology*. Seventh World Conference on Titanium, TMS1993:2689–2696.
27. Wang K, Gustavson L. Microstructure and properties of a new beta titanium alloy, Ti-12Mo-6Zr-2Fe, developed for surgical implants. *ASTM STP*. 1994;1272:76–87.
28. Lalor PA, Shortkroff S, Aberman HM, et al. In vitro biocompatibility studies of Ti-6Al-4V and Ti-Mo-Zr-Fe particles. *ORS Transactions*. 1994;19:850.
29. Goodman SB, Fornasier VL, Kei J. The effects of bulk versus particulate titanium and cobalt chrome alloy implanted into the rabbit tibia. *J Biomed Res*. 1990;24:1539–1549.
30. Roe RJ, Grood E, Shastri R, et al. Effect of radiation sterilization and aging on UHMWPE. *J Biomed Mater Res*. 1981;15:209–230.
31. Streicher R. Influence of ionizing irradiation in air and nitrogen for sterilization of surgical grade polyethylene implants. *Radiat Phys Chem*. 1988;31:693–698.
32. Rimnac C, Wright T, Klein R, et al. Characterization of material properties of ultra high molecular weight polyethylene before and after implantation. *Trans Soc Biomater Implant Retrieval Sympos*. 1992;15:16.
33. U.S. Patents #5,414,049, #5,449,745, #5,543,471.
34. Sun DC, Stark C, Dumbleton JH. The origin of the white band observed in direct compression molded UHMWPE inserts. Trans Twentieth Annual Meeting of the Soc. for Biomaterials. 1994, 121.
35. Sutula LC, Sperling D, Collier J, et al. Symposium III. Hip

Society and Association for Arthritic Hip and Knee Surgery, Orlando Fl., 1995.
36. Furman B, Li S. The effect of long term shelf aging of ultra high molecular weight polyethylene. Trans. Twenty-first Annual Meeting of the Soc. for Biomaterials. 1995, 114.
37. Clough RL, Shalaby SW, eds. *Radiation Effects on Polymers.* ACS Symposium Series; 1991:475.
38. Masri BA, Gomez-Barrena E, Furman B, et al. Comparison of in vivo and in vitro oxidation of Charnley acetabular components. Research: joint replacement Session, Scientific Program, Paper Number 391, American Academy of Orthopaedic Surgeons Annual Meeting, Atlanta, Georgia, 1996.
39. Sun DC, Stark C, Dumbleton JH. *Polymer Preprints.* 1994;35:969–970.
40. McKellop H, Shen FW, Yu YJ, et al. Effect of sterilization method and other modifications on the wear resistance of UHMWPE acetabular cups. Polyethylene Wear in Orthopaedic Implants Workshop, Twenty-third Annual Meeting Soc. for Biomaterials 1997.
41. Taylor G, Gsell R, King R, et al. Stability of N2 packaged gamma irradiated UHMWPE. Trans. Twenty-third Annual Meeting Soc. for Biomaterials 1997, 421.
42. Jahan MS, Wang C, Schwartz G, Davidson JA. Combined chemical and mechanical effects on free radicals in UHMWPE joints during implantation. *J Bio Mat Res.* 1991;25:1005–1017.
43. Higgins J. Improved processing of UHMWPE for orthopaedic bearings. Total Hip Replacement: Back to the Future Symposium, Cambridge, Ma., 1995.
44. Schroeder DW, Pozorski KM. Hip simulator testing of isostatistically molded UHMWPE: effect of ETO and gamma irradiation. Trans. Forty-second Annual Meeting of the Orthopaedic Research Society. 1996;478.
45. Sommerich R, Flynn T, Schmidt MB, et al. The effects of sterilization and contact area and wear rate of UHMWPE. Trans. Forty-second Annual Meeting of the Orthopaedic Research Society. 1996;486.

75
Robotically Assisted Cement Removal

Bill Williamson, William Bargar, and Alan Kalvin

In revision total hip replacement (RTHR) surgery, a failing hip implant, typically cemented, is replaced with a new one by removing the old implant, removing the cement, and fitting a new implant into the enlarged canal broached in the femur. As the installed base of orthopedic implants grows and ages, replacement of existing implants, especially those relying on bone cement for fixation and fit, is steadily increasing. In 1992, 23 000 RTHR procedures were performed in the US, with an annual growth rate of 10%. The average cost per procedure was $23,744 with an average hospital stay of 10.9 days.

RTHR is a difficult procedure fraught with clinical and technical challenges and a high incidence of complications. Femoral cement removal and canal preparation present the most difficulties. The goal is to remove as much of the old cement as possible to facilitate the insertion of the new implant and provide an optimal surface for bone support and interdigitation. Whereas the cement mantle in the proximal area of the canal is visible and relatively easily accessible, the cement mantle and plug in the distal area are hard to see and reach due to the canal depth and bowing of the femur. Removing cement is tedious, time-consuming, and risky, taking on the average between 30 minutes and 2 hours. Femoral canal preparation is more difficult than in a primary case because there is little good bone left and because the required surgical manipulations are more delicate. The reamers typically used tend to follow the old canal, making axis and position corrections virtually impossible. The femur is fractured in about 18% of cases and the surgeon perforates the cortical wall of the femur in another 10% of cases. When errors occur, more time is required to repair the damage, additional blood is lost, and the infection rate increases.

None of the current techniques for cement removal is fully satisfactory. Osteotomes and flexible reamers are difficult to manipulate and have a tendency to follow the old canal. Hand-held high-speed drills cut cement fragments but require fluoroscopy for guidance to avoid perforating the femur walls. New technologies, such as cement softening using an ultrasonically driven tool or the use of lithotripsy to fracture cement, might lower the complication rate but are unlikely to significantly improve accuracy or shorten the procedure.

The growing numbers, greater difficulty, and reduced margin for error make RTHR a natural target for robotics machining to remove old cement and prepare the new cavity.

Method

Our starting point is the ROBODOC,[1,2] Integrated Surgical Systems' (ISS) computer-integrated system for primary hip replacement procedures. ROBODOC was developed clinically by ISS from a prototype developed at IBM Research. Preclinical testing showed an order-of-magnitude improvement in precision and repeatability in preparing the implant cavity as compared to hand-held broaches and reamers. To date about 800 human cases have been performed with very encouraging preliminary results.

In traditional primary total hip replacement (PTHR) procedures, the damaged joint is replaced by a metallic implant inserted into a canal broached in the femur. Using a computed tomography (CT) scan of the hip and femur, the ROBODOC system allows the surgeon to preoperatively plan the procedure by selecting a properly sized implant and positioning it as desired. The corresponding canal is then milled in the femur using a high-speed cutting tool controlled intraoperatively by a robotic arm.

The ROBODOC system consists of an interactive presurgical planning system, called ORTHODOC, and a robotic system for use in the operating room. A ROBODOC PTHR starts with a minor surgical procedure in which three small pins are implanted in the femur. A CT scan of the patient shows the femur and pins, which are used to register the images to the robot. Next, ORTHODOC processes the CT data set, locates the three pins within the CT data set, and allows the surgeon to select three orthogonal planar slices through the 3D image volume. The surgeon then selects a desired implant model and size and interactively positions a model of the implant relative to the CT volumetric images. OR-THODOC superimposes cross-sectional displays of the implant model on the femoral views, allowing detailed examination of bone-implant interfaces. In the operating room, surgery follows the established protocol up to the point at which the femoral head is removed. The femur is then placed into a fixation device and attached to the robot base. The three pins are exposed and located in robot coordinates by a combination of force-compliant guiding and autonomous tactile search by the robot. The system then computes the transformation from CT (planning) to robot (actual) coordinates and machines out the desired shape in the femur while the surgeon follows the progress on an intraoperative display. Once the shape is cut, the robot is moved out of the way and the procedure resumes manually as usual.

Project Overview

To apply the existing ROBODOC technology to revisions it is necessary to accommodate the artifact encountered when producing CT images of metallic implants in bone and to allow sufficient visualization of the cement-bone or implant-bone interface to allow surgeons to define a cut volume that will remove most (or all) of the cement and preserve and prepare the remaining bone for the new implant. For discussion, we will assume the surgeons will want to implant a cementless prosthesis. Therefore, the cut envelope must match the prosthesis envelope in its intended position and orientation, as well as allow for implant insertion.

It is also frequently the case that events can occur intraoperatively that can alter the preoperative plan. These include intraoperative fracture, cement removal problems, and other unanticipated factors. In order to optimize the system, intraoperative imaging registered to a common coordinate system and incorporated into ORTHODOC would be required. This would allow intraoperative modification of the plan in order to take full advantage of ROBODOC's capabilities to accurately remove the cement mantle and prepare the bone for the implant. This ability to use intraoperative imaging is not yet developed and represents a future area of research and development.

Our goals for the project are: (1) elimination of cement removal complications, specifically cortical wall penetration and bone fractures; (2) significant reduction of cement removal labor and time required; (3) improved positioning accuracy and fit of the new implant resulting from precise, high-quality canal milling; and (4) reduction of bone sacrificed to fit the new implant. In addition to the direct patient benefits, these advantages can save costs, both by potentially reducing operating room charges and by shortening hospital stay and recovery time.

Therefore, we have broken down the project into three stages:

1. CT artificial removal
2. Interactive cut volume definition
3. Cement/bone machining

CT Artifact Removal

In revision hip replacement surgery, the presence of an implant in the femur results in blooming and streaking of the CT image (Fig. 75.1). Because metal objects are opaque to x-ray beams in the diagnostic energy range, their scanning yields incomplete projection data. CT images reconstructed from this incomplete data contain artifacts, the extent of which depends on the material type and volume of the implant. Artifacts in CT scans of RTHR patients with metal femoral implants are most marked in the proximal section, where the implant is the thickest. The artifacts make it difficult to determine the boundary between the implant, the cement, and the bone. Since the quality of the CT images is key in determining the quality of the surgical plan, reducing artifact as much as possible is essential.

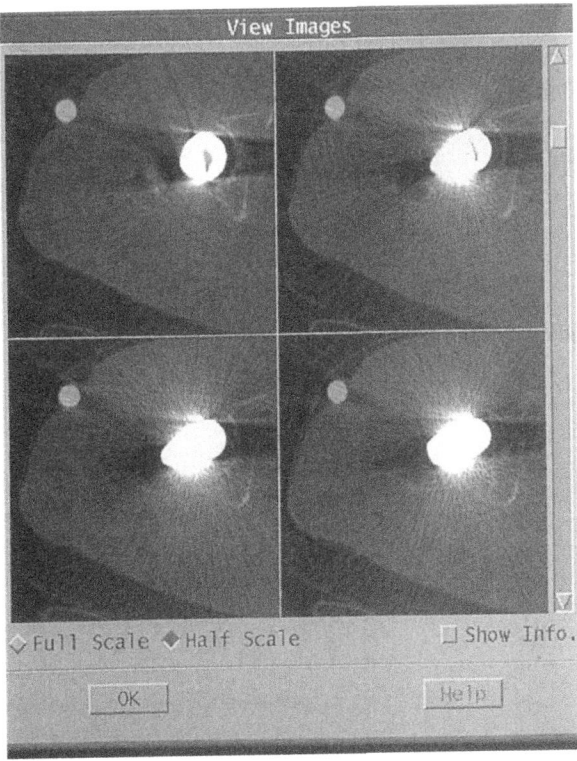

Figure 75.1 Cross-sectional ORTHODOC views of a CT study of a failing implant. (See color insert.)

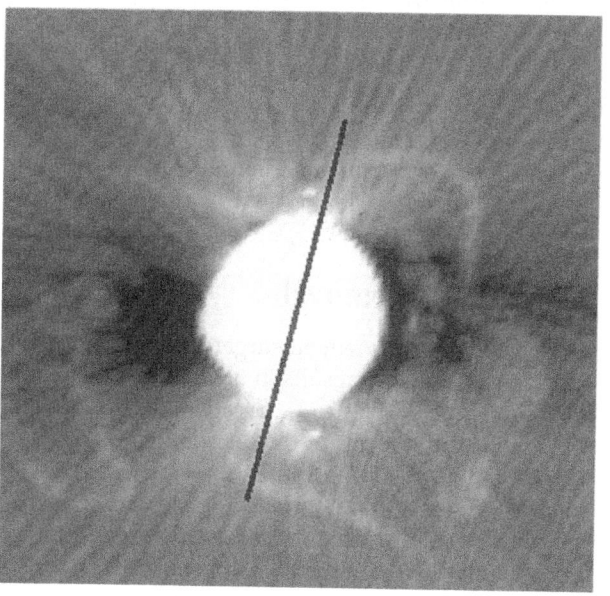 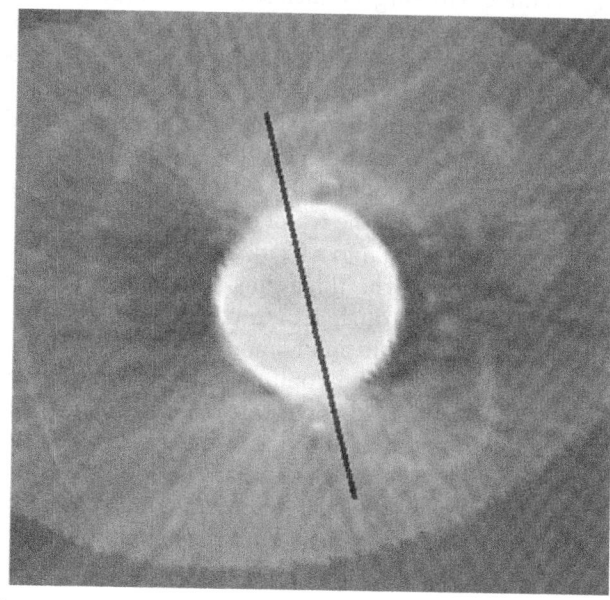

Figure 75.2 A. Original CT axial image of bone with implant. B. Artifact reduced image of bone with implant. (See color insert.)

The best approach for reducing metal-induced CT artifacts is to correct the raw projection (sonogram) data before image reconstruction. Projection data are simulated by forward projecting the corrupted CT images. These simulated projections are then modified to correct for the data missing in the original (true) projections because of the x-ray opacity of metal. Finally, new CT images are reconstructed from the modified projections. Due to limitations imposed by CT manufacturers, access to these projection data is generally problematic. As a practical alternative, we have chosen the simulated projection approach.

Our approach uses "scout" images to improve the modification of simulated projections. Scout images are projection data and have a standard, well-documented, and easily accessible format. We are capturing on the order of 12 to 20 scout images, instead of just a couple (anteroposterior, lateral) as is the current practice. By using the scanning geometries of the scout images to generate simulated projections, and including these pro-

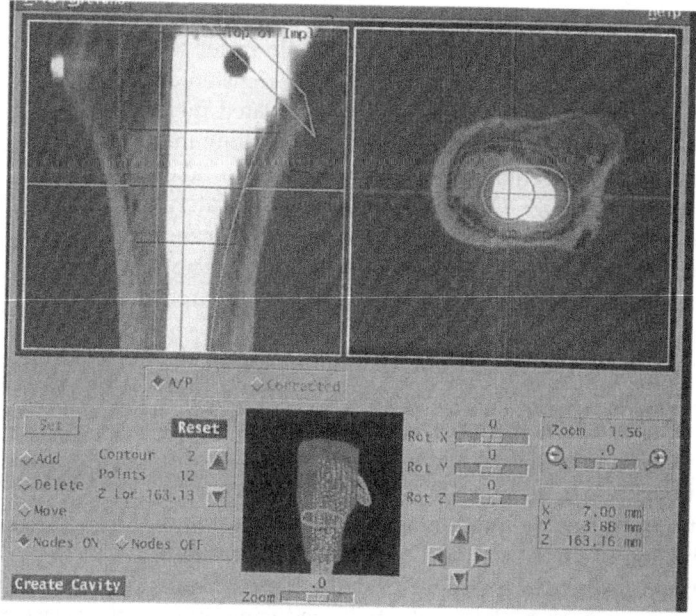

Figure 75.3 Example of user interface surgeon uses to interactively define cut cavity for robot. (See color insert.)

jections within the larger set of all simulated projections, the scout data can be used as "ground-truth" in the modification of the simulated projections (Fig. 75.2). Scout images also have the potential to be useful on their own to reconstruct either 2D or 3D images.[3,4,5] Furthermore, methods developed for image reconstruction from limited views have application in both surgical planning based on 2D x-rays instead of CT images and in 2D/3D registration.

Interactive Cut Volume Definition

The ORTHODOC surgical planning workstation has been further augmented in the area of interactive cut volume definition. The surgeon now plans on separate anteroposterior and transaxial views, which simplifies the process and does not interfere with normal implant selection and placement. The surgeon first segments out the bone cement by creating a contour that defines the bone/cement interface on several computed tomography (CT) slices (see Fig. 75.3). This contour data is fed into a cut path generator algorithm, which outputs a second contour identifying the computed robot cut path based on the cutter diameter. The cut path is created by examining all the contours the user has entered and constructing a cut path that allows for a straight insertion path along the vertical axis. The surgeon can now edit each contour to maximize cement removal and/or minimize the removal of cortical bone.

Future versions of the cut path generator will automatically compute the robot reorientation angle needed to more effectively machine out the user-defined cavity, thus removing the constraint of a "straight line insertion path" imposed by the current system.

We have also begun the process of allowing the surgeon to plan using planar x-rays. This is the typical method of preoperative planning in both primary and revision cases and it permits greater flexibility in the preoperative planning system. A key element in this scenario is registering x-rays to each other, thereby allowing implant movements in one view to be simultaneously reflected in other views. In addition, we must minimize the impact and changes to current clinical practices in obtaining preoperative x-rays.

Cement Machining

We have designed and conducted experiments to simulate as closely as possible bone cement removal. We have tested whether the cutters currently used in RO-BODOC PTHR are adequate to cut bone cement by milling circular shapes in the actual cement used clinically. To determine accuracy, measured cavity diameters were compared to planned, obtaining satisfactory results for shape and position accuracy. In addition, we test for compliance when cutting distally the bone (ie, how distal can we cut bone cement and still achieve the required accuracy?). This testing is necessary in order

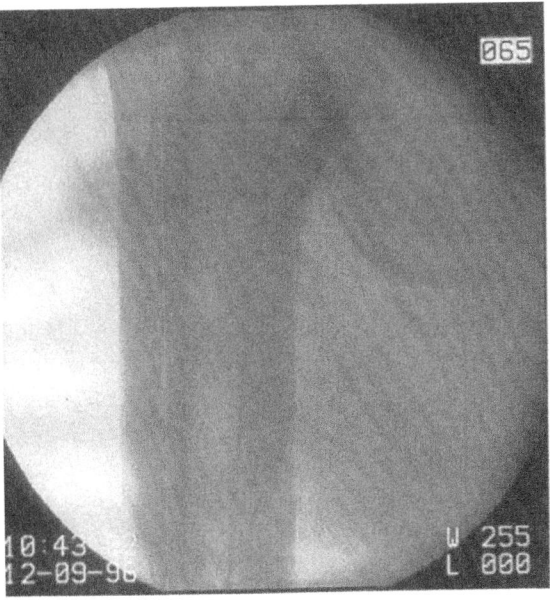
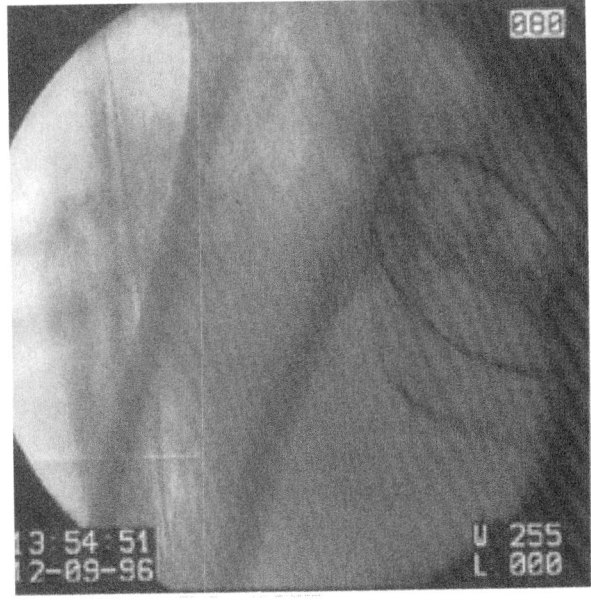

A   B

Figure 75.4 A. Inter-Op fluoroscope after implant removed, cement mantel is still intact. B. Inter-Op fluoroscope after robot removed bone cement. (See color insert.)

to remove the cement plug located deep within the femoral canal. With current instrumentation, the ROBODOC system can cut an implant cavity to a depth of about 225 mm (with a sleeve diameter of 12.5 mm) along the axis of the bone.

Clinical Results

The RTHR applications have been used successfully on several patients at the Berufsgenossenschaftliche Unfallklinik in Frankfurt, Germany. Figure 75.4 shows preoperative plans and the postoperative fluoroscope images.

Conclusion

Our goal is to develop and clinically demonstrate a computer-integrated system to assist surgeons in revision total hip replacement surgery. Preliminary results indicate that the proposed approach is viable. We believe that some of the solutions developed specifically for RTHR will be applicable to many orthopedic and other surgical problems.

References

1. Paul H, Mittelstadt BD, Bargar WL, et al. A surgical robot for total hip replacement surgery, *Proc Of IEEE Int Conf On Robotics and Automation*, France 1992.
2. Taylor RH, Mittelstadt BD, Paul HA, et al. An image-directed robotic system for precise orthopedic surgery, *IEEE Transactions on Robotics and Automation*. 1994;10:(3).
3. Barrett HH. Limited-angle tomography for the nineties. *J Nucl Med*. 1990;31:1688–1692.
4. Inyoue T. Image reconstruction with limited angle projection data. *IEEE Trans Nuclear Science*. 1979;NS-26:2666–2669.
5. Saint-Felix D, Trousset Y, Picard C, et al. In vivo evaluation of a new system for 3D computerized angiography. *Phys Med Biol*. 1994;39:583–595.

Part 8
Medical Malpractice in Revision Hip Surgery

Douglas Danner and Roderick H. Turner

It has been an honor and a privilege to prepare this material with Counselor Danner. Counselor Danner has been a distinguished member of the defense Bar and has served as a practicing attorney, author, and lecturer with his principal focus on medical injury cases. He is past President of The Massachusetts Defense Lawyers Association. He is a Fellow of the America College of Trial Lawyers, and is a member of numerous other legal societies. In his 36 years of experience, he has focused his energies on the defense of malpractice cases and he has written prolifically, including a three-volume treatise,[1] coauthored with L.L. Varn, Esq. and entitled "Medical Malpractice Checklist and Discoveries" directed principally to the legal profession. Some of the material in these three volumes is presented in a shorter book[2] directed principally towards the medical profession, entitled "When Bad Things Happen to Good Doctors: A Malpractice Primer." This 181-page volume is eminently readable and is a very thorough treatment of the malpractice experience from a physician's point of view. I would recommend it highly to all who wish to avoid malpractice litigation, and especially to those with litigation pending.

Much of the material in this chapter is taken directly from Counselor Danner's primer and we are most grateful to the publishers for permission to use some abbreviated portions of this text. The publisher of this primer is Clark Boardman Callaghan, a division of Thomson Information Services, Inc., 50 Broad Street, Rochester, NY 14694. It has been both a pleasure and a valuable working experience to work with Counselor Danner in the preparation of this material.

Part B
Medical Maintenance in Revision Hip Surgery

76
Medical Malpractice in Revision Hip Surgery

Douglas Danner and Roderick H. Turner

Malpractice in Perspective

The American Academy of Orthopedic Surgeons has prepared an in-house publication[3] entitled "Managing Orthopedic Malpractice Risk." While not as thorough a treatise as the Malpractice Primer[2] mentioned above, it does provide some interesting specifics. The core of data on which the AAOS book is based is a survey of 351 orthopedic claims made in recent years in which the outcome of the legal action is known. This claim data was provided by 20 insurance companies covering orthopedic surgeons in multiple states, including New York, California, Massachusetts, Illinois, and many others. All cases had orthopedic code diagnoses and an orthopedist was the defendant in 81.6% of the cases.

The most common primary allegations encountered in the AAOS study were as follows:

1. Poor surgical performances
2. Failure to diagnose the patient's condition
3. Postoperative infection
4. Failure to diagnose or properly manage a complication
5. Technical complications

We should note the lack of informed consent is a very common allegation and proper informed consent is absolutely critical, however informed consent is infrequently the solitary or primary allegation in a medical injury case.

Analysis of the depositions of the 351 claims reveals that in 88.1% of the claims the issue was resolved prior to trial. Of these 351 orthopedic cases, 30.8% were dismissed, 26.2% were withdrawn, and 31.3% were settled. Of the cases that went to court before a jury (usually) or before a judge, the verdicts were 9.1% defense verdict and 2.6% plaintiff verdict.

So the orthopedic surgeon faced with a malpractice suit should be encouraged by the knowledge that there is roughly a 50% chance that the problem will go away, about a 10% change that it will go to formal court, and a 2.6% chance of a guilty verdict.

However, all these reassuring numbers will not be achieved without considerable investment of time, study, and energy. The purpose of this section and the publications mentioned above[2,3] is to guide you in how to invest and commit this time, study, and energy.

Many people erroneously believe that it is the incompetent physician or borderline physician who is the victim of a malpractice suit. This is NOT SO. The specialist or the above-average physician with substantial expertise is a common target of a malpractice suit.

The inescapable truth about medical malpractice is that it cannot be completely prevented. Although immeasurable benefits have been brought to mankind with new diagnostic and therapeutic procedures, the hazards of medical practice have increased enormously. Today even the best trained and most conscientious doctors are finding themselves defendants in malpractice suits. This seems incongruous considering the fact that never before in the history of American medicine has so much sophistication and technology been available in the delivery of health care.

There are many and varied reasons for the increase in malpractice actions. Probably the most important is the disappearance of the close relationship between doctor and patient that once existed in this country. Relatively few general practitioners are sued, particularly those who are friends of their patients. With increasing referral to large or distant medical centers and with the modern "team" approach to the patient, close personal contact between physician and patient is often minimal or virtually lacking. An additional contributing factor to this increase is the rising cost of medical care. High costs may cause people to expect more from their medical care and to be more critical of the care they receive. Public awareness of the "miracles" of modern medicine may also lead to greater expectations from the medical system, making people less willing to tolerate a less than perfect result.

Classically, three factors often combine to initiate a medical malpractice case: an unexpected bad result; a big bill; and a poor relationship among the patient, the patient's family, and the doctor. If you have an early awareness of potential trouble, you may be better able to deal with it appropriately.

Although a malpractice suit isn't something to be taken lightly, if you do find yourself the victim of one, don't let it ruin your practice or your mental or physical well-being. Let the insurance company and the attorneys do the worrying. You should inform yourself regarding what you need to do at each stage, but meanwhile, get on with your life and your medical practice.

A malpractice suit does not mean the end of your practice or professional life, but it does mean that a certain amount of your time and energy over the next months or even years will be spent going over records, talking with lawyers, and preparing the defense of the claim. This is all time that you would undoubtedly rather devote to other things. While every effort will be made to schedule meetings and hearings at your convenience, you will not be able to ignore the ongoing suit. On the other hand, it should not significantly interfere with your practice or your life.

The first involvement will start as soon as you are served with the summons and complaint by the court officer. At that time you should devote the equivalent of several days over several weeks to obtaining and studying legible copies of your office and hospital records. You will find the insurance company claim representative to be very experienced in these matters. The claim representative is readily available to guide you completely and will probably obtain from you a detailed recorded statement setting forth everything you know about your care and treatment of the plaintiff.

Preparation for an attendance at your pretrial oral deposition will require a significant investment of your time, perhaps the equivalent of several days over several weeks.

Finally, trial preparation and the trial itself will take your time. If the case has not been resolved by then, this will consume several days in trial preparation, and then your involvement with the trial may take a few days to a week or more. Since 90% of all cases are resolved prior to the trial, the chances of your involvement at trial are small.

You personally may be worried, distressed, and even furious that in spite of your best efforts, your patient has elected to embarrass you publicly. The traumatic impact of your case presents you with a basic challenge to your intellectual integrity and idealism. Throughout the life of the case, and for the rest of your medical practice, in spite of contrary temptations, we earnestly hope that you will:

1. Continue to practice the best medicine you can as a compassionate and caring professional.
2. Never look at each patient as a potential plaintiff in a malpractice action.
3. Never practice defensive medicine by ordering unnecessary diagnostic studies or consultations if they are not in the patient's best interest.

Legal Principles Underlying Malpractice Litigation

When a physician undertakes the care of a sick or injured patient, the physician does not promise that the patient will be cured or even substantially benefited by treatment. It is, naturally, hoped that the patient will be benefited, but the law recognizes that good results are not always attainable.

Commonly, physicians may become professionally liable for malpractice in one of five ways:

1. Through the physician's own negligence (failing to conform to generally accepted medical practice).
2. Through the negligence of the physician's employees (Respondeat Superior—the employer is liable for harm due to the negligent conduct of employees for actions occurring during or arising out of the employment relationship).
3. Through failing to obtain the informed consent of the patient prior to treatment.
4. Through breaching the physician–patient contractual relationships (for example, by abandoning the patient, disclosing confidential information, or guaranteeing a cure or some other specific result).
5. Through the negligence of the physician's partners.

Malpractice can be simply defined from the legal viewpoint as an unwarranted departure from accepted medical practice that results in an injury to a patient. Medical malpractice cases arise from treatment rendered to a patient, whether in a physician's office, in the hospital setting, or otherwise. The law places upon the physician a duty to conform to the standard of care of the average, qualified practitioner in the same area of medical specialization under the same or similar circumstances.

The physician is not required to accept any patient. The physician may arbitrarily refuse the proffered professional employment. The physician may, moreover, undertake to treat the patient only for a certain ailment or injury, or at a certain place, or for a specified time. However, when a physician does undertake the professional care of a patient, the physician is obligated to provide care that meets the standards of the average qualified physician.

If the doctor practices as a specialist, the doctor will be held to the standard of care of the average qualified member of the profession practicing in the specialty, taking into account the advances in the profession. The doctor is obligated to exercise his or her best judgment as a physician in the care and treatment of the patient. A physician who assumes the duty of any express contract made with the patient may be liable for any breach of that special agreement. For example, a contract for the successful removal of a cataract would be duty distinct from the physician's underlying duty of due care.

The doctor must keep abreast of progress in the profession and utilize accepted and recognized methods of diagnosis and treatment. Any physician who undertakes a method of diagnosis and treatment that is not of a recognized and accepted school of medicine, or that does not have the approval of at least a significant minority of medical practitioners, does so at the risk of liability.

Once a physician accepts any person as a patient, the physician acquires a legal duty to provide care that conforms to accepted standards of medical practice. Negligence is a breach of this duty resulting in harm to the patient.

Four elements must be established by the patient in a given set of circumstances to constitute liability or negligence on the part of the physician:

1. A physician–patient relationship actually existed that would impose a duty on the physician
2. The physician's conduct was negligent, that is, that the physician breached the duty to the patient
3. The patient's negligence was the proximate cause of injury to the patient
4. The patient suffered compensable injury or damage.

An error in judgment is not malpractice. However, a course of action or inaction cannot be excused as a mere error in judgment if it is contrary to the accepted standard of medical care. Physical impairment of the patient alone is not proof that the physician failed to treat the patient in conformity with the commonly accepted standards of medical care. The fact that the plaintiff suffered after treatment by the defendant does not establish negligence on the defendant's part.

Any negligence on the part of the patient, by a patient's act or omission to act, can provide an important defense. Many states follow the comparative negligence rule, whereby negligence on the part of the plaintiff patient diminishes the jury's verdict by the percentage of the plaintiff's negligence found by the jury. If the jury finds that the plaintiff's percentage of the total negligence in the case is 51% or greater, the plaintiff's negligence usually bars the recovery of the plaintiff.

Unique Aspects of Revision Hip Surgery that Enhance the Possibility of Malpractice Litigation

1. Failed earlier procedures make the patient more likely to be disappointed,[4,5] and even hostile.
2. Repeat surgery weakens the bones, muscles, tendons, and other connective tissues.[6-8]
3. The presence of scar from repeated surgery gives inelasticity and fixation to neurovascular structures, especially the sciatic nerve and its components.[9-11]
4. Revision surgery is particularly common in patients with an underlying diagnosis of congenital dysplasia. These patients, in turn, have minimal bone into which to implant new components.[11-15]
5. The incidence of dislocation is two to five times higher in revision surgery than in primary surgery.[16-19]
6. Revision patients tend to be older and have more intercurrent medical problems than do primary hip surgery patients.[20,21]
7. Operating time is longer and blood loss is greater in revision surgery.[22-24]
8. Removal of cemented components or partially bone in-growth components can be technically demanding, and this introduces new surgical steps and new areas for complications.
9. The failure of the earlier surgery introduces a family–patient–physician interface in which the revision surgeon may be interpreted as criticizing the earlier surgeon or surgeons.
10. Implant components in revision surgery are more likely to be complex and/or modular in revision surgery.[25,26,27]

Specific Diagnoses and Areas that Can Lead to Malpractice Litigation in Revision Surgery

1. Peripheral nerve injuries: Peripheral neuropathy is particularly significant because the patient may feel he is worse following surgery than prior to surgery, even if the hip revision went well otherwise. Peripheral nerves are put at greater risk when there is extensive scar, difficult posterior exposure, leg lengthening, and/or dislocation.[10,28,29]
2. Postoperative infection: Here we often encounter the allegation/complaint of "failure to diagnose." If the postoperative hip patient, either primary or revision, has untoward fever, pain, swelling or redness, the surgeon should have a "short fuse" to introduce a needle into the joint.
3. Dislocation: Dislocation is particularly prone to trigger litigation, especially when recurrent or in con-

junction with either nerve injury or questionable component position.[16–18]

4. Deep venous thrombosis: Prophylaxis against DVT has become so standard that it should be used in almost all cases.[30–33] If prophylaxis is not used because of a medical contraindication, this should be documented in the chart and a vena caval filter should be considered, especially in high-risk cases.
5. Anesthetic complications: Anesthetic complications in revision surgery are slightly more common because of longer operative times, blood loss, and requirement for more extensive intraoperative monitoring.
6. Cardiac complications: Same as #5 above.
7. Femoral stem breakage: Stem breakage litigation is usually an issue of product liability, but the surgeon must be sure that the components are of sufficient size and strength.[34]
8. Abdominal complications: These must be diagnosed and treated promptly or they can be grave (especially gall bladder and vascular).
9. Genito-urinary complications: Same as #8 above, especially urinary bladder perforations.[35,36]
10. Plastic surgical complications: The presence of multiple old incisions and ischemic scars make both incision planning and tissue handling very critical.
11. Heterotopic ossification: It is generally agreed that heterotopic bone is more common when repeated surgery is necessary.[37–41] However, it has not been a particularly litigious area.
12. Polyethylene failure: This is undoubtedly the most rapidly growing area of both malpractice and product liability litigation in the field of hip surgery. Suffice it to say here that surgeons performing hip replacement must be absolutely certain that any poly component implanted is "state of the art" as regards quality, manufacturing standards, thickness, and sterilization techniques.[42–49] Product recalls are more common than in the past and hospital employees must respond to them promptly and thoroughly.
13. Vascular injury: Injuries of the iliac-femoral system in revision surgery are usually, although not always, intra-abdominal.[50] Detailed knowledge of intrapelvic structures and osseous anatomy is essential to avoid these complications in revision surgery.
14. Leg length irregularity: This allegation is listed in the AAOS survey.[3] However the authors' experience has been that the leg length inequality complaints are usually encountered in primary hip cases, as these patients usually start with equal leg lengths and have high expectations of remaining equal. Revision patients commonly start with unequal leg lengths and their expectations are more realistic.

Preparing for a Deposition

How to Handle Your Deposition

A deposition is a form of oral testimony taken from a witness under oath—not in court, but conducted in a manner approved by the court. The testimony is taken before a court reporter, reduced to writing, and often used in court at trial. The deposition is a pretrial discovery procedure and is probably the most important way to investigate the facts. The person whose deposition is being taken is called the *deponent*.

The general purposes of a deposition are discovery of facts, impeachment, and preservation of the testimony of a witness. The purpose of a trial is to ascertain the facts and to apply the law to the facts. The jury must know the facts in order to decide between conflicting claims of the plaintiff and the defendant and to decide what, if any, relief should be granted and what, if any, damages should be awarded to the plaintiff. Depositions are generally taken to obtain information that cannot be obtained through counsel's investigation or from the client or other witnesses, and to supplement testimony and evidence obtained from other sources.

Impeachment. A deposition serves the purpose of freezing a witness' story. If the deponent later testifies at the time of trial in any way differently from the deposition testimony, a transcript of the deposition testimony can be used at trial for the purpose of impeachment by showing prior inconsistent testimony. Juries are inclined not to believe witnesses who change their stories.

Preservation of the testimony of a witness. A witness or party who, for one reason or another, might not be available at the time of trial can be deposed and the transcript of the deposition testimony may later be used at trial if the deponent cannot appear to testify at trial.

Learning the identity of witnesses. Examining counsel can require the deponent to state the names and identities of other persons who may be witnesses to the particular occurrence or who may have other information that might be useful. This information may lead to further investigation or depositions.

Facts and issues are narrowed and clarified. Through proper questioning during the deposition, and by conferring with the deponent's counsel after the deposition, complex facts and issues of the case often can be reduced to the few that are really in controversy, thereby saving everyone's time. Each party will learn about the opponent's side of the case.

Evaluating the case for settlement. In most instances, cases that ultimately are settled cannot be properly evaluated for settlement until counsel on both sides have completed taking depositions. Counsel will have an opportunity during the deposition to evaluate the impression that the opposing party is going to make on a jury.

Settlement opportunity. The taking of the deposition is often a convenient opportunity for counsel to discuss the possibility of settlement.

How to Prepare for the Deposition

There is a great difference between a deposition and a trial. The deposition is a one-sided affair that favors the examining party. As the deponent, you are under a general obligation to answer all questions. You will be asked some questions that would not be admissible in court; This permits adequate discovery and pretrial preparation. No judge will be present and your attorney will play a very limited role. It is critical that you remember these two facts. Your defense trial counsel will be listening to every question you are asked and he or she will object to those that are improper. Do not misconstrue his or her silence as a failure to protect your interest.

Your attorney may hold a predeposition conference with you prior to the deposition date. Before attending that conference you should painstakingly and thoroughly review the entire case. Carefully review all documents pertaining to the case. Your attorney may want to advise you about the tougher questions you will be asked. Your attorney may even wish to conduct a "dry run" or play "devil's advocate" with you to ask key questions expected to be asked by the opposing counsel.

The deposition may be conducted anywhere. It will probably be in the office of the examining counsel. The setting will be informal and as relaxed as possible. Usually only you, your counsel, the examining counsel, and a court reporter will be present. The plaintiff can attend, but rarely does. The examining counsel may well be quite friendly, but do not be lulled into a condition of false security. This cordial atmosphere is often created so that you will be more likely to talk more freely.

Prepare mentally and physically for your deposition, which may be exhausting. Get plenty of sleep and rest for a few days before. Make no other plans before or after your deposition; you'll need all your energies to concentrate throughout your deposition.

Twenty Pointers on Deposition Conduct

The most important matter of all is the way in which you answer questions. Read the following pointers now and read them again the night before the deposition.

1. Do not answer a question until you understand it. If the question is unclear, ask examining counsel to repeat it or phrase it in clearer language. The court reporter can also be asked to read back the question.
2. Think about each question before answering it. Do not supply information not requested by the question, even though you may think it is relevant. If examining counsel does not ask you all you know, do not volunteer information, even though the temptation to do so will be great.
3. If you do not know the answer to a question, say "I don't know." Do not feel that just because a question is asked, you are expected to know the answer to it. If you do not recall what is asked about, say "I don't recall."
4. Give factual information in answer to a question only if you have first-hand knowledge of the facts. Do not base your answer upon so-called hearsay information—that is, something someone else said to you—unless you are specifically asked for hearsay information.
5. Do not hide any facts for which you are specifically asked unless you are advised not to answer a question.
6. If an objection is made by your counsel, stop speaking. If you are advised not to answer the question, do not answer it.
7. Unless your lawyer makes an objection and advises you not to answer, you must assume that you are bound to answer if you know the answer.
8. Avoid asking questions in your answers unless you are asking for a clarification of a question. Only the examining counsel can ask questions.
9. Do not try to memorize your answers. Give a factual, straightforward response to the questions.
10. If facts are asked about information you think may be contained in written records, especially medical and hospital records, answer by referring the opposing counsel to those records. If opposing counsel wants your recollection, check it against any records you may have, even if you are sure of the answer.
11. Dress neatly and according to your usual formal habit and style.
12. Exercise courtesy and good manners.
13. Remember that opposing counsel will be evaluating you constantly. From the very moment your appear, you are under observation. You must, therefore, take great care in your appearance, manner, and remarks at all times. This will show opposing counsel that you would impress a jury.
14. Do not look for traps in every question. There are not many trick questions, and if one comes along your counsel may be able to help you out by an objection or other means. In trying to second-guess each question, you will create the appearance of calculation, hesitation, apprehension, or possibly simple stupidity.

15. Do not argue with opposing counsel. Never become angry or hostile. Remain calm and unemotional even if you feel that the opposing attorney is deliberately trying to provoke you. A person who gets emotionally upset loses the ability to think clearly and may give answers that will be regretted later. It is unlikely that you will be insulted or browbeaten, but if this seems to be happening, resist the urge to meet it with similar tactics. Even if the lawyer on the other side is acting outrageously, it will help your case if you maintain an outward appearance that your emotions are under control.
16. Speak up so that all can hear you. Keep your hands away from your mouth. Answer each question with a verbal response; the court reporter transcribing your testimony cannot take down nods or shrugs.
17. The law requires that you testify according to your best memory. If you are uncertain about an answer to a question, indicate this uncertainty in your response. If you have no memory whatsoever on a given point, say so. Do not guess or assume what you now think must have happened. However, if you have no clear recollection of doing a particular act inquired about, but it was your regular standard practice routinely to do such an act, then you may testify that it is your best memory that you did do that act.
18. Do not be afraid to admit that you have had conferences with your lawyer about the case. Every lawyer has conferences with his or her client. If examining counsel asks you "Did your lawyer tell you what to say at this deposition?" you may answer "My lawyer told me to tell the truth." Opposing counsel should not ask you to repeat any conversations between you and your counsel; those conversations are legally privileged and are not subject to disclosure.
19. You can be required to give a simple yes or no answer if you can answer the question that way, but later you will have an opportunity to explain your answer if it needs explanation. If opposing counsel cuts you off in the middle of an important explanation, you should state that you have not finished your answer and request that you be allowed to finish. If this request is denied, your counsel can ask you to amplify your answer during his or her cross-examination.
20. You must fight against showing exasperation, boredom, or fatigue, even though the questioning may be very extensive. You will be protected against unwarranted harassment by your counsel. Let your counsel know, however, if you feel ill or overly tired during the course of the examination. Your counsel can arrange for a short break or, if necessary, the adjournment of the deposition until another day.

The Examining Counsel

As stated above, the examining counsel may have several reasons for taking a deposition. The form of the examiner's questions may identify the use that the transcript will have. For discovery purposes, the questions will be broad and the subjects far-reaching. This will encourage rambling answers that might reveal new facts. Questions will be precise and sharply focused if the deposition is conducted primarily to produce admissible evidence, which is testimony that a judge could allow a jury to hear at trial.

Examining counsel will probably ask many leading questions. A leading question is really a statement of fact that contains the answer and only asks the witness to agree. Counsel is asking you to answer yes to particular words or phrasing. Counsel will try to "put words in your mouth." If any part of the leading question is incorrect, you should not answer yes but make it clear by your answer that you cannot entirely agree.

Most examiners like to proceed in a linear or chronological fashion. However, if the examiner discovers a new area of inquiry, the questioning will ignore chronology and focus on the new material. After this new subject matter is exhausted, the questions will revert to a chronological narrative.

The examiner will try to get responsive answers. Often the same question will be asked in several different ways to pin you down on your response. The examiner will try to force you to be as accurate and precise as you will allow. If you make any statements that are inconsistent with a prior statement you have made, you may not be confronted with the prior statement until trial.

Pitfall Questions

Perhaps the first step taken by examining counsel will be to create a record that shows that you understand the nature of a deposition and the uses to which it can be put. If, at trial, you insist that contradictory testimony was caused by your failure to understand what was transpiring, you can be impeached with this kind of testimony.

It is, of course, not possible to predict what questions you will be asked or in what order they will come. As a rule, the first few questions will seem incidental (name, address, family background, where you practice medicine). The first major series of questions will probably be focused on your education (from college through post-specialty training, if applicable). It is possible that the examiner will go into very great detail on this matter.

At some point early in the deposition, examining counsel will begin a meticulous, often redundant, exhaustive inquiry concerning the events that led to the lawsuit. No detail is too small. Not all questions will seem relevant, not all will be relevant, not all will even be intelligent.

Usually, prior to your deposition, plaintiff's counsel will have obtained a long, detailed narrative statement from your patient, the plaintiff, of every step and procedure that was involved in your patient's medical care and every word that was said during the course of your care of the plaintiff. At your deposition, you may be asked to give a similar statement, which the plaintiff's examining counsel can compare to the plaintiff's version of the facts. You will likely be asked to recount anything and everything that you did or did not do for or to your patient and everything that was said by anyone connected with the case. You will be asked to trace every step of the medical care of your patient, including history, physical examination, differential diagnosis, diagnosis, treatment, prognosis, as continued from day to day, visit by visit, from the first visit to the last. The examining counsel's objective will probably be to completely commit you on every point of fact so that you cannot later testify differently at trial without risking serious impeachment. There are, however, some questions of which you should be especially wary. Among these are:

1. Questions that focus on your patient's records. Often a doctor–patient relationship extends over a decade or more. You may well be asked about treatments unrelated to the one that provoked the malpractice action. Review your entire history of this patient. Prepare a chronology. Be especially sensitive to your earliest knowledge of facts that led to the treatment now under review.
2. Questions that focus on what information you conveyed to the patient, how it was communicated, why, and—most important—what was not communicated to the patient. For example, counsel may ask if prior to the surgery you informed the patient about certain relatively remote risks associated with the specific operation. You may be asked if you were aware of certain risks.
3. Questions about your pretreatment preparation. You may be asked if you consulted textbooks or journals or other doctors about the condition you treated.
4. Questions about the extent of your knowledge about the particular medical situation that gave rise to this case. Have in mind that, as you consult medical treatises to prepare for your deposition, the more you volunteer expert medical information, the more you help plaintiff's counsel. It is preferable not to give plaintiff's counsel any more information than the specific question calls for.
5. Questions about "good medical practice" or "bad medical practice." Concepts of good or bad practice are mostly foreign concepts to the average physician. Questions on medicolegal issues, standards, and concepts and questions asking that the physician judge others should be avoided, if possible. Consideration should be given to the following responses: "I do not understand your question." "You are asking about legal matters beyond my medical knowledge." "I know my area of medical practice but I am unable to give an opinion or judgment on what other physicians may do or not do."
6. Questions containing words with multiple meanings. On the medicolegal issue of causation, the words "inconsistent with" can transform a remote possibility into an apparently common causal relationship, as in vomiting being "consistent with" a spontaneous perforation of the cecum. In cases involving alleged misdiagnosis, certain words and phrases that have different meanings may be used. Your response may be based on what you understood the word to mean, but later opposing counsel may argue your response as proving something different. Whereas opposing counsel wants it to appear that you did think of the plaintiff patient's ultimate diagnosis, opposing counsel may use words like "consider," "think about," "cross your mind," "occur to you" and "mentally include in your differential diagnosis." Thus, whenever a multiple meaning word is used in the question, your answer may be that you are "not sure of the question but as I understand it, my answer is . . . ."
7. Catch-all questions. Watch out for questions that are too broad to answer. You will be asked, "Tell us everything you can about . . ." Keep your answer accurate and truthful, but as brief as possible. You might want to start your answer, "That's a big subject, but briefly . . . ."
8. Hypothetical questions. Of course, there are many questions the physician will find difficult to answer. The toughest are those in which the examining counsel asks you to assume certain facts. These questions will include key words like *assume, supposing, if, what if*, and others that ask for an answer based on facts you will find to be different from the facts known to you about your case.
9. No memory. If you have no memory of particular facts inquired about while you are under cross-examination at your deposition, and if the case is later settled, there will be no serious problem for your defense. However, if the case goes to trial and you later recall the particular facts, you can be effectively impeached and embarrassed by having testified at your deposition that you had no earlier recollection. Thus, on the vital facts of the case, you should prepare for your deposition as if you were giving trial testimony.
10. Answers limited to "yes," "no" or "I cannot answer yes or no." At trial, and possibly at your deposition,

you may be forced to limit your answers to "yes" or "no" or "I cannot answer yes or no."

Do's and Don'ts of Testimony

The following suggestions regarding your testimony are applicable to both your deposition testimony and your trial testimony. Although written for the defendant doctor, this section applies equally to the plaintiff.

General

1. Always tell the truth.
2. Listen carefully to the entire question before you attempt to answer it.
3. If a question is unclear in any way, ask the examining counsel to repeat it or phrase it in clear language. Do not answer any question until you understand it.
4. Prepare you answer before beginning. Be thoughtful and careful—quick answers suggest either that you are not a careful person or that you have rehearsed or memorized your answers.
5. Qualify your answer if that is necessary for you to give an accurate and truthful answer. Qualify your answers only as necessary. Don't allow yourself to be forced into a flat "yes" or "no" answer if a qualified answer is required.
6. Give factual information in answer to a question only if you have knowledge of the facts; otherwise, identify any assumptions you have to make. Do not hide any facts you know that you are specifically asked about.
7. The law requires only that you testify to your best recollection. If you are uncertain about an answer to a question, indicate this uncertainty in your response.
8. Answer only the question asked. Be as concise and as accurate as possible.
9. Do not volunteer more information than is expressly called for in the question. Extraneous information will only hurt your case.
10. Do not look for traps in every question. There are not very many trick questions and, if one comes along, your counsel will try to assist you either by objecting or by some other means.
11. Do not try to "second guess" every question. Although you should be deliberate in your responses. You should avoid creating the appearance of calculation, hesitation, apprehension, or simple stupidity.
12. At trial, if your attorney objects to a question, do not answer it until you hear the judge's ruling.
13. Do not take notes, documents, or reports to the witness stand unless your counsel approves because opposing counsel will be entitled to examine them.
14. Do not communicate with the opponent or opponent's counsel, except as necessary.
15. Do not, under any circumstances, mention "insurance company" or "insurance."

Communication with the Jury

16. Do not talk down to the jurors. They will resent it and their opinion of you will suffer. Remember that, collectively, juries are very intelligent.
17. Be respectful to the jury at all times.
18. Although the jurors may appear at times to be uninformed or bored, remember that they will ultimately decide the case and it is your job to convince them of the correctness of your testimony.
19. Speak directly to the jurors. Look at them if you feel comfortable doing so, rather than at the judge, clerk, reporter, or examining counsel.
20. Do not be pompous or self-satisfied, and do not create the appearance that you are condescending toward the other people in the courtroom.
21. Do not patronize the judge or jury—enhancing their self-esteem will encourage them to decide in your favor.
22. Do not be smug.
23. Speak up so that all can hear you.
24. Speak in an understandable manner using clear and simple terms the jury can understand.

Appearance

25. Do not demonstrate relief, defeat, or triumph; such action may detract from your performance.
26. Take the stand and leave the courtroom deliberately and confidently.
27. Avoid pins or insignias identifying you with any group.
28. Use correct posture. Maintain a professional demeanor. Sit upright, hold your head erect, and try to avoid nervous mannerisms.
29. Dress neatly and in accordance with the importance of the occasion.
30. Be respectful and courteous towards the opponents as well as towards the judge and jury.
31. Control your temper. Anger and hostility towards the opponent—or arguing with the opposing counsel—will jeopardize your testimony.
32. Do not show exasperation, boredom, or fatigue, even though the questioning may be extensive. The object is for you to project an air of professionalism and reasonable confidence that will persuade the jury that you know what you are talking about and that you are correct.
33. Avoid revealing surprise or displeasure at evidence developed during cross-examination.
34. Do not become defensive when cross-examination starts.

35. Be sure your appearance is neat, discreet, composed, compassionate, poised, and expressive.
36. Do not be afraid to correct opposing counsel, particularly if facts are misstated; but correct only when necessary and do so without belligerence or hostility.

Competence and Expertise

37. Be alert—assume all the counsel in the courtroom are as expert as you are in the narrow field involved in the case.
38. Communicate your expertise clearly, concisely, and understandably. Avoid technical language whenever it is possible to communicate your point in "plain English."
39. Do not overstate your expertise or be arrogant; opposing counsel will certainly be aware of your qualifications and experience, and any attempt on your part to go beyond them will make you vulnerable to cross-examination.
40. Acknowledge the limits of your expertise. Be able to say "I don't know" without embarrassment. No single person can be expected to know everything about a particular field.
41. Do not exaggerate. Any attempt to puff up your qualifications or to elaborate the extent of the examination you have made may be exposed.
42. Do not express opinions on cross-examination that you are not qualified to give. Keep your answers within your area of expertise.
43. Be willing to disagree with the so-called "authorities" if you are convinced that they are wrong.
44. Do not guess at an answer, particularly on cross-examination.
45. Do not regard it as an admission of ignorance to indicate that your opinion is not absolutely conclusive. It is in the nature of expert testimony to be less than 100% certain of your conclusions.
46. Do not try to bluff. If you don't know the answer to a question, say so.
47. Be reasonable and fair. Be able to concede gracefully that, with different facts, you might reach a different opinion.
48. Use a confident tone of voice. Be firm, but not aggressive, hostile, or belligerent.
49. Project an air of competence.

Cross-Examination Styles You May See

1. An ingratiating cross-examiner who befriends you and tries to get you to agree to apparently innocuous statements.
2. A cross-examiner who threatens silently, often with a stack of ostensibly authoritative papers or books.
3. An over-dramatic action—your confident responses should show the jury whom to trust.
4. A cross-examiner who pauses after each answer. Once you have finished, do not feel compelled to fill the silence by volunteering information.

Trick or Compromising Questions

1. Compound questions. If one question is buried in another, ask the opposing lawyer to separate them before you answer.
2. Double negatives—the potential for confusion is obvious.
3. Misquotations or mischaracterizations of your prior testimony or publication. Correct even minor deviations.
4. Attempts to introduce intervening or independently sufficient causes within a hypothetical question. If some of the conditions posed deviate from the facts, bring this to counsel's attention.
5. Hypothetical questions that do not contain enough information or the right information to support a conclusion. State that you cannot answer the question as asked.
6. Catch-all, general, broad questions. Keep your answer accurate and truthful and as brief as possible.
7. Be careful to answer the question that a simple yes or no answer may not convey what you mean.
8. Avoid answering a "loaded" question, where you are condemned by whatever answer you give.
9. Knowledge or awareness. Questions like "Did you know that . . . ." or "Were you aware that . . . ." are dangerous because the opposing counsel usually then states a fundamental medical fact or premise that, if the defendant had known or been aware of it, the medical standard would have required him or her to have acted in a particular way, such as doing or not doing a particular act.
10. "Consistent with." In legal terms, "consistent with" means nothing but it is a clever device to convert remote causation to a more likely causal connection. Opposing counsel may try to get you to agree that certain signs or symptoms are consistent with a particular disease or diagnosis.
11. "Fair to say that . . . ." When this phrase is used, you can be quite sure that opposing counsel has no intention of being fair to you but wants to make it look as if he or she is. Try to avoid agreeing by responses such as, "I don't know if that is fair or not," or "That is not how I would characterize it."

"Authoritative" Writings

1. Beware of stating that any particular source is "authoritative"; you may be held, at least in the eyes of the jury, as establishing the absolute correctness of everything said by that "authority."
2. Unless you are prepared to vouch for the truth of any "authority," it is much safer, and probably more commensurate with your views, to explain that a source

may be helpful but is not conclusively binding and not the definitive word in the area.
3. If you are challenged by a source regarded as authoritative, you may—and should—seek to distinguish this case from those referred to in the source material.
4. Request to see any authoritative source that is used by opposing counsel to impeach your testimony.

Challenge Areas to be Expected (and Possible Responses)

1. If you have to make admissions you think are damaging, do so without embarrassment or fuss, and qualify them if you can by your explanation.
2. Reveal to your counsel all derogatory material regarding your background, qualifications, or interest in the case.
3. You may be asked if you have talked with counsel about this case in advance of trial. You may respond that you did talk with counsel, since it is perfectly proper for you to have consulted with your counsel. You may add that your counsel told you to tell the truth.

Leaving the Witness Stand

1. When leaving the stand, do not manifest relief, triumph, or defeat. If you need to breathe a justifiable sigh of relief, save it until you are outside the courtroom.
2. Don't leave too quickly; walk deliberately at a normal pace.
3. Leave the courtroom to avoid recall to the witness stand unless your counsel has instructed you otherwise. Often opposing counsel will think of some additional questions, but if you are no longer available, these questions cannot be asked.

Malpractice Prevention

Physician–Patient Relationship

The single most important factor in preventing malpractice suits is to maintain a good physician-patient relationship. Physicians who take the time to talk with their patient and who are aware of their patient's expectations and fears are far less likely to leave the patient feeling dissatisfied or angry, and are therefore far less likely to have suits filed against them. Be nice to your patients. Show concern for your patients.

Accept only patients you are willing to treat. Because of personality or other characteristics, there may be patients with whom you may find that you can *not* establish a satisfactory therapeutic relationship. It is better if you do not undertake their treatment. Do be careful, however, not to abandon the patient. Referrals to other physicians should be given. If the patient has urgent medical problems, you may want to make it explicit that you will treat those problems only, and then will assist the patient in finding another physician.

Recognize "suit prone" patients and take special care with them. Watch out for:

1. The patient who is overly concerned with money
2. The patient with unusually strong criticism of past doctors
3. The "doctor shopper" patient
4. The suspicious, neurotic, and severe hypochondriasis patient
5. The patient with unrealistic expectations
6. The high risk medical problem patient
7. The overly grateful and obsequious flatterer
8. The demanding and consumerist patient
9. The stubbornly resistant noncomplying patient
10. The intense pain-related compulsive note-taker

Limit your practice size to the number of patients you can treat with appropriate, thorough care. Overwork increases the incidence of mistakes and also tends to tax your attentiveness to your patients and cause them to feel dissatisfied. Fatigue causes accidents, not only on the highway. The added tension associated with not being able to serve your patients on a timely basis is not worth the extra fees, and in the long term may prove much more costly than you ever anticipated.

Don't take on work that you are not fully qualified to handle. Once you assume responsibility for a patient, you must render skill and care in diagnosis and treatment equal to the standard of your colleagues in the same specialty. This may mean referring a patient to a specialist if you do not have the necessary professional skill to treat him.

Be sure that your specialty procedures are performed well within the standard of care. Specialty procedures require specialty education, specialty training, and specialty experience. These procedures are measured against national specialty standards.

Discuss unusual fees with patient prior to treatment. You should arrive at an understanding with the patient on the matter of fees. Misunderstandings about fees, particularly where they involve higher fees than anticipated, frequently result in suits. Indiscretion in billing and use of impractical collection methods as well as unusual or unexpected fees are common triggers for malpractice claims. Avoid them.

Watch your public relations. As a doctor, you are a member of a distinct minority that will be judged, along with you, by your actions. Fulfill you civic responsibilities willingly, including testifying in court when required.

Ongoing Patient Care

See a case through once started; do not abandon the patient. The doctor–patient relationship should be legally and ethically terminated. The practitioners should also advise his patients of any anticipated absence from practice and should recommend, or make available, a qualified substitute.

Schedule an adequate number of follow-up visits until a clear recovery is attained. This is especially important if the patient is not progressing satisfactorily. Be aware also of patients who need ongoing care. In such cases, it may be prudent to notify a "no-show" patient of the potential consequences of his or her actions. You should thoroughly document any careless or neglectful patient, especially where contact is by telephone and potential problems such as with drugs can arise. You should record the problem, your advice, and the patient's response.

Always tell patients to call if the problem worsens or the patient is dissatisfied with his or her progress. This indicates your ongoing interest in the patient and suggests that you are available for explanations or further treatment as deemed necessary by the patient. Document that you have made these statements.

Don't experiment or use more radical procedures than necessary. When you treat a patient, you must not experiment without the patient's explicit and informed consent, and without sufficient reason to believe that such experimentation offers greater potential for benefit to the patient than currently accepted methods of treatment. Avoid using drugs or procedures with which you are not fully familiar. Don't use radical procedures unless more conservative therapy has been tried or has been eliminated for sound reasons.

Referrals

Practice within the limits of your competency; refer to a competent specialist problems outside your expertise.

Patients with whom you cannot establish a satisfactory physician–patient relationship should be referred. These are the patients most likely to bring suit. A constructive way to view this is not that you are unloading your "difficult" patients, but rather that you are trying to help the patient find a physician with whom he or she will be more satisfied or more comfortable.

Refer new patients once your caseload becomes burdensome. Simple refusal to accept a patient may not be sufficient if the patient needs immediate care, and it might not be good community relations.

Consultations

Obtain a consultation when you are uncertain about the diagnosis or treatment, especially when the medical problem is outside of your specialty.

Obtain a consultation when you anticipate an unhappy outcome for the patient. These may be cases which present high risk, or in which the prognosis is given, or in which complications arise.

Obtain a consultation if the patient or his family requests one, or if your handling of the case is being questioned.

Medical History

Take a complete medical history, including all past medical problems and all current symptoms, not just those appearing to relate to the problem for which the patient is seeking treatment.

Document the significant details of the history—positives and negatives. Failure to record negatives is classical and often creates problems, particularly where the plaintiff's attorney will argue, "If it wasn't recorded, it wasn't considered" or "If it wasn't recorded, it wasn't done."

Attempt to obtain records from prior treating physicians and from recent hospitalizations. Document such efforts.

Physical Examination

Make a thorough examination. In any contact with a person seeking treatment, you must spend enough time and attention in examining and diagnosing his or her problems to be able to make a defensible disposition of the case, whether you accept the person as a patient or not.

To protect yourself from liability for error in diagnosis, you must be able to show that you: (1) thoroughly examined the patient; (2) took a proper history; (3) conducted the diagnostic tests and procedures that are currently considered appropriate; and (4) carefully eliminated alternative modes of diagnosis and treatment.

To protect others, including your colleagues, from questions of liability, you should be careful to include a differential diagnosis when the facts permit a reasonable inference that something other than your diagnosis may be valid.

Formulating Diagnoses

Document the reasons for your preliminary diagnosis in your records, and modify, with further documentation, as appropriate.

Don't overlook the possibility of multiple diagnoses.

If the diagnosis is unclear and the treatments for the various possibilities would be very different, obtain a consultation.

Order tests appropriately: simple, inexpensive, and safe tests when they might give useful information; expensive or dangerous tests only when clearly indicated.

Take x-rays in treating suspected fractures. X-rays should usually be taken before and after reduction, immediately following surgical interventions, and postoperatively during healing to check position and progress. Failure to order sufficient x-rays can create tremendous difficulties in defending a malpractice case.

Informed Consent

Always obtain informed consent for any procedure or treatment. Recent surveys of physicians' practices suggest that some are still ignoring the formal aspects of the requirement of informed consent, while others are overreacting by terrifying their patients with a recitation of every possible remote risk and requiring written consent for every small procedure. The best path both for legal protection and for good medical care lies in the middle.

Obtain written consent for all major or risky procedures. Broad, vague blanket consent forms are probably useless legally. The form should state the nature of the procedure or treatment and the major or common risks and complications. To minimize the possibility of this increasing patient alarm or suspicion of liability, regard this as an opportunity to "educate" rather than to "warn" the patient.

Do take extraordinary medicolegal precautions prior to removal of a patient's organs. Organ removal should be conducted only under "ideal" medical and legal conditions. For example, although voluntary nontherapeutic surgical sterilization may be lawful and such operations may be permissible for the purpose of family limitation motivated solely by personal or socioeconomic considerations, it is recommended that for every such procedure the practitioner obtain from the patient and the spouse, if any, a signed, written recognition of: (1) the lack of any guarantee of successful sterilization; (2) the necessity for supplementary contraceptive measures until sterilization can be reasonably assured (particularly after vasectomies); and (3) the risk of tissue breakdown and recanalization and subsequent fertility. You should consult your attorney before agreeing to perform a procedure with clear medicolegal overtones.

If the interests of a third party are involved, obtain that party's written consent also. Examples include amniocentesis or sterilization, in which cases it is prudent to obtain the signature of the patient's spouse.

Informed consent "do's and don'ts:"

1. Recognize that every patient has a strong interest in being free from nonconsensual invasion of his or her bodily integrity.
2. Recognize that it is the prerogative of the patient and not the physician to determine the direction in which the patient's interests lie.
3. Recognize that every competent adult has a right to forego treatment, or even care, if it entails for the patient what appear to be intolerable consequences or risks, even though the patient's sense of values may be unwise in the eyes of the medical profession.
4. Recognize that the knowing exercise of the patient's right to forego treatment requires knowledge of the available options and the risks attendant on each.
5. Recognize that a physician's failure to divulge in a reasonable manner to a competent adult patient sufficient information to enable the patient to make an informed judgment whether to give or withhold consent to a medical or surgical procedure constitutes professional misconduct.
6. Recognize that the physician's privilege to withhold information for therapeutic reasons, such as where sound medical judgment might indicate that disclosure would complicate the patient's medical condition or render the patient unfit for treatment, must be cautiously exercised.
7. Make sure that the patient understands the nature of his or her medical condition.
8. Make sure that the patient understands the nature of the proposed treatment or procedure.
9. Make sure that the patient understands any possible alternative treatment or procedure.
10. Make sure that the patient understands the nature and probability of medically significant risks of the proposed treatment or procedure and any alternative treatment or procedure.
11. Make sure that the patient understands the benefits to be reasonably expected and the chances of success or failure of the proposed and alternative treatments or procedures, including the likely result of no treatment or no procedure.
12. If there is a significant risk of death, serious harm, or the likely irreversibility of the procedure, disclose it.
13. Disclose and document your disclosure of the peculiar risks associated with a specific treatment or procedure.
14. Disclose and document your disclosure of the inability of the physician to predict results, if that is the case.
15. Disclose and document your disclosure of risks to a greater extent when the proposed treatment or procedure is experimental, new, novel, ultrahazardous, capable of altering sexual capacity or fertility, or purely cosmetic in nature.
16. Disclose and document your disclosure of your intent to perform procedures incidental to the principal procedure, such as an appendectomy during a hysterectomy.
17. Make the disclosures yourself and do not expect the nurses or paramedical personnel to make them.

18. Follow the rule that "the greater the risk to the patient, the less the chance of therapeutic benefit to the patient, the more you should explain to the patient."
19. Act as if you or your family were on the receiving end of the treatment or procedure.
20. Record your disclosures and the consent in a permanent way, either by a detailed writing in the medical or hospital records or by using a fully explanatory written consent form.
21. Make sure you fill in the blanks where the operative procedure or proposed treatment should be indicated.
22. Don't say you are going to do a routine operation; none is routine.
23. Don't inform the patient that the treatment or procedure is simple.
24. Don't tell the patient that no complications will occur, because complications may occur.
25. Don't expect to obtain informed consent by merely answering the patient's questions, because the patient won't ask you the right questions.
26. Don't expect a patient's signature on a consent form that was thrust under the patient's nose by a nurse just before the patient was wheeled to the operating room to provide you with a strong defense in a later legal action against you for the patient's lack of informed consent.
27. The use of video informed consent will be discussed in the final section of this chapter, by Dr. David Hungerford. It is important to note that the patient and the family be given ample opportunity to address questions directly to the operating surgeon after viewing the tape. This personal session with the patient and the family is equally important whether the tape is "home-made" by the surgeon or professionally produced.

Records

Medical records are a true paradox: although despised for their necessity, they are cherished for their usefulness. In the courtroom, medical records are witnesses whose memory never dies. The four general purposes of medical records are as follows:

1. Refresh and improve the recollection of the physician or nurse of what he or she has done and what is being planned as to the patient's care.
2. Communicate the important data to all those participating in the patient's care.
3. Bring together in easy grasp all the important patient information regarding the care, the course, and the plan for the present and future of the patient.
4. Create a legal document to record and substantiate a standard of medical care for medicolegal and other possible reviews.

Keep meticulous records and be sure your colleagues, employees, residents, students, and nurses do the same. These records can become your best friend or your worst enemy.

Drugs

It is appropriate to educate patients about their medications, including (1) The name of the drug and what it is supposed to do; (2) How and when to take it; (3) Contraindicated foods, activities or other drugs; (4) The side effects of the drug. Provide written information that a patient can read after leaving the doctor's presence.

Be aware of recommended drug doses and of the information in the *Physician's Desk Reference* or *PDR* and patient package inserts. If deviating from the recommended dosages, document your reasons and monitor the patient particularly carefully.

Know and closely monitor for the side effects and potential reactions of the drugs you prescribe. Warn the patient of what to watch for, and know how to treat any reactions.

Limit the number of refills on prescriptions, especially on controlled drugs and those requiring careful monitoring. Never authorize over the telephone a refill for a prescription not originally written by you. Document all prescriptions, refills, instructions, and warnings to the patient on a medicated flowsheet. Make your prescriptions clear. Encourage pharmacists' questions; they are normally intended to help, not hinder, good patient care.

Obtain, document, and regularly update medical histories from patients, including contraindications to medications. Post medication allergies on patient charts.

Medical Equipment

Check the condition of your equipment. Do this frequently and make use of all available safety devices. Follow established routine for checking the condition of your equipment.

Refresh your memory on the operation of complex and rarely used equipment. Make sure you have a backup for vital equipment, supplies, and people.

Telephone Advice

Avoid diagnosing, prescribing, or instructing over the telephone. If you do diagnose, prescribe, or instruct by telephone, make a complete record, and try to schedule a follow-up visit whenever possible. Try to limit your telephone medical advice to situations in which the patient is well known to you, has a simple problem, and will follow your instructions.

Other Physicians, Assistants, and Delegating Procedures

Be aware of the competence of doctors with whom you affiliate. In some situations, such as your partners who "take calls" for you, you may be liable for their errors.

Assistants should be competent, trained for the procedures they handle, and adequately supervised. Do not delegate medical procedures to students. You should personally supervise procedures performed by students or residents. Be alert to feelings by the patient of being slighted when tasks are delegated.

Use good sense when talking about other doctors. Keep the attending doctor fully informed.

Beware the "Who Butchered You" Syndrome, a subsequent physician who is critical, or appears to be critical, of the defendant doctor's conduct in the presence of the plaintiff or the plaintiff's family.

Have a review system. A good peer review system should be in place in your office, clinic, or hospital to make sure all staff members are up to date and performing at acceptable levels. Make sure all staff members report adverse occurrences, determine underlying causes, and take corrective action.

Representations and Instructions to Patients

Don't promise to cure or give an overly optimistic prognosis. Your promise or guaranty of a cure or of a particular result is grounds for legal action if it is not fulfilled. Therefore, it's better not to be overly optimistic or promise too much to the patient.

Instruct patients carefully. Emphasize the dangers of continuing medication beyond the prescribed period or discontinuing medication prematurely. Special precautionary instructions should be given to those caring for patients, especially for patients who are potentially dangerous or suicidal or who have a communicable disease.

Exercise tact, but be alert for liability problems. A proper professional manner should be maintained at all times toward both the patient and his or her family. An attentive doctor may sense quite early a disturbing undercurrent in the relationship.

Confidentiality

Do not disclose confidential information or publish pictures without the patient's specific consent. Allow no unauthorized persons to be present at an operation or delivery.

Recall that a patient has a right to a copy of his medical records upon presentation of signed authorization and payment for copying services. A patient cannot be denied a copy of his or her records simply because he has failed to pay his bills.

Keep a Bad Situation from Getting Worse

Don't panic if a complaint or accusation is made. There may be a strong temptation to argue, alibi, or even retaliate, but don't do it. Covering up an error by destroying records or other evidence is an even bigger error.

Don't admit fault or become confessional. Speak with extreme caution to the complaining patient. Above all, don't admit that you were at fault. Most physicians do not have the legal background to determine whether they are legally responsible for an untoward result.

Don't disclose insurance policy coverage. It is unwise for you to tell a patient, or the patient's attorney, that you carry professional liability insurance. The mere mention of this fact may plant the seed of a lawsuit in the mind of a dissatisfied patient.

Don't take patients into your confidence in your self-criticism, hindsight, or thinking out loud.

Video Informed Consent for Revision Total Hip Replacement

Patients presenting for revision total hip replacement represent a very heterogeneous group, particularly in degree of difficulty and anticipated outcome. However, the fact is that this group of patients faces a more demanding course with a lower chance of success than they did with their primary arthroplasty. It is therefore extremely important that the patient understand the issues concerning this second intervention. Each of these patients has already undergone a major surgical procedure that has now failed, and they may be somewhat disillusioned about the prospects of revision surgery. Many will also be apprehensive. In practices where significant numbers of these patients are presenting for reoperation, the needs of these patients for resources and information often outstrip the time available from the harried practitioner. The diagnostic group into which these patients are placed is no different than for primary total hip replacement.

For the past 10 years, I have been using a personally made, amateur video tape as a preliminary step in the informed consent process. It is the purpose of this brief narrative to report the results of that experience. The tape I use was shot on a camcorder and edited using two VCRs—no high-tech procedures are involved. One of the keys to the tape's acceptance by the patient is that it is not high-tech, with background music, fades, flips. It basically is a videotape of their surgeon talking to them by way of a medium that allows the use of props and a consistent, thorough coverage of the issues in-

---

This section provided by David Hungerford, M.D.

volved in their impending surgery. The successful video does not include anything more or less than what a surgeon ought to be telling the patient about the surgery on a individual basis. It does, however, allow the use of props and a consistent presentation that covers all of the bases and does form a record of what the patient was shown. The videotape has been a considerable time saver. The videotape runs 23 minutes and allows me to present much more information to the patient than I probably would have time to do in a busy clinical setting. The patient is given paper and pencil to write down any questions or concerns or points they don't understand.

At the conclusion of the viewing, I meet with the patient to go over their concerns. In the past, when giving oral informed consent to the patient, the patients would frequently call in a day or two later and have questions and concerns that they wanted addressed. This rarely happens now. Occasionally a patient will ask if a family member or spouse can come in at a later date to view the tape. The tape is generic for revision total hip replacement and it also includes aspects of the particular hospital in which I practice. The videotape includes an introduction to the basic problem of why hip replacements fail; issues of exposure; the duration of the procedure; blood loss and the use of cell saver, as well as donated blood; the common complications for which the patient is at risk; the hospital course, discharge procedures, and arrangements for follow-up; and the importance of follow-up. I have shared this approach with many colleagues, some of whom have expressed resistance to the idea on the basis that such a technique is too impersonal. Commercial products are available that are much more polished, but I have no experience with them on the basis of that same fear. Because mine is a personal videotape of their surgeon talking to them via video, patients actually seem to count it as time that I spend with them. One of my patients effused to our case manager how well I had addressed her concerns—"He explained everything to me, it was great!". In fact, the only thing that the patient had done was to see the videotape and when she was finished she said that she had no further questions. In her recollection at the time of admission several weeks later, she said that I had answered all her concerns. Far from shortchanging a patient and offering a reduced level of expedited service, the use of videotape allows the time to be spent addressing the patient's real concerns while providing them all the information that they need in order to experience a truly informed consent.

References

1. Danner D, Varn LL. *Medical malpractice: checklists and discoveries*. Rochester, NY: Clark Boardman and Callahan Div. of Thomas Information Services; 1995.
2. Danner D. *When bad things happen to good doctors: a malpractice primer*. 13th ed., Rochester, NY: Clark Boardman and Callahan Div. of Thomson Information Services; 1996.
3. American Academy of Orthopedic Surgeons. Managing orthopedic malpractice risk. Prepared by The Committee on Professional Liability. Rosemont, IL: AAOS; 1996.
4. Gore DR, Murray MP, Gardner GM, Mollinger LA. Comparison of function two years after revision of failed total hip arthroplasty and primary hip arthroplasty. *Clin Orthop*. 1986;208:168–173.
5. Pellicci PM, Wilson PD Jr., Sledge CB, Salvati EA, Ranawat CS, Poss R, et al. Long-term results of revision total hip replacement. A follow-up report. *J Bone Joint Surg Am*. 1985;67:513–516.
6. Malkhani AL, Sim FH, Chao EY. Custom-made segmental femoral replacement prosthesis in revision total hip arthroplasty. *Ortho Clin North Am*. 1993;24:727–733.
7. Hoogland T, Razzano CD, Marks KE, Wilde AH. Rev. of Mueller total hip arthroplasties. *Clin Orthop*. 1981;161:180–185.
8. Kavanagh BF, Fitzgerald RH Jr. Multiple revisions for failed total hip arthroplasty not associated with infection. *J Bone Joint Surg Am*. 1987;69:1144–1149.
9. Schmalzried TP, Amstutz HC, Dorey FJ. Nerve palsy associated with total hip replacement. Risk factors and prognosis. *J Bone Joint Surg Am*. 1991;73:1074–1080.
10. Zechmann JP, Reckling FW. Association of preoperative hip motion and sciatic nerve palsy following total hip arthroplasty. *Clin Orthop*. 1989;241:197–199.
11. Mulroy RD Jr., Harris WH. Failure of acetabular autogenous grafts in total hip arthroplasty. Increasing incidence: a follow-up note. *J Bone Joint Surg Am*. 1990;72:1536–1540.
12. Paavilainen T, Hoikka V, Paavolainen P. Cementless total hip arthroplasty for congenitally dislocated or dysplastic hips. Technique for replacement with a straight femoral component. *Clin Orthop*. 1993;297:71–81.
13. Fredin H, Sanzen L, Sigurdsson B, Unander-Scharin L. Total hip arthroplasty in high congenital dislocation. 21 hips. *J Bone Joint Surg Br*. 1991;73:430–433.
14. Gerber SD, Harris WH. Femoral head autografting to augment acetabular deficiency in patients requiring total hip replacement. A minimum five-year and an average seven-year follow-up study. *J Bone Joint Surg Am*. 1986;68:1241–1248.
15. Marti RK, Schuller HM, van Steijn MJ. Superolateral bone grafting for acetabular deficiency in primary total hip replacement and revision. *J Bone Joint Surg Br*. 1994;76:728–734.
16. Woo RY, Morrey BF. Dislocations after total hip arthroplasty. *J Bone Joint Surg Am*. 1982;64:1295–1306.
17. Grossman P, Braun M, Becker W. [Dislocation following total hip endoprosthesis. Association with surgical approach and other factors]. *Z Orthop Ihre Grezgeb*. 1994;132(6):521–526.
18. Ali Khan MA, Brakenbury PH, Reymonlds IS. Dislocation following total hip replacement. *J Bone Joint Surgery Br*. 1981;63:214–218.
19. Daly PJ, Morrey BF. Operative correction of an unstable total hip arthroplasty. *J Bone Joint Surg Am*. 1992;74:1334–1343.
20. Callaghan JJ, Salvati EA, Pellicci PM, Wilson PD Jr,

Ranawat CS. Results of revision for mechanical failure after cemented total hip replacement, 1979 to 1982. A two to five-year follow-up. *J Bone Joint Surg Am.* 1985;67:1074–1085.

21. Raut W, Wroblewski BM, Siney PD. Revision hip arthroplasty. Can the octogenarian take it? *J Arthroplasty.* 1993;8:401–403.
22. Cone J, Day LJ, Johnson GK, Murray DG, Nelson CL. Blood products: optimal use, conservation, and safety. *Instr Course Lect.* 1990;39:431–434.
23. del Sel H, Brittain G, Wroblewski BM. Blood loss and operation time in the Charnley low friction arthroplasty. *Acta Orthop Scand.* 1981;52:197–200.
24. Semkiw LB, Schurman DJ, Goodman SB, Woolson ST. Postoperative blood salvage using the Cell Saver after total joint arthroplasty. *J Bone Joint Surg Am.* 1989;71:823–827.
25. Pellicci PM, Haas SB. Disassembly of a modular femoral component during closed reduction of the dislocated femoral component. A case report. *J Bone Joint Surg Am.* 1990;72:619–620.
26. Cameron HU. The two- to six-year results with a proximally modular noncemented total hip replacement used in hip revisions. *Clin Orthop.* 1994;298:47–53.
27. Barrack RL, Burke DW, Cook SD, Skinner HB, Harris WH. Complications related to modularity of total hip components. *J Bone Joint Surg Br.* 1993;75:688–692.
28. Nercessian OA, Macaulay W. Peripheral neuropathies following total hip arthroplasty. *J Arthroplasty.* 1994;9:645–651.
29. Johanson NA, Pellicci PM, Tsairis P, Salvati EA. Nerve injury in total hip arthroplasty. *Clin Orthop.* 1983;179:214–222.
30. Woolson ST, Watt JM. Intermittent pneumatic compression to prevent proximal deep venous thrombosis during and after total hip replacement. A prospective, randomized study of compression alone, compression and aspirin, and compression and low-dose warfarin. *J Bone Joint Surg Am.* 1991;73:507–512.
31. Imeperiale TF, Speroff T. A meta-analysis of methods to prevent venous thromboembolism following total hip replacement. *JAMA.* 1994;271:1780–1785.
32. Huo MH, Salvati EA, Sharrock NE, Brien WW, Sculco TP, Pellicci PM, et al. Intraoperative heparin thromboembolic prophylaxis in primary total hip arthroplasty. A prospective, randomized, controlled, clinical trial. *Clin Orthop.* 1992;274:35–46.
33. Lieberman JR, Huo MM, Hanway J, Salvati EA, Sculco TP, Sharrock NE. The prevalence of deep venous thrombosis after total hip arthroplasty with hypotensive epidural anesthesia. *J Bone Joint Surg Am.* 1994;76:341–348.
34. Chao EY, Coventry MB. Fracture of the femoral component after total hip replacement. An analysis of fifty-eight cases. *J Bone Joint Surg Am.* 1981;63:1078–1094.
35. Radford PJ, Thomson DJ. A case of methylmethacrylate bladder stone. *Acta Orthop Scand.* 1989;60:218–219.
36. Tostain J, Gilloz A. [Migration of cement into the bladder after total hip replacement (author's transl)]. *Rev Chir Orthop Reparatrice Appar Mot* 1980;66:391–393.
37. Rockwood PR, Horne JG. Heterotopic ossification following uncemented total hip arthroplasty. *J Arthroplasty.* 1990;5 Suppl:S43–S46.
38. Errico TJ, Fetto JF, Waugh TR. Heterotopic ossification. Incidence and relation to trochanteric osteotomy in 100 total hip arthroplasties. *Clin Orthop.* 1984;190:138–141.
39. Pagnani MJ, Pellicci PM, Salvati EA. Effect of aspirin on heterotopic ossification after total hip arthroplasty in men who have osteoarthrosis. *J Bone Joint Surg Am.* 1991;73:924–929.
40. Pedersen NW, Kristensen SS, Schmidt SA, Pedersen P, Kjaersgaard-Andersen P. Factors associated with heterotopic bone formation following total hip replacement. *Arch Orthop Trauma Surg.* 1989;108:92–95.
41. Warren SB. Heterotopic ossification after total hip replacement. *Orthop Rev.* 1990;19:603–611.
42. Mathiesen EB, Lindgren U, Reinholt FP, Sudmann E. Wear of the acetabular socket. Comparison of polyacetal and polyethylene. *Acta Orthop Scand.* 1986;57:193–196.
43. Cates HE, Faris PM, Keating EM, Ritter MA. Polyethylene wear in cemented metal-backed acetabular cups [see comments]. *J Bone Joint Surg Br.* 1993;75:249–253.
44. Bosco J, Benjamin J, Wallace D. Quantitative and qualitative analysis of polyethylene wear particles in synovial fluid of patients with total knee arthroplasty. A preliminary report. *Clin Orthop.* 1994;309:11–19.
45. Jasty M, Bragdon C, Jiranek W, Chandler H, Maloney W, Harris WH. Etiology of osteolysis around porous-coated cementless total hip arthroplasties. *Clin Orthop.* 1994;308:111–126.
46. Davidson JA. Characteristics of metal and ceramic total hip bearing surfaces and their effect on long-term ultra high molecular weight polyethylene wear. *Clin Orthop.* 1993;294:361–378.
47. Collier JP, Mayor MB, Surprenant VA, Surprenant HP, Dauphinais LA, Jensen RE. The biomechanical problems of polyethylene as a bearing surface. *Clin Orthop.* 1990;261:107–113.
48. Bono JV, Sanford L, Toussaint JT. Severe polyethylene wear in total hip arthroplasty. Observations from retrieved AML. PLUS hip implants with an ACS polyethylene line [see comments]. *J Arthroplasty.* 1994;9:119–125.
49. Tsao A, Mintz L, McRae CR, Stulberg ST, Wright T. Failure of the porous-coated anatomic prosthesis in total knee arthroplasty due to severe polyethylene wear [see comments]. *J Bone Joint Surg Am.* 1993;75:19–26.
50. Aust JC, Bredenberg CE, Murray DG. Mechanisms of arterial injuries associated with total hip replacement. *Arch Surg.* 1981;116:345–349.

Index

NOTE: Page numers in italics refer to illustrations; page numbers followed by the letter *t* refer to tables.

Abduction angle, 34
Abscess, 420–421
Acetabulum
  abduction angle, 34
  acetabular inserts, 1
  acetabular teardrop destruction, 94
  bipolar prosthesis, 298–300
  bone stock loss and grafting
    causes of bony defects, 93
    classification system for
      reconstruction, 94
    correlation of bony defects with
      reconstruction, 93–94
    reconstructive approach by type of
      bony defect, 94, *94–98, 95– 97*
  cavitary deficiencies, 293–296,
    294–295, 330–333, *332*
  determination of hip center, 320–324,
    325, 326
  fractures, 40, 535–536
  loosening of cemented acetabular
    components, 5–6
  posterior deficiencies, 339–347, *340,*
    342–346
  segmental deficiencies, 302–306,
    303–305, 333–336, *333–336*
  structural allografts, 309–319, *310–318*
  templating, 130–132, *131*
  use of cages, 349–355, *350–352,*
    354–355
  use of oblong or modular cups,
    326–329, *327, 328*
Acrylic fragmentation, 6
Acute pain, 78
Addiction, pain medications and, 84–85
Agency for Health Policy and Research
  (AHPR), 554
Airway management, anesthesia and,
  418–419
Allogenieic red blood cell transfusion, 119
Allograft bone, 156–157
Aluminum ceramics, 1
American Academy of Orthopedic
  Surgeons (AAOS)
  classification system for acetabular
    deficiencies, 93, 94
  classification system for femoral
    deficiencies, *100,* 100–102, 101t,
    102t, 112, 113t, 168
  outcome studies and, 554

American Association of Tissue Banks
  (ATTB), 156
Anatomic medullary locking (AML)
  component, 163
Anemia, 419
Anesthesia
  complications
    airway management, 418–419
    cementing and, 420
    dislocation and, 420
    neurologic, 420–421
    headache after regional, 421–422
    hemodilution, 124–125
    hypotensive, 126t–127
    hypothermia and, 423–424
    intraoperative moitoring/IV access
      and, 422–423
    peripheral nerve injuries and, 422
    safety issues in high-risk cases, 127
    toleration of low hematocrit, 127
    venous thromboembolism and, 410
Angina, 425
Angiography, 73, *73*
Ankylosing spondylitis
  heterotopic ossification and, 64–65
  motor weakness and, 524
  pain and, 81
  protrusio acetabuli and, 538
Anterior partial trochanteric osteotomy
  (APTO), 263, *264*
Anterolateral surgical approach,
  270–273, *271, 272*
Anteroposterior (AP) view, 59, *60*
Antibiotics
  diagnosis of infection and, 380–381
  Girdlestone arthroplasty and, 512
  resistance of common staphylococcus
    to, 373
Anticoagulation, 366, 428. *See also*
  Venous thromboembolism,
  Thromboprophylaxis
  cement extrusion, *445,* 445–446, *446*
  diverticulitis and, 443, *444*
Anticonvulsants, 85
Antrectomy, 439
Aortoiliac disease, 50
Apoptosis, 23
Arachnoiditis, 80
Arrhythmia and conduction
  abnormalities, 427–428

Arthritis, 79, 81
  acetabular fractures and, 487
  chondrolysis and, 487
  chronic pain syndrome and, 78
  differential diagnosis of hip pain and,
    79
  heterotopic ossification and, 467–468
  motor weakness and, 523
  nerve injury and, 365
  posttraumatic, 65
  protrusio acetabuli and, 538
  total replacement of joints and, 3
Arthritis Impact measurement Scales
  (AIMS), 556
Arthrography
  diagnosis of infection and, 378
  nuclear, 67
  radionuclide, 73
  signs of loosening and, 5
  use in evaluation, 51, 65–68, *67, 68*
Arthropor-II cup, 323
ASA Difficult Airway Algorithm, 418–419
Aspiration
  Girdlestone arthroplasty and, 509
  infection and, 374, 377–378
  use in evaluation, 51, 65–68, *67, 68*
Aspirin, 438
  heterotopic ossification and, 470
  as thromboprophylaxis after total hip
    arthroplasty and, 407
  as thromboprophylaxis after total
    knee arthroplasty, 409
Atraumatic myositis ossificans
  circumscripta, 464
Austin-Moore prosthesis, 478, 479, 499
Autologous blood, 119
Autologous bone graft, 155–156
Autonomic dysfunction, 79
Avascular necrosis, motor weakness
  and, 523

Bilobed cups, *161,* 161
Biomechanics
  anterior thigh pain, 139
  impingement and dislocation, *140,*
    140–141
  restoration of the joint center,
    139–140, *140*
  forces acting on the hip joint,
    135–136, *136*

Biomechanics (*Contd.*)
  load transmission across the implant–bone interface, 136
    effect of implants on cortical loading, 137–138, *138*
    intramedullary fixation of cementless femoral prostheses, 136–137, *137*
    response of femur to stress-shielding, 138–139
Biomet Modular Acetabular Reconstruction System, 326–328
Biopsy
  diagnosis of infection and, 378
  Girdlestone arthroplasty and, 509
Bipolar prosthesis, 38, 298–300
Birch-Schneider ring, 161, *162*
Bladder stones, 451–452
Bleeding peptic ulcer, 439
Blood management
  anesthesia and, 419
  considerations for, 118–119
  techniques for blood salvage
    hemodilution, 120
    intraoperative, 120
    postoperative reinfusion, 120–121
    preoperative autologous donation, 119
    preoperative use of recombinant human erythropoietin, 121–122
Bone bank/bone graft
  allograft bone, 156–157
  autologous bone graft, 155–156
  osteoinduction/osteoconduction, 155
  primary osteogenesis, 155
  proximal femoral reconstruction allografts, 158
Bone grafting
  acetabular, 309–319, *310–318*
  revision with bone graft, 171, *172*
  revision without bone graft, 172–174
Bone morphogenic protein (BMP), 155
Bone resorption, 6, 7
  biochemical mediators of, 8
Bone scans. *See* Radionuclide imaging
Bone stock loss and allografting
  acetabulum
    causes of bony defects, 93
    classification system for reconstruction, 94
    correlation of bony defects with reconstruction, 93–94
    reconstructive approach by type of bony defect, *94*, 94–98, *95*, *96*
  femur
    AAOS classification system, *100*, 100–102, 101t, 102t, 112, *113*
    bulk solid allografts, 108–110
    cortical strip grafts, 107–108
    revision with impaction grafting and cemented fixation, 106–107
    revision with longer revision stem—diaphyseal fixation only, *103*, 103–104, *105–107*
    revision with longer revision stem with proximal and distal fixation, 102–103, 102t
    revision with long stem and reduction osteotomy of femoral shaft, 41–42, 104–106, *106*
    revision with primary stem, *102*, 102t
  trochanter
    AAOS classification system, 112, *113*
    fixation and hardware for trochanteric osteotomy, 115–117
    modifications in type of osteotomy, 115–117
    nonunion after osteotomy, 113–114
    osteolysis and, 114
    osteopenia and, 114–115
    postoperative care after osteotomy, 116
    preoperative planning for osteotomy, 112
Bretylium, 82
Brooker classification, 466
Broviac central venous catheter, 381
Bulk solid allografts, 108–110
Bupivacaine, 66, 82
Burch-Schneider cage, 335, 336, 340, 345
Bursitis, 268
Butyrophenones, 85

Cages, 349–355, *350–352*, *354–355*
Calcar allografts, 109
Calcar isthmus-to-canal ratio, 158
Calcar resorption, 431
Calcar width, 158
Cameron anterior osteotomy surgical approach, *285*, 285–286
Campylobacter intestinalis, 373
Cancellous autograft, 156
Cancellous bone, 182
Cannulated end mill technique, 154
Carcinomatous neuropathy, 79
Cardiovascular complications
  arrhythmia and conduction abnormalities and, 427–428
  hypertension and, 427
  myocardial disease and, 427
  pacemakers and, 428
  perioperative therapy and intensive care and, 428
  postoperative, 428–429
  preoperative risk assessment and, 425–427, 426t, 427t
  prosthetic heart valves and anticoagulation and, 428
  role of the cardiovascular consultant and, 425
  valvular heart disease and, 427
Catheterization, 449
Caudal oblique view, 59, *60*
Causalgia, 79, 82
Cavitary deficiencies, 112, 293–296, *294–295*, 330–333, *332*
Cefazolin, 379
Cell washing, 120–121
Cement
  anesthesia and, 420
  cemented long-stem femoral components
    indications and rationale, 239, *240*, *241*
    surgical technique, 239–242
  cement within cement revision
    indications, 214, *215*
    results, 215–216
    technique, 214–215
  extrusion, anticoagulation therapy and, *445*, 445–446, *446*
  fixation, situations needing special technical considerations, 208–211, *209–210*
  mantle fractures, 5
  removal tools, 150–151, *151*
Central pain, 79
Cerebral palsy
  Girdlestone arthroplasty and, 508–510
  motor weakness and, 523
Chain-extension, 12
Charcot joints, 475
Charnley, Sir John, 11, 379, 522
Chills, clinical evaluation and, 49
Cholecystectomy, 441
Cholecystitis, 439–441, *440*
Chronic pain, 78
Circumferential proximal femoral deficiency, 158
Classification systems
  AAOS, for acetabular deficiencies, 93, 94
  AAOS, for femoral deficiencies, *100*, 100–102, 101t, 102t, 112, 113t, 168
  Brooker, 466
  heterotopic ossification (HO), 466–467, 469
  nerve injuries, 362–363
  periprosthetic hip infection, 374
  trochanter deficiencies, 112, *113*
Clean air, 371, 379
Clonidine, 85
Closed reduction, dislocation and, 396
Clostridium bifermentans, 373
Cobalt-chrome (Co-Cr), 1–2, 208, 372
Cobalt-chrome-molybdenum (Co-Cr-Mo), 565–566t, *566–567*, 567t
Collagenase, 8
Colonna reconstruction, 382
Color Doppler imaging, 74
Color subtraction arthrography, 65

Index

Committee on Muskuloskeletal Specialty Societies (COMSS), 557
Complex regional pain syndrome (CRPS), 49, 79, 82
Component malposition, as a risk factor, 34
Compression, 363, 365
Compression molding, 12
Computed tomography (CT)
  for acetabular revision surgery, 293
  cavitary deficiencies and, 330
  for diverticulitis, 443
  epidural hematoma and, 421
  for fractures, 41
  genitourinary problems and, 449
  Girdlestone arthroscopy and, 510
  hip aspiration with, 65
  limitations of, 70, 75
  metastatic disease and, 498, 499
  nephrolithiasis and, 450
  nerve injury and, 367
  for perforated ulcer, 438
  preoperative planning and, 144
  protrusio acetabuli and, 539
  robotically assisted cement removal and, 576–580
  templating and, 132
  of urological injury, 455–456, 456
  use in evaluation, 55, 60
Congenital hip dysplasia, motor weakness and, 523
Congestive heart failure, 425, 429
Continuous passive motion, thromboprophylaxis after total knee arthroplasty, 410
Conversion hip replacement, 477
  after failure of surgical treatment of hip fracture, 477–481, 478
  following previous acetabular fracture, 487–488
  following previous femoral osteotomy, 481–487, 482, 483, 484–485
Cornell Hip Rating Questionnaire (CHRQ), 556, 557
Cortical allografts, 157
Cortical autografts, 156
Cortical loading, 137–138, 138
Cortical shaft index, 158
Cortical strip grafts, 107–108
Cortical window, 432, 432–433
Corticosteroid therapy, infection and, 371–372
Costs. See Economic considerations
Coumadin, 421
Courant, R., 562
C-reactive protein (CRP), 50, 81, 375–376, 509
Creeping substitution, 155, 181
Cross-linking, 13, 17, 572
Cross-shear, 14

Cup abduction angle, polyethylene wear and, 14
Cup-Out® pneumatic impact wrench, 149, 149
Cups, oblong or modular, 326–329, 327, 328
Cystography, of urological injury, 456
Cytokines, 2, 8, 27–28
Cytoscopy, 449, 450

Dall Miles Cable Grip System™, 163, 164, 193, 397–398, 531
Debonding, and cemented femoral components, 5, 6
Debridement, 382–383, 459
Debris
  infection and, 372
  wear, 1, 7, 7
Decalcifying, 156
Decision analyses, 555
Degenerative osteoarthritis, 79
Degenerative spondylolisthesis, 49
Depression, 50
Developmental dysplasia of the hip (DDH), 266, 309, 524
Dextran
  as thromboprophylaxis after total hip arthroplasty, 407
  as thromboprophylaxis after total knee arthroplasty, 409
Diabetes, 79, 371–372, 425
Diagnosis Related Groups (DRGs), 545
Dialysis, infection and, 372
Diaphyseal fixation, 103, 103–104, 105–107
Differential diagnosis, of hip pain, 79–81
Diffuse idiopathic skeletal hyperostosis (DISH), 65, 467–468
Digital holography, 75
Digital subtraction arthrography, 65, 67
Diphosphonates, heterotopic ossification and, 470
Direct lateral and vastus slide surgical approach, 251–262, 252–261
Direct lateral approach, 251
Discontinuity, femoral, 101, 112–113
Dislocation, 1, 140, 140–141
  anesthesia and, 420
  cement fixation, 208
  direct lateral and vastus slide approach and, 261
  incidence of, 391
  mechanism of, 32, 391–392
  motor weakness and, 527
  neurological injury and, 365
  nonoperative care for, 36
  operative care for, 36–38, 37, 37t
  perioperative factors, 33–36, 33t
  postoperative factors, 32–36, 33t
  predisposing factors for, 392–395

preoperative factors, 33, 33t
  radiographic evaluation of, 65
  in revision total hip replacement, 202
  timing of, 32
  treatment of, 395–398
Distal fixation
  complications, 221
  patient selection, 217–218
  rationale, 217–218, 219
  results, 221–222
  surgical technique, 219–221, 220
Diverticulitis, anticoagulation therapy and, 443, 444
Dorsal column stimulator, 83
Drill and excavation
  cannulated end mill technique, 154
  end mills, 154, 154
  router technique, 154
Drug dependency, pain medications and, 84–85
Dual-isotope scans, 72
Dual-tracer studies, 72
Duralock cup, 323

Economic considerations, 386, 410–411, 545
Ectopic cement, 50
Eicosinoids, 2
Electromiography, 364, 367
End mills, 154, 154
Endosteal grafting, 176
  results, 180–181
  synthesis of findings, 181–183
  technique
    aftercare, 179–180
    canal preparation, 177
    circumferential restraint, 177–178, 178
    impaction of morsellized allograft, 178, 179
    introduction of cement and pressurization, 178
    introduction of femoral component, 178–179
    occlusion of canal, 177, 177
Endothelial cells, 27
Enterococcus, 373
Entrapment, 36, 79
Epidural anesthesia, 421–422
Equipment
  cement removal tools, 150–151, 151
  component removal, 143–144
    acetabular components, 144
    cemented socket, 144–145
    cementless socket, 145–146
    femoral component, 146–147
  Cup-Out® pneumatic impact wrench, 149, 149
  end mills, 154, 154
  hardware for trochanteric osteotomy, 115–116

Equipment (Contd.)
    operating room environment, 142–143
    preoperative planning and, 142
    stem extractors, 150, *150*
    ultrasonic plug puller, *152*, 152–153
Erythrocyte sedimentation rate (ESR), 50, 81, 375–376, 509
Erythropoietin, 121–122
Escherichia coli, 372–373t
Ethylene oxide (ETO), 17, 156, 572
Euthermia, anesthesia and, 424
Evaluation
    algorithms for the painful total hip arthroplasty
        loose cemented, 52, *54*
        loose cementless, 52, *53*
        lysis without looseness, 56, *56*
        stable cemented, 52, *55*
        stable cementless, 52, *53*
    arthrogram, 51
    aspiration, 51
    clinical
        history, 47–49, *48*
        physical exam, 49
    CT scans, 55
    extrinsic disease and, 49–50
    intraoperative, 52
    laboratory analysis, 50
    nuclear medicine scans, 51–52
    of pain syndromes, 78–87
    radiographic, 50–51, 59–75, *60–64*, *67–75*
Expansile osteolysis, 21
Extended lateral femoral osteotomy surgical approach, 280–283, *281–283*
Extended proximal femoral osteotomy, 486
Extended trochanter osteotomy surgical approach, 277–278, *278*

Faber test, physical exam and, 49
False aneurysm, 443
Femoral nerve, 366–367
Femoral neuralgia, 80
Femur. *See also* Fractures
    abduction angle, 34–35
    bone stock loss and allografting
        AAOS classification system, *100*, 100–102, 101t, 102t, 112, 113t, 168
        bulk solid allografts, 108–110
        cortical strip grafts, 107–108
        revision with impaction grafting and cemented fixation, 106–107
        revision with longer revision stem—diaphyseal fixation only, *103*, 103–104, *105–107*
        revision with longer revision stem with proximal and distal fixation, 102–103, 102t
        revision with long stem and reduction osteotomy of femoral shaft, 104–106, *106*
        revision with primary stem, *102*, 102t
    cemented femoral component, 169–170
    cementless femoral component, 170–171
    circumferential proximal femoral deficiency, 158
    femoral stem in S-ROM (standard range of motion) system, 225–226, *226*, *227*
    intramedullary fixation of cementless femoral prostheses, 136–137, *137*
    loosening of cemented femoral components, 5–6
    proximal femoral reconstruction allografts, 158
    response to stress-shielding, 138–139
    surgical techniques (*See* Surgical approaches, femoral revision)
    templating and, 132–133, *132–133*
Fever
    aseptic loosening and, 4
    clinical evaluation and, 49
Fibrinogenesis, 8
Fibroblasts, 2, 23
Fibromyalgia, 78, 80
Fibronectin, infection and, 372
Fibrous tissue, 6
Finite element analysis (FEA), 562–565, *563*, *564*, *565*
Fit and fill, 224
Fluoroquinolone, 381
Focal uptake, 71
Foreign bodies, infection and, 372
Fourier Transform Infra-red Spectroscopy (FTIR), 570
Fournier's Gangrene, 452
Fractures, 1
    rates, 204, 205t
    diagnosis, 41
    femoral, *41*, 42
    femoral stem
        etiology of, 431
        evaluation of, 432, *432*
        removal of, 432–436
    incidence and etiology, 40, 41t
    long-stem prostheses and, 532, 534t
    nonoperative treatment, 530–531t
    operative treatment, 531–532t, *533*
    periprosthetic acetabular, 535–536, *536*
    periprosthetic femoral fracture classification, 530
    in revision total hip replacement, 202
    treatment options and results, *41*, 41–42

Freezing
    effects on incorporation of segmental cortical allografts, 109
    freeze-drying, 155, 156, 198
    fresh, 155, 156, 198
Frozen section, diagnosis of infection and, 378, 512
Functional Milestones Scale (FMS), 556
Functional Status Index (FSI), 556
Fusion defects, in UHMWPE, 12

Gait
    antalgic, 3
    physical examination and, 49
Gallium, 72
Gamma irradiation, 17
Ganz ring, 335, 336, 350
Gas atomized dispersion strengthened (GADS), 566
Gas plasma sterilization, 17, 571, 572
Gender
    dislocation and, 392
    genitourinary complications and, 448
    heterotopic ossification and, 467
    urinary infection and, 450
Genitourinary complications, 448
    Girdlestone arthroplasty, 508
    intraoperative urogenital injury, 453–455
    kidney and bladder stones, 451–452
    preoperative evaluation, male patient, 448–449
    preoperative urological consultation, 449–451
    radiological imaging and, 455–457
    scrotal abnormality, 452–453
    urinary retention, 451
Giant cells
    foreign body, 25, 27
    multinucleated, 26–27
Girdlestone arthroplasty, 68, 505
    defect, 459–460, *462*
    indications and contraindications for, 506–508, *506–508*
    physical rehabilitation and, 550–552
    preoperative evaluation, 508–510
    preoperative templating, 510–511
    surgical procedure, 511–514
    timing of revision surgery, 510
Gluteus medius syndrome, 80
Glycocalyx, 372, 373
Glycolax, 381
Gouty arthrosis, 79
Graft Augmentation Prosthesis (GAP) reinforcing ring, 350–351, *352*, 352–353
Grafting. *See* Bone bank/bone grafts; Bone grafting; Endosteal grafting
Granulomatous response, 16, 25
Guanethidine, 82

HAQ (Health Assessment
    Questionnaire), 556
Hardware. *See* Equipment
Harris score, 553, 558
Health Status Survey, 556
Heliobactyer pylori, 438
Hematocrit, 127
Hematoma, 366
Hematuria, 449–450
Hemiarthroplasty, 477–478
Hemispheric jumbo cup, 349
Hemodilution, 120, 124–125
Hemorrhage, 443
Heparin, as thromboprophylaxis after
    total hip arthroplasty, 405–407,
    406
Hernias, 50
Herniated nucleus pulposis, 80
Heterotopic bone, direct lateral and
    vastus slide approach and, 261
Heterotopic ossification (HO), 64–65, 464
    biology of, 464–465
    classification of, 466–467, 469
    clinical presentation of, 465–466
    incidence of, 467
    method of fixation and, 468
    presence of existing ectopic bone
        and, 469, *469*
    prior surgery and, 468
    radionuclide imaging and, 70
    risk factors for, 467–468
    surgical approach for, 468
    treatment and prevention of, 469–473
Hiatus hernia, 441
Hickman central venous catheter, 381
Himont, 12
Hip center, 320–324, *325, 326,* 349
Hoechst, 12
Hydroxyapatite, 1
Hypertension, 427, 429
Hyperthermia, infusion of unwashed
    blood and, 121
Hypertrophic osteoarthritis, 65
Hypochondriasis, 50
Hypotensive anesthesia, 126t–127, 419
Hypothermia, and anesthesia, 423–424
Hysteria, 50

Iliopectineal bursitis, 79
Iliopsoas syndrome, 80
Immunohistochemistry, 27
Immunosuppression, infection and, 372
Impaction grafting, 176–183
Impact Mallory-Head, 225
Impact modular total hip implant
    allograft and, 236
    bone preparation, 234–236
    clinical results, 236–237, *237*
    exposure, 234
    trial implantation and leg lengths,
        236, *237*

Impingement, *140,* 140–141
Implant inventory
    acetabulum—cavitary defects
        allograft bone, 160–161
        cementless cups with peripheral
            and/or dome screws, 160, *161*
        lateralized components, 160
        peripheral screws, 160
    acetabulum—massive bone loss, 162
    acetabulum—medial wall defects
        metal-backed hemispheric
            component, 161–162
        protrusio ring, 161–162
        ring-support systems, 162
    acetabulum—pelvic discontinuity,
        162
    acetabulum—segmental defects
        allograft bone, 161
        bilobed cups, *161,* 161
        cemented hemispheric
            components, 161
        cementless hemispheric
            components, 161
        large-fragment, partially threaded
            screws, 161
        ring-stabilized components, 161
    femur
        cemented femoral components,
            162–163
        mild to severe proximal
            metaphyseal deficiencies, 163
    femur— defects below the lesser
        trochanter
        calcar replacing prostheses, 163
        lateralized neck components,
            163–164
    femur—intercalcary defects
        bowed and long stems, *163,* 163
        wires, *163,* 163
    greater trochanter
        bolts, 164
        clamps, 164
        wires, *164,* 164
Implant research
    advances in cobalt-chromium-
        molybdenum and titanium
        implant alloys, 565–568
    advances in UHMWPE technology,
        568–574
    finite element analysis (FEA) and,
        562–565
Indomethacin, heterotopic ossification
    and, 470
Inert packaging, 17, 571
Infection
    algorithm for lysis without looseness,
        56
    arthritides and, 79
    aseptic loosening and, 4
    aspiration and, 68, *68*
    with cement fixation, 204, 205t

classification of, 374, 375t
diagnosis of, 374
    arthrography, 378
    biopsy and reoperation, 378
    frozen section, 378
    hip aspiration, 377–378
    lab tests, 375–376
    radiography, 376–377
    scintigraphy and, 378
economic considerations and, 386
Girdlestone arthroplasty and,
    507–508
microbiology of, 372–373t
operating room sterility and, 371
osteolysis and, 4
prevention of, 378–379
    antibiotics, 380
    clean air, 379
    prophylactics, 379–380
    surgical technique, 380
radiographic evaluation of, 68–70, *69,*
    70
radionuclide imaging and, 70
in revision total hip replacement, 202
routes of, 372–373
sequence of, 371–372
treatment of, 380
    antibiotic supression, 380–381
    surgical, 381–386
urinary, 450–452
Inflammation, 2, 79
Informed consent, 594–595, 596–597
In situ hybridization, 27
Intermittent plantar compression, as
    thromboprophylaxis after total
    hip arthroplasty, 407
Intermittent pneumatic compression
    as thromboprophylaxis after total hip
        arthroplasty, 407
    as thromboprophylaxis after total
        knee arthroplasty, 409–410
Intestinal obstruction, 441–443, *442, 443*
Intraoperative evaluation, 52
Intraoperative trauma, 65
Intravenous polygram (IVP),
    genitourinary problems and, 449
Intravenous regional blockade, 82
Intravenous urography, of urological
    injury, 456
In vitro experiments, *27,* 27–28, *28,* 29t,
    231
Irradiation, 156
Ischemia, 363, 365, 443
Ischial osteolysis, 94
Ischiogluteal bursitis, 79
IWB (Index of Well Being), 555, 556

Judet views, 59, 293, 510, 539
Juvenile rheumatoid arthritis, protrusio
    acetabuli and, 538

Kidney stones, 451–452
Kyphosis, physical exam and, 49

Labeled leucocytes, 72, 72
Laboratory analysis, 50, 81
   diagnosis of infection and, 375–376
   genitourinary complications and, 449
Laceration, 363
Laparoscopy, for cholecystectomy, 441
Larson's scale, 553
Laser technology, 147
Lateral view, 59
Leukocyte scan
   Girdlestone arthroplasty and, 510
   infection and, 376–377
Limb lengthening, 365, 366
Limb length equalization
   anatomic leg length inequality, 492–493
   dislocation and, 395
   functional leg length inequality, 493–496, *493–496*
   Girdlestone arthroplasty and, 506
   nerve injury and, 368–369
   physical exam and, 49
Limp
   clinical evaluation and, 48–49
   direct lateral and vastus slide approach and, 261
Linear osteolysis, 21, 22
Link America partial pelvis replacement, 162
Liverpool approach, heterotopic ossification and, 468
Loosening, 1
   mechanisms of, 5–6
   osteolysis and, 22
   radiographic evaluation of uncemented stems for, 63, *63–64, 64*
   radiographic signs of, 4, *4–5*
   radionuclide imaging and, 70
   symptoms of, 3–4
Low molecular weight heparin
   hematoma formation and, 421
   as thromboprophylaxis after total knee arthroplasty, 408–409
Lumbar facet syndrome, 79
Lumbar lordosis, physical exam and, 49
Lumbar plexitis, 80
Lumbar spondylosis, 49
Lymphatic opacification, 67, 69
Lymphocytes, 25

Magnetic resonance imaging (MRI), 70, 75
   epidural hematoma and, 421
   Girdlestone arthroscopy and, 510
   metastatic disease and, 498, 499
   nerve injury and, 367
Malalignment, femoral, 101, 112–113

Malpractice, 583–584
   legal principles underlying, 584–585
   preparation for a deposition and, 586–590
   prevention of, 592–596
   specific diagnoses that can lead to, 585–586
   testimony and, 590–592
   video informed consent and, 596–597
Mast cells, 27
Mayo hip score, 553–554
McMaster-Toronto Arthritis Patient Preference Disability Questionnaire (MACTAR), 558
Medical Outcomes Study Short Form 36, 556
Medicare, 386, 545
Meralgia paresthetica, 80, 81
Merle d'Aubigné hip score, 558
Meta-analyses, 554–555
Metabolic equivalent (MET), 426, 427t
Metabolic neuropathies, 50
Metal drilling/extraction techniques, 434–436
Metal fatigue, 431
Metalloproteases, 8
Metastatic disease, 498
   evaluation of, 498–499
   treatment of, 499–504, *500, 501,* 502t, 503t
Methylene diphosphonate (MDP), 70
Methylmethacrylate, 1, 64
Microphage, 2
   activation, 23
   inflammatory responses, 6
   particle-stimulated, 27
Microwave thermotherapy (Prostatron), 451
Midas Rex instruments, 434
Migration, in acetabular reconstruction, 94
Minnesota Multiphasic Peronality Inventory (MMPI), 50
Modified Dall surgical approach, 263–265, *264–265*
Modifed Lowenstein, 59, *60*
Modularity, S-ROM system and, 224–225, *225, 230,* 230–231, *231*
Monk soft top prosthesis, 23
Mononeuropathies, 78, 80, 83
Morphine, 420
Morse taper, 182, 192
Motor weakness, 522, *523*
   causes of, 523–526
   implications of, 522–523
   treatment of, 526–528
MTS hip simulator, 572
Mueller O ring, 161
Muller reinforcement ring, 335, 336, 350
Myelomeningocele, motor weakness and, 523–524

Myobacterium tuberculosis, 373
Myocardial disease, 427
Myocardial infarction, 425, 428
Myocardial ischemia, 419, 428–429
Myofascial pain, 78
Myositis, 464
Myositis ossificans progressiva, 464

Naproxyn, heterotopic ossification and, 470
National hip registry, 554, 559
Nephrolithiasis, genitourinary complications and, 450
Nerve conduction velocity, 367
Neurological injury
   anesthesia and, 422
   diagnosis and management, 366–367
   nerve degeneration and regeneration, 362
      clinical diagnosis of, 364
      nerve injury pathology, 362–364
      peripheral nerve morphology, 361–362
   prevention, 368–369
   prognosis, 368
   in revision hip arthroplasty, 364–366
Neuropathic pain, 78
Neuropraxia, 49, 362–363
Neurotmesis, 362–363
New England Baptist Hospital, and efficiency in revision total hip surgery, 545–548
Nickel, 372
Nifedipine, 82
Night sweats, clinical evaluation and, 49
Nitroprusside, 429
Nonradiation sterilization, 571
Nonsteroidal anti-inflammatory medications (NSAIDS), 84, 118, 268, 438, 470
Nonunion, 36
   conventional trochanteric osteotomy and, 269
   dislocation and, 395
   extended trochanteric osteotomy and, 277
   hip fractures and, 477
   proximal femoral osteotomy and, 481
   in revision total hip replacement, 202
Nottingham Health Profile (NHP), 556

Ober test, 496
   physical exam and, 49
Obesity
   conventional trochanteric osteotomy and, 267
   dislocation and, 392
   and external devices, 36
   infection and, 371–372
   polyethylene wear and, 14

Oblique femoral osteotomy, 483
Obturator nerve, 366–367
Obturator neuralgia, 80
Offset of the prosthesis, 526
Ogden plate fixation, 531
Ogilvies syndrome, 442
Oh-Harris™ syringe, 207
Omniflex, 225
One-stage reconstruction, 383, 385t
Onlay strut allographs
　biology of, 185–186
　clinical experience with, 186
　operative technique for, 186, 186–187, 187
Open reduction and internal fixation (ORIF), 41–42, 51, 531–532
Operating room environment, 142–143
Opioids, 84–85
　chronic therapy, 86
　substance abuse history and, 86–87
ORTHODOC, 576–577
Osteoarthritis, protrusio acetabuli and, 538
Osteoblasts, 26
Osteoclasts, multinucleated, 26–27
Osteogenesis imperfecta, protrusio acetabuli and, 538
Osteoinduction/osteoconduction, 155
Osteolysis, 1
　around cemented components, 6–8, 7, 7, 22
　around uncemented components, 8, 8–9, 9, 22, 23
　cement fixation and, 208
　clinical evaluation of, 52–56
　definition and types of, 21, 22t
　incidence of, 22–23
　loss of femoral bone stock in revision, 167
　trochanter and, 114
　wear debris and, 23, 24–25, 25–27, 26
　wear debris and in vitro experiments, 27, 27–29, 28, 29t
Osteomalacia, protrusio acetabuli and, 538
Osteonecrosis, 477, 487
Osteopenia, 114, 267
Outcome studies, 553
　historical perspective, 553–554
　methodology, 554–555
　outcome instruments, 555–557
　in revision total hip arthroplasty, 558–559
　significance of, 559
　in total hip arthroplasty, 557–558
Oxacillin, 379
Oxidation, of UHMWPE, 13

Pacemakers, 428
Paget's disease, 81
　heterotopic ossification and, 470
　protrusio acetabuli and, 538

Pain
　adjunctive medications for, 85
　anterior thigh pain, 139–141, 140
　aseptic loosening and, 3–4
　causes of, 48t
　cementless components and, 8
　differential diagnosis of
　　extra-articular sources of musculoskeletal origin, 79–80
　　extra-articular sources of neuropathic origin, 80
　　intra-articular sources, 79
　　postoperative, 80–81
　evaluation and treatment of, 81
　femoral stem fracture and, 432
　functional leg length inequality and, 494
　Girdlestone arthroplasty and, 506–507
　hemiarthroplasty and, 477–478
　heterotopic ossification (OH) and, 64–65
　infection and, 371, 374
　location of, 48
　medications for
　　NSAIDS, 84
　　opioids, 84–85
　peripheral neuropathies, 83
　postoperative hypertension and, 429
　reflex sympathetic dystrophy, 81–83
　stress fractures and, 41
　treatment challenges and, 86–87
　trochanteric, 268
　types of, 47–48, 78–79
Paralytic ileus, 441–442
Patient-controlled anesthesia (PCA), 420
Patient education
　and nerve injury treatment, 367
　physical rehabilitation and, 550, 552
　and prevention of dislocation, 36
Patient history, 48–49
Patient Outcome Research Teams (PORTs), 554
Patulous host canal, 194
Peptic ulcer disease, 438
Peptococcus asaccharides, 372–373t
Peptococcus magnus, 372–373t
Peptostreptococcus microsphore, 372–373t
Percutaneous nephrostomy, 457
Perforated ulcer, 438–439, 439
Perforation, 204, 205t, 446
Perioperative risk factors, 33–36, 35
Periosteal injury, pain caused by, 79
Peripheral mononeuropathies, 78, 83
Peripheral nerve morphology, 361–362
Peripheral neuropathies, 83, 365
Periprosthetic uptake, 71–72
Peritonitis, 438–439
PFC cup, 323
Phagocytes, facultative, 23
Pharmacodynamics, 84
Pharmacokinetics, 84

Phenothiazines, 85
Phenoxybenzamine, 85
Physical examination, 49
Physical rehabilitation, 549–552
Physical therapy, anatomic leg length inequality, 495
Physician Payment Review Commission (PPRC), 545
Piezo electric effect, 152
Pigmented villonodular synovitis, 79
Piriformis syndrome, 80
Plain film radiography, 60–63, 61–63
Pneumatic plantar compression, 410
Polymethylmethacrylate (PMMA)
　endosteal grafting and, 178, 182
　FDA approval of, 224
　infection and, 372
　metastatic disease treatment and, 499
　ultrasonic removal of, 152
Polytetrafluoroethylene, 5
Postdural puncture headache (PPD), 421–422
Posterior deficiencies, of acetabulum, 339–347, 339t, 340, 340t, 342–346
Posterolateral surgical approach, 247–250, 248, 249
Postherpetic neuralgia, 79, 80
Postoperative care
　for acetabular revision surgery, 295
　for acetabular segmental deficiencies, 305–306
　direct lateral and vastus slide approach and, 260, 260–261, 271
　endosteal grafting and, 179–180
　for Girdlestone arthroplasty, 514
　physical rehabilitation and, 550–552
　for posterior acetabular deficiencies and, 345
　for proximal femoral deficiency, 193–202, 194–201
　structural allografts and, 316–317
　trochanteric osteotomy, 116
Postoperative complications
　anesthesia, 418–424
　cardiac, 425–429, 426t, 427t
　deep venous thromboembolism, 401–413, 402, 403t, 404, 406, 412
　dislocation, 391–399
　femoral stem fracture, 431–436, 432–435
　genitourinary, 448–457, 456
　heterotopic ossification, 464–473, 467, 469, 471, 472
　infection, 371–387, 373t, 375t, 385t
　nerve palsy, 83
　neurological injury, 361–369
　risk factors, 36
　surgical, 438–446, 439, 440, 442–446
　wound, 459–462, 460–462
Post-polio syndrome, motor weakness and, 524

Preoperative planning, 89–91
  abdominal complications, 438
  acetabular revision surgery, 293
  acetabular segmental deficiencies, 302
  anesthesia, 124–128
  biomechanic challenges, *132–138,
    135–141, 140*
  blood management, 118–122
  bone bank/bone graft, *155–158*
  bone stock loss and allografting
    acetabulum, 93–98, *95–97*
    femur, 100–110, *101, 101t, 102t, 103,
      105–108*
    trochanter, 112–116, 113t
  cavitary deficiencies, 330
  distal fixation, 218–219, *219, 220*
  drill and excavation, *154,* 154
  equipment, 142–147, 149
  femoral revison, 168–169
  Girdlestone arthroplasty, 508–510
  hand tools, 150–151, *150–151*
  implant inventory, 160–164, *161–164*
  metastatic disease, 499
  physical rehabilitation, 549–550
  posterior acetabular deficiencies,
    339–340
  protrusio acetabuli, 538–539
  segmental deficiencies, 333
  templating, 129–133, *130–133*
  ultrasonic cement removal, *152,*
    152–153
Preoperative risk factors, 33
Prevention
  dislocation and, 395–396
  functional leg length inequality and,
    496
  of neurological injury, 368–369
  patient education and, 36
Primary exchange arthroplasty, 383
Primary osteogenesis, 155
Propionibacterium acnes, 373
Prospective Payment System (PPS), 545
Prostaglandin-E$_2$, 8
Proteus mirabilis, 373
Protrusio acetabuli, 266
  definition and etiology, 538
  preoperative planning and patient
    evaluation, 538–539
  surgical reconstruction, 539–542
Protrusio ring, 162
Proximal femoral deficiency
  allografts, 189–190, *192*
  reconstruction allografts, 158
    postoperative care for, 193–202,
      194–201
    technique for, 189–193, *190–193*
Proximal sleeve (SPA), 224
Proximal sleeve (ZTT), 224
Pseudoaddiction, pain medications and,
  85
Pseudobursa, 67

Pseudomonas aeruginosa, 373
Psychological factors
  hypochondriasis and, 50
  neurologic complications and, 367
  treatment of pain and, 86
Pubic rami stress fractures, 50
Pulsed Doppler imaging, 74
Pyloroplasty, 439

QALY (quality adjusted life years), 555

Radiation, ionizing, 471–473
Radiofrequency ablation (TUNA),
  urinary, 451
Radiofrequency thermocoagulation of
  the sympathetic chain, 82
Radiography, 59–60, *60*
  for acetabular revision surgery, 293,
    295
  advanced imaging techniques, 73–75,
    74 (See also specific techniques)
  aspiration and arthrography and,
    65–68, *67, 68*
  cavitary deficiencies and, 330
  to detect loosening, 50–51
  diagnosis of infection and, 376–377
  evaluation for heterotopic ossification
    (HO), 64–65
  evaluation of dislocation and, 65
  evaluation of infection with, 68–70,
    69, 70
  evaluation of uncemented stems
    with, *63,* 63–64, *64*
  femoral stem fracture and, 432
  Girdlestone arthroplasty and,
    509–510
  metastatic disease and, 498, 499
  plain film, 60–63, *61–63*
  preoperative planning and, 144
  protrusio acetabuli and, 539
  radionuclide imaging and, 70–73,
    70–73
  reflex sympathetic dystrophy, 82
  retroperitoneal surgical approach
    and, 287
  signs of loosening and, 4
  templating and, 129–130
Radiolucencies, signs of loosening and,
  4, *4*
Radionuclide hepatic aminodiacetic
  acid (HIDA) scanning, 440
Radionuclide imaging, *70–72, 70–73,*
  376–377
  fractures and, 41
  infection and, 376
  reflex sympathetic dystrophy and, 82
  of urological injury, 456
  use in evaluation, 51–52
Radiotherapy, for heterotopic
  ossification, 65
Ram extrusion, 12

Randomized clinical trial (RCT), 554
Range of motion
  heterotopic ossification (OH) and,
    64–65
  physical exam and, 49
Recombinant human erythropoietin,
  121–122
Reflex sympathetic dystrophy (RSD),
  79, 81–83
Research
  implants, 562–574
  outcomes studies, 553–559
Resection arthroplasty, 385–386
Reserpine, 82
Resin, 12
Resource Based Relative Value Scale
  (RBRVS), 545
Retention, urinary, 450, 451
Retrograde pyelogram, genitourinary
  problems and, 449, 457
Retroperitoneal surgical approach,
  287–289, *287–289*
Revision. *See* Femur, revision
Revision total hip arthroplasty, venous
  thromboembolism and, 407–408
Revision total knee arthroplasty,
  venous thromboembolism and,
  410
Rheumatoid arthritis
  anesthesia and, 418
  Girdlestone arthroplasty and,
    507–508
  infection and, 371
  motor weakness and, 523
  neurological injury and, 365
  osteolysis and, 25
  pain and, 79, 81
  protrusio acetabuli and, 538
Richards Modular, 225
Rickets, protrusio acetabuli and, 538
Rifampin, 381
ROBODOC, 576–577
Robotically assisted cement removal
  (RTHR), 576–580
Router technique, 154

Sacroiliac joint dysfunction, 79
Salmonella choleraesuis, 373
Scarpa's triangle, 79
Sciatic nerve, 366, 513
Sciatic neuralgia, 80
Sciatic neuropathy, 49
Scintigraphy. *See* Radionuclide imaging
Scoliosis, physical exam and, 49
Scout images, 578–579
Scrotal enlargement, 452–453
Segmental defects
  acetabulum, 302–306, *303–305*
  femoral, 112
Segmental defects
  onlay grafting, 185–187

use of femoral allografts, 189–202, *190–200*
Sickness Impact Profile (SIP), 556, 558
Silvash total hip system, 224
Singh index, 158
Six minute walk, 556, 558
Skeletal pain, 78
Soft tissue reconstruction, 460–461
Somatosensory evoked potential (SEEP) monitoring, nerve injury and, 369, 513
Sonography. *See* Ultrasound
Spinal osteophytes, heterotopic ossification and, 467–468
Spinal stenosis, motor weakness and, 523–524
Spondylosis, 492
SRN total hip system, 224
S-ROM (stability, range of motion) Oblong Cup system, 163, *164*
   clinical trials for, 231–232
   femoral reconstruction and, 482
   femoral stem in, 225–226, *226, 227*
   history of, 224, *225*
   implantation, 226, *228, 229*
   indications for using, 228–230, *229*
   modularity and, 224–225, *225,* 230, *230–231, 231*
   neck lengths and offset, 226, *228*
   for proximal femoral allografts, 189–190, *192*
   proximal sleeve and, 226
   technique for using, 326–328
Stabilization, 17–18, 572
Staphylococcus aureus, 372–373t, 383, 421
Staphylococcus epidermis, 372–373t
Steinman pin, 492
Stem designs, 136–137, *137*
Stem extractors, 150, *150*
Stenosis
   aortic and mitral, 425
   femoral, 101, 112–113
   spinal, 49, 80, 81
Sterilization methods, 17–18, 142–143, 156, 571
Streptococcus viridans, 373, 383
Stress erosive gastritis, 439
Stress fractures, 41
Stress-shielding, 21, 138–139
   radiographic evaluation of uncemented stems for, *63,* 63–64, *64*
Structural allografts, acetabular, 309–319, *310–318*
Subsidence, 63, *64*
Subtraction arthrography, 65, *67*
Surface finish, 1
Surgical approaches
   for femoral revision
     anterolateral, 270–273, *271, 272*
     Cameron anterior osteotomy, *285,* 285–286
     conventional trochanteric osteotomy, 266–269, *268, 276*
     direct lateral and vastus slide, 251–262, *252–261*
     extended lateral femoral osteotomy, 280–283, *281, 282*
     extended trochanter osteotomy, 277–278, *278*
     modified Dall, 263–265, *264–265*
     posterolateral, 247–250, *248, 249*
     retroperitoneal, 287–289, *287–289*
     trochanter slide, 274–275, *275*
   for Girdlestone arthroplasty, 511–514
   Liverpool approach, heterotopic ossification and, 468
   motor weakness and, 524–526
   rate of dislocation and, 393
   acetabular cup design/degree of head capture, 393–394
   femoral component head size, 394
   head neck ratio and femoral offset, 394
Surgical complications
   abdominal, in the postrevision period
     acute cholecystitis, 439–441, *440*
     bleeding peptic ulcer, 439
     intestinal obstruction, 441–443, *442, 443*
     peptic ulcer disease, 438
     perforated ulcer, 438–439, *439*
     preoperative evaluation, 438
     stress erosive gastritis, 439
   anticoagulation therapy, 443
     cement extrusion, *445,* 445–446, *446*
     diverticulitis, 443, *444*
     instrument perforation, 446, *446*
     technical complications, 443–445, *444, 445*
Surgical (or chemical) sympathectomy, 82–83
Surgical techniques
   Burch-Schneider cage and, 345
   for femoral revision, 165
     cavitary defects—bone grafting, 167–174, *172*
     cavitary defects—endosteal grafting, 176–183, *177–180*
     cemented long-stem femoral revision, 239–242, *240–241*
     cement fixation femoral revision, 204–211, *205–210*
     cement within cement femoral revision, 214–216, *217*
     distal fixation, 217–223, *219–220, 222*
     impact modular total hip implant, 234–238, *237*
     segmental defects—onlay grafting, 185–187
     segmental defects—use of femoral allografts, 189–202, *190–200*
     S-ROM prosthesis, 224–232, *225–231*
   for posterior acetabular allografting and plating, 343–345, *344, 345*
   protrusio acetabuli and, 539–542
Sympathetic blockade, 82
Syngeneic grafts, 109
Synoviocytes, 2
Systemic lupus erythematosus, 79

Technology
   laser, 147
   limitations of, 142
Teflon™, 11, 23
Templating, 129–130, *130*
   acetabulum, 130–132, *131*
   femur, 132–133, *132–133*
Thimerosal, 156
Thomas test, physical exam and, 49
Three stage reconstruction, 385
Thromboprophylaxis
   after total hip arthroplasty
     aspirin, 407
     dextran, 407
     heparin, 405–407, *406*
     intermittent plantar compression, 407
     intermittent pneumatic compression, 407
     warfarin, 403–405
   after total knee arthroplasty
     aspirin, 409
     continuous passive motion, 410
     dextran, 409
     intermittent pneumatic compression, 409–410
     low molecular weight heparin, 408–409
     pneumatic plantar compression, 410
     warfarin, 409
Ti-5Al-2.5Fe, 566
Ti-6Al-7Nb, 566
Ti-6Al-4V, 565, 566–568
Time trade-off technique, 558
Ti-12Mo-6Zr-2Fe (TMZF), 566–567
Tinel's sign, 363
Titanium, 1, 5
Titanium alloys, 566–568t, *568,* 569t
Tolerance, pain medications and, 85
Tomograms, fractures and, 41
Traction, 363–364, *365, 366*
Transesophogeal echocardiographic (TEE) monitoring, 420, 428
Transgluteal lateral approach, 251
Traumatic myositis ossificans circumscripta, 464
TreBay™ bear claw, 150, *150*
Trendelenberg's sign, loosening and, 3
Trendelenberg test, physical exam and, 49

Trephine, 433–434, *434*
Tricyclic antidepressants, 85
Trigger points, for myofascial pain, 79–80
Trilogy cup, 323
Triple-isotope scans, 72
Trochanter
　bone stock loss and allografting
　　fixation and hardware for trochanteric osteotomy, 115–116
　　modifications in type of osteotomy, 115–117
　　nonunion after osteotomy, 113–114
　　osteolysis and, 114
　　osteopenia and, 114–115
　　postoperative care after osteotomy, 116
　　preoperative planning for osteotomy, 112
　extended trochanteric osteotomy, 277–278, *278*
　reattachment of, 193
　transtrochanteric approach
　　evaluation of, 56
　　and nonunion, 36
　trochanteric bursitis, 79
　trochanteric osteotomy surgical approach, 266–269, *268, 276*
　trochanter slide surgical approach, 189, *190*, 274–275, *275*
Tumor invasion, 79
Two-stage reimplantation protocol, 383, 385t

UHMWHDP (ultra-high molecular weight high-density polyethylene), 1, 2. *See also* Wear, polyethylene
　advances in, 568–574, *569, 570,* 571t, *572, 573*
　cross-linking and, 13, 17
　difference from HDP, 12
　manufacture and processing of, 12–13
　oxidation and, 13
　sterilization methods and, 17
　structure of, 12
Ultrasonic system for cement removal, 152–156

Ultrasound, 70, *74,* 74–75, 378, 440, 449
Uncemented stems, radiographic evaluation of, *63,* 63–64, *64*
Ureteral injury/repair, 454–455

Vagotomy, 439
Vanadium, 372
Vancomycin, 379
Varus alignment, 431
Vascular claudication, 50
Vascular viability, radionuclide imaging and, 70
Venous thromboembolism
　anesthesia and, 410
　cost effectiveness and, 410–411
　epidemiology of, 402–403t
　pathogenesis of, 401–402, *402*
　prophylaxis for high-risk patients and, 413
　revision total hip arthroplasty and, 407–408
　revision total knee arthroplasty and, 410
　screening considerations and, 411–413
　thromboprophylaxis after total hip arthroplasty
　　aspirin, 407
　　dextran, 407
　　heparin, 405–407, *406*
　　intermittent plantar compression, 407
　　intermittent pneumatic compression, 407
　　warfarin, 403–405
　thromboprophylaxis after total knee arthroplasty
　　aspirin, 409
　　continuous passive motion, 410
　　dextran, 409
　　intermittent pneumatic compression, 409–410
　　low molecular weight heparin, 408–409
　　pneumatic plantar compression, 410
　　warfarin, 409
Visceral pain, 78

Vitalock cup, 323
Volkmann's canals, 79

Wake-up test, 513
Walderman Link partial pelvis replacement ring, 161, *162*
Wallerian degeneration, 362, *363, 364,* 367
Warfarin
　as thromboprophylaxis after total hip arthroplasty and, 403–405
　as thromboprophylaxis after total knee arthroplasty, 409
Wear
　debris, 1, *7, 7,* 16
　osteolysis and, , 16, 23, 24–25, *24–27, 26*
　polyethylene, 6
　　as a complex mechanism, 12
　　factors affecting, 14–17, *14–17*
　　history of, 11–12
　　mechanism of, 13–14
　　metal-on-metal design and, 11
　　particulate debris, 11
　in vitro experiments and, *27,* 27–28, *28*
Weight bearing, pain from loosening and, 3
Western Ontario at McMaster University Osteoarthritis Index (WOMAC), 556, 558
White band, 13
White blood cell count (WBC), 50, 81
Whitman reconstruction, 382
Wolff's Law, 21, 157
Wound problems, 459, *460, 461*
　infection and, 374
　management of the nonhealing Girdlestone arthroplasty defect, 459–460, *462*
　salvage of the exposed joint prosthesis, 459
　soft tissue reconstruction, 460–461
Wroblewski compression spring device, 396

Zickel nail, 501
Ziegler process, 12
Zirconia ceramics, 1

SPRINGER NATURE

GPSR Compliance

The European Union's (EU) General Product Safety Regulation (GPSR) is a set of rules that requires consumer products to be safe and our obligations to ensure this.

If you have any concerns about our products, you can contact us on ProductSafety@springernature.com

In case Publisher is established outside the EU, the EU authorized representative is:

Springer Nature Customer Service Center GmbH
Europaplatz 3
69115 Heidelberg, Germany

The manufacturer's authorised representative in the EU is Springer Nature Customer Service Centre GmbH, Europaplatz 3, 69115 Heidelberg, Germany. If you have any concerns regarding our products, please contact ProductSafety@springernature.com

Printed and bound by CPI Group (UK) Ltd, Croydon, CR0 4YY
23/03/2026
02076374-0004